Walter J. Christopher, D.V.M.
March, 65

Dr. & Mrs. Walter J. Christopher
236 Sioux Street
Fairlane Trailer Acres
Fayetteville, N. C. 28303

EQUINE
MEDICINE
& SURGERY

EQUINE MEDICINE & SURGERY

A TEXT AND REFERENCE WORK

The Work of Sixty-eight Authors

Edited by

J. F. BONE, B.A., B.S., D.V.M., M.S.

E. J. CATCOTT, D.V.M., Ph.D.

A. A. GABEL, D.V.M., M.Sc.

L. E. JOHNSON, D.V.M., M.Sc.

W. F. RILEY, Jr., D.V.M., M.S.

WITH 379 ILLUSTRATIONS

FIRST EDITION

AMERICAN VETERINARY PUBLICATIONS, INC.

114 NORTH WEST STREET, WHEATON, ILLINOIS

DRAWER KK, SANTA BARBARA, CALIFORNIA

1963

PREFACE

It is customary to describe a medical volume as intended for students and practitioners, but the more satisfactory it is for the one, the less satisfactory it may be for the other. The practitioner may, at any time, see rare and obscure diseases. He will therefore wish to have a comprehensive book to which he can refer. The student, however, must strive to grasp the broad aspects of a subject and a knowledge of common diseases and their treatment. His time is so limited that he cannot afford to seek out the variations of every clinical syndrome, or he will become buried in a mass of details. Ideally, there should be books of reference and books of instruction. Practically, this would be very difficult for a subject like Equine Medicine and Surgery. As this book is intended for both practitioners and students, it inevitably has some dichotomy of purpose. However, a good synthesis of these two objectives can conceivably be placed inside a single binding, and this we have attempted to do.

The prospect of an equine textbook was considered nearly three years ago when it was decided to prepare a small monograph that would be helpful to veterinary students and general practitioners alike. The enthusiastic response to our initial inquiries regarding the need for such a text prompted us to expand our initial concept to include a wider scope of information. Contrary to the dismal predictions of the 1920's, the veterinary profession has not withered away nor has the horse become a rarity. In fact, the future of equine practice throughout the world looks brighter today than it did in the heyday of the draft horse. In terms of number of practitioners involved, capital investment, and monetary value, equine practice is now in a favorable and expanding position. The horse is making a tremendous comeback at a time when sources of scientific information about it are sorely needed. In an effort to alleviate some of the need, this book has been produced.

It has been said that genius is the art of picking brains. If this is so, then this book is a work of genius because 68 teachers, research workers, and practitioners have contributed to its writing, and many others have given helpful advice and criticism. By compiling the contributions of so many it has been possible to assemble current information on an extensive list of topics concerning equine medicine and surgery. At the same time, this procedure precludes the possibility of achieving a uniformity in style throughout the book. Its content has been organized, however, into a format which we hope is orderly and sensible.

The discussions of disease syndromes have been grouped, as much as possible, on the basis of their relationship to a specific etiology. The syndromes without well-defined etiologies have been organized on the basis of their effect on the various physiologic functions. Because of their relative importance in equine practice, separate chapter groupings have been made for the discussions relating to nutrition, lameness, and reproduction.

The separate discussions of disease entities generally refer to etiology, epizootiology, clinical signs, lesions, diagnosis, treatment, and control. Each discussion is aimed to highlight the points of clinical interest. Comprehensiveness in subject matter has been sought, but major emphasis has been placed upon the more commonly encountered clinical problems of equine practice. It also has been our intent to design a book which will be of value to our colleagues abroad, and not exclusively a text for American veterinarians.

It is a pleasure to present this book to the veterinary profession. We feel that it not only fills a gap in our literature which has existed for better than four decades, but it also places between a single set of covers most of the published information on equine disorders. We acknowledge our debt to older authors and workers in the field of equine medicine and surgery, for without their basic contributions and willingness to communicate their work to others, much of the material in these pages would never have become professional knowledge.

J. F. BONE
E. J. CATCOTT

AUTHORS

HAROLD E. AMSTUTZ, D.V.M.
Professor and Head, Department of Veterinary Clinics, School of Veterinary Science and Medicine, Purdue University, Lafayette, Indiana.

E. NORMAN ANDERSON, B.V.Sc., D.V.M.
President, Pinehurst Farms Veterinary Center, Ltd., Consultant in Surgery to the Department of Surgery, University of Manitoba, Pinehurst Farms Veterinary Center, Ltd., Winnipeg, Manitoba, Canada.

ROBERT H. BAKER, D.V.M.
Practitioner, West Covina, California.

RALPH D. BARNER, D.V.M., M.S., PH.D.
Professor, Department of Surgery and Medicine, College of Veterinary Medicine, Michigan State University, East Lansing, Michigan.

EDWARD G. BATTE, B.S., D.V.M., M.S.
Professor and Head, Veterinary Section, North Carolina State College, Raleigh, North Carolina.

VICTOR R. BERLINER, PH.D.
Director, Division of Endocrinology, Ortho Research Foundation, Raritan, New Jersey.

JESSE F. BONE, B.A., B.S., D.V.M., M.S.
Associate Professor, Veterinary Medicine, Oregon State University, Corvallis, Oregon.

CHARLES H. BRIDGES, D.V.M., M.S., PH.D.
Professor and Head of the Department of Veterinary Pathology, School of Veterinary Medicine, A. & M. College of Texas, College Station, Texas.

JOHN W. BRITTON, B.A., D.V.M.
Practitioner, Oakdale, California.

JOHN T. BRYANS, B.S., M.S., PH.D.
Professor, Department of Animal Pathology, Kentucky Agricultural Experiment Station, University of Kentucky, Lexington, Kentucky.

J. F. BULLARD, D.V.M., M.S.
Assistant Dean, Professor of Surgery, School of Veterinary Science and Medicine, Purdue University, Lynn Hall, Lafayette, Indiana.

CHARLES H. BURGER, D.V.M., M.S.
Practitioner, Bakersfield, California.

ROBERT J. BYRNE, D.V.M., M.S.
Associate Professor, Department of Veterinary Science, University of Maryland, College Park, Maryland.

ARTHUR A. CASE, B.S., M.S., D.V.M.
Professor, Veterinary Medicine and Surgery, School of Veterinary Medicine, University of Missouri, Columbia, Missouri.

C. D. COOPER, D.V.M.
Practitioner, Lemoore, California.

HENRY CRESSWELL, V.M.D.
Practitioner, Norristown, Pennsylvania.

TONY J. CUNHA, B.S., M.S., PH.D.
Professor and Head, Department of Animal Science, University of Florida, Gainesville, Florida.

D. K. DETWEILER, V.M.D., M.S.
Professor of Physiology and Director of the Comparative Cardiovascular Studies Unit, School of Veterinary Medicine, University of Pennsylvania, Philadelphia, Pennsylvania.

J. DITCHFIELD, D.V.M.
Diplomate, Bacteriology, Assistant Professor, Ontario Veterinary College, Guelph, Canada. Fellow, Department of Microbiology, School of Hygiene, University of Toronto, Toronto, Canada.

DAVID C. DODD, B.V.Sc.
Diplomate, American College of Veterinary Pathologists. Veterinary Diagnostic Officer, Ruakura Animal Research Station, Department of Agriculture, Hamilton, New Zealand.

E. R. DOLL, B.S., M.A., D.V.M.
Professor, Department of Animal Pathology, Kentucky Agriculture Experiment Station, Lexington, Kentucky.

MURRAY E. FOWLER, B.S., D.V.M.
Assistant Professor of Medicine, Surgery, and Clinics, University of California, Davis, California.

JOHN FRANCIS, D.Sc., M.Sc., F.R.C.V.S.
Professor, Department of Preventive Medicine, University of Queensland, Brisbane, Australia.

ALBERT A. GABEL, D.V.M., M.Sc.
Assistant Professor, Department of Veterinary Surgery and Radiology, College of Veterinary Medicine, The Ohio State University, Columbus, Ohio.

WALTER J. GIBBONS, D.V.M., M.S.
Professor of Large Animal Medicine and Surgery, College of Veterinary Medicine, Auburn University, Auburn, Alabama.

JOVAN GLIGORIJEVIC, D.V.M.
Director, Institute of Radiology and Physiotherapy, Zagreb, Yugoslavia.

FRITZ P. GLUCKSTEIN, B.S., D.V.M.
Veterinary Analyst, Regional Analysis Division, Economic Research Service, U. S. Department of Agriculture, Washington, D. C.

ROBERT PAUL HANSON, PH.D.
Professor of Veterinary Science and Bacteriology, University of Wisconsin, Madison, Wisconsin.

RICHARD C. HERSCHLER, B.S., D.V.M., PH.D.
Assistant Professor, Veterinary Clinics, Purdue University, Lafayette, Indiana.

PAUL E. HOFFMAN, D.V.M.
Assistant Professor, Department of Medicine and Surgery, School of Veterinary Medicine, University of Georgia, Athens, Georgia.

ROBERT A. HOLMES, B.A., B.S., M.S., D.V.M.
Practitioner, Belmont Park, Elmont, New York.

HARVEY H. HOYT, D.V.M., PH.D.
Professor and Head, Department of Veterinary Medicine and Clinics, College of Veterinary Medicine, University of Minnesota, St. Paul, Minnesota.

R. SCOTT JACKSON, B.A., D.V.M.
Resident Veterinarian and Manager, Rancho Los Cerritos, Ontario, California.

L. E. JOHNSON, D.V.M., M.Sc.
Professor, Department of Veterinary Surgery and Radiology, College of Veterinary Medicine, The Ohio State University, Columbus, Ohio.

E. WYNN JONES, M.R.C.V.S., PH.D.
Professor, Veterinary Medicine and Surgery, College of Veterinary Medicine, Oklahoma State University, Stillwater, Oklahoma.

B. W. KINGREY, D.V.M., M.S.
Head, Department of Medicine and Surgery, Director of Clinics, College of Veterinary Medicine, Iowa State University, Ames, Iowa.

NELS KONNERUP, B.S., D.V.M.
Veterinary Analyst, Regional Analysis Division, Economic Research Service, U. S. Department of Agriculture, Washington, D. C.

FRANK KRAL, D.V.M., V.M.D. (h.c.) Docent habilitatus
Professor of Veterinary Medicine, School of Veterinary Medicine, University of Pennsylvania, Philadelphia, Pennsylvania.

J. V. LACROIX, D.V.S.
Practitioner (retired), Evanston, Illinois.

D. G. LEWIS, M.R.C.V.S.
Practitioner, Strood, Kent, England.

PIERRE LIEUX, D.V.M.
Practitioner, Riverside, California.

ALEX LITTLEJOHN, B.V.Sc., M.R.C.V.S.
Research Scholar, Royal (Dick) School of Veterinary Studies, Summerhall, Edinburgh, Scotland.

R. L. LUNDVALL, D.V.M., M.S.
Professor, Veterinary Medicine and Surgery, Iowa State University, Ames, Iowa.

WILLIAM D. MALHERBE, B.V.Sc.
Head, Department of Clinical Pathology, Faculty of Veterinary Science, University of Pretoria, Republic of South Africa.

JOHN P. MANNING, D.V.M., M.S.
Assistant Professor, Department of Veterinary Clinical Medicine, College of Veterinary Medicine, University of Illinois, Urbana, Illinois

FRED C. NEAL, D.V.M., M.S.
Department of Veterinary Research, University of Florida, Gainesville, Florida.

CARL OLSON, B.S., M.S., PH.D., D.V.M.
Chairman, Department of Veterinary Science, University of Wisconsin, Madison, Wisconsin.

DONALD F. PATTERSON, D.VM.
Assistant Professor of Medicine and Clinical Investigator, Comparative Cardiovascular Studies Unit, School of Veterinary Medicine, University of Pennsylvania, Philadelphia, Pennsylvania.

D. POYNTER, B.Sc., PH.D., M.I. BIOLOGY
Department of Parasitology, Veterinary Research Department, Allen & Hansburys, Ltd., Ware Hertfordshire, England.

D. L. PROCTOR, D.V.M.
Practitioner, Lexington, Kentucky.

F. K. RAMSEY, M.S., D.V.M., PH.D.
Professor and Head, Department of Veterinary Pathology, College of Veterinary Medicine, Iowa State University, Ames, Iowa.

WILLIAM O. REED, D.V.M.
Practitioner, Hialeah, Florida, and Elmont, Long Island, New York.

CHARLES H. REID, D.V.M.
Practitioner, Hollywood, California.

R. F. RIEK, M.Sc., D.V.Sc.
Senior Principal Research Officer, Veterinary Parasitology Laboratory, Brisbane, Australia.

R. G. ROLOFSON, B.S., D.V.M.
Practitioner, Colorado Springs, Colorado.

JAMES R. ROONEY, A.B., D.V.M., M.S.
Professor, Department of Animal Pathology, Kentucky Agricultural Experiment Station, University of Kentucky, Lexington, Kentucky.

A. R. SKEWES, D.V.M.
Practitioner, Union Grove, Wisconsin.

J. F. SMITHCORS, D.V.M., PH.D.
Technical Editor, American Veterinary Publications, Santa Barbara, California.

R. H. SMYTHE, M.R.C.V.S.
Practitioner, Nottingham, England.

D. K. SORENSEN, D.V.M., PH.D.
Professor, Department of Veterinary Medicine and Clinics, College of Veterinary Medicine, University of Minnesota, St. Paul, Minnesota.

J. D. STEEL, B.V.Sc.
Senior Lecturer in Veterinary Medicine, Faculty of Veterinary Science, University of Sydney, Sydney, Australia.

C. D. STEIN, V.M.D.
Consultant, Animal Disease Eradication Division, U. S. Department of Agriculture, Washington, D. C.

HARLEY H. SUTTON, D.V.M.
Practitioner, Georgetown, Kentucky.

JAMES L. TEMPLE, D.V.M.
Practitioner, Arcadia, California.

MYRON THOM, D.V.M.
Practitioner, Pasadena, California.

N. W. VAN HOOSEN, D.V.M.
Practitioner, Auburn, Washington.

J. T. VAUGHAN, D.V.M.
Assistant Professor, Department of Large Animal Surgery and Medicine, School of Veterinary Medicine, Auburn University, Auburn, Alabama.

LYMAN R. VAWTER, D.V.M., M.S.
Professor (emeritus), Veterinary Medicine, Oregon State University, Corvallis, Oregon.

WILSON H. WOHLER, JR., D.V.M.
Practitioner, Aledo, Texas.

CONTENTS

CHAPTER 1

THE EXAMINATION

THE PHYSICAL EXAMINATION

The examination of the horse to determine the presence of disease or unsoundness is a matter of trained observation, carried out in a methodical manner. The procedure to be set out in the following pages may give the student the impression that it is a protracted operation which will take a very long time to perform. Although this may appear to be so on paper, in reality, after a little experience, the various stages follow one another quite automatically and a complete examination of a horse, sick, injured or lame, can be conducted in less than a quarter of an hour.

The veterinarian may be asked to examine a horse for a variety of reasons. Usually, he is told the purpose of the examination before he sees the animal, but in certain circumstances, especially when litigation may ensue, it may be necessary, or advisable, to conduct an examination with as little inquiry as possible concerning the reason.

PROCEDURE

When asked to make an examination of a horse which is stabled, as opposed to one in pasture, one should endeavor whenever possible to see the animal "cold," which means that it should not have been taken out of the stable and exercised immediately before your visit. Presuming that the horse is in a box stall and that to see it requires opening the door (in the absence of a grill or window), do so very quietly to cause the horse no alarm. Speak gently to it and stand in the doorway for a few minutes, taking notes of all you see. Observe whether the horse is tied or loose, if it is blanketed or uncovered, and if it wears a halter.

Look at the horse and assess its type and general bodily appearance. Observe whether it looks sleek, recently groomed, free from patches of baldness and rubbing marks—or, whether it is rough, dirty, and obviously un-groomed. Glance at the hoofs and limbs, and under the belly for mudmarks, which indicate that the horse has either worked or exercised recently or has been running outdoors. Next, see if the manger is full and neglected, or partly emptied, and observe if the horse is still chewing roughage. Take notice of the general attitude of the horse, its expression and demeanor. Does it appear bright and lively, inquisitive concerning your presence, or is it standing listless, with head and ears drooping, displaying no interest whatever? Does it show signs of sweating? Observe any indication of colic, or other pain, usually exhibited by pawing the ground, looking round at the belly, and rising and lying down frequently.

Notice whether the horse stands squarely on all 4 feet, if it continually rests one limb, "points a toe," or frequently changes position as it stands. Take particular heed of signs of stamping the feet (usually the hind) upon the floor, or any other evidence of skin irritation such as rubbing. Observe any stiffness in movement or muscular rigidity. Glance at the membrana nictitans and notice if it partly covers the eye when the horse moves or raises its head.

Now pay particular attention to the manner in which the horse handles its limbs. Does it favor any one of them, stand on a toe with the heel raised or knuckle at any of its joints? Can you see any indications of swelling, cuts or abrasions?

Note if there are any fresh feces on the floor of the stall or in the bedding. If there are any, observe their amount and consistency—whether they are scanty, dry and hard, perhaps coated with a dried mucus in the form of a grayish film. If no solid feces are visible look at the horse's tail to observe if it shows signs of recent diarrhea. Look at the walls of the stall for similar evidence. Glance at the manger and hay rack. From where you are standing, do they show indications of having been chewed? Have they recently been painted or covered with tin or zinc?

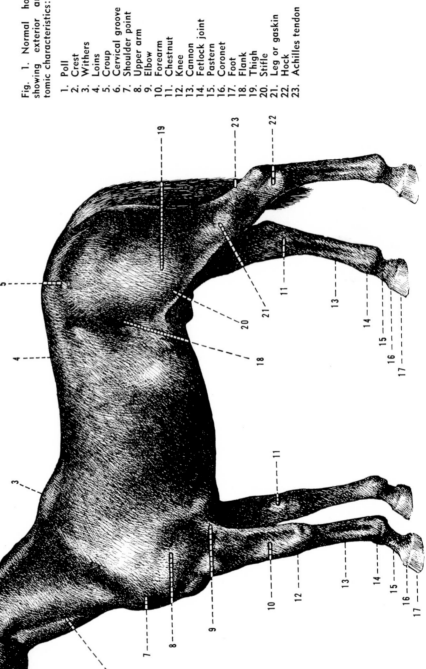

Fig. 1. Normal horse showing exterior anatomic characteristics:

1. Poll
2. Crest
3. Withers
4. Loins
5. Croup
6. Cervical groove
7. Shoulder point
8. Upper arm
9. Elbow
10. Forearm
11. Chestnut
12. Knee
13. Cannon
14. Fetlock joint
15. Pastern
16. Coronet
17. Foot
18. Flank
19. Thigh
20. Stifle
21. Leg or gaskin
22. Hock
23. Achilles tendon

Watch the horse turn around in the stall at your command and note any lameness or stiffness; whether a hock is jerked quickly upward (stringhalt); or if the tail is elevated and quivering as the horse turns. Observe any swelling of a limb; a hindlimb from thigh down, or a forelimb swollen from foot to elbow; listen for the looseness of a shoe evidenced by a "clicking" sound.

Now speak to the horse; walk up alongside of its left shoulder, and pat its neck. If it has no halter ask the attendant to put one on. While he is doing this look in the manger and observe the quantity of food present; observe whether it is dry or damp, and whether it contains wet "quids" of food, chewed and dropped. Smell the food; note its nature and quality.

If the animal is blanketed have the covering removed. Examine the skin surface for any signs of bareness or irritation. Note any skin thickening on either side of the neck which may have been caused by hypodermic injections. Now feel the pulse, count the respirations, note the type of respiration and take the temperature.

PULSE RATE

The pulse may be taken at the submaxillary artery on the inner aspect of the lower ramus of the jaw, immediately before the artery crosses the bone. It may also be taken beneath the forearm where the radial artery travels down behind the radius.

The normal pulse rate of the horse varies from 28 to 42 per minute according to age, temperament, and whether the horse has been at rest for at least several minutes or if it has just been exercised. Being handled by a stranger may raise the pulse rate from 28 to 35 pulsations per minute. Regarding the influence of exercise, the pulse rate corresponds roughly with the degree of hyperpnea. A pulse rate of 40 should fall to 30 within five minutes after fast trotting over 100 yards, but after a gallop it may take a considerable time to regain its normal rate. When a circulatory disturbance is suspected, the horse should be exercised with a stable companion of similar type, and the pulse and respiration rates of the two horses

compared before and after slow and then fast action.

Young horses have a more rapid pulse than old animals. A yearling will register from 40 to 58 a minute in normal health. Often the rapidity of the pulse rate is inverse to body weight. Small ponies at rest, and after light exercise, often have a rate of 40, rising to 50 after trotting. In heavy horses, such as Shires and Clydesdales, the pulse rate more often ranges from 28 to 40 per minute.

BREATHING RATE

The breathing, observed by viewing the flank movements or those of the ribs, should produce from 8 to 12 inspirations a minute in the 6-year-old horse at rest. In horses up to 5 years old the average number may be 14, rising to 16 if moved over once or twice in the stall. In yearlings and 2-year-olds, the number will vary from 10 to 15 inspirations a minute. The nature of the respiratory movement is of great importance. One should look for doubling of the expiratory movement, an effort to empty an emphysematous lung of residual air, characterized by an expiratory movement of the ribs broken by a pause, then followed by a more exaggerated expiratory impulse which may be transmitted through the flank to convey a tremor through the whole body. Any horse exhibiting the slightest indication of double expiration should be stimulated to cough by momentarily compressing the trachea a few inches below the larynx between the thumb and fingers.

One should carefully observe the abdomen along the lower borders of the ribs. In the horse, the normal type of breathing is costo-abdominal, the ribs and abdominal muscles nearly equally sharing in the respiratory movements. When this is not occurring, as when the breathing is abdominal rather than thoracic, a distinct furrow will be observed between the rib cartilages and the lower border of the abdomen. This may result from a painful chest condition, damaged ribs or intercostal muscles, or any painful condition which causes attempts at fixation of the diaphragm. Also such a furrow may result from an increased effort to breathe, and when there is a double expiratory lift of the flanks necessary to counter-balance the loss of elasticity within the emphysematous lungs. The groove which appears at the flank, along the costal arch, is referred to as the "heaves line." This must not be confused with a somewhat similar line sometimes visible in well-conditioned race horses, which have perfectly normal breathing motions.

Auscultation should be performed with a stethoscope. Areas of pulmonary consolidation can be detected mainly by the absence of sound over the affected area, sometimes with a surrounding area of crepitation. In emphysema, a whole selection of adventitious noises are produced, best heard high upon the chest wall.

RECORDING THE TEMPERATURE

Temperature is taken by introducing the thermometer through the anus, taking care not to lose contact with the butt end of the instrument. When the rectum is loaded with feces an effort should be made to keep the mercury end of the thermometer in contact with the rectal lining. The normal equine temperature averages 100 F., with a range of 99.5 to 101.3 F. The latter reading may be regarded as normal in a horse which has been exercised immediately prior to examination. Foals and yearlings may register up to 102 F., especially if nervous, after exercise or excitement, and in hot, humid weather.

Next, have the horse's head turned toward the light and stand in front of it. Look at both eyes and note the presence or absence of discharge. Are the eyes bright and glistening or do they appear dull, grayish, or partly closed? Observe any evident opacity. Separate the eyelids and observe the conjunctiva, noting its color, the degree of congestion of the blood vessels, the nature of any exudate present, and any indication of jaundice.

Place the hand below the chin and raise the jaw. Watch the membrana nictitans to see if it protrudes over the eyeball. Place the right hand, palm downward, on the horse's muzzle to steady the head, then open the left nostril with thumb and index finger, and look at the mucous lining inside the false nostril. Change hands and examine the other nostril. Note any redness, yellowness, nasal discharge, and the presence or absence of petechiae. Examine the nasal septum for signs of ulceration.

Pass the right hand along the inner aspect of each ramus of the lower jaw, noticing any enlargement of the lymphatic glands and any edema of the intermandibular space. Palpate the parotid glands by placing a hand on each gland. Start below the larynx and work upward to the ear while exerting gentle pressure.

Smell the breath for evidence of sinus infection, caries, or retained "quids" of food beneath the cheeks. Pass 2 fingers into the interdental space and open the mouth sufficiently to inspect the tongue and roof of the mouth. Now is a very good time to make a note of the horse's age. After doing this, pass the hand over the poll, noting any enlargement, sinus formation, or evidence of pain upon pressure.

Now, look carefully at the jugular furrow on each side, observing the presence or absence of a jugular pulse. Take particular notice of any thickening of the skin over any part of the furrow which may have resulted from an intravenous injection.

Along the lower part of the neck observe the ridge produced by the cervical vertebrae; notice any enlargement, any difficulty in bending the neck or in getting the head to the ground, and any atrophy of the neck muscles (which may cause the cervical vertebrae to assume prominence). Look at the withers and note any bruising or swelling, fistula formation, or sitfast below the saddle on either side of the back.

Next, stand in front of the horse and compare the 2 shoulders for size, swelling or atrophy. Let your gaze travel down over the sternal region, then down each forelimb in turn, and at both together for comparison. Pay special regard to the feet and coronets. Do they match on either side, and are the feet rounded and of good conformation? Make a note of obvious splints, cracked heels, chipped knees, bowed or thickened tendons, overshot knees, or knuckling at knees or fetlocks. All this can be done visually, without at present resorting to palpation. Glance down the sides, behind the elbows and under the breast for girthgalls. Note any capped elbows or fullness of the sternal region.

Stand 8 feet behind the horse and note the contour of the quarters and the 2 tuber coxae to judge whether they are level. When chronic lameness of a hindlimb exists there is frequently atrophy of the corresponding quarter. Have a forefoot lifted, run the palm of the hand under the thighs and feel the lymphatic glands for soreness or swelling (lymphangitis). Note any hock enlargement, especially "capped hock." Observe any swelling of the fetlocks, cracking of the heels, or signs of greaseheel, particularly in heavy horses. Next lift each foot in turn. Study the sole, its concavity or flatness, note the frogs, and the width at each heel. Observe any undue wear of either branch of the shoe, or at toe or heel. Pay special attention to the flexor tendons and other structures at the back of the cannon bones.

Now have the horse led out very quietly. Place yourself in a safe and convenient location within the stall and watch the horse turn and walk out. Again observe whether the point of either hock jerks upward more than its fellow when the horse turns or whether one hock is raised normally while the other is not. Notice also a tendency to raise one foot from the ground and hold it with a quivering movement before it is again put down.

Now have the horse walked away from you for 30 yards, turned and trotted back. Let it stand a few seconds while you watch how it settles on its feet. Then have it turned again, trotted gently away, and again brought back. Turn the horse in each direction in a short circle—then have it pushed backward 10 yards in a straight line.

By this time, you may have detected lameness, an injury, some abnormality of temperature, pulse or respiration. If so, now is the time to make a more detailed examination of the defect.

Lameness will be considered in another section of the book. Therefore, let us suppose now that you suspect an abdominal disease. You should note whether the abdomen seems to be "tucked-up" or whether it is distended and appears tympanitic. Do not mistake obesity for abdominal distention. We will presume that the manger contains uneaten food and that the horse has a temperature of 103 F. You have looked for feces in the stall and noted whether they are normal in appearance and quantity. If they are semifluid, you can examine some on the spot to see if any evidence of worm infestation is present. If there is no such evidence, you should retain a sample for microscopic examination for eggs and larvae.

When the feces are firm or coated you should make a rectal examination and palpate the large intestines. First, examine the large colon and then move the hand backward and downward to the cecum. Determine whether these portions of the bowel are overloaded with feces, and if gas is present. Remove a handful of feces if any are within reach, and note their consistency.

While the hand is in the rectum palpate the bladder. If you want a sample of the gelding's urine you may place the palm of your hand upon the bladder and maintain a gentle pressure for 1 or 2 minutes; the horse then will stretch and micturate. If the patient is a mare you can at this time palpate the uterus and ovaries.

If the horse appears ill, yet shows no definite indication as to the cause of illness, inquire regarding possible contacts, or possible sources of infection. Get all dates and particulars, the time of the first sign of illness and its nature, together with full particulars regarding diet, the source of drinking water, the nature and amount of work being carried out. Also make tentative inquiries, if it appears advisable, regarding illness among horses known to have been in contact with the patient. Any accidental cause may be investigated. Did the horse obtain access to any edible material or to anything of a poisonous nature? When a horse has been grazing, determine the nature of the herbage, the presence of dangerous plants, sprays, mineral deposits, or polluted streams. If the circumstances warrant further investigation, now is the time to set about a more detailed examination of certain organs.

EXAMINATION OF THE EYES

The eyes of the horse may be examined in a stable provided with a window, or the horse may be brought into a doorway. Standing it in an archway, when one is available, provides ideal lighting during the daylight hours for viewing the eyes. Bright sunlight often masks a slight opacity.

The practitioner should be provided with a black, flat disc (matte surface), about 5 inches in diameter, fitted with a handle. The reflection of the matte surface upon the cornea removes unwanted shadows and allows regulation of the amount of daylight entering the eye. It also provides a contrast between the natural appearance of the cornea and that of any abnormalities on its surface, or within its substance. The eyes of healthy horses are examined best after exercise when the pupils are naturally dilated.

The practitioner should have observed already any swelling of the eyelids, and the presence or absence of discharge from the conjunctival sac. In addition, he should notice any lacerations or incomplete closure of eyelids due to faulty healing of previous lacerations. The eyelids can be parted to examine the conjunctival sac, noting the presence of foreign bodies, papular swellings, neoplastic growths, or abnormalities of the membrana nictitans.

When superficial injury to the cornea is suspected the instillation of a 2% fluorescein solution (preferably with the consent of the owner) will aid the discovery of surface opacities, and after a short interval the dye will appear at the corresponding punctum within the nostril, if the lacrimal canal is patent. It is wise to make an examination of the depths of the eye before using the dye which may temporarily interfere with examination of the lens, if a corneal abrasion exists.

Before using fluorescein, one should observe the degree of pupillary dilation in both eyes simultaneously, under precisely similar conditions of lighting. By alternately closing one eyelid and releasing it, the reactions of the pupil to light may be studied. Remember that both pupils should be equally dilated.

Observe the supra-orbital fossa to see if it is well-filled with postorbital fat, or if it is hollow. Compare the state of the fossa with the bodily condition of the horse. If the latter is fat and the fossa (especially if one only) is hollow, there may be some abnormality in the size of the eyeball, its muscular attachments, or its nerve supply. Look below the pupil into the anterior chamber within the cornea. An accumulation of grayish or yellowish material (hypopyon) at this site represents purulent exudate either from the ciliary body, the iris, or from a penetrating corneal ulcer or wound. In the horse, it may be associated with periodic ophthalmia. Small grayish-white dots or spots on the cornea may represent chronic inflammatory changes and be composed of cells deposited from the aqueous humor on the deep layer of the cornea. They indicate an existing inflammation of the ciliary body (cyclitis).

The sclerae may be examined by opening the lids and tilting the head into various positions. The healthy sclera is white and glistening, but in old horses it may appear yellowish or rust-colored, with a yellowish deposit of lipoid material. In the normal eye, the circle of blood vessels within the sclera surrounding the corneal margin is not visible, but inflammatory changes in some other part of the eye may cause its appearance as a vascular ring.

To make an examination of the corneal surface, anterior chamber, lens, and the fundus of the eye by artificial illumination, one darkens the stall or examines the eye at night. The instruments employed are an electric ophthalmoscope and a flashlight. The glass of the flashlight should be covered with a piece of black paper in which a narrow slit has been made. Then the light may be used either for direct or oblique illumination of the eye, and can be rotated to get the best effect from the slit beam.

Oblique illumination gives a good view of the cornea, iris, and anterior chamber of the eye. The ophthalmoscope enables one to view the outer surface of the cornea and conjunctiva, using a +20 lens, or whichever lens best suits the person employing it.

The lenses on the ophthalmoscope run from −10 to +20 diopters, and can be rotated in succession, so that different degrees of refraction pass between the eye of the observer and the eye observed. Each lens varies by 0.5D to 1D, according to the make of instrument. On one side of the disc the lenses are minus, on the other side plus. If the examiner wears bifocal glasses he must be careful to view through the same segment of his glasses.

It is better to focus first on the fundus of the eye and try to obtain a clear view of the optic disc, which in the horse lies low in the fundus. If the examiner is tall he may look down at the disc, but if short he will need to stand on a stool. If when looking at the fundus and the optic disc the visible structures appear to be perfectly clear, without any interruption, there probably is no cataract present. However, to detect small opacities of the lens it is better to use a parallactic method.

One may have found by examination of the optic disc that a degree of obstruction to the passage of light rays exists in some portion of the lens. To further examine the cataract, one focuses on the corneal surface and then rotates the lens disc to the +15 lens through which the lens surface may be seen. Further decreases of 0.5D afford a better idea of the location of the opacity, whether anterior, posterior, or contained in the lens nucleus. The size of the opacity can also be appreciated. One must remember that small cataracts may cause little effect on visual function. Much depends on their position in the lens. One that lies dead center does not always cause the worst defect of vision as can be shown by placing confetti-like pieces of paper on different parts of a camera lens. However, cataract always constitutes an unsoundness.

EXAMINATION OF THE EARS

Observe the position of the ears at rest and during movement. Excessive aural movement may be one sign of defective vision. Whenever the horse focuses both eyes on an object the ears usually prick forward. When one ear tends to lop over, notice whether the upper eyelid of the same side tends to droop. If it does, there may be a nerve injury or, rarely, a psammoma.

EXAMINATION OF THE TEETH

The examination of teeth requires an oral speculum and a flashlight. A blindfold over the horse's eyes may facilitate handling. The tongue should be brought through the interdental space and held covered by a cloth, taking care not to pull sufficiently upon it to tear the frenum. With the speculum in place, the flashlight should be used to carefully examine the molar teeth. Observe the presence of irregular or "wavy" dental surfaces, or the absence of a molar with a corresponding increase in growth of the opposite tooth. Caries usually can be suspected from the odor which exudes.

EXAMINATION OF THE HEART

The heart should be auscultated while the horse is in the box stall and at rest, then again after exercise. The subsidence of the increased number of beats harmonizes with the lowering of the pulse rate, and it is only necessary to determine how long it requires to attain a normal pulse after strenuous exercise. All extrasystoles or irregularities should disappear after exercise if they are unimportant.

The stethoscope will aid in detection of a great many abnormalities of the heart. When any are evident, it is advisable to have the heart examined by electrocardiography, especially in the case of race horses. With the stethoscope, the apex beat can be heard over the ribs behind the elbow, but to cover the whole of the cardiac region it is advisable to have the left foreleg held forward.

The size of the heart can be ascertained reasonably well, and the presence of dilation detected by auscultation. Irregularity, evidenced by missing beats, double systole, brachycardia and tachycardia should be observed. Determining the time required by the heart to return to the original number of beats after fast exercise, provides useful evidence regarding its working efficiency. Irregular action of the heart while the horse is at rest should disappear after a gentle 50-yard trot.

By the time the veterinarian has completed an examination in this manner he should know a great deal about the patient. It has truthfully been remarked that the veterinarian of years ago usually knew practically everything about the horse by the time he had it walked from its stall. This sort of knowledge requires experience and a background of "horse sense," which in modern times is not so easy to acquire. By following the directions given and examining every horse available, it may rapidly be accumulated by an observant pupil.

EXAMINATION FOR SOUNDNESS

To describe in detail the procedure relating to the examination of horses of various types prior to sale or purchase, would require a volume of its own. In the space available, it will be possible only to point out what must always be looked for, what to avoid, and the things which must never be overlooked.

Horses are examined professionally for a variety of reasons. They may be stallions to be purchased for stud, mares intended for riding, driving or jumping, and in all probability with a view to subsequent breeding. They may be yearlings intended later for training, or they may be ponies intended for the use of children. In addition, we still have a number of horses used for heavy work, and we have polo ponies. However, the majority of the horses a veterinary practitioner is called upon to examine are those intended for racing or breeding, or hunting.

The first question to be asked is "What constitutes soundness and unsoundness?" Before attempting to answer this question categorically we must realize that a completely sound horse is a rarity, and there are variations in the degree of unsoundness. Some defects may be trivial but nevertheless constitute unsoundness.

The legal definition of unsoundness in Great Britain is based on the judgment of Baron Park (1842) who declared:

"The rule as to soundness is that if at the time of sale the horse has any disease which actually does diminish the natural usefulness of the animal, so as to make him less capable of work of any description, or which in its ordinary progress will diminish the natural usefulness of the animal, or if the horse has either from disease or accident undergone any alteration of structure that either actually does at the time or in its ordinary effects will diminish the natural usefulness of the horse, such a horse is unsound."

[The existence of any disease or condition which impairs the animal's usefulness, present or future, or any alteration of structure caused by past disease or injury which impairs use-fulness, will cause a horse to be classed as unsound. Soundness, likewise, is related to the anticipated use of the horse and for this reason more than one definition of soundness will apply to a specific circumstance. Although the assessment of soundness in the horse may be based upon law, as it is in England, many other countries, including the United States, have no legal definition of soundness. In these, the evaluation of soundness is a contractual relationship between veterinarian and client. Although no legal definitions exist, there are specific concepts of soundness which are usually applied.—Editor.]

Defects which must always be regarded as constituting unsoundness include:

(a) Interference with respiration, such as may result from chronic cough, pulmonary emphysema, or any tendency to whistle or roar. Blowing and snorting, when produced voluntarily and not as the result of overfatness, need not be considered as unsoundness.

(b) Dental defects which interfere with grazing or proper mastication; overshot and undershot mouths.

(c) Faults and vices such as shivering, stringhalt, weaving, crib-biting and wind-sucking.

(d) Blindness or deafness.

(e) Any spinal abnormality or any nervous disorder interfering with the full use of muscles.

(f) Failure or inability to lie in the stable. This may be difficult to detect on a single examination. Similarly, a horse which habitually kicks in harness, or one which jibs may be regarded as unsound, although it may be difficult for a veterinarian to recognize these vices unless he sees the animal at work.

(g) Certain bursal enlargements constitute unsoundness. A distention of one of the bursae of the ligamentum nuchae, at poll or withers, even when not producing obvious inconvenience, is a definite unsoundness. Many horses exhibiting windgalls, or even distention of the synovial capsule of the knee joint, without lameness, may be accepted as sound, and will in all probability retain their full usefulness. But a horse suffering from a synovial distention of the hock joint, such as a thoroughpin or bog spavin, is unsound, although the defect may never interfere with the usefulness of the animal. Whenever a minor defect, such as a windgall, is recognized but is not regarded as causing unsoundness, its existence should invariably be noted in the veterinary certificate, with or without comment regarding prognosis.

(h) All varieties of arthritis, ostitis, or acute periostitis constitute unsoundness. A horse with a ringbone or a spavin is unsound, whatever the future may hold for it, and, similarly, a sidebone constitutes an unsoundness, especially in a light horse, regardless of the fact that most aged horses have some degree of calcification of the lateral cartilages, which may never cause lameness or inconvenience. Any defect of the navicular bone is an unsoundness. Although one is justified in certifying that a horse shows signs suggestive of the presence of navicular disease, one would be unwise to assert that the disease was present, unless it previously was confirmed by x-ray examination.

(i) Laminitis, seedy-toe, canker, and all chronic foot conditions constitute unsoundness, even when they do not cause lameness. Contracted feet, false quarter, keratoma, sandcrack (until it has grown out), render a horse unsound.

(j) Permanent changes in the superficial and deep flexor tendons or in synovial sheaths; changes in the suspensory and check ligaments, or in the plantar ligament (curb), cause unsoundness. A horse with curbs may remain free from lameness for some time but, nevertheless, this does not warrant its being described as sound.

(k) Many minor injuries in a hunter are ascribed to "wear and tear," and although they should be mentioned in a certificate, they need not be classed as unsoundness, unless they interfere with usefulness or might reasonably do so at a later date. They include a missing incisor tooth in a steeplechaser, slightly chipped knees or fetlocks in a hunter or a stallion, small fibrous thickenings of the skin of the knees and fetlocks, and small wounds which have healed leaving a visible scar. All of these and many other similar defects can be entered in the certificate as "identification marks."

A horse which has recovered successfully from a roaring operation creates a problem. If a scar remains in the operative area with characteristic adhesion of the skin and the underlying laryngeal fascia, the fact should be mentioned in the certificate, but it is unwise to assert quite unreservedly, that such a horse had been subjected to surgery without better evidence.

The British Ministry of Agriculture and Fisheries has listed the following defects as disqualifying a stallion for license under the Horse Breeding Acts, 1918 and 1948: Clinical evidence of glanders, farcy, dourine, epizootic lymphangitis, mange, tuberculosis, or other contagious or infectious diseases. The stallion must be free from the following diseases and defects: cataract, sidebone, bone spavin, roaring, navicular disease, stringhalt, whistling, defective genital organs (as cryptorchidism), shivering and ringbone. The veterinarian must indicate that the animal: (a) is not lame, (b) is lame, but not sufficiently to interfere with its usefulness as a stallion, (c) or is sufficiently lame to interfere with its usefulness as a stallion.

Ringbone is considered to include articular or periarticular ringbone, and any bony growth that partly or completely surrounds the pastern or pedal joints. It is not intended to be applied to well-defined, isolated exostoses at the fetlock.

It is essential to develop a complete routine of examination to be carried out to the last detail. One must use eyes and fingers, look at every part of the body in turn, and run the hands and fingers over every joint and tendon in ordered sequence.

The worst method of examining a horse is to list a selection of unsoundness, e.g., spavin, ringbone, faulty molar teeth, and to jump from one part of the horse's anatomy to the other with no set order. By starting at the head and ending at the tail, remembering that a horse has 2 sides to its body, and particularly that it owns 4 feet, one is less likely to overlook any part of the body, or any form of unsoundness.

IDENTIFICATION

The first entry to make in one's notebook is an accurate description of the animal, one which will enable another owner, or another veterinarian, to identify it without likelihood of another animal's being substituted without his knowledge. Age, breed, sex, height, color and markings should be entered in this order. Any identifying features, as tattoos or nonpigmented irises, should then be noted. The Royal College of Veterinary Surgeons has recommended a type of certificate form, and has issued a list of colors of horses, and how they should be described in a certificate. The college advocates a form carrying an outline of both sides of a horse, upon which the markings can be drawn in their correct shape and position.

MEASURING

Height should never be guessed. The measuring stick used should be accurate, fitted with a spirit level and shod with metal. All 4 legs of the horse must be perpendicular to the ground, the forelegs in line. The poll shall not be lower than the highest point of the withers when the measurement is taken. Measurements should be recorded as "with" or "without shoes." Ordinary shoes permit a ½ inch allowance, but no allowance should be made for tips, plates or Charlier shoes.

Smooth concrete is the best material on which to stand the horse to be measured. The concrete must be level for if the hindfeet are ½ inch lower than the forefeet this will be reflected at the withers.

AGE

The following notes are not intended to be a treatise on the dentition of equines but merely to indicate a few of the more obvious characteristics of the teeth of various animals as an indication of their age.

All veterinarians have received some instruction concerning dentition. As a guide to age, dentition can be accepted only within certain limits, as it is not infallible. Animals differ in the nature of their teeth, the thickness of the enamel, and the hardness of the dentine, as well as in the nature of the food they eat and the water they drink. Horses which graze on very short pasture, particularly on sandy

or gravelly soil, will wear their teeth much more rapidly than those fed on a loamy soil with richer foliage, and much faster than horses kept indoors and fed on crushed oats, bran and hay.

THE TEETH OF THE HORSE

The horse, mule, and ass normally have 6 incisor teeth, consisting of 2 centrals, 2 laterals, and 2 corner teeth. Although veterinarians and horse-owners almost invariably use this terminology, one may use the terms: first, second and third pairs of incisors. There are 6 cheek teeth on either side of each jaw, make up of 3 premolars and 3 molars. The 3 premolars become changed for permanent premolars.

At birth there are 2 central incisors. These may not appear until the seventh or tenth day. At 4 to 6 weeks the lateral incisors appear. At 6 to 9 months the corner incisors appear. At 1 year, all 6 temporary incisors are present but only the centrals show marked wear of their tables. The corners are sharp and shell-like. At 2 years, all incisors show wear of their tables. The infundibulum will have disappeared from centrals and laterals, and possibly from the corners.

At 2½ years, the central incisors are loose or shed. A 3 years, the 2 permanent centrals have erupted and are in wear. At 3½ years, the temporary laterals are shed. At 4 years the laterals are in wear. At 4½ years the corner temporary incisors are shed. At 5 years the corner incisors are in wear. Both at 2 years and 5 years, there will be a full set of incisors: temporary at 2 years, permanent at 5 years.

Temporary incisors appear rather fragile and shell-like. They are smaller than permanent incisors. Their biting edges tend to curl over, like the edges of a shell, and they are pear-shaped, with an appreciable neck next to the gum. At 1 year, the temporary incisors are close together, but at 2 years, the jaw has widened and there may be slight gaps between the teeth, especially near the gums.

On a great many occasions, 2-year-olds have been mistaken for 5-year-olds, and vice versa. A 2-year-old when well-housed, fed, and groomed, may in appearance resemble a 5-

year-old externally on first sight, but to the practiced eye the state of development usually is more evident in the 5-year-old. The tail of a 2-year-old usually is shorter than that of a 5-year-old, reaching to just above or level with the hocks. In a 5-year-old, it usually reaches to well below the hocks. Even this is a variable feature and, in any case, tails may be pulled or trimmed. Tails also are apt to grow faster with good feeding and housing.

If any real doubt about age is experienced, the solution lies in an examination of the cheek teeth. At birth, the foal carries 3 cheek teeth: all temporary premolars which later will be cast and exchanged for permanent premolars. At 1 year of age, there are 4 cheek teeth: the 3 premolars and the first permanent molar. At 2 years old the colt or filly has 5 cheek teeth: 3 premolars and the first and second molars. At 4 to 5 years old it has 6 cheek teeth: 3 permanent premolars and all 3 molars.

A supernumerary premolar, the so-called "wolf tooth," may appear in front of the first premolar, at 5 to 6 months.

The canine teeth usually are present only in the male, though rudimentary ones are quite common in the female. These appear at 3½ to 4 years and are fully developed at 4½-5 years. They will be absent in a 2-year-old. At first they are grooved on their inner surfaces, but this groove will wear away by the seventh year.

The age of horses from 5 years upward is not so easy to judge accurately. The incisors at 6 years meet at a right angle in a well-formed mouth, with no forward inclination. After this age they commence to incline progressively in a forward direction with the years, until at 20 years they meet at an acute angle, and at 25 to 30 they are almost horizontally placed.

The table surfaces of the incisors serve as a guide from 6 years onward. After 7 to 8 years a horse is somewhat unjustly referred to as aged. Each permanent incisor carries on its table a dark, depressed ring known as the infundibulum. The dark ring is surrounded by a light-colored ring of enamel. At 6 years, the infundibulum has worn away, but a trace of enamel may remain. At 7 years, the infundibulum has disappeared from the centrals and laterals, apart from a trace of enamel. At 8 years, the infundibulum has disappeared from all of the incisors.

Later, due to wearing away of the crowns of the incisor teeth, a central mark appears in the tables due to exposure of the pulp cavity. The time of its appearance is a little variable and will depend upon feeding conditions and the quality of the teeth. Usually at 8 years, it appears in the central incisors. Usually at 9 years, it appears in the lateral incisors. Usually at 10 to 12, it is present in all the incisors. The shape of the tables varies from oval to triangular and then to round as the horse becomes older. In the horse up to 7 years, the tables are oval. At 9 years, the table surfaces of the centrals are triangular. In the horse at 10 years, the laterals show triangular table surfaces. At 11 years, the corners show triangular table surfaces. After 13 years, the tables become rounded with a central pulp mark. At an advanced age, the tables again become oval, but this time from front to back.

The corner incisor tooth does not wear evenly throughout its surface, so that a projection, or hook, develops at its posterior edge, and as the tooth wears from front to back without reducing the length of the hook, one gets the impression that the tooth carries a projection downward from its rear edge. This hook and accompanying notch first appear at 7 years. At 8 years, the hook has worn away somewhat, and by 8½ to 9 years the incisor surface is again level. At 11 years, the hook reappears and the notch becomes successively deeper, so that by 13 years it is very noticeable. After this, it usually persists throughout life.

Galvayne's groove is a well-marked longitudinal groove which first appears as a notch at the outer side of each upper corner tooth just below the gum. As the animal ages, the groove travels down the tooth as a narrow longitudinal furrow, often stained yellow or brown. It makes its appearance at 10 years; earlier in occasional cases. It reaches half-way down the tooth at 15 years. It has reached the bottom of the tooth at 20 years. At 25 years, it has disappeared from the upper half of the tooth. At 30 years it has disappeared completely.

PROCEDURE FOR EXAMINATION

Endeavor always to examine the horse before it has been exercised. Many horses come out of the stable slightly lame, but fail to show lameness after a preliminary "warming-up."

Similarly, after the completion of the examination, shut the horse in the box for a half-hour at least, before having it led out and trotted once more, to make sure that lameness has not followed the gallop carried out for examination of the horse's breathing pattern.

Feet: In the examination for soundness, the feet must be given very careful attention. Place yourself in front of the horse, which should stand on concrete or on a perfectly level area. Study the size and outline of each foot from the front, then from the side, and finally from the rear. Make sure that each pair matches exactly in every respect. One should be the complete replica of the other of the pair after due allowance is made for right and left. Later in the examination you should have the shoes removed and make an examination for corns. Nobody can examine a horse's feet thoroughly if its shoes are on. Look carefully at the outline of the hoof quarters, soles, and heels. Note the frog and bars, then decide whether one heel is narrower than the other or whether the foot shows any sign of contraction. Don't forget that both feet may be contracted.

A contracted foot usually is one which supports less weight at all times than its fellow, and there usually is a reason for this fact. Very often a light hammer, correctly used, will give some indication by the percussion feel, the percussion note, and the reaction of the horse whether or not a soreness or unsoundness exists. The shape of the foot, the wear at the toes and quarters, also will provide valuable information.

Respirations and Heart Action: Not every veterinarian can ride a horse to examine it, nor is it always wise to do so. The rule is—when riding the horse one should use the widest space available, and when having it ridden by someone else, select the smallest space compatible with an efficient gallop.

If it is decided to longe the horse, select ground which is not slippery. Have the animal cantered for a period on a rope lead rather than galloped, and then change the direction of travel. Cantering on a lead in a small circle tests the wind better than galloping in a wide field. Following this, turn the horse in short circles, watching its movement and noticing hock flexion in particular, then have the animal backed by hand for about 15 yards.

The best routine procedure is to examine in the following order: In the stable check the pulse, temperature, and respiration. Examine the heart. Examine the eyes first in the stable, then in the doorway. Measure the height on a level surface. Examine for age, also examine the molar teeth. Have the horse taken out, noticing its movements. Stand the horse squarely in the yard. Walk around it, studying the animal from the front, back, and either side.

Have the horse walked away, trotted back, then trotted away, walked back. Repeat if necessary. Commence examination at the head. Proceed down neck and withers, ribs, quarters, tail, and beneath tail. Return to the left forelimb. Examine it from withers to ground, carefully palpating every joint and tendon and examining these visually from every angle. Stand in front of the horse and, commencing at the shoulders, compare the 2 limbs and the feet. Then go to the other side and examine the right forelimb from the withers to the ground.

Proceed to the hindlimb. Stand behind the horse and compare its quarters, pin bones, hocks, tendons, and feet. Examine the left hindlimb in detail. Examine the right hindlimb in detail. Trot horse up and down once more. Proceed to the examination of respirations. Directly after this, re-examine the heart and note how long it takes to return to normal rate.

Now shut the horse in its box. After at least a half-hour take it out again and make a further examination for lameness by trotting it up and down, as before. Keep a close eye on hock action, excessive or diminished flexion. Again check the heart.

After you have completed your outdoor examination, have the shoes removed and make a further close inspection of the feet, searching for corns, seedy-toe, false quarter, horn tumor, and sandcrack. It always is a good practice to scrub the hooves with a hard brush. This removes any "filling" and makes inspection of the foot much easier. Trim out each heel inside and outside, and between the bar and wall in a search for corns, removing thin wafers of horn with a suitable foot knife. If a corn is present the deeper layers will show a reddish stain in a recent case, varying to yellowish or violet in a corn which has existed for some length of time. Never forget to look for a corn. Much litigation has arisen from such omission. Before leaving the premises make careful notes of all your findings but divulge nothing until you have completed your certificate.

R. H. SMYTHE

[Parts of the procedure which has been described reflect the fact that the examination for soundness in Great Britain is regulated by established legal concepts.]

RADIOGRAPHIC EXAMINATION OF THE LEGS

Radiography is a valuable aid to a correct diagnosis. Its value is based on the practitioner's knowledge of the "apparently normal." Unfortunately, many of the subtle changes which may have significance are not well-understood nor illustrated. The illustrations of the radiographs presented in this book are of gross conditions selected because of their photographic reproducibility. It is not meant to imply that lesser pathology is of little or no significance. To the contrary, it is in the beginning stages of disease that correct radiographic interpretation has its greatest value.

There are 2 great deficiencies in large animal radiography. The first, and more important, is the lack of good illustrative radiographs of the "normal" or nearly normal anatomy of the legs. This deficiency places the burden of differential interpretation upon the experience of the practitioner. Second, the size of the large animal prevents the application of many of the usual radiographic technics. Special equipment and technics are necessary to cope with the problems of penetration and definition presented by great bulk.

The first deficiency may be mitigated by duplicating the radiographic view with an actual skeletal reference. Such a reference supplies a low-cost source of information about the normal and also eliminates confusing impressions arising from the appearance of superimposed shadows.

The second deficiency of great size need not concern us here as the legs of the light horse are not appreciably larger than those of a man.

The purpose of this discussion is to mention radiographic evidence of some of the more common conditions affecting the legs of the horse. Most soft tissue lesions have been ignored. These lesions do not radiograph well and are best diagnosed by careful visual and digital examination, and attention to the history of the case.

Any discussion of radiographic methods necessarily will include reference to the standard technics. These have been described at length by Carlson, but a few words covering the basic requirements are, nevertheless, in order.[1]

EQUIPMENT

Any 110-volt portable machine of 10 milliampere, 80 kilovolt, and $\frac{1}{8}$ to $\frac{1}{4}$ second timing capacities is satisfactory. Lesser rated machines may be used but with a reduced latitude of operation. The point of portability is stressed for many obvious reasons but among the most important is the saving of time which their use permits. Also, rapid compensation can be made with portable equipment for any movement of the horse prior to the actual taking of the radiograph.

TECHNIC

Two right angle views always are necessary. Other angle views may be added. It is false economy to use a single view technic. The radiograph reduces 3 dimensions to 2 dimensions. A single view leaves one dimension unaccounted for; all dimensions should be viewed.

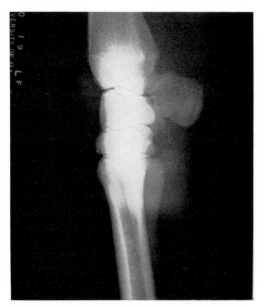

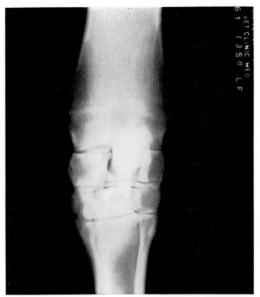

Fig. 2. "Normal" lateral view of the carpus.

Fig. 3. "Normal" A.P. view of the carpus.

The problem of motion by the patient which destroys definition of the image in the developed radiograph can largely be solved by patience, quick reflexes, and by purposeful distraction of the horse. Whistling or humming will satisfactorily mask the click of the timer.

Radiation exposure of the practitioner is to be avoided. The client's exposure to ionizing radiation normally is much less than that of the veterinarian. He usually is willing to hold the cassette. It is proper to supply him with leaded gloves. There also are several inexpensive props which eliminate the necessity for anyone to hold the cassette.[2]

Determination of proper settings on the x-ray machine may be made in a number of ways. Carlson recommends the formulation of a technic chart. This method is time-consuming and probably is not practical for the occasional user of x-ray equipment. Nor does the application of recommended settings consider the peculiarities of each machine. There are several helpful procedures, however, which may be employed satisfactorily: 1. Use cassettes containing high speed intensifying screens and Royal Blue film (Kodak), and 2, begin with a time setting of ¼ second, 10 ma., and 70 kvp (kilovoltage peak), and a 30-inch film-focal distance.[3] A certain amount of trial and error is

inherent in this recommendation because it does not take into consideration the thickness of the part to be radiographed. The thicker parts of the legs, such as the hock, carpus, and fetlock require more penetrating rays for proper visualization of all parts. An additional 5 kvp will supply this penetration. However, this procedure will not fit all situations. An anterior-posterior view of the fetlock will best show the proximal sesamoid bones if the remainder of the fetlock is purposely overexposed and is too dark for good contrast. Likewise, the distal sesamoid, or navicular bone, will best be visualized by overexposure of the remainder of the area. A general procedure to follow is to stabilize 3 of the 4 variable factors. These 3 are milliamperage, exposure time, and distance from the x-ray tube to the film; vary only the kilovoltage.[4]

An additional consideration is that of "line drop," or a fall in line voltage. Most small machines do not meter the line drop which occurs under many farm conditions. This drop in line voltage may be as much as 20 volts between the house and the barn, and it may vary with the time of day. It is better to purposely overexpose the film, and by careful developing to salvage a suitably diagnostic radiograph than to repeat the call. It readily is apparent that no one exposure will satisfactorily accomplish the desired results. The use of the aforementioned technic, however, will result in fewer radiographs retaken, and reduce the attempts to diagnose from films improperly exposed. Only diagnostic radiographs have any value.

A radiograph is a permanent record of a shadow and the record is only as good as its identification. Each radiograph should be permanently marked with the client's name, the date, and the identity of the leg, *i.e.* John Smith or a case number, 1-1-62–RR (right rear). If the part radiographed is symmetrical, an additional mark indicating medial or lateral is necessary.

The radiograph is possible only because the subject matter through which the x-rays pass is largely space. The atoms of matter are so arranged as to leave great expanses of distance between their various particles. It is through these spaces that the x-rays pass.

The standard right angle views recommended in radiographing the legs of the horse are designated on the basis of the direction taken by the x-rays. A lateral view is produced by directing the x-ray tube toward the leg with the cassette held against the medial aspect of the leg. An anterior-posterior view (A.P.) is produced by directing the x-ray tube toward the leg with the cassette held against the posterior portion of the leg. The radiograph is referred to as a lateral, A.P., or oblique on the basis of the angle which the x-rays took to reach the plate.

The developing and processing of exposed films is an integral part of the total effort. Failure at this point can destroy an otherwise excellent radiograph obtained with perfect exposure and positioning. The developing solutions must be fresh. Kodak's handbook describes several good methods, and is available on request.[3]

Developing time can be varied. Under hospital conditions, a maximum time of 5 minutes at 68 F. is recommended. The degree of development should be such that the black portion of the radiographs will not allow recognition of anything placed beneath it and the light source. If the radiographs were obtained by an overexposure technic, a preset time developing technic cannot be used. The radiographs will have to be lifted from the developing solutions and examined in safe light to determine the proper degree of development. This technic is not without pitfalls and uniformity is difficult, if not impossible. It is, however, practical rather than to make an additional call.

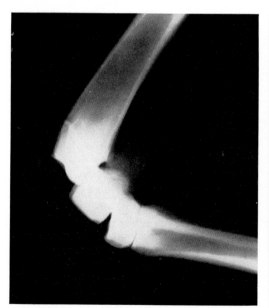

Fig. 4. "Normal" flexed lateral view of the carpus.

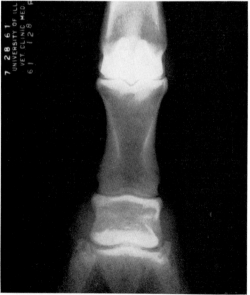

Fig. 5. "Normal" fetlock, pastern, and coffin joints, A.P. view.

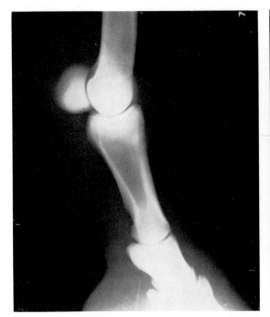

Fig. 6. "Normal" fetlock, pastern, coffin joints, lateral view.

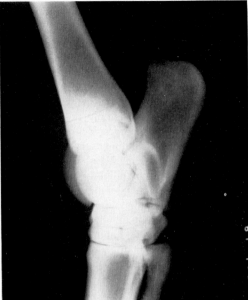

Fig. 7. "Normal" hock, lateral view.

INTERPRETATION

Radiographic detection of any changes in bone depends upon variations of the contour or in the density. These changes may be the result of physiologic atrophy, or pathologic destruction or production of bone.

Fractures produce changes in both contour and density. The fracture line is visualized most often as a dark line; however, a compression fracture will show as a white line indicating increased bone density. The type of fracture most difficult to recognize is the subperiosteal crack which often cannot be seen without the aid of a magnifying glass. Even then, a great degree of care must be exercised because of the many "apparently normal" aberrations seen in the internal structure of the leg bones of horses.

There are 5 locations from which bony pathologic processes may arise. These locations and an example of an originating process are:

1. Periosteum—sarcoma.
2. Cortex—osteoma.
3. Medullary canal—osteomyelitis.
4. Epiphysis—rickets.
5. Articular surface—infectious arthritis.

There are 5 points to consider when analyzing a bone lesion: 1. Bone production or destruction, 2, expansion of bone, 3, condition of the cortex, 4, invasion of soft tissue by bone, and 5, atrophy of bone.

It cannot be emphasized too often that recognition of these changes depends on a knowledge of the normal structure, or a readily available skeletal reference. The reference bone may be held in such a manner as to duplicate the radiographic view and thus may be used for comparison.

Bone production will be visualized as a change in the normal bony outline. Periostitis, ostitis, and tumors serve as good examples. The inner layer of the periosteum is the chief bone-forming structure, and any evidence of periosteal change is good evidence of new bone production.

Destruction of bone occurs most often as a result of bony infections, and is visualized as darkened areas in the radiograph.

Expansion of bone is seen as a result of a centrally growing tumor, or more commonly in the condition known as "bucked shins."

Change in the condition of the cortex is a response to pressures, irritations or atrophy. Cortical changes are more often visualized in the horse's legs as a result of infections. Such infections generally follow a compound fracture and cause osteomyelitis and osteitis. Thinning of the cortex is seen in rickets.

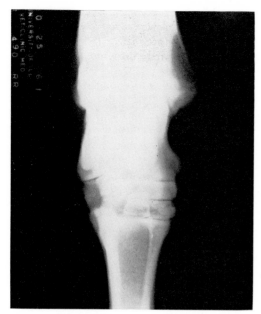

Fig. 8. "Normal" hock, A.P. view.

Invasion refers to penetration of new bony growth into soft tissue. Osteophytic projections into ligaments or tendons are common examples of bony invasion.

Atrophy of bone occurs most often as a result of disuse. Demineralization apparently follows reduced activity of the part and the accompanying reduction of the blood supply. A history of a long-standing lameness which produced a marked degree of inactivity frequently is associated with bone atrophy. A completely immobilized fracture also is subject to normal atrophy. This condition is most evident when radiographs of opposing legs are compared.

Interpretation of radiographs may be improved by several procedures. The radiograph can be viewed while wet and when dry. Often the dry radiograph reveals more clearly the subtle and minute changes. Two types of light source should be used routinely. The usual practice of using the radiographic view box as well as the use of a spotlight is recommended. The spotlight enables visualization of the overexposed areas and emphasizes the outline of soft tissue areas. The radiograph should be viewed from several distances. A magnifying glass will aid in close examination of a part.

It often is the very small, beginning lesion which escapes notice, or to which no significance is attached. If this type of lesion is the only one found and its location is compatible with the type of lameness presented, it should never be discounted. These so-called insignificant lesions are more often present at the edges of a joint surface. They often are referred to as "lipping." These calcium or bony deposits may appear to be "free" from the cortex and apparently suspended in space, or they actually may be a lesion of the bony cortex. The deposits which appear free are embedded in the joint capsule. Gradual enlargement of the deposit is the usual rule. The deposits which appear as a "lipping" at the edge of the articulating surfaces involve the periosteum. Any evidence of periosteal reaction is evidence of bony growth.

Perhaps the most difficult interpretation for the occasional viewer of radiographs is the identification of the acute lesion as opposed to the chronic. Bony changes take place more slowly than soft tissue changes. A radiographic examination of an injury or lameness within a few days of its occurrence does not allow enough time for most bony changes to occur. Several weeks are necessary for the development of changes which can be visualized radiographically. Early radiographic interpretation should be restricted to the discovery of fractures. In the acute or first stages of a bony lesion, the periosteum will have a fuzzy appearance and a darkened area will be apparent between it and the bony cortex. This same lesion in the chronic or quiet stage will appear irregular, but the outline will be clear and well-defined.

It should be remembered that radiographic consultation is available at all veterinary colleges. Though it may not be feasible or even possible to send the patient, good radiographs can be mailed at a nominal cost.

J. P. MANNING

REFERENCES

1. Carlson, W. D.: Veterinary Radiology. Lea & Febiger, Philadelphia, Pa., 1961.
2. Williams, F. L.: Radiology Laboratory Manual for Veterinarians. W. F. Lester Company, Pullman, Wash., 1959.
3. Kodak, Eastman Co.: The Fundamentals of Radiography. Eastman Kodak Co., Medical Division, Rochester, N. Y., 1960.
4. Banks, W.C.: J.A.V.M.A., 135 (1959) 467-470.

TRANSRECTAL AND TRANSVAGINAL RADIOGRAPHY

INTRODUCTION

The diagnostic use of x-rays in large domestic animals represents one of the greater unsolved roentgenologic problems. Until recently, whole anatomic regions have remained beyond the reach of x-ray technics. Large masses of muscle and the enormous diameters of some organs have rendered roentgenoscopy and roentgenography difficult or seemingly impossible. Clinicians have been particularly interested in the pelvic area and the lumbosacral portion of the spinal column, but diagnostic procedures in these regions have been generally confined to rectal and vaginal palpation since the massive musculature and skeletal structures in this area predicate against x-ray penetration. Radiologic illustration of these areas would be a valuable aid to more accurate diagnosis. A great number of surgical and therapeutic procedures likewise would be facilitated by adequate x-ray films.

In an effort to solve some of these problems and improve diagnostic methods for studying pathology of the posterior region, transrectal and transvaginal roentgenography was attempted. Analysis of the anatomic structures of this area revealed that intervening muscular and skeletal masses would be reduced 50% or more by this procedure, and would greatly facilitate roentgenologic presentation. No insuperable difficulties of film placement were anticipated in the use of the rectal or vaginal lumen, as this aspect of the problem was analogous to the use of the oral cavity for dental roentgenography. Cassette design, however, was recognized to be a distinct, and possibly a troublesome, problem.

The idea of transrectal roentgenography has been considered for several years. Little has apparently been done, however, in perfecting either technic or methodology. Visnyakov[2] stated that the pelvic area of large animals can only be demonstrated roentgenographically via the transrectal approach. His method involved manual emptying of the rectum and the insertion of a 12 x 18 cm. film wrapped in black, paraffin-impregnated paper. The film

corners were rounded to prevent injury to the patient. No data were given about the results obtained.

Alksnis[1] reported three methods of transrectal radiography: 1. By means of film without a fluorescent, intensifying screen, or folia, 2, by means of film and folia, and 3, by means of film and folia enclosed in a metal cassette. His first method was satisfactory for foals. The second method gave 2 satisfactory pictures from larger animals, but the third method failed because the metal cassettes were unsuitable for rectal introduction. In his summary, he discussed the need for special foliae and casettes.

MATERIALS AND METHODS

Our work on transrectal radiography began in 1947. It was recognized at the outset that a properly designed cassette was the key point in the practical solution of the problem. The use of film alone either with or without folia was attended with erratic results and without practical significance. Furthermore, the benefit of a folia is problematic in uncassetted film since close apposition of film and folia cannot be maintained, and this condition is essential for a good photograph. It was evident that this problem could be solved only through the use of special films or with a properly designed cassette. The employment of special films was disregarded for technologic reasons and attention was focussed on the cassette.

To be effective, the cassette should satisfy certain criteria. It must be noninjurious to the mucous membranes of the rectum and vagina. It should be flexible to conform to the shape of the rectal or vaginal wall, and the folia should adhere to the film under all conditions of flexion.

Basing our studies upon these criteria, all metallic or other hard cassettes were discarded at the outset. Measurements of the anal opening following spinal anesthesia and local anesthesia of the anal sphincters revealed that maximum anal diameters fell within the range of 8 to 12 centimeters. Since the cassette would have to remain within these limits, and since a hard cassette could not be enlarged once it had passed into the more dilatable rectal lumen, it was obvious that metal would not satisfy either the technical or anatomic requirements.

It was decided that rubber or rubberized cloth was the most suitable material for the cassette since it is flexible and harmless to the rectal and vaginal mucosa. Its flexibility facilitates passage through the anal or vaginal opening, and once inside, its size and shape can be adjusted readily to the anterior or posterior portions. The rubber not only protects the folia but allows it to be held in close apposition to the film by applying a slight vacuum to the closed case. After appropriate negative pressure has been obtained, the walls of the

the area to be roentgenographed. Cassettes of 3 sizes are employed: 16 x 30 cm. for radiography of the sacrum, 10 x 30 cm. for radiography of the lumbar vertebrae, and 14 x 20 cm. for general radiography in the pelvic region.

The fact that the rectum becomes narrower anteriorly results in the cassette's remaining bent during radiography of the lumbar region. Through trial, it has been established to what extent bending adversely affects the clarity and accuracy of the roentgenogram. Highly arched bendings of the film should be avoided by using a narrower cassette.

The animal is prepared for radiography by

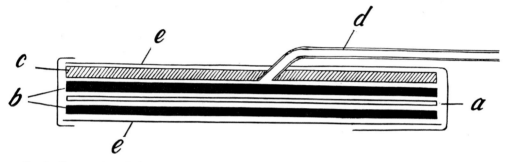

Fig. 9. Cross-section of the cassette: a, film; b, flexible folia (intensifying screen); c, leaded rubber; d, rubber tube; e, outer wall of the case.

cassette collapse upon the film and folia and hold them firmly together. In a vacuumized case, the film can be bent freely without changing the relationship of film and folia. The vacuum need not be high; oral aspiration is sufficient if a pump is not available.

The cassette's final design is a rectangular sack of rubberized cloth the front edge of which is somewhat rounded. A piece of leaded rubber is first placed in the cassette to protect the hand from radiation during fixation in the rectum. The film, together with its flexible folia, is placed above the leaded rubber. The cassette is then closed with adhesive tape and vacuum applied to collapse the walls against the film. The thickness of the filled case is about 1 cm., which is advantageous in that it prevents too abrupt bending and consequent breaking of the folia or film (Fig. 9).

The size of the cassette varies with the size of the animal, the projected location of the film within the rectal or vaginal cavities, and

injecting a caudal anesthetic until relaxation of the anus occurs. The rectum is then emptied and the bladder evacuated. Roentgenography should not be performed when the bladder is full. Enemas or laxatives are not indicated.

The anus is opened with an anal dilator and the rolled cassette, lubricated with oil, is inserted into the rectum. Further manipulation of the cassette is done intrarectally. For anterior radiography, the dilator is left in place since it tends to suppress peristalsis, and also makes further handling easier. For posterior radiography, when the cassette may be partially in the anal region, the dilator is removed. The cassette is fixed, oriented, and centered by hand within the rectum, and is straightened as much as possible before being held against the part to be photographed.

Transrectal radiography of the pelvis and lumbosacral regions of the spinal column only can be performed regionally because of site and film limitations. Therefore, the pelvic re-

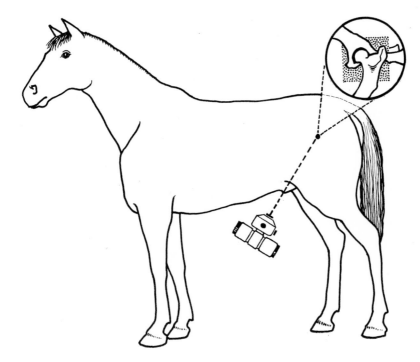

Fig. 10. Transrectal radiography of the coxofemoral joint showing position of the x-ray tube.

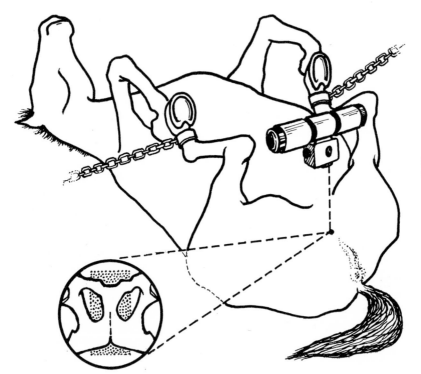

Fig. 11. Transvaginal radiography of the pelvic floor.

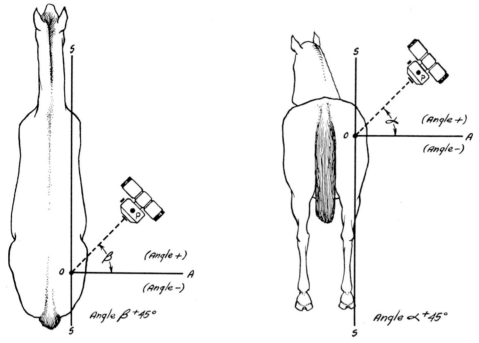

Fig. 12. Positioning for radiography of pelvic structures.

gion is divided into seven regions based on anatomic and clinical considerations:

(1) The coxofemoral joint (Fig. 10).
(2) The sacroiliac joint.
(3) The tuber coxae.
(4) The pelvic floor.
(5) The sacrum.
(6) The tuber ischii.
(7) The lumbar vertebrae.

Transvaginal radiography also is feasible. It is particularly indicated for radiography of the posterior ventral parts of the pelvic region; specifically, the coxofemoral joint, the tuber ischii, the body of the ischium, and the floor of the pelvis (Fig. 11).

All roentgenograms except those of the pelvic floor are taken with the animal in a standing position. The direction of the primary beam is perpendicular to the plane of the cassette and is oriented by means of two angles. These are established in the following manner. An imaginary sagittal plane (S) is constructed through the object (O). A perpendicular to this plane is drawn from the object, forming the line AO. A second line OP is drawn from the object through the focal spot (P) on the anode of the x-ray tube. The angle AOP, when lying in the vertical plane, forms the angle alpha (α) and when in the horizontal plane forms the angle beta (β). The perpendicular AO represents the baseline in both cases. Angles dorsal or anterior to the baseline are expressed in positive terms (*e.g.*, +50°) and where posterior or ventral to the baseline are expressed in negative terms (*e.g.*, —50°). The length of the line AO is immaterial. Vertical angles (angle alpha) and horizontal angles (angle beta) can then be combined to give exact positioning of the axis of the primary beam in relation to the object. The focal distance PO is variable and is calculated for the conditions under which each exposure is made (Fig. 12).

For instance, a roentgenogram of the tuber coxae taken at an angle alpha +40° and angle beta +60° at a focal distance of 25 centimeters would position the x-ray tube 25 centimeters anterodorsally to the tuber coxae with the beam directed posteroventromedially. A similar radiograph taken at angle alpha —40° and angle beta —60° and 25 centimeter focal distance would position the x-ray tube 25 cm.

ventroposteriorly to the tuber coxae with the beam directed anterodorsomedially.

Appraisal of Technic

Analyses of radiographs taken via the transrectal and transvaginal approaches show that this method of radiography is suitable for use in large domestic animals. Although species and individual differences exist in the morphology of the pelvic cavity, the technic can be adjusted to obtain reasonably clear pictures. The significance of this method in large animal practice is obvious. It is an effective diagnostic tool that should prove to be of value to the practitioner since standard x-ray tubes can be used to achieve thoroughly practical results.

The transvaginal approach, due to the anatomic structures and relationships in this area, can be used only to delineate a limited number of regions. The minimal bending of the cassette results in a better picture, however. With the exception of the tuber coxae and the lumbar region, this technic is completely satisfactorily, and in the excepted regions it is adequate. In lumbar radiography, however, Alksnis' assertion that aortic pulsation interferes with obtaining a satisfactory roentgenogram was not substantiated by our experience.

The technical difficulties in determining angular data and the design of a proper cassette were severe. The problem of the cassette is still not completely solved. Their present designs are far from perfect, especially in regard to the methods used to close the cassette. Also, the flexibility of the case cannot be fully utilized because of the tendency of the fluorescent folia to crack when bent too severely. These technical problems, however, could easily be solved by those who have greater facilities (Fig. 13).

J. Gligorijevic

REFERENCES

1. Alksnis, A.: Deutsche Tieräztl. Wochenschrift **51** (1943) 49.
2. Višnjakov, A.: Veterinarnaja rentgenologija, Moskva, 1940.
3. Gligorijević, J.: Veterinarski arhiv **18** (3/4) (1948) 53-72, (Zagreb).

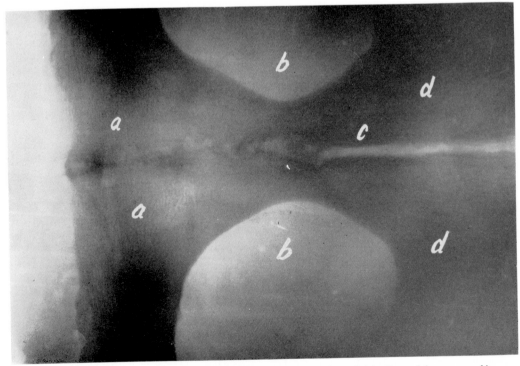

Fig. 13. Radiograph (negative print) obtained by transrectal technic. Pelvic floor of horse: a, pubis; b, obturator foramen; c, symphysis pelvis; d, ischium.

THE POSTMORTEM EXAMINATION

Introduction

Much useful information can be gathered from a postmortem examination but only if it is done in a logical manner and with an intelligent approach. It probably is better not to do one than to make a cursory examination of the organs of the peritoneal and thoracic cavities and then draw some hasty uninformed conclusions. This operation should be approached with a completely open mind as it is not wise to try to fit the findings to preconceived ideas of what abnormalities are present. It is not always possible to make a complete examination, so one at least should not neglect to examine systems or organs which the clinical signs have indicated may be affected.

General Considerations

If the animal has to be destroyed, choose a method which will cause little change or damage to organs and tissues. Preferably, give an intravenous injection. A supersaturated solution of magnesium sulfate administered as quickly as possible is both cheap and effective and causes a minimum of change. Above all, do not resort to shooting an animal in the head unless unavoidable, and certainly not if examination of the brain is indicated. This may seem axiomatic but it is by no means unknown for veterinarians to shoot an animal, and then submit the head for examination of the brain.

If the animal has died, carry out the autopsy as soon as possible after death. Autolytic and putrefactive changes make identification and interpretation of lesions more difficult as they advance.

Certain general principles should be understood by anyone who desires to glean information from a necropsy examination, and some of these are now discussed.

Rigor mortis is a change which occurs in skeletal, cardiac, and smooth muscles. It occurs within 2 to 4 hours after death and lasts for 48 to 96 hours. Fever or increased muscular activity before death causes more rapid appearance and disappearance of rigor. Before rigor sets in, the muscles, particularly cardiac and smooth muscle, seem soft and flabby. The heart appears dilated and filled with blood but this is normal. After rigor, the heart is contracted and firm and much of the blood has been expressed from the ventricles, especially the left. The urinary bladder contracts with rigor and is therefore usually empty after this develops.

Edema, hemorrhage, and thrombus formation are vital processes and cannot occur after death. It is true that blood can run from cut vessels and does clot after death but a thrombus is attached to the wall of a blood vessel, and a clot is not.

Congestion is a term which must be used with extreme caution and never at all unless one is certain that more blood than normal is present. One frequently reads of congested lungs, stomach, intestines, meninges and other organs when in fact the amount of blood present is in most cases normal. The lymph nodes of young animals normally are large and pale and the follicular pattern is not as distinct as in adults.

In describing the findings, one should use only terms whose meaning is clearly and widely known. Lesions should be described in terms of size, shape, location, color and consistency. By using these criteria and descriptive terms, anyone reading the record will understand it, but if reference is made to size in terms of an orange or football some may not know what is meant. Likewise, rather than say a lesion was on the back, describe its location in the skin on the left side about an inch from the midline and between the third and fourth lumbar vertebrae.

One can learn to recognize the abnormal only by knowing the normal so be certain that as many normals as possible have been seen before stating that a normal variation is a lesion.

Technic

A thorough external examination is made first, paying attention to the state of the hair, skin, feet, and in particular to the natural orifices, joints, mucous membrane of the mouth, and conjunctiva. Look for local and diffuse swellings and external parasites.

For the dissection, the carcass is always placed on the left side and the prosector operates with the head to his right. Raise the right foreleg and insert the knife into the axilla. All future knife cuts are now made from the inside toward the skin surface. The leg is separated from its muscle attachments to the body and laid back flat on the ground or floor. The skin over the right side of the neck, thorax, and abdomen is then reflected from the ventral to the dorsal midline. The incision is continued above the prepuce or mammary gland and the hindleg is laid back in a similar manner to the foreleg. In this process, the acetabular joint is opened and any abnormality of the synovia and articular surfaces should be noted. The synovia normally is clear, slightly yellow, and viscous. Infection may cause turbidity, formation of fibrin flakes and strands, inflammation of the synovial membrane, and irregularities of the smooth articular surfaces. Evidence of infection here is most likely to be seen in very young animals, and it usually incriminates the umbilical vessels as the portal of entry.

After reflecting the limbs, the axillary and prefemoral lymph nodes are incised and examined. In male animals, the external genitalia and, in females, the mammary gland and nodes are examined at this time. Excess fluid within the cavity of the scrotal tunics is indicative of the presence of similar fluid in the peritoneal cavity since these cavities are connected. The testes are cut longitudinally and then examined by means of several transverse incisions. (Both testes normally are in the scrotum at birth or shortly thereafter.) Epithelial tumors, both benign and malignant, often are seen on the prepuce and penis.

The abdominal and thoracic cavities are now opened. Commencing near the xiphoid process, cut through the wall of the abdomen close and parallel to the posterior arch of the ribs. During this procedure the knife point should not be placed inside the abdomen, otherwise some of the viscera will certainly be punctured, and result in contamination of the cavity and unnecessary artifacts. When the dorsal limit is reached the cut is continued to the pubis, then ventrally to the midline so that a large flap has been made of the abdominal wall. Now grasp the posterior edge of the thoracic wall at about the middle of the costal arch and raise it so that the diaphragm is stretched taut. Make a small cut through the diaphragm into the pleural cavity as close to the attachment to the ribs as possible. Normally, air will rush into the thoracic cavity, causing the lungs to collapse and the diaphragm to bulge posteriorly. Failure of this to occur means that the pleural space is occupied or that air is unable to escape from the lungs, suggesting such things as pleural effusion, pulmonary emphysema, some obstruction to the main air passages, or that the lungs are filled with fluid. Continue the incision along the attachment as far as the middorsal and midventral lines.

The thoracic wall is now removed by using a pair of large rib shears to cut through the ribs close to the sternum from the last to first rib and then in the same order close to the vertebral attachment. Finally, free the wall from the diaphragm leaving the latter as complete as possible and still attached in the carcass. Note the condition of the parietal pleura, and then free one of the longer ribs from the intercostal muscles on each side and break it in the middle to test the quality of the bone. This will be difficult or impossible in adult animals with normal bone. The ribs normally should break with a distinct snap. A rib which bends before breaking, especially in a young animal, suggests faulty nutrition.

Proceed now to examine the abdomen. Look for excess fluid in the peritoneal cavity, displacement and symmetry of the viscera and make certain that all organs are present. Check for the pancreas, spleen, liver, and 2 of all paired organs. In males, it may be necessary to look for an undescended testicle. If this is not done these organs may be damaged, destroyed or even lost during removal of the alimentary tract, particularly if there should be adhesions which make this operation difficult. Using the rib shears, cut through the pubis on each side to the obturator foramen, and then from the foramen through the ischium. Dissect away the floor of the pelvic girdle which is freed by this operation (Fig. 14).

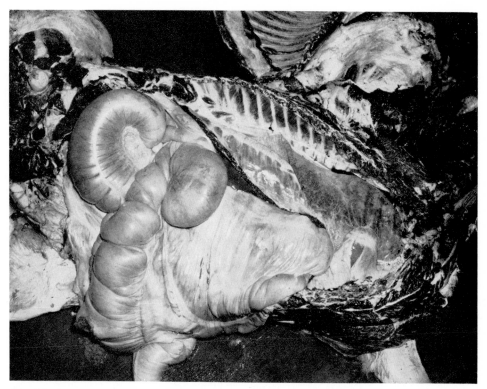

Fig. 14. Carcass on left side. Viscera exposed after removal of right abdominal and thoracic wall.
(Photo by H. Connor. Courtesy, Washington State University.)

Now, examine the pancreas, then grasp the small intestine approximately at the middle and free it from its mesenteric attachment forward to the duodenum and posteriorly to the colon. This is done by pulling firmly on the intestine with one hand and making short quick strokes with the knife blade held as close as possible to the intestine and almost at right angles to it. Before freeing the duodenum see that there is no obstruction to the bile duct.

Now, grasp the esophagus firmly at its entrance to the stomach and sever it close to the diaphragm. Lift the stomach clear of the carcass, taking care not to spill any contents into the abdomen. The rest of the tract is likewise lifted clear and laid aside. The cecum and colon are freed back to the pelvic inlet.

The spleen and liver are then removed, examined, and incised liberally. Fibrous tags are often found attached to the surface of these organs; they are often caused by the larvae of *Strongylus edentatus*. The kidneys are now removed but left attached to the ureter. The adrenals can be examined now but it is preferable to leave them attached to the kidneys. The rectum and anus plus the entire genitourinary tract are removed as a unit.

Make a cross section of the adrenals and note the color and ratio of cortex to medulla. Cut each kidney longitudinally in half, and strip off the capsule in order to see the surface clearly. Large, cortical, hemorrhagic infarcts often are seen in the kidneys of foals; the cause is unknown. Open and inspect the ureters, bladder, and urethra. The urine of the horse contains much mucus, and a few hours after death it becomes turbid because of desquamated epithelial cells. This often is incorrectly interpreted as pyuria, and a false diagnosis of pyelitis or cystitis may be made.

Open the genital tract from the vulva through the vagina, cervix, and uterus. Inspect the ovaries for follicles, cysts, atrophy, and tumors, and the oviducts for obstruction or other lesions. In males, observe the accessory sex organs. One should note here that the ovary of the mare is very firm and fibrous, and normally contains several cysts.

The thoracic organs are examined next. Observe the heart and lungs *in situ* and note the presence of excess fluid or adhesions. Reflect the skin from the side of the face, then free the tongue and pull it back. The buccal cavity can now be inspected. While keeping tension on the tongue cut through the cartilaginous hyoid articulations and free the tongue, larynx, trachea, and esophagus back to the thoracic inlet. Continue in the same manner, freeing the lungs and heart and also the esophagus and aorta back to the diaphragm where they are severed. These organs now are examined as a single unit without detaching any part. Examine the tongue grossly, then make several cross sections and inspect the musculature. Examine the thyroid, parathyroids and thymus glands and then open the full length of the esophagus. Note the symmetry and consistency of the lungs, inspect the bronchial nodes, then open the larynx, trachea, and several of the bronchi out to the pleura. Any local swellings or areas of firmness are incised. Marked con-

gestion and edema often are seen together with frothy fluid in the air passages but this usually is associated with terminal heart failure.

Examination of the heart is done without detaching it from the lungs and anterior viscera. With the tongue on the prosector's left, cut through the right ventricular wall from the pulmonary artery to the posterior vena cava along the interventricular septum and inspect the valves and endocardial surface. To examine the left chambers, make a vertical cut through the middle of the left ventricular wall and left atrium. After inspecting as before, insert the point of the knife under the anterior cusp of the atrioventricular valve up into the aorta and cut outward to expose this vessel and its valves. The vessels and septa are examined for anomalies and the cardiac muscle is incised for inspection (Fig. 15).

The parietal peritoneum, pleura, and diaphragm now can be inspected without obstruction. Because of the frequent occurrence and importance of verminous arterial thrombi caused by *Strongylus vulgaris* larvae, special attention should always be paid to the aorta and its branches. In the horse, the most

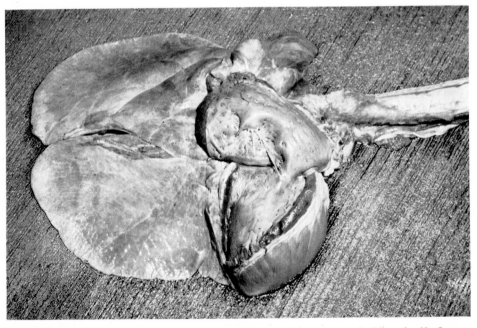

Fig. 15. Heart and lungs with the chambers on right side of heart exposed. (Photo by H. Connor. Courtesy, Washington State University.)

probable cause of almost any lesion of the abdominal organs is verminous arterial thrombosis. Such a statement as this is somewhat sweeping, but at least if the prosector has this in mind he should not fail to find a thrombus when one is present.

Some of the joints should be examined, especially in young animals, because localization of infection in the lower limb joints and tendon sheaths is not uncommon. As a routine, open the stifle and shoulder joints and in the young always inspect the hock and knee joints and the adjacent synovial tendon sheaths.

Reflect the skin and muscle from the head and look for any evidence of trauma. If there are clinical signs consistent with a lesion of the central nervous system it is advisable to collect at this time a sample of the cerebrospinal fluid and perform Pandy's test** for globulin content. To do this, remove the dorsal cervical muscles to expose the atlanto-occipital joint. With a syringe and needle, puncture the membrane in the midline and insert the needle just far enough to place its opening within the subdural space, and withdraw the fluid. This test is usually only of value in an autopsy of a fresh carcass. If, through faulty technic, blood is drawn into the syringe, the sample is of no value.

The cord now is severed at the atlanto-occipital level and the head removed. To expose the brain, 3 saw cuts are required. The first cut is transverse behind the orbits and the other 2 extend on each side from this cut to just inside the occipital condyles. Make these cuts as nearly vertical as possible. The section of calvarium between the cuts can now be removed. The dura is freed from the dorsum of the brain and then while holding the head upright, carefully sever the cranial nerves and let the brain slip out. Examine the dura and internal surfaces and remove the pituitary gland. Small tumors (chromophobe adenomas) often are found in this gland in old horses. The brain can be transversely sliced at intervals of about 1 cm. or a single slice is made into the lateral ventricles and the whole piece put into

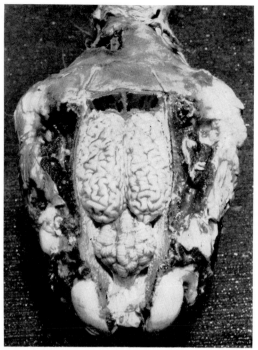

Fig. 16. Section of calvarium removed to show brain *in situ*. (Photo by H. Connor. Courtesy, Washington State University.)

a large jar of formalin for later examination. Masses of cholesterol (cholesteatoma) often are present in the choroid plexuses but are of no special significance (Fig. 16).

The final system to be examined is the gastrointestinal tract. The stomach is opened along the greater curvature, then the intestinal tract is exposed from the duodenum to anus. If circumstances do not permit such a complete examination, open and examine the intestinal tract in several places at regularly spaced intervals.

Depending on the case, it may be necessary to alter the technic and to examine systems which usually are neglected. The operator may have to examine the skeletal muscles, eyes, spinal cord, or feet but one can be guided in reference to this by the clinical findings.

Lesions and suspected areas of pathology are preserved in 10% aqueous formalin. The tissue slices must be no more than 1 cm. thick and there should be 10 times as much formalin as tissue.

The record is best written in the same order as the autopsy was done. It is not necessary

***
**Add 1 drop of cerebrospinal fluid to 4 to 5 ml. of a clear saturated solution of phenol. A cloudy precipitate forms in a few seconds if it is strongly positive (++++) or a slight turbidity develops within 30 seconds if weakly positive (+).

to make interpretations on the report but it is important to remember to adhere to description in terms of size, shape, color, consistency, and location.

D. C. DODD

NOTES ON EUTHANASIA

Performing euthanasia can be a most harrowing and unrewarding experience for the veterinarian concerned. Particularly is this so around a race track when large numbers of people immediately appear on the scene. The veterinarian must decide quickly if euthanasia is to be performed, and then do it in a rapid and efficient manner. I have used most of the commercial products prepared for this purpose and have found none that were entirely satisfactory, especially in regard to the quantity of material required to euthanatize a horse. After experimenting with numerous products and drugs I have adopted the following formula:

Strychnine sulfate   —100 grains
50 ml. sucostrin chloride—100 mg. per ml.
Q.S. nicotine sulfate   —100 ml.

This preparation has been used routinely in our practice at race tracks, horse shows, and wherever it was necessary to destroy an animal. A 10 ml. dose given intravenously with a 16-gauge needle appears to be sufficient for animals of all sizes. Its action is instantaneous and is not accompanied by struggling.

We have never been criticized by an observer since using this preparation and method to perform euthanasia. It was once feared that the sucostrin chloride in the mixture might deteriorate. I have used the same bottle carried in the car during all kinds of weather for more than a year, however, and the solution appears to retain its effectiveness. I feel that its great advantage is its rapidly fatal action with such a small dose.

E. N. ANDERSON

Saturated solutions of either chloral hydrate or magnesium sulfate cause the death of horses quickly and with little struggle. When used for animals already recumbent they should be injected intravenously, as rapidly as possible, using a 14-gauge needle and an intravenous outfit. To lay an animal down in a small area prior to euthanasia, succinylcholine is recommended for intravenous injection at 3 times its usual dose. As horses often survive quite high doses of succinylcholine, a saturated solution of chloral hydrate is administered as soon as the animal is down and until death occurs.

If drugs are not available and the horse, preferably, is recumbent, another procedure for euthanasia is to sever the aorta at its termination with a small knife which is carried into the rectum. The large pelvic arteries may be severed alternatively.

It should be noted that horses are very sensitive to electric current. Their euthanasia by exposure to lethal currents has been used satisfactorily at a number of the veterinary colleges in the United States.

A. A. GABEL

CHAPTER 2

RESTRAINT AND ANESTHESIA

FUNDAMENTALS OF PHYSICAL RESTRAINT

Despite all the science that has been introduced into equine practice, restraint of the species remains chiefly an art. Virtually a lifetime of experience, including knowledge gleaned from the experience of others, is barely enough to enable a man to cope with the many problems of restraint. This is considerably more of a problem with horses than with most other species of large animals since they must inevitably be handled as individuals. Through proper application of the principles of restraint man is placed on equal footing with the horse, and often equal consideration is given to the animal's protection from undue restraint or injury. The risk of personal injury is greatly exaggerated in the minds of the neophyte practitioner, but is there nevertheless. It is mitigated only by one's increasing knowledge of and ability to apply the principles of restraint.

With these thoughts in mind, detailed descriptions of equipment and procedures are precluded. The objective here is to introduce these principles of horsemanship and restraint so necessary to the successful conduct of equine practice.

HORSEMANSHIP

The proper application of restraint first requires a knowledge of "the nature of the beast," an acquaintance with the species. This may be said for the use of any method. What distinguishes mere restraint from its most effective counterpart is a second but no less important requirement which we refer to as horsemanship. This implies an understanding of the psychology of the animal, and by taking advantage of this, one can use the equine's instinctive behavior and individual temperament to advantage. The horse practitioner must have confidence, and the animal's being suspicious by nature makes this important.

Horsemanship comes with experience, but the newcomer asks, "What can I do in the meantime?" In the first place, he would do well to copy the quiet and deliberate approach of the veteran. Many novices reveal their lack of confidence by being overly cautious; that is, by spending too much time in a hesitant approach while the horse becomes increasingly distrustful. One's approach should be direct and to the point, while at the same time avoiding unnecessary or hurried actions; any sudden movements are apt to be misinterpreted by the horse as threatening.

Self-confidence alone is not enough. One should also possess (or attempt to acquire) a generous measure of self-discipline. There are many times when you must be firm in dealing with a horse or mule, particularly in the case of the spoiled or contrary individual, in order to gain his attention and respect. On the other hand if you overindulge your temper, instead of winning the animal's respect, you will have produced fear, quite as dangerous an emotion as malice. The old saying of "patience is a virtue" is never so true as when dealing with dumb animals.

Horsemanship also implies an ability to quickly and accurately assess the variety of temperaments encountered in the many breeds and types. The ability to determine which animals can and which cannot be trusted provides an additional advantage. Regardless of what reputation a breed or type may have, all equine temperaments may be roughly grouped into 3 categories: 1, The unbroken animal which merely is ignorant of the ways and intentions of man and usually is free of any vices or bad habits, 2, the trained and trusted (within the limits of his training) individual, and 3, the spoiled animal possessing either a bad disposition, bad habits or both. Allowances must be made for the first category, and those unwise in the training of equines may be at a disadvantage here. The second group obviously is the most appreciated. The last group requires closer examination.

As to what actually spoils a horse, we may point to management or disease. Man usually is the common denominator in both instances.

Horses nearly always reflect the temperament of their owners or handlers, and once a horse is spoiled his handling and subsequent education become difficult, but not always impossible, tasks. One should strive to handle the animal in such a way as to leave him easier to manage at succeeding times, and to conscientiously avoid making his disposition worse. This especially is so when handling young or untrained individuals since bad habits are easy to acquire, but difficult to break.

Selection of the Restraint Method

At the risk of oversimplification, one general rule can be applied to the restraint of equines. The amount of restraint necessary is in inverse proportion to the amount of handling the animal has received; bear in mind such factors as patience and temperament. Probably the most useful tools in breaking equines and giving a man the amount of confidence needed to handle them are a feed bucket, a grooming brush, and a hoof pick. Other knowledge will be acquired during the use of these 3 items.

Several considerations in arriving at a choice of the restraint method are enumerated in the following:

1. The individual's temperament:

In addition to what has already been said regarding this subject, it should be added that what works for one horse may be contraindicated for another purely on the basis of temperament. This being so, the knowledge of a variety of approaches or restraint methods becomes necessary.

2. Age:

This particularly applies to the problems of foal and yearling restraint and to the aged horse.

3. Size and physical condition:

Restraint procedures may vary when dealing with light horse breeds and the heavy or draft types. Also, the ever-increasing number of ponies warrant special consideration. The physical condition of the individual may be an added factor.

4. Anatomic location involved:

The area of the body as well as the extent of involvement must be considered in deciding if restraint should be applied locally or generally.

5. Anticipated duration of procedure:

The time required determines whether the animal should be restrained by purely physical means or by chemical agents; such considerations also guide the use of short-term or long-term anesthetics, the use of casting harness or operating table, etc.

6. Sensitivity of the part:

This consideration also involves any expected excitement on the part of the patient and possible risk to the operator. One is required to choose among sedatives, tranquilizers, local anesthetic agents, general anesthetics, or a combination of several methods. Humane technic always should be given first priority.

7. Self limitations:

Personal limitations as well as those of equipment and facilities must be considered.

8. Professional responsibilities and liabilities:

Upon accepting a case for diagnosis, treatment, etc. one also assumes a certain degree of responsibility for the animal's well-being. This includes responsibility for injuries, exhaustion, and complications that may result from either the poor choice or the incorrect application of a restraint method.

9. Trained assistants:

The successful implementation of many procedures, whether basic or advanced, often requires specially trained or experienced personnel. The undertaking of such operations without this help is a handicap and may jeopardize the outcome of the procedure or even the life of the patient.

RESTRAINT EQUIPMENT AND METHODS

This discussion of the methods of restraint will be confined to a few high points, including common errors made by the inexperienced.

Halter and Lead

At the top of the list of restraint equipment is the halter and lead, or shank as it may be called. Just as a rider conveys his wishes or commands to the horse's head via the reins, a handler on the ground uses the halter and lead for the same purpose. The man restraining the head has the most important job of any of the assistants. From that position he is best able to predict or determine what the horse may do, and be best able to control the horse's actions. This is done in a variety of ways and usually a combination of several at the same time. The assistant first endeavors to divert the horse's attention by "entertaining" the head. He may jangle the lead, talk to the horse, and tug lightly at his halter. When necessary, he takes more definite action, such as pulling the head hard around to the side to wheel the hindquarters away from the operator and prevent his being kicked. This action requires that the assistant always stand on the same side of the horse as the operator. The same is done to prevent a horse from biting or to throw him off balance if he should strike, or rear and paw with the front legs.

The man on the head should be careful to devote his entire attention to the job at hand. He should avoid abusing the horse and should limit his efforts to distract or soothe the animal to what is necessary. It is a good rule to always hold a horse by a lead; avoid holding him by the halter alone as one has less control over the horse, and should the animal resist or attempt to pull away, it is necessary to either relinquish control immediately or risk having a hand trapped in the halter—a dangerous position.

A horse should be led from the near, or left, side. One should stand just behind the animal's head and to the side of the left shoulder and take a short length of lead in the right hand. An important thing to remember is never to attempt to lead a horse by standing in front facing him and pulling on the lead rope. Always face in the direction you desire to go, and if the horse resists, have an assistant coax the animal from the rear. Few men can win a tug of war with a horse. If you should be alone and the same thing occurs, the horse can be pulled first to one side and then to the other until forward movement is established. A loop of rope, such as a lariat, can be passed over the hindquarters and thence forward through the halter to exert a pull directly from behind. The majority of balky horses, whether halter-broken to lead or just stubborn, will respond

nicely to this urging. Still another alternative is to back the horse if the distance to cover is short, such as through a doorway. Sometimes an animal can be led blindfolded when it would ordinarily balk.

There are many types of halters. The most common ones in use are the leather halter and the rope halter. Leather halters though varying widely in quality are all of the same basic construction. They have the advantage of permitting maximum use of the chain shank, as well as adapting readily to special devices such as cross-ties, side-sticks, neck cradles, bibs, halter twitches, and the like. They are, however, more expensive than rope halters and not as strong. For these reasons, the rope halters constructed of braided cotton or nylon are very popular, particularly for use with the farm-and western-types of horses.

Special halter types include the heavy, reinforced table halters for confinement to operating tables, and the dental halter with a rigid loop of steel incorporated into the nose band. Both of these have D-rings at the 4 quadrants of the nose band as well as on the crown piece behind the poll. These enable one to secure the head from any and all directions. The rigid nose band in the dental halter provides ample space to open the jaws of the horse for dental surgery without encroaching on the cheeks.

The list could be lengthened to mention the stallion bridle, lounging caveson, Tennessee grass halters, stable and track halters, and so on; but it is important to end with a word of caution. This is directed at the use of cow halters and temporary rope halters on horses. These last 2 are both "draw" halters, that is they constrict around the head and/or muzzle when tightened. This can cause serious injury, especially if the horse is tied up and begins to pull against the tie. Painful trauma to the nasal bones and passages, along with hemorrhage and asphyxia, have resulted from such negligence. If it is necessary to improvise, either take a knot in the lead rope where it slips, or avoid tying a horse by such a halter.

There are 2 types of leads: the rope lead and the leather-chain shank. Here again, each has certain advantages. The rope lead is cheaper and stronger, and it permits the horse to be tied to a stationary object. The chain shank, on the other hand, should never be used to tie a horse, but it can be used for more effective restraint by passing the chain portion over the horse's muzzle, through the mouth, under the jaw, or over the gum of the incisors. A common mistake is the overuse of the chain. Once a horse has been abused by it, he may resent being led or handled with one.

Regarding the subject of tying a horse, one should never leave a strange horse alone when tied because he may become excited and on finding himself attached to a stationary object, may struggle to become free. This is a hazardous situation as the horse is quite likely to become injured or to injure persons nearby. One should never attempt to do anything to a horse that is tied. This includes such seemingly minor operations as examining the incisor teeth, looking at an eye, taking the pulse, etc. Many horses use the slighest excuse to sit back on their halters, invariably breaking a piece of tack. These are called "halter-breakers" and frequently cannot be tied at all.

The particular halter or lead to be used usually is selected on the basis of expense, strength, or degree of restraint required. The purpose for all is the same—to control the head of the horse.

The Twitch

This method of restraint consists of causing pressure on the labial nerves and hence an unnatural sensation to a sensitive area of the head in order to divert the animal's attention from some other procedure. This is done most simply by grasping the upper lip firmly in the hand and squeezing, shaking, or twisting it. Almost the same effect may be obtained by using the lower lip or the ear, being careful not to produce injury. There actually is little danger of injuring the lips or ears by such manual restraint. The advantages are that this method affords a small amount of diversion for a short time and can be employed readily on any occasion. This frequently is all that is

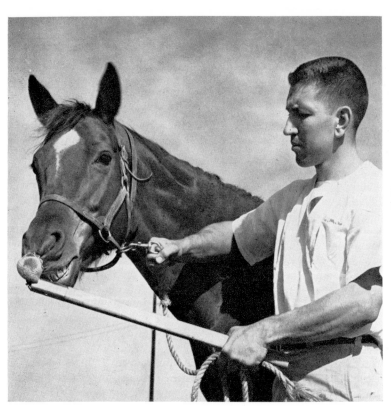

Fig. 1. Position of operator when applying chain twitch.

necessary for the examination of a wound, administration of an injection, taking the temperature, obtaining a fecal specimen, etc.

For greater restraint over a prolonged period, one can apply either a rope twitch (most severe) or chain twitch (most effective—if used correctly) usually to the upper lip and occasionally the lower lip. Such twitches should not be used on the ear because of the danger of breaking a conchal cartilage or damaging a nerve to cause a lop ear or, equally as bad, a head-shy horse.

Concerning the proper use of the twitch, a few special remarks are in order. First, one should realize that there are some horses which never should be twitched. These individuals, through overuse of the twitch or some painful experience in the past, greatly resent the twitch and fight it, even after it is applied. Learn to recognize those animals and choose some alternate method. Second, a twitch functions best when it is applied as needed. Its effect is greatest when first applied and is lost if the lip becomes numb; therefore, be sure to alternate the pressure of the loop around the lip, so that its maximum effect occurs at the moment needed, and when this is past, relax the pressure enough to allow sensitivity and circulation to return. In order to prevent injury to the mucous membrane or gum, care should be taken to fold the lip on itself so that only skin surface is in contact with the loop.

A word of caution is warranted concerning the the use of short-handled twitches; some horses may strike, or rear and paw even when the twitch is on. A short handle places one in a dangerous position as it doesn't provide the length needed to hold it. For this reason many experienced men prefer to make their own rope twitches using a strong, hickory handle of approximately 36 to 40 inches in length. I believe this is the optimum length and better than many of the commercial twitches.

Often it becomes the duty of one man to hold the horse's lead rope and twitch. This man should stand at the side of the horse's shoulder on the same side as the operator (Fig. 1). This allows him to perform his job and at the same time removes him from range of the front feet. If this location is not convenient, the next best place is directly in front of the horse's head in such a position as to be able to move backward or to either side.

Other types of twitches include a metal screw clamp, "humane twitch" (Fig. 2), and the halter twitch, a loop of rope with a snap in one end. The loop is twisted around the lip and the other end snapped into a halter ring. These 2 types can be used if there is no assistant to hold the twitch. Twitches for ponies must be modified somewhat in size of loop and rope. Nylon parachute cord or a small diameter, cotton cord work well for this purpose. Whichever is used, one should be careful to show some regard for the horse and not use the twitch abusively.

War Bridles, Gags, and Barnacles

This is a very old group of restraint devices which have been largely abandoned in recent years due to their potential severity. They are, however, alternatives which can be resorted

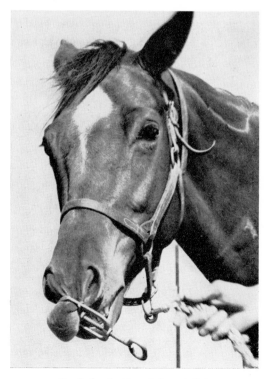

Fig. 2. Application of clamp twitch.

to when dealing with vicious or unmanageable animals. Barnacles can replace the twitch for quick restraint for special purposes, such as passing a stomach tube.

War bridles and gags consist of slip loops of small diameter, braided cotton rope (as sash cord) taken through the mouth or around the jaw and behind the ears. A simple gag exerts pressure on the corners of the mouth and the back of the head. A Magner's war bridle has a loop around the lower jaw with the rope passed around the off-side of the head and back through the jaw loop on the near side. The Yankee war bridle is a slip loop placed around the head and passing over the gum of the upper incisors. A combination of the last 2 types employs a jaw loop with a bight of rope passed around the back of the head and the long end of the rope passed over the gum of the upper incisors and through the bight on the near side of the head. These are all quite severe and must be used with discretion.

A barnacle is a hinged pair of handles (wooden or metal) which clamps the lip in the same manner as the twitch. These are quite handy and can be constructed easily from a pair of worn-out hoof nippers by simply cutting off the jaws, leaving the hinged handles.

TAIL RESTRAINT

This usually is employed for 1 or more of 3 reasons: 1. To get the tail out of the way for a genitourinary procedure, 2, to discourage kicking, and 3, to prevent the animal from collapsing on its hind parts. This may be accomplished by hand or by a rope tied to the end of the tail. The tail may be pulled by hand to one side to give access to the perineal regions when no more restraint is required, or preferably, it can be pulled upward and held forcefully over the back in such a manner as to discourage kicking. This requires a second assistant to hold the tail in both hands while the operator performs his job.

When placing a horse on an operating table, doing a standing castration, vaginal spay, etc., a rope is tied to the end of the tail and then passed over a side wall, ceiling joist, table side, or overhead ring. The end of the rope is held by the second assistant. This restrains against kicking and helps prevent the horse from going down, as frequently happens at such times due to pain, anesthesia, or profound tranquilization. It is important to note, however, that the tail rope is held and never tied to a stationary object if the horse is standing. An exception is when the horse is secured to an operating table by the table halter and body straps as well as the tail rope. The tail also serves as a good handle in helping a horse to his feet; make sure that he first is standing on the forelimbs, of course.

Tail restraint can be used to further advantage in subduing unmanageable ponies, foals, and weanlings. This often can be done by one man, with an arm around the animal's breast or a hand across the muzzle or in the halter and the other hand holding the tail over the back. An unruly weanling or pony can be caught and held in this manner even without the aid of a halter. This may be all the restraint necessary for intubation and worming, collection of fecal samples, or other short-term procedures. Bear in mind, however, that the tail is not indestructible and reasonable care should be taken when using this method.

RESTRAINT OF FOALS

In restraining the young foal or weanling which has not been halter-broken (even though he may be wearing one), never do so by catching his halter or applying a halter and then attempting to hold him by such. His immediate reaction is to rear and invariably he falls backward, striking his head or neck. Thus a simple procedure may result in a mortal wound. It is much preferred to corner the foal in a smooth-walled box stall, free of buckets, tubs, sharp edges or other hazards, with the mare standing close by, restrained by an assistant. Then, the foal can be cradled in the arms, one around the neck or breast and the other around the rump. On larger, more obstreperous foals, the hand around the hindquarters can be moved to the tail and by applying tail restraint (over the back) and leaning over the back of the foal, he usually can be well-managed.

A common mistake is to separate the mare and foal for one reason or another. The abandoned foal often will become panic-stricken and unless confined to a completely safe place may inflict self-injuries ranging from lacerations and contusions to broken bones. It cannot be emphasized too strongly that care must be exercised when restraining the young and unreasonable patient.

RESTRAINT IN STALLS

By taking advantage of surroundings familiar to the animal, certain procedures often can be carried out with greater ease and in a quieter manner in the individual's stall. This includes such routine jobs as passing a stomach tube, dressing teeth, examining the eyes, medicating a wound, etc. Usually the best position for both assistant and operator is the center of the stall, or at least toward the center with the horse restrained or led alongside a wall. By doing this, if the horse becomes excited or unruly, one can maintain a safe position by walking the horse in a circle around the perimeter of the stall. At the same time the operator keeps to the inside (normally the left) shoulder of the horse. With a short hold taken on the lead shank and with the elbow of the same arm placed squarely against the side of the horse's neck, it is possible to keep his head turned toward you and at the same time keep his hindquarters turned away from you.

The stall also provides a safe place for performing examinations of the hind parts, such as rectal examinations on mares. To do this, the animal is backed into the doorway of the stall so that the hindquarters are even with or just inside the stall door. It is particularly convenient if the door is located on the left side of the stall as entered. Then, the mare can be held with her near side along the adjacent wall as you work from around the corner just outside the door. If the doorway is too wide, the stall door can be closed to the optimum size if of the sliding type. One can then work from the side of the stall wall or door while standing in the hallway.

The darkened stall is an excellent place for examining the eyes, since there is no outside diffusion of light, and there usually is a minimum of other distractions.

The stall also is the best place for doing routine standing castrations. The footing is good, a solid wall prevents the horse from sticking a foot through it (as can be the case if using a lot fence), and the tail rope can be pulled over the top of the wall to further restrain the horse. The animal is pushed against the side of the stall wall, often with the hind end in a corner, and then restrained for castration by simultaneous use of twitch and tail restraint. There is less pain, and consequently, less restraint is necessary if a nerve block of the spermatic cord and a local anesthetic are administered prior to surgery.

In addition to the foregoing, the size and construction of a stall are important in the application of other restraint methods, such as cross-ties, slinging, recovery from anesthesia, and the use of special restraint methods.

RAISING THE FEET AND LEGS

The manner in which this task is performed depends largely on the degree to which the animal has been previously handled. For the horse that has had daily grooming care there is no problem, as he usually will assist one by picking up his feet. For the animal whose feet have never been handled, much less shod, picking them up may amount to breaking the horse. If physical force alone is not enough, one can employ sedatives or tranquilizers, the twitch, a sideline, or other devices. Regardless of the temperament of the horse, the general approach is the same. First, have a reliable assistant at the head and have the horse standing on all 4 legs so that he can readily shift his weight to 3. Then, starting at the horse's shoulder, let your whereabouts and intentions be known to the horse. If the front leg is to be raised, move the hand down the leg to the fetlock and pinch the volar digital nerves just above this joint. This usually induces the horse to pick up the foot. Some animals require more forceful means, such as inducing flexion of the carpus with your knee while abducting the leg, but the average horse will submit to the first method.

Raising and holding the hindfeet offer slightly more of a problem and here again, the man at the head and a careful approach are important. The horse that cannot be handled behind usually will give advance warnings by moving away from you, feinting with the hindleg that is being approached, or merely taking the weight off the leg so that he can kick at any time. Assuming that the horse can be handled, the approach here differs from that used for the front leg in that the hand nearest the horse is kept on the animal's tuber coxae while the other travels down the leg to the cannon bone and then draws the leg forward. The hock and toe are flexed and held in that position when the leg is raised. This partially restricts voluntary movement of that leg by the horse. The leg is held by cradling the hock and distal part of the limb in a girdle formed by passing the arm nearest the horse over and around the hock and grasping the foot in a flexed position. The cannon of the horse's leg is propped on the inside of the thigh that is nearest the horse. Then one can use the other hand to clean the foot, trim, or perform whatever job is necessary (Fig. 3). The operator's stance should be stable so that he is not thrown off balance by any struggling of the horse. When releasing the leg, the procedure is reversed; the near hand is passed to the horse's tuber coxae and used to push oneself to the front of the horse.

Another important point is that when close to the animal's hind parts, one usually is in a safer position when close to its side. This greatly reduces the distance to travel and thus the time required to move out of line of a possible kick. These precautions are required primarily for a strange horse or one which cannot be trusted. Animals which are safe require only a fraction of the time and effort in doing the same job. As an example, many race horses are perfectly accustomed to having all 4 feet examined and cleaned daily from just the left side (working from under and across when raising the right feet).

Occasionally a front foot is raised and held so as to prevent a horse from kicking with the hindfeet. This is done by raising the front foot on the same side on which one is working. This is based on the fact that if a horse raises

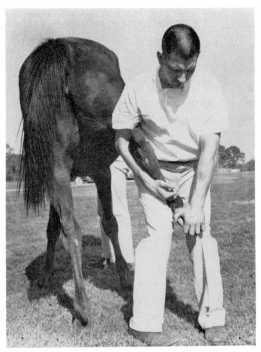

Fig. 3. Position for examination or treatment of hindfoot.

a second leg to kick with, he cannot stand very well unless the 2 on the ground are diagonally opposed. Hence, if the left front leg was raised, the horse would not be so able to kick with the left rear leg since his main support would depend upon the right front and left rear legs. In holding up a front foot to deprive the horse of one leg, don't hold it so firmly that you support him with your own legs. Sometimes a front leg is strapped up as in restraint of a mare during breeding. The strap should be arranged, however, so that it can be released quickly in the event of a struggle. If unable to free her leg, the mare may cast herself. Tying a hindleg involves the use of a single rope sideline. This does not permit as careful examination of the foot, but may discourage kicking. For the resistant individual, tranquilizers and sedatives are indicated.

SLINGS

As a general rule, slings are indicated when the animal, once raised to a standing height and position, can and will support, or partially support, his own weight at least part of the time. If he will not support his weight, the animal is preferably left lying in a deep bed of clean, dry straw and turned or lifted at regular intervals. There are times when a sling is used only temporarily to raise a weak animal to his feet, after which he can stand and move independently. There are animals that have tolerated a sling well for a period of many weeks (fracture cases), but in such instances the individual is able to bear his own weight, standing free of the sling for lengthy periods. For an animal to hang in a sling constantly is to consign him to certain death.

There are many poor slings and a few good ones. The major objection is poor construction of poor quality materials. A good sturdy sling, easily adjusted, is a prized possession. There are relatively few occasions for its use, but when it is needed, nothing else will suffice.

STOCKS

These vary widely in construction and versatility but all are used to simplify treatment of the standing animal by closely restricting his movements. They are of particular use in dental procedures, minor surgery, some major surgery, physiotherapy, radiotherapy, and various examination procedures.

The use of a kick-board in conjunction with stocks enables one to work around the rear of a standing horse in relative safety. This is a barricade constructed of either oak boards or heavy, marine plywood with reinforced backing. It operates on the same principle as a half Dutch door, and is slipped into the stocks behind the horse. It is approximately 40 inches high and wide enough to brace against the uprights of the stocks. The side facing the horse should be smooth or even padded and the top edge covered to protect him. It should be tied to the stocks with ropes passed through rings on the back side to keep it from falling forward against the horse. The horse should be backed fairly close against it, and the operator works from behind. Aside from the exceptional horse that gets one leg over the board, the operator is safe from being kicked. The kick-board is used in doing urethrotomies,

perineal and recto-vaginal repairs, caudal myotomies, occasionally Caslick operations, and examinations that cannot be accomplished in the stall for some special reason. For all their good features, stocks are potentially dangerous in that an excited or unruly animal can cause serious injury to himself. Care must be taken to reduce pain and excitement with local anesthetics and tranquilizers.

Though stocks ordinarily are constructed of heavy wooden timbers or steel pipe, occasionally rope stocks are used. Some horses cannot be handled safely in stationary stocks and, of course, they are not always on hand. Much as the driving harness on a cart horse or the gear on a mule seems to exert a psychologic advantage, rope stocks may perform the same function. One type which is particularly effective in discouraging a horse from rearing is known as the hippo-harness, also referred to as Sigler's method of restraint. A single rope, 30 to 40 feet in length, is doubled across the withers, passing an end to each side. A half-hitch is taken around each forearm, passing back to the hindlegs where a half-hitch is taken around each gaskin, and then back up to cross at the loins. The ends are pulled tight and either tied (for quick release) or held by 2 assistants. This has been found to be very successful even in horses that could not be twitched.

CASTING METHODS

Equipment varies widely but all operate on 1 of 2 different principles: one type flexes the hindlegs and sits the horse down before he is cast on his side (for example, double rope sidelines, Stroup, and Tramp harnesses); the second type pulls on all 4 legs at once (as the Baker, Danish, and English or Conkey type hobbles). Personal experience has influenced my opinion that the first type is the safer for casting a horse to the ground because it minimizes the danger of injuring knees or striking the head. Also, there is less risk of a broken back or other serious injury with the first type (Fig. 4).

When the animal is on the ground, harness types may again be divided into 2 categories. Those which bind the legs in a flexed and

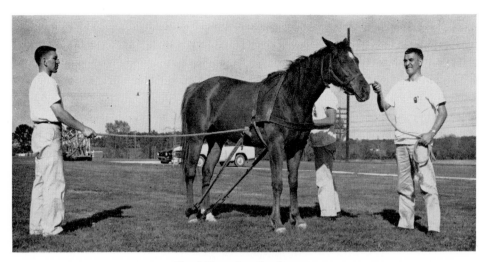

Fig. 4. Type of casting harness.

somewhat abducted position are the most common. These are ideal for castrations, cryptorchid operations, ventral midline procedures, or those requiring sternal recumbency. However, the second type enjoys certain advantages too. These are the ones which pull all 4 feet together with the legs extended and adducted, as the English hobbles. These are used somewhat less for castration but are better for any procedures done in lateral recumbency, as laparotomy and extensive dental procedures where a table is unavailable. They are of particular value in restraining the feet and legs of the animal that already is down and anesthetized—such as when transporting a horse from the operating table to the recovery area.

The simplest type is the double rope sideline, using 60 feet of ½-inch soft cotton rope, which usually will suffice for a versatile casting harness. Leather hobbles for the hindlegs also are desirable. If, however, one has many horses to cast, he soon appreciates the advantages of a strong, adjustable leather harness. Regardless of limitations or aforementioned indications, as one becomes more familiar with the use of a particular harness, its versatility and applications will increase correspondingly for that individual.

When it becomes necessary to cast foals or ponies for various procedures, casting harnesses seldom are used. Either rope sidelines are improvised, or the animal is anesthetized and

laid down. A very simple method of casting ponies and foals is suitable for all but the larger or older individuals. It requires little or no apparatus other than a halter, and practically no sedation except as may be needed to quiet an excited animal. Standing at the side of the animal and leaning over its back, one hand grasps the halter and pulls the head around slightly while the other hand grasps the tail as it is passed forward between the hindlegs and to the flank of the opposite side from which you are standing. Then by pulling upward and backward, using your knees somewhat as a fulcrum, the animal is upset and lowered to the ground. This can be done quite gently and restraint maintained with one man on the head and one holding the tail between the legs. For procedures not requiring a general anesthetic, the patient is back on his feet as soon as released, and with no sedative hangover.

For any casting procedure it always is wise to sedate or tranquilize the animal sufficiently to reduce or eliminate the undesirable struggling associated with such an operation. This is indicated from a humane standpoint as well as to reduce the risk of physical injury to both patient and operator. The ease of restraint and smooth recovery further justify the use of such chemical agents. In addition, many animals are cast solely by the use of certain chemical agents, such as pentothal, chloral hydrate-magnesium sulfate, and succinylcholine chloride. Used properly, these agents are relatively safe and achieve the objective of casting with a minimum of struggle or effort.

OPERATING TABLES

There are many types of operating tables, varying widely in construction, special features, materials, and versatility. The most expensive are constructed of stainless steel, operate by hydraulic pressure, raise and lower into the floor, and tilt in 2 planes. The most inexpensive usually are homemade affairs of wooden construction and operate only in 1 plane. Some commercial tables of sturdy wooden construction have the added feature of being mounted on wheels and are portable. Considering the number of models available, operating tables are economically feasible for most practitioners. They do offer very definite advantages for well-controlled and aseptic surgery.

There are 2 procedures for confining the animal to the table. For the type which tilts to vertical and does not lower into the floor, the horse is premedicated with a tranquilizer and/or sedative agent, then led alongside and tied to the table by head ropes, a tail rope, 2 body bands, and a rope on the inside front foot. The ropes and bands are positioned and as much slack removed as possible without letting the horse feel the presence or the tug of the attachments. Then, at a signal and in one smooth, synchronized operation, the horse is lifted. All slack is removed and the ropes are secured instantly, so that if a brief struggle ensues the horse cannot move out of position. This is a necessary procedure to prevent injury. If done properly there is very little struggle with practically no danger to horse or assistants. The table is tilted to horizontal, the horse is repositioned on the table, all 4 legs are tied down, and all the slack is taken out of the other ropes. Then general or local anesthesia is begun preparatory to the surgery.

Protective padding is imperative. The entire table surface should be padded; if this is not possible, a wide area under the head and another under the body should be padded. This is necessary to prevent bruising of the bony prominences, but far more important is protection against injury of the superficial nerves and sensory organs. Such injuries include brain concussion, damage to eyes, ears, and the facial and radial nerves.

Of equal importance and perhaps greater occurrence are the nerve injuries produced by the animal's straining and kicking against insufficiently padded hobbles or leg ropes. Most of these injuries involve the hindlegs and cause paralysis of the digital extensors. When the horse gets to his feet on recovering from anesthesia, he is observed to knuckle on one or both hindlegs. The interference may be sufficient to prevent him from rising until the legs are splinted in extension. Although the majority of cases recover spontaneously in a few days, it is much better to prevent this by padding with a thick layer of cotton, burlap, or foam rubber before applying the leg ropes or hobbles. This also eliminates rope burns and bruised quarters. An alternate method involves the use of large diameter, soft cotton or soft nylon rope hobbles that serve the dual purpose of padding and restraint. Due to the thickness required these cannot be used on some tables but where applicable they are highly desirable.

One other form of nerve injury that occurs infrequently as a result of certain recumbent procedures is femoral nerve paralysis. This flaccid paralysis of the hindlimb, comparable to radial paralysis of the forelimb, may be caused by overstretching the nerve on the medial thigh. This in turn can be caused by stretching and abducting (in extension) the hindleg. Bearing this in mind, any procedures requiring such strained positions of the hindleg should be done with care and for short duration.

These same precautions should be observed with the use of casting harnesses.

Whether the animal is cast or put on an operating table, the head should be held in the extended position, since if it is flexed, partial obstruction of the airway occurs.

The horse may be removed by either tilting the table back to vertical and letting him walk away, or if he is still anesthetized, by hobbling his legs and sliding him off the horizontal table onto a cart.

When using a table which lowers flush with the floor, the horse is cast and anesthetized on a protective mat on the table surface or he may be "dropped" with succinylcholine chloride, then bound down and anesthetized completely before raising the table to standard height. To release the horse, the table is lowered into the floor, then the animal is unbound and allowed to get up naturally.

SPECIAL RESTRAINT METHODS AND DEVICES

These include a miscellany of things not discussed previously. Of interest are the devices for preventing a horse from chewing or licking wounds and dressings on the legs. Neck cradles permit freedom in the stall while keeping the horse from the front legs. For the occasional animal that learns to "cheat" on the cradle (by propping a front foot on the side of the stall until he can reach the leg with his mouth) a leather bib can be attached to the underside of the halter extending forward under the muzzle. If only a hindleg is involved, a side-stick run from a side-ring in a surcingle to a halter ring is sufficient to restrict the reach and allow still greater freedom.

When these devices are not available, or fail to work, the reliable cross-tie always can be employed. This prevents any freedom in the stall, that is, the horse cannot lie down or move any further than to reach feed and water placed before him. It does, however, keep him from removing bandages or irritating wounds with his mouth, which justifies this method of restraint. It is applied most easily by hooking 2 leads in opposite sides (cheek rings) of the halter and tying them short across the corner of the stall, usually over the feed bunk. If the horse is in a narrow slip or tie stall he can be tied across the stall. This may necessitate watering by hand several times a day.

Even in cross-ties, an occasional horse will find a way to irritate a wound, such as rubbing it on the ropes of the cross-tie or on the feed tub or water bucket. For these animals, an overhead swivel tie, consisting of a rope dropped from a beam, ring, or slide wire is snapped into the nose band of the halter. This includes a swivel to prevent twisting the rope. If hooked in the crown piece of the halter, the horse may slip it over the back of his head. The horse cannot lie down, but is allowed greater freedom than by the cross-tie. Hay can be conveniently located in a hay net suspended in front of the animal.

Other devices, such as hoods and blinds, are useful both to protect the head from injury and in moving a balky horse. Blinds also may be used to delay a horse's getting up directly when recovering from anesthesia, that is, before he has recovered sufficiently to stand alone.

Breeding hobbles are constructed of either rope or leather, but operate on the same principle. The restraining ropes extend from a neck or breast collar, between the forelegs and to the hocks or pasterns of the hindlegs. Such hobbles prevent a mare from kicking the stallion and protect the assistants near the hindquarters. They also can be used to protect a clinician performing a rectal examination or any operation around the hind parts. When applied, one always should take care to adjust the hobbles properly to prevent any slack whatsoever, and also provide for their immediate release in case of such emergencies as the stallion catching a leg in one of the ropes, the mare becoming cast, etc.

In conclusion, regardless of the method used, the skillful and most effective application of restraint requires a knowledge of the species and a true understanding of horsemanship. Then, if one endeavors to master the principles involved, he can choose or devise the necessary methods to suit any situation.

J. T. VAUGHAN

Acknowledgment: Much of the material in this discussion appeared in the article, "An Introduction to Equine Restraint," by J. T. Vaughan, which appeared in Auburn Vet. 14: Spring (1960) 147-156.

ADDITIONAL NOTES ON PHYSICAL RESTRAINT

INTRODUCTION

These comments will be confined to the restraint of mature animals, it being presumed that most veterinarians realize that submissive behavior should not be expected of untrained, young horses. The rule for "infants" is unhurried, firm, and kind handling.

The proper restraint of mature horses is an art and should be defined as "the ability to render an animal—wild or domestic—amenable to handling and/or treatment, without abuse to the animal and with safety to the handler." Time was when the veterinarian was primarily a "horse-man," had farm or ranch experience as a boy, had ridden and driven horses, and thus was more or less educated in the art of handling horses before acquiring a veterinary education.

Then—and now—veterinarians were rated by the finesse with which the animal was approached and handled. The ability to judge an animal's disposition and to make a quick appraisal enables an operator to know at once what to expect and how to handle any situation quietly but firmly. Crude methods which are simply an exhibition of brute force cannot be considered intelligent horse-handling. Employment of such methods necessitates that treatment be done only while a mental and physical truce is in effect on both sides, and therefore, treatment must necessarily be hurried and perhaps not complete. If restraint is attempted on a brute force basis, the animal often will overcome man simply because the animal has more strength. An exception may be taken to the indefensible argument that—"if one cannot handle him, he's better off dead." This remark is indicative of a man unfit to practice good restraint. Fortunately, the majority of veterinarians today are well-equipped mentally and physically to practice restraint of animals in a dignified manner that is gratifying to witness.

This being the day of ataractics or tranquilizers, it is becoming fashionable to use these drugs in every situation in which the timidity of the operator is the motivating influence. Tranquilizers may enable one to secure a result, but their use has certain disadvantages. They do nothing for the animal's education nor do they improve the operator's skill in handling horses. No lesson has been given; no conditioned reflex nor impression has been left upon the animal. The horse will, in the future under the same conditions, react in the same way and have to be controlled in

the same manner; whereas, if handled with proper finesse without the assistance of drugs, animals may be so conditioned that undesirable behavior probably will not be demonstrated again.

RESTRAINT EQUIPMENT

Revolutionary as this may seem, in the hands of a skilled operator working under rural conditions, about the only restraint equipment necessary is a twitch, a soft cord, ⅛ to ¼″ wide and 20′ long, and a soft cotton rope ¾″ wide, 25′ long, plus 1 or 2 hobbles to avoid burns. Ninety percent of horse restraint can be accomplished with this equipment. Exceptions might be made in the cases of a vicious, unpredictable stallion or a nymphomaniac mare. In such cases restraint is more difficult; the procedure takes longer and can be hazardous. Professional trainers of "bad" horses realize this, and since these animals are dangerous castration often is the only advisable solution.

Custom and good restraint technic have decreed that a twitch should be part of the veterinarian's armamentarium. A ring twitch, in our experience, is preferable to a stick twitch. This is made of a simple iron ring, 7″ in diameter, formed of ⅜″ round bar stock, having threaded through it a double loop of ordinary sash cord. This double loop is large enough only to allow passage of the hand with the fingers apart. This allows the operator to grasp the horse's nose in the proper place for the twitch's application which is midway between the cornu of the alar cartilages and the margin of the upper lip (Fig. 5). Placed too high the twitch interferes with breathing and causes resentment; placed too low it includes only the thickened margin of the upper lip. This is painful and can enrage the animal.

Nicety of application of the twitch is an art. In my hands neither tongs nor chains have the flexibility of the cord-ring twitch and the same finesse of application cannot be practiced with them as with the ring twitch. The average stick-twitch loop is too large and twisting it is inconvenient. A resentful animal, by striking, often will put its foot and leg over the stick and when this happens, the twitcher finds

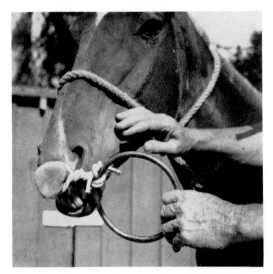

Fig. 5. Application of ring twitch.

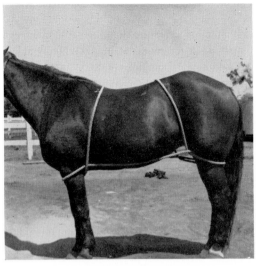

Fig. 6. The hippo lasso or harness.

himself in the position of trying to support the front end of the animal by means of a lever which has one end attached to the animal's nose. This added weight enrages him and the striking continues until the twitcher is forced to release the twitch, leaving a plunging animal swinging a club attached to its upper lip. This is dangerous both to the operator and animal. Then the entire procedure must be repeated, only this time the twitcher has on his hands an animal conditioned to rebel.

This situation does not occur with the cord-ring twitch. By passing the hand through the ring, its application is faster, the hold on the lip can be better judged, and its use can easily be varied with circumstances. By reversing the procedure the twitch can be removed in a manner which automatically places the hand in the right position to rub the animal's nose as the twitch slides down the arm.

Since the ring and cord loop are small, the rare escapee cannot club either himself or the handler, and can quickly divest himself of the twitch without the more serious prospects of

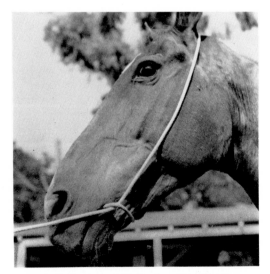

Fig. 7. One type of "Indian" or "War" bridle.

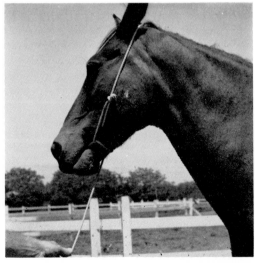

Fig. 8. Another type of "Indian" or "War" bridle.

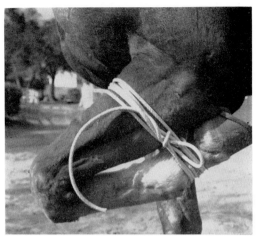

Fig. 9. Foreleg restraint. Put slip-loop around pastern, wind several wraps around forearm, and on last wrap bring rope between forearm and heel to secure with 2 hitches around 2 different strands of rope. Leave rope end free.

injury associated with the use of the stick twitch.

The word, twitch, has the same derivation as the word, twist, and that is exactly how one should be handled. It should be applied by twisting. It is not and should not be used to either pull or push the animal's head—a common mistake which reflects poor acquaintance with the proper procedure. The cord-ring type of twitch can be successfully applied to an ear without fear of damage, provided the application is close to the head. We have yet to

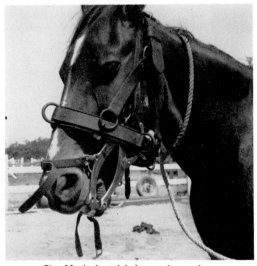

Fig. 10. A dental halter and speculum.

see a damaged ear from judicious use of such restraint. It also is perfectly feasible to apply a twitch to the lower lip when for some reason the upper lip cannot be used.

Accompanying illustrations (Fig. 6-10) demonstrate certain other applications of the basic equipment used for restraint of equines. Their supplementation by stocks, operating tables, and such equipment is of great help when available.

C. H. REID

DRUGS USED IN RESTRAINT

SEDATIVES

Sedatives should be used if a horse needs to be quieted prior to a standing operation in which local anesthesia is used, or prior to other procedures which may cause slight or momentary pain (for example, placing a needle into a joint). Physical restraint of standing horses can be used following sedatives.

Sedatives or tranquilizers often are used prior to restraining horses with a casting harness or putting them on an operating table. If the animal is given a sedative and restrained, local anesthetics can be used to perform some operations. The advantage of this method is that the animal is able to walk as soon as the operation is finished provided the dose of drug is kept low. The disadvantage of the method, especially in prolonged or delicate surgery, is that struggling may: 1. Cause poor surgical technic. 2. Cause contamination of the surgical field. 3. Cause occasional deaths due to "cardiac failure."[9,10] 4. Cause occasional cases of azoturia.[11,12]

Since sedatives may interfere with the swallowing reflex, animals should not be permitted to eat or drink for several hours after administration of the drug.

Chloral Hydrate: Chloral hydrate is a good sedative in horses because it reduces the response to pain, in spite of evidence that it is a poor analgesic in other species. It makes an animal less likely to kick, strike or attempt to escape; if any of these actions are attempted, they usually are less forceful.

Intravenous administration is preferred because chloral hydrate can be given "to effect" by this route. When a 7% solution (35 Gm.

chloral hydrate crystals made up to 500 ml.) is used, the dose and speed of injection can be regulated conveniently. If any of the drug should accidentally be injected perivascularly, less serious inflammation will result than if a more concentrated solution is used. (See Chapter 3 for ways to prevent perivascular injection.) It is best to administer the solution "to effect." Two-thirds of the estimated dose can be given as fast as it will flow through the intravenous outfit and a 14-gauge needle; then the infusion should be interrupted for 2 to 3 minutes. More is then given if needed. To determine the effect of the dose already given, the horse can be pushed in the region of the tuber coxae. If the horse "gives" easily or stumbles, he has had enough. Doses should not be given to make the animal become very unsteady or "go down" (become recumbent). Although the dose required for good sedation depends on the physical condition and temperament of the animal, it usually is about 300 ml. of 7% chloral hydrate solution for a 1,000-pound mature horse.

An oral dose of 5 Gm. of chloral hydrate per 100-pounds can be used.[13] When administered per os the drug should be diluted in a quart or more of cold water and given by stomach tube.[14] Horses will not drink chloral hydrate solutions unless they are very thirsty. If a solution of chloral hydrate is administered by drenching, irritation of the upper alimentary tract may occur, or inhalation of the drug may result in serious inflammation of the respiratory tract. Gelatin capsules containing the drug may break or be dissolved in the pharynx and cause severe pharyngitis. A disadvantage of oral administration is that sedation occurs only after 20 or 30 minutes, and the degree of depression is more variable than after intravenous injection.[13,14]

Chloral Hydrate Combined with Other Drugs: Chloral hydrate 12% with magnesium sulfate 6% or chloral hydrate 21 Gm. (328 grains), magnesium sulfate 11 Gm. (164 grains) and pentobarbital sodium (Nembutal: Abbott Labs.), 5 Gm. (75 grains) made up to 500 ml. have been used successfully as sedatives.[15,16] Many veterinarians give one of these products "to effect" or give a conservative calculated dose; then if needed, they administer an additional dose 5 to 10 minutes later.

Pentobarbital Sodium: There is a danger of the horse's becoming excited following injection of pentobarbital sodium for sedation, especially if a high dose is used. The dose which has been recommended in horses weighing 1,000 pounds is 1.0 Gm. (15 grains).[1] Slow, intravenous injection to effect is preferred. Not more than 5 ml. (1 grain per 1 ml.) should be administered at any one time.

NARCOTICS

Narcotics, effective for relief of pain, have not been used widely in horses. They sometimes are indicated in horses with fractures, those suffering from other extensive trauma and in severe cases of intestinal colic. Meperidine hydrochloride (Demerol: Winthrop Labs.) is the narcotic which has been used most successfully in horses. The dose is 0.5 to 2 mg. per pound, administered intravenously and slowly. Methadone hydrochloride (Dolophine: Eli Lilly and Co.) should not be used because of the marked excitement which occurs sometimes.

TRANQUILIZERS

Tranquilizers are useful in controlling hyperexcitable and nervous horses. These drugs have little effect on the cerebral cortex when compared to sedatives. Their mechanism of action is complex and is not yet thoroughly understood.[17] Horses which are tranquilized seem to become sleepy and less responsive to usual happenings in their environment. However, they can be aroused and may even react more violently than they would have before administration of the tranquilizer if they are subjected to strong or unusual stimuli, especially painful ones. These drugs are not sedatives nor analgesics. If painful procedures are attempted following their administration, horses may react violently and injure themselves or persons working with them. Tranquilizers should not be used in horses in danger of surgical shock as they have a hypotensive effect.

Tranquilizers can be used on horses which are difficult to handle prior to doing procedures which are not painful, such as taking radiographs, passing a stomach tube, or shoeing. They are useful in prolapsing the penis for examination or cleaning. Tranquilizers also are being used prior to shipping or as an aid in training horses. The use of these agents prior to anesthesia will be discussed later in this chapter.

Advantages of tranquilizers compared to those of chloral hydrate or the sedative mixtures containing chloral hydrate are: 1. Several of them can be administered intramuscularly if a horse is so wild that an intravenous injection cannot be given, 2, horses will eat several of the tranquilizers in feed, 3, horses can be permitted to eat and drink following their administration, 4, the period of action of most tranquilizers is longer than that of the sedatives. (This can be a disadvantage under some conditions.)

Disadvantages of tranquilizers compared to those of chloral hydrate sedation are: 1. Horses sometimes react more violently to painful stimuli than they would have before administration of the drug, 2, tranquilizers have a slower onset of action; therefore, it is difficult to give them "to effect." Moreover, time is lost if one waits until they have taken full effect before doing a procedure, 3, there is a variable response to a given dose by individual horses of the same breed, age, weight, and temperament, 4, several veterinarians have noted that horses seem to be less affected by tranquilizers if they become excited prior to administration of the drug.[18,19]

A number of reports discuss the untoward effects in horses with the use of some of the individual tranquilizers and the relatively few such effects with others.[20,21,22,23,24,25] Most likely, some of the serious reactions with the safer drugs have been due to the accidental intracarotid injection of the drugs which can occur quite easily if a small-gauge needle is used for injection.[26] The resistance of the small-gauge needle slows the flow of blood making it difficult to determine whether it is in the jugular vein or carotid artery (See Chapter 3). The animal becomes violent 2 to 5 seconds after starting the injection and usually goes down. Death results sometimes. Rapid injection has been mentioned as a cause of reactions and death, but this is doubtful since it takes up to 10 or 20 minutes for tranquilizers to produce their full effect. Lundvall concluded that an anaphylactic reaction occurred in one case.[21] Deaths have occurred due to animals struggling against restraint for long periods following administration of tranquilizers.

Promazine Hydrochloride (Promazine: Ft. Dodge Labs.) (Sparine: Wyeth Labs.): Promazine probably is used more in horses than any of the other tranquilizers. There is less variation in response with this drug than with others. A few reports have recorded the untoward effects following the use of promazine.[21,40] Some of the complications are due to an occasional animal going down when high doses are used, and some probably are due to accidental intracarotid injection.[26]

If intravenous injection is possible this route of administration is preferred since the drug will become effective sooner than by other routes. The effect can be seen within 3 to 5 minutes, although maximum effect apparently does not occur until about 20 minutes after injection. In the normal standing horse, the maximum hypotensive effect occurs approximately 20 minutes after injection.[27] The intravenous dose of promazine recommended is up to 0.33 mg./pound. If doses much higher than this are used, an occasional animal will go down, although doses up to 1.0 mg. per pound usually will not cause untoward effects.

Intramuscular injection also is effective, but the delay before maximum effect of the drug occurs is longer. A dose of 0.33 to 0.5 mg. per pound is recommended by this route.

Oral promazine is available. Such a preparation can be dispensed, especially for use prior to loading and transporting or for breaking and training horses. The manufacturers recommend that 0.3 to 1.25 mg./pound of body weight be used. The best dosage should be determined for each animal, starting with a low dose. The effect of the drug can be seen 45 to 60 minutes after administration, with maximum effect in 1 to 2 hours. The duration of effect usually continues for 4 to 8 hours, and some animals remain calm for up to 24 hours. The persons using this drug should be warned that increasing the dose may not increase the effectiveness of the drug and that high doses may cause horses to go down.

Chloropromazine Hydrochloride (Thorazine, T.M. Reg.: Smith, Kline and French Labs., distributed by Pitman-Moore Co.): Chloropromazine was one of the first tranquilizers used in horses. The dose usually used is 0.1 mg./pound intravenously, and up to 0.5 mg./pound sometimes is used intramuscularly. The drug still is being used although it sometimes causes a tendency toward aimless walking and there have been reports of "panic reactions" following its use.[20,22,23,24] It is thought that this may result from the distress of the feeling of weakness since the "horses sink slowly down on their haunches before plunging forward and becoming excited."[20,22] In one case, Hall concluded that hypotension was not associated with the reaction.[20] Perhaps these reactions are a result of giving a dose which is too great for the individual animal.

Propiopromazine Hydrochloride (Tranvet: Abbott Labs.): Propiopromazine is a more recently developed, potent tranquilizer which is effective in horses. Duration of action is longer than with the other tranquilizers commonly used in horses. A dose of 0.05 to 0.1 mg./pound given intravenously or intramuscularly is recommended. The manufacturer recommends that the lower dose be used in Standardbred and Thoroughbred horses. The response to this drug appears to vary with the individual animal. If high doses of the drug are used, the horses may go down or if, subsequently, general anesthesia is used, the horses may remain recumbent for long periods.

Acepromazine Maleate (Atrovet: Ayerst, McKenna and Harrison Ltd.): Early reports on the use of acepromazine in horses have been favorable.[19,28] The dose recommended by the manufacturer is 25 mg./1,000 pounds intravenously, 50 to 200 mg./1,000 pounds intramuscularly, or 60 to 120 mg./1,000 pounds orally. Acepromazine has not been distributed to veterinarians in the United States.

Triflupromazine Hydrochloride (Vetame: E. R. Squibb & Sons): Triflupromazine has been recommended for use in horses at a dose of 10 to 15 mg./100 pounds given intravenously or intramuscularly up to a maximum total dose of 100 mg. The package insert warns: "Some horses may respond with temporary motor activity such as determined trotting. If they are allowed to trot on a lead, this quickly passes and tranquilization sets in."

Others: It is recommended that perphenazine (Trilafon: Schering Corp.), and isobutrazine, (Diquel: Jensen-Salsbery Labs.), should not be used in horses because of the excitement which sometimes occurs. Convulsions often occur if moderately high doses of perphenazine are administered to horses.[25]

Succinycholine Restraint (Sucostrin: Squibb & Sons), (Anectine: Burroughs Wellcome): The use of succinylcholine hydrochloride (suxamethonium) to cause recumbency in horses has become popular because the horses usually go down quietly about 20 to 30 seconds after the injection and little or no assistance is required. The dose required usually is 4 to 5 mg./100 pounds intravenously. If the horse fails to go down, the total calculated dose should be increased 4 to 8 mg. in mature horses on the next injection which can be given 5 minutes later. Muscular twitching (fasciculation) usually is observed soon after the injection is given and before the animal falls. If twitching occurs but the horse does not go down, a slightly higher dose should cause the animal to fall on the next injection. The head should be pulled to one side as the horse falls to prevent injury to the lips or incisor teeth, since the head may drop quickly. Horses usually are able to get up and stand 5 to 10 minutes after the injection is given.

A period of apnea varying from a few seconds to several minutes occurs after the animal falls. Artificial respiration (see section later in this chapter) should be used to oxygenate the animal if breathing stops for more than a minute or if cyanosis occurs. The use of anticholinesterase drugs and respiratory stimulants is countraindicated following succinylcholine. There is danger of prolonged periods of apnea and death occurring if doses are administered repeatedly to prolong recumbency, especially if artificial respiration is not given.

Minor surgery such as castration often is done while the horse is immobilized following injection of succinylcholine. Horses which have been given only succinylcholine are fully conscious but unable to respond to painful stimuli. For this reason Hansson, who did much of the early work with the agent, recommended that a sedative dose of pentobarbital sodium be administered with succinylcholine.[29,30] Other sedatives given before or with succinylcholine would probably be effective. Local anesthesia can be used prior to administration of succinylcholine to prevent pain. Also, as soon as breathing starts following casting with succinylcholine, anesthesia can be induced using intravenous or inhalation technics.

Succinylcholine should be stored at refrigeration temperature. Long exposure to higher temperatures will reduce its potency. Care should be used to avoid contamination with blood, since its effectiveness is reduced by the cholinesterase in the blood. It should not be mixed with thiopental sodium or other alkaline solutions.

Tachycardia and cardiac arrythmias occur in horses restrained with succinylcholine, probably due to anoxia. Succinylcholine does not appear to have a direct effect on blood pressure in horses.[31] Subendocardial hemorrhages of the myocardium have been described in horses killed following the use of succinylcholine.[32,33] The lesions were more severe in the animals given 3 times the usual dose.[32] Since the lesions probably are caused by anoxia, it is recommended that the dose be kept to a minimum and artificial respiration be used if apnea occurs.[32] The hemorrhages produced by the use of succinylcholine are similar to the agonal hemorrhages resulting from exsanguination of animals given no drugs.[33] The lesions probably are quickly resolved in healthy horses.[33]

Malnourished, aged or debilitated horses, especially those with cardiac or liver disease, are poor risks for the use of succinylcholine. It also is dangerous to use it in horses with respiratory disease and those with disturbed electrolyte balance.[9] It should not be used in animals which have been exposed to or treated with organic phosphorus insecticides or other agents which lower serum cholinesterase. Procaine or other agents which compete with succinylcholine for cholinesterase could be dangerous if administered intravenously or if large doses were used prior to injection of succinylcholine.[34,35]

A. A. GABEL

GENERAL ANESTHESIA

During surgical anesthesia (Stage 3 of general anesthesia) the animal does not perceive pain, and there is an absence of reflex response to painful stimuli. It is safest to use the lightest possible plane of surgical anesthesia which produces satisfactory conditions for surgery. Until recently, it was usual to rely upon a single drug to produce anesthesia. When only one drug is used, the dose is increased to deepen or prolong anesthesia; therefore, the period of recovery often is prolonged, even in operations of average length, because a large quantity of the drug is required. Also, if a deep plane of anesthesia is required there may be danger of severe respiratory depression and death. The trend is now toward the use of several agents, either mixed together or better, one followed by others in logical sequence. The advantages of these methods are that the average length of recovery time is shorter and the margin of safety is greater, because most drugs are detoxified or are made ineffective by different physiologic mechanisms. Some tranquilizers have been effective in minimizing induction and emergence excitement. Recently, intravenous agents have been used for induction, and inhalation agents for the maintenance of anesthesia. When this combination is used induction and recovery are rapid and free of struggling.

PREANESTHETIC PREPARATION

Physical Examination: A general examination should be done prior to anesthesia, with special emphasis on examination of the respiratory and cardiovascular systems, since safe anesthesia requires an adequate supply of oxygen to the vital organs, especially the higher nervous centers. It is essential to recognize hypofunction or decreased reserve of the respiratory and/or cardiovascular system prior to the induction of anesthesia, in order that they can be compensated for if possible, and so the owner can be warned of the danger.

Respiratory System: The nature and rate of respiration should be noted before and after exercise if the animal can be exercised safely. The respiratory system should be auscultated. The throat and nostrils should be examined. Lesions of the respiratory system which limit the exchange of oxygen, carbon dioxide, and anesthetic gases or vapors include: 1. Respiratory obstructions including laryngeal edema and paralysis, 2, alveolar emphysema (broken wind) and other conditions which reduce effective ventilation or increase dead space, 3, atelectasis, consolidation, or abdominal distention, which cause decreased vital capacity, 4, abnormal or reduced surface for the exchange of gases between the blood and alveolar air due to pulmonary edema, congestion, and inflammation.

Cardiovascular System: The heart should be auscultated before and, if possible, after exercise to determine whether the rhythm is normal and whether there are murmurs which may (or may not) indicate valvular lesions. The pulse should be checked, and the skin examined for coldness and clamminess if the history suggests surgical shock. The legs and dependent parts of the body should be observed for edema, and the mucous membranes should be examined for evidence of anemia or icterus. Other examinations or laboratory determinations may be indicated if abnormalities are suspected.

If a systemic infection or toxemia exists, there may be secondary myocardial damage with reduced cardiac efficiency or peripheral pooling of blood and tissue fluid with consequent reduction in rate of venous return. In these circumstances, the anesthetic risk is markedly increased.

Diet: Some veterinarians routinely fast animals for periods of 12 to 72 hours prior to the induction of anesthesia. Many now believe, however, that fasting is not necessary in horses, since regurgitation is not a problem. Nevertheless, if the digestive tract contains a large amount of ingesta, diaphragmatic action may be somewhat limited and the danger of rupture of the stomach or colon may be increased

when the animal is cast, or during stormy recovery. Long periods of fasting often are done prior to ovariectomy and cryptorchidectomy to decrease visceral pressure during manipulation in the abdomen. Long periods of fasting may decrease the ability of the liver to resist the toxic effects of chloroform, and perhaps other anesthetic agents. This may increase the risk of anesthesia and/or prolong the recovery time. It is wise to use a diet high in carbohydrates prior to anesthesia and surgery to increase the glycogen reserve. The bulk in the diet should be reduced for several days prior to planned abdominal surgery, but the caloric intake should be maintained or increased if possible.

Preanesthetic Medication: Drugs are often administered prior to anesthesia to facilitate its induction and maintenance and to reduce recovery time and the amount of struggling on recovery. Goals of premedication should be to: 1. Calm nervous or restless animals, 2, potentiate the anesthetic agents used, 3, reduce respiratory and salivary secretions if an anesthetic agent which stimulates these secretions is to be used. Drugs commonly used to achieve these goals include the phenothiazine-derived tranquilizers, sedatives, meperidine, and atropine.

Tranquilizers: Several of the tranquilizers are effective in calming horses prior to induction of anesthesia and they minimize excitement and struggling during recovery. Tranquilizers should not be used in animals with a history suggesting surgical shock, or in those showing signs of surgical shock. Promazine hydrochloride has been used more than the other tranquilizers as a preanesthetic agent. The response of horses to promazine as a preanesthetic agent is good more consistently than their response to other tranquilizers which have been evaluated extensively. As a preanesthetic agent it reduces the dose of chloral hydrate required for anesthesia by 33 or 40% or more,[36,37,38,39] shortens the recovery period,[19,36,38,39] and reduces struggling during recovery.[38,40] A dose of from 0.25 to 0.5 mg./pound generally is used. The intravenous route is recommended since the maximum effect then occurs about 20 minutes following injection. It has been shown that recovery time is significantly shorter if 0.33 mg./pound is given, compared to 0.5 mg./pound, if chloral hydrate (0.33 ml. of a 7% solution/pound), followed by thiopental sodium (Pentothal: Abbott Labs.) "to effect" is used to induce and maintain anesthesia.[41]

Other tranquilizers which have been recommended as preanesthetic agents are: chloropromazine, propiopromazine, acepromazine maleate and triflupromazine.

Preanesthetic sedation can be achieved by chloral hydrate administered either orally or intravenously. Chloral hydrate 12% with magnesium sulfate 6% or chloral hydrate 21 Gm. (328 grains), magnesium sulfate 11 Gm. (164 grains) and pentobarbital sodium 5 Gm. (75 grains) made up to 500 ml. also can be used.

Narcotics: Meperidine hydrochloride may be used as a premedicant in cases of intestinal colic requiring surgical intervention. Not only does it have a mild atropine-like action, but it also is an analgesic and spasmolytic. A dose of 0.5 to 2 mg./pound usually is adequate. If desired it can be used with a tranquilizer. The chief disadvantage of this drug is its depressing effect upon the respiratory center. Therefore, the use of narcotics with large doses of barbiturates or chloral hydrate is undesirable.

Atropine: When irritating inhalation anesthetic agents are used, control of excessive salivary and respiratory secretions is necessary. This usually is accomplished by the parenteral use of atropine sulfate (0.02 mg./pound). Atropine inhibits secretions which might interfere with ventilation or which might be aspirated into the lungs. It also lessens the chance of laryngeal spasm, a factor of importance when horses are intubated. The disadvantage of the use of atropine is its interference with pupillary reflex. It is the opinion of some workers that atropine is indicated specifically prior to chloroform anesthesia, because in large doses it prevents reflex vagal inhibition of the heart. It is probable, however, that death during chloroform anesthesia results more frequently from ventricular fibrillation or direct myocardial depression.

If a period of deep anesthesia of more than 15 to 20 minutes is anticipated, a bland oint-ment should be applied to the eyes to prevent drying of the corneas.

STAGES AND SIGNS OF ANESTHESIA

As anesthesia is induced, the animal reacts in a specific, characteristic pattern. The recognition of the signs and stages of anesthesia is important for the animal's safety (Table 1). In 1937, Guedel described the stages and planes of ether anesthesia in man.[42] The stages are: 1. Prenarcosis, also called sedation, hypnosis, or analgesia, 2, narcosis, also called the stage of uninhibited response, involuntary movement, delirium or excitement, 3, surgical anesthesia, 4, medullary (respiratory) paralysis. Recovery is but a reversal of these stages. Deep surgical anesthesia seldom is required, and the stage of medullary paralysis always should be avoided. Four planes of surgical anesthesia (Stage 3) are recognized. (Some authors describe light, medium and deep surgical anesthesia.) Attempts have been made to apply the stages and planes of anesthesia to animals, including the horse, but the stages of anesthesia in the horse are not as clearly demarcated as in man, and the signs of anesthesia vary with the preanesthetic and anesthetic agents used.

Stage 1: Behavior during Stage 1 varies with the animal's temperament and the anesthetic agent used. Sometimes there is unrest initially or even excitement. The initial onset of drug action sometimes causes apprehension. Excitement will be accentuated by excessive restraint and by the use of inhalation anesthetic agents. If induction of anesthesia is started with the horse standing, it usually will stand quietly but may become incoordinated. The response to painful stimuli usually is reduced. If the animal is recumbent (after being cast or being put on an operating table) care should be taken that this stage is not confused with surgical anesthesia. The horse may lie quietly, apparently relaxed, with regular respirations which often are deeper than normal, and the eyes may be closed. A careful examination will reveal dilated pupils and active reflexes; painful stimuli evoke response.

Stage 2: As the onset of anesthesia progresses Stage 1 gradually merges into Stage

Table 1.—Stages of Anesthesia

Signs or Reflexes	Stage 1 Prenarcosis (Sedation)	Stage 2 Narcosis (Uninhibited Response)	Stage 3 Surgical Anesthesia Plane 1	2	3	4
Respiratory	Normal	Irregular. May have reflex apnea. Become deeper as approach surgical anesthesia.	Progressive depression of rate and depth, varying with anesthetic agent. Occurs earliest with barbiturates, latest with ether.			
Cardiovascular		Accelerated	Steady rate and rhythm. Usually faster than normal. Varies with anesthetic agent.			Tachycardia Bradycardia Arrhythmias
		Arrhythmias especially when stimulated.				
Eye: Nystagmus		Usually present	Usually present			
Corneal					Absent	
Pupil		Dilation and Reflex	Constricted————→		Progressive————→ dilation	
Palpebral	Normal	Sometimes spontaneous rhythmic blinking	Progressive Absent———————————————→ depression			
Lacrimation			Progressive drying, especially with ether.			
Laryngeal			Absent, adequate depression for intubation.			
Equilibrium		Lost——————————————————————————————————————→				
Muscle Tone: General	Normal	Increased	Progressive decrease varying with anesthetic agent used.			
Anal sphincter tone			Progressive decrease————————→ Relaxed			
Anal sphincter reflex			Progressive suppression————————→ Absent			
Bladder sphincter tone						Dribbling of urine.

2 with no clear-cut demarcation between them. As induction progresses to Stage 2, the animal loses its ability to stand. This stage is characterized by the loss of upper motor neuron control. When this control is suppressed or released, reflexes become more primitive and exaggerated. The animal should not be stimulated while in this stage. Wright states that such stimulation, in addition to causing excitement and struggling, may even cause cardiac failure.[9,10] Struggling and excitement during this stage occur less frequently when a tranquilizer is used before induction of anesthesia. A sign of disturbed postural reflexes, in addition to the inability to stand, is the onset of a slow, synchronous, horizontal rolling of the eyeballs (nystagmus). As the degree of depression increases, the movement of the eyes usually becomes more rapid. Oscillations may be as frequent as 50 per minute. Spontaneous blinking, synchronous with the nystagmus, sometimes is present during this stage. The ears also will twitch occasionally. As anesthesia becomes deeper the range of movement of the eyeballs usually decreases, but the frequency often increases until only a flickering movement can be observed. During recovery from anesthesia, the frequency of nystagmus

may increase when the animal struggles. The incidence, constancy and nature of nystagmus depend on the preanesthetic and anesthetic agents used. This sign should not be depended upon as an indication of the depth of anesthesia, because it may be present or absent at any time the horse is in Stage 2 or light surgical anesthesia (Stage 3).

Stage 3: In surgical anesthesia the animal does not perceive nor respond to painful stimuli.

Response to painful stimuli first is absent in Plane 1. Respiration varies with the anesthetic agent used but usually is deep, and the rate usually is between 6 and 12 per minute. The rhythm and depth of respiration usually are regular, but may be irregular if barbiturates are used. Nystagmus often is present in this plane of anesthesia, but it may be fast and weak. Tapping the zygomatic area causes the horse to blink (palpebral or eyelid reflex). The anal and corneal reflexes are strong. (Careless or excessive touching of the cornea to check the corneal reflex may cause keratitis.) The pupil usually is constricted, but there may be slight additional constriction if a bright light is directed into the eye. (The pupil is dilated throughout anesthesia if atropine has been administered.) The opiates also affect the pupillary reaction, and chlorpromazine has been reported to cause constriction of the pupil.[43] Horses sometimes move slightly during Plane 1 of surgical anesthesia with chloral hydrate, intravenous ether, or promazine, chloral hydrate and thiobarbiturates, and probably with other agents.[11,41] These movements are independent of surgical stimuli, *e.g.*, they sometimes occur while no painful manipulations are being done, just before or after painful stimulation which causes no response. The cause of these movements probably is release of spinal motor reflexes after inhibition by higher centers due to the action of the anesthetic agents on the higher centers. These slight movements usually do not interfere with surgery, but are a signal for administration of more of the anesthetic agent to maintain anesthesia. They are helpful in maintaining light anesthesia when an untrained layman must give the anesthetic agent at the command of the surgeon.

In Plane 2, the respirations are regular, usually not as deep, and are often slower than in Plane 1. Skeletal muscle relaxation is marked. The tone of the anal sphincter is decreased, but it will contract if stimulated. Nystagmus does not occur in this or lower planes of anesthesia. The pupil is constricted unless drugs which cause dilation have been used. The palpebral reflex usually is absent. (It may be present during ether anesthesia.) The corneal reflex is weak, and is absent in lower Plane 2 anesthesia. The eyelids may be closed or open. They frequently are open during ether or halothane anesthesia.

In Plane 3, the depth of respiration usually decreases, and the respiratory movements generally become less smooth. As intercostal paralysis develops, the chest movements tend to follow slightly those of the diaphragm. Skeletal muscles are very relaxed. The anal sphincter has little tone, but will respond to stimulation. The pupil is partially dilated and there is a slow, weak response to bright light. Corneal and palpebral reflexes are absent.

The deepest plane of surgical anesthesia, Plane 4, always should be avoided since death due to paralysis of the medullary centers may occur if anesthesia is carried slightly deeper. Respiration is severely depressed. The rate often is less than 4 per minute and breathing is shallow. Inspiration is short and gaspy since the thoracic muscles are paralyzed and breathing is entirely diaphragmatic. This type of respiration also may occur during the use of large doses of muscle relaxants. If rebreathing equipment is being used, there is progressive inflation of the reservoir bag indicating low oxygen consumption. Pulse rate usually is increased, but with halothane anesthesia progressive slowing of the heart occurs as deeper anesthesia develops. The strength of the pulse usually decreases in deep anesthesia. Often there is less hemorrhage at the operative site due to low blood pressure. Cyanosis and the dark color of blood and tissue at the operative site develop if insufficient oxygen is being transported to the tissues. The pupils are dilated and fail to respond to light. Ocular reflexes are absent. The anal reflex is absent and the sphincter relaxes. Relaxation of the bladder sphincter may permit dribbling of urine; this also may occur in Plane 3.

Stage 4 (Medullary (Respiratory) Paralysis): The pupils are dilated and will not respond to light. All reflexes are absent. Respiration stops and vasomotor collapse occurs; death soon follows.

Recovery: Recovery is but a return through the stages which the animal passed during induction of anesthesia. Since recovery depends upon the distribution of drugs within the tissues, their elimination and/or detoxification, this process is slower, and Stages 2 and 1 are more obvious. No attempt should be made to make the animal rise before it is able to do so. Operations performed upon the limbs, especially when locomotor function is partially limited, require that the animal remain recumbent for a longer period of time. Emergence struggling is more frequent in animals which have not received preanesthetic tranquilizers and in animals stimulated or excessively restrained during recovery.

The length and nature of the recovery depend on the drug or drugs used. Recovery is rapid with most of the inhalation anesthetic agents since they are excreted rapidly, unchanged. The recovery rate from inhalation agents varies inversely with their solubility in the blood and tissue fluid. For example, recovery from ether anesthesia is much slower than recovery from halothane or cyclopropane anesthesia. With most anesthetic agents, the recovery time is affected by their distribution to body tissues, and with some by the total amount of drug administered and by occurrence of the acute tolerance phenomena. (See the section on thiobarbiturates.)

It is unwise to inject dextrose solutions during the recovery period since the "glucose effect" may cause return to a deeper stage of anesthesia and prolong the recovery time.[44,45] This phenomenon was observed in one case following anesthesia of a horse with promazine, chloral hydrate and thiopental.

Following general anesthesia, animals should not be permitted to eat or drink until they are fully recovered, since they may aspirate feed and/or water.

A. A. GABEL
E. W. JONES

SAFETY

The lightest plane of surgical anesthesia (Stage 3) which produces suitable operating conditions obviously is safest. As little drug as is necessary should be used to attain these conditions. Plane 1 of surgical anesthesia is adequate for most operations, but certain ones require deeper anesthesia, for example those around the head (especially of the eye). Lack of muscular relaxation seldom is a problem in equine surgery if the animal is in surgical anesthesia.[10] However, a deeper plane of surgical anesthesia or the use of muscular relaxants may be used for some abdominal or orthopedic surgery.

The rate, depth, and character of respiration are important guides in regulating the depth of anesthesia. If inhalation anesthesia is being used, changes in degree of filling of the rebreathing bag indicate changes in the minute volume, and often the depth of anesthesia. The color of the mucous membranes, the color of the tissue at the operative site, and the rate and strength of the pulse also should be watched. A widely dilated pupil which will not respond to light should be a cause for concern since it may be a result of hypoxia or deep anesthesia. The spontaneous movements described in Plane 1 of surgical anesthesia are helpful in maintaining light anesthesia. A cardiac monitor can be used to indicate the electrical activity of the heart. Unfortunately, this does not always reflect the function of the cardiovascular system. Furthermore, in most cases in which animals are taken to Stage 4 anesthesia, respiration stops before the heart stops. Observations in dogs and man indicate that a cardiac monitor is not reliable for evaluating the functional competence of the heart when there is severe hypotension and barbiturate depression.[46]

INDUCTION OF ANESTHESIA

Horses usually are cast or secured on an operating table before surgical anesthesia is induced (see section on restraint). Preanesthetic use of tranquilizers and/or sedatives makes these procedures easier and safer. A good method, if the horse is to be cast, is to place the casting harness on the horse after the preanesthetic tranquilizer has taken effect, then administer, during 2 to 4 minutes, a dose of chloral hydrate or one of the chloral hydrate mixtures sufficient to cause the animal to fall soon after the injection is finished.

The use of "rapid injection" thiobarbiturates to induce anesthesia is discussed under intravenous anesthesia. Restraint is not needed with this method.

Succinylcholine can be used to put the horse down. It is best to restrain the animal as soon as it falls and to induce anesthesia when respirations become satisfactory. Induction can be done with intravenous agents or with a rapid-acting inhalant agent such as halothane.[47,48,49]

Whenever a horse is recumbent, especially when under anesthesia, the head should be held in the extended position. If the neck is flexed, the airway is partially obstructed.

MAINTENANCE OF ANESTHESIA

For short operations an agent can be selected which will maintain anesthesia for the duration of the operation. For example, preanesthetic tranquilization plus induction to Plane 2 of anesthesia with chloral hydrate, magnesium sulfate, and pentobarbital sodium may provide 15 to 30 minutes of surgical anesthesia. There is a tendency to induce anesthesia to too great a depth in order to prolong the effect and avoid additional maintenance doses. Additional drug may be required either by inhalation or by injection, to maintain surgical anesthesia beyond the duration of effect of the induction dose. Additional large doses, especially if given in haste, can lead to overdosage, respiratory failure, and even death.

INTRAVENOUS ANESTHESIA

Intravenous anesthesia is more practical than the inhalation method for the veterinarian who operates in the field away from hospital facilities. The equipment is less expensive and more easily transported. (See Chapter 3 for safe methods of injecting the intravenous anesthetic agents. Many of them cause inflammation if injected perivascularly).

INTRAVENOUS ANESTHETIC AGENTS

Chloral Hydrate: The experimental use of chloral hydrate in horses was described in 1875.[49] Clinical use of intravenous chloral hydrate anesthesia was developed during the 1930's.[9] The drug continues to be used extensively in horses.[9,10,19] It is safe, if given "to effect," to produce light anesthesia. If deep anesthesia is produced, respiratory depression may occur and the margin of safety is narrow. Chloral hydrate undoubtedly is the most practical anesthetic agent available at the present time if only one drug is used. Some of the chloral hydrate is detoxified by metabolism and a small part is excreted unchanged.[51,52] Contrary to earlier theory, there is little evidence that chloral hydrate anesthesia causes serious liver degeneration.[13] No degeneration was detected in the livers of 18 horses examined following 2½ hours of chloral hydrate anesthesia. Euthanasia was performed at the termination of anesthesia.[12]

The disadvantages of chloral hydrate anesthesia are the prolonged recovery period and occasional violence during recovery.[9,10,38] If a single injection "to effect" is used to produce deep narcosis (Stage 2 anesthesia) horses usually will be able to stand about an hour after the injection is given, but if a short period of surgical anesthesia (Stage 3) is achieved the horse usually will not rise before 1½ or 2 hours.[9] Supplementation of chloral hydrate anesthesia with thiopental sodium or pentobarbital sodium has been described.[9] If promazine is given as a preanesthetic agent, the dose of chloral hydrate and the recovery time will be decreased by about 40%, and there seldom will be struggling on recovery.[19,36,38,39,40]

Chloral Hydrate 12% and Magnesium Sulfate 6%: Reflexes are depressed more at lower doses than with chloral hydrate alone.[53] The margin of safety may be greater than with chloral hydrate alone. This combination of drugs is less irritating than chloral hydrate if injected perivascularly.[53] The use of promazine as a preanesthetic agent causes recovery to be shorter and quiet.

Chloral Hydrate, Magnesium Sulfate, and Pentobarbital Sodium: The formula used is chloral hydrate 21 Gm. (328 grains), magnesium sulfate 11 Gm. (164 grains) and pentobarbital sodium 5 Gm. (75 grains), made up to 500 ml. This combination gives a quiet induction and recovery, and the margin of safety is greater than with chloral hydrate alone.[15,16] Less struggling occurs during recovery and the recovery period is shorter than with chloral hydrate alone.[15,16] Promazine is useful as a preanesthetic agent with this combination.

Pentobarbital Sodium: This agent is unsatisfactory for general anesthesia because of the long recovery period and amount of struggling on recovery.[16] It has been used on foals in which, because of their size, it can be controlled. Its use to prolong chloral hydrate anesthesia has been described.[9,10]

Thiobarbiturates: Two drugs in this group, thiopental sodium and thiamylal sodium (Surital: Parke, Davis & Co.) have had considerable use in horses.

With any anesthetic agent the stage of anesthesia is related to the concentration in the brain. Since there is little blood-brain barrier to thiobarbiturates, equilibrium between the blood and brain levels is reached quickly.[54,55,56] Onset of action occurs as soon as the dose, administered intravenously, is delivered to the brain (15 to 20 seconds).[54,55,56] Mark *et al.*, state that if these drugs are given "to effect" this prompt onset of action is a safety factor, "since there is less likelihood of gross overdose with such a drug than with one whose action is delayed, other things being equal."[55]

Most anesthetic agents used intravenously are effective until they are inactivated or detoxified by being metabolized or by being excreted, but the effectiveness of the thiobarbiturates decreases rapidly because the drug concentration in blood is rapidly lost to the lean body mass and especially to fat.[56,57] If small additional injections are used to maintain anesthesia, smaller or less frequent injections are required as the period of anesthesia progresses, since the drug accumulates in the storage tissues. Following the last injection, the plasma concentration of the thiobarbiturate quickly falls to a level below that which produces anesthesia, unless a large total dose has been administered. The storage tissues maintain a low plasma level while the drug is metabolized at a rate of about 10 to 15% per hour by the liver, and probably the kidney and muscle.[58,59] If large total doses (more than 4 or 5 mg. per pound) of thiobarbiturates are administered, recovery is prolonged since a high concentration occurs in the storage tissue which maintains a high blood level for a longer period.[41,56,60] The accumulation of the thiobarbiturates in the tissue is much more important in reducing their effective blood level than is that of other anesthetic agents.

Laryngospasm rarely occurs in horses but occasionally is seen when thiopental sodium is used in horses. There is less laryngospasm with thialbarbitone sodium (Kemithal: Ft. Dodge Labs.), or thiamylal sodium. Occasionally laryngospasm has been encountered with the use of pentobarbital sodium/thiopental sodium mixture (Combuthal: Abbott Labs.) in foals.

Rapid injection of too much barbiturate probably reduces the cardiac contractile force and causes a decrease in blood pressure. In man, even slow injection often causes a decrease in blood pressure.[61]

An increase in diastolic blood pressure occurred in horses during slow induction of anesthesia with thiopental sodium following preanesthetic administration of chloral hydrate or promazine.[11] Slow injection of thiobarbiturates in dogs and monkeys sometimes causes an increase in blood pressure due to vasoconstriction in the spleen, kidneys and extremities.[62,63,64,65] Perhaps a similar response occurs in horses. In man, there usually is vasodilatation with compensation by the heart to maintain blood pressure.[60]

The rapid intravenous injection of 4 to 6.5 mg./pound of thiopental sodium causes horses to collapse in 15 to 20 seconds. They seldom fall hard, but sink slowly, then roll to one side. A man holding the lead rope and a man holding the tail can ease and control the fall. After falling, horses take 1 to 2 breaths, then a brief period of apnea follows (usually 10 to 80 seconds). When breathing recommences it often is irregular in rate and depth. The duration of anesthesia is from 2 to 20 minutes and the horse usually is able to regain its feet in from 20 to 60 minutes after the injection.[66] Similar results are obtained with thiamylal sodium.[69] Violence and incoordination have been reported during recovery from thiopental sodium.[9,10,67,68] If an effective dose of thialbarbitone sodium is injected rapidly, the hazard of apnea is great.[13] Death seldom occurs with this method of injecting thiopental sodium in healthy horses even if their weight is overestimated, but there is great danger in animals with respiratory or cardiovascular disease. There is less danger of severe respiratory depression and death when the thiobarbiturates are injected slowly "to effect" rather than by the rapid injection method.[41]

It appears that acute tolerance to thiobarbiturates occurs in horses.[9,41] It can be avoided by injecting them slowly following the use of preanesthetic tranquilizers, sedation and restraint. Acute tolerance is the phenomenon by which the brain becomes tolerant to the effect of the thiobarbiturate, due to a high concentration in the blood and brain sometime during anesthesia, usually at induction.[41,60,70] The peak level attained appears to be the principal factor in determining the plasma level of thiobarbiturate at which the patient awakens.[60,70] The higher the peak level of thiobarbiturate, the higher the concentration required to maintain anesthesia. In one group of human patients, anesthesia was induced with 3 to 4 mg./kg of thiopental sodium and a second group was induced with 6 to 8 mg./kg. One-half as much total thiopental sodium was required to maintain the former group in anesthesia for 60 minutes compared to the latter group.[70] Avoidance of acute tolerance results in longer periods of anesthesia per unit of thiobarbiturate used. But more important, the time from the end of surgical anesthesia until the animal is able to stand appears to be shorter in relation to the length of the period of surgical anesthesia if thiobarbiturates are injected slowly "to effect," compared to the rapid injection method. It appears that a horse is able to stand only when a certain low plasma level of thiobarbiturate is reached, whether or not acute tolerance has occurred.[41,71]

Methohexital: Methohexital (Brevane: Corn States Labs.), has proved to be dangerous in horses. Convulsions and sometimes death have occurred during light anesthesia.

Promazine and Barbiturates: In 19 cases, 0.25 mg./pound of promazine was administered intravenously 20 minutes prior to rapid injection of thiopental sodium (3.74 mg./pound); an average of 6.5 minutes of anesthesia was produced.[71] The horses were able to stand within an average of 45.8 minutes after the injection. In 24 cases, a mixture of thiopental sodium and pentobarbital sodium was injected (3.64 mg./pound) instead of thiopental sodium; an average of 8.3 minutes of anesthesia was produced and the average time until the horses were able to stand was 33.5 minutes. Differences between the periods of anesthesia and recovery times were not statistically significant. "The anesthesia achieved by this technique was easily and rapidly induced, restraint was not required, and recovery was rapid and occurred without emergence excitement or struggling."[71]

Promazine, Chloral Hydrate, and Thiobarbiturates: This combination of agents was used 23 times to produce anesthesia on experimental horses, and on 82 consecutive surgery cases requiring general anesthesia.[41] Promazine, 0.33 mg. or 0.5 mg./pound was administered intravenously. Ten minutes later 0.33 ml. of 7% chloral hydrate per pound was administered intravenously and the horse was cast. Additional chloral hydrate up to a total dose of 0.5 ml./pound was administered in the clinical trials when it was required to prevent struggling during preparation for surgery. Plastic tubing was inserted into the jugular vein so an untrained assistant could give intravenous thiopental sodium or thiamylal sodium at the command of the surgeon. In mature horses, 5 ml. of a 3% solution of the thiobarbiturate was injected at 30 to 60 second intervals until surgical anesthesia was reached and additional doses were given as needed to maintain anesthesia during surgery.

In 23 experimental trials and 28 consecutive clinical trials, surgical anesthesia was maintained for an average of 57 minutes and the animals stood within an average of 42 minutes after surgical anesthesia ended. An average of 2 Gm. of thiobarbiturate per animal (2.7 mg. per pound) was required.

Excellent anesthesia was maintained and there was no struggling on recovery. Three animals attempted to rise before they were able, but there was no violent or incoordinated movement in their attempts to rise. No complications or deaths occurred during anesthesia or recovery, even in poor risk patients.

No observable difference in the nature of anesthesia or recovery was noted, nor was there any statistically significant difference in the length of recovery or in the vital signs in 7 trials in which the effect of thiamylal sodium was compared to that of thiopental sodium. The same animals and the same doses of promazine and chloral hydrate were used on different days.

The average time from the end of surgical anesthesia until standing was significantly shorter, at the 95% confidence level (analysis of variance), in the animals given the lower dose of promazine.

The probable reasons for the relatively long periods of anesthesia from these small total doses of drugs are: 1. The logical order of drug injection, 2, the additive effect of the anesthetic agents or perhaps synergism, 3, the avoidance of acute tolerance.

The drugs are given in a logical order: e.g., the drug with the longest period of activity is given first and the shortest acting one is given last. By the time the period of anesthesia and surgery is finished, part of the promazine has been inactivated, but much of it still is active and keeps the animal quiet during recovery. Much of the small dose of chloral hydrate which has been given before anesthesia is induced, has been detoxified. The thiobarbiturates have a short period of activity since the blood concentration is lost rapidly to the lean body mass and to the fat.[56,57]

The anesthetic effects of the drugs used are additive and it has been stated that there is synergistic action between phenothiazine-derived tranquilizers and thiobarbiturates, and between chloral hydrate and thiobarbiturates.[60,72] Promazine potentiates the action of anesthetic agents.[38,73,74] Thiopental has been used following chloral hydrate to reduce the amount of that drug required to maintain anesthesia.[9,10]

Since small doses of each of the drugs are required for anesthesia, the margin of safety with the combination of drugs should be safer than anesthesia with one of the drugs alone. Detoxication or inactivation of each of the drugs is by a different mechanism.[51,52,57,59,75] The combined respiratory depressing effect of the drugs is less than if a large dose of one drug was used. Promazine has little or no respiratory depressing effect at the dosage used.[71,76] There is less danger of severe respiratory depression and death when the thiobarbiturate is injected slowly "to effect" than when it is administered by the rapid injection method.[41]

Intravenous Ether: "The margin of safety with intravenous ether appears to be rather narrow." This anesthetic method appears to be less safe than others. "Another disadvantage of the method is that considerable time is needed to prepare the large quantity of ether-sodium chloride solution required."[11,12]

MUSCLE RELAXANTS DURING GENERAL ANESTHESIA

There is seldom a need for the use of muscular relaxants in horses during surgical anesthesia.[10] They have been used for better muscular relaxation with light anesthesia in orthopedic and abdominal surgery. They usually are of little help in reducing fractures if there is excessive myotatic reflex caused by injury to muscles (commonly called contracture).[9] If they are used to reduce articular luxations, the luxation is more likely to recur.[9] Large doses of muscular relaxants often cause severe respiratory depression or apnea. In these cases, artificial respiration must be used to oxygenate the animal until spontaneous respirations return.[77]

Succinylcholine Chloride: Intravenous infusion of a 0.2% solution of succinylcholine chloride at a rate of about 4 to 5 ml. per minute has been used along with intravenous or inhalation anesthesia to produce sustained muscular relaxation without respiratory arrest.[31]

If apnea develops at any time, the infusion should be stopped until spontaneous respirations return, then infusion should be started at a slower rate.

D-Tubocurarine: It was found that a single injection of ⅜ units/pound of curare caused paralysis of the skeletal muscles in 5 of 10 horses (caused them to fall) but that higher doses caused toxic effects (apnea).[78] D-Tubocurarine at a dose of 20 units per 100 pounds has been used with thiamylal sodium by "rapid injection."[69] Recovery is reported to be less violent if the curare is not used. Curare also can be injected slowly "to effect" during anesthesia.

A. A. GABEL

INHALATION ANESTHESIA

There has been interest in inhalation anesthesia in horses for many years, but until recently the only inhalation methods used to any extent were open-method chloroform and the use of ether with auto-inhalation type vaporizers.[79]

DELIVERY OF INHALATION
ANESTHETIC AGENTS

To achieve an anesthetic concentration in the brain by inhalation technics it is necessary to deliver an adequate concentration of the anesthetic agent to the animal, provide an adequate concentration to the alveoli, have efficient exchange between alveoli and blood, and deliver the anesthetic agent to the brain efficiently.

DELIVERY OF ADEQUATE CONCENTRATION OF
ANESTHETIC AGENT TO THE ANIMAL

Equipment for inhalation anesthesia is described subsequently. Delivery of the requisite concentration of anesthetic agent in oxygen or air presents no problem when a gas such as cyclopropane is used. Adjustment of the appropriate flow meters is all that is necessary. Volatile anesthetic agents must be vaporized in concentrations suitable for induction. The efficiency of vaporizers varies with: 1. The temperature of the anesthetic agent, 2, the rate of gas flow, 3, the relation of the gas flow to the anesthetic agent.

1. Temperature of the Anesthetic Agent: Other factors being constant, the vapor concentration varies directly with the temperature of the liquid. When a liquid is vaporized, cooling results. Cooling is undesirable because it slows evaporation and the concentration of the anesthetic vapor decreases. This cooling often causes vaporization to fall below the level required for anesthesia, especially with ether.[81] Cooling can be minimized by using anesthetic agents at room temperature, not refrigeration temperature; avoiding unnecessary vaporization by using a rebreathing system; using an anesthetic container which efficiently exchanges heat with its environment (large outside surface of the vaporizer, and construction of conductive material as copper will help; glass is a poor conductor); and supplying an external heat source such as a water bath or chemical heat source. Fire or electric heat sources should be avoided because of explosion hazards. Warm water often is used but the use of a chemical such as calcium chloride hexahydrate is more efficient. A closed circuit with CO_2 absorption maintains and generates heat.

2. Rate of Gas Flow: The more rapid the gas flow, the greater the anesthetic concentration unless there is evaporative cooling. Flow of gas causes an increased rate of evaporative cooling. The high rate of gas flow necessary for the horse, as compared with man and smaller animals, and the consequent cooling and fall in anesthetic vapor concentration, explain the difficulty of using inhalation ether for anesthesia in the horse.

3. Relation of Gas Flow to the Anesthetic Agent: The greater the surface area and duration of contact of gas with anesthetic liquid, the more efficient the vaporization. A bubble vaporizer emitting very small gas bubbles is therefore most efficient, the vapor concentration being greatest when the vaporizer is full. Less vaporization occurs when gases merely flow over the surface of a liquid. This principle is used in vaporizers in which the animal breathes over the anesthetic agent. In this way, vaporization varies with the activity of the respiratory system and tends to stabilize the depth of anesthesia. The surface area of contact in inhalers can be increased by the use of baffles, wicks, or an increase in size of the container.

ALVEOLAR CONCENTRATION OF ANESTHETIC AGENT

Provided sufficient anesthetic gas or vapor is being delivered to the horse, the rapid buildup of an alveolar concentration depends upon adequate respiratory movement. Effective minute volume (the amount of air reaching the alveoli each minute) is reduced by central respiratory depression due to high doses of drugs such as barbiturates, chloral hydrate, and meperidine, and by disease of the respiratory tract. Also of significance are partial obstruction in laryngeal paralysis, and alveolar emphysema. Respiratory efficiency also is decreased by inhibition of the normal movements of the thoracic cage by restraint, lateral recumbency, and abdominal distention. Increased dead space due to chronic alveolar emphysema (heaves) or increased mechanical dead space during the use of too large a mask also decreases gas exchange. The use of an endotracheal tube improves the effective ventilation by reducing the dead space. Uptake of anesthetic agents is hastened by efficient pulmonary ventilation or hyperventilation.

EXCHANGE BETWEEN THE ALVEOLI AND BLOOD

As the anesthetic agent reaches the alveolar air, it crosses the alveolar capillary membrane into the blood. Exchange between alveoli and adjacent capillaries depends on the nature of the diffusing surface, the pulmonary circulation, and the solubility of the anesthetic. Diffusion is reduced by pneumonia, atelectasis, emphysema, congestion, edema, and fibrosis.

A gas or vapor which is relatively insoluble in blood and tissue fluid (cyclopropane or halothane) quickly reaches equilibrium in the inspired air, alveoli, and blood. Induction and recovery therefore are rapid.

It is important to remember that factors influencing exchange and uptake of anesthetic gas and vapors also influence the exchange of O_2 and CO_2.

DISTRIBUTION OF ANESTHETIC AGENT IN THE BLOOD

Delivery of the anesthetic agent to the brain is dependent on adequate function of the cardiovascular system, and is similar to these factors which influence the distribution of intravenous anesthetics.

EQUIPMENT FOR ADMINISTERING INHALANT ANESTHETIC AGENTS

Inhalant anesthetic agents can be administered by the open or semiopen method, the draw-over method, or the semiclosed or closed method with CO_2 absorption.

Open Method: The open or semiopen method usually is used to administer chloroform to the horse. This is the only anesthetic agent which can be used satisfactorily by this technic. (It will not vaporize in cold weather.) Petrolatum should be applied to protect the nasal mucosa. The horse usually is cast and restrained before induction is started.[14] However, some veterinarians tie the horse to a tree, or other "safe" fixed object, place a burlap "mask" over the nose and pour chloroform onto the mask. The mask is removed as soon as the horse falls to prevent too deep a plane of anesthesia. Short operations often can be done before sensations return. If the horse is cast prior to induction, the mask, burlap, or towel is placed over the nose, and the anesthetic agent is dripped onto the towel or poured onto a sponge which is placed into the mask. The mask should be arranged so that all the inspired air passes through it, and the dead space of the mask should be limited to facilitate induction.

Advantages of this method include portability of equipment, inexpensiveness, and ease of administration. Its disadvantages are uneven anesthesia due to variation in anesthetic concentrations, wastefulness, possible damage to the nasal mucosa, and untoward effects associated with the use of chloroform.

Draw-over Method: In this technic, the animal inhales over the anesthetic agent and exhales through an expiratory valve. This type of vaporizer can be incorporated in a closed system.

Semiclosed and Closed Technics: These methods necessitate a controlled supply of oxygen as well as anesthetic agent. A reservoir bag, a mask or endotracheal tube, and an exhalation valve are used. Carbon dioxide absorption is necessary.

The closed system is based upon the idea that if sufficient oxygen is supplied to satisfy metabolic requirements and carbon dioxide is absorbed, the same mixture of gases or vapors can be used repeatedly. Such a system requires an oxygen supply with a pressure regulator and flow meter, and a cylinder of anesthetic agent with a pressure regulator and appropriate flow meters if gases are used, or a vaporizer if volatile anesthetic agents are used.

Oxygen Supply

A cylinder of oxygen and a pressure regulator and flow meter are needed to supply oxygen. If portability is not desired, a K or H cylinder is the most economical. For ease of handling, an E cylinder is preferable. This size provides sufficient O_2 for ½ to 1 hour of anesthesia with enough oxygen for emergency resuscitation. A flowmeter calibrated from 0 to 15 liters/minute is satisfactory. The basal oxygen requirement of the horse usually is between 2 and 4 liters per minute.

Supply of Anesthetic Gases

Nitrous oxide is supplied in cylinders the size of those used for oxygen. A pressure regulator and a nitrous oxide flowmeter calibrated from 0 to 15 liters/minute are needed. Cyclopropane cylinders do not require a pressure regulator. Because of its potency, a more sensitive flowmeter is needed; one graduated from 0 to 5 liters/minute is satisfactory.

Vaporizers

For ether, a bubble-type vaporizer or a draw-over inhaler can be used. Bubble-type vaporizers used in equine anesthetic systems include the AVR (National Cylinder Gas Division of Chemetron Corp., Chicago, Ill.) and Boyle's (British Oxygen Co., London, England). A draw-over vaporizer (inhaler) incorporated in a closed-circuit, circle system has been found most satisfactory for the administration of ether.

Because halothane is both potent and expensive, vaporizers providing known concentrations of halothane vapor have been designed for human use. Examples include the FNS (Ft. Dodge Labs., Ft. Dodge, Iowa) and the Cyprane (Cyprane Ltd., Keighly, England) which provide concentrations in the range of 0 to 5%. In these vaporizers, the gas flows over the surface of the liquid. A thermostat may be incorporated to maintain constant vapor concentrations despite temperature changes. However, the AVR and the Boyle's vaporizers appear to be most satisfactory when using halothane in horses.

Reservoir Bag

The reservoir bag is needed to accommodate the volume fluctuations as the horse breathes in the closed system. If flammable or explosive anesthetic agents (such as ether or cyclopropane) are used, the bag should be of conductive rubber. The neck of the bag should be larger than the tracheal lumen of the largest horse likely to be anesthetized. It is desirable but not essential that the bag should have an opening at the bottom for drainage of condensate.

The bag size should permit use in a partially inflated condition. Respiratory tidal changes should not cause collapse or overdistention of the bag. Too large a bag slows the ability to change the concentration of anesthetic agent due to the large volume of the system. The respiratory excursions are not readily apparent, their character is difficult to evaluate, and the anesthetic agent is wasted. Too small a bag results in collapse during inspiration and overdistention during exhalation. Satisfactory bag sizes for the horse range from 20 to 60 liters. The large animal unit in Fig. 12 has an adjustable bag.

CARBON DIOXIDE ABSORBER

In any system in which expired air is re-breathed for more than a few minutes it is necessary to remove the CO_2 which accumulates. Soda-lime or baralyme is used to do this. Soda-lime is a mixture of 90% calcium hydroxide with 5% sodium hydroxide, with silicates added to prevent powdering. Baralyme (which is less caustic and produces less heat than soda-lime) is 80% calcium hydroxide with 20% barium hydroxide.[82] Absorbent mixtures usually contain an indicator which changes color as soon as the absorptive capacity is depleted. Exhaustion of the soda-lime or baralyme and, therefore, accumulation of carbon dioxide, is indicated by increased depth of respirations and capillary oozing at the surgical site.[82] Convulsions and death will occur if the CO_2 concentration in the system is allowed to continue to increase. Blood pressure rise occurs, followed eventually by its decline and an acceleration of pulse.

The absorbent is supplied in 4 to 8 mesh-size granules which permit optimal absorption of CO_2 with minimal resistance to the flow of air. For maximum efficiency the air space between and within the absorbent granules should not be less than the tidal volume of the animal. The air space in one pound of 4 to 8 mesh granular absorbent is approximately 400 ml. Since the tidal volume of the average resting horse ranges from 2 to 5 liters, the amount of absorbent in an equine closed circuit system should not be less than 10 lbs. For efficient utilization of the absorbent, it should be contained within a cylindrical canister the length of which is 1.5 times the diameter.[83]

MASK AND ENDOTRACHEAL TUBES

Masks should be airtight with minimal air space. If they do not fit tightly, the anesthetic agent is wasted and the anesthetic concentration is diluted; resuscitation by manual compression of the reservoir bag is difficult. Excessive air space within the mask increases dead space, reduces respiratory efficiency, and allows the accumulation of carbon dioxide. An adjustable exhalation valve should be fitted to the mask or mask adapter to permit variation of the degree of rebreathing and flushing of the system should this become necessary.

When there is danger of aspiration of blood or other fluid, or when operations are to be performed on the head region, a cuffed endotracheal tube should be used. Endotracheal tubes up to 1.5 inches in diameter and from 20 to 40 inches in length can be obtained. Adapters to attach the endotracheal tube to the anesthetic machine should not be of a smaller diameter than the lumen of the tube. An endotracheal tube allows less dead space than a mask.

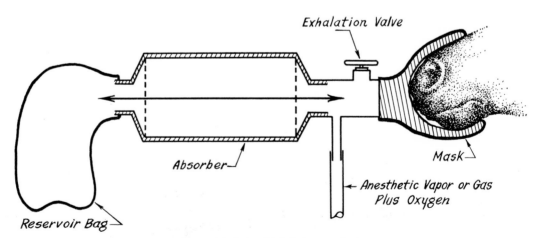

Fig. 11. "To and fro" closed inhalation anesthetic system.

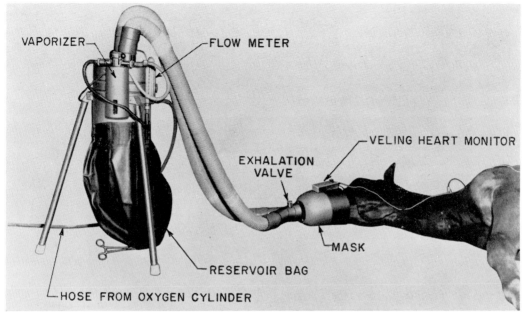

VAPORIZER—   —FLOW METER

—VELING HEART MONITOR

EXHALATION
VALVE

—MASK

—RESERVOIR BAG

—HOSE FROM OXYGEN CYLINDER

Fig. 12. "Circle" closed inhalation anesthetic system.

An endotracheal tube should be passed through a speculum in the mouth. A small wooden speculum is convenient. A small amount of water-soluble lubricating jelly can be applied to the end of the tube. If local anesthetic ointment is applied to the tube, there is less likely to be a cough reflex if anesthesia becomes light. A disadvantage is that the animal is more likely to aspirate feed or water if he is allowed access to them while the local anesthetic agent is in effect. The concavity of the curved tube should be down (against the tongue). The tube should be gently but quickly inserted through the larynx during inspiration.

ASSEMBLY OF EQUIPMENT

The equipment for the closed anesthetic method may be assembled as a "to and fro" system or as a "circle" system.

The "to and fro" system (Fig. 11) consists of a mask or endotracheal tube separated from a reservoir bag by an absorber. Gases pass through the canister both during expiration and inspiration. Fresh oxygen with or without anesthetic gas or vapor is added to the system via an inlet close to the mask. To minimize

dead space, the CO_2 absorber must be as close to the animal as possible in this type of unit. This arrangement is inconvenient; and heated gases resulting from the chemical reaction in the CO_2 absorber flow directly to the horse; this is often objectionable during long operations. Incorporation of an inhaler-type vaporizer is difficult in this unit; therefore, it is usual to rely upon the maintenance gas flow for vaporization.

In the circle system (Fig. 12), expiratory and inspiratory hoses about 4 to 5 ft. long are used between the mask and the remainder of the equipment.[84,85,86] Flap valves or other suitable valves with minimum flow resistance insure a one-way gas flow. Mechanical dead space in such a unit is only the space between the bifurcation of the hose and the animal. Equipment other than the mask or endotracheal tube and adapter for attachment of the hoses can be moved a short distance from the animal and an inhaler type vaporizer can be used. In the circle system, the exhaled gases pass from the mask or endotracheal tube via the expiratory hose to the absorber, through the absorbent to a reservoir bag from whence they return via the inspiratory hose back to the mask. During this last phase of the circle, part of the gases can be passed through an anesthetic vaporizer. Oxygen required by the animal and additional anesthetic gas also can be added in the system at this point.

With either system, negative then positive pressure develops during each complete respiratory cycle. The pressure changes vary with the flow resistance within the system. Excessive pressures interfere with pulmonary circulation and respiratory exchange and cause shallow respiration. Aperture sizes, canister shape and size, the length and type of connecting hose, the nature of the valves, and the size of the absorbent granules influence resistance and therefore pressures within the system. Apertures should be as wide as possible and under no circumstances should they be smaller than the diameter of the trachea. The smallest internal diameter of apertures and hoses in equipment for general equine use should not be less than 2 inches.

If ether or other explosive agents are to be used in the assembled equipment, all parts should be conductive, thereby permitting grounding of the entire anesthetic unit and overcoming the accumulation of static charges.

Induction Using Inhalation Agents

Cyclopropane, halothane, and chloroform are inhalation anesthetic agents which can be used to induce anesthesia rapidly. Induction is less rapid when ether is used. Prior to induction, premedication is desirable to increase the safety margin, to facilitate induction, and to reduce the amount of anesthetic agent required. Because it is necessary to use a mask or endotracheal tube, restraint in the recumbent position is necessary.

Before induction, the closed system anesthetic equipment is tested for leaks by filling the reservoir bag with oxygen, occluding the gas exit, and compressing the bag. The bag is half-filled with oxygen, the exhalation valve closed, and the mask applied or endotracheal tube inserted. The gas flow is adjusted to maintain partial inflation of the reservoir bag. If cyclopropane is used, the flow rate should equal that of oxygen (0.5 to 2 liters per minute) thereby providing a 50% mixture. If a volatile anesthetic agent is used, the oxygen flow should be in the range of 0.5 to 4 liters per minute. If ether is used, the vaporizer should be fully on. Increasing the anesthetic concentration within the system can be accelerated by opening the exhalation valve and compressing the bag to remove the residual oxygen. The gas flow rate should be increased during this time so that adequate gas is available for inspiration. When induction is almost complete, the anesthetic concentration should be reduced gradually to maintenance levels.

Maintenance Using Inhalation Agents

As soon as anesthesia is induced the anesthetic equipment, if not used for induction and already in place, is applied. The oxygen flow is set to maintain partial inflation of the bag. The flow of anesthetic agent is adjusted to maintain the correct depth of anesthesia. If a bubble vaporizer is used, it usually must be set to produce a fine stream of bubbles when using halothane or chloroform, but usually it must be one-half to fully on for ether. If a "tight" closed system is being used, it may be necessary to shut off halothane for several minutes up to one-half hour after the desired depth of anesthesia is stabilized. Ten to 20% cyclopropane usually is adequate; it may be necessary to turn it off for short periods. Nitrous oxide requires higher concentrations, usually between 50 and 80%, and it may need to be supplemented with a volatile anesthetic agent. If less than 20% of the gas in the system is oxygen, hypoxia may occur.

Inhalation Anesthetic Agents

Chloroform: Until recent years chloroform paralleled chloral hydrate in popularity as an equine anesthetic agent. Induction in other species requires 2 to 4% chloroform vapor; 1.5% is adequate for maintenance. Concentration requirements for the horse are not available. The usual method of administration is discussed under "open method." Only chloroform from newly opened containers should be used.

The respiratory center is depressed; respiratory arrest due to overdosage is accompanied by severe circulatory embarrassment so that artificial respiration may not revive the animal.

A progressive increase in depth of chloroform anesthesia causes a fall in blood pressure due to depression of the vasomotor center, the myocardium, and the vascular musculature. Chloroform has a marked propensity to produce cardiac arrhythmias, especially during induction and light anesthesia. Cardiac function may become ineffective due to direct myocardial depression, ventricular fibrillation or possibly vagal inhibition. These complications are likely to be initiated by sudden changes in vapor concentration, epinephrine release, and by increased blood CO_2 associated with hypoventilation.

Liver and to some extent kidney degeneration is a common complication following chloroform anesthesia, especially after prolonged use and in pregnant or malnourished animals. Hypoxia also is a factor in causing the degeneration. Chloroform should not be used in pregnant mares since it may cause abortion due to placental separation. The onset of respiration by the newborn is not adversely affected if the dam is anesthetized with chloroform for delivery.

Despite the disadvantages of chloroform, some workers are of the opinion that it deserves further consideration, especially when induction is achieved with other drugs and pulmonary ventilation and oxygenation are adequate.[9]

Ether (Di-ethyl ether): Ether vapor is 2.5 times as heavy as air and is highly flammable and explosive in both air and oxygen throughout the useful concentration range. On exposure to air, it is slowly oxidized to peroxides, which are respiratory irritants; therefore, only freshly opened "ether for anesthesia" should be used. In man, a 10 to 12% vapor is required for induction and 4 to 6% for maintenance of anesthesia.[58] Anesthesia cannot be attained in horses with the use of the open drop method of ether administration. Efficient induction and maintenance are difficult, especially in large animals, because of the need for high initial concentrations and the rapid fall in vapor concentration due to evaporative cooling. One part of ether is soluble in 12 parts of water. The long induction and recovery periods with ether anesthesia are caused by the great solubility of ether in blood and other body fluids.[62] During induction, a large amount of ether goes into body fluids causing a delay in the blood concentration reaching the level required for anesthesia. Following ether anesthesia (especially long periods) the blood level is maintained by the ether in the body fluids. Ether is excreted unchanged from the lungs.

The irritant effect of ether causes an increased flow of mucus and reflexly stimulates respiration. Pulmonary ventilation, therefore, initially is increased; decreased ventilation occurs only in the deeper planes of surgical anesthesia. An overdose causes respiratory failure before cardiac arrest; therefore, artificial respiration will revive most animals which are overdosed.

The heart rate is accelerated initially due to epinephrine release (sympathetic stimulation). In deeper planes of anesthesia, the heart rate is relatively unchanged. In laboratory animals, the blood pressure, after initial elevation due to sympathetic stimulation, falls in deep surgical anesthesia. This is caused by depression of vascular and skeletal muscular tone, reduced cardiac output, and depression of the vasomotor center.

Ether is relatively nontoxic and produces good relaxation without undue respiratory depression. Since it has a curare-like effect at the myoneural junction, muscle relaxant agents must be used with extreme care when ether is used for anesthesia.[62] Recovery from ether anesthesia usually is free from struggling.

Halothane (Fluothane: Ayerst Labs. Halsan: Fort Dodge Labs.): The anesthetic action of halothane in the horse was first reported in 1957.[87] It has been used clinically.[49,87,88,89] Chemically, it is very similar to chloroform. It is a heavy colorless liquid, not miscible with water, not flammable nor explosive, and stable in contact with baralyme and soda-lime. It is decomposed by light unless stabilized by 0.01% thymol and stored in amber bottles. In the presence of moisture, it corrodes tin and aluminum.

Halothane is a very effective anesthetic agent, being 4 to 5 times as potent as di-ethyl ether and twice as potent as chloroform.[9] Induction in other species is accomplished with 2 to 4% halothane vapor, and maintenance requires 1 to 2%. Values, however, are not available for the horse. Because the brain absorbs only small amounts of halothane and because the solubility in body fluids is low, induction and recovery are more rapid than with either chloroform or ether.

In man, myocardial contractile force and blood pressure fall in proportion to the concentration of vapor inhaled.[90] Hypotension is due mainly to the effect of the drug on the heart and to vasodilatation. Myocardial sensitivity to epinephrine is reported, although cardiac arrhythmias are observed only during deep anesthesia. Slowing of the heart usually occurs in proportion to the depth of anesthesia. There usually is less capillary oozing than with the use of other general anesthetic agents. This effect is not related to severe hypotension.[91,92] In spite of the hypotensive effect, halothane may help prevent surgical shock.[91]

Halothane is a respiratory depressant. It has been shown to produce decreased pulmonary ventilation in the horse with a consistent increase in the plasma CO_2. It is not a bronchial irritant and secretions are not stimulated.

Unlike chloroform, halothane does not damage the liver and kidney. Muscle relaxation is good. Overdose is manifested by progressive hypotension, respiratory depression and respiratory failure.[9,82]

Cyclopropane: Cyclopropane was first used in equine anesthesia in 1946.[98] It is a colorless gas about 1½ times as heavy as air. Since it is easily liquefied at room temperatures under a pressure of 5 atmospheres, it can be stored in light alloy cylinders and a reducing valve is not needed. It is very explosive when mixed with oxygen or air. It is a potent anesthetic agent resembling ether in its effect. However, it is less irritating to the respiratory tract and causes more depression to the respiratory center. It is excreted unchanged, and provides fair muscular relaxation. It does not cause liver damage but tends to produce cardiac irregularities. Because of its cost and because it is explosive, cyclopropane should be used only in closed-circuit machines.

Nitrous Oxide: Nitrous oxide was one of the first anesthetic agents used in man, but its use in the horse was not possible until the development of a closed circuit gas machine for large animals, because it is relatively impotent. It is of value in equine anesthesia only when used with other anesthetic agents. It is a nonirritating gas which is neither flammable nor explosive. One investigator recommends that nitrous oxide not be used in horses because of evidence of circulatory shock (diffusion anoxia) during recovery.[99]

E. W. JONES

COMPLICATIONS OF GENERAL ANESTHESIA

Complications are uncommon if animals are examined prior to anesthesia and any deficiencies compensated for if possible, if a reliable combination of drugs and method of administration are used, and if signs of anesthesia are used to maintain the lightest possible plane of surgical anesthesia which will give adequate conditions for the surgery being performed.

OVERDOSING

The most common complication in equine anesthesia is overdosing caused either by not using the signs of anesthesia to control the depth of anesthesia, or if an intravenous method is being used, taking the animal to a very deep plane of anesthesia with one injection in an attempt to produce a period of anesthesia long enough for completion of the operation. (If plastic tubing is used (Chapter 3), an untrained assistant can give injections as needed to maintain anesthesia.)

Since respiration almost always stops before the cardiovascular system becomes ineffective, the most important treatment of animals which have been overdosed with anesthetic agents is to make sure the airway is clear and to perform artificial respiration, preferably with oxygen (see following section). The administration of the anesthetic agent should be stopped; if a closed-system, inhalation anesthesia is being used, the anesthetic gas or vapor should quickly be flushed from the system and 100% oxygen should be used to rapidly fill the system. If the heart continues to beat, efficient artificial respiration usually will result in re-establishment of spontaneous respiration. Analeptics are of little value.

RESPIRATORY COMPLICATIONS

Obstruction: Partial obstruction causes inadequate tidal air exchange in relation to the respiratory effort. It is apparent especially when a closed system is used for inhalation anesthesia since excursions of the reservoir bag are small. Abdominal movement is excessive and the respiration often is noisy. In complete obstruction, the strong diaphragmatic movement and excessive negative pressure within the chest cause decreased size of the thoracic cage and, at the same time, the abdomen bulges. If there is inadequate gaseous exchange, cyanosis may be observed, but it may not be apparent if the animal is receiving oxygen. Accumulating CO_2 elevates blood pressure and increases capillary oozing. If partial obstruction occurs when inhalation anesthesia is being used, delivery of anesthetic agent to the lungs is impeded causing prolongation of induction, or during maintenance the depth of anesthesia may become lighter. Prolonged obstruction may cause pulmonary edema.

Respiratory obstruction in the horse may result from: the head being held in an abnormal position, laryngeal edema, paralysis or spasm of the larynx, obstructive lesions of the nasal sinuses or pharynx, or it may be caused by secretions, blood or exudate in the airway.

The hazards of obstruction should be anticipated whenever possible and an endotracheal tube used. If an endotracheal tube is not at hand, a tracheotomy should be done. Partial obstruction of the airway by the soft palate usually is characterized by sonorous respirations and usually is not serious; however, it can be corrected by passing a ½ to ¾"-diameter tube via the nostril on the lower side as far as the pharynx. Alternatively, a tube can be passed via the mouth into the pharynx. This method also is of value in instances of nasal obstruction. Whatever the obstruction, a free airway should be established immediately, either by use of an endotracheal tube, nasopharyngeal tube, oropharyngeal tube or a tracheal tube. Fluids should be removed by suction either through the endotracheal tube or tracheal tube.

Disturbances of Respiratory Rate and Rhythm: These disturbances occur commonly in the horse, especially during deep intravenous anesthesia. Rapid breathing may occur during light anesthesia, especially when ether is being used or when there is an accumulation of CO_2 in a closed system. An increase in respiratory rate also may be observed during painful surgical stimulation. Slow breathing usually results from deep anesthesia and may be accentuated by the use of meperidine or barbiturates. Although very slow breathing, especially during deep anesthesia, is undesirable, a respiratory rate as slow as 2 to 4 per minute should not cause undue concern as long as respirations are deep and cyanosis does not occur. Often when the respirations are slow during anesthesia, they also are irregular. The use of analeptics may increase pulmonary ventilation but may accentuate the irregular rhythm.

Apnea (Cessation of Breathing): Brief apnea occurs during rapid induction with barbiturates. Reflex apnea may occur briefly during induction with ether or chloroform or during insertion of an endotracheal tube when the animal is inadequately anesthetized. Apnea of short duration also is common during restraint or relaxation produced with succinylcholine. Apnea due to hyperventilation and resultant hypocarbia is of little importance in the equine but can occur if automatic resuscitation is being used, especially during the prolonged use of muscle relaxants.

Persistent apnea obviously is hazardous and quickly fatal. Every effort should be made to recognize the cause immediately, but in any case the presence of a free airway should be established, artificial respiration commenced, and oxygen administered if it is available.

In cases of severe respiratory depression or apnea, analeptics sometimes are given in addition to artificial respiration. These drugs may increase pulmonary ventilation and stimulate the central nervous system.

Amphetamine is sympathomimetic and a cerebral cortical and medullary stimulant. Overdosage causes hyperexcitability. Dosage is 100 mg. or more by slow intravenous injection to effect.

Pentylenetetrazol (Metrazol) causes stimulation of the central nervous system, especially the medulla and midbrain. In high dosage it is a convulsant. Experience with this drug indicates that the suggested dosage is of little value in anesthetic emergencies. The indicated dose depends upon the degree of depression, and it should be administered slowly intravenously. Doses as high as 100 ml. of 10% solution have been used. When apparent, the action is immediate; the respirations increase in rate and depth, the pulse is accelerated, and transient muscle tremors develop. Reflexes such as the palpebral and anal may return or become more active. The action is not permanent, the initial depression soon recurring. The action is more prolonged after several doses.

CARDIOVASCULAR COMPLICATIONS

Surgical Shock: The horse appears to be very susceptible to shock associated with trauma or intestinal obstruction. In cases of acute intestinal obstruction, progressive hemoconcentration is rapid. Death may occur within a few hours. Obstructions in similar locations in other species usually are not so rapidly fatal. The signs of surgical shock include skin which is cold to the touch, rapid weak pulse, and often sweating and depression. Shock is serious during anesthesia because it is likely that the shock will be accentuated during the course of the anesthetic period by the surgical procedure. It reduces the dose of anesthetic agent required.

It is essential that anesthesia be considered with these facts in mind and that the following general procedure be adopted.

1. Initiate therapy for shock prior to induction and continue it during maintenance of anesthesia. Treatment should include the use of blood, plasma, or plasma expanders. Antibiotics should be administered to overcome possible endotoxic shock, especially in cases of intestinal obstruction.

2. Preanesthetic sedatives and anesthetic agents should be selected to minimize additional circulatory embarrassment. Tranquilizers should not be given. Light inhalation anesthesia is preferable since recovery will be rapid and respiratory depression minimal. If intravenous anesthesia is used, care should be taken to avoid overdosage since less than the normal amounts of the agents usually will be required.

3. Pulmonary ventilation should be efficient. Circulatory embarrassment causes defective O_2 supply to and CO_2 elimination from the tissues. The lungs should be well-supplied with oxygen since the circulation already is inadequate and further anoxia to the vascular system will cause more dilation and loss of plasma fluid to the extravascular space.

Cardiac Irregularities: Serious cardiac irregularities which may terminate with ventricular fibrillation are most likely to occur during anesthesia with chloroform, cyclopropane or halothane. Ether is less likely to cause serious arrhythmias. The use of epinephrine likely will intensify arrhythmias. If serious irregularities occur, it is best to stop administration of the anesthetic agent and, if necessary, continue anesthesia with agents less likely to affect cardiac function. Ventricular fibrillation can be detected only if electrocardiographic equipment is available to monitor the electrical activity of the heart. If it is not possible to defibrillate the heart electrically, an attempt can be made to inject 20 ml. of 1% procaine solution into the left ventricle.

Cardiac Arrest: Primary cardiac arrest (not caused by shock or toxemia) seldom occurs in horses except following cessation of respiration due to overdose of an anesthetic agent. Other causes which have been suggested for cardiac arrest are pathology of the heart prior to anesthesia, or possibly vago-vagal reflex during light anesthesia, especially during hypoxia or hypercarbia. This reflex may result from manipulation of peritoneum or mesentery, inhalation of strong anesthetic vapors, intubation or stimulation when the animal is not in surgical anesthesia.

If cardiac arrest occurs, artificial respiration with oxygen should be started immediately if it is not already being done. In an attempt to start the heart, 2 to 5 ml. of 10% calcium chloride or 1 ml. of 1:1000 epinephrine can be injected into the left ventricle.

Delayed Complications: Complications due to general anesthesia may arise after recovery. They include degeneration of the liver and other parenchymal organs and disease of the respiratory system.

It is doubtful whether degeneration of parenchymal organs is of major importance in the horse. Chloroform is the main offender in causing degeneration of the liver and kidney. The livers of pregnant and malnourished animals are especially susceptible to damage. It also is probable that hypoxia during anesthesia causes degeneration to be more severe. Although chloral hydrate was at one time thought to cause liver degeneration, recent studies indicate that it produces little change in the liver.[12,13] Based on the action of other anesthetic agents in other species, it is unlikely that other agents cause liver damage in horses.

The most common respiratory complication following anesthesia is pneumonia caused by the aspiration of secretions, exudate or blood. This may occur if an agent which is irritating to the respiratory mucous membranes, such as chloroform, is used without preanesthetic atropine. Pulmonary edema or alveolar emphysema may occur rarely.

ARTIFICIAL RESPIRATION (RESUSCITATION AND ASSISTED PULMONARY VENTILATION)

Artificial respiration is indicated in cases of respiratory depression or failure due to overdosage of an anesthetic agent, the use of large doses of muscle relaxants and in newborn foals which fail to breathe adequately.

Clear Airway: The head should be extended. An endotracheal tube, tracheal tube or nasopharyngeal tube may be used as an aid in insuring a clear airway.

When an endotracheal tube is used, it should be as large as will pass into the trachea, and an inflatable cuff should be used. A mouth speculum should be used to prevent the horse from biting the tube. If an intranasal or nasopharyngeal tube is used it should be large enough to provide a snug fit in the nostril. The tube should be well-lubricated and the other nostril and the mouth must be occluded if the lungs are to be inflated with positive pressure. It is possible, although rarely necessary, to pass an endotracheal tube via the nasal route. A mask can be used in giving artificial respiration, but it does not insure a free airway. The mask, of course, must fit the face without leaks and should be as small as possible to reduce the dead space. Should nasal obstruction or the position of the soft palate impede

resuscitation, a nasopharyngeal or oropharyngeal tube can be used, and the mask applied over it.

SUPPLYING OXYGEN TO THE LUNGS

Manual Methods: Lateral compression of the thorax by intermittently applying pressure will cause some exchange of air. The pressure should be applied 6 to 10 times per minute and should be forceful enough to cause as great an excursion of the thorax as possible. The method, however, is inefficient and the operator soon tires.

The following technic has also been described: "Stand at the back of the horse (which usually is lying in a lateral recumbent position). Grasp the skin of the abdomen at the mid line and pull up, noting that the viscera are pressed into the thorax. Release abruptly. The viscera rebound, pulling the diaphragm posteriorly."[34] This method requires a great deal of strength and is tiring.

Free-flowing oxygen administered with a nasopharyngeal tube can be administered along with artificial respiration but this method of oxygen therapy is inefficient. If a tube is passed into the trachea almost to its bifurcation, diffusion of oxygen from the end of the tube to the lungs will oxygenate a horse which is not breathing.[93] If the tube is passed into a bronchus there is danger of lung damage.

A demand flow system can be used to supply oxygen, but it is useful only if the animal is breathing or if one of the given methods is used to produce respiratory movements. A cuffed endotracheal tube mask or "closed" nasal tube is required. During expiration, the flow of oxygen is stopped by the demand flow valve.

Positive Pressure Methods: It is possible to apply intermittent positive pressure in foals and ponies by blowing on a cuffed endotracheal, or a nasopharyngeal tube if leakage from the nostrils and mouth is prevented, while pressure is being applied. A simple bellows may be used in a similar way.[94] Compressed air, or preferably oxygen also can be used to intermittently inflate the lungs. A regulator valve is necessary to control the flow of gas. The lungs should be inflated to produce visible respiratory excursions, but great caution should be used to prevent overinflation and serious injury. Between periods of inflation, the oxygen supply hose is removed to permit passive relaxation of the thorax (expiration). There is more danger of overinflation if the "tube system" is closed tightly. This method is unsatisfactory for long periods of artificial respiration since it requires continuous cautious effort.

When a closed circuit gas machine is in use, intermittent positive pressure can be applied by manual compression of the reservoir bag. This method of applying artificial respiration to horses for long periods is tiring also.

Automatic Resuscitators: With either the volume-rate type or pressure-regulated type resuscitator, compressed air or oxygen can be used, but oxygen is most efficient.

The volume-rate resuscitator, such as the Knight-Wood type (Arnold & Sons, Veterinary Instruments, Ltd. London, England), is operated at a rate determined by the setting of the electrically controlled interrupter. The depth of respiration can be controlled by changing the gas flow rate or by changing the frequency of the interruptions. As this type resuscitator is not controlled by pressure change, overinflation of the lungs is possible because the volume delivered is not influenced by high pressure in the system. A gas flow of at least 30 liters per minute is necessary for the average mature horse.

Pressure-regulated resuscitators, such as the Stanton (Chemetron, Chicago, Ill.) and Seeler (Globe Industries, Inc., Dayton, Ohio) automatically switch from the positive to the negative phase of the cycle when a certain pressure is reached (usually 15 mm. to 35 mm. of Hg.), and switch again to the positive phase when the pressure is reduced to about −3 to −5 mm. Hg. Such a resuscitator should be equipped with a "manual over-ride" for greater usefulness. These resuscitators adjust to any degree of respiratory effort by the animal and do not "work against" these efforts. They will operate for long periods with little attention, without danger of overinflation of the lungs. With such resuscitators 50 liters or more of gas per minute are required in mature horses.

A. A. Gabel and E. W. Jones

LOCAL ANESTHESIA

Local anesthesia was introduced in 1884 with the use of cocaine. Substitutes for this relatively toxic drug were developed early in the nineteen hundred's.

Local anesthesia may be produced by: 1. Topical or surface application, 2, infiltration of the anesthetic agent directly into the surgical site, 3, field block, in which the anesthetic agent is injected around the surgical site, so nerves supplying the site are anesthetized, 4, nerve block, in which the drug is injected into or near the nerves supplying the area, or 5, epidural block, in which the nerve roots are blocked in the vertebral canal.

Depending upon the location and the surgical procedure to be done, anesthesia induced by these methods may be used alone or in conjunction with the use of a sedative, with the animal either standing or recumbent.

Drugs Used for Local Anesthesia

Drugs commonly used as local anesthetic agents in horses include procaine hydrochloride (Novocain), lidocaine hydrochloride (Xylocaine or Lignocaine), hexylcaine hydrochloride (Cyclaine), butacaine sulphate (Butyn sulphate, tetracaine hydrochloride (Pontocaine), piperocaine hydrochloride (Metycaine), and proparacaine hydrochloride (Ophthaine). The last 4 drugs are used primarily for topical anesthesia.

Procaine, the most widely employed local anesthetic agent, usually is used as a 2% solution for infiltration anesthesia and as a 2% or 4% solution for conduction (nerve block) anesthesia.

Lidocaine (Xylocaine) is 2 to 3 times as potent as procaine. One-half to 2% solutions are used for infiltration and 1 or 2% solutions are used for conduction anesthesia. Two to 5% solutions produce topical anesthesia. Lidocaine has a more rapid action and longer duration of effect than procaine.

A 1% solution of hexylcaine (Cyclaine) is several times more effective than a 1% solution of procaine for conduction anesthesia. It has a longer duration of action. One or 2% solutions are used for conduction anesthesia and 5% for topical. It has a topical anesthetic effect almost equal to that of cocaine.

With the exception of cocaine (a vasoconstrictor) and lidocaine (no effect) local anesthetic drugs are vasodilators.[62,100] Vasoconstricting agents, such as epinephrine, 1-norepinephrine (Levarevenol) or neosynephrine, often are added to delay absorption of the anesthetic agent and to prolong its effect. Since toxicity depends upon the rate of absorption and rate of detoxification (chiefly by the liver), the addition of a vasoconstrictor also increases the margin of safety. Usually 1:50,000 to 1:200,-000 epinephrine is used. The lowest of these concentrations probably will produce maximal vasoconstriction, but because of instability of epinephrine, the higher concentrations sometimes are used, especially in ready-prepared solutions.[62]

Hyaluronidase causes wider diffusion of the anesthetic agent, resulting in a larger area being desensitized if the infiltration method is used. Effective anesthesia often develops more rapidly. However, the duration of anesthesia usually is shortened unless a vasoconstrictor is used also. Hyaluronidase generally is used at the rate of one turbidity unit per milliliter. With the use of the local infiltration method, a combination of epinephrine and hyaluronidase with procaine increases the duration of anesthesia almost 5 times and doubles the area anesthetized.[101] The effect of hyaluronidase in anesthetic solutions used for nerve blocks is less apparent, although it appears that less anesthetic agent is required to produce an adequate nerve block, and the onset of action occurs sooner. Hyaluronidase cannot be used as a substitute for accurate technic since fascial planes act as barriers to solutions containing it.

Absolute ethyl alcohol occasionally is injected into a nerve to relieve a painful condition which is incurable. For good results, the nerve must be isolated and the injection made directly into the nerve. The nerve tissue beyond the injection site is destroyed and sensation returns only if and when regeneration occurs. This treatment is an alternative to neurectomy.

Aseptic precautions should be taken when local anesthetics are injected. Sterile solutions and injection equipment should be used. In-jection should not be made into tissue showing signs of inflammation. Trauma will cause more inflammation and if infection is present it may be spread mechanically. Hyaluronidase will increase the spread of infection. Also, it is difficult to produce local anesthesia in an area of acute inflammation because the tissue pH is low.[35] If an infected area is to be operated on, it is wiser to do a nerve block some distance proximal to the site or to use general anesthesia.

Although the equine species appear to be less affected by the toxicity of the commonly used local anesthetic agents than are primates, only as much anesthetic agent as necessary should be used. Care should be taken to avoid injection of large amounts of local anesthetic agents into blood vessels.

TOPICAL (SURFACE) ANESTHETIC AGENT

Topical agents are used mainly in the eye and on mucous membranes. They are used to anesthetize the mucous membrane of the larynx when "roaring operations" are done on conscious horses. The agent often used for this purpose is butyn sulphate.[95] Topical agents satisfactory for use in the eye include Butyn sulphate, Pontocaine, Metycaine and Ophthaine in 0.5 to 5% solutions.

INFILTRATION ANESTHESIA

Numerous injections of small volumes of a relatively dilute, suitable, local anesthetic agent are made throughout the area to be anesthetized. If skin wheals are made before injecting deeper structures, and the anesthetic agent is injected as the needle is advanced, there should be little pain evidenced by the animal. Undamaged needles should be used to prevent breakage, and as small a gauge as possible should be used to minimize trauma. Since horses are prone to inflammation and edema in response to trauma, it should be prevented and a minimum amount of local anesthetic agent should be used. Infiltration anesthesia commonly is used in minor surgery, for suturing wounds and for therapeutic cautery (firing) of small areas.

Field Block Anesthesia

A field block is done by injecting a local anesthetic agent into the skin and deeper tissue around, but not at, the site of the operation. Infiltration of the soft tissue around an extremity to produce anesthesia distal to that point also is an example of a field block.

Nerve Block Anesthesia

Nerves are blocked by injecting an anesthetic agent along their course. Numerous nerve blocks are used to produce regional anesthesia of areas of the head and limbs of the horse. It is important to know the anatomy of the region and to use the bony landmarks to locate the injection site.[96] It is best to desensitize the skin at the site with a wheal of local anesthetic agent before placing the needle when doing nerve blocks. It is best to aspirate before injecting at a nerve site to prevent the injection of a large quantity of local anesthetic agent into a blood vessel. Time must be allowed for nerve block anesthesia to become effective.

Nerve Blocks of the Head Region

Nerve blocks of the head region include the infra-orbital, the mandibular and the supra-orbital blocks.

Infra-orbital Block: The infra-orbital block is useful for surgery of the upper lips and the nostrils. It can be used for trephining the maxillary sinuses and extracting the upper incisors and cheek teeth.

The infra-orbital nerve is a branch of the maxillary division of the fifth cranial nerve and is entirely sensory. From the pterygopalatine fossa, it passes into the infra-orbital canal within which it gives branches to the upper molars, canine and incisor teeth, and to their alveoli and gums. After it emerges from the infra-orbital foramen, it supplies sensation to the upper lip and cheek, the nostrils, and the lower half of the face.

Depending on the area to be anesthetized, the nerve may be blocked as it crosses the pterygopalatine fossa, within the infra-orbital canal or as it emerges from the canal.

To block the nerve at the pterygopalatine fossa, the needle should penetrate the skin at a point about 1 inch ventral to the lateral canthus of the eye and just below the facial crest. Direct the 4-inch, 18-gauge needle medially, slightly dorsally and upward along the posterior surface of the maxillary tuberosity until it reaches the perpendicular plate of the palatine bone in the region of the maxillary foramen. Inject about 10 ml. of a suitable local anesthetic agent. Blood flow from the needle during insertion indicates puncture of the maxillary artery or the vena reflexa. If this occurs, the point of the needle is too far ventral or posterior.

The infra-orbital foramen is located halfway along and 1 inch dorsal to a line connecting the nasal notch and the anterior end of the facial crest. With the use of this location as a guide, the foramen can be located accurately by palpation. A 2- or 3-inch, 18- or 20-gauge needle is passed through the skin about 1 inch anterior to the foramen and then into the canal for about 1 inch. Five ml. of local anesthetic agent usually is adequate. Another method is to make a perineural injection at the point where the nerve emerges from the foramen.

Mandibular Alveolar Block: The mandibular alveolar block can be used for surgery of the mandible, the lower molars, incisors and lower lip. The nerve usually is blocked at the point of entry into the mandibular canal. The lower lip and incisors are adequately anesthetized when the nerve is blocked at the mental foramen as it leaves the mandibular canal.

The alveolar branch of the mandibular division of the fifth cranial nerve enters the mandibular canal via the mandibular foramen which is located on the medial aspect of the mandible beneath the pterygoid muscle. Within the mandibular canal, branches are given off to the teeth and alveoli. After emerging from the canal via the mental foramen, the nerve supplies the lower lip.

This block may be performed at the mandibular foramen or the mental foramen, depending on the area of anesthesia required.

The mandibular foramen is located on the medial side of the mandible at the intersection of a line which is a continuation of the anterior border of the supra-orbital process passing vertically down from the lateral canthus of the eye, with a line which is a continuation of the occlusal (table) surface of the lower molars. A 5-inch, 18-gauge needle is inserted at the ventral border of the mandible below the foramen and passed upward against the medial surface of the ramus of the mandible for the distance necessary to reach the intersection of the guide lines. This distance should be marked on the needle prior to insertion. Ten to 20 ml. of a local anesthetic agent is then deposited in this region.

The mental foramen is located beneath the tendon of the depressor muscle of the lower lip on the lateral aspect of the ramus of the mandible at the middle of the interdental space. The nerve can be palpated leaving the foramen if the tendon is displaced slightly. The needle is inserted at this location into the foramen and 5 ml. of a local anesthetic agent is injected.

Supra-orbital (Frontal) Nerve Block: The indication for this block is surgery of the upper eyelid and part of the forehead.

The supra-orbital nerve, a terminal branch of the ophthalmic division of the fifth cranial nerve, emerges from the orbit via the supra-orbital foramen in the supra-orbital process and innervates the upper lid and part of the frontal area. The auriculo-palpebral branch of the facial nerve and the lacrimal branch of the trigeminal nerve join with the supra-orbital nerve in supplying the area.

These nerves can be blocked by introducing a 20-gauge needle ½ inch into the supra-orbital foramen, which can easily be palpated in the supra-orbital process.

NERVE BLOCKS OF THE LIMBS

Nerve blocks of the equine limb include the median, the ulnar, the musculocutaneous, the tibial, the deep peroneal, the volars and plantars, and the posterior digitals. Nerve block should always be done prior to doing a neurectomy or alcohol nerve block, to determine whether the treatment will relieve the pain.

Median Nerve Block: The median nerve block, when combined with blocking of the

ulnar and musculocutaneous nerves is useful in doing surgery distal to the carpus. Lameness can be diagnosed in the carpal region if an animal remains lame following volar nerve blocks but goes sound when these 3 nerves are blocked. The nerve may be blocked when performing a median neurectomy.[9]

The median nerve supplies branches to the deep digital flexor and flexor carpi radialis muscles; the remainder is sensory, supplying an interosseus branch to the radius and ulna and terminating in the medial and lateral volar nerves. The nerve passes across the medial aspect of the elbow adjacent to the collateral ligament and beneath the posterior superficial pectoral muscle and the antibrachial fascia. It then passes into the groove bounded by the posterior border of the radius cranially, the belly of the flexor carpi radialis caudally, and the caudal superficial pectoral and deep fascia superficially.

The nerve can be blocked as it crosses the medial aspect of the elbow joint where it sometimes can be palpated, or better, approximately 2 inches below the elbow joint adjacent to the caudal surface of the radius. A 2-inch, 18-gauge needle enters the skin at the posterior border of the radius at the lower edge of the posterior superficial pectoral muscle. It is directed medially and somewhat upward to penetrate the superficial pectoral muscle and deep fascia. The posterior surface of the radius helps to indicate the necessary depth of the needle. Fifteen ml. of local anesthetic agent usually is adequate.

Ulnar Nerve Block: This block is used for minor surgery of the anterolateral aspects of the radial, carpal, and metacarpal areas and in conjunction with median and musculocutaneous blocks as indicated in the foregoing.

The nerve provides muscular branches to the superficial digital flexor, the flexor carpi ulnaris, and the ulnar head of the deep digital flexor. It sends a cutaneous branch to the skin at the lateral and posterior aspects of the radius and the anterolateral aspects of the carpus. In the distal third of the forearm the nerve lies between the flexor carpi ulnaris and the ulnaris lateralis and bifurcates to form superficial and deep branches. The former supplies the dorso-lateral surface of the carpus and the latter joins the lateral branch of the median, forming the lateral volar nerve.

The injection site is about one hand's breadth (4 inches) above the accessory carpal bone between the ulnaris lateralis and the flexor carpi ulnaris. The needle should be inserted just through the fascial layer, a depth of less than 1 inch.

Musculocutaneous Nerve Block: The musculocutaneous nerve block often is used along with blocks of the median and ulnar nerves.

This nerve sends branches to the biceps brachii and coracobrachialis muscles after which it continues as a cutaneous nerve down the craniomedial surface of the forearm. The nerve emerges between the palpable distal ends of biceps and brachialis muscles. It may be palpated cranial to the cephalic vein, proximal to the junction of the cephalic and accessory cephalic veins, near the medial border of the extensor carpi radialis. Distally, the nerve divides into several branches, accompanying the cephalic and accessory cephalic veins.

Infiltrate the nerve at the site at which it may be palpated, or make a linear subfascial block across the course of the cephalic and accessory cephalic veins on the internal aspect of limb half-way between elbow and carpus.

Tibial Nerve Block: Indications for this block appear to be limited. It may assist in anesthesia of the hock, especially the caudomedial part.

The tibial nerve is a continuation of the sciatic passing between the 2 heads of the gastrocnemius muscle, providing innervation to the flexors of the digit and extensors of the hock. It then divides into the medial and lateral plantar to supply, in conjunction with the peroneal, the distal part of the limb. At the usual point at which the nerve is blocked, a hand's breadth above the tuber calcis, it lies in loose connective tissue between the fascia of the deep flexor cranially and the tarsal tendon of the semitendinosis and biceps femoris caudomedially.

Palpate the nerve, which approaches ¼ inch in diameter, about 1 hand's breadth (4 inches) proximal to tuber calcis on the caudomedial aspect of deep digital flexor. Inject 10 to 15 ml. of local anesthetic agent around the nerve in this area.

Deep Peroneal Nerve Block: Applications for this block are limited; it may be used to assist anesthesia of the limb in conjunction with tibial nerve blocks where plantar blocks are not adequate. However, a considerable portion of the distal limb, including the tarsus, is supplied by the superficial peroneal and saphenous nerves. The deep peroneal supplies twigs to the joint capsules.

The peroneal nerve which descends from the sciatic deviates cranio-laterally and divides into the superficial and deep branches. The former innervates the skin of the lateral surface of the tarsus and metatarsus, and the latter branch supplies the cranio-lateral surface of the tarsus and metatarsus. At the site of injection, about 4 inches above the tibiotarsal joint, the nerve lies between the long and lateral extensors of the digit and cranial to the septum between these muscles. The superficial peroneal is located in this same groove but external to the fascial sheath around the extensors.

Locate the groove between the long and lateral digital extensors about 4 inches proximal to the tibial tarsal joint. Insert a 2-inch, 18- or 20-gauge needle through skin and fascia in a posteromedial direction, anterior to the intermuscular septum between the long and lateral digital extensors. The nerve lies at a depth of approximately 1½ inches in an average sized horse. Inject 10 to 20 ml. of local anesthetic agent. The superficial branch may be blocked by infiltration in the same site prior to penetration of the fascia.

Volar and Plantar Nerve Blocks: These blocks are employed for surgery of the extremity and to assist in the diagnosis of lameness.

The medial and lateral volar nerves are terminal branches of the median nerve. In addition, the lateral volar nerve is joined by the terminal branch of the ulnar nerve at the level of the accessory carpal bone beneath the tendon of the flexor carpi ulnaris. In the carpal region the medial nerve passes through the carpal arch adjacent to the deep flexor, and the lateral nerve passes distal and laterally from the accessory carpal bone in the annular ligament until it reaches a lateral position relative to the deep flexor tendon similar to the medial branch. Throughout the metacarpal region, the nerves lie on the dorsolateral and dorsomedial aspects of the deep flexor tendon and are accompanied by the metacarpal arteries and veins. The lateral artery is smaller. The nerves lie caudal to the blood vessels. At about the middle of the metacarpus, the medial nerve supplies a branch which passes obliquely distal and lateral behind the flexor tendons to anastomose with the lateral volar nerve just above the distal ends of the second and fourth metacarpal bones.

Each volar nerve divides at the level of the proximal sesamoids into dorsal, middle, and posterior branches. The dorsal branch ramifies in the dorsal surface of the fetlock and pastern and innervates most of the proximal interphalangeal and part of the distal interphalangeal and the metacarpalphalangeal joint capsules. The middle branch, which is inconstant, passes distally between the artery and veins, and partially innervates the corium, the lateral cartilage, and the pastern joint capsule. The posterior branch, the posterior digital nerve, is the largest of the branches; it passes distally on the posterior surface of the digital artery in the groove between the first and second phalanx and the deep flexor tendon.

The plantar nerves in the hindlimb originate from the tibial nerve and are distributed in a similar manner.

The volar and plantar nerves can be blocked at high or low sites. The midmetacarpal and midmetatarsal regions should be avoided since the block is likely to be incomplete due to the anastomotic branch passing from the medial to lateral branch. Whichever site is used, the block may be performed with the limb in a weight-bearing or flexed position. It is preferable to insert the needle in a proximal direction, so that movement by the animal tends to be away from the direction of the needle so it is less likely to be broken. A 20-gauge, 1-inch needle and 5 to 10 ml. of local anesthetic agent usually are adequate.

The low site, which is most often used, is located in the groove between the deep flexor tendon and the suspensory ligament about 2 inches above the fetlock joint, just above the bifurcation of the nerves. If blood is aspirated on insertion of the needle, it should be redirected to a more caudal position. A block at this level will anesthetize the hoof region, the pastern joint, and the skin up to a plane through the fetlock joint.[97]

At the high site, 3 or 4 inches below the carpus (above the anastomatic branch), the nerves lie dorsolateral and dorsomedial to the deep flexor tendon, beneath the fascia which covers the flexor tendons and suspensory ligaments. In order for anesthesia to result, the injection must be beneath this fascia. If the anesthetic agent is injected outside the fascia, subcutaneous swelling can be seen and felt. A successful block will give anesthesia of the digit from the fetlock down. Usually, there also will be anesthesia of the digital synovial sheath, but not the flexor tendons within it.[97] Slight local edema, which is a frequent complication of volar and plantar nerve blocks is reduced to a minimum by the application of a bandage for 24 to 48 hours after the injection.

Posterior Digital Nerve Block: Since the area anesthetized is restricted to the posterior (caudal) half of the foot, use of this block is limited to the diagnosis of lameness in this region, especially navicular disease.

The nerve usually is blocked at the middle of the pastern in the groove between the tensed deep flexor tendon and the first phalanx. The nerve lies immediately in front of the edge of the tendon.

The nerve may be palpated and blocked on the lateral aspect of the fetlock as it passes over the joint.

EPIDURAL ANESTHESIA

Epidural (peridural or extradural) anesthesia is obtained by blocking the spinal nerves in the epidural space as they emerge from the meninges. Epidural injections usually are given between Cy 1 and Cy 2 in the horse. The amount injected usually is kept small, so the animal remains standing. After casting, larger doses can be used to extend anesthesia to the posterior abdominal area, but there is danger of horses injuring themselves during recovery from such doses which cause them to lose control of their rear legs. Injection at the lumbosacral junction also has been described but it is dangerous since an accidental massive "true spinal" may result in death of the animal.[97]

Indications: Uses of this technic include surgical procedures involving the tail, perineum, vulva, anus, vagina, and rectum. In patients which are poor risks for general anesthesia, the animal may be cast and larger doses may be used for surgery on the hindlegs or posterior abdomen.

Anatomy: The posterior part of the spinal cord tapers to a point, the conus medullaris, in the posterior lumbar region. The conus medullaris is prolonged for a short distance as the filum terminale. This terminal part of the spinal cord and the meninges extends only to the midsacral region, but the sacral and coccygeal nerves continue back in the spinal canal. The combined sacral and coccygeal nerves about the conus medullaris and filum terminale are termed the cauda equina. Surrounding this structure, within the spinal canal, is loose fatty tissue. The spinal canal terminates in the region of the fourth coccygeal vertebra.

Technic: The site of injection is the first intercoccygeal space since Cy 1 usually is fused with the sacrum. Figure 13 shows 2 ways that the needle can be placed when giving an epidural. The point of injection can be located by palpation while manipulating the tail. It is approximately 1 to 2 inches cranial to the most proximal long tail hairs, and is at the level of the caudal fold when the tail is elevated. A 2- or 3-inch, 18-gauge needle is inserted downward and forward at an angle of about 30° from vertical (perpendicular to the contour of the croup) exactly at the midline. Penetration through the interarcuate ligament between the vertebral arches usually can be felt. The floor of spinal canal offers firm resistance to the needle point. If the needle is directed off the midline or if it is directed nearly vertically so it passes into the intervertebral space, anesthesia will not result. A second method of introducing the needle is to have it enter the skin about one inch caudal to the junction of Cy 1 and Cy 2 near the first tail hairs. In this case the direction of the needle is downward and forward at an angle of 30° with horizontal.

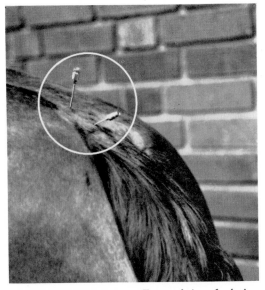

Fig. 13. Epidural injection. Two technics of placing the needle through the intervertebral space between Cy 1 and Cy 2. Courtesy of A. A. Gabel, D.V.M.

When this method is used, the needle passes cranially into the spinal canal and there is less chance of it going into the intervertebral space. When the needle is correctly placed there is little resistance to injection.

If the surgical procedure is to be done standing, care should be taken to avoid large doses which will cause ataxia or falling. When there is doubt about the dose to be used, it is best to err toward underdosage. The needle can be left in place and additional anesthetic agent given later if needed. Maximum effect with procaine occurs about 10 minutes after injection. Varying with the surgical procedure to be done and size of the animal, from 3 to 25 ml. of 2% procaine or its equivalent is used. Most mature 1,000-pound horses will not fall if 15 ml. of 2% procaine is used. If more extensive (more anterior or cranial) epidural anesthesia is required, the animal should be cast, since considerable ataxia, staggering, and excitement result when an epidural block is used to cast the animal. If large doses are used it may be necessary to restrain the animal until it regains the use of its rear legs. When epidural anesthesia is administered in the animal in lateral recumbency, the nerves emerging on the "upper side" may be unaffected; therefore, it is wise to put the animal on the side to be operated when doing the epidural, then turn the animal onto its other side about 10 minutes later.

The addition of epinephrine to the anesthetic solution prolongs its action in epidurals. The addition of hyaluronidase may make results erratic and unpredictable. Occasionally, a horse is found in which despite the repeated use of good technic in doing epidural injections, only partial anesthesia or irregular areas of anesthesia will develop. This is true especially if epidural anesthesia has been used on the animal several times before.

As anesthesia as far anterior as the anterior lumbar region is rarely used, hypotension and resulting shock due to blocking of the vasomotor nerves probably seldom occur in horses.

E. W. JONES

REFERENCES

1. Frank, E. R.: Veterinary Surgery. 6th ed. Burgess Publishing Company, Minneapolis, Minn. 1959.
2. Leahy, J. R., and Barrow, P.: Restraint of Animals. Cornell Campus Store, Inc. Ithaca, N. Y., 1953.
3. McGee, W. R.: Veterinary Notebook, The Blood-Horse, Lexington, Ky., 1958.
4. Powers, J. C., Jr.: Practitioner, Ocala, Fla., Personal communication, 1962.
5. Raker, C. W.: Head, Large Animal Clinic, University of Pennsylvania School of Veterinary Medicine, Philadelphia. Personal communication, 1958.
6. Schell, Cynthia T.: Walk, Trot, Gallop. Published by the author, Auburn, Ala., 1957.
7. Schell, F. G.: Head, Large Animal Clinic, Auburn University School of Veterinary Medicine, Auburn, Ala. Personal communication.
8. White, G. R.: Restraint of Domestic Animals. Published by the author, Nashville, Tenn., 1912.
9. Wright, J. G. and Hall, L. W.: Veterinary Anesthesia and Analgesia. 5th ed. Williams & Wilkins Co., Baltimore, Md., 1961.
10. Wright, J. G.: Anesthesia and narcosis in the horse. Vet. Rec. 70 (1958) 329-336.
11. Gabel, Albert A.: Intravenous ether anesthesia in equine animals. Am. J. Vet. Research 89 (1961) 720-730.
12. Gabel, Albert A.: Intravenous ether anesthesia in equines. Thesis. The Ohio State University, Columbus, 1959.
13. Jones, L. M.: Veterinary Pharmacology and Therapeutics, 2nd ed. Iowa State College Press, Ames, 1957.
14. Guard, W. F.: Surgical Principles and Technics. Published by the author, 2274 Yorkshire Rd., Columbus 21, Ohio, 1953.
15. Millenbruck, E. W. and Wallinga, M. H.: A newly developed anesthetic for horses. J.A.V.M.A. 108 (1946) 146-151.
16. Millenbruck, E. W.: A newly developed anesthetic for large animals. J.A.V.M.A. 112 (1948) 345-347.
17. Shaw, D. L. and Page, J. A.: A three-year review of the pharmacologic properties and clinical performance of promazine. Current Therap. Res. 2 (1960) 199-226.
18. Cherry, D. R.: Problems encountered in light horse practice. Can. Vet. J. 1 (1960) 537-542.
19. Panel report on sedation and anesthesia of horses. Mod. Vet. Prac. 40 (Nov. 1959) 45-47.
20. Hall, L. W.: The effect of chloropromazine on the cardiovascular system of the conscious horse. Vet. Rec. 72 (1960) 85-87.
21. Lundvall, R. L.: An unusual case of anaphylaxis in a pony. Vet. Med. 54 (1959) 346-347.
22. Owen, L. N. and Neal, P. A.: Sedation with chloropromazine in the horse. Vet. Record 69 (1957) 413.

23. Travernor, W. D.: Anesthetic procedures in the larger domesticated animals. Proc. of Royal Soc. Med. 53 (9) (1960) 717-720.
24. Turbes, C. C.: Chlorpromazine in cattle and horses. Allied Vet. 24 (1958) 3-7.
25. Williams, R. C. and Young, J. E.: Professional and therapeutic rationale of tranquilizers. Vet. Med. 53 (1958) 127-131.
26. Gabel, Albert A.: Accidental intra-carotid artery injection. J.A.V.M.A. In preparation.
27. Gabel, Albert A., Hamlin, R., and Smith, C. R.: The effect of promazine and chloral hydrate on the cardiovascular system of standing horses. In preparation.
28. Ford, R. W.: Tranquilizers to control vice in horses. Quest. and Ans. Mod. Vet. Pract. 40 (1959) 61.
29. Hansson, C. H.: Succinylcholine iodide as a muscular relaxant in veterinary surgery. J.A.V.M.A. 128 (1956) 287-291.
30. Hansson, C. H. and Edlund, H.: Experimentella undersokningar och klinisha erfarenheter av succinylcholinjodid (celocurin) ur Veterinarmedicinsk syhpunkt. Nord. Vet. Med. 6 (1954) 671-686.
31. Belling, T. H. and Booth, N. H.: "Studies on the pharmacodynamics of succinylcholine chloride in the horse." J.A.V.M.A. 126 (1955) 37-42.
32. Larson, L. H., Loomis, L. N. and Steel, J. D.: Muscular relaxants and cardiovascular damage with specific reference to succinylcholine chloride. Austral. Vet. J. 35 (1959) 269-275.
33. Tavernor, W. D.: The effect of succinylcholine chloride on the heart of the horse. Vet. Rec. 72 (1960) 569-572.
34. Squibb, E. R. & Sons: Package Insert Sucostrin Chloride, Veterinary. E. R. Squibb & Sons, New York, N. Y.
35. Goodman, L. S. and Gillman, A.: The Pharmacological Basis of Therapeutics, 2nd ed. The MacMillan Co., New York, N. Y. 1956.
36. Dawson, H. A., Lickfeldt, W. E. and Biengle, L. A.: Promazine in equine practice. J.A.V.M.A. 135 (1959) 69-71.
37. Raker, C. W. and English, B.: Promazine and its pharmacological and clinical effects in horses. J.A.V.M.A. 134 (1959) 19-23.
38. Raker, C. W. and Sayers, A. C.: Promazine as a preanesthetic agent in horses. J.A.V.M.A. 134 (1959) 23-24.
39. Shultz, C. W.: Tranquilizers in large animal medicine. Vet. Med. 53 (1958) 73-76.
40. Gorman, T. N.: Promazine hydrochloride in equine practice. J.A.V.M.A. 134 (1959) 464-466.
41. Gabel, Albert A.: Promazine, chloral hydrate and ultra-short-acting barbiturates anesthesia in horses. J.A.V.M.A. 140 (1962) 564-571.
42. Guedel, A. E.: Inhalation Anesthesia, 2nd ed. The MacMillan Co. New York, N. Y. 1951.
43. Robinson, M.: Tranquilizers in veterinary practice. Austral. Vet. J. 36 (1960) 127-132.
44. Lamson, P. D., Craig, M. E. and Hobdy, C. J.: The potentiation of barbiturate anesthesia by glucose, intermediate metabolites and certain other substances J. Pharm. and Exp. Therap. 103 (1951) 460-470.
45. Richards, R. K. and Taylor, J. O.: Some factors influencing distribution, metabolism and action of barbiturates: A Review. Anesthesiology 17 (1956) 414-458.
46. Booth, N. H.: Evaluation of a cardiac monitor. J.A.V.M.A. 140 (1962) 664-668.
47. Larsen, L. H.: Recent developments in anesthetics and muscle relaxants. N. Z. Vet. J. 6 (1958) 61-75.
48. Neal, P. A. and Wright, J. G.: The use of succinylcholine chloride as a casting agent in the horse prior to induction of general anesthesia. Vet. Rec. 71 (1959) 731-735.
49. Allen, C. and Reed, W. O.: Inhalation anesthesia. Proc. Amer. Equine Pract. Assn. Conv., Dec. 1959.
50. Marcenac and Lemetager: Contribution a l'e'ted de l'anesthesia a l'hydrate de chloral par voie veineuse chez les equides. Bull. Acad. Vet. France 3 (1930) 141-146.
51. Owens, A. H. and Marshall, E. K.: Further studies on the metabolic fate of chloral hydrate and trichloroethanol. Bull. Johns Hopkins Hosp. 97 (1955) 321.
52. Payne, L. C.: Detoxification of chloral hydrate. Am. J. Vet. Research 15 (1954) 468-471.
53. Danks, A. G.: Anesthesia in horses and swine. Cornell Vet. 33 (1943) 344-346.
54. Butler, T. C.: The rate of penetration of barbituric acid derivatives into the brain. J. Pharm. & Exp. Ther. 100 (1950) 219-226.

55. Mark, L. C., Burns, J. J., Ines Campones, C., Ngai, S. H., Trousof, Natalie, Papper, E. M., Brodie, B. B.: The passage of thiopental into brain. J. Pharmacol. and Exper. Therap. **119** (1957) 35-38.

56. Mark, L. C., Burns, J. J., Brodie, B. B. and Papper, E. M.: Clinical applications of studies of the physiologic disposition of thiopental. New York J. Med., **56** (1956) 2819-2822.

57. Brodie, B. B., Bernstein, E. and Mark, L. C.: The role of body fat in limiting the duration of action of thiopental. J. Pharmacol. and Exp. Therap. **105** (1952) 421.

58. Schwartz, H., Ngai, S. H. and Papper, E. M.: Manual of Anesthesiology. Charles C Thomas, Springfield, Ill. 1957.

59. Brodie, B. B., Mark, L. C., Papper, E. M., Lief, P. A., Bernstein, E. and Rovenstine, E. A.: The fate of thiopental in man and a method for its estimation in biological materials. J. Pharmacol. & Exp. Therap. **98** (1950) 85-96.

60. Dundee, J. W.: Thiopentone and Other Thiobarbiturates. E. S. Livingstone Ltd., Edinburgh and London, 1956.

61. Collins, V. J.: Evaluation of pentothal anesthesia after twenty years: Its use and abuse. Bull. New York Acad. Med. **31** (1955) 438-445.

62. Drill, Victor, A.: Pharmacology in Medicine, 2nd ed. McGraw Hill Book Co., New York, N. Y. 1958.

63. Gruber, C. M., Gruber, C. M. Jr., and Lee, K. S.: A study of the effects of the thiobarbiturates on the cardiovascular system. Arch. Int. Pharmocodyn. **91** (1952) 461-488.

64. Gruber, C. M., Haury, V. G. and Gruber, C. M. Jr.: The cardiac arrythmia characteristic effect of the thiobarbiturates as influenced by changes in arterial blood pressure. J. Pharmacol. & Exp. Therap. **63** (1938) 193-213.

65. Sollman, T.: Pharmacology. 8th ed. W. B. Saunders Co., Philadelphia, Pa., 1957.

66. Longley, E. O.: Thiopentone (Penothal) sodium as a general anesthetic in the horse. Vet. Rec. **62** (1950) 17-20.

67. Ford, E. H.: Some observations on the use of thiopentone in large animals. Vet. Rec. **63** (1951) 636-638.

68. Henderson, W. M. and Brooksby, J. B.: Thiopentone as an anesthetic in the horse. Vet. Rec. **62** (1950) 38.

69. Riley, W. F.: Practical procedures in horse practice, proceedings AVMA 89th Annual Meeting, 1952.

70. Dundee, J. W., Price, H. L. and Dripps, R. D.: Acute tolerance to thiopentone in man. Brit. J. Anaesthesia **28** (1956) 344-352.

71. Jones, E. W., Johnson, L., and Heinze, C. D.: Thiopental sodium anesthesia in the horse—a rapid injection technique. J.A.V.M.A. **137** (1960) 119-122.

72. Dundee, J. W., and Scott, W. E. B.: Effect of phenothiazine derivatives on thiobarbiturate narcosis. Current Research in Anesth. and Analg. **37** (1958) 12-19.

73. Bosio, S.: Risultati e considerazioni sull'impiego del talofen (promazina base) quale preanestetico e potenziatore dell'anestesia. Min. Anest. **25** (1959) 84-88.

74. Dobkin, A. B.: Potentiation of thiopental anesthesia by derivatives and analogue of phenothiazine. Anesthesiology **21** (1960) 292-296.

75. Walkenstein, S. S., and Seifter, J.: Fate, distribution and excretion of P 35 promazine. J. of Pharm. & Exp. Therap. **125** (1959) 329-336.

76. Krantz, J. C. and Carr, C. J.: The Pharmacologic Principles of Medical Practice, 4th ed. Williams & Wilkins Co., Baltimore, Md., 1958.

77. Hall, L. W.: The use of muscle relaxant drugs in equine anesthesia. 1961 Meeting of European Professors of Veterinary Surgery Abst. Mod. Vet. Prac. **56** (1961) 35-36.

78. Booth, N. H. and Rankin, A. D.: Studies of the pharmacodynamics of curare in the horse. Am. J. Vet. Research **14** (1953) 51-56.

79. Henkels, P.: Die Zur Zeit technik der reflexlosen, leicht stener barn Pferden narkose fur Klinik und Aussenpraxis. Deuts. Tierarzt. Wschr. **46** (1938) 801-804.

80. Jones, E. W.: General anesthesia in the horse. Thesis, Cornell University, Ithaca, N. Y. 1950.

81. Dripps, R. D., Eckenhoff, J. E. and Vandam, L. D.: Introduction to Anesthesia—The Principles of Safe Practice, 2nd ed. W. B. Saunders Co., Philadelphia, Pa. 1961.

82. Lee, J. Alfred: A Synopsis of Anesthesia, 4th ed. Williams and Wilkins Co., Baltimore, Md. 1959.

83. Evans, F. T. and Gray, T. C.: General Anesthesia, Vol. I & II, Butterworth & Co. Ltd., London, England, 1959.

84. Jones, E. Wynn: Equine anesthesia—maintenance by inhalation techniques. J.A.V.M.A. **139** (1961) 785-790.

85. Hansson, C. H. and Johannisson, D.: Inhalation anesthesia with automatic artificial respiration during succinylcholine relaxation in large animals Nord. Vet.-Med. **10** (1958) 469.

86. Weaver, B. M. Q.: An apparatus for inhalation anesthesia in large animals. Vet. Rec. **72** (1960) 1121.

87. Hall, L. W.: Bromochlorotrifluoroethane (Fluothane): a new volatile anesthetic agent. Vet. Rec., **69** (1957) 615-618.

88. Fisher, E. W. and Jennings, S.: The use of "Fluothane" in horses and cattle. Vet. Rec.: **70** (1958) 567-618.

89. Jones, E. W., Vasko, K. A., Hamm, D., and Griffith, R. W.: Equine general anesthesia—use of halothane for maintenance. J.A.V.M.A. **140** (1962) 148-153.

90. Bloodwell, R. D., Brown, R. C., Christenson, G. R., Goldberg, L. I., and Morrow, A. G.: The effect of Fluothane on myocardial contractile force in man. Anesth. & Analg. **40** (1961) 352-361.

91. Hartung, L.: Fluothane in thoracic surgery: a study of 500 cases. Anesth. & Analg., **15** (1958) 932-946.

92. Ausheman, H. M. and Adam, A.: Fluothane: a new nonexplosive volatile anesthetic agent. South. M. J., **52** (1959) 46-52.

93. Rankin, A. D.: Personal communication. The Squibb Institute of Medical Research, New Brunswick, N. J. 1962.

94. Rankin, A. D. et al.: Artificial respiration in large animals, J.A.V.M.A. **120** (1952) 196.

95. Churchill, E. A. and Delahanty, D. D.: Panel—Respiratory problems of horses; their diagnosis and treatment. Proceedings 6th Annual American Assn. of Equine Practitioners Convention (1960) 119-131.

96. Sisson, S. and Grossman, J. D.: The Anatomy of the Domestic Animals, 4th ed. W. B. Saunders Company, Philadelphia, Pa. 1953.

97. Astra: Xylocaine[R] in Veterinary Anesthesia (a motion picture). A/B Astra Sodertalje, Sweden. Available from Jensen-Salsbery Laboratories, Inc., Box 167, Kansas City 41, Missouri.

98. Loquidice, C. N., and Aranes, G. M.: La Anastesia por gases en los Animals Domesticos. (1946) Universidad Nacional de la Plata, Facultad de Medicina Veterinaire.

99. Hansson, C. H. and Johannisson, D.: Inhalation anesthesia with automatic artificial respiration during succinylcholine relaxation in large animals. Nord. Vet.-Med. **10** (1958) 469.

100. Lee, J. Alfred: A Synopsis of Anesthesia. 4th ed. Williams & Wilkins Co., Baltimore, Md., 1959.

101. Kirby, C. K., Eckenhoff, J. E., and Looby, J. P.: The use of hyaluronidase with local anesthetic agents in surgery and dentistry. Ann. N. Y. Acad. Sci. **52** (1950) 1166. Cited by Jones, L. Meyer: Veterinary Pharmacology and Therapeutics. 2nd ed., Iowa State College Press, Ames, 224, 1957.

ADMINISTRATION OF MEDICINE

(INCLUDING BLOOD TRANSFUSION AND FLUID AND ELECTROLYTE THERAPY)

In administering medicine to horses, a confident, deft approach to the animal and the judicious use of as little restraint as possible are easiest and safest. Severe methods of restraint on a nervous animal may do him more harm than the medication can do him good. A horse which has been kept in a box stall usually can be medicated most easily in its stall since it is less likely to become excited there than in less familiar surroundings. Naturally, the route of administration chosen depends on the medicine to be given, the speed of onset and duration of action required, the economy, the temperament of the animal, and the skill of the person administering the medicine.

ORAL ADMINISTRATION OF MEDICINE

With Water or Feed

Medicines which can be given in feed or water include: vitamin-mineral supplements, drugs for control of parasites, oral tranquilizers, oral electrolytes, and many others.

Animals which are difficult to medicate, especially ponies and foals, can be dosed easily if the medicine can be made into an electuary by mixing a medicine in powdered form with corn syrup, honey or molasses. Sugar can be mixed with liquid or semiliquid medicines to make an electuary. The sticky mixture can then be placed on the animal's tongue, teeth, and lips and usually is eaten readily.

Stomach Tube

The correct use of the stomach tube is a safe, professional method of giving liquid medication. The nasal route usually is preferred for passing a stomach tube. Choosing a tube of the right size is important. Plastic or rubber tubes up to a ¾-inch outside diameter can be used in adults, and sizes down to ⅜-inch diameter are available for ponies and foals. Sometimes even smaller improvised tubes such as male horse catheters are required in ponies and foals. Attempts to force a tube which is too large can cause damage to the turbinate bones. Relatively stiff tubes are preferred by many veterinarians since very limber ones tend to curl or kink in the pharyngeal region and sometimes come back out the same nostril, the opposite nostril or the mouth. When tubes become very stiff because of cold weather, they should be softened with warm water before an attempt is made to pass them. Some plastic tubes do not become stiff when cold. The end of the tube should be beveled and smooth with no rough place or nicks (such as often results from animals chewing on tubes) because irritation of the nasal mucosa may cause pain and hemorrhage. Many veterinarians like to have a mark on the stomach tube indicating the distance from the nostril to the esophageal opening (16 inches in the average horse) and another mark indicating when the tube reaches the stomach (5½ feet in the average horse).

If the animal will eat, a little grain can be given to him before passing the tube to lubricate the pharynx and esophagus with saliva in order to make the passage of the tube easier. The end of the tube can be lubricated with water, mineral oil or lubricating jelly to facilitate its passage. In order to pass the tube quickly and efficiently, the animal can be backed into the corner of the stall and the assistant should hold the head firmly by the halter lead, and if necessary, with a twitch also. Many veterinarians routinely use a twitch on the horse's nose while passing the tube to prevent movement of the head. If the horse moves his head violently as the tube passes the ventral turbinate bone, the tube may hit and damage the turbinates.

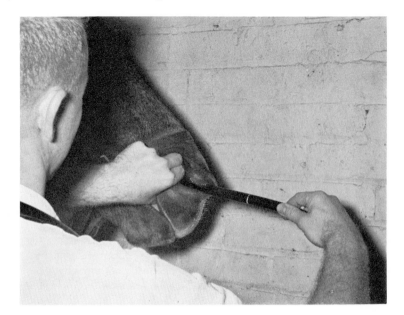

Fig. 1. Passing a stomach tube. The left thumb is placed in the right upper interdental space and the tube is held on the floor of the nasal cavity, against the nasal septum.

Most right-handed operators find it easiest to pass the tube through the right nostril as shown in Fig. 1. The left thumb is placed in the right upper interdental space and the fingers of the left hand hold the tube on the floor of the nasal cavity, against the nasal septum.[1] The curved end of the tube should be kept deflected downward as it is passed. (Stomach tubes can be carried in a coil approximately 12 inches in diameter to keep them curved.) The tube is then advanced until it strikes the pharynx and simultaneously with the first swallow, it is advanced into the esophagus. (Swallowing usually occurs when the end of the tube touches the pharynx.) If the tube enters the esophagus there will be moderate resistance as it is "grasped" by the esophagus. Each time the horse swallows, the tube can be advanced. It should never be forced since it may bow upward and damage the turbinate bones. It should always be held against the floor of the nasal cavity as it is advanced to prevent injury to the turbinates. The operator should always determine that the tube is passing into the esophagus by both seeing and feeling it. If necessary, he can alternately advance and withdraw it several times while determining its location. The tube usually is found in the esophagus in the left jugular furrow, but the esophagus may be on or to the right of the midline. Care must be taken that the carotid artery pulse, or the swallowing contractions of the esophagus, are not mistaken for the end of the tube. If the tube can be advanced very easily after being pushed beyond the pharynx, it probably is in the trachea. This can be verified usually by "feeling the tube rattle" in the trachea by shaking gently the throat or larynx. The operator should not assume that it is in the esophagus if it cannot be "felt" in the trachea since it may be curled back in the nasal passage or mouth. It must be in the esophagus before the medicine is administered!

A stomach pump or funnel may be used to give medicine through a tube. Water should be used to rinse medicines from the tube. It should be thoroughly drained to prevent loss of water in the laryngeal region as the tube is removed. Some veterinarians "blow out" the tube before removing it and some hold a finger over the end of the tube while it is being removed. The tube should be held on the floor of the nasal cavity as it is removed and it should be removed slowly to prevent its end from hitting the ventral turbinate bone as it is withdrawn. If the tube is difficult to withdraw, it should not be forced; it should be manipulated slowly and gently. Passing the stomach tube through the nostril is an easy, safe technic if details of the method are followed.

Passing a stomach tube through the nostril usually causes the horse to resist less than when passing it through the mouth, especially if the tube must be kept in place several minutes while medicine is given. If the tube is passed through the mouth a speculum is needed to prevent the animal's chewing it.

DRENCHING

A danger of inhalation pneumonia always is present when liquid medicines are administered orally (drenching). Also it is difficult to dose accurately by drenching, since some of the medicine usually is lost. Attendants should be given careful instructions when they use this method. Oily, bland, tasteless medicines are dangerous as a drench since they can easily pass into the trachea. Animals with pharyngitis and those which may have partial pharyngeal paralysis or other cause of difficult swallowing should not be drenched. Be especially cautious with animals which are semicomatose, have encephalitis, forage poisoning, botulism, strangles, and purpura hemorrhagica. Horses should not be drenched through the nostrils because there is more danger of inhalation than if the oral route is used, and the nasal mucous membrane may be irritated.

When a horse is drenched, a dose syringe, or plastic or strong glass bottle with a long smooth neck, can be used. Small quantities should be diluted so that a large fraction of the dose is not lost, and to prevent irritating the mucous membranes if the medicine is irritating. Suspensions should be shaken before their administration.

The horse's head should be held up so that the front of the face is horizontal or only slightly higher. If it is held higher, the horse may have difficulty in swallowing. If the head cannot be held up by hand, a rope can be attached to the face band of the halter, and the rope put through an overhead pulley or over a beam or rafter (Fig. 2 and 3). Some one should hold the rope so the horse's head can be lowered quickly. It should not be tied to a fixed object.

If necessary, the person giving the medicine can stand on a bale of straw or some other object in order that he can reach the head more easily. If a bottle is used, its mouth should be introduced into the interdental space just in front of the first cheek teeth. The base of the bottle is kept down until the mouth of the bottle is in the horse's mouth, Fig. 2; then it is raised to allow about 4 ounces of the liquid to enter the mouth, Fig. 3. The bottle is then removed until the horse swallows. This method is repeated until all of the medicine has been given. If the horse coughs or accidentally bites off the end of the bottle, its head should be lowered immediately. Inhalation of the medicine may occur if it is poured into the horse's mouth rapidly while he is being forced to hold up his head.

BOLETS, PILLS AND CAPSULES

Medicaments in bolets, pills or capsules can be given orally, either by hand or with a balling gun. However, if a balling gun is used carelessly, the pharynx may be injured. Serious pharyngitis may result if capsules containing irritating medicines break in the pharynx, or lodge there and dissolve. The use of large bolets, pills, and capsules is dangerous in ponies and foals because they may become lodged in the esophagus.

To ball a horse by hand, it is best to withdraw the tongue by grasping it with one hand, to pull it to one side, between the upper and lower cheek teeth, and to place the moistened bolet, pill or capsule as far back on the tongue as possible. When the tongue is released, the bolet is carried into the back of the mouth. The mouth should then be held closed until the horse swallows. The head should be held in the normal position; if it is held high, the horse may have difficulty swallowing. If the balling gun is used, it is best to grasp the tongue as described before, to introduce the balling gun between the incisor teeth, and to discharge the bolet on the base of the tongue. If the balling gun is introduced into the back of the pharynx, the animal may gag and "cough out" the bolet. A strong balling gun with a head that will not come off and one which cannot be bitten off should be used.

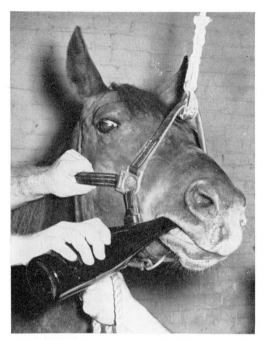

Fig. 2. Drenching. The head should be held a little higher than it appears in the picture.

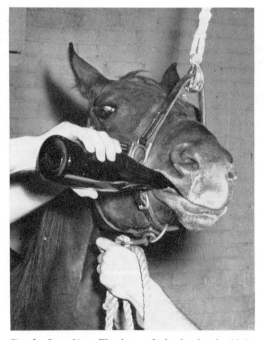

Fig. 3. Drenching. The base of the bottle should be raised after the mouth of the bottle is in the horse's mouth to allow about 4 ounces of the liquid to enter the mouth. The bottle should be removed until the horse swallows; this is repeated until all of the medicine has been given.

Unfortunate cases have been reported in which the head of the balling gun became lodged in the esophagus.

PARENTERAL ADMINISTRATION OF MEDICINE

Advantages of parenteral administration, depending on the route and material used, are the more rapid onset of action, the longer duration of action, the economy in some cases (less drug is needed to attain adequate blood and tissue levels), and the ease of administration.

Ideally, a sterile syringe should be used for each injection. Disposable plastic syringes and metal syringe carriers are useful. A practical way to carry a variety of needles is to place them in a glass jar partly filled with an alcoholic antiseptic, so that one desired for an injection can be obtained easily with a forceps. A pad should be put in the bottom of the jar to prevent the needles' movement and their becoming dulled. At the end of the day, the needles which have been used can be returned to the jar after cleaning and inspecting them. Naturally, sharp needles make parenteral injections easier to perform and less painful to the animal. Needles that have been damaged by bending or that have become loose at the hubs should not be used because they may break.

If, in spite of these precautions, a needle is broken while beneath the skin or in a muscle, it should be removed immediately. Broken needles migrate since the point offers less resistance to the tissue than the broken end. The exact location of the needle should be noted as soon as it breaks. If a skin incision is required, the skin should be prepared thoroughly for surgery. If it is difficult to locate a needle which has been left in extremities for several days or weeks, radiographs are helpful. Sometimes is is both unnecessary and unwise to attempt to remove a broken needle which has been left deep in the tissue if it is not near vital structures and is not causing difficulty.

Antiseptic precaution should be used when giving injections. Merely wetting an injection site with an antiseptic probably is no better than using no preparation of the site. For routine injections, the site should be rubbed thoroughly with an alcoholic antiseptic to remove dirt which is loosened and put into solution with the antiseptic. It is best not to clip the area for routine injections since a stubble is left which may be carried beneath the skin as the needle is inserted. If a joint capsule or the subarachnoid space is to be invaded with a needle, preparation of the skin should be the same as that used in major surgery. Injections should not be made where the harness or saddle touches the animal.

Subcutaneous Injection

A suitable site for subcutaneous injections is the middle of the side of the neck where the skin is loose. An 18- or 20-gauge, one-inch needle is recommended. After an area is prepared for injection a fold of skin should be raised and the needle inserted, with the syringe attached, into the end of the fold. The needle can be held beneath the skin between the thumb and fingers as the injection is made. Raising a fold of skin minimizes the animal's response to the needle and prevents injecting the medication intradermally or beneath the fascia. It probably is best not to "fan the needle" or massage the area after the injection is made because of the additional trauma caused.[2]

Intramuscular Injection

Intramuscular injections should be made into the belly of a muscle; nerves, vessels and bony prominences should be avoided. Sites often used for intramuscular injections are the gluteal, pectoral, and triceps muscles and the lateral muscles of the neck. Some veterinarians prefer to inject race horses, especially those in training, in the neck, for if myositis occurs it will less likely affect their performance. Show horses often are injected in the pectoral muscles. This dependent area has a tendency to show more swelling than the other sites mentioned if the injectable preparation causes inflammation. Swelling due to inflammation seldom can be seen in the gluteal area. The triceps should not be used in horses which will be harnessed or saddled within the following few weeks.

An 18- or 20-gauge needle is satisfactory for most intramuscular injections. The length of the needle depends on the size of the patient's muscle. After the injection site is prepared, the site of the injection should be touched and the needle inserted. The syringe is attached and if blood cannot be aspirated by pulling on the plunger, the injection is made. Not more than 20 ml. should be injected at one site but if the material is at all irritating it is better to use less than this amount at any one site.

Intravenous Injection

Solutions for intravenous injections should be warmed to near body temperature. Solutions which are cloudy or have particles suspended in them should not be used. Drugs should not be mixed if a precipitate is produced or any deleterious chemical or biologic effect results.

The jugular vein is used for most intravenous injections in the equine species. Needles for intravenous injection should be at least 2 inches long, so that the point can be inserted at least one inch into the lumen of the vein. If a very small-gauge needle is used for intravenous injection it may be difficult to tell when the vein has been entered and whether the needle is in the vein during the injection. This especially is true if the blood is viscous due to dehydration or toxemia. The danger of using a small-gauge needle is that the injection can be made accidentally into the carotid artery.[3] The resistance of a small-gauge needle slows the flow of blood and the arterial blood may be mistaken for venous blood.

Before the needle is inserted through the skin, be sure that it is directly over the vein. Figures 4 and 10 show ways that the vein can be distended and the skin tensed to make placing the needle into the vein easier. It may be necessary to put a tourniquet around the neck to "hold off" both veins if the horse's neck is heavily muscled (Fig. 28). The needle should be grasped in such a way that the operator can control it (Fig. 4 or 10). It should be pushed through the skin, keeping it perpendicular to the plane of the skin until blood flows from the needle, then about one inch of

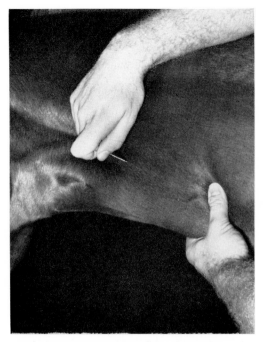

Fig. 4. Intravenous injection. Grasp the needle so that it is easily controlled and "hold off" the vein. In this case both jugular veins are being "held off."

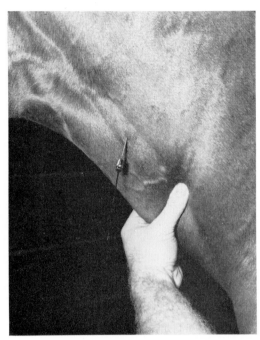

Fig. 5. Intravenous injection. The needle has been directed into the vein perpendicular to the plane of the skin. Blood flows freely from the needle.

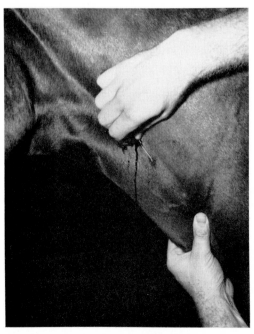

Fig. 6. Intravenous injection. The needle is directed down the lumen of the vein by grasping the hub and holding it near the skin surface while advancing it.

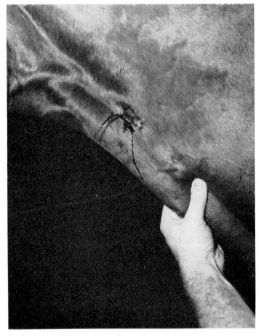

Fig. 7. Intravenous injection. The needle is in place. Blood should flow freely when the vein is "held off."

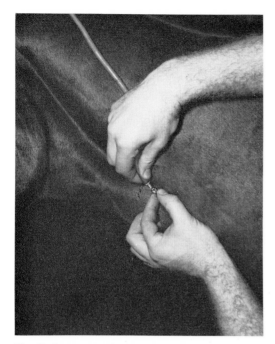

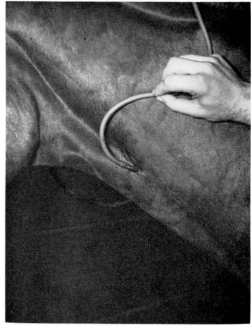

Fig. 8. Intravenous injection. The needle should be held firmly while the intravenous outfit is attached so that the needle is not advanced through the wall of the vein.

Fig. 9. Intravenous injection. Tubing of the intravenous outfit should be held in such a way that the needle is not pulled out of the vein if the horse moves.

it is beneath the skin (Fig. 5 and 11). If blood does not flow freely from the needle, one of the following is the cause: The needle has gone either dorsal or ventral to the vein; it has not reached deeply enough; it has passed through the vein; or the needle, due to being improperly sharpened, is occluded by a plug of skin. If blood does not flow after the needle point is one inch beneath the skin, the operator should observe where the point is and make the necessary correction without withdrawing the needle from the skin. After the needle has been withdrawn ¼ inch or so, the blood often will flow; if it does not, the needle should be redirected toward the vein. After the needle is in the vein, it should be inserted more deeply into the vein by directing it cephalad ("up"), Fig. 12, or caudad ("down"), Fig. 6 in the lumen of the vein. At least one inch of the needle should be in the lumen of the vein before the injection is made. The author prefers to direct the needle with the flow of blood (caudad) because this prevents the injected material from seeping around the injection site, since the material is discharged beyond

the site. Those who direct the needle toward the flow of blood (cephalad), argue that the injected material is dispersed more thoroughly and is less likely to irritate the intima of the vein if their method is used.

The method of inserting of plastic tubing into the veins of animals to permit continuous or repeated injections is shown in Fig. 14 and 15.[4] The method is useful during surgical procedures requiring general anesthesia since an assistant can be directed by the veterinarian to give additional anesthetic agent as needed, without danger of extravascular injection. The method also is useful for rapid injection of irritating drugs.[1] An attempt never should be made to remove the tubing while the cannula needle is still in the vein because the tubing may be cut off inside the vein by the bevel of the needle. If the tubing becomes stuck in the needle, the needle and tubing should be removed together and the procedure repeated. A needle, preferably a blunt one, can be used to adapt a syringe or intravenous outfit (simplex) to the tubing. A clamp on the intravenous outfit may be used to control the

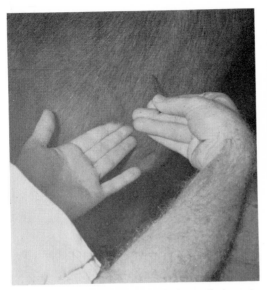

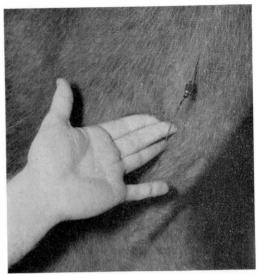

Fig. 10. Intravenous injection. This is another way to grasp the needle and "hold off" the vein.

Fig. 11. Intravenous injection. The needle is directed into the vein perpendicular to the plane of the skin.

rate of flow and a drip chamber may be placed below the clamp so that the rate of flow can be visualized. A commercial sterile intravenous catheter (Bardic, Deseret Intercath: C. R. Bard, Inc., Summit, New Jersey) can be used in a similar manner. A tomcat catheter or similar long blunt needle can be used inside a cannula needle in the same way to prevent perivascular injection. In this case, the cannula needle is left in place until the catheter is removed.

After the needle has been placed in a vein, a syringe can be attached to make the injection if a small quantity of nonirritating medicine is to be injected. It is recommended that irritating materials such as chloral hydrate, barbiturates, broad spectrum antibiotics, and sulfas not be given with a syringe attached directly to a needle in a vein. If the animal moves during the injection, part of the drug may be injected perivascularly. As a consequence, inflammation of the neck may occur and the skin and tissue around the vein may slough. These drugs should be administered as dilute solutions with an intravenous outfit or with a length of plastic tubing or tomcat catheter inserted into the vein.

Before an intravenous outfit is attached to a needle, the medicine should be allowed to

gravitate into the tubing to force out any air. A small quantity of the solution should be allowed to rinse any antiseptic left in the tubing. If the horse is frightened by the bottle's being held in the air, have the man holding the halter lead cover its eyes on the side on which the injection is being made. The needle should be held while the adapter of the intravenous outfit is attached to prevent the needle's being advanced through the wall of the vein. (Fig. 8). Figures 9 and 13 show a way to hold the tubing to prevent removing the needle from the vein if the animal moves during the injection. After a small quantity of medicine has been injected, it is wise to see if the needle is still in the vein. Blood will flow from the needle if the adapter of the intravenous outfit is removed from the needle and the vein is "held off" (Fig. 7). If the medicine must be given slowly, the bottle should be raised occasionally to see if it still will flow freely by observing the rapid bubbling. This is an advantage of using a relatively large-gauge needle. Another way to check whether the needle is in the vein is to use an intravenous outfit with a plastic observation tube near the attachment to the needle (Fig. 13). The bottle can be lowered occasionally to see if the blood appears in the tubing. Throughout the period of

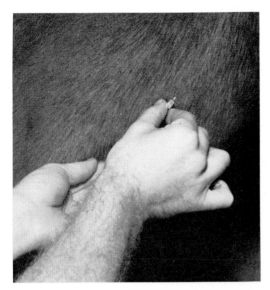

Fig. 12. Intravenous injection. The needle is directed up the lumen of the vein by grasping the hub and holding it near the skin surface while advancing it.

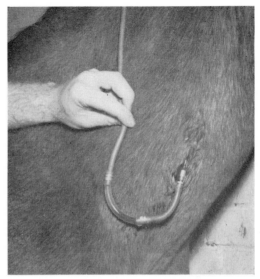

Fig. 13. Intravenous injection. This intravenous out-fit has a section of clear plastic tubing. If the bottle of medicine is lowered, blood should appear in the tubing if the needle is in the vein.

injection, the site should be observed for swelling.

The intravenous outfit should be rinsed thoroughly with water, followed by an alcoholic antiseptic as soon as the injection is finished. An intravenous outfit can be kept in a clean, dry container or a jar of alcoholic antiseptic.

If a quantity of irritating drug is thought to to have been injected perivascularly (blood will not flow from the needle following an injection) the needle should be left in place and 0.9% sodium chloride solution in a quantity approximately 5 times as great as the quantity of drug thought to have been injected perivascularly, should be injected. The saline will dilute the drug and prevent much of the inflammation that would otherwise result. Hyaluronidase also may be used.

INTRADERMAL INJECTION

The intradermal injection is used in doing the Mallein test. Site of the injection should be ¼ inch from the margin of the lower lid, midway between the medial and lateral canthus. The back of the hand can be rested against the nose to prevent injury to the eye if the horse moves its head quickly.

INTRATHECAL INJECTION

Injections have been made into the cerebral spinal fluid at the lumbosacral area, or between the atlas and axis for the treatment of tetanus and other diseases of the central nervous system. These technics also are useful for obtaining samples of cerebrospinal fluid. The site of puncture should be prepared as for major surgery. The site for lumbosacral puncture is located where a line between the tuber coxae crosses the midline. An 18- or 20-gauge needle, or cannula with stilet, 4 to 6 inches long is pushed downward and slightly forward, on the median plane, until it passes through the dura mater into the subarachroid space. "Temporary blocking of the jugular veins will assist in causing the spinal fluid to flow through the needle."[1] Caution should be used with either technic to prevent injury to the spinal cord.

INTRA-ARTICULAR INJECTION

Intra-articular injections are useful in treating some cases of arthritis. (Intra-articular injection of adrenocortical steroids or their synthetic analogues suppresses the inflammation of arthritis. Pain is relieved, but unfortunately,

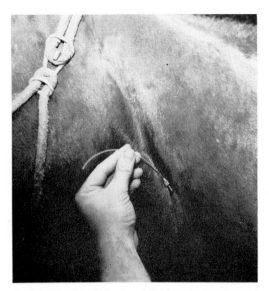

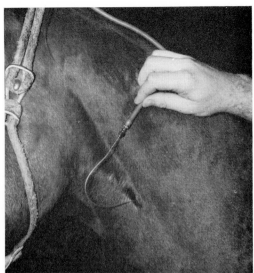

Fig. 14. Plastic tubing placed in the vein for repeated or continuous intravenous injection. A needle (preferably a thin-walled needle) is put in the vein in the usual manner and part of a length of tubing is passed into it. The tubing should never be removed while the needle is in the vein since the bevel of the needle may shear off part of the tubing in the vein.

Fig. 15. Plastic tubing in vein. The needle has been pulled over the tubing and a smaller gauge needle (preferably a blunt one) is used as an adapter for the intravenous outfit or syringe.

if the patient continues to be exercised, permanent severe damage to the joint may occur.) Arthrocentesis (puncture of a joint) also is useful for obtaining a sample of synovial fluid for macroscopic and laboratory examination, or to relieve increased intra-articular pressure.[5] The intra-articular injection of potent or concentrated solutions of local anesthetic agents to temporarily relieve the pain of arthritis has been described as being useful in confirming diagnoses of arthritis.[6,7]

Before arthrocentesis is done, the skin at the site should be prepared as for major surgery, and the needles and syringes should be heat-sterilized to minimize the risk of introducing infection into the joint. When possible, tendons and their sheaths should be avoided to prevent trauma to them and to help prevent breaking the needle should the horse move the limb while it is in place.[5] Care also should be taken to avoid trauma to articular surfaces with the point of the needle.[5] An 18-gauge needle is satisfactory for most arthrocenteses.

A few seconds after the needle enters a joint, a few drops of synovial fluid may drip from the needle, especially if the needle is tapped gently or the joint is moved slightly. A sterile syringe may be used to gently as-

pirate a sample for examination, or to reduce the amount of fluid in the joint prior to an injection. If the plunger of the syringe is withdrawn too rapidly or forcibly, a small, villous portion of the synovial membrane may be drawn into the needle, resulting in the needle becoming occluded.[5]

Figures 16 through 24 show the technic recommended for arthrocentesis of the joints of horses' limbs. A movie showing these technics is available.[6]

OTHER PARENTERAL ROUTES

The intraperitoneal and intrathoracic routes should not be used in horses. Punctures of the medullary cavities of bones have little clinical usefulness in horses.

MISCELLANEOUS ROUTES OF ADMINISTERING MEDICINE

CONJUNCTIVAL INSTILLATION

The conjunctival route of administering drugs in horses has little use. The conjunctival installation of mallein has given less reliable results than the intradermal method.

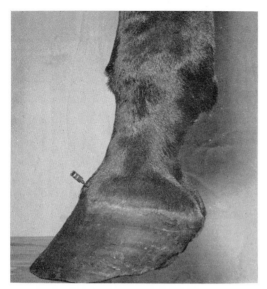

Fig. 16. Arthrocentesis of the coffin joint. The joint should be extended during the puncture. It is convenient to support the foot on a box or block. The needle enters the skin at a point ⅓ inch above the coronary band and ⅓ inch off the middle sagittal plane of the hoof. The needle is directed downward and toward the middle sagittal plane as shown.

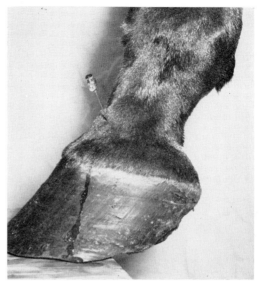

Fig. 17. Arthrocentesis of the pastern joint. This joint should be extended during the puncture and the foot can be supported on a box or block. It probably is easiest to enter this joint at a site ½ inch off the middle sagittal plane of the leg, on a line between the medial and lateral eminences of the distal end of the first phalanx where the collateral ligaments attach. The needle is directed downward and toward the middle sagittal plane as shown.

INSTILLATION INTO THE RESPIRATORY TRACT

Nasal instillation of rhinopneumonitis virus is being used to expose animals to produce immunity.[9] Injection directly into the trachea, between the tracheal rings, has little usefulness.

INHALATION THERAPY

Inhalation therapy includes the use of oxygen, aerosols, and medicated steam. Oxygen therapy can save animals by supplying more oxygen to the vital cells of the body (especially the brain) during anoxia. It is useful in saving newborn animals which fail to breathe properly, as well as in pneumonia and edema of the lungs, and in cases of inadvertent overdosage of anesthetics or muscle relaxing agents. (See chapter 2 on anesthesia.)

Oxygen can be administered to horses with an improvised oxygen tent, a nasal catheter or a therapy mask. A convenient tent for a foal is a nearly airtight plastic or glass container. Oxygen can be supplied to the container with a hose from a reducing valve on an oxygen tank. If available, a flow meter can

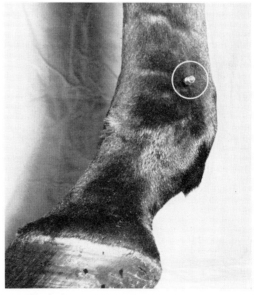

Fig. 18. Arthrocentesis of the fetlock joint. This puncture is best done with the horse standing. The needle is introduced directly into the part of the joint capsule which can be palpated in the triangular space formed by the distal end of the third metacarpal (cannon) bone in front of the suspensory ligament and behind the proximal sesamoid bones distally.

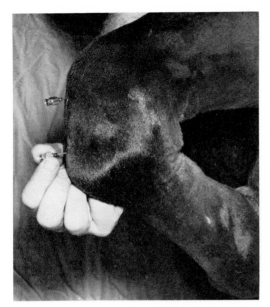

Fig. 19. Arthrocentesis of the carpal joints. It is best to have the carpus flexed to make the joint cavities readily accessible. The needles are placed directly into the joints (radiocarpal and intercarpal) as shown, at sites on the medial-anterior aspect of the joints, between the tendons of the extensor carpi obliquus and the extensor carpi radialis. These sites are readily palpable. As the joints are entered there is usually a faint sucking sound due to negative pressure. Injections are not made into the distal joint since it is arthrodial and communicates with the middle or intercarpal joint.

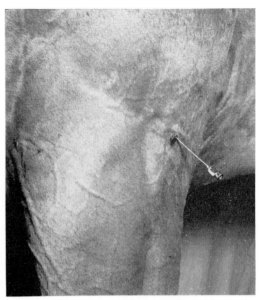

Fig. 20. Arthrocentesis of the elbow joint. To locate the site for this puncture, palpate the lateral ligament of the elbow joint and its attachments to the humerus and radius. The needle penetrates the skin just anterior or posterior to the ligament of the transverse plane (of the limb) located between the middle and lower ⅓ of the ligament, and is directed medially and slightly upward. A needle at least 2 inches long is required.

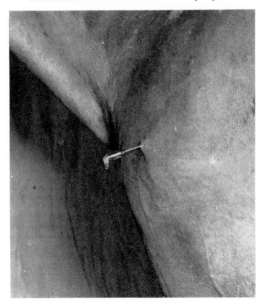

Fig. 21. Arthrocentesis of the shoulder joint. The anterior and posterior parts of the lateral tuberosity of the proximal end of the humerus are palpated. The puncture is made between them. The needle is directed somewhat posteriorly and slightly upward as it is introduced medially. A needle at least 5 inches long is needed in large horses.

be used. There probably is more danger of explosion with oxygen tents than with other methods.[10]

A size-10 endotracheal tube or comparable plastic tube can be used as a nasal catheter. An inflatable cuff or tape can be used to hold it in place.[10] A bland lubricating jelly should be used on the tube and cuff, and it should be moved to the opposite nostril at least every 12 hours to prevent irritation of the nasal mucosa.

Therapy masks usually include a reservoir bag and an exhalation valve. They may frighten the horse and sometimes are difficult to keep in place.

Oxygen flow rates of 4 to 30 L/minute usually are used in adult animals. Except for very short periods of administration, oxygen should be humidified. This is done by placing a humidifier or nebulizer containing water in the line between the flow meter and the horse.

Therapeutic aerosols of antibiotics and adrenocortical steroids have been used in treating respiratory infections of horses. Treatments can be given for 15 to 30 minutes 1 to 3 times

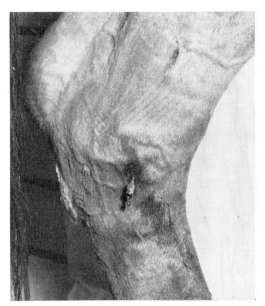

Fig. 22. Arthrocentesis of the hock (tibiotarsal) joint. The best site for puncture is between the extensor tendons and the medial ligaments (anterior part of the medial side of the leg). The saphenous vein should be avoided.

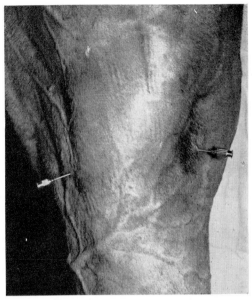

Fig. 23. Arthrocentesis of the stifle joint. The stifle joint has three synovial sacs: a very large one at the femoropatellar articulation, and smaller ones medial and lateral in the femorotibial articulation. Usually the medial, and sometimes the lateral sac, communicates with the femoro-patellar sac.[8] The illustration shows the lateral sac entered between the lateral patellar ligament and the lateral femorotibial ligament. The medial sac has been punctured just behind the medial patellar ligament, well in front of the medial femorotibial ligament. Two-inch needles are satisfactory.

daily. Particles must be smaller than one micron for an aerosol to be stable. Wetting agents have been used to aid in the elimination of respiratory secretions.

Prior to the introduction of modern chemotherapeutic agents, the use of medicated steam was popular in treating respiratory infections. Medicated steam can be generated in a tight room, or in the bottom of a long grain bag into which the horse's nose is inserted.[11]

ENEMAS

Rectal injection seldom is used except to stimulate evacuation of the large intestine. Some veterinarians and owners insist that every foal born be given an enema. This is necessary in some foals for evacuation of meconium. Drugs have been used by this route to treat inflammation of the rectum and to attempt to destroy parasites found there. Sedatives have been administered to horses by this route, but the method is not recommended.

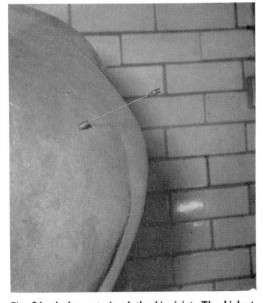

Fig. 24. Arthrocentesis of the hip joint. The highest, most posterior part of the trochanter major and its lateral, more ventral and anterior part are palpated. The needle enters the skin between these points. It is directed medially and somewhat anteriorly through a cannula (to reduce skin resistance). A needle 8 inches long is required in large horses.

Care always should be taken to avoid injury to the rectum. The risk and incidence of injury are high in newborn foals. If the rectum is ruptured, peritonitis and death will result. Long, hard tubes or catheters and syringes with long nozzles should not be used in giving enemas. It is unnecessary and dangerous to forcefully work even a soft tube back and forth in the rectum. In foals, a soft plastic tube with a guard which permits entry of only about 2 inches of the tube is safest. It is well to lubricate the enema tube before inserting it. Gravity is safer than the use of positive pressure for flowing the fluid into the rectum. There is danger of rupturing the rectum or large intestine if a large quantity of fluid is forced into the rectum under pressure, especially if return flow around the tube is occluded.

Instillation into the Female Reproductive Tract

Although many veterinarians consider the procedure to be useless or even harmful, the vagina can be medicated by insufflation or douching. Sanitary procedure always should be used when medication is instilled into the uterus. An insemination rod can be directed through the cervix by visualizing it through a vaginal speculum, or the hand and arm covered with a glove and sleeve can take a catheter through the vagina and direct it into the cervix.

Other Routes

Medicines can be injected into the urinary tract for bactericidal action, local antisepsis, or local anesthetic action. Medicine also can be applied to the skin for these effects or to cause counterirritation.

BLOOD TRANSFUSION

Blood transfusion is an effective treatment for many critically ill animals. This treatment often is not used because the veterinarian feels he will not be paid for his time. If the owner is not familiar with the use of blood transfusions in animals, it is wise to explain their value to him and prepare him to pay a fair fee for the service.

Intravenous injection of whole blood or plasma increases the blood volume and supplies antibodies, electrolytes, nutrients, and blood elements essential for correcting hemorrhagic diseases. In anemia, whole blood will raise the erythrocyte count and the oxygen carrying capacity of the recipient's blood. Blood transfusion is indicated in cases of serious blood loss due to trauma, shock, septicemia (navel ill), severe gastrointestinal or respiratory diseases, purpura hemorrhagica, severe burns and neonatal isoerythrolysis (hemolytic icterus).[12] Many chronically ill or debilitated animals will not respond to blood transfusions; cases for blood transfusion should be selected carefully.

Selecting a Donor

Although the first blood transfusion administered to a horse seldom will cause severe illness or death if the blood is incompatible since the level of normally occurring antibodies is generally low, cross-matching should be done if possible.[13,14,15,16] If the previous transfusion history of the animal is unknown or vague, it is unwise to give a transfusion without cross-matching.[13] Any hemolysis due to incompatibility will stress the animal because of the loss of erythrocytes, and the spleen, liver, and reticuloendothelial system will have to dispose of the lysed blood cells and hemoglobin. Lower nephron nephrosis occurs if the hemolysis is extensive.[17] The first sign of a transfusion reaction is uneasiness. The animal may flex each of the hindlegs in turn, yawn several times, and hold its head down. Breathing may become shallow and rapid or the animal may hold its breath. In severe reactions, defecation and micturation occur and the horse may fall over.[15] Excessive hemorrhage may occur following such transfusion reactions.[18]

The second and subsequent transfusions of incompatible blood containing the same antigen or antigens are more likely to cause serious reactions.[13] Several days must elapse after the first transfusion before antibodies are produced. Cross-matching always should be done before giving a transfusion to foals with hemolytic icterus. It also should be done before giving a transfusion (especially repeated transfusions) to a female which may be used for breedings, since injecting her with antigens not contained in her erythrocytes may cause her to produce antibodies and increase her chance of later producing a foal with hemolytic icterus. If she has borne an incompatible foal, there is greater probability that she already has antibodies; consequently, there is a greater chance of serious transfusion reaction. Antibodies can develop as a result of immunization with vaccines prepared from equine tissues.[19]

If it is impossible to cross-match the blood prior to transfusion, some veterinarians suggest that it is safer to use animals of a different breed or of a different bloodline as a donor. Although minor incompatibilities (donor's serum agglutinates recipient's cells) are less likely to be serious than major incompatibilities, there is less chance of their occurring if the following animals are avoided as donors: 1. Horses which have received transfusions with blood which was not cross-matched or was known to contain antigens not found in its erythrocytes. 2. Mares which have produced foals with hemolytic icterus. 3. Horses which have received vaccines of equine origin.

Healthy, mature horses should be chosen as donors. If possible an animal which has recovered completely from the disease, if an infectious disease is being treated, should be used since beneficial antibodies may have developed during the illness. The prospective donor should be examined; at least the temperature ought to be taken and the mucous membranes examined for normal color. Preference should be given to donors with high hematocrit and hemoglobin if these determinations are done.

CROSS-MATCHING TECHNIC

Uniformity in nomenclature of antigens in horse erythrocytes has not been established.[12,13,20] Commercial antiserum for typing is not currently available. Because of "incomplete" antibodies no simple cross-matching test is entirely reliable in revealing all the antibodies in horse blood.[12,21] A test similar to the Coombs' Test, which requires the use of rabbit, antihorse globulin serum, is needed to reveal the "incomplete" antibodies.[22]

The following cross-matching test is more reliable than macroscopic plate or tube tests, since weak agglutinations often occur which cannot be recognized macroscopically.[23] Blood samples are collected from the recipient and several prospective donors. The clots are allowed to separate, or a centrifuge may be used to separate them from the serum. The serum is removed from each sample to labeled tubes. A suspension of erythrocytes is made from the blood of each animal by resuspending cells from the clot in several ml. of saline. This can easily be done by transferring the cells with an applicator stick. The cell suspension should be of such concentration that it looks like thin tomato juice. One drop of the cell suspension and 2 drops of the serum are added to a test tube for each test: donor cells plus recipient serum (major test) and donor serum plus recipient cells (minor test). The tubes are incubated for 5 to 8 minutes in a 37 F.-water bath or for 30 minutes at room temperature. The tubes then are centrifuged at about 1,000 rpm for one minute. They then are jarred sharply to resuspend the cells by hitting the hand containing the tubes against a solid object. A strong agglutination can be detected macroscopically. The contents of the tubes then should be placed on a slide and examined microscopically at 100 x magnification. Cover slips are not used. If there is doubt whether agglutination has occurred, the slide should be tipped from side to side for a few minutes. If agglutination is occurring, it will become stronger; if not, any clumps not due to agglutination which have formed will "break-up." Figures 25, 26, and 27 show strong agglutination, weak agglutination, and a negative test.

In our laboratory somewhat less than ½ of random combinations of animals cross-matched, both the major and minor tests are negative.[23] It is recommended that both tests be negative before transfusing the blood. Reactions occurring on the minor test are less serious, since the serum of the donor, which contains the antibodies, is diluted in the en-

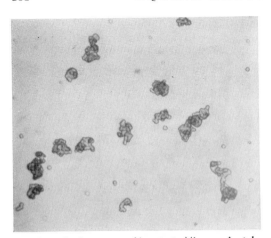

Fig. 25. Blood cross-matching test. Microscopic tube agglutination test—strong agglutination.

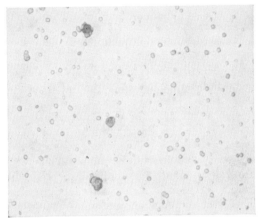

Fig. 26. Blood cross-matching test. Microscopic tube agglutination test—weak agglutination.

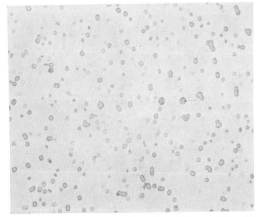

Fig. 27. Blood cross-matching test. Microscopic tube agglutination test—negative. Note the orderly stacking of erythrocytes in a rouleau (common in horse blood) compared to the random clumping in agglutination.

tire blood volume of the recipient and less agglutination and hemolysis are likely to occur than if the donor's cells are agglutinated by the recipient's serum (major reaction). If a more suitable donor is not available, a donor which shows reaction on the minor test may be used.

Rarely, a phenomenon known as autoagglutination occurs, especially in animals which are anemic or those affected by virus disease. When it occurs, the recipient cells are agglutinated by its own serum *in vitro*. In these cases, prospective donor's cells usually show some agglutination on the minor test since autoagglutinins in the recipient's serum agglutinate them. A donor which shows a weak minor reaction must be used.

Any veterinarian, hospital laboratory, or private laboratory can run such a cross-match test.

DIRECT BLOOD TRANSFUSION

Direct blood transfusion is uncommonly used. The disadvantages of the direct blood transfusion method are that fibrin and clots tend to plug the syringe, and the donor and recipient must be brought close together. It is no more beneficial than the indirect method.[18] If the direct transfusion method is used, a 12-or 14-gauge, 2-inch needle should be used in both the donor and recipient. The needle should be directed cephalad in the donor and the veins of the donor should be distended by using a tourniquet around the neck. Tubing 5 to 6 feet long from the donor to a standard 40-ml. Shikles syringe and from the syringe to the recipient should be filled with sodium citrate solution before the transfusion is started, to exclude air from the system and to prevent clotting.[16] The citrate then can be discarded before attaching the tubing to the needle in the recipient's vein.

INDIRECT BLOOD TRANSFUSIONS

The indirect method of blood transfusion is recommended. Horse blood seldom needs to be stored, but if it is, aseptic precautions should be used in collecting and handling it, and antibiotics (one Gm. of streptomycin and one million units of penicillin per gallon of blood) can be used to aid in preventing bacterial growth.[24] A.C.D. solution is a better anticoagulant solution than sodium citrate if blood is to be stored.[25] Four liters can be collected safely from a mature, healthy 1,000-pound horse, but if 8 liters (2 gallons) is removed, the horse may sweat and show signs of weakness.[18] The usual way to collect blood is to distend the jugular vein by using a tourniquet and introduce a 12-or 10-gauge needle into the jugular vein (Fig. 28). If a 10-gauge needle is used, one gallon of blood can be collected in from 6 to 10 minutes. Bleeding trocars which will permit the passage of a 3/16-inch tubing into the vein sometimes are used to save time if a large quantity of blood is to be collected.[26] The blood can be collected in gallon jugs (for mature horses) or in 500-ml. bottles (for foals). The inside of the container should be wet with the sodium citrate solution before starting the collection and the container should be aggitated constantly by a circular motion to keep the blood and citrate well-mixed. Equipment used to handle blood should be chemically clean but need not be sterile if the transfusion is given within minutes after collecting the blood. Commercially available sodium citrate should be used as directed. A 4% solution can be prepared by putting 20 Gm. of sodium citrate in a bottle and adding 500 ml. of water. To make a final dilution of 0.4% sodium citrate, 400 ml. of this solution is put into each gallon jug, and 50 ml. is put in each 500 ml. bottle. Commercial blood collection sets are available for collecting blood for transfusion, but they are expensive when large quantities of blood must be collected for transfusion to mature animals.

A method using vacuum produced in a one-gallon polyethylene jug to speed up the collection of blood has been described.[27] An intravenous outfit with the tubing-type air vent is attached to the bottle and the vent clamped. The bottle then is collapsed and the end of the intravenous tubing is attached to the needle in the donor's vein. Another system to speed the collection of blood is to use a one-gallon aspirator bottle which is connected to the needle in the donor's vein and to a pressure-vacuum pump.[28] Either of these methods also

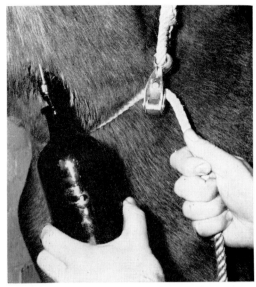

Fig. 28. Collecting blood for transfusion. A tourniquet is used to "hold off" both jugular veins. A 10- or 12-gauge needle is inserted into the vein and directed toward the head. A short length of siliconized tubing can be used to direct the flow of blood into the bottle (not being used in this picture). A gallon of blood can be collected in 6 to 10 minutes with a 10-gauge needle.

may be used to speed the administration of blood by using positive pressure. A Shikles outfit also can be used for positive pressure. Caution must be used with these methods since rapid injections can be dangerous. Also, air may inadvertently be injected into the vein if the container is tipped or becomes empty and pressure continues to be applied.

Although it is possible to give too large a quantity of blood, more often too little is given too late in the course of disease. The smallest effective dose in a mature horse is 4 liters (1 gallon) and 2 gallons are almost always indicated. The blood volume of a horse is about 9% of the body weight.[29] Up to 20% of the blood volume can be given safely at one time to an animal which has not lost blood by hemorrhage, if it is given slowly, but most veterinarians prefer to give no more than this at one time.[30] Additional blood can be given at 12-hour intervals as indicated. Larger volumes can be given in cases of blood loss. Twenty percent of the blood volume in a 1,000-pound horse is approximately 2½ gallons. A 100-pound foal usually can be given 2 pints of blood if there has been no blood loss.

In exchange transfusions of foals with hemolytic icterus, up to 10 pints of blood may be given, but during the transfusion blood must be withdrawn from the foal either simultaneously or intermittently, and discarded. It is best to start transfusing before withdrawing blood from the foal and eventually to administer 2 to 3 pints more blood than is withdrawn and discarded. If more than 20% of the blood volume of the animal is given rapidly (for example, following hemorrhage) by the indirect transfusion method, calcium gluconate should be administered slowly through a different intravenous needle, since the citrate will "bind" free calcium in the animal's blood.

Blood should be strained before it is administered. A filter-type transfusion apparatus can be used, or if one is not available, sterile gauze can be placed over the mouth of the bottle before the intravenous outfit is placed on it. An intravenous outfit with a tubing-type air vent should be used to prevent air entering when gauze is used as a strainer on the bottle top. Blood also can be strained by placing a metal screen over a funnel and pouring the blood through it into another vessel. Clotting on the screen can be prevented by first wetting it with sodium citrate solution. If blood must be given very slowly or the veterinarian wishes to leave an attendant in charge, the plastic tubing method of giving injections, Fig. 14 and 15, can be used. Because of its viscosity, blood flow through such tubing is slow. Equipment used for blood transfusion must be cleaned immediately after use.

Blood to replace reduced blood volume, e.g., in shock or following hemorrhage, can be given rapidly. However, rapid injection or large doses of blood are especially dangerous in animals with pulmonary or cardiovascular disease and in other debilitated animals. It is well to auscultate the heart and lungs (for pulmonary edema) and check the pulse (estimate relative blood pressure) periodically while transfusing these animals. In mature animals there usually is no untoward effect due to speed of transfusion if a 14-gauge needle is used and the bottle or jug of blood is suspended not more than 3 feet above the injection site. In foals, a 16-gauge needle will limit the flow satisfactorily if pressure is not used and the container is suspended not more than one foot above the injection site. The recommended rates of injection of blood are as slow as 40 ml. per minute in horses and as fast as 720 ml. per minute (with positive pressure) in mature cattle.[31,26]

PLASMA TRANSFUSION

Plasma is approximately equal to blood in treatment of conditions in which blood volume, but not erythrocytes, are deficient. Blood volume decrease is a more serious factor than erythrocyte loss in many conditions, including surgical shock. An advantage of plasma over blood is that there is little risk of transfusion reaction. Plasma easily can be produced by drawing blood into a container with sodium citrate as for transfusion, centrifuging it, and removing the plasma. If a large quantity is required, it can be obtained by leaving the container of blood stand in a refrigerator for at least 12 hours, for good yield, then aspirating the plasma from the top of the container with a siphon or a large syringe. The yield of plasma is a little less than ½ the volume of blood collected.

Plasma substitutes seldom are used in large animals because of their cost and the relative ease of transfusing blood or plasma. Serious reactions have been reported in horses following the use of dextran.[15]

FLUID AND ELECTROLYTE THERAPY

Fluid therapy is important in the treatment of many diseases. Any animal which fails to eat and drink needs oral or parenteral fluid and electrolyte therapy. Although a limited number of articles have been written on fluid therapy in large animals, there are little data on the subject from which to scientifically draw conclusions. Many recommendations must be based on knowledge of the effects of similar diseases of man and other species, taking into consideration the difference of the horse from these species. The common deficits and imbalances of fluid and electrolytes will be considered along with specific treatment for deficits; then treatment in general will be discussed.

Ideally, abnormal losses of fluid and electrolytes which occurred prior to the start of treatment (deficit), continuing abnormal losses, and continuing normal losses should be replaced. Elkinton and Danowsky point out that there are several ways to determine the state of hydration and the electrolyte needs of patients:[32] 1. The history of the illness. For example, if there has been diarrhea, for how long and how severe? 2. Physical examination to determine the state of hydration. 3. Experience with and knowledge of this and similar diseases. 4. Laboratory findings, especially hematocrit, hemoglobin, urinalysis, and concentration of electrolyte ions in the serum. If a veterinarian has a good practical knowledge of physiology, he can use the first 3 of these. Often laboratory findings also can be used. The normal physiologic values (Table 1) are useful in treating fluid and electrolyte imbalances when laboratory determinations can be done. The concentration of electrolyte ion is best expressed in milliequivalents/liter (mEq per/L).[33,34] Expressing the ion concentrations in mEq/L is superior to the use of a weight per volume system since ions combine on an atom per atom basis; their atomic weights and valence must be considered when relating one to another.[33] It is found that 1 Gm. of NaCl equals 17 mEq of Na^+ and 17 mEq of Cl^-. One gram of KCl equals 13 mEq of K^+ and 13 mEq of Cl^-.

It is suggested that the reader review the physiology of water and electrolytes.[29]

DEHYDRATION

The most common cause of simple dehydration, without electrolyte deficiency or change in electrolyte balance, is the lack of water intake. This can result either from the animal's not being given water or the animal's refusing to, or being unable to drink. It has been stated that horses require 10 to 12 gallons of water per day in addition to the water obtained from food intake and metabolic oxidation.[29] More or considerably less than this may be required depending on the weather and the activity of the animal. It commonly is stated that 3% of the body weight will be lost before one can determine by clinical signs that

Table 1.—Normal Blood and Urine Values of the Horse Useful in Fluid and Electrolyte Therapy

Blood:

Serum sodium	*149 (146–152) mEq/L
Serum potassium	*3.3 (2.7–3.5) mEq/L
Serum calcium	*5.5 (5–6.5)　mEq/L
Serum magnesium	*(1.5–2.1)　mEq/L
Plasma chloride	*102 (98–106)　mEq/L
Plasma bicarbonate	**28.6　mEq/L
	*23.0　mEq/L
CO_2 combining power	**64 Vol. %
	*51.5 Vol. %
pH	*7.2–7.55
Hematocrit	Heavy horses 34–46%
	Light horses 36–48%
Hemoglobin	Heavy horses 10–14%
	Light horses 12–16%
Serum protein	**6.5 Gm./100 ml.

Urine:

Specific gravity	1.040
pH	8

*Spector, W. S.: Handbook of Biological Data. W. B. Saunders Co., Philadelphia and London (1956):53.

**Dukes, H. H.: The Physiology of Domestic Animals. 7th Ed. Comstock Publishing Associates, Ithaca, N. Y., 1955.

dehydration is occurring.[35] Therefore, a horse which weighs 1,100 pounds can lose about 4 gallons of body fluid before dehydration is noticed clinically. A useful method of determining the state of body dehydration is to raise a fold of skin and see how quickly it returns to place. When 3% of the body weight is lost, the skin is slightly dry and tight. When 6% of the body weight has been lost due to dehydration, the eyes are sunken; there is a markedly dry, tight skin; the mucous membranes and cornea are dry.[36] Most animals die due to dehydration when about 20 to 25% of the body weight is lost.[30]

Dehydrated animals have small amounts of concentrated urine (high specific gravity) if renal function is not impaired. Hemoglobin, hematocrit, and plasma protein values are elevated before dehydration can be seen clinically, and the concentration of all of the electrolyte ions becomes elevated if the dehydration is severe and there is not proportionate loss of electrolytes.[37,38] Changes in hematocrit or hemoglobin are useful in evaluating treatment. Care must be used in evaluating laboratory findings. For example, if an anemic animal becomes dehydrated, the hematocrit and hemoglobin values may be in the normal range.

Treatment of simple dehydration is, of course, to permit the animal to drink water, or if the animal is unable to drink or will not drink, a stomach tube can be used to administer the water. If a stomach tube cannot be passed due to an esophageal lesion, intravenous treatment can be used to maintain the animal. From data on other species it is calculated that a 1,000-pound horse at rest in cool weather requires approximately 2½ to 3½ gallons of 5% dextrose intravenously daily for maintenance of hydration if he is unable to drink water.[34,39,40,41,42,43,44] This will not satisfy the nutritive requirements, however, and electrolytes will be required if the animal is not eating.

If an animal is severely overhydrated and lacks electrolytes, central nervous system disturbance will occur. Overhydration is not likely to occur unless large quantites of water are given by stomach tube or large quantities of isotonic dextrose are injected. Overhydration of horses seldom occurs.

Dehydration and Electrolyte Loss

Electrolyte loss usually accompanies dehydration in animals which are sick. Animals which are not drinking enough water usually are not eating enough to supply their needs for electrolytes. Many diseases cause additional loss of electrolytes. Daily electrolyte determinations help in estimating the electrolyte needs of sick animals.[45] Little application of electrolyte determinations has been used in sick horses; therefore, it is necessary to evaluate findings from these determinations on knowledge from other species. Sometimes, in spite of an electrolyte deficit, the serum electrolyte concentration will be elevated if there is a greater deficit of water than of electrolyte. It is hoped that the following discussion of electrolyte imbalance problems will help veterinarians in estimating electrolyte needs.

Sodium and Chloride Loss

When there is a deficit of sodium (Na) there usually is a deficit of chloride (Cl) and also a deficit of extracellular water.[32] The deficit of these extracellular ions often is greater than the deficit of water, especially if the animal has been drinking but not eating. The signs associated with severe sodium loss are rapid, thready pulse, and cold, clammy extremities due to peripheral vascular collapse. The most important cause of sodium loss in the horse is loss of fluid from the body surface, and from body openings, especially due to diarrhea. Burns cause a loss of water, sodium, chloride, protein and blood cells.

A horse at moderate work loses 50 to 60 Gm. NaCl per day in sweat and 35 Gm. in urine.[46] From these data and from information on other species, it is estimated that a horse at rest in cool weather requires 50 Gm. NaCl to replace normal daily loss.[32,40,43,44,46] This 850 mEq of Na^+ and Cl^- could be supplied by about 6 liters (1½ gallon) of 0.9% NaCl solution, "physiologic saline." If a deficit is present when treatment is started or if there is a continuing abnormal loss, a larger amount will be needed. This treatment would not replace the loss of other electrolytes. Postoperatively animals tend to retain NaCl, so perhaps somewhat less than this amount would be needed in these cases.[44] Excessive amounts of NaCl solutions should not be injected postoperatively.[43]

Animals suffering from heat exhaustion usually have a deficit of water and sodium chloride. If the animal is permitted to drink water, the relative lack of sodium chloride becomes worse. The animal should be permitted to eat free salt. Intravenous 0.9% sodium chloride solution or 0.9% sodium chloride with 5% dextrose should be administered slowly to animals seriously affected. Hypertonic solutions (up to 5%) of sodium chloride administered very slowly intravenously may be more beneficial if the animal has been drinking water.

Anhydrosis in race horses in the tropics has been successfully treated with intravenous sodium chloride solutions followed by forced feeding of salt in the grain daily.[47] However, Lord states that the only successful treatment of the condition is putting the horses in air-conditioned stalls.[48]

Excessive sodium retention almost always is accompanied by retention of water. Peripheral or pulmonary edema, which is the most important sign of sodium and water retention, may be associated with severe liver, kidney or cardiovascular disease.

ACID-BASE BALANCE

The hydrogen ion (H^+) concentration(pH) of body fluid is maintained by buffer systems, the most important of which is the following:[29]

$$HCl + NaHCO_3 \rightleftarrows NaCl + H_2CO_3$$

| Strong | Buffer | Neutral | Weak |
| Acid | Salt | Salt | Acid |

Respiration plays a major role in controlling the pH of body fluids since the concentration of carbonic acid (H_2CO_3) is proportional to plasma carbon dioxide (CO_2) tension (partial pressure). If the CO_2 tension and, therefore, H_2CO_3 concentration are reduced due to hyperventilation, respiratory alkalosis occurs; but if their concentration increases due to hypoventilation, respiratory acidosis occurs. The plasma concentration of bicarbonate or CO_2 combining power indicates the acid-base balance of an animal (the plasma bicarbonate concentration $\times$ 2.24 = the CO_2 combining power). Low bicarbonate concentration indicates acidosis, and high bicarbonate indicates alkalosis. Blood and other body fluids change pH only slightly except in severe disturbances.

Metabolic acidosis is the term used to indicate relative decrease in fixed cation (Na^+ is the most important one) in relation to fixed anion (Cl^- is the most important one). In metabolic alkalosis, the opposite imbalance occurs. The kidney is important in maintaining the condition of the buffer systems by selective excretion and reabsorption of fixed anions and cations.

Excessive sodium and potassium loss in relation to the amount of chloride lost due to diarrhea, or due to loss of saliva through an esophageal fistula, may result in acidosis. Acidosis will be intensified by the injection of sodium chloride solution, since the ratio of Na^+ to Cl^- ion in the solution is 1:1 but the ratio in the body fluid is approximately 1.5:1. The excess Cl^- displaces CO_2. Starvation, or renal insufficiency resulting in retention of organic acids (uncommon in horses) also can cause acidosis.[34,49] Signs often seen in animals with acidosis are depression, disorientation, weakness, and rapid breathing. In addition to the plasma bicarbonate concentration being lower than normal, the urine pH usually is lower than normal (more acid).

Intravenous injection of lactated Ringer's solution or replacement solutions containing lactate or acetate ions (Table 2) are indicated in diarrhea. In cases of severe acidosis and potassium loss, solutions containing up to 55 mEq of lactate or acetate and up to 17 mEq of potassium are more beneficial than lactated Ringer's solution (Table 2). Lactate or acetate is metabolized rapidly and replaced by bicarbonate. Potassium and calcium, which also are lost in diarrhea, are supplied by these solutions. Young animals with diarrhea develop acidosis and potassium deficit more rapidly than mature animals. Their body surface per pound of body weight and their metabolic rate is greater than that of mature animals, and their kidneys do not conserve cations as well.[49] A suggested daily dose of one of these solutions for a moderately dehydrated foal is 5 to 10 ml./pound per day. If only one visit per day can be made to treat the foal, it is best to inject the solution slowly, using the plastic tubing method, Fig. 14 and 15, or one-half of the solution may be given subcutaneously. Oral buffer salt solutions such as sodium bicarbonate may be helpful in treating acidosis, but no work has been reported on this in horses.

Alkalosis probably seldom occurs in horses since they seldom vomit. Vomiting is the usual cause of Cl^- depletion which causes alkalosis in other species. Prolonged, intensive therapy with potassium-deficient solutions or with solutions supplying alkaline ions (bicarbonate, lactate or acetate) can cause alkalosis.[34,49]

POTASSIUM

Potassium (K) is probably the most neglected ion in electrolyte treatment due to the

Table 2.—Useful Fluid and Electrolyte Solutions

Solutions*	Gm./L.	mEq./L. Cations	mEq./L. Anions	Calories	Tonicity
Sodium chloride (0.9% NaCl)	9.0	154 Na	154 Cl	—	Isotonic
Sodium chloride (5% NaCl)	50.0	855 Na	855 Cl	—	Hypertonic
Dextrose 2½% in 0.45% NaCl	25 Dextrose 4.5 NaCl	77 Na	77 Cl	85	Isotonic
Dextrose 5% in 0.22% NaCl	50 Dextrose 2.25 NaCl	38.5 Na	38.5 Cl	170	Hypertonic
Dextrose 5% in 0.9% NaCl	50 Dextrose 9.0 NaCl	154 Na	154 Cl	170	Hypertonic
Dextrose 5% in water	50 Dextrose	—	—	170	Isotonic
Dextrose 10% in water	100 Dextrose	—	—	340	Hypertonic
Ringer's solution	8.6 NaCl 0.3 KCl 0.33 CaCl₂	147 Na 4 K 5 Ca	156 Cl	—	Isotonic
Dextrose 5% in Ringer's solution	8.6 NaCl 0.3 KCl 0.33 CaCl₂	147 Na 4 K 5 Ca	156 Cl	170	Hypertonic
Dextrose 10% in Ringer's solution	8.6 NaCl 0.3 KCl 0.33 CaCl₂	147 Na 4 K 5 Ca	156 Cl	340	Hypertonic
Ringer's lactate solution	6.0 NaCl 0.3 KCl 0.2 CaCl₂ 3.1 Na lactate	131 Na 4 K 3 Ca	110 Cl 28 lactate	—	Isotonic
Dextrose 2½% in half-strength Ringer's lactate	25 Dextrose 3.0 NaCl 0.15 KCl 0.1 CaCl₂ 1.5 Na lactate	65 Na 2 K 1 Ca	54 Cl 14 lactate	85	Isotonic
Commercial preparations formulated to correct losses due to diarrhea, sometimes called "balanced" solutions (with or without dextrose)	Various salts are used to give concentrations of ions indicated	140± Na up to 10 Ca up to 17 K up to 6.4 Mg.	103± Cl up to 55 lactate or acetate	±	Isotonic or hypertonic if with dextrose

*Concentrated solutions can be obtained which can be mixed with distilled water to make the desired solutions.

common practice of using "physiologic saline" which contains only Na⁺ and Cl⁻. This treatment often does more harm than good since potassium is further depleted by sodium diuresis. The kidney conserves potassium poorly. It is the cation found in highest concentration in the cell. Based on man's normal requirements for potassium, a normal, mature 1,000-pound horse probably needs between 200 and 450 mEq per day.[32,41,44,50]

The most common cause of potassium deficit is lack of intake due to the animal's not eating. This is very important postoperatively since additional potassium is needed for the "building up" of protein in healing, and potassium loss may be abnormally high postoperatively due to cell destruction. Potassium

loss accompanies persistent diarrhea. Potassium deficit also is associated with abnormal renal function and alkalosis, which are uncommon in horses. If large amounts of sodium are administered, potassium can be depleted.[43,50] Treatment with ACTH or adrenocortical steroids increases excretion of K⁺ and retention of Na⁺. Low serum potassium levels cause disturbances of neuromuscular physiology. Signs of potassium depletion are muscle weakness, tremors, anorexia, and gastrointestinal stasis. Studies on man and other animals show that electrocardiographic changes also occur.

The serum concentration of potassium does not always reflect the potassium balance; much of the body potassium can be lost before the serum level decreases.[32,51] Reasons that the serum level of potassium may be normal or even elevated when potassium deficit exists are: 1. Potassium may shift from cellular to extracellular fluid. 2. A greater depletion of extracellular water than potassium may occur. 3. There may be kidney or adrenal cortical disease. Care should be taken to prevent hemolysis of samples collected for potassium determination, since the potassium freed by the cells will cause inaccurate (high) values. Small-gauge needles should not be used since they may cause trauma to blood cells, and only clean, dry syringes and test tubes should be used. When serum potassium levels are low, a deficit usually exists.[44,52] Acidosis often is associated with potassium deficit, and the concentration of chloride in the urine often is high.[34]

Oral electrolyte solutions, lactated Ringer's solution, Ringer's solution, and many commercial replacement preparations (Table 2) are sources of potassium. Potassium should not be administered if renal function is not adequate, since selective excretion by the kidney is the only way an imbalance of fixed ions can be corrected. If there is oliguria or anuria due to a fluid volume deficit, water should be administered orally or a hydrating solution should be given intravenously to promote more normal renal function. Examples of such hydrating solutions are 5% dextrose, 5% dextrose in 0.225% sodium chloride or 2½% dextrose in 0.45% sodium chloride. When a high serum level of K^+ is attained by rapid intravenous injection, or due to injection of K^+ in an animal with poor renal function, muscle weakness and cardiac arrhythmias may occur. If very high serum levels are reached, ventricular fibrillation or cardiac arrest may occur. It may be dangerous to inject solutions with concentrations greater than those listed in Table 2. Injection rate should be as slow as is practical and the heart should be auscultated periodically during injection. As it is with other drugs, the immediate response of the animal is related to serum concentration of the electrolyte, not to the total body concentration of the electrolyte.

CALCIUM

Although acute hypocalcemia is not common in horses, occasionally postparturient tetany occurs. Mares may become recumbent and have tetanic spasms. They respond well to slow intravenous injection of 20% calcium gluconate. Calcium is used by some veterinarians to treat "toxemia." Calcium injections should be given slowly since there is danger of cardiac arrhythmias or even cardiac arrest. It is well to auscultate the heart during the injection.

TREATMENT OF FLUID AND ELECTROLYTE IMBALANCE

Each horse is an individual problem and should be treated individually. Before starting treatment of fluid and electrolyte imbalance, an estimate should be made of the deficits which already have developed. A plan of therapy should be made to replace this deficit, the continuing normal loss, and continuing abnormal loss (for example, loss due to diarrhea). Each day the treatment should be adjusted to the needs, which can be estimated by signs, weight of the animal, and laboratory data if available.[33,44,45,50]

ORAL ROUTE

The oral route often is overlooked in fluid and electrolyte therapy. It is recognized universally as being superior to parenteral routes.[53] If a mistake is made in estimating the animal's needs, there probably is less danger of doing harm by overtreating with an oral electrolyte than by injecting excessive amounts of an electrolyte parenterally.[44] Materials for oral treatment usually are less expensive and less time is required to administer oral preparations than injectables.

Unless there is pharyngeal paralysis or an esophageal lesion, the animal should be tempted to eat palatable, nutritious feed, since feed is the natural source of electrolytes. Loose sodium chloride or dilute oral electrolyte solutions may be offered to the animal to attempt to replace deficits.

If an animal cannot or will not eat or drink, or cannot be permitted to eat or drink because of a mouth lesion, a stomach tube can be passed and fluids, electrolytes and if possible nutrients (syrups, milk, milk substitutes, eggs, thin cereal gruels, and vitamin-mineral supplements) can be supplied this way.[45,54]

Depending on the deficits, a 1,000-pound horse can be given from 25 to 75 Gm. NaCl and from 10 to 25 Gm. KCl or an equivalent amount of a commercial oral electrolyte in several gallons of water twice daily by stomach tube. It probably is best to use enough water to make the solution isotonic or somewhat hypotonic. About one gallon of water is required with each 40 Gm. of NaCl to make an isotonic solution. Potassium should not be administered unless the kidneys are functioning adequately. If the animal is eating or being nourished by stomach tube, the feed probably will supply the maintenance requirements of electrolytes.

The following is a daily maintenance ration for a 1,000-pound mature horse at rest (the ration will pass through a funnel and stomach tube when added to water): Wheat flour 3 pounds, soybean flour 2¼ pounds, alfalfa leaf meal 1½ pounds, dry nonfat milk ⅓ pound, corn oil 3 tablespoonfuls, and molasses 1¼ pints. A vitamin-mineral supplement and/or electrolytes may be added to these ingredients if they have been depleted previously. Approximately the minimum energy requirement is supplied, but more than the minimum requirement of protein is provided by this ration. The extra protein may be beneficial in horses which are suffering from tissue damage or those which are debilitated and need protein for tissue repair. It is recommended that one-half of this ration be mixed with 2½ to 5 gallons of warm water (so it will mix more readily), and that this be given twice daily. (It is unwise to put more than 5 gallons of fluid into the stomach of a 1,000-pound horse at one time with a stomach tube.) If the horse can be permitted to drink, additional water can be offered continuously. (Some horses will drink the mixture if they can be permitted to eat soft feeds.) One-half of this ration in 2½ gallons of water was administered twice each day for 6 days by stomach tube

to 3 horses weighing about 1,000 pounds. The weather was cold and the horses were not exercised. The horses would not drink additional water offered to them. There was no significant change in the following determinations done on 2 of the horses prior to the trial and on the third and sixth days of the trial: hematocrit, hemoglobin, plasma protein and serum sodium, potassium and chloride. There also was little change in these determinations on a horse with pharyngeal paralysis maintained on this ration for 10 days, when he was unable to swallow. The ration was administered to 3 other animals for an average of 3 days following oral surgery. After a few days on the ration, the fecal material became green and had the consistency of cow manure. Diarrhea or impaction did not occur in any of the 7 horses except in one yearling colt which developed diarrhea due to salmonella enteritis.

PARENTERAL ADMINISTRATION

Parenteral therapy should be used in those cases in which esophageal lesions make it unwise to feed the animal or to pass a stomach tube. This method of therapy also is best when absorption from the gastrointestinal tract is seriously impaired due to gastroenteritis. Animals in critical condition, such as those with heat exhaustion, should be given therapy intravenously to obtain as rapid a response as possible. An animal with tetanus often can be treated more safely by the intravenous route than by using a stomach tube. The use of oral and intravenous therapy often can be combined.

Intravenous injection is the only parenteral route recommended for fluid therapy in horses, but it may be necessary to use the subcutaneous route sometimes in foals which require large volumes of fluid if only one visit can be made to treat the foal each day and the continuous infusion method, Fig. 14 and 15, cannot be used. Hypertonic solutions should not be given subcutaneously in dehydrated animals since more fluids will be drawn out of the circulation prior to absorption.

The danger of injecting electrolytes in animals with poor renal function has been discussed in the section on potassium. The solutions in Table 2 should not be given at a rate greater than the rate recommended for administration of blood (see section of blood transfusions). (The 5% solution of sodium chloride, which seldom is indicated except in some cases of heat exhaustion, should be given even more slowly and cautiously.) It is wise to auscultate the heart periodically during any injection.

It is unnecessary to keep a large number of different intravenous solutions on hand. Almost any animal needing fluid and electrolyte therapy can be treated adequately with one or a combination of the following solutions: 0.9% sodium chloride, 5% dextrose, 5% dextrose in Ringer's solution and one of the preparations formulated to correct losses due to diarrhea (Table 2).

It is impossible to supply sufficient nutrients intravenously to maintain a horse for long periods with preparations now available. Dextrose most commonly is used as a 5% solution, but a 10% solution can be used to supply more calories if the solution is injected slowly to prevent diuresis due to the dextrose, and the loss of dextrose into the urine. In a 1,000-pound horse, the rate of injection of a 10% solution if it is to be entirely utilized, should not exceed 2,200 ml. per hour, since dextrose probably is metabolized at a rate of about 0.22 Gm./pound per hour.[30] Therefore, unless the continuous infusion method is used, Fig. 14 and 15, 5% dextrose solution is more practical. If more than 75 Gm. of dextrose is injected intravenously in an "average-sized" horse in 15 minutes some is lost in the urine.[55] Once an animal shows improvement in hydration and begins to eat and drink, dextrose injection probably should be limited or discontinued to avoid interference with return to eating and drinking. Dextrose solutions which are very hypertonic, including up to 50% solutions, sometimes are used to "detoxify" animals. These solutions may do more harm than good in dehydrated animals, since they remove more fluid from the cells and may cause diuresis.[30] The use of 50% dextrose probably is seldom indicated in horses.

Dilute solutions of ethyl alcohol have been used intravenously in man to supply energy, but their use has not been reported in horses. Fat emulsions for intravenous injection have been developed. These products supply much more energy (calories) per unit of volume than 5 or 10% dextrose. There has been no report of their use in horses.

Protein hydrolysates have been recommended for use parenterally in large animals. The recommended doses would supply only a fraction of the daily maintenance requirement of protein for a mature horse. (Only 30 to 60% of the protein in most of these products was found to be retained in dogs.[39]) Allergic responses sometimes occur when some of these products are administered parenterally to horses. For mature horses, the oral treatment with less expensive protein seems to be more practical. B-complex vitamins should be given parenterally to animals which cannot eat or be fed with a stomach tube for several days, since the supply of these vitamins soon is depleted in animals which are not eating.

If it were necessary to maintain a 1,000-pound horse for several days on intravenous fluids and nutrients, the amounts required would make it impractical. To demonstrate the magnitude of the problem, the solutions needed to supply the daily nutritional requirements are listed (replacement of previous and current abnormal loss is not being considered):[46]

1½ gallons 10% dextrose in Ringer's solution.
2 gallons 10% dextrose.
1½ gallons 10% protein hydrolysate in 5% dextrose (safety of injecting large quantities of these products is doubtful).
A fat emulsion to supply at least 1500 additional calories (if these products prove to be safe in horses).
Vitamins.

Injection would have to be slow throughout the day, in order that the cardiovascular system not be overloaded and in order that the nutrients could be utilized to best advantage.

A. A. GABEL

REFERENCES

1. Guard, W. F.: Surgical Principles and Technics. W. F. Guard, 2274 Yorkshire Rd., Columbus 21, Ohio, 1953.

2. Armistead, W. W.: Canine Medicine, 2nd ed. 43 Authors. American Veterinary Publications, Inc. Santa Barbara, California, 1959.

3. Gabel, Albert A.: Accidental intra-carotid injection. J.A.V.M.A. In preparation.

4. Kingma, F. J.: A technique for the slow infusion of fluids, J.A.V.M.A. 117 (1950) 403.

5. VanPelt, R. W.: Arthrocentesis of the equine carpus. Vet. Med. 55 (1960) 30-34.

6. Astra: Xylocaine[R] in Veterinary Anesthesia (A movie) A/B Astra Sodertalje, Sweden. Available from Jensen-Salsbery Laboratories, Inc. Box 167, Kansas City 41, Missouri.

7. Science Report: Diseases of the joints—diagnosis and treatment. Mod. Vet. Prac. 39 (1958) 28-32.

8. Sisson, S. and Grossman, J. D.: The Anatomy of Domestic Animals. 4th Ed. W. B. Saunders Co., Philadelphia, Pa. 1953.

9. Doll, E. R.: Immunization against viral rhinopneumonitis of horses with live virus propagated in hamsters. J.A.V.M.A. 139 (1961) 1324-1330.

10. Kowalczyk, T.: Method pipes oxygen to ailing animals. Maryland Vet. 1 (1960) 15.

11. U.S. Dept. Agriculture: Diseases of the Horse. U.S. Gov't Printing Office, Washington, D.C., 1942.

12. Bruner, D. W., Doll, E. R., Hull, F. E. and Kinkaid, A. S.: Further studies on hemolytic icterus in foals. Am.J.Vet.Research. 11 (1950) 22-25.

13. Ferguson, L. C.: The Blood Groups in Animals. Advances in Veterinary Science, Academic Press, New York, N.Y. 1955: 106-137.

14. Bruner, D. W. and Doll, E. R.: Blood groups in horses (Indian system): their value in transfusion and neonatal isoerythrolysis, Cornell Vet. 43 (1953) 217-221.

15. Archer, R. K. and Franks, D.: Blood transfusion in veterinary practice. Vet. Rec. 73 (1960) 657-661.

16. Coffee, W. M.: Blood transfusion in large animals, J.A.V.M.A. 115 (1949) 165.

17. Smith, H. A. and Jones, T. C.: Veterinary Pathology. Lea & Febiger, Philadelphia, Pa., 1957.

18. Irwin, D. G. H.: A survey of blood transfusion in veterinary medicine. JSAVMA 29 (1958) 281-293.

19. Doll, E. R. et al.: The influence of equine fetal tissue vaccine upon hemagglutination activity of mare serum: its relation to hemolytic icterus of newborn foals. Cornell Vet. 42 (1952) 495-505.

20. Gilman, M. A., Schwarz, A. and Wallerstein, H.: Immunohemalologic studies of the Thoroughbred horse, Am.J.Vet.Research. 21 (1960) 393-396.

21. Equine Research Station, Newmarket, England: Blood transfusions in the foal, Quest. and Ans. Mod. Vet. Prac. 41 (1960) 54.

22. Coombs, R. R. A., Mourant, A. E., and Race, R. R.: Detection of weak and incomplete Rh agglutinogens. Lancet 249 (1945) 15-16.

23. Loeb, W. F.: Personal communication. College of Veterinary Medicine, Ohio State University, Columbus.

24. Schalm, O. W.: Cattle Diseases (57 authors), American Veterinary Publications, Inc., Santa Barbara, Calif., 1956.

25. Grace, Oliver D.: Blood transfusions and parenteral fluid therapy. Vet. Med. 51 (1956) 175-179.

26. Kroger, L. M.: Blood transfusion in cattle under range conditions. Proceedings AVMA Meeting 1954, p. 377-379.

27. Jen-Sal Laboratories: New blood transfusion method, Jen-Sal J. 37 (1954) 4-5.

28. Simpson, C. F., Sanders, D. A. and French, R. B.: A technic for the collection and transfusion of blood in cattle, J.A.V.M.A., 120 (1952) 17.

29. Dukes, H. H.: The Physiology of Domestic Animals. 7th Ed., Comstock Publishing Associates, Ithaca, N. Y., 1955.

30. Jones, L. M.: Veterinary Pharmacology and Therapeutics, 2nd ed., Iowa State University Press, Ames, 1957.

31. Quin, A. H.: A technic for blood transfusion, Vet. Med. 56 (1961) 435.

32. Elkinton, J. R. and Danowski, T. S.: The Body Fluids. The Williams and Wilkins Company, Baltimore, Md., 1955.

33. Helmer, O. M.: Symposium on parenteral fluids, nutrition and electrolytes. The milliequivalent as a unit of measure in the interpretation and correction of electrolyte disturbances. Minnesota Med. (supp.) 38 (1955) 1-3.

34. Benjamin, Maxine M.: Outline of Clinical Pathology. 2nd Ed., The Iowa State University Press, Ames, 1961.

35. O'Donnell, Frank A.: A review of fundamentals in fluid therapy. Haver-Lockhart Messenger 41 (1961) 34-35.

36. Meier, H.: Parenteral fluid therapy. Mod. Vet. Prac. 39 (1958) 44-54.

37. Burch, J. E.: Fluid therapy in the horse. Proc. Sixth Annual Am. Assn. of Equine Pract. Assn. Conv., Dec., 1960.

38. Roberts, R. M.: Fluid and electrolyte imbalance. Rocky Mt. Vet. 6 (1958) 8-11.

39. Abbott Laboratories: A practical approach to fluid therapy in veterinary medicine. Abbott Laboratories, North Chicago, Ill., 1958.

40. Abbott Laboratories: Fluids and electrolytes. Abbott Laboratories, North Chicago, Ill., 1960.

41. Brooks, S. M.: Basic Facts of Body Water and Ions. Springer Publishing Co., Inc., New York 10, N.Y., 1960.

42. Freeman, A.: Fluid therapy in large animals. Rocky Mt. Vet., 5 (1957) 6 and 22-28.

43. Talbot, N. B.: Homeostatic limits to safe parenteral fluid therapy. New Eng. J. Med. 248 (1953) 1100-1108.

44. Tovey, G. H.: Technique of Fluid Balance. 2nd ed., Charles C Thomas, Springfield, Ill. 1960.

45. Jastremski, M., and Fenebee, J. W.: Fluid replacement in the treatment of dehydration from diarrhea in the horse. J.A.V.M.A. 128 (1956) 153-155.

46. Committee on Animal Nutrition: Nutrient Requirements of Horses. National Academy of Sciences—National Research Council Publication 912, Washington, D.C., 1961.

47. Gilyard, R. J.: Chronic anhidrosis with lowered blood chlorides in race horses. Cornell Vet. 34 (1944) 332-336.

48. Lord, W. E.: Thoroughbred practice in the tropics. Proc. Sixth Annual Amer. Assn. of Equine Pract. Convention, Dec., 1960.

49. Baxter Laboratories, Inc.: Fluid therapy handbook. Baxter Laboratories, Inc. Morton Grove, Ill., 1960.

50. Hardy, J. D.: Fluid Therapy. Lea & Febiger, Philadelphia, Pa., 1954.

51. McSherry, B. and Gringer, I.: Disturbance in acid-base balance and electrolytes in calf diarrhea. A report of eighteen cases. Am.J.Vet.Research. 57 (1954) 535-541.

52. Statland, H.: Fluid and Electrolytes in Practice. 2nd ed., J. B. Lippincott Co., Philadelphia, Pa. 1957.

53. Mead Johnson & Co.: Fluid Therapy Handbook. Mead Johnson & Co., Evansville, Ind., 1957.

54. Frank, E. R.: Veterinary Surgery. 6th ed., Burgess Publishing Co., Minneapolis 15, Minn., 1959.

55. Link, R. P.: Glucose tolerance in horses, J.A.V.M.A., 97 (1940) 261-262.

CHAPTER 4

VIRAL DISEASES

EPITHELIOTROPIC VIRAL DISEASES

GENERAL COMMENT

Vesicular stomatitis, equine cutaneous papilloma, and equine sarcoid are the only epitheliotropic viral diseases generally recognized in the horse in the United States. Horse pox is frequently mentioned in the European literature, but its occurrence in the United States has not been authenticated. Coital exanthema is rarely seen in the United States and its etiology is not clearly established. Though some strains of the virus of vesicular exanthema may infect the horse it is not regarded as a natural

healed. Though this is not recognized as a naturally occurring disease it should be kept in mind that the horse is susceptible to at least some strains.

EQUINE CUTANEOUS PAPILLOMATOSIS

This is an infectious disease[3] of horses up to 3 years of age.[4] The papillomas, or warts, commonly appear on the nose and about the lips as small, elevated, circumscribed, keratinizing masses up to 10 mm. in diameter (Fig. 1). The number of warts may vary from 2 or 3 to as many as a hundred or more, covering

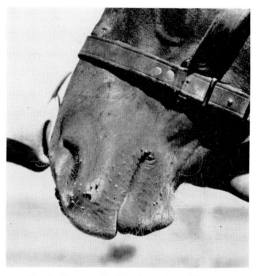 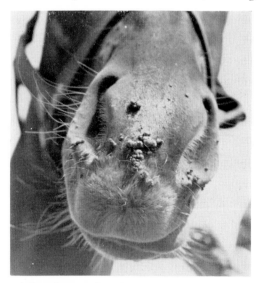

Fig. 1. Front and side view of papillomas on nose and lips of a yearling Quarter horse. They had appeared 60 days before. One month later the warts had nearly disappeared.

disease of the horse.[1] Crawford[2] applied vesicular exanthema virus to the scarified tongue of horses. In 16 to 20 hours there was elevation of temperature which returned to normal in a few hours. The epithelium at the inoculation site became thickened and gray-yellow in color. The lesion did not spread and vesicles did not form. The affected epithelium became detached and there was excess salivation. Feed was refused because of soreness of the tongue. Within a week from inoculation the lesions

the entire muzzle. Occasionally, when only a few warts develop, they may grow to a relatively larger size. The disease is self-limiting, and the warts disappear within about 3 months from the time they are first noted. If they are allowed to regress on their own accord, they cause the animal little inconvenience and disappear without leaving scars. Surgical removal is usually not necessary, and if done, care should be taken to avoid causing scar tissue.

The disease is caused by a filtrable virus

which appears to be infectious only for horses. Calves, lambs, dogs, rabbits, and guinea pigs are resistant to the causative agent of equine cutaneous papilloma. The disease can be transmitted to young susceptible horses by intradermal injection or exposure of scarified skin with the virus. Infective material placed on intact skin does not produce the disease. The incubation period, that is the time from exposure to appearance of papilloma, is 2 to 3 months.

Although the exact mechanism of transmission of the disease is not known, it appears quite likely that the virus usually gains entrance through small wounds or abrasions of the skin. The common location about the nose and muzzle suggests that the playful habit of colts in "nuzzling" various things and objects would lead to breaks of the skin and introduction of the virus. Such things as halters and curry combs, contaminated following contact with infected animals, may spread the virus. The disease usually is transmitted by an animal in which the infection is either in the active or incubative stage of the disease. The virus is relatively resistant and may contaminate fences, mangers, and the walls of stables. How long the virus may live under such conditions is not known. There is evidence[5] that cattle may become infected from contact with

fences and feed bunks contaminated with the virus of bovine cutaneous papillomatosis.

Treatment: Treatment is usually unnecessary if it is clearly explained to the owner that the condition is self-limiting. The animal will be immune upon recovery from papillomatosis. Vaccine therapy is not indicated, especially with wart vaccines derived from other species, since the virus of equine cutaneous papillomatosis is known to occur only in the horse. Surgical removal of warts from the horse is not necessary unless there are cosmetic reasons. Even then, it is wise to avoid surgical interference early in the course of the disease. Surgical removal of bovine warts early in the disease often will result in stimulating the growth of remaining warts and cause recurrence of others.[6]

If equine papillomatosis is a problem in a horse-breeding establishment, consideration should be given to thoroughly cleaning the paddock, fences, and stable followed by disinfection to destroy the virus. A strong lye or formaldehyde solution should be satisfactory. This should be done with due consideration of the source of infective material from active or incubative cases of the disease in the young stock. Under some conditions, prophylactic immunization would be advisable, using a formalin-treated suspension of warts from infected

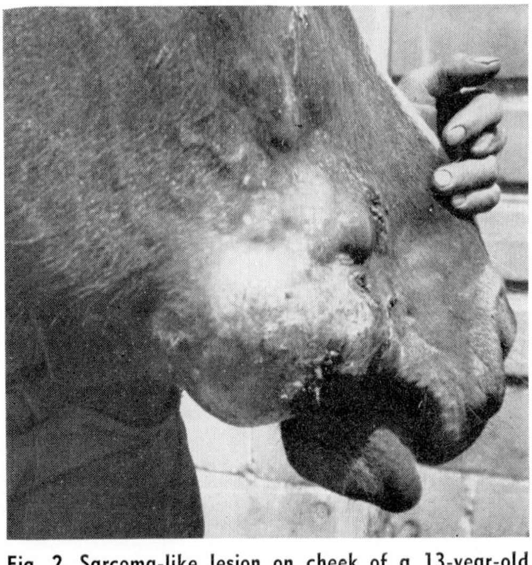

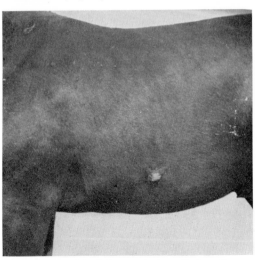

Fig. 2. Sarcoma-like lesion on cheek of a 13-year-old horse. Recurrence of tumor that had been removed 3 years previously. The tumor contained abscesses which drained through fistulous tracts to openings in the skin.

Fig. 3. Sarcoma-like lesions on body wall of an 8-year-old mule. This growth was removed and specimen is illustrated in Fig. 4 and 5. Histology of the tumor is illustrated in Fig. 6 and 7.

colts of the same band as a vaccine. Such a program of prophylactic immunization has been used in herds of dairy cattle where cutaneous papillomatosis is common. Calves have been protected adequately with a small (5 ml. of 10% ground wart suspension) subcutaneous dose given at 3 to 6 weeks of age.

SARCOMA-LIKE LESIONS OF THE SKIN

Sarcoma-like lesions of the skin of horses apparently are caused by the virus of bovine cutaneous papillomatosis. This condition was recognized as a clinical entity by Jackson[7] in South Africa, and is called equine "sarcoid." About the same time, workers in North Africa[8,9,10] recognized the disease, but called it a Schwann tumor, believing it to arise from Schwann sheath cells of nerves. It was suspected of having a viral etiology and spread by rubbing an affected part of the body against unaffected skin. Sarcomatous lesions have been produced in the skin of horses with the virus of bovine cutaneous papillomatosis, and warts have been produced in the skin of cattle with material from this disease in the horse. Equine "sarcoid" may occur more commonly than it is diagnosed because there is no simple way to recognize the presence of virus. The diagnosis cannot be made on the basis of histologic appearance only, but must take into account the location of the lesions and the history of the case. For example, Runnells and Benbrook[11] reported 90 cases of sarcoma from horses and mules. In 76 instances the lesion was located where equine "sarcoid" might be expected. Local recurrence was recorded in 11 cases, and there may have been more as the records were considered incomplete. The virus of this disease might also be the stimulus for some of the so-called "exuberant granulation reactions" not uncommonly seen during the healing of wounds in equine skin.

Equine "sarcoids" usually start as an isolated, single growth on the leg, head, shoulder, pectoral region or sides of the body (Fig. 2 and 3). The initial lesion may resemble a papilloma, since there is an initial proliferation of epithelium as well as connective tissue (Fig. 4). Soon the fibroblastic growth develops more rapidly, and the epithelium becomes thin, breaks, and an ulcer may be formed. As the tumor increases in size bacterial infection with associated inflammatory changes may occur. The growths are very firm and fibrous, (Fig. 5 and 6) and histologically have the appearance of a fibrosarcoma (Fig. 7, 8 and 9).

In natural cases of the disease that are called to the veterinarian's attention, the tumors show progressive growth and are often multiple and scattered over the body. They tend to recur at the site from which they have been removed.[12]

In the experimental form of the disease, a growth is usually apparent 3 to 4 weeks after intradermal inoculation of the virus of bovine cutaneous papillomatosis.[13] The growth at first is covered with hair, later the epithelial elements of the skin (hair follicles, glands, and epidermis) disappear, leaving a raw surface. In some animals the growth regresses in 1 to 8 months. If the scarified skin of experimental animals is inoculated with the virus a similar pattern follows and, in addition, there is an initial stimulation of epidermis. Surgical removal of the experimentally induced lesion early in its development is nearly always followed by recurrence of the growth.

Treatment: These are difficult cases to handle and the results usually are unsatisfactory. Although the sarcoma-like lesions have never been known to metastasize to the internal organs, the persistent tumor mass with its covering of skin is unsightly and objectionable. Surgical removal may or may not be successful. The experimentally induced lesions may actually be stimulated by surgical interference early in the course of the disease, and this fact should be borne in mind when considering an individual case. The growth rate of the tumor nodules can be determined by measurement at intervals to form a basis for deciding whether the growth is slow or rapid. The rate of growth in typical experimental cases is indicated in Fig. 10 and illustrates what can be expected. If the lesion is so located that it is not subject to trauma nor does not interfere with the harness, it should not be disturbed. If the lesion must be surgically removed, it should be done after the growth has reached its maximum size or is beginning to regress.

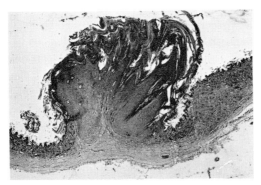

Fig. 4. Initial lesion of equine "sarcoid" in which the growth resembles a wart with stimulation of epithelium. This occurred on the breast of the 13-year-old horse shown in Fig. 2.

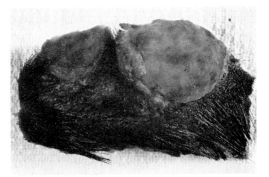

Fig. 5. Exterior surface of lesion in Fig. 3 showing loss of hair over the 2 large nodules of tumor.

The sarcoma-like lesions can occur in horses, mules or donkeys of most any age. Horses more than 20 years old have been found susceptible to the bovine cutaneous papilloma agent.

A typical case history will illustrate the course of the disease. A 6 year-old mule developed a nodular tumor mass, 8 cm. by 10 cm., with surrounding, smaller, satellite nodules on the right lateral surface of the anterior third of the neck near the base of the ear. This lesion was removed surgically and then recurred, reaching a size of about 8 cm. in 3 months. It was removed again and recurred. Five months later the growth again had reached such a size that it was removed a

third time. Recurrence again occurred at the edge of the scar and was still growing slowly when the mule was destroyed about 7 months later. A second tumor nodule, 5 cm. in diameter, was present on the internal surface of the right ear, and was removed at the time of the initial surgery. It recurred to such an extent that about one-third of the ear was removed 8 months later. Recurrence again developed and the tumor covered the remaining internal surface of the ear at the time of necropsy. A third growth developed on the left side of the animal 8 months after the initial surgery, and when removed it measured 10 cm. by 12 cm. (Fig. 2, 4 and 5). The operative wound healed readily, and the tumor

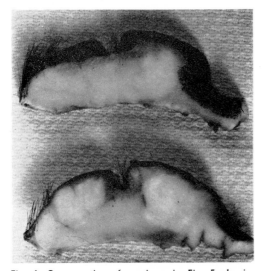

Fig. 6. Cross section of specimen in Fig. 5 showing depth of the growth.

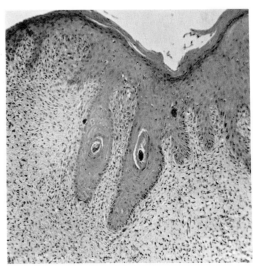

Fig. 7. Sarcoma-like growth replacing normal structures of skin and showing irregularity of overlying epithelium. Section from tumor shown in Fig. 2, 5, and 6. X 80.

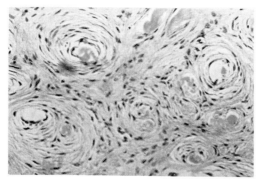

Fig. 8. Section from same tumor as Fig. 7 but showing whole growth pattern of fibroblasts causing tumor to resemble a Schwann tumor. X 160.

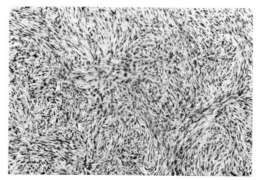

Fig. 9. Section from another skin tumor on animal illustrated in Fig. 3. This shows a marked resemblance to fibrosarcoma. X 120.

did not recur. A fourth tumor was observed initially about 9 months after the original surgery. It was located on the left side of the animal and measured about 1 cm. in diameter. Six months later it had become 2.5 by 3 cm. in size and was removed, but it developed again. In another 6 weeks it again measured 2.5 cm. in diameter. About 6 weeks before the animal was destroyed, a fifth small nodule was found in the middle of the back (Fig. 8).

This case illustrates the succession of tumor nodules that can develop and the frustrations associated with their surgical removal.

C. OLSON

REFERENCES

1. Madin, S. H., and Traum, J.: Vesicular exanthema of swine. Bact. Rev. 19 (1955) 6-19.
2. Crawford, A. B.: Experimental vesicular exanthema of swine. Proc. 40th Annual Meeting of the U.S. Livestock Sanitary Assn. J.A.V.M.A. 110 (1937) 380-395.

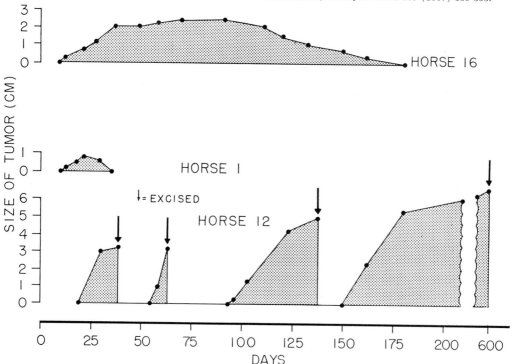

Fig. 10. Diagrammatic representation of rate of growth of sarcomas induced in skin of experimental horses. Each dot represents a point of observation. The record for horse 16 is typical of the results obtained. The record for horse 1 indicates a small, short-liver tumor in the skin of this animal. This was an unusual result. The record for horse 12 indicates the unusually large size of the sarcoma induced in this animal and the recurrence of growth following excision of the mass at 3 different times.

3. Cadeac: Sur la Transmission expérimentale des papillomes des diverses espéces. Bull. Soc. Sc. Vet., I. Lyon 4 (1901) 280-286.

4. Cook, R. H., and Olson, C.: Experimental transmission of cutaneous papilloma of the horse. Amer. J. Path. 27 (1951) 1087-1097.

5. Bagdonas, V., and Olson, C.: Observations on the epizootiology of cutaneous papillomatosis (warts) of cattle. J.A.V.M.A. 122 (1953) 393-397.

6. Olson, C., and Skidmore, L. V.: Therapy of experimentally produced bovine cutaneous papillomatosis with vaccines and excision. J.A.V.M.A. 135 (1959) 339-343.

7. Jackson, C.: The Incidence and Pathology of Tumors of Domesticated Animals in South Africa. Onderstepoort J. Vet. Sci. and Animal Indust., 6 (1936) 1-460.

8. Lafargue, V., Montpellier, J., and Jacquemin: Un cas de schanno-sarcome du scrotum du mulet. Rev. Med. Vét. (Toulouse), 88 (1936) 452-457.

9. Montpellier, J., Badens, P., and Dieuzeide, R.: Tumeurs schwanniennes cutanées du mulet. Rev. Med. Vét. (Toulouse), 89 (1937) 216-224.

10. Montpellier, J., Dieuzeide, R., and Badens, P.: Greffe d'une tumeur schwannienne chez le mulet. Acad. Vét. de France Bull., 12 (1939) 91.

11. Runnells, R. A., and Benbrook, E. A.: Connective Tissue Tumors of Horses and Mules. Am. J. Vet. Res., 2 (1941) 427-430.

12. Olson, C.: Equine sarcoid, a cutaneous neoplasm. Amer. J. Vet. Res. 9 (1948) 333-341.

13. Olson, C., and Cook, R. H.: Cutaneous sarcoma-like lesions of the horse caused by the agent of bovine papilloma. Proc. Soc. Exp. Biol. and Med 77 (1951) 281-284.

VIRAL PAPULAR DERMATITIS

This condition possibly is a variant form of horse pox, although it has been described as a separate disease entity. It consists of firm papular swellings which do not form vesicles or pustules. The lesions become encrusted within 1 week after their appearance, leaving circumscribed hairless areas. There is no apparent systemic effect and no local pruritus. The lesions may appear anywhere upon the body. The cause is an epitheliotropic virus that can be grown on chorioallantic membranes of chick embryos. The disease has been reported from the United States, Australia, and New Zealand. It occurs principally in saddled horses and the lesions tend to localize around the girth, thus preventing the animals being used with a saddle. The course is approximately 3 weeks. The therapy to date is symptomatic, and has been relatively ineffective. Since the virus is quite resistant and will persist for a considerable time on equipment and fomites, careful disinfection of harness, other equipment, and stalls is necessary.

J. F. BONE

REFERENCE

1. New Zeal. Vet. J. 8 (1960) 92.

VESICULAR STOMATITIS

Vesicular stomatitis is an epitheliotropic disease of horses, cattle, and swine. Two similar but distinct viruses induce the macules, vesicles, and erosions which appear successively in the mucous membranes of the mouth or on the skin of the foot. Rarely is there mortality or serious sequelae; for this reason the disease is treated lightly by some authorities. The economic significance of vesicular stomatitis lies in its ability to effectively disable an animal for 1 to 2 weeks. During this period the animal should not be moved to other premises or sent to market. Lactation may cease. For many owners, failure of lactation or restriction of movement at an inopportune time can mean great financial loss.

Vesicular stomatitis has existed in America for many years. However, it was in Africa that Theiler (1901) first recognized it in horses and described the disease as a clinical entity. Later, in 1916 after a French veterinarian (Jacoulet, 1915) reported vesicular stomatitis in horses shipped from the United States and Canada, it was belatedly recognized in America (Teidebold et al., 1916; Gregg et al., 1917). The virus etiology of the disease was established by Cotton in 1926; and in the following year, he demonstrated that there were two serologic types of the virus (Cotton, 1927).

Etiology: The two serologically distinct viruses which produce clinically indistinguishable disease are named after the states in which they were first isolated, New Jersey and Indiana. Galloway and Elford (1933) estimated the size of the two viruses to be 70 to 100 $m\mu$ on the basis of filtration experiments. Chow et al. (1954) examined the virus with an electron microscope and observed that the rod-shaped particles averaged 60 $m\mu$ in diameter and 210 $m\mu$ in length. Bradish et al. (1956) photographed the rod-shaped particles and gave the dimensions as 69 $m\mu$ × 175 $m\mu$. As almost all viruses attacking animals are spheres or ellipsoids, vesicular stomatitis virus is unique in its shape.

The physical properties of the virus are similar to those of other animal viruses (Olitsky, 1927). At a temperature of 56 C. (132

F.) activity is retained for 10 to 20 minutes and at 37 C. (98 F.) for 3 to 4 days. At refrigeration temperatures (6 C. or 42 F.) the infectivity of the virus persists for 1 to 2 months, and when frozen (−20 C. or −4 F.) it may remain viable more than a year. Sunlight and ultraviolet light are harmful to the virus, and even visible light is reported to be detrimental (Bradish *et al.*, 1956). The effectiveness of certain disinfectants under laboratory conditions is given in Table 1. The viruses of vesicular stomatitis can resist action of physical and chemical agents longer in the presence of certain body substances and fluids. Inactivation times obtained in the laboratory with partially purified preparations may be inadequate if decontamination of virus in saliva, blood or feces is desired. For this reason it is best to use a longer period or a heavier treatment than has been reported to result in inactivation.

Propagation of the virus in the laboratory has made possible studies on morphology, serology, and physical properties of the virus. Vesicular stomatitis virus is readily cultivated in guinea pigs, mice, chicken embryos, and tissue cultures. Mature guinea pigs are inoculated in the foot pad epithelium; and if virus is present in the inoculum, vesicles develop in approximately 48 hours (Wagener, 1932). Virus can be harvested from the foot pad vesicles. Mature mice are inoculated in the cerebrum and within 3 days become hypersensitive, incoordinated, and paralytic (Cox and Olitsky, 1933; Cunha, *et al.*, 1955). Death results on the third to the fifth day. Suckling mice develop a fatal infection irrespective of the route by which the virus is introduced. The virus is recovered from the brain of both mature and suckling mice.

When chicken embryos are inoculated into the allantoic chamber, death results in 24 to 48 hours (Burnet and Galloway, 1934; Karstad and Hanson, 1958). Large amounts of virus are contained in the allantoic fluids. Several kinds of tissue cultures will support growth of the virus, including chicken fibroblasts, bovine kidney cells, human HeLa cells and guinea pig kidney cells (Bachrach *et al.*, 1955; Fellowes *et al.*, 1956; McClain and Hackett, 1958). In all instances the virus is cytopathic.

Table 1.—Activity of Disinfectants on Vesicular Stomatitis Virus

DISINFECTANT	DILUTION OF COMMERCIAL PREPARATION	
	Percent inactivating virus in 15 minutes	Percent failing to inactivate
Lye	not determined	3%
Therapogen	20%	2%
Septisol	2%	1%
Formalin	1%	not determined
Crestal fluid	1%	0.5%
Wescodyne	0.5%	0.3%
Roccal	0.5%	0.3%
B-K powder	0.1%	not determined

Tissue culture propagated virus may be recovered from the supernatant fluids.

Species Susceptibility: All horses that do not have antibodies to vesicular stomatitis are believed to be susceptible. In various epizootics 30 to 95% of the exposed animals have become clinically infected (Gregg *et al.*, 1917; Heiny, 1945). Inapparent infections may have occurred in the remainder (Brandly *et al.*, 1951). Gregg *et al.* (1917) observed that horses were more susceptible than mules, and mules more susceptible than burros. Differences in susceptibility among breeds of horses or horses of various ages are not on record (Burton, 1917); however, cattle increase in susceptibility with age, calves being more resistant than mature animals, while swine decrease in susceptibility, young pigs being infected more readily than adults.

Clinical Signs: The incubation period following natural and experimental exposure is 1 to 3 days (Hanson, 1952). Usually the first sign of the disease is pytalism; saliva dribbles from the lips and can be seen on the food. The rectal temperature may rise to 104 F., but usually the fever lasts only a few hours. The animal becomes somewhat depressed. Water is taken rather copiously but feed consumption is reduced because of inability to eat, rather than inappetence. The lesions in the mouth are found on the mucous membranes of the lips and the tongue. The vesicles on the tongue usually coalesce before rupturing and, as a result, the erosion may sometimes cover half of the surface. The wound appears deep, raw, and bleeding with shreds of dead epithelium at the margin. The persistence of pytalism co-incides with the severity of the tongue lesions.

On the foot, the vesicles appear on the coronary band. Pressure on the hoof results in pain and causes the animal to limp. Separation of the hoof wall from its underlying structure has been reported, and the result has been loss of the entire hoof (Heiny, 1945). Long after healing, the site of the lesion may be apparent from the ring of connective tissue which forms during the repair process. Both foot and mouth lesions may be observed in a single animal.

The pathogenesis of this infection has not been studied in the horse. Presumably it follows the pattern described for the pig (Chow and McNutt, 1953). In this species, the virus enters through an abrasion in the epithelium. Exposed cells are penetrated, and the virus multiplies within them and is released in a matter of a few hours. Since the virus can generalize in natural cases and often generalizes if it is inoculated intravenously (Cotton, 1926), there must be a transitory viremia even though virus has rarely been detected in the blood. The macular and papular stages are ephemeral and rarely seen in natural cases. Even the vesicle which varies in diameter from a few millimeters to 3 centimeters ruptures so rapidly, particularly where the epithelium is delicate or where the surface is subject to trauma, that it may not be observed (Brandly et al., 1951). In some instances, the vesicle may persist as long as 24 hours. Usually, the rectal temperature falls when rupture occurs and the amount of saliva produced increases. The animal is least inclined to feed at this time because of the painfulness of mastication.

Lesions: The first sign of change visible microscopically is separation of the epithelial cells in the Malpighian layer (Chow and Mc-Nutt, 1953). The intercellular bridges between the prickle cells are stretched by edematous fluid which accumulates in the intercellular spaces, forming small vacuoles. A large number of small vacuoles give the appearance of swelling, evident on the surface as a macule. As neighboring vacuoles become confluent, a transparent bleb, the vesicle, can be seen on the surface. At this point multilocular, intercellular edema is scattered throughout the thickened Malpighian layer. Atop the vesicle is a thin layer of spongiotic epithelial tissue and keratinized cells. Deeper cells disarranged by the intercellular edema suffer degenerative changes characterized by the disappearance of the protoplasmic intercellular bridges and gradual loss of cytoplasm. Nuclear pyknosis and karyolysis are evident. The process extends downward into the dermis, disrupting and infiltrating the basal cell layer. There may be edema and hemorrhage in the dermal papillae, engorgement of the lymph and blood vessels, and perivascular leukocytic infiltration.

The specific pathology of vesicular stomatitis is limited to the epithelial tissues. Secondary infection may follow, and mixed infections are possible. Radeleff (1949) reported from Texas what was probably a mixed infection. Several horses suffering from vesicular stomatitis developed a central nervous system disturbance. A mare and her colt displayed similar signs: violent seizures, profuse sweating, a respiration rate that rose to 45, a pulse that varied from 20 to 120, and a rectal temperature of 104 F. The colt died. Virus was not isolated from these animals.

Frank et al. (1945) experimentally induced a similar fatal disease in horses which he had inoculated intracerebrally with vesicular stomatitis virus, New Jersey type. In 1955, the U. S. Public Health Service received a brain from a cow that was presumed to have died from rabies. Rabies virus was not demonstrated. Although antisera to the agent isolated would neutralize the New Jersey type vesicular stomatitis, antisera prepared to vesicular stomatitis would not neutralize the agent. This is what one would expect if the disease were caused by a mixed infection. The possibility that vesicular stomatitis can act synergistically with other infections and produce fatal disease of cattle and horses needs further study.

Immunity: Within 10 days to 2 weeks after development of infection in horses, neutralizing and complement fixing antibodies may be detected in blood (Hanson, 1952; Bankowski and Kummer, 1955; Jenney et al., 1958). The titer of both increase for 2 to 4 weeks and then persist at a high level, with some variations, for many months. The complement fixing titer has been observed to disappear before the neutralizing titer in cattle and swine (Mulhern,

1958). The persistence of either in horses has not been determined. Horses are refractory to re-exposure a month after infection; and though the immunity has been broken by introducing large quantities of virus, it appears to be reasonably firm.

In the enzootic areas of Georgia and South Carolina, clinical cases of vesicular stomatitis in horses are seldom seen (Hanson and Karstad, 1959). Presumably, the animals become immune as colts, possibly while they are still carrying a measure of antibody from the mare. All individuals which have been tested from that area have been shown to have neutralizing antibodies, and it has not been possible to find a horse that is susceptible to experimental infection. Neutralizing antibodies have been shown to persist in cattle that have been isolated from the disease for 7 years. Persistence in horses is likely to be as long. There is no evidence that horses which have recovered from a given serotype can be naturally reinfected by that serotype. There is no cross immunity between the two virus infections, nor is there cross serologic reaction as measured by the neutralization or complement fixation tests (Brooksby, 1948). On the other hand, using the Ouchterlony precipitation test in gel, it has been possible to show that a common antigen is possessed by New Jersey and Indiana vesicular stomatitis viruses (Myers, 1961).

Host Range: Vesicular stomatitis virus has been isolated from diseased horses, cattle, and hogs. Ample serologic evidence of natural infection of these species as well as of man has been obtained. Infection of sheep and dogs has been suspected upon clinical grounds but has not been confirmed on the basis of serology (Hanson, 1952). Serologic studies, on the other hand, have revealed that several wild animals, the white-tailed deer, feral swine, raccoon, and the bobcat, frequently are infected in regions where the disease is enzootic (Karstad *et al.*, 1956).

Most of the human infections which have been studied have been those of laboratory workers. The virus has been isolated on 2 occasions and the serologic response measured for more than a hundred cases (Fellowes *et al.*, 1955). The disease resembles influenza in that it is marked by fever and chills and severe muscular pains. Mucosal lesions may be observed but usually are absent. In some enzootic areas, such as southern Georgia, up to 25% of the population tested possessed significant antibody titers (Hanson and Karstad, 1959).

The experimental host range of vesicular stomatitis includes 6 rodent-like animals: mouse, rat, guinea pig, chinchilla, rabbits, hamster; 2 carnivores: raccoon and ferret; and 2 primates: the rhesus and cynomologus monkeys and the domestic chicken (Olitsky, 1927; Fellowes *et al.*, 1955). In these experimental animals, clinical disease, if it is induced, is either epitheliotropic following intradermal injection or neurotropic when inoculation is intracerebral. Aerosols and nasal sprays have produced disease in young mice, chinchillas, and ferrets. Contact transmission has been observed only among young pigs and adult ferrets.

Epizootiology: On the basis of the historical epizootics of vesicular stomatitis, it is quite apparent that the disease does not spread at random through the population of susceptible animals in the United States. Spread is also independent of population density. Certain topographic features seem to favor dissemination. Heiny (1945) pointed out that in Colorado the disease spread along streams rather than along commercial arteries of traffic. This was also true in the Middle West in 1937 and 1949. The disease, for the most part, has been restricted to areas in which streams and wetlands are relatively abundant. It has occurred most frequently among animals in wooded pastures.

The seasonal incidence of the disease is equally striking. On the basis of a tabulation of all reported cases of vesicular stomatitis by month over a 30-year-period, 90% occurred in August and September. Few cases have occurred in July and October. Only rarely in the United States is the disease seen as early as April or as late as November. Cases are more apt to be seen earlier and later in the states bordering the Gulf of Mexico than in states near the Canadian border.

In Georgia, sentinel swine did not become infected before April or after October (Hanson and Karstad, 1959). During the summer the disease could be detected by setting out susceptible sentinel swine when clinical cases were not observed in livestock in any of the adjoining counties. Even further south where there is no frost, as in Mexico, Venezuela, and Colombia, the disease though seen every year has not been seen during all months of the year. Camargo (1954) reported, on the basis of several years of observation in Mexico, that the disease is confined almost entirely to the rainy season.

Vesicular stomatitis appears to have a reservoir in frost-free areas of America and from these centers the disease spreads northward as opportunity permits during the warm months, invading only those regions in which conditions for transmission are satisfactory. The epizootic factors seem to include forest cover, proximity to wetlands, and the presence of susceptible animals.

The disease can be considered enzootic as it exists in warm climates where it reappears annually and where a portion of the susceptible animal population always possesses antibodies. The disease is epizootic in cold climates where it appears irregularly and where the susceptible animals usually are free of antibodies. Infections of wildlife, man, and swine are characteristic of areas in which the disease is enzootic. In the epizootic areas, the infection is recognized primarily as a clinical disease of horses and cattle.

Transmission among cattle and horses was once believed to occur by contact. Theiler in 1901 was first to point out that the disease was transmitted with difficulty or not at all, even when animals were in close contact, unless abrasions were present in or around the mouth. Cotton in his description of the 1926 New Jersey outbreak and Heiny in his observations on Colorado outbreaks pointed out that it often is impossible to explain dissemination by contact. The many field observations of seasonal prevalence, of the rapid spread along water courses, and of failure to spread in open pasture and stables suggest that a vector is instrumental in the transmission of the disease.

Ferris *et al.* demonstrated, in 1954, that vesicular stomatitis virus could be transmitted under laboratory conditions by several species of biting Diptera. Transmission in each instance was mechanical. The biting parts, con-taminated while feeding on a infected animal, were capable of transmitting the virus for a period of 3 or 4 days to a susceptible individual. The insects which Ferris used successfully included mosquitoes, stable flies, and horse flies.

In the period since that time, attempts made to isolate virus from insects captured in enzootic areas have been unsuccessful. Isolation of virus has not been attempted from insects captured during an epizootic.

Roberts *et al.* (1956) studied the population of potential vectors in the area in Wisconsin in which two epizootics had occurred. He showed that the population varied from year to year in respect to species composition and numbers. Some species which were abundant in the spring of one year would be found in large numbers only in the fall of another year. Some species increased in numbers over the 3 years of study and others decreased. The insects which might be vectors of the virus were not distributed evenly in the study area. Wetland pastures had a very different insect population than did dryland pastures. The presence or absence of tree cover in the pasture also modified the population.

Diagnosis: Presumptive diagnosis of vesicular stomatitis of horses on clinical grounds is not difficult. Other viral or bacterial infections do not produce in horses a similar set of signs and lesions. Cattle and swine are susceptible to foot-and-mouth disease and vesicular exanthema, entities that are clinically indistinguishable from vesicular stomatitis. Foot-and-mouth disease does not affect horses, and vesicular exanthema was found to be infective for them only on one occasion. Subsequent isolates have not been shown to be pathogenic for horses. Caustic substances and photosensitivity may produce lesions in horses which simulate those of vesicular stomatitis. Usually the history would be sufficient to distinguish noninfectious and infectious diseases.

A diagnosis of vesicular stomatitis is confirmed by isolation of the virus or demonstration of an increase in specific antibody (Table 2). A bit of epithelium, saliva or vesicular fluid from an infected horse contains enough virus to infect susceptible laboratory hosts. Either chicken embryo or the mouse is satisfactory (Karstad and Hanson, 1958). The presence of virus in suspected material usually can be determined within 48 to 72 hours. Identification of the isolate would be dependent upon further study, such as determination of its host range or its serologic identity. If vesicular fluid is available, rapid identification of vesicular stomatitis can be made by using it as an antigen in a complement fixation test (Jenney et al., 1958). A properly equipped laboratory can make the diagnosis in a matter of a few hours.

Animals that recover from vesicular stomatitis infection possess antibodies to the virus which may be detected in several ways. The neutralization test is sensitive and dependable. Sera to be tested are mixed with a quantity of virus and inoculated into a susceptible host. If antibodies are present, the virus is neutralized and the host survives. If antibodies are not present, the virus produces its characteristic lesion. The test is quantitative. From 1,000 to 10,000 neutralizing doses are usually possessed by convalescent animals a month after infection.

The complement fixation test can be used to detect antibodies. Several alternate procedures have been studied and are employed in some laboratories to detect antibodies to vesicular stomatitis virus.

Prevention and Control: Treatment of vesicular stomatitis is symptomatic. The animal should be made as comfortable as possible and provided with plenty of water and soft feed. If there is indication of a complicating infection, proper therapeutic procedures should be utilized. Ordinarily, recovery is prompt and complete.

Holbrook and Geleta (1957) have studied the possibility of preparing a killed vesicular stomatitis virus vaccine for use in swine. Intramuscular inoculation of cattle with live virus usually results in an inapparent infection and a long-lasting immunity. Planned exposure of cattle is practiced in some enzootic areas to avoid disease complications during lactation. Neither killed nor live virus has been tried with the intent to immunize horses. One might suspect that the horse, which is apparently more susceptible than the cow, would develop clinical disease if live virus were given. Owners

Table 2.—Diagnosis of Vesicular Stomatitis by Isolation of the Virus

Laboratory Host	Procedure	Result
Tissue culture	Inoculate 0.1 ml. on chicken fibroblasts grown on glass.	Virus induces cytopathogenic effect in 2 to 3 days.
Chicken embryo	Inoculate 0.1 ml. into allantoic sac of 8-day embryo.	Virus kills the embryo in 3 to 4 days.
Mouse	Inoculate 0.03 ml. intracerebrally in 3-week-old mice.	Virus induces paralysis and death in 2 to 3 days.
Chicken	Inoculate 0.03 ml. into the tongue epithelium.	Virus induces the development of a vesicle on the tongue in 1 to 2 days.
Guinea pig	Inoculate 0.03 ml. intradermally in the foot pad.	Virus induces the development of a vesicle on the foot pad in 2 to 4 days.

who move horses in and out of areas in which the disease is active might consider seriously the use of a killed virus vaccine.

Prevention of vesicular stomatitis has been based primarily on management. An animal which is kept stabled and protected from attack by insects apparently has little chance of becoming infected even in an area in which the disease is being transmitted. Animals on open, upland pastures apparently have much less chance developing the disease than those in lowland, wooded pastures.

R. P. Hanson

REFERENCES

Bachrach, H. L., Callis, J. J. and Hess, W. R.: The growth and cytopathogenicity of vesicular stomatitis virus in tissue culture. J. Immunol. 75 (1955) 186.

Bankowski, R. A. and Kummer, M. B.: Vesicular stomatitis and vesicular exanthema differentiation by complement fixation. Amer. J. Vet. Res. 16 (1955) 374.

Bradish, C. J., Brooksby, J. B. and Dillon, J. F., Jr.: Biophysical studies of the virus system of vesicular stomatitis. J. Gen. Microbiol. 14 (1956) 290.

Brandly, C. A., Hanson, R. P. and Chow, T. L.: Vesicular stomatitis with particular reference to the 1949 Wisconsin epizootic. Proc. Book, 88th Ann. Meet. A. V. M. A., (1951) p. 61.

Brooksby, J. B.: Vesicular stomatitis and foot-and-mouth disease differentiation by complement fixation. Proc. Soc. Exper. Biol. and Med. 67 (1948) 254.

Burnet, F. M., and Galloway, I. A.: The propagation of the virus of vesicular stomatitis in the chorioallantoic membranes of the developing hen's egg. Brit. J. Exper. Path. 15 (1934) 105.

Burton, A. C.: Stomatitis contagiosa in horses. Vet. J. **73** (1917) 234.

Camargo, N. C.: A contribution to the study of vesicular stomatitis in Mexico. U. S. Livestock San. Assn. **58** (1954) 379.

Chow, T. L., Chow, Fuho and Hanson, R. P.: Morphology of vesicular stomatitis virus. J. Bact. **68** (1954) 724.

Chow, T. L. and McNutt, S. H.: Pathological changes of experimental vesicular stomatitis of swine. Amer. J. Vet. Res. **14** (1953) 420.

Cotton, W. E.: The causal agent of vesicular stomatitis proved to be a filter-passing virus. J.A.V.M.A. **70** (1926) 168.

Cotton, W. E.: Vesicular stomatitis. Vet. Med. **22** (1927) 169.

Cox, H. R. and Olitsky, P. K.: Neutrotropism of vesicular stomatitis virus. Proc. Soc. Exper. Biol. and Med. **30** (1933) 653.

Cunha, R. G., Eichhorn, E. A. and Mata, F. O.: Differentiation between foot-and-mouth disease and vesicular stomatitis viruses by means of mouse inoculation. Amer. J. Vet. Res. **16** (1955) 472.

Fellowes, O. N., Dimopoullos, G. T. and Callis, J. J.: Isolation of vesicular stomatitis virus from an infected laboratory worker. Amer. J. Vet. Res. **16** (1955) 623.

Fellowes, O. N., Dimopoullos, G. T., Tessler, J., Hess, W. R., Vardaman, T. H. and Callis, J. J.: Comparative titrations of vesicular stomatitis in various animal species and in tissue culture. Amer. J. Vet. Res. **27** (1956) 799.

Ferris, D., Hanson, R. P., Dicke, R. J. and Roberts, R. H.: Experimental transmission of vesicular stomatitis virus by Diptera. J. Infec. Dis. **96** (1955) 184.

Frank, A. H., Appleby, A. and Seibold, H. R.: Experimental intracerebral infection of horses, cattle and sheep with the virus of vesicular stomatitis. Amer. J. Vet. Res. **6** (1945) 28.

Galloway, I. A. and Elford, W. J.: The differentiation of the virus of vesicular stomatitis from the virus of foot-and mouth disease by filtration. Brit. J. Exptl. Path. **14** (1933) 400.

Gregg, J., McGuire, F. X., Glover, G. J., Gillespie, A. and Gregory, G.: Vesicular stomatitis contagiosa. Amer. J. Vet. Med. **12** (1917) 221.

Hanson, R. P.: The natural history of vesicular stomatitis virus. Bact. Rev. **16** (1952) 179.

Hanson, R. P., Rasmussen, A. F., Brandly, C. A. and Brown, J. W.: Human infection with the virus of vesicular stomatitis. J. Lab. and Clin. Med. **36** (1950) 754.

Hanson, R. P. and Karstad, L.: Feral swine as a reservoir of vesicular stomatitis virus in southeastern United States. Proc. U. S. Livestock San. Assn. **62** (1959) 309.

Heiny, F.: Vesicular stomatitis in cattle and horses in Colorado. No. Amer. Vet. **26** (1945) 726.

Holbrook, A. A. and Geleta, J. N.: Vesicular stomatitis immunization with inactivated vaccines of chicken embryo origin. U. S. Livestock San. Assn. **61** (1957) 308.

Holbrook, A. A. and Patterson, W. C.: The use of chickens in the differential diagnosis of vesicular exanthema and vesicular stomatitis. J.A.V.M.A. **131** (1957) 196.

Jacoulet, M.: Au sujet d'une stomatite érosive de nature indéterminée (chez le cheval). Bull. soc. cent. med. vet. **68** (1915) 576.

Jenney, E. W., Mott, L. O. and Traub, E.: Serological studies with the virus of vesicular stomatitis. I. Typing of vesicular stomatitis by complement fixation. Amer. J. Vet. Res. **19** (1958) 993.

Karstad, L. H., Adams, E. V., Hanson, R. P. and Ferris, D. H.: Evidence for the role of wildlife in epizootics of vesicular stomatitis. J.A.V.M.A. **129** (1956) 95.

Karstad, L. H. and Hanson, R. P.: Primary isolation and comparative titrations of five field strains of vesicular stomatitis virus in chicken embryos, hogs and mice. Amer. J. Vet. Res. **19** (1958) 233.

Lamb, C. G.: Discussion. J.A.V.M.A. **52** (1918) 419.

McClain, M. E. and Hackett, A. J.: A comparative study of the growth of vesicular stomatitis virus in the tissue culture systems. J. Immunol. **80** (1958) 356.

Mulhern, F. J.: Report of the committee on vesicular diseases. Proc. U. S. Livestock San. Assn. **63** (1958) 346.

Myers, W. L.: Some immunochemical aspects of vesicular stomatitis virus infection. Doctoral thesis, University of Wisconsin (1961).

Olitsky, P. K.: Physical, chemical and biological studies on virus of vesicular stomatitis of horses. J. Exper. Med. **45** (1927) 969.

Patterson, W. C., Holbrook, A. A., Hopkins, S. R. and Songer, J. R.: The effect of chemical and physical agents on the viruses of vesicular stomatitis and vesicular exanthema. Proc. U. S. Livestock San. Assn. **62** (1958) 294.

Radeleff, R. D.: Clinical encephalitis occurring during an outbreak of vesicular stomatitis in horses. Vet. Med. **44** (1949) 494.

Roberts, R. H., Dicke, R. J., Hanson, R. P. and Ferris, D. H.: Potential insect vectors of vesicular stomatitis in Wisconsin. J. Infec. Dis. **98** (1956) 121.

Shahan, M. S.: Effect of temperature, phenol and crystal violet on vesicular stomatitis virus. Amer. J. Vet. Res. **7** (1946) 27.

Skinner, H. H.: Infection of chickens and chick embryos with the viruses of foot-and-mouth disease and of vesicular stomatitis. Nature (London) **174** (1954) 1052.

Spencer, J. S.: Communication from Noiceiter, Maryland. Amer. Farmer **8** (1826) 283.

Teidebold, T. C., Mather, C. S. and Merrillat, L. A.: Gangrenous glossitis of horses. U. S. Livestock San. Assn. **20** (1916) 29.

Theiler, S.: Eine contagiöse Stomatitis des Pferds in Süd-Afrika. Deut. tierärztl. Wochschr. **9** (1901) 131.

Wagener, K.: Foot-and-mouth disease and vesicular stomatitis. J.A.V.M.A. **80** (1932) 39.

NEUROTROPIC VIRAL DISEASES

Among the important neurotropic viral diseases of the horse are the arthropod-borne encephalitides, rabies and Borna disease. The arthropod-borne encephalitides include the three equine types found in North and South America, *viz.*, eastern, western, and Venezuelan equine encephalomyelitis as well as Japanese encephalitis which affects horses in the Far East. Borna disease, frequently referred to as a type of equine encephalitis, is immunologically unrelated to the arthropod-borne encephalitides, and, as far as is known, is not transmitted naturally by arthropod vectors. Rabies also is distinct from the other neurotropic viral diseases and is spread to horses by the bite of other animals.

THE ARTHROPOD-BORNE VIRAL ENCEPHALITIDES

The term, arthropod-borne encephalitides, was first suggested in 1943 by Hammond and Reeves to designate those neurotropic viral diseases transmitted in nature by insect vectors. This group includes the Venezuelan, eastern, and western types of equine encephalomyelitis as well as St. Louis encephalitis, Japanese encephalitis, and Russian spring-summer encephalitis. Later, Casals, using a variety of serologic tests, established a classification scheme which included the arthropod-borne encephalitides as well as a number of other viral diseases not necessarily affecting the nervous system.[1] Casals used the term, Arbor viruses, to designate the members included in his classification scheme. Thus far, there are

Table 3.—Representative Members of Groups A and B Arbor Viruses

GROUP A:	GROUP B:
Venezuelan Equine Encephalomyelitis	Japanese Encephalitis
Eastern Equine Encephalomyelitis	St. Louis Encephalitis
Western Equine Encephalomyelitis	Russian Spring-Summer Encephalitis
Semliki Forest	Louping Ill
Sindbis	Yellow Fever

three major groups of Arbor viruses. Members from Groups A and B are listed in Table 3. Other groups of Arbor viruses include the causative agents of Rift Valley Fever, Colorado Tick Fever and California encephalitis. Within groups, cross relationships between individual members can be demonstrated by use of hemagglutination-inhibition and neutralization tests. This relationship within groups is most pronounced in Group B. In Group A, on the other hand, there are less cross-reactions, although it now appears that the viruses causing Venezuelan and eastern equine encephalomyelitis are immunologically closer than was once realized.[2] Western equine encephalomyelitis virus appears to be distinct from those causing eastern and Venezuelan equine encephalomyelitis, but it is immunologically related to Sindbis virus.[3]

Public Health Significance: In certain areas of the world, the arthropod-borne encephalitides are significant causes of human disease and death. Among the four major types which affect both horses and man, Japanese encephalitis and western equine encephalomyelitis cause the most serious public health problems. Eastern equine encephalomyelitis is a rarity in man, considering both the clinically recognizable form and inapparent infections. Although Venezuelan equine encephalomyelitis is not an uncommon infection of man in South America, fortunately, it is rarely a fatal disease.

Epizootiology: Although there are still many gaps in our knowledge of the epizootiology and epidemiology of the arthropod-borne encephalitides, a generally accepted pattern has emerged as a result of extensive ecologic studies on representative members of the group. It generally is accepted that Japanese encephalitis and western equine encephalomyelitis are transmitted from infected mosquitoes to birds. The virus multiplies in the avian

hosts and, for a few days, the birds serve as a source of infection for mosquitoes which feed on their blood. If the mosquito which feeds on an infected bird is a biologic vector, the virus will multiply in its body and appear finally in the salivary glands. Presumably, the infected mosquito then transmits the virus to other vertebrate hosts during probing action at the time of feeding. If the mosquito's victim happens to be a susceptible vertebrate, such as a horse or a man, the resulting infection may lead to disease of the central nervous system.

The epizootiology of eastern equine encephalomyelitis is not as well understood as that of Japanese encephalitis or western equine encephalomyelitis. Although it is generally accepted that birds and mosquitoes are involved, a single consistent pattern of infection has not yet emerged.

Even less is known about the epizootiology of Venezuelan equine encephalomyelitis. Presumably, mosquitoes are the chief vectors of this infection, but there are some doubts as to the chief reservoirs of the virus. Furthermore, contact infection between animals is possible.

Role of the Horse: Although both eastern and western equine encephalomyelitis were recognized as virus diseases during horse plagues occurring in the early 1930's in the United States, the first investigators pointed out that horses were not the common source of infection and that the disease was not highly communicable. Therefore, the appellation "equine" was not used to imply that the horse spread the disease, but simply to indicate that horses were the chief victims, which probably is still true today.

In general, it can be said that horses, like man, do not perpetuate eastern equine encephalomyelitis, western equine encephalomyelitis or Japanese encephalitis. The horse is probably a complete "dead-end" in the case of western equine encephalomyelitis. Possibly, the same is true of Japanese encephalitis, although experimental transmission from one horse to another via infected mosquitoes has been accomplished.[4] In the case of eastern equine encephalomyelitis, viremia is a rather consistent finding in the infected horse. Therefore, it is possible that under certain circumstances, the horse could serve as a source of infection for mosquitoes, but it should be emphasized that these situations are rare.

Eastern Equine Encephalomyelitis

History, Distribution and Incidence: Eastern equine encephalomyelitis (blind staggers, eastern encephalitis, eastern viral encephalomyelitis) was observed and described in horses as early as 1831 in Massachusetts. In all probability, eastern equine encephalomyelitis existed as an infection in North American wildlife prior to introduction into the New World of the modern horse by early European settlers. The disease has occurred along the Atlantic coast and in the states bordering the Gulf of Mexico in epizootic proportions, particularly in 1900, 1901, 1933, 1938, 1947, 1956, and 1959. The reported incidence of infectious equine encephalomyelitis has been recorded by the U. S. Department of Agriculture since 1938, but these figures do not separate the incidence of eastern and western equine encephalomyelitis. From my personal experience in accumulating and comparing estimates of the incidence of the disease with official figures, it appears that there is a tendency to underestimate losses due to this entity.

Eastern equine encephalomyelitis occurs most frequently in pastured animals during the summer and they may die or disappear without notification of a veterinarian or the proper livestock control authorities. In some instances, not all suspected or confirmed cases are reported to the U.S.D.A. in time for their annual report. For example, although the U.S.D.A. reported only 8,800 cases of infectious equine encephalomyelitis in horses, ponies, and mules for the United States in 1947, a careful analysis by the State of Louisiana revealed that there had been more than 14,000 cases in Louisiana alone that year, most of them presumably of the eastern type.[5]

The designation "eastern" does not serve accurately as a descriptive term for the geographic distribution of the disease. Eastern equine encephalomyelitis has been confirmed in horses in Canada, Mexico, South and Central America, and in island areas of the Caribbean as well as in southwestern sections of the United States. Furthermore, the virus of eastern equine encephalomyelitis reportedly has occurred in the Philippine Islands in monkeys.[6]

Epizootiology: The epizootiology of eastern equine encephalomyelitis is not well-understood. According to evidence thus far advanced, there are two cycles of infection which involve birds and mosquitoes. The first, or sylvan cycle, involves a fresh-water swamp mosquito, *Culiseta melanura,* and various swamp-dwelling birds along the Atlantic Coast and the Gulf of Mexico. In some way, the virus is kept alive or maintained year after year without doing any appreciable harm to man or beast. During some years, however, the infection spreads from this woodland cycle and "spills over" to other birds, most probably small commensal birds such as the English sparrow and cardinal. From these birds, the infection is spread further by other mosquitoes which attack horses, man, and other vertebrates. It is this explosive type of multiplication that accounts for epizootics and epidemics of the disease. Man is probably a dead-end host and the same might be said for horses, although, under certain circumstances, unvaccinated horses could serve to amplify and enhance viral activity, particularly in the presence of large numbers of easily infected mosquitoes.

The Virus: The virus of eastern equine encephalomyelitis is quite small, measuring about 40-60 mμ. It has a wide host range and is adaptable to a variety of living organisms and tissue culture systems. Eastern equine encephalomyelitis virus is highly pathogenic for guinea pigs, mice, rabbits, day-old chicks, and embryonating eggs. Antigens for hemagglutination-inhibition and complement fixation tests can be prepared readily from tissues, eggs and tissue culture fluids infected with the virus.

Clinical Signs in Horses: To the practitioner observing an early case of eastern equine encephalomyelitis, the most obvious signs are marked depression and a high fever. The course of the disease is short—usually not more than 2 to 3 days elapse before death. Cutaneous reflexes are diminished. Drooping of the lower lip, oscillation of the eyeballs, a distinct reluctance to move and a marked incoordination, particularly on turning, are other characteristic signs. Animals are quite apt to act in a bizarre way during final stages of the disease, and are known to have walked through the sides of buildings, to have knocked down walls, and to have climbed to the top of woodpiles and other obstacles. Once recumbent and unable to rise, an animal may dig a trench in the ground by a continuous running motion with its front legs.

Prognosis: The prognosis in eastern equine encephalomyelitis is extremely poor, since the mortality in clinically recognized cases is 90% and permanent brain damage is common in those animals which survive. Occasionally, however, affected horses make a complete recovery.[7]

Diagnosis: Along with clinical findings, one must consider the place and time of occurrence of the case. The current appearance of other cases in the region also would aid in establishing a provisional diagnosis. Obviously, the laboratory confirmation of early cases in a particular area would assist greatly state livestock control authorities and public health officials as well as practicing veterinarians. By confirming early-season cases of eastern equine encephalomyelitis, the lives of other horses could be saved if information were to be disseminated quickly and immunization procedures instituted. Though it is true that several weeks are required for commercial vaccines to induce good protection, the incidence of late-season cases might be reduced.

Even for the experienced veterinary practitioner, sporadic cases of eastern equine encephalomyelitis pose a problem in differential diagnosis. Among other diseases that might be confused with eastern equine encephalomyelitis are botulism, rabies, and tetanus. Although reports of listeriosis in horses are rare, this disease should also be considered. Still another

syndrome that could be confused with eastern equine encephalomyelitis, or western equine encephalomyelitis for that matter, is the condition initially called "X-disease" of horses. This disease chiefly involves the liver, but the affected animals often exhibit signs indistinguishable from the equine encephalitides. It is of interest that a significant number of cases of "toxic hepatitis," similar to "X-disease," were seen in the Philadelphia area in 1959. Among the many cases of hepatitis, one of eastern equine encephalomyelitis was separated from the others by careful laboratory studies.[8] The cause of equine "X-disease" is still unknown although workers in 1938 associated many of the cases with the use of serum-virus immunization against equine encephalomyelitis.

From the practitioner's point of view, every effort should be made to obtain laboratory confirmation of early cases of eastern equine encephalomyelitis. There are two chief methods of accomplishing this: (1) through examination of serial serum samples from affected animals, and (2) examination of brain from horses which die or must be killed.

To accomplish serologic confirmation, one must obtain serum samples during the first time the affected animal is seen and several days to 2 weeks later. Admittedly, this is rarely possible in cases of eastern equine encephalomyelitis since affected animals usually die 2 to 3 days after the early signs are noted. A rise in titer in the paired serum samples is considered confirmation of eastern equine encephalomyelitis. It also should be noted that animals dying of eastern equine encephalomyelitis almost invariably have hemagglutination-inhibition titers as well as detectable neutralization antibody. Although examination of single serum samples has limited value, it has been our experience that a negative hemagglutination-inhibition test on an acutely sick animal will almost always rule out eastern equine encephalomyelitis.

Although removal and processing of the brain for laboratory examination is a tedious undertaking, the reasons for establishing an early diagnosis are nevertheless compelling. In removing the brain, the operator should wear heavy rubber gloves and take extreme precautions in handling saws, knives, and axes. It should be emphasized that a puncture wound by a splinter of contaminated bone could have grave consequences. A good description of the technic for removing the brain of a horse may be found in Chapter 1.[9]

Histologic examination of the brain of suspected horses is conducted to determine the presence of characteristic microscopic lesions. The isolation and identification of eastern equine encephalomyelitis virus is, of course, the final and indisputable confirmation of the disease. There are times, however, when the histopathologic examination strongly suggests eastern equine encephalomyelitis and yet the virus cannot be isolated from the brain. This is true especially in those cases which linger for more than 3 or 4 days before dying or being killed. Under these circumstances, positive histologic findings could only furnish a presumptive diagnosis which could be strengthened further by positive serologic findings.

It is unfortunate that many state livestock diagnostic facilities do not examine serum or brain specimens for eastern equine encephalomyelitis; therefore, veterinarians must often rely on public health laboratories and other agencies. If specimens are submitted to public health laboratories during a busy period, the animal specimens might receive a low priority. It is the opinion of the author that regional cooperative laboratories involving groups of states could best handle this problem. To be ready for any contingency, the laboratory should have trained, properly immunized personnel, and a dependable source of animals. Other essential requirements include stock strains of virus and immune sera, as well as capabilities for producing antigens and conducting serologic tests.

A detailed description of laboratory methods for confirmation of equine encephalitis is given elsewhere.[10]

Treatment: Since so few affected animals survive the disease, there is little information available on the best means of treatment. Suffice it to say that all means possible should be used to keep the animal comfortable, protect it from injury, and maintain body fluid levels. The use of saline laxatives may also be indicated.

There is little scientific basis for the use of specific immune serums in treating the disease, although some clinical reports indicate otherwise. As pointed out before, by the time clinical signs of disease appear, there is also neutralizing antibody present in the circulating blood. It is evident that the virus is capable of multiplying in the brain and producing damage despite the presence of circulating antibody. Therefore, the parenteral administration of immune serum can do little to mitigate the disease.

Prevention and Control: Annual immunization of horses and other equine species is recommended in all areas having a history of epizootics. Animals which may be moved to or through epizootic or enzootic areas during the encephalitis season also should be immunized.

Although annual springtime vaccination is generally recommended, this could just as well be done in the northeastern United States in June or early July. Further, horse owners on the fringe of enzootic areas could be advised of the relatively low risk and have their animals immunized only in the threat of a widespread epizootic.

In view of the fact that eastern and western equine encephalomyelitis viruses are not restricted geographically as once thought, bivalent vaccines, which protect against both virus types, are to be recommended. Commercial vaccines are administered intradermally in 2 doses at 7 to 10 day intervals. If the manufacturer's recommendations are carefully followed, there are very few sequelae from vaccination and, more important, the vaccine is effective in preventing the disease.

The use of specific immune serum in protecting animals which might be exposed to the virus may be indicated under certain circumstances. However, this serum is no longer readily available.

In the face of an epizootic of eastern equine encephalomyelitis, every effort should be made to protect susceptible animals from mosquitoes and biting flies. Significantly, stabled horses and those at race tracks are not affected often. Application of mosquito control methods is recommended strongly during transportation of animals.

There seems little scientific basis for restricting the movement of horses during an epizootic of eastern equine encephalomyelitis. In the first place, infected horses rarely have enough virus in their blood to infect mosquitoes (with the possible exception of the salt marsh mosquito, *Aedes sollicitans*). Secondly, it would require an unusual set of circumstances to have an infected horse transported to a disease-free area and serve as a source of virus for the indigenous mosquito population. More than likely, the biologic factors favorable for the perpetuation of the eastern equine encephalomyelitis virus exist only in certain areas of the United States and introduction of an infected vertebrate into an unsuitable region would result in an end to activity of the virus.

In summary, control of eastern equine encephalomyelitis hinges on vaccination of susceptible horses which may become exposed to the infection and protection of animals from potential vectors during an epizootic period.

WESTERN EQUINE ENCEPHALOMYELITIS (WESTERN ENCEPHALITIS)

As with other diseases indigenous to the New World, the history of western equine encephalomyelitis is obscured by lack of early reports and documentation. What was probably western equine encephalomyelitis was described in the latter part of the nineteenth century and through the early part of this century. In 1930, a highly fatal disease of horses and mules in the San Joaquin Valley of California was found due to a filtrable virus. Subsequent studies proved that this virus was unrelated to the agent of Borna disease, the cause of equine encephalitis in Germany. When the causative agent of equine encephalomyelitis along the eastern cost of the United States was revealed in 1933, it soon was established that this agent differed from the virus causing equine encephalomyelitis in California and other western states.

Western equine encephalomyelitis is found primarily in the western and midwestern United States. In at least a few states, among them Texas and Louisiana, both eastern and western equine encephalomyelitis have been found in horses. The virus of western equine encephalomyelitis has been recovered from birds in New Jersey[11] but there is no evidence that human or animal disease has resulted from its presence there. Reports of finding western equine encephalomyelitis in Czechoslovakia await further confirmation.[12]

The significance of western equine encephalomyelitis is evident from the fact that more than 100,000 horses were affected in the 1938 outbreak. Despite the drop in horse population due to farm mechanization, the disease remains a serious threat to the valuable farm animals which remain, as well as to light horses and ponies. The unpredictable nature of the arthropod-borne encephalitides justifies continued research and vigilance concerning these diseases.

Public Health Aspects: Western equine encephalomyelitis is a considerably greater public health problem than the eastern type. Outbreaks of the disease in man have been more numerous and more severe. The horse is strictly a dead-end host in the western equine encephalomyelitis cycle since blood-virus levels in infected horses are either undetectable or insignificant. Therefore, public health aspects of the problem are unrelated to the horse. The urgent need for reporting and confirming early cases in horses is based on the fact that public health officials could be alerted for possible human infections. Thus, the horse may be considered a sentinel for the disease by serving as an early warning to man of its presence and activity.

The Virus: The virus of western equine encephalomyelitis resembles that of eastern equine encephalomyelitis in so many respects that a detailed discussion of it is unwarranted here. Suffice it to say that it is a member of the "A" group of Arbor viruses. On the basis of cross-protection tests, it is not related to the virus of eastern equine encephalomyelitis. However, there are a few subtle relationships detected when hemagglutination-inhibition and complement fixation studies are used to compare these two viruses. Of all the group A viruses, western equine encephalomyelitis is most closely related to Sindbis,[3] which, as nearly as can be ascertained, causes no disease in horses. The possible application of this relationship as an immunologic procedure merits investigation.

The epizootiology and epidemiology of western equine encephalomyelitis have been investigated rather extensively and are better understood than is the natural history of eastern equine encephalomyelitis. It is well-established that the mosquito, *Culex tarsalis*, is the chief vector of western equine encephalomyelitis. Probably wild birds are the primary reservoir of the virus during an epizootic but the agent of western equine encephalomyelitis has also been found in wild mammals and even reptiles. As stated previously, the horse may be safely considered a dead-end host. Though it seems clear that wild birds are the chief reservoirs of western equine encephalomyelitis virus, it is not certain which species of avian hosts are primarily involved or whether one could substitute for another depending on the locality.

Clinical Pathology: What has been said concerning the clinical pathologic aspects of eastern equine encephalomyelitis could just as well be said for the western type. The chief difference is that the expected mortality is about 50% for western equine encephalomyelitis but 90% for eastern equine encephalomyelitis. Therefore, practicing veterinarians in the western United States may expect to see and treat more cases of western equine encephalomyelitis than their colleagues on the East Coast engaged in a similar practice. Since many cases might be milder and more prolonged, western practitioners have a greater opportunity to study and utilize for future reference the more subtle neurologic changes associated with the disease.

The pathologic changes encountered in western and eastern equine encephalomyelitis are much the same. If there are differences, they are the result of a more prolonged course in western equine encephalomyelitis. Thus, lesions would be longer in forming than those seen in the short fulminating cases of eastern equine encephalomyelitis.

Diagnosis: Here again, diagnosis is based on clinical findings, location of cases, time of year, weather conditions, and prevalence of potential insect vectors. In making a differential diagnosis, one should consider the same diseases as discussed for eastern equine encephalomyelitis. One might be influenced by the presence or absence of rabies in the area, or conditions associated with moldy corn poisoning and botulism. Dr. Karl Meyer has suggested that the term "forage poisoning" be restricted to sickness in animals in which it has been possible to establish an inseparable relationship between the feed containing a poisonous substance and the intoxication following its ingestion.

Prognosis: The mortality of western equine encephalomyelitis in horses is about 50%. Prognosis usually is unfavorable when a state of prostration has been reached. Cases showing profound prostration are to be considered hopeless.

Treatment: The fact that about half of the horses with western equine encephalomyelitis will survive justifies a greater effort in treatment than for those having eastern equine encephalomyelitis. Although there seems to be little scientific basis for administering specific immune serum, even in early cases, there are reports in the literature describing its benefits in western equine encephalomyelitis.[13] Immune serum as a prophylactic measure may be justified in a limited number of instances.

In treating clinical cases of either western or eastern equine encephalomyelitis, the same basic principles apply. It should be emphasized that there is no specific drug, antibiotic or biologic product known to influence the course of this disease. Therefore, supportive treatment based on the physical state of the affected horse is the only rational therapy. In addition to maintaining proper fluid and electrolyte balance, protecting the animal from injury and attempting to lower the fever, it is further indicated that the animal be kept standing. If this is not possible, it should be maintained in the sternal position. Animals in lateral recumbency should be turned over from time to time in order to prevent pulmonary congestion and pneumonia.

Early investigators of western equine encephalomyelitis collaborating with practitioners in Colorado, Nevada, and other western states suggested the use of a supportive device. The apparatus is a combination of wooden stocks and a canvas sling. The padded chest and rump boards and convenient feed and water racks are features worth consideration when treating cases of the equine encephalitides as well as other severely disabling diseases of the horse.

Prevention and Control: Annual immunization against western equine encephalomyelitis is the most satisfactory means of controlling the disease. Protection of horses from potential insect vectors during an epizootic also is indicated. It should be emphasized that these measures will serve to reduce the number of cases of western equine encephalomyelitis in horses but will have no effect on the total amount of virus activity in a given area. The survival and perpetuation of western equine encephalomyelitis virus is dependent on existing ecologic conditions including the type and number of insect vectors and avian reservoirs. Control measures, therefore, should be based on the assumption that western equine encephalomyelitis virus has existed for a long time in the western hemisphere and can be expected to remain indefinitely; and that horses play no role in perpetuating the infection and protective measures are designed only for their own well-being.

VENEZUELAN EQUINE ENCEPHALOMYELITIS (PESTA LOCA)

A third member of Casals' group A Arbor viruses is the virus of Venezuelan equine encephalomyelitis. The disease is confined chiefly to South and Central America, although there is some evidence that Venezuelan equine encephalomyelitis is more widespread than first believed. Venezuelan equine encephalomyelitis is a serious disease of horses in Latin America and its particular effect is felt in areas where horses are used for transportation and agricultural uses. The disease also affects humans although it usually does not involve the central nervous system and the mortality rate in man fortunately is low.

Venezuelan equine encephalomyelitis differs from eastern equine encephalomyelitis and western equine encephalomyelitis inasmuch as affected animals may die of a fulminating, systemic disease before distinct central nervous signs are manifested. Another significant fact worthy of mention is that blood-virus levels in infected equines are sufficiently high to infect potential arthropod vectors. For this reason, the horse may be considered a reservoir of the virus, at least during epizootic periods. The danger of introducing infected horses into the United States has been stressed by the U. S. Livestock Sanitary Association.[14]

Epizootiology: The epizootiology of Venezuelan equine encephalomyelitis has not been studied extensively. Birds and horses which are exposed to the virus develop high blood-virus levels. A number of arthropods are capable of transmitting Venezuelan equine encephalomyelitis virus from host to host. Among them are *Mansonia titillans, Aedes taeniorhyncus* and *Culex quinquefasciatus.*[14,15,16]

Venezuelan equine encephalomyelitis is unique among the arthropod-borne encephalitides in that contact infection between horses is possible.[17]

Clinical Pathology: As previously indicated, the disease may appear in equines as either an encephalitis or a severe, fulminating disease affecting the hemopoietic tissues and blood vessels. Onset of the disease is marked by fever and depression. Neurologic signs similar to those observed in eastern and western equine encephalomyelitis may follow soon. Subnormal temperatures are observed prior to death. Diarrhea is a frequent sign in experimentally infected horses.

There are few significant gross pathologic changes to be seen in fatal cases of Venezuelan equine encephalomyelitis. The location and extent of microscopic changes depend on the affected organs. The blood-forming organs, pancreas, and kidney, are the chief organs affected in those animals dying of the nonencephalitic infections. The virus can be isolated from these organs at the time of death. Detailed descriptions of the histopathologic changes may be found elsewhere.[17] In horses which have died from encephalitis, marked vascular changes are noted in the brain and quite possibly such cases could be differentiated microscopically from fatal cases of eastern and western equine encephalomyelitis.

Diagnosis: Diagnosis of Venezuelan equine encephalomyelitis presents a number of problems to the veterinary practitioner. The varied clinical manifestations increase the spectrum of diseases to be considered in making a differential diagnosis. In making a differential diagnosis of the encephalitic form of disease, one would be faced with the same considerations cited for eastern and western equine encephalomyelitis. It should be pointed out that eastern and western equine encephalomyelitis viruses exist in areas where Venezuelan equine encephalomyelitis is prevalent also and laboratory confirmation is necessary to identify the causative agent. The acute fulminating case of Venezuelan equine encephalomyelitis presents a different type of problem to the practitioner. Among diseases to be considered in making a differential diagnosis are purpura, African horsesickness, and possibly, equine infectious anemia and leptospirosis. Laboratory confirmation is essential in differentiating these conditions.

The principles previously outlined for laboratory confirmation of eastern and western equine encephalomyelitis apply as well to Venezuelan equine encephalomyelitis. However, it should be pointed out that the clinical manifestations should be a guide in the selection and processing of tissues for laboratory examination. The risk of handling infected tissues and blood from dead animals also is considerably greater than for the North American types of equine encephalomyelitis.

There are few laboratories prepared to handle Venezuelan equine encephalomyelitis virus. Most of them could not handle infected horse brains or tissues without soon infecting all their personnel. Suspected cases, therefore, should be reported to the appropriate public health or disease control authorities for proper disposition.

Prognosis: Prognosis generally is poor, particularly for those animals which go down and cannot stand without support.

Treatment: The same basic principles of treatment outlined for other Arbor virus infections would apply to Venezuelan equine encephalomyelitis.

Prevention and Control: Since this disease is of foreign origin, it is suggested that the reader consult other sources for comprehensive information. A discussion of the control of Venezuelan equine encephalomyelitis is given elsewhere.[14]

JAPANESE ENCEPHALITIS
(Japanese B Encephalitis)

Japanese encephalitis is a member of the B group of the Arbor viruses and is widespread throughout the Far East. The virus of Japanese encephalitis causes an encephalitis in man and horses. It also may cause abortion in pregnant swine, but does not produce encephalitis or any other manifestation of disease in adult pigs.

Japanese encephalitis is a significant public health problem in Japan, Korea, and other parts of the Orient. The incidence of Japanese encephalitis in horses in Japan from 1950 to 1958 has varied from a high of 669 cases in 1950 to a low of 21 cases in 1953.

The virus shows many biologic characteristics common to the other Arbor viruses. It differs from the North American equine Arbor viruses in that it is not pathogenic for day-old chicks, or for that matter, any avian host. Japanese encephalitis virus does, however, infect birds and induces a viremia sufficiently high to infect mosquitoes.

Japanese encephalitis is transmitted to man and horses by the bite of infected mosquitoes. On the basis of epidemiologic studies and laboratory transmission experiments, it is believed that *Culex tritaeniorhynchus* is the chief vector of Japanese encephalitis in Japan. The avian hosts of the virus in Japan probably are wading birds such as egrets and herons. More than likely, the horse is a dead-end host in the ecology of Japanese encephalitis.

The clinical-pathologic aspects of Japanese encephalitis in the horse are similar to those of the arthropod-borne encephalitides. There probably are more subclinical cases of Japanese encephalitis in horses than frank cases of the disease. The mortality in Japanese encephalitis-affected horses is low compared to the North American types of equine encephalomyelitis. Pathologic changes due to disease are similar to those seen in western and eastern equine encephalomyelitis.

The aspects of the disease involving diagnosis and control are beyond the scope of this text. Suffice it to say, that if the disease is suspected in an animal recently introduced into the United States, the veterinarian involved should immediately notify the local, state or federal animal disease control authorities.

BORNA DISEASE

Although Borna disease is a type of equine encephalomyelitis, it is not one of the arthropod-borne encephalitides. The disease has occurred for many years in central Europe and may appear during any season. In this respect, it differs from the arthropod-borne encephalitides which occur most frequently in late summer. The mode of transmission of Borna disease is obscure, but quite possibly the digestive tract is a portal of entry.

The clinical-pathologic picture of Borna disease resembles that seen in the North American types of infectious equine encephalitis. However, the incubation period of Borna disease is at least 4 weeks, in contrast to the shorter period observed in other types of equine encephalomyelitis. The disease has a course of 1 to 3 weeks and mortality generally is high. A characteristic inclusion, the Joest body, is observed in the ganglion cells in brains of animals dead from Borna disease.

Sheep also are affected by the virus of Borna disease. Rabbits are highly susceptible to the virus and, for this reason, are preferred in the laboratory for isolation studies.

Horses can be immunized against this disease.[18] Further discussion of the immunizing action and control measures is beyond the scope of this publication.

RABIES (LYSSA, HYDROPHOBIA)

General Comment: Rabies is a disease of antiquity and is found throughout the world. Although the disease generally is enzootic in nature, occasionally it may approach epizootic proportions. Rabies is an important public health problem since the disease invariably is fatal in man and because of the severe immunization procedure indicated for people exposed to the bite of rabid or potentially rabid animals. The virus is carried in the salivary glands of rabid animals and is spread to man and other animals as the result of virus-contaminated bite wounds. Dogs and certain wild animals are the chief spreaders of the infection. The horse can be considered a dead-end host in the chain of rabies infections. A summary of the incidence of equine rabies in the United States from 1950 to 1960 is given in Table 4.

The Virus: Rabies is caused by a filtrable virus and was one of the earliest viruses to be recognized as such. The classic studies of Louis Pasteur on rabies prophylaxis in man are familiar to everyone and need no review here.

The virus is small, measuring 100-150 mμ in diameter, and all mammals are susceptible to its effects. Rabies virus has a predilection

Table 4.—Reported Incidence of Rabies in the United States (Compiled by the U. S. Department of Agriculture)

YEAR	NO. OF HORSE CASES	NO. OF DOG CASES	NO. OF HUMAN CASES	OTHER ANIMALS*	TOTAL/YR.
1950	33	4,979	9	2,889	7,910
1951	34	5,194	14	2,780	8,022
1952	38	5,261	21	3,133	8,453
1953	21	5,688	14	3,144	8,867
1954	29	4,083	8	3,162	7,282
1955	33	2,657	5	3,149	5,844
1956	30	2,592	10	3,214	5,846
1957	24	1,908	6	3,070	5,008
1958	31	1,643	6	3,134	4,814
1959	22	1,124	6	2,965	4,117
1960	36	697	2	2,693	3,428
Total	331	35,826	101	33,333	69,591

*Other animals includes cattle, sheep, swine, cats, goats, and miscellaneous species.

for the central nervous system and the salivary glands, and it is from these tissues in rabid animals that the virus can be isolated.

Epizootiology: Although much emphasis was originally placed on the role of the dog in the spread of rabies, recent work has shown a new and more perplexing reservoir in wildlife. Among those wild animals which may play an important part in maintaining the virus in nature are skunks, foxes, and certain species of bats.

Clinical Pathology: The incubation period of rabies in horses is from 3 weeks to 3 months. The earliest manifestations of the disease are increased excitability and viciousness. An inflammatory reaction may appear at the site of the original bite inflicted by the rabid animal. Affected horses may bite or tear their own flesh at this site. As the disease progresses, the horse may show paroxysms of aggressive behavior. Tremors and muscular spasms become evident. In the final stages, the hindlimbs become paralyzed, dysphagia and convulsions ensue, and death follows. The pulse and respirations are increased in frequency from the onset of clinical signs until death.

As might be expected, the significant postmortem lesions in equine rabies are found in the brain. There are no prominent macroscopic lesions found in the central nervous system. Histopathologic changes in the brain are indicative of an encephalitis. The presence of Negri bodies, which are spherically shaped eosinophilic bodies found in the cytoplasm of the neurons, is considered diagnostic for rabies. However, failure to demonstrate Negri bodies does not rule out rabies, and it is considered essential to carry out mouse-inoculation tests as a confirmatory measure.

Diagnosis: Provisional diagnosis of rabies is based on clinical findings. As in the case of other infectious diseases, the veterinarian's early provisional diagnosis will be guided by the prevalence of the disease in the area, the presence of infected dogs, foxes, and other wildlife, and a history of the horse's having been bitten. In making a differential diagnosis, tetanus and equine encephalomyelitis are among the other diseases to be considered. Again, early clinical signs of aggressiveness, self-inflicted wounds, and eating of wood,

straw or other such material would lead one to suspect rabies.

Laboratory Confirmation: Laboratory confirmation is of vital importance to animal disease control and public health authorities. If rabies is suspected in an affected horse, the animal should be isolated and kept alive as long as possible. When terminal, if the animal must be killed, this is best done by pithing, not by gun-shot. The head of the suspect horse should be packed in wet ice and sent to the laboratory along with a complete case history.

Since so much has been written on laboratory confirmation of rabies, a detailed description of laboratory technics is unwarranted here. In addition to the standard references books on virological methods, a World Health Organization monograph published in 1954 is highly recommended.[19]

Prognosis: Once clinical signs of rabies appear in an animal, the disease is invariably fatal.

Treatment: None.

Prevention and Control: Unfortunately, there is little information on routine immunization of horses against rabies. The relatively small number of equine cases in the United States probably does not indicate such procedures. Prevention of rabies in horses is more dependent upon suppression of the disease in dogs and wildlife.

It is evident that horses can be successfully immunized against rabies by the use of killed vaccines of brain origin, since this procedure is used in the initial phases of hyperimmune serum production. In this process, horses are given an initial dose of 40 ml. of phenolized rabbit brain vaccine. A second and third dose of 80 and 120 ml., respectively, is given at weekly intervals following the first dose. The horses are then given subcutaneous injections of living, fixed virus and evidently withstand this challenge. High titered immune serum is produced by this immunization procedure.

There is little information available on the use of attenuated vaccines for the active immunization of horses against rabies. It is suggested that veterinarians wishing more information on this subject get in touch with the producers of these vaccines.

It is not a common or generally recommended procedure to treat horses once they have been exposed to the bite of a rabid animal. If the biting incident is discovered early enough, the wound should be cauterized with nitric acid and immunization instituted immediately. There also may be benefit from the use of large doses of hyperimmune serum as an adjunct to postexposure vaccination. The practitioner would be well-advised to consult with the animal disease control officer in his state with regard to handling such cases since it would involve prolonged quarantine of the exposed horse.

R. J. BYRNE

REFERENCES

1. Casals, J. and Brown, L. V. Hemagglutination with arthropod-borne viruses. J. Exptl. Med. **99** (1954) 429-449.
2. Hearn, H. J. Jr. Cross-protection between Venezuelan equine encephalomyelitis and eastern equine encephalomyelitis virus. Proc. Soc. Exptl. Biol. Med. **107** (1961) 607.
3. Parks, J. J. and Price, W. H. Studies on immunologic overlap among certain arthropod-borne viruses. 1. Cross-protection relationships among group A viruses. Am. J. Hyg. **67** (1958) 187-206.
4. Gould, D. J. and Byrne, R. J. Transmission of Japanese encephalitis virus to horses by the mosquito Culex tritaeniorhyncus Giles. Manuscript in preparation.
5. Oglesby, W. T. Outbreak of infectious equine encephalomyelitis in Louisiana. J.A.V.M.A. **113** (1948, 1947) 267-270.
6. Mace, D. L., Ott, R. L. and Cortez, F. S. Evidence of the presence of equine encephalomyelitis virus in Philippine animals. Bull. U. S. Army Med. Dept. **9** (1949) 504-507.
7. Devine, E. H. and Byrne, R. J. A laboratory case of viral encephalitis (equine type) in a horse in which the animal completely recovered from the disease. Cornell Vet. **50** (1960) 494-496.
8. Lose, M. P., Hetrick, F. M., Elliot, G. A. and Byrne, R. J. A laboratory-confirmed case of virus encephalitis (eastern equine type) in a horse in Pennsylvania. Cornell Vet. **50** (1960) 440-444.
9. Jones, T. C. and Gleiser, C. A. Veterinary Necropsy Procedures. (1954) J. B. Lippincott, Philadelphia, Pa.
10. Byrne, R. J. Laboratory confirmation of equine encephalomyelitis. (1958) U. S. Livestock Assoc. Proceedings, 62nd Annl. Mtg., 1-6.
11. Holden, P. Recovery of western equine encephalomyelitis virus from naturally infected English sparrows of New Jersey. Proc. Soc. Exptl. Biol. Med. **88** (1955) 490-492.
12. Albrecht, P. Natural foci of the western type of North American equine encephalomyelitis (WEE) in Czechoslovakia. III. Morphology of experimental infection with Czechoslovak strains of equine encephalomyelitis. Acta Virol., Eng. Ed., Praha. **1** (1957) 188-197.
13. Records, E. and Vawter, L. R. Equine encephalomyelitis antiserum. J.A.V.M.A. **82** (1933) 608.
14. Todd, F. A. Foreign Animal Diseases. (1954) Report of Committee of the U. S. Livestock San. Assn.
15. Gilyard. Bul. U. S. Army Med. Dept. **75** (1944) 96. (Quoted from: Hagan, W. A. and Bruner, D. W. 1961. The Infectious Diseases of Domestic Animals. Fourth Ed., Comstock Publishing Associates, Ithaca, N. Y., p. 816.)
16. Chamberlain, R. W., Sikes, R. K. and Nelson, D. B. Infection of Mansonia perturbans and Psorophora ferox with Venezuelan equine encephalomyelitis virus. Proc. Soc. Exptl. Biol. Med. **91** (1956) 215-216.
17. Kissling, R. E., Chamberlain, R. W., Nelson, D. B. and Stamm, D. D. Venezuelan equine encephalomyelitis in horses. Am. J. Hyg. **63** (1956) 274-287.
18. Zwick, Seifried and Witte. Arch. f. Tierheilk. **59** (1929) 511. (Quoted from: Hagan, W. A. and Bruner, D. W. 1961. The Infectious Diseases of Domestic Animals. Fourth Ed., Comstock Publishing Associates, Ithaca, N. Y., p. 816.)
19. Laboratory Techniques in Rabies, World Health Organization, Geneva, 1954.

PANTROPIC VIRAL DISEASES

AFRICAN HORSESICKNESS

African horsesickness, an acute or subacute febrile and seasonal viral infection of equines, until recently considered a disease enzootic in certain African areas, spread explosively in 1959 and 1960 to vast areas of the Middle East and Asia. The disease is spread by *Culicoides* spp. (biting midges or gnats) and cannot be transmitted by direct contact.[2,5,20]

Horses are fully susceptible to the disease, while mules and donkeys are variably more resistant. The clinical course and lesions vary according to the 4 forms in which the disease may be manifested, but in all cases a distinct febrile reaction is noted. Mortality among horses in severe outbreaks may exceed 90%. Mules and donkeys may suffer serious debility but losses are less spectacular.[3,12,19]

History: According to Henning,[12] references to a disease in parts of Africa identifiable as horsesickness were made as early as the Second Century, A.D. Evidently, the disease existed in an unidentified reservoir host for no equines existed in the Cape area of South Africa until the first white settlers imported horses early in the Eighteenth Century. These animals were soon affected extensively by a disease referred to in the area as "perreziekte" or "pardeziekte." There was early recognition that weather conditions influenced the course of the disease and it was later determined that the incidence increased in years of high rainfall and consequent insect activity. Likewise, it was noted that insect dormancy associated with frost resulted in disappearance of the disease.[12]

In the enzootic areas of Africa the disease has appeared in modern times in cyclic waves of intensity varying from 10 to 20 years—a situation associated with development of natural immunity among the equine population to several immunogenically distinct strains of the virus and periodic resurgence of certain highly invasive virus strains.[4,12]

After the development of an attenuated neurotropic virus vaccine in South Africa in about 1935, annual vaccination in this particular area has significantly reduced the consequences of the disease.[4,10,12] However, in other areas where vaccination is periodically neglected, large-scale incidence causes serious losses.[4,12]

In retrospect, African horsesickness probably was responsible for Livingstone and other early explorers finding it necessary to travel on foot or to use oxen for transport.[12] Likewise, the disease may be responsible in part for continuation of primitive agricultural practices common in middle Africa.

The occasional outbreak of the disease in North Africa and the Middle East until recently has been a temporary problem since the disease apparently had not become established or found a suitable permanent reservoir host.[2]

Current Distribution: Horsesickness now appears capable of existing permanently in any area of the world where the principal insect vectors, *Culicoides,* are found. After the disease penetrated the Persian Gulf area of Iran and Pakistan in 1959, it became quiescent in the winter of 1959-60. A wave of cases broke out in the spring of 1960, spread westward through the Middle East to the eastern Mediterranean and to the island of Cyprus, then eastward through India where climatic conditions favored its persisting throughout the 1960-61 winter months.[20,25,26] By the end of 1961, Indian authorities had determined that despite a sharp increase in infection rate during the last quarter of that year, the total losses for 1961 were about a third those of 1960. However, the mortality rate among affected animals remained nearly 90%—about the same as in 1960. Reduction in the number of animals affected is considered at least in part a result of artificially or naturally induced immunity.

Extension in and beyond the infected eastern two-thirds of Turkey has occurred only once during 1961 when a small focus of infection appeared in the region of Izmir near the Mediterranean coast. This extension of the disease within an area heretofore considered free was apparently controlled by isolation and revaccination of equines in the affected vicinity. [19,20,21,22,26,27]

Etiology and Pathogenicity: The causative agent of horsesickness is a viscerotropic virus found in the blood, tissue fluids, serous exudates and various internal organs of equines. The virus occurs in the blood from the onset of the febrile reaction and persists there no longer than 30 days. Under ordinary circumstances, the virus is only moderately resistant to drying and heating, but it may remain viable for as long as 2 years in putrified blood. Theiler believed, however, that putrefactive organisms interfered with infectivity.[12]

African researchers have proved the plurality of strains and determined that immunity acquired against one will not necessarily protect against heterologous strains. Several strains of the virus, all approximately 50 millimicrons in size, have been identified, and these currently fall into 8 immunogenic groups. Typing strains was first accomplished by Alexander,[1] 1935-36, and Alexander and Mason, 1941,[3] by neutralization tests in mice utilizing equine antiserum.[12] McIntosh,[9] 1955, found rabbit hyperimmune serum more sensitive in intracerebral serum neutralization tests in mice. Using this method he was able to define 42 virus strains which could be grouped in seven immunological types.[9,10] Later an eighth group was identified, and the Middle East strain may yet prove to be another entity.[13,20]

Equines are the only animals naturally affected by this virus. Various other animals including dogs, goats, ferrets, mice, guinea pigs, and rats may be experimentally infected. Dogs have been fatally infected through ingestion of meat from infected carcasses. Mules are less seriously affected and donkeys are relatively resistant in most areas, with the South African donkey showing the highest degree of resistance. The ferret is susceptible by inoculation, and is a useful animal in isolating virus strains.[9,10,12]

The Razi Institute in Iran has reported serologic evidence of African horsesickness in two human cases. Although the role of humans as carriers or susceptibles is inconclusive, this preliminary study indicates the need for further research to define the status of other host species.

Foals of immune dams are resistant, possibly through ingestion of antibodies in the colostral milk. Antibodies disappear in the foal at about 6 to 9 months of age.[12]

Transmission: African horsesickness is not transmitted directly. Early experiments involving direct association of sick and healthy horses, protected from insects, failed to produce the disease. The disease can be transmitted readily by intravenous injection of virulent blood, less easily by subcutaneous injection, and orally only when massive doses of virulent material are administered.[5,12,19,20]

Various insects have been incriminated, but there is overwhelming evidence that *Culicoides* are the principal vectors of African horsesickness. This confirmed earlier views that *Culicoides* were the probable vectors; views based on observations that animals stabled at night and protected against the night-flying, biting midges were not affected in areas of enzootic infection. Studies also tended to eliminate certain other insects on the basis of ecologic and environmental factors which indicated that many were not active during outbreak periods.[12]

There appears to be little possibility of intercontinental introduction of the disease through shipment of horses if they are vaccinated, quarantined at point of embarkation, shipped by sea, and again quarantined in insectproof enclosures at port of entry. However, transmission of the disease in aircraft carrying either an infected vector or host is very possible, and quite probably the mode of infection in the Middle East outbreak.[12,19,20,21]

Clinical Signs: Many early descriptions of the disease parallel modern clinical observations. Theiler beginning in 1921 described 4 distinct forms of the disease. 1. The pulmonary or acute form commonly known as Dunkop in South Africa; 2. The cardiac form, Dikkop; 3. The mixed form; and 4. Horsesickness fever.

The incubation period generally is short in natural infection, but is commonly 5 to 7 days with a range of 48 hours to 21 days in experimentally induced infection. An intermittent fever reaching 105 to 106 F. about 24-72 hours after the onset of the febrile reaction is common in all forms of the disease.[12]

Detailed pathologic aspects of this disease are discussed in a paper presented at the 98th Annual American Veterinary Medical Association Meeting in Detroit, and a slide study set is available at the Armed Forces Institute of Pathology at The Walter Reed Army Medical Center in Washington, D.C. A color film of the disease in Iran and the Middle East has been prepared by the U.S. Dept. of Agriculture and is now ready for distribution.

1. The pulmonary, or acute form (Dunkop), as in Africa in the past, is a common form of the disease seen in the current virulent outbreaks. The incubation period is relatively short—3 to 5 days—and distinct symptoms of acute pulmonary edema often are apparent in the terminal stages. At the onset of the disease the only obvious symptoms may be an acute febrile reaction with the temperature reaching 105 to 106 F. within 2 to 3 days. The appetite remains good and animals may continue to eat or show a desire for food after breathing becomes difficult and severe coughing is apparent. As paroxysms of coughing develop, animals generally discharge quantities of yellowish serous fluid and froth. After the signs of coughing and dyspnea appear, the head and neck are distended, ears droop, and severe sweating occurs. Finally the animal may choke, then sway, stagger, and fall. Although the voluminous discharge of fluid may not be obvious until the terminal stages, in most fatal cases the animal appears to literally drown in its own fluid secretion. Rarely, less severe signs occur with inactivity and severe dyspnea being the dominant symptoms. Recovery may follow but dyspnea is apparent for a considerable period.[6,12,20]

2. The cardiac form (Dikkop) generally is considered a subacute form of the disease. It may occur in either natural outbreaks or in cases of immunity-breaks by overriding infection with different strains of the virus. Incubation periods are variable, depending on the virulence of the virus, but generally are 5 to 7 days in acute cases, and as long as 3 weeks in milder ones. The febrile reaction generally develops more slowly and persists for a longer period than in the pulmonary form. Swellings

in the region of the head and neck, particularly in the temporal fossae, as well as edema of the eyelids and lips, are relatively constant symptoms. These swellings may extend to the region of the chest. A more rapid course of the disease generally produces more pronounced edematous swelling. Petechiae are often observed on the undersurface of the tongue, and the mucous membranes of the mouth and tongue often appear bluish. Cardiac symptoms reflecting hydropericarditis and endocarditis occur and there may be signs of pulmonary edema. Manifestation of abdominal pain and restlessness is common. Recovery from this form of the disease is more common than from the pulmonary form, but the convalescent period of survivors generally is longer.[6,12] Fig. 11, 12, 13.

3. The mixed form rarely is diagnosed as such during life and generally occurs as a result of mixed strain infections or as a result of unusual susceptibility to immunization with polyvalent vaccines. Animals may succumb to respiratory or cardiac afflictions described in the preceeding forms of the disease with the combined lesions apparent only on postmortem examination.[12]

4. Horsesickness fever is a mild and frequently overlooked form of the disease. The incubation period varies from less than 5 days to as long as a month. The temperature rises to above 105 F. in 1 to 3 days, dropping to normal within 3 days. Symptoms of illness are slight with inappetence, slight conjunctivitis, accelerated pulse and labored breathing the only apparent reactions. Horsesickness fever is generally seen in Africa in horses and mules undergoing immunization or in animals in which immunity is partially dissipated. However, immunization reactions in donkeys in the Middle East have produced the more severe symptoms characteristic of the other forms of the disease. In Africa, it is reported to be the only form of the disease that can be artificially produced in the donkey and Angora goat.[2,12]

Diagnosis: The locale of the disease can no longer be relied upon as a factor in diagnosis of this disease. Permanent establishment in the Middle East and parts of Asia, hitherto thought not to be areas conducive to perpetuation of African horsesickness, indicates that this disease, like bluetongue, may infect any region where *Culicoides* occur.[19,20,21]

Diagnosis by clinical signs is quite possible in areas where experience with the disease has resulted in familiarity on the part of veterinarians with the gross symptoms and lesions. However, the multiplicity of virus strains, the various forms in which the disease appears, and the subclinical manifestations make a confirmed laboratory diagnosis absolutely essential. Such diagnosis is readily accomplished in

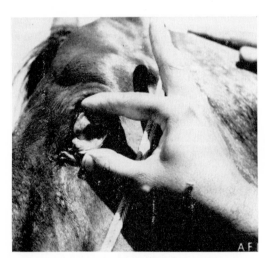

Fig. 11. African horsesickness showing edema of the conjunctiva. Photo from Armed Forces Institute of Pathology, Washington, D. C.

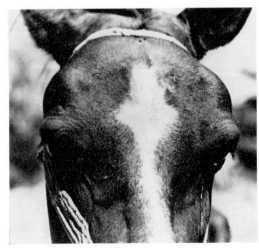

Fig. 12. African horsesickness showing edema of the supraorbital fossae and epiphora. Photo from Information Service, government of Cyprus.

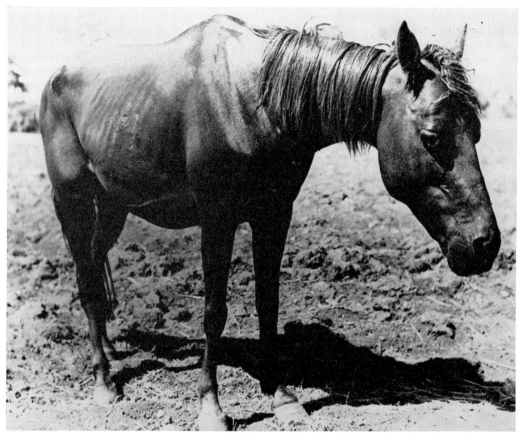

Fig. 13. African horsesickness, typical attitude. Note edema of supraorbital fossae, lateral aspect of face, and abdominal area. Photo from Information Service, government of Cyprus.

properly equipped laboratories by serum neutralization tests in mice or by complement fixation tests. The complement fixation test is less type-specific, but is nevertheless a useful tool in rapid diagnosis.[9,10,12]

In areas where concurrent infections, such as babesiasis and equine infectious anemia appear, differentiation through the usual tests for these diseases should be carried out.[12]

Immunity: Immunity to African horsesickness is relative. A solid immunity produced by infection or immunization to one or more strains does not necessarily produce complete immunity against exposure to other strains. For practical purposes, polyvalent vaccines containing sufficient virus concentration of at least 7 separate virus strains protect equines against the disease. The antigenic behavior of the Middle East virus, however, indicates that this strain, as soon as adequate neurotropic attenuation is reached, should also be included in the vaccines used in the newly affected areas. A peculiar situation—a high degree of susceptibility in the Middle East donkey to the polyvalent vaccine—indicates that this animal may be more susceptible than the South African donkey and that it may be necessary to eliminate certain South African strains of virus from the vaccine for this class of equines or to attenuate the Middle East strain to a point where it no longer produces severe vaccinal reaction.[2,10,12,13,20]

In South Africa natural infection followed by recovery has generally resulted in solid immunity. However, occasional breakdowns are attributed to infection by a new strain to which the animal has not previously been exposed.[12] The development of immunity to African horsesickness is relatively slow. After inoculation of an attenuated neurotropic adapted virus, neutralizing antibodies may not be significantly detectable for 20 days and a high antibody titer may not be reached for 6 months or more.[12] Nevertheless, immunity of high order apparently is established shortly after the appearance of neutralizing antibodies unless overriding exposure to a particular virus strain is encountered. Both the experiences in South Africa and those of the Middle East demonstrate that application of polyvalent, neurotropic-adapted vaccine produces a practical immunity against the disease. The effective level of attenuation for certain species of animals in some regions remains in doubt, but experimental work promises a solution to this problem. In South Africa, the consistent annual vaccination of approximately 20% of the horse population has produced adequate protection against the disease.[3,10,12,20]

The Vaccine: Modern African horsesickness vaccine is produced by serial intracerebral propagation of the virus in mouse brains. At about the 100th serial passage each of the 7 or 8 antigenically different virus strains is sufficiently attenuated to produce an effective vaccine. Pooled quantities of the separate neurotropically adapted strains are incorporated into a freeze dried vaccine. These pooled strain vaccines generally provide adequate immunity. The 7 South African strains are incorporated in the vaccine now produced and used in the Middle East. Since the strain isolated in this area does not conform serologically in all respects to any of the 7 or possibly 8 immunogenically separate strains of South Africa, it has been suggested that this strain be neurotropically adapted and included in the vaccine now used in newly affected countries. In several of the infected areas of the Middle East the forminalized spleen vaccine, similar to that used in South Africa before development of the mouse brain vaccine, was used to some extent in emergencies. This vaccine provided only partial protection, and the immunity was of short duration.[10,12,13,20,21]

Control: Aside from prevention through vaccination, the methods for controlling the disease are removal of animals from areas where the transmitting biting insects are active, night stabling, and use of insecticides or insect repellents. Such precautions are only partially effective since the range of the vector is quite wide and it is capable of penetrating even fine mesh screens and is relatively resistant to insecticides or insect repellents.[12,20]

The extensive spread of the disease in the Middle East and Asia provides evidence of the problems involved in its confinement. Apparently, only restricted movement of animals, careful prevention of introduction of infected vectors, and a wide natural barrier prevent its spread to any area where the natural or reservoir host exists. The possibility that the disease is permanently established in the Middle East and Asia is very likely, and its extension from these areas to new ones is a constant threat. The experiences in the recently infected Middle Eastern areas prove the necessity for constant vigilance, effective control over movement of animals from infected areas, and adequate preparation in assuring availability of vaccines. A policy of vaccinating all equines in affected zones within a 10-mile radius of international airports and seaports has been recommended constantly as an essential element in preventing further spread to outside unaffected areas. It is also recognized that extending the immunization in infected countries to the widest possible extent reduces the chances for further spread of the disease.

The economic significance of African horsesickness is quite obvious since the past experiences in Africa and the current situation in the Middle East and Asia indicate that the disease cannot be eradicated readily even by intensive application of highly effective vaccines. The solution to the problem of continuous vaccination in affected areas lies in finding and eliminating or controlling the unknown reservoir.[12,13,19,20,21,22]

N. M. Konnerup
F. P. Gluckstein

REFERENCES

1. Alexander, R. A. Studies on the neurotropic virus of horsesickness, VI. Propagation in the developing chick embryo. Onderstepoort J., **11** (1938), 9-19.
2. Alexander, R. A. The 1944 epizootic of horsesickness in the Middle East. Onderstepoort J., **23** (1948), 77-92.
3. Alexander, R. A. and Mason, J. H. Studies on the neurotropic virus of horsesickness, VII. Transmitted immunity. Onderstepoort J., **16** (1941), 19-32.

4. Alexander, R. A., Neitz, W. O. and DuToit, P. J. Horsesickness immunization of horses and mules in the field during the season 1934-1935, with a description of the technique of preparation of polyvalent mouse neurotropic vaccine. Onderstepoort J., 7 (1936), 17-30.

5. DuToit, R. M. The Transmission of bluetongue and horsesickness by Culicoides. Onderstepoort J., 19 (1944), 7-16.

6. Piercy, S. E. Some observations on African horsesickness including an account of an outbreak amongst dogs. E. Afr. Agric. J., 17 (1951), 62-64.

7. Polson, A. The particle size of African horsesickness virus. Onderstepoort J., 16 (1941), 33-50.

8. Polson, A. and Dent, J. The rate of inactivation by ultra-violet irradiation as a means of distinguishing horsesickness virus. Brit. J. Exp. Path., 31 (1950), 1-4.

9. McIntosh, B. M. Complement fixation with horsesickness viruses. Onderstepoort J., 27 (1956), 165-169.

10. McIntosh, B. M. Immunological types of horsesickness virus and their significance in immunization. Onderstepoort J., 27 (1958), 465-538.

11. United Nations, Food and Agriculture Organization. Animal Health Yearbook 1960. Rome, 1961.

12. Henning, M. W. Animal Diseases in South Africa. 3rd ed. South Africa, Central News Agency, Ltd., 1956.

13. Haig, D., Report to the Government of Turkey on the production of African horsesickness vaccine. Food and Agriculture Organization of the United Nations. Rome, 1961.

14. Kesteven, K. V. L. Report to Food and Agriculture Organization Council. Food and Agriculture Organization of the United Nations. Rome, 1961.

15. Seal, John R. Special reports on African horsesickness in the Middle East and Asia. Naval Medical Research Unit III. Cairo, 1960.

16. Piercy, S. E. The menace of African horsesickness. New Scientist (217), London, January 1961.

17. Maurer, Fred D. Exotic diseases on the move. Guest editorial, J.A.V.M.A. 138 (1961), 214-215.

18. Maurer, Fred D. African horsesickness, J.A.V.M.A. 138 (1961), 15-16.

19. Food and Agriculture Organization. Report on African horsesickness. Held at Beirut. Food and Agriculture Organization of the United Nations. Rome, 1961.

20. Food and Agriculture Organization/International Office of Epizootics. Report of the FAO/OIE. Emergency meeting on African horsesickness and African swine fever. Held in Paris. Food and Agriculture Organization of the United Nations. Rome, 1961.

21. Food and Agriculture Organization/International Office of Epizootics. Draft report of the FAO/OIE International meeting on emerging diseases. Held in Ankara. Ankara, 1961.

22. Food and Agriculture Organization Veterinary Staff: Personal communications, 1961.

23. Maurer, Fred D.: Personal Communications, 1961.

24. Wilkins, Howard: Personal Communications, 1961.

25. Food and Agriculture Organization of the United Nations. Report to the Government of India on Horsesickness Control and Foot and Mouth Disease Investigations, Rome, 1962.

26. United States Department of Agriculture. Foreign Agriculture Service Despatch No. Agr.-54, African Horse Sickness in India—Status through December 31, 1961. New Delhi, 1962.

27. United States Department of State, Incoming Airgram No. A-282. Abstract from Istanbul Press, September 26, 1961 on Horse Plague in Eastern Turkey. Ankara, October 3, 1961.

EQUINE INFECTIOUS ANEMIA

Equine infectious anemia, or swamp fever, is an acute or chronic disease of equine animals (horses, mules, and donkeys). It is characterized principally by intermittent fever, marked depression, progressive weakness, loss of weight, edema, and anemia of a transitory or progressive type.

History: The disease was first reported from Europe in 1843 and now has a worldwide distribution. In addition to Canada and the United States, the disease exists in certain well-defined areas in Germany, Switzerland, Sweden, Norway, Finland, Yugoslavia, Hungary, Russia, Japan, and sections of northern Africa. In recent years outbreaks have been reported from Uruguay and Venezuela, South America.

In North America, in about 1880, equine infectious anemia was first recognized as a specific disease of horses in Canada. The disease has existed for at least 70 years in the United States. Suspected outbreaks have been reported from 42 of the 50 States. Its prevalence in the United States has been declining with the substitution of motorized equipment for horsepower in industry, agriculture, and the Army, but it is still of grave concern the world over to the establishments that handle large numbers of horses.

Etiology: The filtrable virus which causes the disease may persist in an infected animal for years. It is believed to be present in the blood and body tissues of affected animals at all times and may be eliminated with some of the secretions or excretions, such as the milk, semen, saliva, ocular and nasal secretions, urine, and feces.

Despite reports to the contrary, the virus is restricted to solipeds. It has not been cultivated *in vitro* and cannot reproduce itself consistently in animals other than equines.

The carrier animal, which remains a source of infection for susceptible animals during its lifetime, appears to be the chief factor determining the survival of the virus in nature.

The virus shows considerable resistance against disinfectants, heating, freezing, and drying. It may retain its virulence for several months in infected dried blood protected from sunlight, and in frozen, infected tissue for at least 9 months.

Epizootiology: The disease has been experimentally transmitted by injection of minute amounts of virulent blood and by the bite of the stable fly, horsefly, Anopheles and Psorophora mosquitoes, and the biting louse. The transmission of the virus by insects is purely mechanical. Although the disease may be transmitted by these means, and by the ingestion of contaminated material, the common method of its spread under natural conditions is not known definitely. The most certain method of transmission, however, is the injection of virulent blood into or under the skin either by insect vectors or accidentally, and it therefore appears that it is more apt to be disseminated by this means than by ordinary contact.

Ordinarily the disease spreads slowly and sporadically, but it may occur in epizootic form in a large group of susceptible horses following the introduction of carriers, especially when circumstances are favorable for its transmission, such as abundance of bloodsucking flies and the use of unsterilized hypodermic needles and other surgical instruments. Outbreaks of this nature have occurred at biologic institutions, army posts, race tracks, and breeding farms.

Clinical Signs: The clinical signs of infectious anemia are variable and depend largely on the form of the disease. It may occur as an acute, rapidly fatal disease or more commonly as a chronic affection, characterized by intermittent attacks of fever, loss of weight, progressive weakness, marked depression, and dropsical swellings of the lower parts of the body and legs. The disease also may exist in a subclinical form in which no clinical signs are apparent, though the affected animal carries virulent virus in the blood stream. The incubation period, usually about 12 to 15 days, may vary from a few days to 3 months or longer.

In the acute form the onset is sudden, being characterized by a rise in temperature which usually goes to about 105 F. and may reach 108 F. The affected animal may show a high continuous fever or frequent, intermittent febrile attacks which rapidly terminate in death. More commonly the attacks decrease in frequency and intensity, resulting in the subacute or chronic type of the disease (Fig. 14).

Other signs which may occur during the course of the disease include inappetence, accelerated pulse, marked depression, incoordination, weakness of the hindquarters, frequent shifting of the body weight from one leg to another, frequent micturition, congestion and yellowish discoloration of the conjunctiva, sublingual and nasal petechial hemorrhages, and decrease in the number of red blood corpuscles.

Following the intermittent febrile attacks, which usually last 3 to 5 days, the temperature and red cell count usually return to normal and the animal appears well except for a loss of weight. Occasionally, however, the initial attack will persist until the animal dies.

The subacute and chronic forms of the disease differ from the acute in that the febrile attacks are less severe and the intervals between them are longer. The subacute cases may terminate in death during or following one of the attacks, or the reactions may grow less frequent, the animal finally becoming a chronic case or a clinically recovered carrier. In general, the chronic form is manifested by unthriftiness, marked depression, muscular weakness, emaciation, and edema of the dependent parts.

As the disease progresses, evidence of anemia may develop, the red corpuscle count may be extremely low, the blood may appear thin and watery, there may be a marked increase in the sedimentation rate of the red blood cells, and in the later stages the visible mucous membranes may become pallid. The pulse may be slow and weak, the heart action may become irregular, and a jugular pulse may be visible.

The inactive, or latent, form of the disease may follow the initial attack, but it usually is preceded by several attacks of fever. This form is observed in animals that apparently have recovered from the acute, subacute, or chronic types of the disease. Animals affected with the disease in the latent form show no clinical signs and are known as clinically recovered carriers. The temperature remains normal, and there is no reduction in the red corpuscles or any sign of disease for a period of years, yet the infectious agent remains present in the blood stream and other tissues, and may be eliminated in body excretions. Such animals obviously are a menace to other horses that may be near them, since they are reservoirs of infection that usually go unrecognized and uncontrolled. The inactive form of the disease may, however, become active at any time and present all the characteristics of the acute or subacute form. Unusually hard work or any debilitating influence may reactivate the infection.

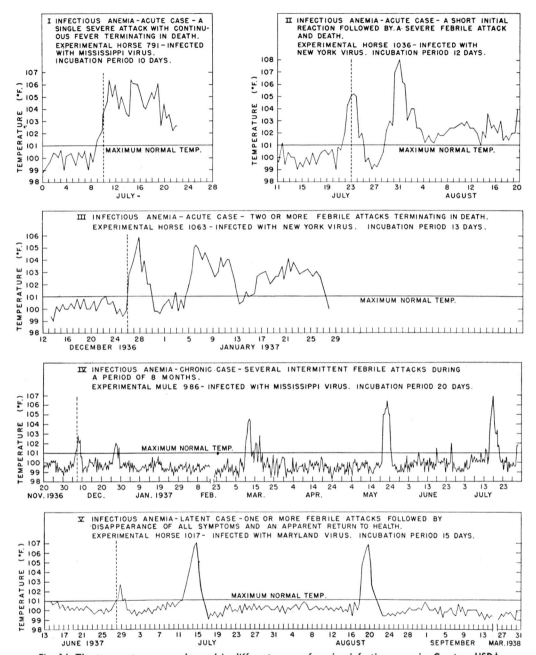

Fig. 14. The temperature curve observed in different cases of equine infectious anemia. Courtesy USDA.

Lesions: The pathologic alterations may be very well-marked and plainly visible (in some cases so pronounced as to be striking), or they may be so slight as to escape detection except by persons having considerable experience with the disease. In acute cases, the most constant lesions are petechial and ecchymotic hemorrhages on surfaces of the major parenchymatous organs and on the serous and mucous membranes. There also may be enlargement of the heart, spleen, liver, and kidneys (Fig. 15).

In subacute and chronic cases, the lesions seen in acute cases are observed in varying de-

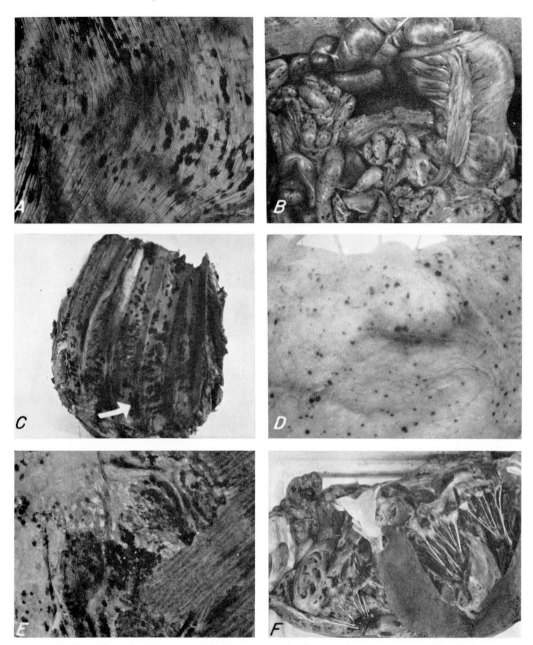

Fig. 15. Hemorrhagic lesions in acute infectious anemia. A—Abdominal surface of diaphragm. B—Serous surface of intestines. C—Pleura. D—Mucous surface of bladder. E—Myocardium. F—Endocardium. Courtesy of the Animal Disease and Parasite Research Division, Agricultural Research Service, U. S. Department of Agriculture.

grees together with emaciation, pale mucous membranes, and gelatinous infiltration of fat tissue. In cases with a history of several febrile attacks the liver may be greatly enlarged, hard and friable, and on histologic examina-

tion reveals a heavy deposition of hemosiderin and round cell infiltration with characteristic nodular formation. The latter feature is of diagnostic importance.

In carriers and chronic cases of a mild type,

little or no anatomic alteration is observed at necropsy.

Diagnosis: The inoculation test is the only reliable means of diagnosis that is now recognized. In carrying out this test young, healthy horses from nonenzootic areas are inoculated with filtered blood serum of the suspected case. The test horses are held under observation in an isolated unit for 60 days, and temperatures are recorded twice daily. A tentative diagnosis based on history, clinical signs, and a series of blood examinations can be made in active cases with some certainty. The postmortem and microscopic findings in deceased animals furnish additional supportive evidence on which to base a diagnosis.

Infectious anemia also should be suspected when the history of an outbreak indicates that several horses in a group suddenly develop signs of an unusual malady with no apparent cause. Such outbreaks may occur in any assemblage of horses from widely scattered areas for races, horse shows, county fairs and rodeos, or following the introduction of new horses into establishments maintaining large numbers of horses, such as biologic institutions and breeding farms. Suspicion is maintained when the outbreak is characterized by such early symptoms as anorexia, depression, muscular weakness, loss of flesh, and a sharp increase in body temperature without any previous respiratory or intestinal disorder, and when only a few of the affected horses die during or following the initial attack, while most of the others appear to recover in about a week, but subsequently develop similar febrile attacks.

A clinical diagnosis of infectious anemia should be confirmed by the inoculation test, especially if a large number of horses are involved. Infectious anemia in the inactive form is ordinarily not detected, since no clinical symptoms are present to cause suspicion.

In acute cases occurring in the field, animals may die before the usual train of symptoms develop. The disease in the acute form may be confused with anthrax, influenza, purpura hemorrhagica, or acute equine encephalomyelitis. In the subacute and chronic forms, it may be mistaken for trypanosomiasis (dourine, murrina, and surra), leukemia, neoplasms, nutritional anemias, or a heavy infestation with strongyles. The possibility that some of those maladies may be the source of the trouble can be eliminated by laboratory examination.

The use of laboratory criteria for diagnosis is of limited value. Hematologic tests for evidence of anemia, if positive, may add supportive evidence to a clinical diagnosis. Likewise, microscopic examination of the hepatic tissues of a horse that has died of infectious anemia also may show characteristic changes which aid in confirming a tentative diagnosis. However, results obtained with many different types of laboratory tests, which have been advocated for diagnosis of the disease, frequently are indefinite or nonspecific and, therefore, undependable.

Treatment and Control: No specific treatment or method of vaccination has been developed for infectious anemia. Numerous drugs, dyes, chemicals, and antibiotics have been used for treatment with unsatisfactory results. Affected animals in areas where the disease is enzootic appear to develop some tolerance to the malady. Many of the animals in such localities are affected with a mild chronic form of the disease and, if handled with care, can perform a limited amount of work. Veterinarians in these areas employ supportive treatment to improve affected animals' condition. Arsenical compounds (mainly sodium cacodylate) are given intravenously at regular intervals for this purpose. Additional treatments include injection of liver extract, blood transfusions, rest, elimination of intestinal parasites, and an abundance of good food. Such treatment produces some clinical improvement, but it has no lasting value, the animals remain infected, are subject to fever, and may be virus carriers.

Though no systematic program for the control of infectious anemia can be undertaken until a definite and practical means for identifying chronic carriers is developed, the following measures constitute the most effective means known to prevent spread of the infection. When a definite diagnosis of infectious anemia has been made, it is advisable, if practicable, to destroy the animal and dispose of the carcass by cremation or deep burial. This method of control has been followed in small, isolated outbreaks and in establishments keeping large numbers of horses, and it has been effective. This method is impracticable, however, in areas where the disease is widely distributed and exists chiefly in a mild chronic form.

Infected animals should be isolated from healthy animals. Flies and mosquitoes should be controlled. Only horses known to be free from the disease should be used as donors for blood transfusions and all antiserums of equine origin intended for treatment of horses should be heated to destroy the virus. Companies operating under government license are now required to heat all antiserums prepared from horses to 58 to 59 C. (136.4 to 138.2 F.) for an hour to destroy any infectious anemia virus which they may contain.

The common use of equipment that may produce skin abrasions or absorb body secretions or excretions is to be avoided. Surgical instruments, particularly hypodermic and bleeding needles, tattooing instruments, and syringes should be cleaned and sterilized before being used on each animal. Stables in which infected animals have been kept should be cleaned and disinfected.

The shipment of susceptible horses into enzootic areas, or the introduction of horses from infected localities into clean areas, should be avoided. In places where large numbers of horses are assembled from various parts of the country, such as race tracks, horse shows, and county fairs, it is advisable that all horses be kept in separate, clean, well-ventilated stalls free from flies, and fed and watered from separate containers.

C. D. STEIN

EQUINE INFLUENZA

Equine influenza is an acute, febrile disease of the horse caused by a myxovirus having properties of the Type A influenza viruses.

History: Epizootic outbreaks of an undifferentiated respiratory disease occurred in Sweden in 1955 and 1956.[1] The clinical signs were similar to those described in veterinary textbooks for undifferentiated influenza. Serologic studies on the horses revealed development of complement fixing antibody against the soluble antigens of several Type A strains of influenza virus. A similar disease appeared in horses at a meeting in Dresden in the spring of 1956.[2] The disease had spread extensively over Eastern Europe by midsummer; a large outbreak occurred in Czechoslovakia where it was studied by veterinary and medical investigators. A new myxovirus was isolated by Sovinova et al.[3] and described as being similar to the Type A influenza viruses.

Etiology: Equine influenza is caused by a myxovirus identified as A/equi/Prague/56.[3] The virus shares soluble antigens with the Type A influenza viruses of man and swine.[3] It is morphologically similar to the influenza viruses.[5] Its hemagglutination spectrum is similar to that of the A/Asian/57 strains.[4] The virus propagates in the amnion of chicken embryos, after which it is adaptable to allantoic cultivation.[3] Experimental host ranges are similar to those of the other influenza viruses. There is no cross reaction with other influenza viruses in hemagglutination inhibition tests.[4] The disease is transmitted rapidly by aerosolized secretions, direct contact, and indirectly by contamination of food, water and equipment.

Distribution: Since it is a newly identified disease, little is known of its distribution. In addition to its occurrence in Sweden and Czechoslovakia, a serologic survey conducted under the auspices of the World Health Organization[6] revealed evidence of the occurrence of the disease in Rumania, Denmark, Finland, the Federal Republic of Germany, Japan, Poland, The Netherlands, the Soviet Union and possibly Australia. An independent survey in America[7] revealed a high percentage of horses with hemagglutination inhibition antibody against A/equi/Prague/56. This evidence indicates that either the A-equi or a related virus occurs in America, but differential titers in acute phase and convalescent serums or recovery of virus have not been reported.

Clinical Signs: The clinical signs are quite similar to those described in standard accounts of undifferentiated "equine influenza." The incubation period varies from 2 to 10 days. The disease is initiated by fever, serous rhinitis, apathy, loss of appetite, and fatigue. Body temperature may reach 106 F. and fever persists 2 to 10 days. Pulse and respiratory rates are increased. The nasal mucosa is congested. Fever is accompanied by a dry cough, which becomes moist later and is accompanied by a mucinous or mucopurulent discharge from the nostrils. Recovery occurs in 1 to 2 weeks in the absence of complications. Horses worked during the febrile period may develop bronchitis or pneumonia. Fatality from uncomplicated infection has not been recorded. No lesions have been described.

Treatment: Antibacterial drugs do not influence the course of the viral infection. Complete rest aids in preventing complications, as may antibacterial therapy during the febrile and convalescent period. The duration of immunity is not known. No vaccines are available.

E. R. DOLL

REFERENCES

1. Heller, L., Espmark, A., and Viriden, P.: Immunological Relationship Between Infectious Cough in Horses and Human Influenza A. Archiv fur die Gesamte Virusforchung. 7 (1956) 120-124.
2. Steele, J. A.: Animal Influenza. Amer. Rev. Resp. Dis. 83 (1961) 41-46.
3. Sovinova, O., Tumova, B., Pouska, F., and Nemec, J.: Isolation of a Virus Causing Respiratory Disease of Horses. Acta. Virologica, 2 (1958) 52-61.
4. Tumova, B., and Fiserova-Sovinova, O.: Properties of Influenza Viruses A/Asia/57 and A/equi/Prague/56. 1. Agglutination of Red Blood Cells. Bull. Wld. Hlth. Org., Art. 789, January 1959.
5. Sovinova, O., and Ludvik, J.: Elektronoptika Studie Viru A/equi/Praha/56. C. S. Epidemiologie, Mikrobiologie and Immunologie, 7 (1958) 6-8.
6. Kaplan, M. M., and Payne, M.: Serological Survey in Animals for Type A Influenza in Relation to the 1957 Pandemic. Bull. Wld. Hlth. Org., 20 (1959) 465-488.
7. Doll, E. R.: Influenza of Horses. Amer. Rev. Resp. Dis., 83 (1961) 48-50.

VIRAL ARTERITIS

Viral arteritis is an acute infectious disease characterized by fever, leukopenia, catarrhal inflammation of the mucosa of the respiratory and digestive tracts, and often by conjunctivitis, palpebral edema, and edema of the legs. Histopathologically, it is characterized by degeneration and necrosis of the media of small muscular arteries. Abortion is frequent when pregnant mares are infected.

History: The name, viral arteritis, was proposed by Doll et al.[1] in 1957 for the disease resulting from experimental infection by a virus recovered from an equine fetus. The disease was characterized clinically,[1,4] pathologically,[2] hematologically,[3] and immunologically,[1] and by these means was distinguished from rhinopneumonitis. The name is based on a specific lesion occurring in the media of small muscular arteries. The clinical signs and gross lesions of arteritis, and also those of rhinopneumonitis, have been recorded for a century or longer in accounts of influenza, distemper, epizootic cellulitis, pinkeye, and shipping fever. The arteritis virus appears to have caused those "forms of influenza" identified as pinkeye, epizootic cellulitis, acute septicemic, enteric, and acute pulmonary. The rhinopneumonitis virus evidently has caused disease regarded as mild, uncomplicated influenza. Specific identification of mild "influenza" caused by the rhinopneumonitis virus was recorded by Manninger and Csontos[5] and Manninger[6] in accounts of equine virus abortion, and by Jones et al.[7] in accounts on equine influenza.

New terminology was proposed because the two viruses produced distinctly different symptoms and lesions in horses, were immunogenically distinct, each caused abortion, each had different experimental host ranges, and neither were related to the viruses causing influenza in man and swine.[1,8] Further justification for a change in terminology was provided by the isolation of an A-type influenza virus from horses by Sovinova et al.,[9] who proposed that the disease be identified as equine influenza.

Distribution: The clinical signs and gross lesions recorded in accounts of equine influenza indicate that the arteritis virus has had worldwide distribution. It likely caused the panzootic in America in 1872-73, and subsequent epizootics. A report by Dale and Dollahite[10] indicates that viral arteritis was encountered in New York in 1939. Current distribution of the disease is not apparent. It occurs sporadically in the United States. Outbreaks have been identified by isolation and identification of the arteritis virus in Ohio, Indiana, California, Pennsylvania, and Kentucky since 1953.

Etiology: The arteritis virus is filtrable through Selas 02 and Seitz EK filters. It is retained by ultrafine membrane filters with a

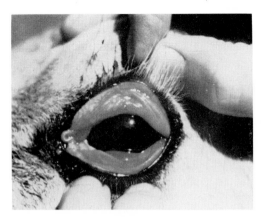

Fig. 16. Viral arteritis. Congestion, edema, and hemorrhage of the conjunctiva.

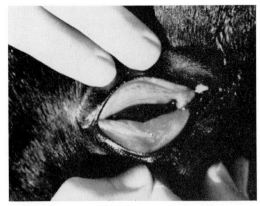

Fig. 17. Viral arteritis. Congestion, edema, hemorrhage, and icteric discoloration of conjunctiva with purulent exudate from secondary bacterial infection.

porosity of 80 to 200 millimicrons. It is not inactivated by penicillin or streptomycin. It is viable up to 7 years when frozen at −4.0 F. in whole organs. It does not produce discernible infection in chicken embryos, rabbits, guinea pigs, mice, hamsters, or Mongolian gerbils. It does not agglutinate erythrocytes of the horse, cow, sheep, guinea pig, chicken, rabbit, hamster, or mouse. The virus propagates in primary monolayer cultures of equine kidney, in which it causes rapid and complete necrosis without forming inclusion bodies. Infectivity titers in equine kidney cultures reach 10^6 to 10^8 per ml. Pathogenicity for horses is reduced by serial passage in tissue cultures. The virus is inactivated at 132.8 F. in 30 minutes and at 98.6 F. in 3 days.[11]

Virus is present in the nasal secretions, saliva, blood, semen, and probably in the feces and urine during the febrile period. It is present in the spleen and blood of horses that die 5 to 7 days after infection, and in the tissues of aborted fetuses. Persistent transmission by the semen, through coitus, was recorded by Schofield[12] and Hutyra and Marek.[13] The disease is transmissible by direct contact, by fomites, by aerosolized secretions, and by nasal, oral, and parenteral inoculation. Equidae are the only known natural hosts. How the virus is perpetuated between outbreaks has not been established. Horses are immunized by natural or artificial infection but the quality and duration of immunity have not been established. A few horses re-exposed after one year showed no clinical signs. Virus neutralizing antibody is demonstrable by tissue culture technics.

Clinical Signs: The incubation period varies from 2 to 10 days. The disease is initiated by fever and a serous discharge from the nostrils. The signs are extremely variable and in very mild cases are closely replicated by rhinopneumonitis, the A-equi influenza virus, and other respiratory infections of obscure etiology. Constant, early signs are fever, leukopenia, excessive lacrimation, serous nasal discharge, congestion of the nasal mucosa, and conjunctivitis (Fig. 16 & 17). Frequent signs are palpebral edema (Fig. 18), dyspnea with an expiratory lift, generalized weakness, depression, reduced sensation, anorexia, colic, diarrhea, loss of weight, and dehydration. Less frequent signs are keratitis, photophobia, icterus, and edema of the legs (Fig. 19), abdomen, mammary gland, scrotum and sheath.

In experimental subjects, the signs appear within 1 to 8 days after inoculation and persist for 2 to 14 days. The pulse and respiratory rates are increased. Temperatures vary from 103 to 106.5 F. Morning remissions are frequent early in the febrile period. Fever persists for 1 to 12 days. A panleukopenia occurs concurrently with fever. The total leukocyte curve is biphasic in adult horses, resulting from a temporary rise in neutrophils 4 to 7 days after onset. Lymphocytes are affected more severely than neutrophils, and are depressed throughout the febrile period. Erythrocytes are unaffected except for their hemoconcentration resulting from dehydration.

In typical cases, the temperature and leukocyte counts become stabilized in normal ranges and other signs are resolved in 7 to 14 days after onset. Longer periods may be required for resolution of edema of the palpebrae and legs. Recovery may be delayed in subjects with severe pulmonary and enteric disturbance.

A multiplicity of forms may be observed. Some horses manifest only an asymptomatic, transient, febrile reaction. The pinkeye form, with conjunctivitis, palpebral edema, excessive lacrimation, and photophobia may be the only overt manifestation in some horses. Others exhibit principally the cellulitis syndrome with edema of the legs, mammary gland and scrotum. Some horses show respiratory signs chiefly, others principally colic and diarrhea, and others a fulminating infection with high fever, early prostration, and a fatal issue within 4 to 7 days. The forms result from effects on certain tissues or organs, rather than selective affinities of virus strains. All forms may be produced experimentally with a single virus.

Abortion occurs late in the febrile period or early in the convalescent period. Abortion occurs within 7 to 14 days after experimental inoculation of pregnant mares. In natural outbreaks, 50 to 80% of mares may abort.

The disease is more severe in pregnant than in barren mares, more severe in weanlings and aged mares than in young adults, and more severe in poorly nourished, poorly fleshed, heavily parasitized horses than in well-nourished, healthy individuals. Mortality is negligible in natural outbreaks.

Lesions: The specific, basic lesion is a degeneration and necrosis of the media of small muscular arteries, which is followed by edema and infiltration by leukocytes. The arterial lesions are found in all parts of the body, and are most prevalent in organs showing extensive gross changes. The lesions occur in arteries with a well-developed muscular layer, principally those with a diameter of 0.5 mm. or

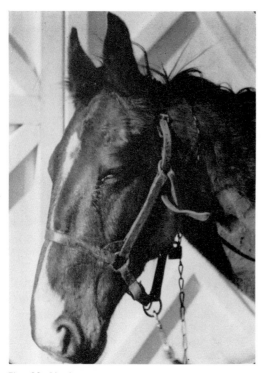

Fig. 18. Viral arteritis. Depressed attitude, palpebral edema, photophobia, and epiphora.

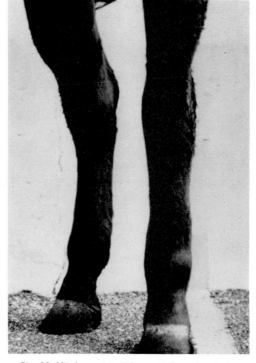

Fig. 19. Viral arteritis. Edema of the pelvic limbs.

slightly more. The earliest change is necrosis of the smooth muscle cells, manifested by loss of nuclei and replacement of cytoplasm with eosinophilic, hyaline material (Fig. 20). This change is accompanied or followed by edema and the appearance of leukocytes in the adventitia (Fig. 21). The media soon is partially or completely replaced by lymphocytes (Fig. 22). Surrounding tissue becomes edematous and infiltrated by lymphocytes. The endothelium and intima usually are intact.

Damage to the arteries results in static circulation, thrombosis, and infarction. The most striking gross lesions are edema, congestion, hemorrhage, and effusion of fluid into the pleural and peritoneal cavities, which may con-

veloping a mucopurulent conjunctivitis. Infrequently, a flocculent precipitate develops in the aqueous humor. It clears spontaneously in 4 to 6 weeks.

Diagnosis: Clinical diagnosis may not be possible on individual cases. In an outbreak affecting several horses, the characteristic signs of fever, leukopenia, serous inflammation of the respiratory tract, conjunctivitis, palpebral edema, excessive lacrimation, photophobia, and edema of the legs usually occur in some or many horses. The respiratory, enteric, and general signs aid in diagnosis. Gross lesions and the presence of characteristic microscopic lesions in the arteries aid in confirming diagnosis in fatal cases. Virus may be recovered from

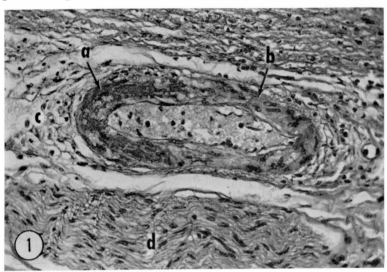

Fig. 20. Early necrotic changes in the media of an artery in the adrenal capsule. Note hyaline material (a) replacing muscle cells which remain in other parts of the media (b) Edema and lymphocytes are seen in the adventitia (c) Normal nerve fiber at (d) AFIP 707824 X 210. H and E stain.

tain from a slight excess to 2 gallons of serumlike fluid containing fibrin clots. Petechial hemorrhages on the serous surfaces and congestion and simple degenerative changes of the solid viscera are the only lesions in peracute cases. Edema is observed in the mediastinal tissues, mesentery, sublumbar tissues, in the small intestine, cecum, and colon, and in the uterus of pregnant mares. The mucosal surface of the intestines is congested and hemorrhagic, with inflammation varying from a simple catarrh to a diffuse diphtheritic condition. The lungs are congested, emphysematous, and edematous. The upper respiratory mucosa is congested and contains petechial hemorrhages. Keratitis is infrequent, except in subjects de-

nasal swabs or washings during the febrile period by inoculating primary monolayer cultures of equine kidney, and subsequently identified by neutralization tests. The disease may be transmitted by blood transfusion during the febrile period and identification made by cross protection challenges. Neutralization tests on paired acute phase and convalescent serums aid in confirming diagnosis. Virus may be recovered from the spleen of horses that die of acute disease and is identified by neutralization and cross protection tests.

Differentiation of fetal arteritis from fetal rhinopneumonitis is not difficult. Abortion from arteritis is not likely to occur without simultaneous clinical disease among other horses

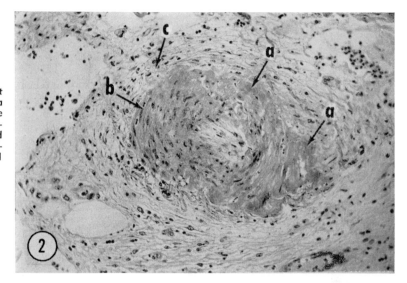

Fig. 21. Early involvement of an artery in the medulla of a lymph node. Hyaline necrosis at (a) intact muscle cells at (b) edema and lymphocytes in the adventitia (c) AFIP 707831 X 160. H and E stain.

on the premises. Abortion from rhinopneumonitis virus is not associated with concurrent clinical disease of mares or other horses. Edema of the lungs and effusion of fluid into the body cavities of fetuses occurs in each disease, but is more prevalent and more severe in rhinopneumonitis. Hepatic necrosis does not occur in fetal arteritis. The arteritis virus does not produce inclusion bodies. The arterial lesions have not been observed in fetuses. Fetuses infected with arteritis virus often die *in utero* and become autolyzed before being expelled. The virus may be recovered from the spleen or lungs of aborted fetuses and identi-

fied by neutralization tests in tissue culture, by reproduction of typical disease in horses, and by cross protection tests.

Sequelae: Arteritis may be complicated by any of the bacterial infections and sequelae common to the shipping fever diseases, as rhinitis, pharyngitis, laryngitis, pneumonia, pleuritis, protracted diarrhea, nephritis, or myocardial damage. Complications are infrequent in stabled farm horses, but may occur readily in horses at hard work or among those in large groups where conditions and stress are favorable for dissemination of secondary infections.

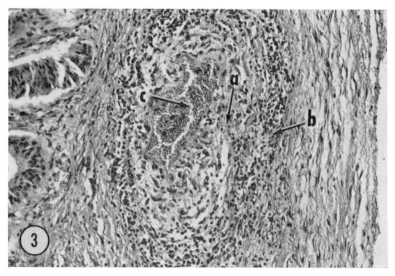

Fig. 22. Artery in adrenal capsule. Extensive necrosis of muscle cells with infiltration of lymphocytes both in media (a) and adventitia (b). The intima is outlined by the erythrocytes in the lumen (c) AFIP 707822 X 155. H and E stain.

Prevention and Control: No vaccines are available for immunization. Introduction of the disease may be prevented by isolation of new receipts. Outbreaks may be interrupted by strict isolation of horses, controlled movement of laborers and equipment, and sanitary disposal of refuse. New cases may continue appearing for 4 to 6 weeks after introduction of the disease on a farm. Precautions should continue for 4 to 6 weeks after the last clinical case. Infected and exposed stallions should not be used for breeding. The disease is transmitted by semen through coitus during the febrile and convalescent period. Stallions may be sterile for 2 weeks or longer following onset. They should be withheld from breeding for 3 to 4 weeks. On return to service, the mares served should be observed closely to determine if virus persists and is being transmitted in the semen.

Treatment: The virus is not affected by antibiotics or sulfonamides and there is no evidence that either influences the course of the viral infection. Antibacterial therapy may aid in suppressing or preventing secondary infection. Absolute rest should be provided for 3 to 4 weeks after symptoms subside, especially for subjects showing severe respiratory or enteric involvement. Return to work should be gradual. Comfortable quarters, palatable feed, and supportive and symptomatic therapy aid in recovery.

E. R. DOLL

REFERENCES

1. Doll, E. R., Bryans, J. T., McCollum, W. H., and Crowe, M. E. W.: Isolation of a Filterable Agent Causing Arteritis of Horses and Abortion by Mares. Its Differentiation from the Equine Abortion (Influenza) Virus. Cornell Vet., **47** (1957) 4-41.
2. Jones, T. C., Doll, E. R., and Bryans, J. T.: The Lesions of Equine Viral Arteritis. Cornell Vet., **47** (1957) 52-68.
3. Bryans, J. T., Doll, E. R., Crowe, M. E. W., and McCollum, W. H.: The Blood Picture and Thermal Reaction in Experimental Viral Arteritis of Horses. Cornell Vet., **47** (1957) 42-52.
4. Doll, E. R., Knappenberger, R. E., and Bryans, J. T.: An Outbreak of Abortion Caused by the Equine Arteritis Virus. Cornell Vet., **47** (1957) 69-75.
5. Manninger, R., and Csontos, J.: Virusabortus der Stuten. Dtsch. Tierarztl. Wschr. 49 (1941) 105-108.
6. Manninger, R.: Studies on Infectious Abortion in Mares due to a Filterable Virus. Acta. Vet. Hungarica **1** (1949) 1-11.
7. Jones, T. C., Gleiser, C. A., Maurer, F. D., Hale, M. W., and Roby, T. O.: Transmission and Immunization Studies on Equine Influenza. Am. J. Vet. Res., 9 (1948) 243-253.
8. Doll, E. R., McCollum, W. H., Bryans, J. T., and Crowe, E. W.: Serological Differentiation of the Equine Abortion Virus from the Human and Swine Influenza, Mumps, and Newcastle Disease Viruses. Am. J. Vet. Res., **17** (1956) 262-266.
9. Sovinova, O., Tumova, B., Pouska, F., and Nemec, J.: Isolation of a Virus Causing Respiratory Disease of Horses. Acta Virologica 1 (1958) 52-61.
10. Dale, C. N., and Dollahite, J. W.: Experimental Transmission of Equine Influenza. J.A.V.M.A. 95 (1939) 534-535.
11. Schofield, F. W.: A Report of Two Outbreaks of Equine Influenza Due to Virus Carriers (Stallions). Ann. Rept. Dept. of Agr., Ontario, 1937.
12. Hutyra, F., and Marek, J.: Special Pathology and Therapeutics of Diseases of Domestic Animals. Alexander Eger, Chicago, 1938.

VIRAL RHINOPNEUMONITIS

Rhinopneumonitis is an acute viral infection characterized by fever, leukopenia, and catarrhal inflammation of the respiratory tract. The viral disease predisposes to secondary bacterial infection which affects various parts of the respiratory tract. Abortion is often a serious sequel when pregnant mares are infected.

History: The abortion sequel of rhinopneumonitis was described by Dimock et al.[1,2] in 1932 as equine virus abortion. Subsequent reports by Dimock et al.[3,4,5] described lesions in equine fetuses, experimental transmission and epizootiologic patterns, but did not relate the abortions to previous febrile, respiratory disease of horses. Manninger and Csontos[6] and Manninger[7] in 1942 and 1949 reported occurrence of equine virus abortion in Hungary, and in transmission trials observed that experimental subjects developed a febrile respiratory catarrh which they regarded as mild equine influenza. Virus abortion was regarded as a sequel of equine influenza. Jones et al.[8] reported a respiratory disease regarded as equine influenza. A virus recovered by them and designated as equine influenza virus was studied in comparison with equine abortion virus by Doll et al.[9,10,11,12,13] The equine influenza virus isolated by Jones et al.[8] was identical with equine abortion viruses found in the United States. The two viruses produced identical reactions in susceptible horses, gave reciprocal reactions in cross protection, serum neutralization and complement fixation tests, and produced identical lesions in equine fetuses, hamsters, and chicken embryos.

Doll et al.[14] in 1957, reported a comparative study of the equine abortion virus and another virus recovered from horses. Each virus produced a disease compatible with recorded descriptions of equine influenza. The viruses are not related serologically, produce distinctly different clinical signs and lesions in horses, have different experimental host ranges, and each causes abortion. They are not related to the influenza viruses affecting man and swine.[14],[15] It was proposed that use of the terms, influenza and virus abortion, be discontinued for diseases caused by the two viruses. Rhinopneumonitis was proposed for the name of the disease caused by the abortion virus of Dimock *et al.*[2],[5] and/or the influenza virus of Jones *et al.*[8] Viral arteritis was proposed for the name of the disease caused by the second virus causing febrile disease and abortion. The changes in nomenclature are supported by recovery of an A-type influenza virus from horses by Sovinova *et al.*,[16] who propose that the disease caused by this virus be identified as equine influenza.

The diseases caused by the rhinopneumonitis virus and the arteritis virus have been described for many years as equine influenza. The accounts of Law,[17] Huidekoper,[18] Hutyra and Marek[19] and many others record clinical signs and lesions obviously resulting from separate infection by each virus. The relation of the A-type influenza virus to the equine respiratory diseases described in these accounts cannot be appraised.

Distribution: Abortions caused by the rhinopneumonitis virus have been identified in 22 states and in Canada. Characteristic respiratory disease occurs wherever horses are raised or assembled in appreciable numbers. Rhinopneumonitis abortions have occurred in nearly all countries of Europe, Russia, Japan, and South America. Abortions have not been reported from England or Australia, but typical respiratory disease occurs and serologic tests indicate presence of the virus.

Host Range: Equidae are the only known natural hosts. Experimentally the virus may be propagated in hamsters,[20] chicken embryos,[21] guinea pigs,[22] mice,[23] a variety of tissues in Maitland cultures,[24] in HeLa cells,[25] and in cell cultures of equine,[26],[27] bovine,[28] porcine,[28] and ovine kidney.[28]

Epizootiology: Rhinopneumonitis occurs enzootically on farms in areas of concentrated horse breeding. A relatively uniform pattern is observed in central Kentucky, where both respiratory and abortion manifestations have been studied. Respiratory disease is observed almost exclusively in young horses, either on farms or when they are assembled for sale or training. Most farms in the area have outbreaks of rhinopneumonitis in the fall or early winter, especially in October, November, and December. The outbreaks in young horses often are associated with weaning and assembling in winter quarters. Mares on the farms have no overt signs of disease at this time, but infection may be demonstrated by serologic tests. The disease spreads rapidly within a stable or training area with all horses becoming infected within a few days or weeks.

Abortions have been observed in every month except July and August. They are most prevalent in midwinter and early spring. Of 700 abortions recorded in Kentucky, 15% occurred in January, 24% in February, 29% in March, and 18% in April. Abortion may occur from the fifth month of gestation to full term. Some foals infected prenatally are born alive at full term. Data on 623 abortions show 11% occurring in the eighth month, 30% in the ninth month, 36% in the tenth month, and 19% in the eleventh month. The data indicate a relation between age of the fetus and occurrence of abortion, but the breeding period of mares and the enzootic pattern in young horses have an important influence on the seasonal incidence and age of the fetus at the time of abortion.

The incubation time between nasal inoculation and abortion varies from 3 weeks to 4 months, establishing that the infection which results in abortion is coincident with the earlier enzootic infection of young horses on the farms. The virus spreads readily by direct contact, fomites, and aerosolized secretions. Virus may spread from one mare that aborts to others but in most outbreaks the evidence indicates that nearly all mares on the premises were infected 1 to 4 months before the first abortions occur.

The disease occurs annually in young horses on many farms that have no introduction of new horses, suggesting the presence of carriers among adult horses. The regularity of outbreaks when young susceptible horses are assembled also indicates a carrier state, but this has not been established conclusively. Outbreaks are frequent when susceptible horses

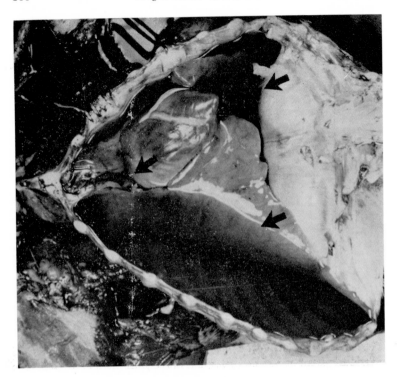

Fig. 23. Fetal rhinopneu-
monitis. Excessive fluid in
the pleural cavity and
edema of the lungs.

are assembled for sales, in yards, in training areas, at race meets or shows, and in military establishments.

Etiology: The virus is filtrable without appreciable loss of titer through Seitz, Selas, fritted glass, Jenkins, and Berkefeld filters. The particle size indicated by electron microscopy[29] varies from 100 to 200 millimicrons, averaging about 170 millimicrons. Morphologically, the particle is rounded, sometimes flattened, and may have a tail structure about 50 millimicrons in diameter and up to twice the particle size in length. Infective particles pass through ultrafine membrane filters with a porosity range of 10 to 50 millimicrons.[30]

The virus survives 2 to 3 years when frozen in whole organs, or in suspension in 20% serum or 10% peptone broths at −4.0 F. It may be lyophilized without loss of titer. The virus is inactive after 2 weeks when dried at room temperature on wood, glass, metal and rope, but may survive 4 to 7 weeks when dried in horsehair or oily burlap. It is present in nasal exudates, expectora, blood, and possibly in the feces during the acute febrile period. It is abundant in the extra-fetal membranes and

fluids and in all tissues of aborted fetuses. Horses may be infected by contact exposure, or inoculation by intranasal, oral, intratracheal, conjunctival, or parenteral routes.

Clinical Signs: The incubation period varies from 2 to 10 days. Primary infection of fully susceptible horses is manifested by fever and a serous discharge from the nostrils. Temperatures may reach 106 F. and fever persists for 1 to 7 days in uncomplicated cases. Fever may be diphasic. Afternoon temperatures usually are higher than morning readings. Leukopenia occurs in parallel with fever. Both neutrophils and lymphocytes are depressed during the first 2 days of fever. Lymphocytes return to normal levels in 2 to 4 days and neutrophils regain normal levels in 5 to 9 days. Feed and water consumption may be reduced but often is unaffected. Mild congestion of the nasal mucous membranes is observed and there may be palpable edema of the mandibular lymph nodes. Enteritis and diarrhea, edema of the legs, and tendovaginitis are infrequent in uncomplicated cases. General depression is slight in horses kept at rest. All signs are exacerbated by forced exercise or work. Recovery is complete in 1 to 2 weeks unless complications develop.

Reinfection may occur at intervals of 4 to 5 months or longer. These subsequent infections are usually asymptomatic, afebrile, and do not result in complications, especially in adult horses on breeding farms. The effect of reinfection on horses in racing or subjected to hard work is not known.

The secondary, asymptomatic virus infection is characteristic of the disease among broodmares. Most purebred horses acquire the disease numerous times on the farm or during training and racing. Subsequent infections, after return to the stud, produce no overt signs, but the virus may invade the fetus and cause abortion. There are no signs of impending abortion. Mares go into labor and expel the fetus quite rapidly. The placenta usually is expelled with the fetus or soon thereafter. The genital tract involutes as following normal parturition. Future breeding performance is not impaired. Mares aborting from virus infection may experience any of the complications associated with foaling or abortion from other causes. Abortion occurs from 3 weeks to 4 months after infection of the mare.

A paralytic syndrome occurs infrequently when pregnant mares are infected. The paralysis is associated with a virus-infected fetus *in utero*. First signs are incoordination of the pelvic limbs, which may progress to paraplegia. Mares may recover if abortion occurs, or is induced, in the early stages.

Foals may be born alive near or at full term with prenatal infection. Often these foals are weak, unable to stand, and exhibit severe respiratory distress. Others stand and may suckle but are weak, febrile, dyspneic, and sometimes icteric. Death usually occurs in a few hours to 3 or 4 days. Bacterial complications and pneumonia ensue frequently.

Lesions: Specific mortality in young or adult horses from proven uncomplicated infection by the rhinopneumonitis virus has not been recorded or observed by the author. Jones et al.[8] recorded lesions resulting from uncomplicated virus infection of horses killed during transmission trials. The lesions included edema, congestion, and petechial hemorrhages

in the upper respiratory mucosae, edema of the mandibular and pharyngeal lymph nodes, and interstitial pneumonitis and pulmonary edema. Inclusion bodies were not observed.

Characteristic lesions occur in most, but not all, aborted fetuses. Diagnostic gross lesions are excessive fluid in the pleural cavity, edema of the lungs, and focal necrosis of the liver. The pleural transudate may be absent or present in quantities up to 2 liters (Fig. 23). It is slightly turbid, has the color of serum, and is almost never tinged with hemoglobin. Edema of the lungs is evident by separation of the interlobular septa, rigidity, firmness and pitting on pressure (Fig. 24). The pulmonary and thoracic lesions are less prevalent in subjects aborted near full term, but are present in 80 to 90% of aborted fetuses. Hepatic lesions are small foci of necrosis varying in size from pinpoint to 3 millimeters in diameter (Fig. 25). They are seen under the capsule of the liver. The number of foci vary from a few to hundreds. Gross hepatic lesions occur in about 75% of fetuses.

Other lesions are hemorrhages on the mucous membranes of the upper respiratory tract, the oral cavity, and digestive tract. Hemorrhages may be absent, or vary from a few petechiae to diffuse hemorrhage. Edema of the pharyngeal tissues is frequent. Lymph nodes throughout the body may be congested and edematous. The placenta has no characteristic lesions, but is sometimes edematous. The inner surfaces of the amnion and foot pads often are stained yellow from passage of meconium.

Intranuclear inclusion bodies may be found in several tissues of aborted fetuses, but occur most frequently in the liver and lungs. The inclusion bodies are amphophilic early in development but tend to be acidophilic in the late stages of development. Inclusion bodies occur in hepatic cells in any part of the liver, but are most readily found in or bordering foci of necrosis (Fig. 26 & 27). Inclusion bodies occur in the epithelium of small bronchioles, terminal bronchioles, and alveoli (Fig. 28). Lungs often are extremely edematous with extensive necrosis of the bronchiolar and alveolar epithelium. Inclusion bodies may be found in any lymphoid tissue, in which there often is an extensive necrosis of lymphocytes (Fig. 29).

Diagnosis: Clinical diagnosis may be made presumptively from occurrence of a contagious respiratory catarrh accompanied by fever and leukopenia. The viral phase often is unobserved, and presence of disease is apparent only after development of secondary bacterial infection. The respiratory and systemic infection may be diagnosed by either complement fixation[31] or serum neutralization tests[32] on paired serums, one obtained during the acute phase and a second obtained 2 to 3 weeks after fever subsides. Serologic tests on single samples of serum are of no value because of

static or have receded. Paired serums obtained after abortion show static or receding titers.

Diagnosis may be made from gross lesions in 80 to 90% of aborted fetuses. Accuracy is improved by histologic examination with demonstration of intranuclear inclusion bodies in the hepatic cells, bronchiolar and alveolar epithelium, and lymphoid tissues. A few virus-infected fetuses are encountered in which inclusion bodies cannot be demonstrated. Virus may be isolated from these in primary cultures of equine kidney and identified by neutralization tests. The virus-infected fetus usually is living when abortion is initiated. The fresh condition of the cadaver is important in differ-

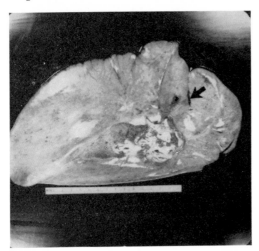

Fig. 24. Fetal rhinopneumonitis. Edema of the lung evident from separation of interlobular septa, excessive weight, firmness, and loss of elasticity.

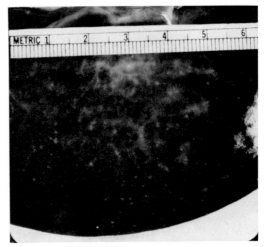

Fig. 25. Fetal rhinopneumonitis. Subcapsular foci of necrosis in the liver.

the extremely wide prevalence of the disease. The virus may be isolated from nasal swabs or washings during the acute febrile period in primary monolayer cultures of equine kidney,[27] and identified by presence of inclusion bodies and neutralization tests. The disease may be identified in horses by transmission and subsequent protection or serologic tests.

Serologic tests on the serum of mares that abort are of no value in diagnosing the cause of abortion. Infection of the mare causes development of both virus neutralizing and complement fixing antibody. These reach their highest titers in 2 to 3 weeks after infection. Abortion occurs 1 to 4 months after infection of the mare, at which time serum titers are

ential diagnosis. Fetuses that die and become autolyzed *in utero*, with diffusion of hemoglobin into the tissues and sanguineous fluids into the body cavities rarely are infected with rhinopneumonitis virus. The septic appearance, autolysis, and acrid odor common to fetuses with bacterial infections do not occur in virus-infected fetuses.

Complications: In the experimental disease, complications seldom occur and nearly always are limited to a mucopurulent rhinitis and pharyngitis. A similar course occurs on farms in confirmed disease of young horses, in which the secondary rhinitis and pharyngitis are more frequent and are associated with a mucopurulent nasal exudate and cough. These signs usually subside spontaneously in 1 to 3

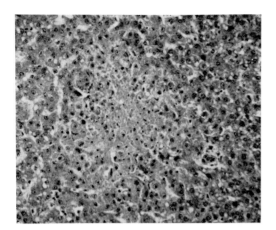

Fig. 26. Fetal rhinopneumonitis. Focal necrosis of hepatic cells. X 120.

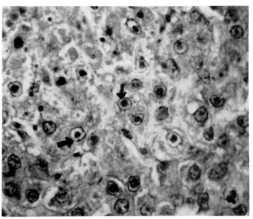

Fig. 27. Fetal rhinopneumonitis. Intranuclear bodies in hepatic cells at the border of a foci of necrosis. X 400.

weeks. Some cases of mucopurulent rhinitis in young horses persist for 1 to 2 months or longer, but the etiology is obscure.

Persistent coughing may follow rhinopneumonitis of horses in training or racing, but the relation of the virus to the race track cough in America or the epizootic cough in Europe has not been established. Pneumonia and pleuritis are infrequent complications in horses on farms, but are common in horses at hard work and those assembled in large groups in yards and remount depots. Hemolytic *Streptococci* are the predominant secondary invaders. *E. coli, Staphylococci, Shigella equuli,* and *Pseudomonas* spp. are recovered frequently, especially from exudates in the upper respiratory tract. Enteritis and diarrhea may occur, prob-

ably as a secondary infection or excitation of latent enteric infections. Horses with protracted pneumonia may develop circulatory complications. Streptococcic infections of joints and tendon sheaths may develop.

Immunity: Natural or induced infection is followed by development of antibody and temporary refractivity to reinfection. Virus neutralizing antibody persists, but after a period of 3 to 6 months horses may be reinfected by nasal inoculation. The reinfection is usually asymptomatic, afebrile, and causes no hematologic disturbance. Occasionally, horses experiencing reinfection have a transient serous nasal discharge and a fever of 1 to 2 degrees lasting from a few hours to 1 or 2 days. Immunity that protects against infection of the fetus per-

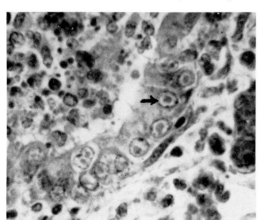

Fig. 28. Fetal rhinopneumonitis. Intranuclear inclusion bodies in the bronchial epithelium. X 600.

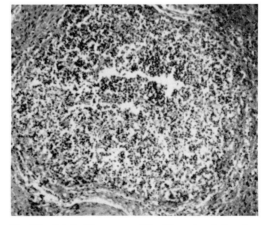

Fig. 29. Fetal rhinopneumonitis. Necrosis of lymphocytes in a Malpighian body of the spleen. X 120.

sists longer, but is variable and not complete. Mares have aborted from virus infection in consecutive pregnancies with intervals of 7 to 11 months between abortions. Experimentally, mares have been infected and the fetus aborted within 4 months after previous experience with live virus. Such mares have high levels of virus neutralizing antibody, but in some manner the virus reaches the fetus. Antigenic variation in the virus has not been demonstrated.

Prevention and Control: Isolation and sanitary procedures do not preclude introduction of the virus by possible carriers. Such procedures are of value for preventing introduction of the virus by infected animals or those in incubative stages. The period of infectivity in active cases is not known, but the course of clinical recovery and development of antibody indicates that isolation for 3 weeks should be adequate. Mares which abort apparently shed virus only with the fetus and for a few days thereafter from the genital tract. The mare which aborts should be cleaned and moved to an isolated area for 2 weeks. The fetus and placenta should be removed in a way that excludes exposure of other horses. The stall and bedding should be soaked with a strong creosote disinfectant and left undisturbed for a week or longer before cleaned.

Several killed virus vaccines have been employed without evident influence on the general incidence of abortions or on the course of outbreaks. Killed vaccines do not establish serviceable resistance to respiratory infection of young horses. A resistant population may be maintained by frequent planned inoculation with live virus slightly modified by passage in hamsters. Inoculations are made by intranasal instillation of the virus twice annually, once early in July and again early in October. The dose is 3 ml. containing 3×10^6 hamster LD_{50} per ml. All horses of each sex and all ages should be inoculated. Such a planned inoculation program should be initiated only in July. This timing takes advantage of the apparent refractivity to abortion during early pregnancy and provides for additional stimulation before the frequent epizootics that occur in the late fall and winter. The inoculations are not recommended late in pregnancy or during the course of outbreaks.

The planned infection program does not entirely prevent abortion from rhinopneumonitis virus, but apparently provides serviceable protection against explosive outbreaks. About 1% of pregnant mares in planned inoculation programs have aborted from infection by native virus. The hamster modified virus also retains a potential for causing abortion. About 0.5% of 2,000 mares aborted from infection of the fetus by this virus. The inoculation program is recommended in areas where the disease is enzootic and serious outbreaks of abortions occur annually. It is essential that the inoculations be made consistently, twice annually, because of the short duration of immunity.

Young horses on farms receive inoculations as sucklings in the summer, as weanlings in the fall, and again as yearlings the following summer. The 3 inoculations with live virus do not provide permanent immunity, but a state of resistance is acquired and subsequent reinfections are quite mild or asymptomatic. Young horses in training have been inoculated without serious interruption of training programs.

The first inoculation of young horses may cause a fever of 1 to 3 F. for 1 to 3 days and a serous rhinitis. The vaccine virus is inconsistently transmissible between horses in close contact. Precautions should be taken to prevent dissemination for 3 weeks following inoculation.

Treatment: The course of the virus infection is not altered by antibiotics or other antibacterial drugs. Secondary bacterial complications may be prevented by antibacterial therapy during and subsequent to the febrile period. Such therapy is most rational for horses in training, racing, or in large acquisitions in which secondary complications may seriously impair the future use of the horse. It is seldom desirable for young horses on farms, except for those with protracted fever or pneumonic complications. The most important part in care of horses infected during the training or racing season is to provide complete rest or only light exercise for a period of 2 to 3 weeks after fever subsides to permit healing of the respiratory mucosa. The rest period avoids complications, especially protracted cough. Treatment of prenatally infected foals born alive at or near full term is usually unsuccessful.

E. R. Doll

REFERENCES

1. Dimock, W. W., and Edwards, P. R.: Infections of fetuses and foals. Bulletin 333 (1932), Ky. Agr. Exp. Sta.
2. Dimock, W. W., and Edwards, P. R.: Is there a filterable virus abortion in mares? Suppl., Bulletin 333 (1933), Ky. Agr. Exp. Sta.
3. Dimock, W. W., and Edwards, P. R.: The differential diagnosis of equine abortion with special reference to a hitherto undescribed form of epizootic abortion of mares. Cornell Vet., 26 (1936) 231-240.
4. Dimock, W. W.: The diagnosis of virus abortion in mares. J.A.V.M.A., 96 (1940) 665-666.
5. Dimock, W. W., Edwards, P. R., and Bruner D. W.: Equine virus abortion. Bulletin 426 (1942), Ky. Agr. Exp. Sta.
6. Manninger, R., and Csontos, J.: Equine virus abortus der stuten. Dtsch. tieraztl. Wschr. 49 (1941) 105-108.
7. Manninger, R.: Studies on infectious abortion in mares due to a filterable virus. Acta. Vet. Hungarica 1 (1949) 1-11.
8. Jones, T. C., Gleiser, C. A., Maurer, F. D., Hale, M. W., and Roby, T. O.: Transmission and immunization studies on equine influenza. Am. J. Vet. Res., 9 (1948) 243-253.
9. Doll, E. R., and Kintner, J. H.: A comparative study of the equine abortion and equine influenza viruses. Cornell Vet., 44 (1954) 355-367.
10. Doll, E. R., Wallace, M. E., and Richards, M. G.: Thermal, hematological, and serological responses of weaning horses following inoculation with equine abortion virus. Its similarity to equine influenza. Cornell Vet., 44 (1954) 181-190.
11. Doll, E. R., Richards, M. G., and Wallace, M. E.: Adaptation of equine abortion virus to suckling Syrian hamsters. Cornell Vet., 43 (1953) 551-588.
12. Doll, E. R., Richards, M. G., and Wallace, M. E.: Cultivation of equine influenza virus in suckling Syrian hamsters. Its similarity to the equine abortion virus. Cornell Vet., 44 (1954) 133-138.
13. Doll, E. R., and Wallace, M. E.: Cultivation of the equine abortion and equine influenza viruses on the chorioallantoic membrane of chicken embryos. Cornell Vet., 44 (1954) 453-461.
14. Doll, E. R., Bryans, J. T., McCollum, W. H., and Crowe, E. W.: Isolation of a filterable agent causing arteritis of horses and abortion by mares. Its differentiation from the equine abortion virus. Cornell Vet., 47 (1957) 3-41.
15. Doll, E. R., McCollum, W. H., Bryans, J. T., and Crowe, E. W.: Serological differentiation of the equine abortion virus from the human and swine influenza, mumps, and Newcastle disease viruses. Am. J. Vet. Res., 17 (1956) 262-266.
16. Sovinova, O., Tumova, B., Pouska, F., and Nemec, J.: Isolation of a virus causing respiratory disease in horses. Acta. Virologica 1 (1958) 52-61.
17. Law, J.: Textbook of Veterinary Medicine. 3rd Ed., Ithaca, N. Y. The Author, 1911, Vol. IV.
18. Huidekoper, R. S.: Diseases of the horse. Special Report. U. S. Dept. of Agr., 498, 1911.
19. Hutyra, F., and Marek, J.: Special pathology and therapeutics of diseases of domestic animals. Chicago, Alexander Eger, 1938.
20. Doll, E. R., Bryans, J. T., McCollum, W. H., and Crowe, E. W.: Propagation of equine abortion virus in Syrian hamsters. Cornell Vet., 46 (1956) 68-82.
21. Doll, E. R., McCollum, W. H., Bryans, J. T., and Crowe, E. W.: Propagation of equine abortion virus in the embryonated chicken egg. Cornell Vet., 46 (1956) 97-108.
22. Semerdjiev, B.: Susceptibility of guinea pigs to the equine abortion virus. Ministry of Agric. and Forest. Annals of Vet. Virus Res. Inst., Sofia, 1 (1958) 103-115.
23. Kaschula, V. R., Beaudette, F., and Bryne, R. J.: The adaptation of equine influenza virus to infant mice by the intratracheal route. Cornell Vet., 47 (1957) 137-142.
24. Randall, C. C., Ryden, F. W., Doll, E. R., and Schell, F. S.: Cultivation of equine abortion virus in fetal horse tissue in vitro. Am. J. Path., 29 (1953) 139-153.
25. Randall, C. C.: Adaptation of equine abortion virus to HeLa Cells. Proc. Soc. Exp. Biol., N. Y., 95 (1957) 508-510.
26. Shimizu, T., Ishizaki, R., Kuno, Y., Ishii, S., and Matumoto, M.: Propagation of equine abortion virus in horse kidney tissue culture. Jap. J. Expt'l. Med. 27 (1957) 175-180.
27. McCollum, W. H.: Personal communication.
28. McCollum, W. H.: Personal communication.
29. Sharp, D. G., and Bracken, E. C.: Quantitation and morphology of equine abortion virus in hamsters. Virology, 10 (1960) 419-431.
30. McCollum, W. H., Doll, E. R., and Bryans, J. T.: Agglutination of horse erythrocytes by tissue extracts from hamsters infected with equine abortion virus. Am. J. Vet. Res., 17 (1956) 267-270.
31. Doll, E. R., McCollum, W. H., Wallace, E. W., Bryans, J. T., and Richards, M. G.: Complement-fixation reactions in equine virus abortion. Am. J. Vet. Res., 14 (1953) 40-45.
32. Doll, E. R., Crowe, M. E., McCollum, W. H., and Bryans, J. T.: In vitro serum neutralization of hamster propagated equine rhinopneumonitis virus. Cornell Vet., 49 (1959) 28-33.

INFECTIOUS EQUINE BRONCHIOLITIS (INFECTIOUS EQUINE COUGHING)

This clinical entity was reported to have occurred epizootically in Great Britain in 1954, and again in 1960. British authors have identified this condition by the ambiguous term, Infectious Equine Coughing.[1,2] It is desirable to distinguish this infection from other entities characterized by coughing if it is determined subsequently that a specific and distinct etiology exists. The entity should be identified, at least for the present, by a term related to its characteristic lesions.

Etiology: The natural history of the disease indicates that a readily transmitted, infectious agent is the precipitating cause. Miller has stated that a cellulotropic virus probably is responsible for the early signs of the disease.[1] Since clinical improvement in prolonged syndromes has been related to antibiotic therapy it may be presumed that secondary bacterial infection occurs occasionally.

Clinical Signs: The clinical syndrome is characterized by frequent paroxysms of harsh, dry coughing, the origin of which appears to be deep-seated. The onset frequently coincides with recent exposure to groups of stabled animals. The coughing syndrome has been observed to spread rapidly among horses of all ages. Elevation of temperature is neither consistent nor marked, although elevations to 104 F. have been observed. The fever generally subsides within 3 to 4 days, but it may persist as long as 2 weeks. Affected animals show little depression and complications are not common. Infrequent sequelae include nasal catarrh, excessive lacrimation, bronchitis, and bronchopneumonia.

Complete clinical recovery is usual and most horses apparently develop some degree of immunity.

Treatment: Affected animals generally recover spontaneously when confined to clean, warm, and dry quarters. Persistent cases may benefit from antibiotic therapy. Recovered animals should be returned gradually to full activity.

—EDITORS

REFERENCES

1. Miller, W. C.: Infectious (epidemic) equine coughing. Vet. Rec. 72 (44), (1960) 954-955.
2. Reynolds, E. Brayley: Infectious equine coughing. Vet. Rec. 72 (47), (1960) 1064.

CHAPTER 5

BACTERIAL AND SPIROCHETAL DISEASES

ANTHRAX

Anthrax is an acute, infectious septicemia which occurs in virtually all mammals. It is produced by a specific organism, *Bacillus anthracis*, and in most cases is characterized by a rapidly fatal course. The horse, though susceptible, is not as easily infected as cattle and sheep but is somewhat more easily infected than man and swine.

Etiology: Bacillus anthracis is a gram-positive, nonmotile, spore-forming, encapsulated rod occurring ordinarily in chains, but occasionally singly or paired. The individual bacillus is a cylindrical rod with square or slightly concave ends, approximately 1 to 1.2 μ in diameter and 3 to 8 μ in length. The capsule can be demonstrated by special stains, and the spores are egg-shaped and located centrally within the body of the bacillus. Spores ordinarily are not found in organisms obtained from recently dead animals although the capsule in such cases is demonstrated readily. In culture, the organism loses its capsule unless it is incubated in an atmosphere containing 10% carbon dioxide.

In the presence of high oxygen levels, favorable humidity and temperature, *Bacillus anthracis* sporulates readily. The spores are extraordinarily resistant to temperature, dessication, and the damaging effects of time. They may retain their viability for upward of 25 years in reasonably favorable environments or in the soil. Due to the fact that 15 minutes' boiling is required to kill spores, it is inadvisable to sterilize anthrax-contaminated substances by boiling in open vessels as the steam may carry viable spores. Perhaps the best disinfectant for anthrax-contaminated material is a 1:1000 solution of mercuric chloride to which 0.5% hydrochloric acid is added. A 10% formalin solution will kill spores in 15 minutes at room temperature. In colder areas, more time must be allowed for sterilization. A freshly prepared 5% sodium hydroxide solution also is suitable for destroying spores.

The vegetative form of the organism is not particularly resistant. It rapidly is destroyed by decomposition in unopened carcasses and may be killed by repeated freezing and thawing. One should always assume, however, that the organism is in the sporulated state and proceed accordingly.

Distribution and Transmission: Although anthrax has a world-wide distribution, it appears to be particularly prevalent in countries without organized control of animal diseases. In countries which have adequate veterinary programs, the disease is relatively infrequent. Nevertheless, even these countries will contain enzootic areas in which the disease persists. Anthrax will tend to be epizootic in areas which have neutral or slightly alkaline soils. In certain of these areas, particularly those which are subject to periodic flooding or are swampy, the organisms may survive for long periods and produce epizootics during the summer and early fall of each year. Generally, an epizootic occurs during hot, humid weather or after heavy rainfalls following periods of drought. Sporadic outbreaks, however, may occur at any time.

The disease may be spread by infected feed and water, vectors, and fomites. Pasture lands can remain contaminated for years, and hay taken from such areas has been shown to transmit the disease. Contaminated water from such establishments as tanneries, rendering and fertilizer plants has been shown to be a source of anthrax. Carnivorous animals and birds may contract anthrax by feeding on dead carcasses and spread the disease via their feces. Blood-sucking arthropods have been incriminated in the spread of the disease among animals. Horses appear to contract the disease as the result of grazing on infected pastures, although feed additives, water, vectors, and fomites have been incriminated in scattered cases.

Clinical Signs: The signs of anthrax are those of a septicemia. Three forms of the disease may occur: an apoplectic form, an acute form, and a subacute form. Apoplectic, or peracute, syndromes occur ordinarily at the beginning of an epizootic and are characterized by sudden onset and a rapidly fatal course. The signs are similar to those of cerebral apoplexy, *i.e.*, staggering, dyspnea, muscular tremors, collapse, convulsions, and death. Massive hemorrhages characteristic of the acute and subacute forms ordinarily are not present. The disease may appear suddenly without any previous indication of illness, and animals may die before treatment can be undertaken.

The subacute and acute forms are characterized by a marked rise in body temperature (up to 107 F.) followed by a period of excitement that merges into depression, respiratory distress, stupor, staggering, convulsions, coma, and death. During the course of the disease, bloody discharges may issue from the body openings, and edematous swellings may appear in various portions of the body. Pregnant animals may abort. Fever, shivering, colic, anorexia, depression, muscular weakness, bloody diarrhea, and swellings involving the external genitalia, the lower abdomen, chest, and the neck may be seen. The acute form usually terminates in death within 48 hours, but the subacute form may persist for 3 to 5 days. Those cases which do not die within this period may recover.

Occasionally, a chronic form of the disease is seen in which local lesions appear that are confined to the tongue and throat. These are concomitant with swelling and bloodstained, frothy discharges from the mouth or nose. Death in these cases results from suffocation. A relatively large percentage of chronic cases will recover. Some, however, will retain the infection in the cervical lymph nodes. A cutaneous form can occur when anthrax organisms are deposited in wounds or abrasions of the skin. This occurs particularly in animals which have been vaccinated, and the disease takes a form similar to malignant carbuncle in man.

Lesions: The lesions of anthrax are those of septicemia. The animal bloats readily and bloody discharges may be oozing from the body openings. The blood fails to clot and has a dark, somewhat tarry appearance. Subcutaneous hemorrhages are common, as are large areas of clear or bloodtinged gelatinous exu-

date similarly located. The spleen is enlarged and dark in color, and the splenic pulp is soft and semifluid in consistency. Liver, kidneys, and lymph nodes usually are hemorrhagic, congested and enlarged. Rigor mortis is either absent or incomplete.

Diagnosis: Anthrax should be suspected when animals die suddenly in or near areas where the disease has appeared previously. Diagnosis based on clinical signs may be difficult in new areas, particularly when the apoplectic form occurs. Anthrax also may be confused with sudden deaths resulting from lead poisoning, sunstroke, malignant edema, hemorrhagic septicemia, purpura hemorrhagica, acute swamp fever, colic, and lightning stroke.

Tentative diagnosis always should be confirmed by laboratory examination. It is inadvisable to open the carcass as the organisms present in the blood will sporulate and form a focus of infection that can persist for years. Specimens for laboratory examination should be obtained as soon after death as possible. Blood smears, cotton swabs, or gauze saturated with a blood sample collected aseptically should be taken, placed in clean glass containers, labeled "suspected anthrax," and sent to the diagnostic laboratory in a sealed metal container. Ears, if taken, must be handled properly if they are to be of any use. The ear should be removed from the lower side of the head, packed in borax, and shipped by the fastest possible means to the laboratory.

Laboratory facilities should be utilized to the fullest extent for the diagnosis of anthrax. It is an unnecessary risk to necropsy animals which are suspected to have died of anthrax. A laboratory diagnosis may be made with direct smears from the suspected material, inoculation of culture media, followed by animal inoculation (preferably guinea pigs or mice) or by the Ascoli precipitation test. The Ascoli test can be applied with either cultured or naturally infected material. In some cases, contaminated samples can be cleared by suspending a small amount of the material in a 1 to 2% phenol-saline solution for one hour, and then culturing.

Treatment and Prophylaxis: Vaccination with appropriate vaccines constitutes safe and effective prophylaxis in most cases. Occasionally, postvaccinal reactions will occur which must be handled like natural outbreaks. The strength of the vaccines will vary according to the virulence of the organism in endemic areas. Ordinarily, No. 1 and 2 spore vaccines will cause little reaction, but No. 3 and 4 vaccines may produce severe reactions in horses which, as a species, are fairly susceptible to the disease. Double or triple vaccination with spore vaccines of increasing strength may be needed to produce a solid immunity in certain areas. Doses are given at 10- to 14-day intervals. Alum-precipitated or saponized vaccines generally are used today and are administered subcutaneously. The duration of immunity is, for practical purposes, one year. In some severely infected areas booster injections may be required 4 to 6 months after the initial vaccination.

Treatment today generally involves the administration of large quantities of antibiotics and nursing care. Such treatment may be supplemented with doses of 50 to 100 ml. of antianthrax serum if the disease is encountered in the early stages. Doses of from 3 to 12 million units of penicillin have been reported to be effective. Terramycin, intravenously, also has been shown to have curative effect. Penicillin has been used as a prophylactic measure in lieu of vaccination in animals exposed to the disease.

Control: Control depends upon destroying infected carcasses by burning and/or burial in quicklime, strict quarantine, disinfection of the area surrounding the carcass, control of insects and other vectors, and destruction of contaminated manure, bedding, and fomites. Sick animals should be isolated for treatment, and healthy animals should be administered prophylactic treatment and immobilized.

REFERENCES

1. Bailey: J.A.V.M.A. **122** (1953) 305.
2. Bailey: J.A.V.M.A. **124** (1954) 296.
3. Bergey, D. H., *et al.*: Manual of Determinative Bacteriology. 7th ed. Williams and Wilkins, Baltimore, Md., 1957.
4. Bone, J. F.: No. Am. Vet. **38** (1957) 12A-38A.
5. Bryan: Am. Jour. Vet. Res. **14** (1953) 328.
6. Burdon: Jour. Bact. **25** (1956) 71.
7. Editorial: No. Am. Vet. **33** (1952) 450.
8. Hagan, W. A., and Bruner, D. W.: The Infectious Diseases of Domestic Animals. 4th ed. Comstock Publishing Associates, Ithaca, N.Y., 1961.
9. Jirina, K.: Mh. Vet. Med. Prague. **15** (1960) 382-383.
10. Johnson and Percival: J.A.V.M.A. **127** (1955) 142.
11. McGoughey and St. George: Vet. Rec. **67** (1955) 132.
12. Merchant, I. A., and Packer, R. A.: Veterinary Bacteriology and Virology. 6th ed. Iowa St. Univ. Press, Ames. 1961.
13. Merck Veterinary Manual: 2nd ed. Merck and Co., Rahway, N. J. (1961).
14. Stein: No. Am. Vet. **33** (1952) 420.
15. Stein and Van Ness: Vet. Med. **50** (1955) 579.
16. Sugg: J.A.V.M.A. **113** (1948) 467.
17. Topley, W. W. C., Wilson, G. S., and Miles, A. A.: The Principles of Bacteriology and Immunity. 4th ed. Williams and Wilkins, Baltimore, Md., 1955.
18. Umeno and Nobata: J. Jap. Soc. Vet. Sci. **17** (1938) 87.

GLANDERS

Glanders is a specific disease produced by the microorganism, *Malleomyces mallei*. It is one of the oldest known diseases of horses. Reference to it in the literature dates back several centuries before Christ. At one time, it occurred commonly throughout most of the world, but now has either been eradicated or effectively controlled in most countries with good veterinary service. The present low prevalence of the disease in developed countries is due to several factors. Fewer horses are used for transportation and for work. As a result, the chance of exposure to infection is reduced. Common watering troughs, proved factors in the spread of glanders, have been eliminated from cities. Knowledge of sanitation and disease control methods has improved. More competent veterinary service is available and its employment is wider since the horse has become a pet. In addition, federal, state, and local public health activities in disease control have contributed to the decreased incidence of glanders.

It should be remembered, however, that glanders is not eradicated. It still is prevalent in many regions of the world, and through rapid transport of animals from one region to another the disease could make its appearance at any time in an area which hitherto has not been affected. The mallein test should be employed on horses at regular intervals to insure its early recognition should infection occur. Since the disease is chronic, glanders may exist for a considerable period of time before characteristic lesions develop.

The disease is transmissible to man and ordinarily is fatal when acquired. Human infection usually is acquired through breaks in the skin or abrasions which come in contact with glanders exudate.

Morphology: *Malleomyces mallei* is a slender, nonmotile, noncapsulated, nonsporulating, poorly staining, gram-negative rod with rounded ends. It varies in size from 0.3 to 0.5μ in width and 1.5 to 5μ in length. Old cultures are pleomorphic and may be composed of forms which range from coccoid to extremely long-branched filaments. Many cells, especially the filaments, show beading and may have minute vacuoles in the cytoplasm. The organism is aerobic and facultatively anaerobic. It grows well on most common laboratory media when incubated at a temperature of 37 C.

A characteristic growth occurs on potatoes. After 48 hours' incubation, a yellowish, viscid, semitransparent growth takes place giving the colonies a "honey-drop" appearance. The cultures gradually turn a deep mahogany color and the potato media is oxidized to a brownish-green.

Clinical Signs: Three forms of the disease are recognized—the pulmonary, nasal, and cutaneous. The pulmonary form is the most insidious. Often no appreciable external evidence is shown in the early stages, and the animal may go for several months without any noticeable impairment of health. Later, however, the horse's general condition becomes poor and there is evidence of pneumonia. Occasionally, in early cases of pulmonary glanders, the horse may show pneumonic signs.

In nasal glanders, the disease ordinarily starts with a unilateral nasal discharge and may be mistaken for rhinitis or strangles. The discharge becomes more copious and purulent as the disease progresses, and may become bi-lateral. Small gray to yellow nodules appear in the lower portion of the nasal cavity. These latter lesions form ulcers with raised irregular borders, which when healed form a stellate scar. The submaxillary glands invariably are involved and may rupture, leaving a crater-shaped ulcer (Fig. 1).

In cutaneous glanders, nodules are found in the skin, subcutaneous tissues, and lymph nodes. The lymphatic channels between infected nodes appear as thickened cords. The nodes ultimately become necrotic, rupture, and after discharging yellowish-gray pus, develop deep, crater-shaped ulcers which bleed easily and are slow to heal (Fig. 2).

Regardless of the form glanders assumes, a postmortem examination almost invariably will reveal lesions in the lungs. The spleen and liver frequently are involved. The regional lymph nodes of affected organs and tissues ordinarily are severely diseased (Fig. 3).

Diagnosis: *Malleomyces mallei* can be demonstrated readily in fresh lesions, but it often is difficult to demonstrate the organism in older lesions. Diagnosis is based upon the mallein test or identification of the causative organism. The male guinea pig is used for the laboratory diagnosis of glanders. An intraperitoneal injection is made using a small amount of the suspected material. If *Malleomyces mallei* is present, an orchitis develops within 3 or 4 days, and with 96 hours thereafter the testicles will abscess and rupture. Before the glands rupture, it is advisable to destroy the animal. Cultures are made from the glandular exudate which should be obtained under aseptic condi-

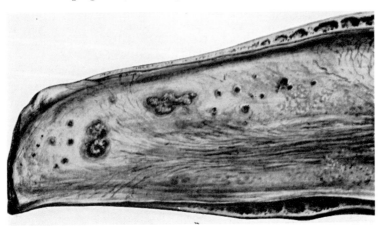

Fig. 1. Ulceration and ecchymotic hemorrhages of nasal septum in horse with glanders.

tions. In addition to testicular involvement, inoculated guinea pigs show lesions in the liver, spleen, pancreas, lungs and other viscera.

Early recognition of glanders can be accomplished with the mallein test, which is a cutaneous reaction similar to that occurring in tuberculosis. The ophthalmic test presently is the procedure of choice for quick diagnosis. It involves the introduction of mallein in either fluid or tablet form under the eyelid. A positive reaction is an intense reddening and pruritus accompanied by a purulent exudate within 6 to 8 hours.

A modification of this test, the palpebral test, is the officially recognized test for glanders. Mallein is injected into the skin close to the edge of the lower eyelid. A positive reaction characterized by extensive edema, congestion of the conjunctiva, and a mucopurulent exudate appears within 36 hours.

Control: The organism is not particularly resistant. Natural dessication and sunlight kill it readily. A number of disinfectants, including roccal, iodine, and mercuric chloride are highly effective. Lysol and phenol apparently are ineffective. The organism can remain viable in water for at least 4 weeks. Some sensitivity has been shown to streptomycin and to systemic sulfonamides, but cures have not been achieved through their use. The organism is a poor antigen, and an effective vaccine has not yet been produced. Prophylaxis depends upon early detection and destruction of affected animals.

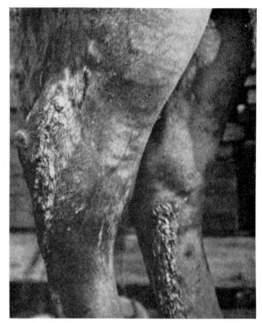

Fig. 2. Cutaneous glanders or Farcy. Courtesy of Cornell University Press.

REFERENCES

1. Ackerman, A. B., *et al.:* Proc. A.V.M.A. (1913) 291.
2. Breed, R. S., *et al.:* Bergey's Manual of Determinative Bacteriology. 7th ed. Williams and Wilkins Co., Baltimore, Md., 1957.
3. Hagan, W. A., and Bruner, D. W.: The Infectious Diseases of Domestic Animals. 4th ed. Comstock Publishing Associates, Ithaca, N. Y., 1961.
4. Hart, G. H.: J.A.V.M.A. 49 (1916) 659.
5. Merchant, I. A., and Packer, R. A.: Veterinary Bacteriology and Virology. 6th ed. Iowa State University Press, Ames, 1961.
6. Merck Veterinary Manual: 2nd ed. Merck & Co., Rahway, N. Y., 1961.
7. M'Fadyean, J.: J. Comp. Path. & Therap. 9 (1896) 322.
8. M'Fadyean, J.: J. Comp. Path. & Therap. 13 (1900) 55.
9. M'Fadyean, J.: J. Comp. Path. & Therap. 17 (1904) 295.

Fig. 3. Pulmonary lesions of glanders. Nodules and hemorrhages indicate diffuse involvement: A, fibrosed nodule, B, caseated cavity, C, hemorrhage, D, early caseation, E, extended hemorrhage.

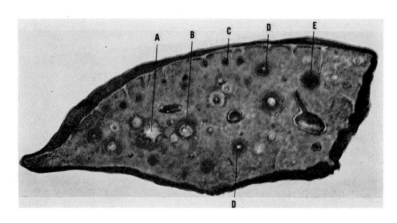

10. M'Fadyean, J.: Comp. Path. & Therap. 18 (1905) 23.
11. Miller, W. R., et al.: Bact. 55 (1948) 115.
12. Miller, W. R., et al.: J. Bact. 55 (1948) 127.
13. Minnett, F. C.: A System of Bact. 5 (1929) 13-55.
14. Mohler, J. R., and Eichhorn, A.: U.S.D.A.-B.A.I. Bull. 136, 1911.
15. Mohler, J. R., and Eichhorn, A.: Proc. A.V.M.A. (1913) 650.
16. Wilson, G. S., and Miles, A. A.: Topley and Wilson's Principles of Bacteriology and Immunity. 4th ed. Williams and Wilkins Co., Baltimore, Md., 1955.
17. Toyoshima, T., and Shibuya, V.: J. Jap. Soc. Vet. Sci. 16 (1937) 136-153.

LISTERIOSIS

Listeriosis is of interest partially because the organism was discovered subsequent to 1900 and actually identified after 1930. It is proof that all pathogens were not discovered in the heyday of bacteriology during the latter portion of the 19th century.

The single species, *Listeria monocytogenes,* has an extraordinarily wide distribution among animals. It appears microscopically as a small, gram-positive, occasionally bipolar rod that is motile, nonacidfast, nonencapsulated and non-sporulating. Filamentous forms occur in some cultures, but the majority of organisms occur singly, or in parallel, or "Y"-shaped pairs. Peritrichous flagella may or may not be present. The rod-like forms measure 0.5μ in width by 1.0 to 2.0μ in length.

There are scant reports in the literature of proven *Listeria* infections in horses, but the disease apparently follows the classic pattern for other species in that a mononuclear leukocytosis is present. The disease is mentioned here only because it has been reported and because it has a potential of infection which is as yet unrealized. Listeriosis in horses has been reported from Norway, Germany, France, and Russia. As yet no other sections of the world have reported infections in horses.

The organism can produce encephalitis. It presents little problem (at least in other species) unless the brain is involved. The clinical signs include ataxia, anorexia, polydipsia, cachexia, and collapse.

The means of transmission of this infection are not definitely known. There is strong circumstantial evidence that Listeriosis is a contact infection. The organisms have been isolated from milk and have been shown to be transferred directly from one animal to another. Completely satisfactory therapeutic agents have not been found. Since the damage is confined principally to the brain, it is difficult to develop a therapeutic concentration of antibiotics or sulfonamides in this area, due to the blood-brain barrier. Sulfonamides and penicillin are useful if given early in the course of the disease. However, in horses, the disease has not yet been characterized sufficiently, and treatment therefore may be administered too late to be effective. Since the signs produced by *Listeria monocytogenes* may be confused with those of other encephalitides, the only certain method of diagnosis is isolation and identification of the organism.

REFERENCES

1. Breed, R. S., et al: Bergey's Manual of Determinative Bacteriology and Immunity. 4th ed. Williams and Wilkins Co., Baltimore, Md., 1955.
2. Berlin, M.: Bull. Acad. Vet. Fr. 19:176, 1946.
3. Grini, O.: Norsk. Vet. Tidsskr. Nr. 3-1943.
4. Hagan, W. A., and Bruner, D. W.: The Infectious Diseases of Domestic Animals. 4th ed., Comstock Publishing Associates, Ithaca, N. Y., 1961.
5. Krage, P.: Berl. u. Munch. Tierarzl. Wschr. Jan. 21:30-31, 1944.
6. Merchant, I. A., and Packer, R. A.: Veterinary Bacteriology and Virology, 6th ed. Iowa State University Press, Ames.
7. Merck Veterinary Manual, 2nd ed., Merck and Co., Rahway, N. J., 1961.
8. Svenkerud, R. R.: Norsk. Vet. Tidsskr. Nr. 9, 1948 60:321.
9. Wilson, G. S., and Miles, A. A.: Topley and Wilson's Principles of Bacteriology and Immunity. 4th ed. Williams and Wilkins Co., Baltimore, Md., 1955.

MELIOIDOSIS

This condition is produced by the organism, *Malleomyces pseudomallei.* The lesions are similar to those of glanders. The causative organism is a short, motile, gram-negative, aerobic rod which forms a heavy cream-colored growth on potato media. Infection results in caseous nodule formation in virtually any or all body tissues except the brain. The nodules may coalesce to form large caseous masses or break down to form abscesses. The only certain method of diagnosis is isolation and identification of the causative organism. The disease is principally pathogenic for rabbits and guinea pigs, but can infect horses, cats, dogs, sheep, goats, swine and man. The mortality rate approaches 100%. It has not been widely reported in the horse. Sulfonamides and members of the tetracycline group of antibiotics have been employed in treatment.

REFERENCES

1. Fletcher, W.: A System of Bact. **5**:56-66, Med. Res. Council (London) 1929.
2. Merchant, I. A. and Packer, R. A.: Veterinary Bacteriology and Virology. 6th ed. Iowa State University Press, Ames, 1961.
3. Hagen, W. A. and Bruner, D. W.: The Infectious Diseases of Domestic Animals. 4th ed. Comstock Publishing Associates, Ithaca, N. Y., 1961.
4. Sutmöller, P., *et al.*: J.A.V.M.A. **130** (1957) 415.
5. Stanton, A. T., *et al.*: J. Hyg. **26** (1927) 33.
6. Miller, W. R., *et al.*: J. Bact. **55** (1948) 115.
7. Ibid, **55** (1948) 127.
8. Breed, R. S., *et al.*: Bergey's Manual of Determinative Bacteriology. 7th ed. Williams and Wilkins Co., Baltimore, Md., 1957.

STAPHYLOCOCCOSIS (Botryomycosis)

A granulomatous disease of horses known as botryomycosis is the result of staphylococcal infection. *Staphylococcus aureus* has been isolated in pure culture from lesions of this condition. At one time, the disease was thought to be caused by a fungus. Botryomycosis usually appears in male animals after castration and localizes in the stump of the spermatic cord. The cord becomes greatly enlarged, sclerosed and small pockets of pus are found interspersed within a mass of granulomatous tissue. Within the purulent exudate, small granules similar to those found in actinomycotic lesions are present. When crushed, these yield pure masses of staphylococci embedded in a matrix.

A similar condition has been noted in the udders of mares and has been referred to as botryomycotic mastitis which is a less virulent form of simple staphylococcal mastitis. One or both mammae are hard and enlarged but are not particularly hot nor painful. Milk production is reduced or absent. The udder contains closely packed, roughly spherical granulomatous areas about a centimeter in diameter. The extent of the affected area is variable. In severe cases, it may include the entire gland. Inside each granuloma is a zone of granulation tissue similar to that occurring in actinomycosis or actinobacillosis. Within the granulation tissue there are several small abscesses and within these are "rosettes" which are packed with staphylococci. Diagnosis is relatively certain from gross examination, and cultural examination of lesions will yield pure *Staphylococcus aureus*.

A third form of botryomycosis occurs as multiple skin lesions consisting of spherical granulomatous nodules ranging from minute size up to 1 inch in diameter. The lesions may or may not rupture to the surface. The general arrangement of the proliferative growth is the same as that found in botryomycotic mastitis, and cultural characteristics of the lesion are identical.

Treatment: Treatment of spermatic cord and skin lesions is surgical. The affected tissue is excised and the animal placed upon appropriate antibiotics for a period of at least 12 days subsequent to surgery. Treatment of the mastitic form is ineffective, the organisms being so well-protected by surrounding tissue that it is virtually impossible to inactivate them.

REFERENCES

1. M'Fadyean: J. Comp. Path. and Therap. **32** (1919) 73.
2. Morrison, S. M., *et al.*: Publ. Health Rep. **76** (8) (1961) 673-677.
3. Hagan, W. A. and Bruner, D. W.: The Infectious Diseases of Domestic Animals. 4th ed. Comstock Publishing Associates, Ithaca, N. Y., 1961.
4. Herzog, M.: Disease Producing Microorganisms. Lea & Febiger, Philadelphia, Pa., 1910.
5. Wilson, G. S. and Miles, A. A.: Topley and Wilson's Principles of Bacteriology and Immunity. 4th ed. Williams and Wilkins Co., Baltimore, Md., 1955.

STRANGLES (DISTEMPER)

Strangles, or distemper, is an acute contagious disease of horses which appears as a mucopurulent inflammation of the nasal and pharyngeal mucous membranes together with abscessation of the regional lymphatics. Occasionally, the disease may spread to other portions of the body. *Streptococcus equi* is considered to be the principal cause of strangles although a second organism, *Streptococcus equisimilis,* has been isolated from cases of a disease clinically indistinguishable from strangles.

Characteristics of the Organism: The causative organism, *Streptococcus equi* or *Streptococcus equisimilis,* does not differ appreciably from other members of the streptococcus group. It occurs in long chains that can be found, virtually in pure culture, in the nasal exudate, or in pus from lesions. Short chains occasionally may be observed and capsules may at times be demonstrated. The organism is gram-positive but tends to decolorize readily. Although *Streptococcus equi* is more resistant to heat than other members of the streptococcal group, this resistance is not excessive. It is killed easily by boiling or by exposure to 70 C. temperature for 10 minutes. Common disinfectants readily destroy the organism. It is more resistant to disinfectants and to drying when present in purulent exudates. The organism belongs to Lancefield's group C. A presumptive bacteriologic diagnosis may be made by identification of streptococci from lesions characteristic of the disease.

Clinical Signs: Signs include a rise in temperature to about 104 to 106 F., increased respiratory rate, depression and anorexia, and inflammation of the nasal mucosa. It is accompanied initially by a catarrhal discharge which is quickly followed by swelling of the submaxillary and pharyngeal lymph nodes, which may later abscess and rupture. As the lymph nodes enlarge, the overlying skin becomes necrotic, denuded of hair, and finally ruptures, releasing large quantities of creamy yellow pus. A laryngitis and cough may develop concomitantly with the lymph node abscessation. The infection may spread along lymph channels to the posterior cervical and mediastinal lymph nodes in which case the disease may become fatal. Ordinarily, however, the infection remains localized in the tissues of the head and anterior cervical region. Once the abscesses stop draining, the temperature rapidly returns to normal. Continuous high fever may indicate internal abscess formation.

Generally, the disease runs a somewhat similar course among all animals infected in a given area. The most dramatic outbreaks occur in horses assembled in large groups such as at race tracks, sales, or horse meets. Younger animals are more susceptible, but cases may appear in older animals which have not been previously exposed, or in animals whose resistance has decreased over a period of years. Factors which reduce the resistance and vitality of the horse, such as exposure to inclement weather, transport fatigue, or viral infections will cause an increased incidence of strangles.

Lesions: The mucous membrane of the respiratory tract shows edema and hemorrhage and may have a mucopurulent exudate on the surface. Abscess formation in the submaxillary and pharyngeal lymph nodes is a fairly constant lesion. Rarely, the mediastinal and mesenteric lymph nodes may be involved, and in some cases metastatic abscesses may be found in the joints or in the visceral organs such as lungs, liver, kidneys, and spleen.

Diagnosis and Prognosis: Strangles usually can be diagnosed from history and clinical signs. However, isolation and identification of *Streptococcus equi* or *Streptococcus equisimilis* from the nasal discharge is helpful in confirming clinical diagnosis. Horses which show unilateral nasal discharge should be regarded with suspicion. Differential diagnosis should include the possibility of glanders. In uncomplicated cases, the prognosis for strangles usually is good since the mortality is less than 2%. In complicated cases involving spread of the disease through the lymphatics, the prognosis will depend upon the individual animal and its response to treatment.

Prophylaxis and Treatment: Since Streptococcus is a fair antigen, the injection of animals with bacterin containing killed *Strep. equi* will help raise the level of immunity and possibly prevent the disease. The use of bacterins, however, is not always beneficial. If given during an outbreak, they may result in an increased number of cases due to stimulation of a "negative phase" wherein the animal is more susceptible to the disease than it would ordinarily be.

During an outbreak, sound sanitary measures are indicated to prevent spread of the infection. Common watering troughs should not be used. Affected animals should be isolated, and their temperatures should be taken at least twice daily. All animals showing elevated temperature should be isolated. Rest is essential and affected horses should be protected from cold, drafts and inclement weather. Stables should be cleaned, and the contaminated bedding burned. Mild antiseptic washes can be used to remove crusted discharges about the head. Antibiotics such as penicillin, penicillin-streptomycin, and tetracyclines should be given in therapeutic doses. The use of antibiotics may be attended by a regression of signs, but in cases where involvement of the lymphatics is pronounced, abscessation and rupture of the nodes may occur 1 or 2 weeks after antibiotic treatment has been discontinued. In these cases, the lesions should be lanced, drained, and the animal given supportive treatment to discourage the possibility of pneumonia. Of the sulfonamides, sulfamerazine and sulfamethazine have been found effective.

Treatment should be continued until the animal's temperature returns to normal. Prompt therapy often will result in preventing abscess formation. Abscessed lymph nodes should be treated topically by applying hot packs and counterirritant ointments until the abscess localizes, at which time it should be drained surgically. If dyspnea is severe it may be necessary to perform a tracheotomy to prevent suffocation.

REFERENCES

1. Bazely, P. L.: Austr. Vet. J. **18** (1940) 189-94.
2. Bazely, P. L.: Austr. Vet. J. **19** (1941) 62-85.
3. Bazely, P. L. Austr. Vet. J. **20** (1942) 141-155.
4. Breed, R. S., *et al.*: Bergey's Manual of Determinative Bacteriology. 7th ed. Williams and Wilkins Co., Baltimore, Md., 1957.
5. Dimock, W. W. and Edwards, P. R.: Kentucky Agric. Sta. Bull. 338, 1933.
6. Hagan, W. A. and Bruner, D. W.: The Infectious Diseases of Domestic Animals. 4th ed. Comstock Publishing Associates, Ithaca, N. Y., 1961.
7. Merchant, I. A. and Packer, R. A. Veterinary Bacteriology and Virology. 6th ed. Iowa State University Press, Ames, 1961.
8. Merck Veterinary Manual. 2nd ed. Merck and Co., Rahway, N. J., 1961.
9. Wilson, G. S. and Miles, A. A.: Topley and Wilson's Principles of Bacteriology and Immunity. 4th ed. Williams and Wilkins Co., Baltimore, Md., 1955.

TULAREMIA

Infection of horses with *Pasteurella tularensis* is rare, but the organism has been isolated from foals dying with pneumonic signs in endemic tularemia areas which were tick-infested and contained infected sheep. The blood of affected sheep has been found to be capable of infecting horses. In foals, the disease apparently starts as a septicemia which later localizes in the lungs. Since the organism is capable of infecting man, care should be taken in examining and handling infected animals.

Pasteurella tularensis is a small, nonmotile, gram-negative, pleomorphic rod measuring 0.2 to 13 microns in diameter to 0.7 to 3.0 microns in length. The culture form is oval or coccoid and the organism is nonmotile and nonspore-forming. The bacterium stains unevenly with most common dyes and smears from animal tissues will show the presence of bipolar forms when stained with methylene blue or carbol fuchsin. The organism is killed in 10 minutes by exposure to 58 C. and can be destroyed readily by most common disinfectants. It will remain viable for several years when preserved in tissues immersed in glycerine and kept at −14 C. Chlortetracycline, oxytetracycline, and various sulfonamides have been shown to be effective in the treatment of this infection.

Diagnosis is made by isolation and identification of the causative organism.

REFERENCE

1. Claus, K.: J. of Bact. **78** (1959) 294-295.

ULCERATIVE LYMPHANGITIS

Etiology: Ulcerative lymphangitis is produced by a specific organism, *Corynebacterium pseudotuberculosis*. *Corynebacterium pseudotuberculosis* is a gram-positive, nonmotile, nonencapsulated coccoidal to filamentous rod 0.5 to 0.6μ wide 1 to 3μ in length that stains unevenly, giving a somewhat beaded appearance. The organism tends to form clumps or palisade arrangements. In natural infections, corynebacteria show marked pleomorphism, but when grown on artificial media, the organism tends to be uniformly coccoid. *Corynebacterium pseudotuberculosis* is not particularly resistant and is destroyed readily by the common germicides, or by boiling or autoclaving. It is a fair antigen, and bacterins made from the organsm will produce a fairly good immunity that will last for about 1 year.

Clinical Signs: In the horse the disease is confined to the lymphatics of the limbs, particularly the hindlimbs. The vessels and regional lymph nodes show nodules, ulceration, and inflammation, producing a syndrome resembling the cutaneous form of glanders. The condition ordinarily is seen in the region of the fetlock, but occasionally involves the upper portions of the limb. Nodules form along the lymph vessels and may enlarge up to 1 inch in diameter. On palpation, these nodes initially are hard and insensitive, but later soften, become painful, and finally rupture. The pus from a ruptured node is greenish-white and blood-tinged. The onset of the disease is slow and usually appears as a painful swelling of the lower portions of both hindlimbs. Initially, marked involvement of the lymph nodes is absent.

Diagnosis: Since this condition is similar to glanders, care should be taken in the diagnosis. The organism should be isolated and identified, preferably by a diagnostic laboratory.

Treatment: Good results have been obtained by i.v. injection of 2 mg. oxytetracycline per pound of body weight once daily for 5 days. Ulcers can be treated with oxytetracycline ointment after preliminary clipping and cleansing of the affected area.

REFERENCES

1. Breed, R. S., *et al.*: Bergey's Manual of Determinative Bacteriology. 7th ed. Williams and Wilkins Co., Baltimore, Md., 1957.
2. Dafaala, E. N., *et al.*: Sudan J. Vet. Sci. An. Husb. 1 (1) (1961) 26-30.
3. Hagan, W. A., and Bruner, D. W.: The Infectious Diseases of Domestic Animals. 4th ed., Comstock Publishing Associates, Ithaca, N. Y., 1961.
4. Hughes, J. P., and Biberstein, E. L.: J.A.V.M.A. 135 (1959) 559.
5. Merchant, I. A, and Packer, R. A.: Veterinary Bacteriology and Virology. 6th ed. Iowa State University Press, Ames, 1961.
6. Merck Veterinary Manual, 2nd ed., Merck and Co., Rahway, N. J., 1961.
7. Wilson, G. S., and Miles, A. A.: Topley and Wilson's Principles of Bacteriology and Immunity. 4th ed. Williams and Wilkins Co., Baltimore, Md., 1955.

LEPTOSPIROSIS

History: Nieschulz and Wawo-Roentoe were the first to demonstrate the susceptibility of the horse to leptospiral infection. They infected a 5-month-old foal by intravenous inoculation of a virulent culture of *Leptospira icterohemorrhagiae* that had been isolated from a case of Weil's disease. Following an incubation period of 5 days, the foal's temperature was elevated and leptospira were recovered in culture from its blood and urine. The animal made an uneventful recovery. Leptospirae could not be cultured from the urine beyond the 13th day after inoculation. A second foal was inoculated with blood taken during the febrile stage from

the first animal. The disease in this foal was rapidly fatal.

Equine leptospirosis, also called water fever and caused by a serotype related to *L. grippotyphosa*, was described in Russia by Lubashenko and Novikova. They recorded 111 cases during a period of 6 years. Mortality was as high as 66% in certain outbreaks. Two isolations of leptospira were made in a group of 28 cases examined bacteriologically. The disease was reproduced by inoculation. The same serotype was implicated in concurrent outbreaks of disease in cattle and foxes. The equine disease was characterized by an elevated temperature of 2 to 3 days' duration, petechiation of the visible mucosae, icterus, a patchy alopecia, and a hemogram indicating a progressive hemolytic anemia.

Well-documented cases of equine leptospirosis recognized in the United States were reported by Roberts, York, and Robinson. They isolated *L. pomona* from horses involved in an outbreak of septicemic disease on a small farm near Ithaca, New York, in the spring of 1952. The signs of infection described by them included elevated temperature, depression, inappetence, and icterus. One mare in this band foaled prematurely. The foal became icteric and died at 48 hours of age. Routine bacteriologic examinations at necropsy were negative and neonatal isoerythrolysis was ruled out by blood compatability tests. Although leptospira were not demonstrated to be the cause of death it seems highly probable that such was the case. The source of the infection on this farm was not determined. Although the disease was diagnosed by blood culture or serology in 9 of 16 horses, cattle and dogs on the farm showed no signs of infection and serologic tests established that they were free of serum agglutinins.

A second case of equine *L. pomona* infection was reported from the same area in 1954. The signs of disease in a mare were similar to those described by Roberts *et al.* Two cows, a heifer, and a second horse quartered in the same small barn with the infected mare remained free of disease during an observation period of 3 months. Negative serologic findings obtained by examination of the serum of the other animals established that the infection neither originated from nor spread to them from the infected mare.

Zaharija reported the occurrence of sporadic cases of *L. pomona* infection in horses quartered with cattle and swine in Croatian villages near Zagreb, Yugoslavia. He recorded a syndrome closely similar to that described in the United States with the additional observation that several infected animals exhibited an urticaria. *Leptospira pomona* was recovered from the blood of these horses and a transient leptospiruria was detected in 3 cases. Swine were implicated as the source of the infection. The signs were reported to be quite mild, recovery ensuing in 5 to 7 days.

A case of equine abortion due to *L. pomona* infection was reported by Wellington, Farris, and Stevenson in Australia. It has been suggested that *L. pomona* infection is responsible for outbreaks of abortion in mares, but the evidence presented for these claims is of a rather tenuous nature.

Leptospiral infection has been accused of responsibility for a form of equine staggers (Schweinsberger disease). It has been suggested that equine infectious anemia is a leptospiral disease and there is a voluminous amount of serologic data in the literature suggesting a causal relationship between leptospirosis and equine periodic ophthalmia. The evidence for leptospirosis as a cause of staggers and infectious anemia is unacceptable. A more detailed discussion of the relationship of leptospiral infection to periodic ophthalmia is provided elsewhere in this volume (see Chapter 15).

Diagnosis: Leptospirosis of horses is an acute febrile disease characterized by a progressive hemolytic anemia. The results of serologic surveys seem to indicate that the infection is not uncommon in horses and that the majority of cases are clinically inapparent.

Leptospira pomona infection of mature horses produces fever lasting for 3 to 5 days with a temperature peak of 103 to 106 F., inappetence, and mild depression. The occurrence of grossly recognizable icterus depends upon the severity of the hemolytic anemia. The hemogram reveals a leukocytosis due to neutrophilia. The leptospiremic stage of the infection lasts from 2 to 5 days and is terminated with the appearance of serum agglutinins at the seventh or eighth day after onset. Recovery is rapid and without complication. Bacteriologic diagnosis may be accomplished by blood culture during the early febrile stage. *Leptospira pomona* is cultivable from the blood for 3 to 5 days during fever. Microscopic examination of wet or dried blood smears is a worthless procedure.

The alternative method for definitive diagnosis is performance of serologic tests using paired samples. A serum sample taken early in the febrile stage will contain no agglutinins for the serotype involved. A second serum sample taken a week following disappearance of fever will agglutinate the organism to high titer. It is well to consider in interpretation of the results of serologic tests that leptospiral agglutinins may persist in high titer in the serum of infected horses for more than 2 years. A single serum sample taken for examination after the acute stage is therefore of little diagnostic significance.

Treatment and Prophylaxis: Equine leptospirosis caused by *L. pomona* is a self-limiting disease. Roberts *et al.* administered penicillin (3,000,000 units) and streptomycin (3 Gm.) daily for 2 days in their cases, with apparent good results. The chronic carrier state in horses does not appear to occur but *L. pomona* has been cultured from the urine of infected horses and cases of the disease should be isolated for several weeks following the acute stage. Although outbreaks of abortion in mares due to *L. pomona* infection have not been proved to occur it should be kept in mind that *L. pomona* infection in a band of pregnant animals is quite likely to produce abortion. There are no controlled data available which support the use of Leptospira bacterin in horses, but it is reasonable to assume that the modern bacterins produced for use in cattle may be applied to advantage in preventing the spread of *L. Pomona* infection in horses.

REFERENCES

1. Bryans, John T.: Studies on equine leptospirosis. Cornell Vet., **45** (1955) 16.
2. Hall, C. E. and Bryans, John T.: A case of leptospirosis in a horse. Cornell Vet., **44** (1954) 345.
3. Lubashenko, S. V. and Novikova, L. S.: Symptoms, diagnosis, prophylaxis and therapy of equine leptospirosis. Veterinarija **24** (1947) 7. Abst. J.A.V.M.A. **112** 352.
4. Lubashenko, S. V. and Novikova, L S.: Leptospirosis in horses. Veterinarija **24** (1947) 11. Abst. J.A.V.M.A. **112**:161.

5. Nieschulz, O. and Wawo-Roentoe, F. K.: Over experimentele infecties van Paarden met *Leptospira icterohaemorrhagiae*. Tijdschr. v. Diergeneesk. **57** (1930) 282.

6. Roberts, S. J., York, C. J. and Robinson, J. W.: An outbreak of leptospirosis in horses on a small farm. J.A.V.M.A. **121** (1952) 237.

7. Zaharija, I.: Klinicki podaci o *Leptospirosis pomona* u konja. Veterinarsk. Arhiva **23** (1953) 318.

8. Zaharija, I.: *Leptospirosis pomona* u konja ustanovljena god. 1951. u. Hrvatskoj. Veterinarsk. Arhiva **23** (1953) 297.

SALMONELLOSIS

Salmonella infections are a cause of infectious abortion in mares, septicemia, omphalophlebitis and pyoarthritis in foals, and colitis in horses of all ages. Excluding the infection caused by *Salmonella abortus-equi* which occurs almost exclusively in horses, equine disease produced by Salmonellae is clinically, pathologically, and bacteriologically closely similar to disease produced by this group of bacteria in other animals.

Clinical Signs and Diagnosis: Colitis caused by Salmonellae is characteristically a disease of the young animal. The highest incidence and most severe cases occur in foals ranging in age from 2 weeks to 4 months. Acute salmonellosis in older animals usually, but not uniformly, is associated with a more or less severe form of stress. This may be in the form of transport exhaustion, the administration of gastrointestinal irritants, heavy parasitic infestation, or following rigorous purgative medication for threatened founder.

The signs of salmonella colitis in foals consist of fever, diarrhea, and progressive dehydration. The body temperature reaches 103 to 106 F. Diarrhea first manifests itself as a watery discharge. The initial diarrhea commonly is followed by a transient period of apparent constipation. Diarrhea recurs and becomes persistent. The fluid feces contain large amounts of mucous. They exude a pronounced but not characteristic fetid odor. Other clinical signs vary in severity, colic may or may not be evident, and foals that are not prostrate nurse willingly. Diarrhea persists for 5 to 10 days in foals that recover. The infection may become quickly septicemic in very young foals, producing fatal issue in 24 to 36 hours after the first apparent illness. Pyoarthritis is not uncommonly a sequel to the diarrheal disease. The mortality rate in foals infected by *S. typhimurium* may be as high as 50%. Animals 4 months of age or older are, in general, less severely affected.

Although rapidly fatal disease occurs in mature animals, the majority of infections in this age group are mild in character. The signs of infection in mature horses may range from no more than elevation of body temperature (101 to 103 F.), inappetence, and a softening of the feces, to a frank, febrile, mucous diarrhea.

Definitive diagnosis of salmonella colitis may be accomplished only by bacteriologic methods. Fresh fecal samples should be submitted to a laboratory with a request for examination for Salmonellae. In watery diarrhea, samples may be taken by passing a cotton swab into the rectum or collecting fecal discharge in a screw-capped glass container.

Salmonella abortus-equi infection in mares is contracted by ingestion of contaminated material. Pregnant mares may abort at any stage of gestation but abortion most commonly occurs between the fourth and eighth months. The aborting mare may show no signs of illness or may have fever with a rise in body temperature to 104 F., colic, diarrhea, and a purulent vaginal discharge. Examination of the fetal membranes will reveal a diffuse, hemorrhagic placentitis. The chorion is edematous and necrotic areas represented by dirty gray, thickened plaques are present. The pleural and peritoneal cavities of the fetus contain an excessive amount of cloudy or hemoglobin-tinged fluid and a hemorrhagic gastroenteritis commonly is seen. None of the grossly observable lesions are in any way specific for *S. abortus-equi* infection. Streptococci and other bacteria produce comparable gross lesions in the equine placenta and fetus.

The diagnosis of *S. abortus-equi* abortion must be made by bacteriologic methods. The causative organism is cultivated readily on ordinary laboratory media from fetal organs and from the placenta. It also may be obtained by culture of the cervix of an aborting mare. The organism remains present in the cervical discharge from only a few days to as long as 3 weeks, therefore cervical cultures for diagnostic purposes should be obtained as early as possible following abortion.

Cultures obtained from aborting mares or fetuses should be submitted to a laboratory equipped for exact identification of the organisms obtained. If cultures are not available, diagnosis may be accomplished by serologic methods. For this purpose, serum from aborting mares should be tested for "H" agglutinins against *S. abortus-equi* cultures. Low titers of these agglutinins commonly are present in the serum of normal horses but serum samples taken from *S. abortus-equi*-infected, aborting mares usually show an appreciably high titer. Serum samples for this examination should be obtained 7 to 14 days after abortion occurs.

Foals may be born alive from *S. abortus-equi*-infected mares. These may be weak, emaciated animals which die of septicemia within hours after birth. Other foals may appear completely normal but within a few days show purulent navel infection, pyoarthritis or both. Pyoarthritis may not develop until 2 or 3 weeks following birth. Infection of the navel may produce septicemic death or joint infection. *S. abortus-equi* infection of foals also may produce diarrheal disease entirely similar to that produced by other Salmonellae.

The majority of mares aborting from *S. abortus-equi* infection rid themselves of the organism readily. The inflammation of the genital tract is rapidly resolved and reproductive function is not impaired. It is important to ascertain that such mares are entirely free of infection before breeding. No mare with an unresolved metritis or cervicitis should be bred. Not only is the opportunity for a successful pregnancy greatly lessened in these animals, but the danger of infecting the stallion is an important consideration. Aborting mares should be examined by culture of the cervix to insure that the causative organism of abortion is not present.

Epizootiology: Although a number of salmonella serotypes are capable of causing equine disease, 3 types, *S. abortus-equi, S. typhimurium,* and *S. enteritidis,* are those most commonly implicated in this country. *S. abortus-equi* has rarely been isolated from animals other than Equidae. *S. enteritidis* is most commonly associated with rodent infection. The droppings of mice and rats may contaminate animal feeds, thereby transmitting the infection. *S. typhimurium* is one of the most ubiquitous serotypes. This organism occurs and produces disease in a wide range of species. The production of manifest infection by the types of Salmonellae involved in equine disease depends upon several factors some of which are known. Animals in robust health, including foals, may ingest these organisms and become asymptomatic intestinal carriers. Foals from farms having outbreaks of *S. enteritidis* infection have been shown to remain carriers for more than a year. The carrier state may occur without the production of any overt disease. Indirect but convincing evidence for the carrier state in older horses is contained in descriptions of salmonella colitis precipitated by administration of gastrointestinal irritants.

Carrier horses are responsible for maintenance of the infection on individual premises, outbreaks being conditioned by contact of carriers with susceptible individuals which are, in the majority of cases, young foals. It is not uncommon for an outbreak of salmonella infection to occur in the foaling barn. The initial infection may be contracted by the foal of a carrier mare and be spread by attendants or utensils to several other foals in the barn. Salmonella live for long periods of time in feces. The improper disposal of fecal material from infected animals or failure to thoroughly clean and disinfect contaminated stalls may be responsible for spread and maintenance of the disease on farms.

Salmonella abortus-equi infection may cause abortion in a high percentage of previously healthy, pregnant mares. This organism is a host-adapted serotype and may possess properties that enable it to invade more readily than do other serotypes found in equine infections. The intestinal carrier state with this serotype occurs among horses. It is highly probable that the stress of pregnancy constitutes a factor conditioning the invasiveness of this organism and producing abortion. The fact that the fetal membranes, fluids, and vaginal discharge of aborting mares contain large numbers of organisms, enchances their opportunity to spread to mares in direct or indirect contact with these materials.

Pathogenesis and Therapy: Salmonella infection produces a necrotizing colitis. This is characterized by severe hyperemia, hemorrhage, and necrosis of the mucosal epithelium and lamina propria. Myriad abscesses are produced by invasion of the solitary lymph follicles, and thrombosis of submucosal blood vessels contributes to development of venous stasis and edema. The organism is cultivated readily from the intestinal tract and from the colic lymph nodes but not from other organs nor from the blood in most fatal cases. Blood cultures taken during the febrile stage of the disease are negative. The infection therefore in the majority of cases is confined to the gut. Invasion of the blood stream undoubtedly occurs, especially in S. abortus-equi infection, but the bacteremia probably is quite transient and large numbers of the organisms are not present in the blood stream at any time. If this were not the case, it is difficult to understand the subclinical or mild illness that occurs in many S. abortus-equi-infected mares and in many horses infected by other serotypes.

The nature of the disease requires therapy directed toward elimination of the causative organism from its most vulnerable position in the intestinal mucosa before the more advanced destructive processes of the infection take place. This requires the use of an antibiotic to which this group of bacteria are susceptible and which can be maintained in effective concentration in the intestine. Several compounds, among which are the nitrofurans and neomycin sulfate, meet these requirements. These compounds should be administered by mouth and should be given often enough to maintain therapeutic levels. Parenteral antibiotics should be used as adjunctives. Animals with severe diarrhea require intravenous fluid therapy. A few foals and older animals that make an apparently satisfactory recovery will be found to be mildly to severely anemic. Blood transfusion is indicated for these animals, especially foals. This procedure often results in a dramatic and lasting improvement in the activity and physical appearance of the animal.

Control and Prophylaxis: Salmonellosis may be transmitted by fomites and every precaution should be taken to prevent contamination of feed and water supplies. Infected animals should be isolated and the manure and bedding disposed of by burning. Fly and rodent control

should be practiced. Grain should be stored in verminproof bins. Attendants should be made aware of the possibility of carrying the infection to other horses and should be instructed in proper sanitary procedures.

Carrier animals constitute a threat to each new crop of foals. The results of attempts to effect a cure of carrier horses by administration of prolonged courses of antibiotics or by vaccination with autogenous bacterins provide no encouragement that this may be accomplished.

The use of a killed bacterin for prevention of S. abortus-equi infection should be a routine practice on breeding farms. S. abortus-equi abortion seems to have disappeared in the United States. Though no controlled experimental data are available to assess the role of vaccination in control of this disease, practical experience indicates that use of the bacterin is a valuable prophylactic measure.

A killed bacterin containing S. typhimurium and S. enteritidis has been used in horses on breeding farms where salmonellosis is a problem in foals. This bacterin produces agglutinin titers in vaccinated animals that are equal to or in most cases higher than those resulting from natural infection. It seems to be of value for limiting outbreaks of the disease and for preventing the recurrence of salmonellosis caused by these serotypes in subsequent crops of foals. Farms not using bacterin have experienced repeated outbreaks of disease due to a single serotype. Those farms using bacterin have not had recurrences.

The S. abortus-equi bacterin is administered to mares in a 3-dose course during the fall of each year. The combined bacterin is given in a 2-dose course to all horses on farms experiencing the disease. A single dose is administered to all previously immunized foaling mares in December of each year. This is done for the purpose of providing the highest practical level of colostral antibody to newborn foals. Foals are given a course of bacterin at 2 months of age. An exact serologic identification of salmonella serotypes involved in any outbreak of diarrheal disease is a requisite for the employment of bacterin. No benefit would accrue from use of bacterin for control of disease caused by serotypes antigenically distinct from those contained in the bacterin.

J. T. Bryans

REFERENCES

1. Bryans, J. T., Fallon, E. H., and Shephard, B. P.: Equine Salmonellosis. Cornell Vet. **51** (1961) 468.
2. Dimock, W. W., Edwards, P. R. and Bruner, D. W.: The occurrence of paratyphoid infection in horses following treatment for internal parasites. Cornell Vet. **30** (1940) 319.
3. Edwards, P. R.: Salmonella aertryke in colitis of foals. J. Inf. Dis. **54** (1934) 85.
4. Edwards, P. R. and Ewing, W. H.: Identification of Enterobacteriaceae. Burgess, Minneapolis. (1955).

ACTINOBACILLOSIS

Actinobacillosis is an infectious disease characterized by acute, fulminating infection of newborn foals and acute or subacute disease of older horses, often with localization in joints or tendon sheaths. The disease has been identified as Shigellosis, sleeper foals, dummy foals, wanderers, viscosum infection, joint-ill, and pyosepticemia of the newborn.

Etiology: The causal organism is *Actinobacillus equuli;* other names used are *Shigella equirulis, Bacillus nephritidis equi, Bacterium viscosum equi, Bacterium pyosepticum equi, Shigella viscosa,* and *Shigella equuli.*[1] The morphology, cultural characteristics, and serology of the organism were studied by Edwards.[3] Rough mucoid, smooth mucoid, transitional, and dwarf strains may be recovered directly from infected tissues. Rough mucoid strains are most frequently isolated. Recognition of variants is important in diagnosis. The organism is extremely diverse in its serologic characteristics. Specific serodiagnostic tests appear impractical. *A. equi* is a gram-negative, nonmotile, pleomorphic rod occurring as single rods, short chains, or long filaments. It grows readily on ordinary culture media. Cultures must be transferred at intervals of 5 to 7 days unless a special semisolid medium is used.[6]

Pathogenicity: Actinobacillosis is principally a disease of young foals. Dimock et al.[2] found that *A. equuli* caused death of 31% of 810 foals examined in Kentucky. It caused death of 46% of 550 foals having bacterial or viral infections. Of 254 foals infected by *A. equuli,* 31% died on the first day of life, 15% on the second, and 12% on the third, with 72% dying within the first week. Foals less than 48 hours old have acute, fulminating septicemias with no obvious tendency for localization. Foals 3 days to 2 weeks old have septicemias with obvious localizations in the kidneys and joints. Those 2 weeks to 2 months old often have localizations in joints and the course is less acute. In horses more than 2 months old, the disease most frequently is initiated as a localized infection of a verminous aneurysm of the anterior mesenteric artery. Infective emboli are dispersed through radicles of the artery, resulting in pyoembolic abscesses, infarction, and septicemia. Localized infections may occur in the lungs, kidneys, or sinuses. Dual infection with *A. equuli* and streptococci occurs frequently in newborn foals.

A. equuli is an inhabitant of the mucous membranes of the pharynx and intestinal tract of clinically healthy horses. It was recovered from intestinal contents by Laudien,[5] from the tonsillar area of 49 of 67 horses by Jarmai,[4] and from the tonsils and taste buds of 10 of 12 horses by Dimock et al.[2] The foal's dam or its immediate environment are the likely source of infection.

Writers on the disease have had a tendency to regard infection as occurring prenatally, a concept that is open to serious question. Prenatal infections may and do occur, but definitely established cases are very few in number. *A. equuli* infection has been detected in only 7 of 3,346 aborted fetuses examined in Kentucky, and in none of 600 foals delivered dead at term. Its appearance in cervical cultures of mares with metritis or cervicitis is so rare that it cannot be regarded as a factor in etiology of these diseases. The rarity of abortion from *A. equuli* infection conforms with the infrequency of its association with cervicitis and metritis. Conversely, streptococci, staphylococci, and coliform organisms which often are associated with cervicitis and metritis cause abortion with relatively greater frequency. These organisms are recoverable from uterine secretions following delivery of a prenatally infected foal. *A. equuli* seldom is recovered from uterine secretions of mares whose foals die of the disease at 1 to 2 days old.

Many foals that succumb from *A. equuli* infection are ill at birth or soon afterward.

This early illness has been regarded as evidence of prenatal infection. If true, the infection likely occurs immediately prepartum. It is quite improbable that the organism could invade the fetus, remain quiescent for any period, and then produce a fulminating septicemia after delivery of a live foal. Since the advent of effective antibacterial therapy, such foals often are completely sterilized from the time of expulsion by saturation with multiple antibiotics, but many die with complete absence of any sign or lesion indicating infection. A constant lesion of newborn foals is an enteritis, indicating that infection is acquired by ingestion and that the intestinal tract is the primary site of the infectious process. Pathogenesis in the newborn foal appears to involve the weak, debilitated, or incompletely developed individuals with defensive mechanisms unprepared for external environment. Such a foal succumbs to infection by organisms capable of causing rapidly developing, acute disease, and which are widely prevalent in its environment. A. equuli is the most frequent invader and is followed in order by streptococci and coliform organisms.

The mode of infection in older horses is obscure. Dimock et al.[2] reported presence of A. equuli in verminous aneurysms with complete absence of evidence of infection elsewhere. They theorize that the organism may be carried to the site by larvae of Strongylus vulgaris.

Clinical Signs: Foals often are ill at birth or develop illness within the first 48 hours. Two general syndromes occur, the sleeper and the dummy. The sleeper case lies in a semicomatose condition, does not rise, occasionally makes feeble movements, and frequently dies within 24 hours. The dummy type is stronger, arises, wanders aimlessly about the stall, refuses to nurse, eventually collapses in a semicomatose state, and usually dies on the second or third day. Other foals appear quite normal at birth and develop signs on the second or third day or later.

The illness is characterized by rapid onset, extreme prostration, and rapid fatality. Pulse and respiratory rates are increased. The temperature may reach 104 F. or higher but frequently falls below normal before death. Soreness and lameness may be observed. Joints of the limbs usually are not visibly or palpably affected during the first 48 hours after birth. Foals developing signs on the third day or later often have soreness and swelling of one or more joints of the legs. Chronically infected joints without signs of systemic illness occur in foals more than 2 weeks old.

Lesions: Foals less than 2 days old have an enteritis and lesions of septicemic infection. The leg joints seldom are visibly affected, but A. equuli may be recovered from the joint cavity. Foals dying on the second day have similar lesions with more pronounced involvement of the joints. In addition to septicemic lesions and arthritis, foals 3 days old or older usually have multiple pyoembolic abscesses in the cortex of the kidney, corresponding in distribution with the glomeruli (Fig. 4). The articular surfaces are not eroded. The joint capsule and supporting tissues are edematous, congested, and contain small hemorrhages. The joint fluids are yellow or amber in color, reduced in viscosity, turbid, and sometimes contain small flocculi of fibrinous material.

All joints often are involved in very young foals. Articular infections tend to be localized to one or a few joints in older foals. The disease in foals more than 2 months old, which usually arises from infection of a verminous aneurysm, is initiated by colic, high fever, and signs of septicemia, which are followed by rapid prostration and early death.

Diagnosis: Clinical signs are not specific for infection by A. equuli. They are replicated by infection with streptococci, coliform organisms, Klebsiella spp., and rhinopneumonitis virus. The last often is confused with septicemias of the newborn since nearly all of them acquire complicating infection by A. equuli or streptococci. The sleeper and dummy syndromes are quite characteristic, but they also are associated with streptococcic and coliform infections. Lesions of septicemia, enteritis, and accompanying involvement of multiple joints justify considering a diagnosis of A. equuli infection. Multiple pyoembolic abscesses in the renal cortex are essentially a specific lesion of A. equuli infection of newborn foals (Fig. 1). In absence of this lesion, definitive diag-

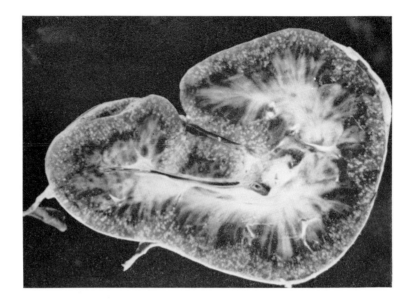

Fig. 4. Multiple abscesses in the renal cortex of a 3-day-old foal.

nosis may be made only by cultural examination.

Prevention: Since *A. equuli* is widely prevalent as a normal inhabitant of the oral cavity, pharynx, and intestinal tract, foaling cannot be accomplished in an environment free of the organism. Usual cleanliness and care of the newborn should be practiced to reduce chances of infection and to avoid stressing the foal unnecessarily. Immunoprophylaxis is not practical because of antigenic diversity of *A. equuli.*

Treatment: Experience in Kentucky has shown that in foals less than 7 days old, infection and death from *A. equuli* exceed the same from other microorganisms by a ratio of 3 to 1. It is prudent, therefore, not to discount the possibility of actinobacillosis in either diagnosis or selection of treatment for foals less than 7 days old. Artificial feeding often is necessary. It should be initiated early and special effort should be made to utilize all of the mare's colostrum. Transfusion with the dam's blood is a traditional treatment and is beneficial as a supportive measure. Dehydration, which often occurs, should be corrected by use of electrolytes and dextrose. Amino acid solutions are beneficial. Sulfonamide therapy is less effective than antibiotics. Streptomycin, 1 Gm. initially, followed by 0.5 Gm. at 3-hour intervals, is very effective. As it is not possible to differentiate consistently streptococcosis

from actinobacillosis, penicillin should be included in treatment when streptomycin is used. Oxytetracycline, 2 to 4 mg./lb. daily in divided doses and tetracycline, 2 mg./lb. daily in divided doses, may be employed. Persistent infections in joints or localized infection of joints in older foals may yield to injection of antibiotics directly into the joint. Antibiotic therapy should be continued for 1 or 2 days after clinical signs subside and temperature returns to normal.

Anthrax is an acute, infectious septicemia in newborn foals. Therapy is initiated immediately after the foal is born, and to be dependably effective must be continued 2 to 4 days. A single injection of an antibiotic often does not provide the desired protection. When employed routinely, prophylactic use of antibiotics may be expected to be beneficial, preventing or eliminating bacterial infection in 3 to 4% of newborn foals.

E. R. DOLL

REFERENCES

1. Bergey's Manual of Determinative Bacteriology, 7th ed., Williams & Wilkins Co., Baltimore, Md., 1957.
2. Dimock, W. W., Edwards, P. R., and Bruner, D. W.: Infections of Fetuses and Foals, Ky. Agr. Exp. Sta., Bulletin 509, 1947.
3. Edwards, P. R.: Studies on *Shigella equirulis*. Ky. Agr. Exp. Sta. Bulletin 320, 1931.
4. Jarmai, K.: Viskossptkamien bei alteren Fohlen und erwachsenen Pferden. Dtsh. Tierarztl. Wchr. **37** (1929) 517.
5. Laudein, L. Quoted by Dimock *et al.* (3).
6. McCollum, W. H., and Doll, E. R. A medium for maintaining the viability of Shigella equuli cultures. Cornell Vet. **41** (1951) 11.

TUBERCULOSIS

Occurrence: The occurrence of tuberculosis in horses depends largely on their exposure to tubercular cattle. A prevalence rate of 0.2% has been recorded, but it usually is much lower. Of 75 strains of tuberculosis bacilli isolated from horses, 69 were bovine, 5 avian, and 1 human.

Clinical Signs: The course of the disease in horses appears to be invariably of a chronic character, and usually the first sign observed is loss of condition, in spite of a normal appetite and abundance of food. In a large proportion of cases, stiffness of the neck is an added and very characteristic sign. In many instances, this stiffness is so pronounced that it cannot escape notice, but it may be overlooked when the horse is not examined with a view to its detection. It is not certain whether the changes in the bones causing this stiffness are true tuberculous lesions.

Polyuria frequently is present during the last stage of the disease. As a rule there is no nasal discharge, but in very rare cases the schneiderian membrane is the seat of lesions, and in a few animals the submaxillary lymph nodes are enlarged and indurated with or without nasal lesions. The final stage, when the disease is allowed to run its course, is marked by fever and a steadily increasing respiratory rate, up to 40 or more per minute. These signs furnish evidence that the disease has become generalized, and that a multitude of miliary tubercles are developing in the lungs. The route of infection usually is by ingestion, but may sometimes be respiratory.

Gross and Microscopic Lesions: One of the outstanding features of tuberculosis in the horse is the frequency with which the lesions, other than the final miliary tubercles, assume a tumor-like appearance. This is best exemplified by lesions in the spleen and mesenteric lymph nodes. The spleen may be enlarged to 10 times the normal size owing to the development in it of rounded growths; there may be simultaneous enlargement of the mesenteric lymph nodes (in one observed case the mass weighed 25 kg.). The individual lymph nodes then are no longer recognizable, but appear as a mass of more or less confluent, tumor-like growths.

As a rule, these tumor-like lesions have a firm, semifibroid consistency, their cut surface is white or yellowish-white and is devoid of any appearance suggesting necrosis or caseation. They never are encapsulated, and the boundary where they meet the splenic pulp usually is more or less irregular. Although this is the most common character of the lesions in the spleen and mesenteric lymph nodes, there are cases in which some of them have undergone pronounced central softening, resulting in the formation of material resembling thick pus. In still other cases which are comparatively rare, necrosis without softening has occurred and has been followed by distinct calcification.

The miliary lesions resulting from the dissemination of bacilli by the blood stream are distributed evenly throughout lung tissue, but often are not seen in other organs. As a rule, the lung literally is crammed with lesions, but the number varies in different cases and their size is inversely proportional to the number. This is explained by the fact that when the lesions are very numerous death may result within a few weeks, but when they occupy less lung tissue the horse may survive longer and the tubercles may attain a diameter of 5 or 6 mm. before death occurs.

The increase in size of lymph nodes in advanced cases is due to the enormous cellular proliferation and to fibrillar increase. Even in long-standing lesions, the capsule may show little or no evidence of fibrous thickening or of pericapsular inflammation, but in other nodes it may be grossly fibrosed. The lesions in lymph nodes may affect both the cortex and medulla, depending on the stage of development. In the early phase, the striking feature is cellular infiltration of the sinuses (benign sinus reticulosis of Robb-Smith), which might easily be mistaken for a nonspecific effect and certainly could not be assumed by histologic examination alone to be due to a mycobacterial infection. The peripheral cortical and medullary sinuses may be packed with epithelioid cells, and giant cells of the Langhans type may be quite numerous.

The germ centers of the lymph nodes may be undisturbed or, at the most, a few may contain small conglomerations of epithelioid and giant cells. Necrosis and caseation may be absent. The grossly enlarged and fibrous nodes, which so often are observed, present a different picture. The normal lymphoid architecture may be largely destroyed and replaced by small and often confluent tubercular follicles. There may be small areas of necrosis and, rarely, some central caseation. These follicles are composed of a central mass of closely packed epithelioid cells, which are of the same histiocytic type seen packing the sinuses. Polymorphonuclear leukocytes may be absent unless there is tissue necrosis; lymphocytes are not numerous and do not form a peripheral barrier as seen in the classical tubercle. Giant cells (Langhans type) may be numerous but are not present in every tubercle and show great variation in size, shape, and number and location of nuclei; many appear to have coalesced to form almost syncytial masses. The cells of these tubercular follicles form a rather heterogeneous collection in the midst of a fibrillar reticulum with numerous fibroblasts. In some other lymph nodes, the appearance of compact confluent lesions may not be so evident; the epithelioid cells lie in a more loose framework and the cytoplasm may not be clear. This appearance might be due to postmortem autolysis.

Diagnosis: The subcutaneous tuberculin test appears to be reliable in horses, but many nontuberculous horses react to an intradermal injection of mammalian and avian tuberculin. The intrapalpebral tuberculin test may be more reliable.

An interesting feature of equine tuberculosis is that approximately 40% of the bovine strains isolated from horses have a lowered virulence for laboratory animals. The same is true of strains of tuberculosis bacilli isolated from lupus in man. The cases from which these strains with lowered virulence are isolated may, however, be severe and progressive.

J. FRANCIS

REFERENCE

Francis, J.: Tuberculosis in Animals and Man (1958). Cassell & Co. Ltd., London. The Williams and Wilkins Company, Baltimore, Md.

CLOSTRIDIAL DISEASES

Distribution: Clostridial diseases of the horse, with the exception of tetanus, are not a major problem for veterinarians or horsemen. Although the horse may become infected with malignant edema and botulism, these diseases are relatively rare and do not present such problems as the ever-present threat of tetanus. The genus, Clostridium, is composed of a large number of gram-positive, rod-shaped, spore-forming, anaerobic bacteria. Most of these occur in the soil. The pathogenic species produce disease principally through the action of their exotoxins upon body tissues. The distribution of clostridia is world-wide and the organisms occur wherever animals are raised. In the spore state, they are highly resistant to environmental damage or disinfectants, and may be introduced readily into new areas by the movement of animals or animal products, or by birds or predatory animals.

Where pathogenic clostridia may be introduced, the locality should be considered permanently infected and the disease expected to appear again and again in susceptible livestock. There always is the possibility of subclinical infections that may be inapparent until circumstances cause the disease to appear in a clinical form.

Etiology: Clostridia may enter the body by several routes, the commonest being via the digestive tract or through breaks in the skin. The diseases which they produce usually are fulminating, with high fever, depression, and a rapid course often terminating in death. Since the number of clostridial diseases in horses is limited, and their clinical features sufficiently peculiar, they readily are recognized by the diagnostician. As in other species, clostridial diseases usually are fatal for horses unless rigorous treatment is given promptly.

All of the pathogenic species of clostridia produce toxins. The destructive action of clostridial toxins in susceptible animals may be due to several separate antigenic components. Since bacterial metabolism involves a complex system of enzyme actions, and toxins that are the products of bacterial metabolism, these substances ordinarily do not appear in laboratory cultures until active growth has been in progress for some time.

Pathogenesis: Knowledge of the action and methods for identification of the various components of bacterial toxins have been expanded through developments in enzyme chemistry. As many as 6 antigenic components have been found in clostridial toxins, which include lethal toxin, hemolytic and necrotizing toxins. Hemolytic action, to a variable degree, is a feature of all edema-producing species of clostridia. Capillary damage, resulting in local hemorrhage, seems to be the result of the solvent of collagenase on supporting and connective tissue, which aids in producing muscular disintegration.

A spreading factor, hyaluronidase, also is produced by clostridia, and may be responsible for the extension of infection into distant tissues. Emphysema arising from bacterial growth contributes to tissue disruption and gas formation. A localized necrotizing action on tissues is produced by one of the toxic components. The lethal effect of clostridial infections apparently is due to a combination of their toxins affecting vital tissues and cells of the host.

Identification: Serologic and/or biochemic methods must be used to identify toxins and their components. The classic method of identifying an individual species by morphologic, cultural, physiologic, and pathogenic features is standard procedure, but it is not entirely applicable in the case of the clostridia since it does not definitely identify the type of organism in regard to its toxin.

All members of the genus, Clostridium, are large, gram-positive, anaerobic, spore-forming rods. The spores usually are oval and may be located centrally, terminally, or eccentrically along the rod, depending on the species. The vegetative forms found in the tissues of infected animals occur singly, in pairs, or in chains. Morphology, cultural characteristics, clinical signs, lesions and toxin types are used to differentiate the species. The diseases produced by clostridia are infectious but not contagious. The vegetative state of the organism is relatively susceptible to disinfectants and drugs but the spore state is very resistant and may live for long periods in the soil and be acquired by susceptible animals from fecal contamination of soil or vegetation, as wound infection or by ingestion. In general, clostridial infections do not assume epizootic proportions although they remain a constant threat to animals.

Because of the very rapid course of clostridial infections, treatment must be started as soon as possible and should employ every means available to save the life of the infected animal. Although many drugs suppress bacterial growth in the patient, they have little or no effect on the toxins which cause the damage. Circumstances may justify the use of specific antitoxins in the treatment or temporary prophylaxis of clostridial diseases where immediate neutralizing effect or protection is needed.

TETANUS

Tetanus is a toxemia produced by *Clostridium tetani* and is characterized by spasmodic, tonic contractions of striated muscles. The disease is world-wide in distribution but it is more common in areas which have been put to agricultural use for considerable periods of time. The disease also is more common in warmer climates.

Morphology: Clostridium tetani is a long, slender rod 0.4 to 0.6 microns in diameter by 2 to 5 microns in length. It may occur in long filaments or in shorter rods. The ends of the organism are rounded. In young cultures and infected material, the vegetative organism appears singly or in short chains which are sluggishly motile by means of peritrichous flagellae. Spores form in cultures after 24 to 48 hours of incubation. The spores are 2 to 3 times the diameter of the cell and are located terminally, which gives the cells a "drum stick" or "tennis racket" appearance. In old cultures, rods and filaments disappear, leaving spherical spores. The organism is gram-positive when young and stains readily with ordinary aniline dyes. Older cultures tend to be gram-negative.

Isolation in pure culture is difficult. Heating of material taken from animals to 80 C., and subsequently inoculating the material into broth may be required for isolation. The organism grows well in liquid media to which finely divided particles of meat are added.

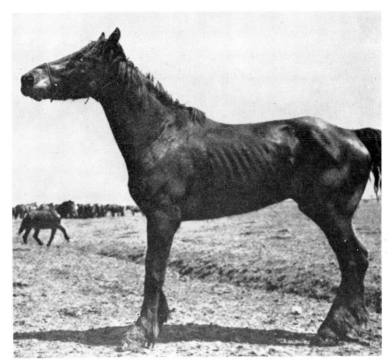

Fig. 5. Characteristic appearance of horse with tetanus. Courtesy of W. E. Jennings, D.V.M.

Pathogenesis: Clostridium tetani apparently exists normally in the intestinal tract of horses and is found in large quantities in equine feces. Infections occur as a result of contaminated wounds. Puncture wounds or lacerations such as those produced by nails and splinters are the types which form the most favorable environment for growth of the organism. Superficial and clean wounds rarely become infected. Unless toxin is present, washed spores will not germinate in living tissue but are ingested and destroyed by phagocytes. The toxin is necessary to produce a local necrosis and a favorable medium for spore germination. In natural infections, foreign material, soil and the character of the wound may produce the same effect. Local death of tissue such as occurs in contaminated, traumatized, anaerobic wounds furnishes a suitable medium for growth and multiplication of the tetanus organisms.

Umbilical infections may occur in the newborn. The vegetative forms of *Clostridium tetani* produce a neurotoxin which is absorbed through the motor end plates of the muscles and apparently passes along the motor nerves to motor cells of the ventral horn of the spinal cord before general signs of the disease appear. A central and a peripheral effect has been noted. The peripheral effect results from absorption of the toxin by the motor end plates. The central effect arises from poisoning of the motor centers. There is some controversy about whether or not the blood vascular system is involved in toxin transport. The bacterial infection ordinarily remains localized.

Clinical Signs: The incubation period varies from 1 to a reported 4 months although it is possible that an intercurrent infection may account for this latter interval. At first, there is a localized stiffness usually involving the muscles of the jaw, the hindlimbs and rarely of the muscles in the region of the infection. After 24 hours, the signs become generalized and pronounced, with hyperesthesia and tonic spasms, probably due to the neurotoxin's effect upon motor nerve centers. Consciousness apparently is not affected. Reflexes are increased and the animal shows systemic response to point stimuli. Muscle spasms of the head cause difficulty in prehension and mastication. The tail is stiff and extended, the limbs are fixed in extension, and the ears are erect. Frequently there is a prolapse of the nictitating membrane. Locomotion is difficult. Spasms of the neck and back muscles cause extension of the head and neck, and the extensor spasms cause the typical "saw-horse" stance. Sweating, disturbance of circulation and respiration, increased heart action, rapid breathing and congestion of the mucous membranes are common. The temperature will rise as high as 108 F. toward the end of a fatal attack as the result of brain damage and derangement of the temperature regulation center in the hypothalamus. In mild attacks, pulse and temperature remain normal. Mortality averages about 80% of infected horses, and recovery is slow, requiring a convalescent period of 3 to 6 weeks (Fig. 5).

Treatment and Prophylaxis: Necrotic tissue should be removed surgically, if practical, and drainage established in the wound area. Cleanliness is essential. Instruments should be sterilized before use. Prophylaxis may be obtained either by injection of tetanus toxoid or tetanus antitoxin. In the horse, the injection of tetanus antitoxin is attended with no particular danger of foreign protein shock since the antitoxin ordinarily is obtained from horse serum. Antitoxin provides a passive immunity which will endure for approximately 2 weeks. If signs of tetanus are present, the antitoxin may be administered at a level of 100,000 to 200,000 units or more. However, this is useful only if given early in the course of the disease.

Active immunization is accomplished through the use of tetanus toxoid. Two doses should be given at 6-week intervals followed by booster injections annually. If wound infections occur in vaccinated animals, it is wise to give a dose of tetanus toxoid as the rise in antitoxin titer will occur more promptly than the development of clinical signs.

In clinical cases, the use of tranquilizing drugs has been shown to have some beneficial effect in reducing the extent and severity of muscular spasms. Penicillin has been recommended in conjunction with antitoxin, and the broad spectrum antibiotics (oxytetracycline, chlortetracycline and chloramphenicol) also have been used effectively. Cases of tetanus should be confined in quiet, darkened box stalls with feeding and watering devices placed high enough so that the animal is capable of

gaining access to them without lowering the head. Support by slinging should be given whenever possible. In severe cases, it is mandatory.

MALIGNANT EDEMA

Malignant edema is an acute, fatal disease which may be contracted by horses, and which is characterized by formation of local areas of swelling, edema, hemorrhage and gas production. The disease is caused by *Clostridium septicum,* a gram-positive, anaerobic, noncapsulated, motile rod approximately 0.6 to 0.8 microns in diameter by 3 to 8 microns in length. In culture, it may appear singly or in short chains. In animal exudates and infected tissues, it occurs in long chains. The individual rod has rounded ends and peritrichous flagellae. The spores are oval and located toward the center of the rod, giving the bacillus a "snowshoe" shape. The organism does not stain uniformly, and granules can be observed in one or both ends of the cell when it is stained with methylene blue. Old cultures tend to decolorize. It grows well in meat infusion medium and forms colonies on blood agar which are surrounded by a hemolytic zone. Surface colonies on agar media have a gray or bluish-gray color and are opaque at the center. The organism has a world-wide distribution and is a common inhabitant of the soil. Endemic regions have variable amounts of soil contamination and the organism persists for long periods of time. It is not known whether it actively multiplies in the soil or merely exists in the spore state.

Pathogenesis: Clostridium septicum gains entrance into the body via traumatic injuries or abrasions of the skin, or may unknowingly be injected into animals during various surgical or inoculation procedures, *e.g.,* infection may follow castration. Horses may become infected as a result of other field operations if aseptic technic is not followed.

Clinical Signs: The clinical signs and lesions usually appear 2 to 4 days after the organism gains entrance to the body. An edematous, pitting swelling forms which primarily involves the subcutaneous tissue and has little or no gas formation. The lesion spreads rapidly, is infiltrated with large quantities of gelatinous exudate, and may become emphysematous. Bloodtinged fluid may escape at the point of the wound, or may be obtained by aspiration. Lameness, fever, increased pulse rate, congestion of the conjunctiva, and marked toxemia ordinarily appear in that order, and are terminated by death in 1 to 4 days after development of the signs.

Genital infections may occur in connection with parturition and are characterized by an edematous, dark red swelling of the vulva and vaginal mucosa. The lesions may spread downward along the thighs. Infections subsequent to castration cause extensive subcutaneous edema which may spread along the abdomen and medial aspects of the thighs. The swellings tend to follow the subcutaneous connective tissue but may also extend along the intermuscular fascia causing dark, hemorrhagic coloration to the associated muscle. Affected muscle usually is dark red but contains little or no gas. Diagnosis is based upon the appearance of characteristic signs and lesions and a history of local injury. Organisms may be obtained from aspiration of the lesions, and microscopic identification of the bacterium can be used to confirm the diagnosis.

Treatment and Prophylaxis: Treatment involves the parenteral administration of large doses of broad spectrum antibiotics, or penicillin-streptomycin (at least 2 to 3 million units daily). Surgical drainage and aeration by deep incision as done in gas gangrene infections of man probably are not indicated under farm conditions. *Clostridium septicum* is a good antigen and immunization may be obtained through the use of bacterins. The toxin produced is of moderate potency but antitoxins are not potent enough to be of value in treating wound infections. Some possible adjuvant effect may be obtained through use of *Clostridium septicum-Clostridium chauvoei* bacterin, even though horses are not susceptible to *Clostridium chauvoei* infection.

BOTULISM

Botulism is caused by ingestion of food containing toxins of *Clostridium botulinum*. It is not an infectious disease but rather an intoxi-cation, and the toxins must be present in the food before ingestion in order for the disease to occur. *Clostridium botulinum* may be found in the intestinal tracts of healthy animals, but if they die the organisms may multiply and produce toxins in the carcass. The bacterium is a common soil organism and this probably is the source of contamination of most foodstuffs.

Botulism is pathogenic to horses although reported cases are not too numerous. It is incriminated in the so-called "forage poisoning" syndrome, and has been isolated from silage and hay. Hays or silage which contain the decomposed bodies of rodents frequently may be inoculated with *Clostridium botulinum*. It is probable that the disease has been diagnosed erroneously, but it is equally probable that a number of cases of botulism in horses have escaped detection.

Clinical Signs: There are 5 principal types of toxin produced by *Clostridium botulinum*. They are identified as A, B, C, D, and E. Domestic animals may be poisoned with any of the 5 types. Botulism is characterized by signs of a locomotor paralysis, general weakness, and difficulty in prehension, chewing and swallowing. The tongue and pharynx become completely paralyzed and swallowing becomes impossible. Death ordinarily results from respiratory paralysis. Dysfunction is confined almost entirely to the nervous system although histologic changes have not been shown. No characteristic lesions are found at postmortem. There may be general hyperemia and hemorrhages in the lungs. Microscopic thrombosis, pulmonary edema, pericardial and epicardial hemorrhages, and hyperemia of the gastric mucosa have been observed, but are not constant nor pathognomonic for the disease.

Diagnosis: A positive diagnosis of botulism only can be made by demonstrating the toxin of *Clostridium botulinum* in material in the digestive tract. The demonstration of toxin in water and feed is circumstantial, but in ingesta it is conclusive. Demonstration can best be accomplished by injecting a filtrate of suspected material into a series of mice and guinea pigs, some of which have received simultaneous injections of antitoxins against particular toxin types. This type of protection test not only identifies the organism but also the toxin produced. The demonstration of *Clostridium botulinum* is of small value since the organism may be found in the intestines or in feed without toxin production.

Treatment: Although immunizing toxoids are available, these have not been used to any great extent in horses due to the infrequency of the disease. Emergency treatment involves use of rapid-acting purgatives, such as the cholinergic drugs. The best method of controlling this disease is preventing animals' access to spoiled foods, or foods which are suspected or shown to contain the organism and its toxin.

L. R. Vawter

REFERENCES FOR TETANUS

1. Abel, J. J., *et al.:* Johns Hopkins Hosp. Bull. **63** (1938) 373.
2. Breed, R. S., *et al.:* Bergey's Manual of Determinative Bacteriology. 7th ed. Williams and Wilkins Co., Baltimore, Md. 1957.
3. Chang and Weinstein: Proc. Soc. Exp. Biol. and Med. **94** (1957) 431.
4. Chodnik, J. S., *et al.:* Vet. Rec. **71** (1959) 904-908.
5. Cottereau, P., *et al.:* Rev. Med. Vet. 111. **23** (1960) 682-686.
6. Dawley, S. E.: Can. Vet. J. **12** (1960) 563-564.
7. Friedemann, V., *et al.:* J. Immunol. **40** (1941) 325.
8. Hagan, W. A., and Bruner, D. W.: The Infectious Diseases of Domestic Animals. 4th ed., Comstock Publishing Associates, Ithaca, N. Y., 1961.
9. Lundvall, R. L.: J.A.V.M.A. **132** (1958) 254.
10. Marie, A.: Ann. l'Inst. Past. **11** (1897) 591.
11. Merchant, I. A., and Packer, R. A.: Veterinary Bacteriology and Virology. 6th ed. Iowa State University Press, Ames 1961.
12. Merck Veterinary Manual, 2nd ed., Merck and Co., Rahway, N. J. 1961.
13. Nicolaier A.: Deutsch. Med. Wehnschr. **10** (1884) 842.
14. Nielsen and Rowsell: J.A.V.M.A. **128** (1956) 59.
15. Owen, L. N., *et al.:* Vet. Rec. **71** (1959) 61.
16. Pillemer, L., *et al.:* Science **103** (1946) 614.
17. Ramon, G., and Lemetayer, E.: Comp. rend. Soc. Biol. (Paris) **106** (1931) 21.
18. Rossdale, P. D., and Scarnall, J.: Vet. Rec. **73** (8) (1961) 184-185.
19. Wilson, G. S., and Miles, A. A.: Topley and Wilson's Principles of Bacteriology and Immunity. 4th ed. Williams and Wilkins, Baltimore, Md. 1955.
21. Tulloch, W. J.: J. Hyg. (Cambridge) **18** (1919-20) 103.

REFERENCES FOR MALIGNANT EDEMA

1. Breed, R. S., *et al.:* Bergey's Manual of Determinative Bacteriology. 7th ed. Williams and Wilkins Co., Baltimore, Md. 1957.
2. Hagan, W. A., and Bruner, D. W.: The Infectious Diseases of Domestic Animals. 4th ed., Comstock Publishing Associates, Ithaca, N. Y. 1961.
3. Merchant, I. A., and Packer, R. A.: Veterinary Bacteriology and Virology. 6th ed. Iowa State University Press, Ames, 1961.
4. Merck Veterinary Manual, 2nd ed., Merck and Co., Rahway, N. J. 1961.
5. Smith: Introduction to Pathogenic Anaerobes. University of Chicago Press, Chicago, Ill., 1954, p. 147.
6. Wilson, G. S., and Miles, A. A.: Topley and Wilson's Principles of Bacteriology and Immunity. 4th ed. Williams and Wilkins Co., Baltimore, Md. 1955.
7. Warrack, Bidwell, and Oakley: J. Path. and Bact. **63** (1951) 293.

REFERENCES FOR BOTULISM

1. Bennetts and Hall: J. Agr. (West. Austral.) **14** (1937) 381.
2. Breed, R. S., *et al.:* Bergey's Manual of Determinative Bacteriology. Williams and Wilkins Co., Baltimore, Md. 1957.
3. Buckley and Shippen: J.A.V.M.A. **50** (1917) 809.
4. Graham and Brueckner: J. Bact. **4** (1919) 1.
5. Hagan, W. A., and Bruner, D. W.: The Infectious Diseases of Domestic Animals. 4th ed., Comstock Publishing Associates, Ithaca, N. Y. 1961.
6. Larsen, Nicholes, and Gebhardt: Am. J. Vet. Research **26** (1955) 573.
7. Merchant, I. A., and Packer, R. A.: Veterinary Bacteriology and Virology. 6th ed. Iowa State University Press, Ames. 1961.
8. Meyer, K. F., and Dubovsky, B.: J. Inf. Dis. **31** (1922) 559.
9. Meyer, K. F., and Dubovsky, B.: J. Inf. Dis. **31** (1922) 641.
10. Merck Veterinary Manual, 2nd ed., Merck and Co., Rahway, N. J. 1961.
11. Theiler and Robinson: Zeitschr. f. Infektionskr. Haustiere **31** (1927) 165.
12. Wilson, G. S., and Miles, A. A.: Topley and Wilson's Principles of Bacteriology and Immunity. 4th ed. Williams and Wilkins Co., Baltimore, Md. 1955.
13. White, P. G., and Appleton, G. S.: J.A.V.M.A. **137** (11) (1960) 652-653.

CHAPTER 6

MYCOTIC DISEASES

SYSTEMIC MYCOSES

INTRODUCTION

The objective of this section is to describe the clinical and mycologic features of systemic fungus infections of the horse. Not all the reported infections will be covered because many of these have been isolated cases, and others are shrouded in the mists of antiquity or ambiguity. Only the mycoses encountered in North America will be included with one important exception—epizootic lymphangitis.

For many years fungus infections were considered to be more of interest than importance, and a diagnosed case was surrounded by all the pomp, circumstance, and exuberance of a Royal birth. Now the pendulum has swung far to the left and the mycologist is receiving more attention than he is honestly worth. This may be due to the momentous strides made in the treatment and control of bacterial disease; the common use of broad spectrum antibiotics, steroids, and folic acid antagonists in treatment; or perhaps just the interest of a small group of workers in the field of mycology.

Artificially the systemic fungus infections may be divided into two broad groups: those infections found in the subcutaneous tissues, and those found as disseminated infections of the internal organs. Many of the systemic mycoses exhibit both forms in their disease spectrum.

Although some of the deep-seated fungus infections are found endemically in certain parts of the continent (for example, histoplasmosis and coccidioidomycosis) individual cases may be found far away from the supposed endemic area. Shifting populations and travel play a large part in the appearance of these diseases in areas where they are completely unsuspected, and, consequently, undiagnosed.

A definite diagnosis of a systemic fungus infection cannot be made without the aid of a laboratory since the organism must be demonstrated in tissue and cultured before one can say that the case in question is a fungus infec-

tion. For this reason, a brief description of the fungus in the laboratory will be included in the following discussions.

SPOROTRICHOSIS

Etiology: The causative organism of sporotrichosis is *Sporotrichum schenckii,* and this fungus, like so many of the systemic fungi, is diphasic. In pus and necrotic tissue, single celled, cigar-shaped bodies may be seen within neutrophils, although they may be quite difficult to demonstrate in such material. On glucose cystine blood agar at 37 C. the organism grows as a creamy, soft, yeast-like colony. Microscopic examination of this colony will show many of the cigar-shaped bodies, similar to the ones seen occasionally in pus.

On Sabouraud's agar, at room temperature, the fungus produces a true mycelial colony, at first white and soft but later becoming tan, or dark brown and leathery. The center of the colony is raised, and radial grooves extend from it out to the flat periphery. Microscopically this type of colony shows a fine, branching, septate mycelium bearing pear-shaped condidia in daisy-like clusters along their length.

The organism is pathogenic for white male rats, young male hamsters, and mice when injected intraperitoneally.

Epizootiology: The natural habitat of *Sporotrichum schenckii* is the external surface of various plants and woods. The disease is world-wide in distribution and is a common mycosis of the horse in North America.

Infection in the horse results from inoculation of the fungus through the skin into the subcutaneous tissue. This may result from injury due to plant barbs, thorns, or splinters of wood. The spores of the organism gain access into the body and are converted into a yeast-like state. Invasion of the regional lymphatics is rapid but the disease rarely becomes disseminated to internal organs.

Clinical Signs: Two forms of the disease have

been described. The first type (which appears to be the classic picture) is that of an ulcerative lymphangitis. Progressing from the node closest to the inoculation site, infection spreads rapidly to involve other nodes in the lymphatic chain. This leads to the appearance of a long string of beads in the affected area. Eventually the nodes rupture and ulcers form. From these ulcers a thin sanguineous pus exudes. Very little temperature rise is noted and the condition is usually limited to one animal. If the disease is allowed to progress emaciation becomes noticeable. The course of the disease is chronic and may last for months.

The second form of the disease is that of multiple, subcutaneous nodules which do not follow any set pattern of distribution, do not involve the lymphatics, do not ulcerate, and are freely movable on palpation.

Diagnosis: Diagnosis of the condition must necessarily include the isolation of the causative fungus in the laboratory. Pus from discharging ulcers or a biopsy of a subcutaneous nodule should be submitted for examination. It is useful to ask the laboratory to examine the specimen for the presence of *Sporotrichum schenkii* since the organism may take a week or more to grow and plates may be discarded in the laboratory before this time has elapsed. Microscopic examination of the specimen is not very useful; cultures must be made before the organism can be identified.

Treatment: Sporotrichosis responds well to intravenous or oral administration of iodides. Sodium or potassium iodide may be given at a continuous low level dosage, or in increasing doses until evidence of iodism appears. There is no practical control of the disease.

EPIZOOTIC LYMPHANGITIS

Etiology: The most distressing fungus disease of the horse is epizootic lymphangitis. This disease, caused by *Histoplasma farciminosum*, has followed the horse from continent to continent, inflicting great casualties among horse populations wherever it has appeared.

In tissue, the organism appears as oval, budding yeasts, 3 to 4 microns in diameter. One pole tends to be more pointed than the other; there is a clear, unstained halo around them

and giant cells packed with the fungus are present. They closely resemble *H. capsulatum.*

On Francis-cystine-blood agar at room temperature, a heaped-up, wrinkled, gray colony appears. Microscopically, this is observed to consist of short, thick, septate mycelia containing round or oval chlamydospores.

The organism may be converted to the yeast stage by cultivation on Francis' agar at 37 C. in the presence of 15 to 20% carbon dioxide. The fungus appears similar under the microscope to the form seen in tissue except for the variation in size. Under an atmosphere of less than 15% carbon dioxide, the mycelial stage always is seen.

Epizootiology: Presumably *H. farciminosum* is found occurring in nature, although the saprophytic form has not been described as yet. The infection may be transmitted from animal to animal by various means: by direct contact or by soil, gates and fences, harness, brushes, and combs. Nasal and ocular discharges often are incriminated in the spread of the disease, both by direct contact and also by contamination of stable and pasture flies.

The disease was world-wide in distribution but, at the present time, is confined to the eastern European continent and Asia. Epizootic lymphangitis is not found in North America.

Although the route of entry seems to be through abrasions in the skin, the incidence of pulmonary infections indicates that inhalation of the organism (undoubtedly in its true fungal stage) is a method of invasion. Thus clinical signs depend upon the mode of introduction into the horse. It must be noted that a major part of systematic work on *H. farciminosum* was done at the dawn of modern mycology and that present-day methods of epizootiology would add immeasurably to our knowledge of the disease.

Clinical Signs: The incubation period is about 2 months. Typically there are nodules under the skin which follow the lymph channels. These nodules develop into abscesses containing a thick, yellow, oily pus. The abscesses break down into chronic indurated ulcers with a pink, shiny, and inverted border. The commonest sites are those exposed to injury: the lower limbs, the periorbital areas, the thighs,

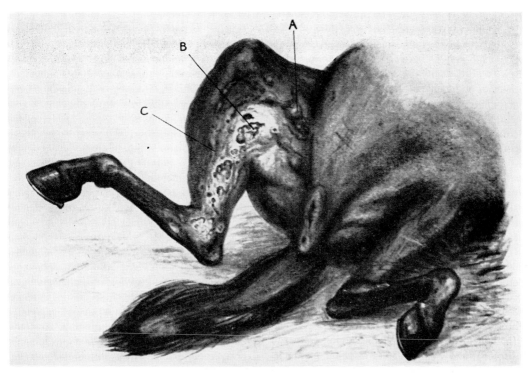

Fig. 1. Lesions of epizootic lymphangitis: A, abscess in formation; B, ulceration at sites of ruptured abscesses; C, enlarged lymph channel.

and areas previously debilitated by harness galls (Fig. 1).

"Often the first sign is a small nodule that develops into a pustule, which if not quickly diagnosed and treated is followed by a second or a chain of pustules along the line of the involved lymphatic vessel and cording of the vessel."[8] Lesions also may be found on the mucous membranes of the mouth, nostrils, and genitalia. At necropsy these lesions may be found to extend into the larynx, trachea, or deeper tissues. Active infection of the pulmonary system is evidenced by dyspnea, a thick yellow discharge, and lung abscessation. In some cases asymptomatic pulmonary infection is demonstrated at necropsy.

In the majority of cases anorexia, a rise in temperature, and debilitation are observed only in the terminal stages of the disease.

Small cutaneous abscesses often are associated with deep pockets of purulent material. Such cases appear as cutaneous ulcers which are refractive to treatment, and often simulate buried foreign bodies. Spread of the infection

usually is rapid. This may tend to incriminate a common source of infection rather than contagion when one considers the long incubation period. This rapid transmission may also be attributed to an increase in virulence of the fungus on passage through horses.

Diagnosis: Specimens must be submitted to a diagnostic laboratory with the request for fungus examination before the disease can be differentiated from glanders, sporotrichosis, or "leeches."

Lesions: The infected lymphatics are corded and thickened and any remaining lymph is thick and cheesy. Ulcers are found along the paths of the affected lymph channels; these ulcers open to the skin and are round with raised and inverted lips.

Erosions of the mucous membranes are found and these may be deep enough to expose cartilage and bone, especially in the nasal passages. Pulmonary lesions appear as nodules which are filled with a thick, purulent exudate. These lesions also may be present in the liver and spleen.

Treatment and Control: There is no economical, effective treatment for epizootic lymphangitis at the present time. In the past, surgical excision of affected areas, in the early stages of the disease, plus intravenous injections of mercury or iodides were claimed to arrest the disease. Most of the cases were diagnosed clinically, however, and it is difficult to determine whether the disease treated truly was epizootic lymphangitis.

Recent work by Russians would indicate that vaccination with formalized cultures of *Histoplasma farciminosum* leads to a long and durable immunity against the disease. Localized treatment of lesions by serum and vaccine injections also was claimed to be effective.

Control of the disease first requires its recognition and second, consideration of its modes of transmission. A clinical diagnosis must be confirmed by laboratory evidence. Fly control, thorough disinfection of all instruments, brushes, and harness, incineration of dressings (and, if at all possible, horses dying from the disease), and the nonuse of infected paddocks for at least 6 months are important in the control of the disease.

STREPTOTHRICOSIS

Etiology: Equine streptothricosis is caused by an organism related to the group of "higher" fungi known as actinomycetes. The classification of the fungus is poorly defined but it probably represents a bridge between true fungi and bacteria. At the present time it is loosely called *Dermatophilus* species.

The fungus will grow on blood agar and appears as a rough, brown colony which looks like a drop of applesauce. Gram or Giemsa stained smears from isolated colonies and from skin scrapings reveal blue filamentous organisms which fragment into robust coccoid elements. Quite often the coccoid elements predominate in skin scrapings. The fungus produces urease, is catalase-positive, and ferments glucose, arabinose, and inositol. It is sensitive to most, if not all, common antibiotics.

Epizootiology: It appears that most cases of streptothricosis follow wetting and abrasion of the skin. The organism may be a plant parasite, or saprophyte, or may exist as part of

the normal flora of the hair coat. It probably is introduced into the skin following an abrasion. Little is actually known of the transmission or contagiousness of the disease but it seems to be of low order.

Clinical Signs: In a recent paper, Bentinck-Smith reviewed the clinical manifestations of the disease in conjunction with a description of 6 cases seen in New York State. In addition, he described 9 other cases which occurred in New York and Vermont. For a full description, the reader is referred to his paper.[2]

The disease is confined to the skin and subcutaneous tissues. The first sign noted is a small patch of lifeless hair. This is plucked easily and usually carries with it a piece of scabby skin. When the scab is removed, a thin, sanguineous, and purulent surface is exposed. Scabs may slough leaving an area of normal skin beneath. Hair will grow back on these areas. There is no pruritus, but affected areas are very tender in the acute stages of the illness. Most of the lesions appear over the back and rump.

Treatment and Control: The lesions respond to drying of the skin, removal of loose scabs, scrubbing with soap and water, and application of fungicidal ointments, preferably mild ointments. Due to the sensitivity of the organism to antibiotics, lotions or ointments containing these agents also may be used.

Effective control appears to be related to improvement of the stabling, and the prevention of excessive dampness and abrasions of the skin.

MYCETOMAS

Etiology: Mycetomas of the horse are due to a number of normally saprophytic fungi which are introduced into wounds of the lower legs, feet, and face. Because the etiology is so varied it is impossible to describe all the fungi responsible for this condition. Perhaps a notable exception is the fungus, *Hyphomyces destruens,* which recently has been described by Bridges and Emmons.[3] They were able to recover this organism from 8 of 23 cases of mycetoma in Texas and Florida, and they give an excellent description of its characteristics. (See discussion in this chapter.)

Epizootiology: Saprophytic fungi from the

soil and vegetation enter cuts or puncture wounds on the feet, legs, or face of the horse and produce granulomas of the skin. The granulomas slowly progress to destroy bone, cartilage, and skin.

Mycetomas are common in tropical and subtropical climates and are known locally as "leeches" in southern United States and as "bursati" or "kunkers" in Asia.

Clinical Signs: Bridges and Emmons prefer to distinguish between "mycetoma" and "phycomycosis." The differentiation, however, is based upon mycologic and pathologic findings as the clinical signs are identical. To avoid confusion this section entitled, "mycetomas," includes both the phycomycoses and mycetomas.

The outstanding sign of a mycetoma is excessive granulation tissue surrounding a previous injury. The lesion drains purulent material from numerous sinus tracts and appears dirty, ulcerated, and massive in relation to the normal surrounding tissues. Spread of the process is slow but inflexible. Severe destruction of bone, cartilage, and tissue will result if immediate steps are not taken to diagnose and treat the disease.

A biopsy of the affected area must be submitted to a laboratory for mycologic examination. It is best (as it is in all suspected fungus infections) to divide the specimen and submit one portion in formalin and the other on ice; and to send both portions as rapidly as possible to the laboratory. The specimen on ice may be conveniently placed inside a clean glass container and then immersed in another container packed with ice. Both must be tightly sealed and watertight. Many laboratories will provide, on request, special containers for fungus specimens.

Lesions: White scar tissue which contains numerous small, yellow, irregular masses is almost pathognomonic of mycetoma. The necrotic areas stand out sharply from the fibrous tissue and often can be shelled out of the lesion. The fungi themselves often are difficult to demonstrate microscopically, and special stains may be required before they can be demonstrated. Culture of these organisms from lesions is not sufficient. They must be seen in

tissue and grown before one can ascribe disease to them.

Treatment and Control: Surgical removal of as much of the granulating mass as possible plus systemic iodides offers the only solution to the problem of mycetomas at present. The prognosis always should be guarded. Local applications of mild fungicides also should be used.

Control, again, requires prompt attention to cuts and abrasions.

Rare or Infrequently Recognized Fungus Infections

Histoplasmosis, North American blastomycosis, actinomycosis, and coccidiodomycosis also have been described as diseases of the horse. Most of these reports have followed necropsies, since the onset and signs are so insidious that they usually defy clinical diagnosis. If a disease is not suspected it cannot be included in a differential diagnosis. Although a great many horses are undoubtedly infected with *Histoplasma capsulatum* and *Coccidioides immitis* every year, most of these infections are asymptomatic and thus go unrecognized. The interested reader is referred to the selected references at the end of this section.

J. DITCHFIELD

REFERENCES

1 Benbrook, E. A., Bryant, J. B., and Saunders, L. Z.; A case of blastomycosis in the horse. J.A.V.M.A. **112** (1948) 475.

2. Bentinck-Smith, J., Fox, F. H., and Baker, D. W.: Equine dermatitis (cutaneous Streptothricosis) infection with *Dermatophilus* in the United States. Cornell Vet. **51** (1961).

3. Bridges, C. H., and Emmons, C. W.: A Phycomycosis of horses caused by *Hyphomyces destruens*. J.A.V.M.A. **138** (1961) 579.

4. Bullen, J. J.: The yeast like form of *Cryptococcus farminosus* (Rivolta) (H. farciminosum). J. Path. Bact. **61** (1949) 117.

5. Burns, R. H. G. and Simmons, G. C.: A case of Actinomycotic infection in a horse. Australian Vet. J. **28** (1952) 81.

6. Jones, T. C. and Maurer, F. C.: Sporotrichosis in horses. Case report. Bull. U. S. Army Med. Dept. **74** (1944) 63.

7. Menges, R. W.: Histoplasmin sensitivity in animals. Cornell Vet. **44** (1953) 21.

8. Plunkett, J. J.: Epizootic lymphangitis. J. Royal Army Vet. Corps. **20** (1949) 94.

9. Richman, H.: Histoplasmosis in a colt. No. Am. Vet. **29** (1948) 710.

10. Saunders, L. Z.: Systemic fungus infections in animals: a review. Cornell Vet. **38** (1948) 213.

11. Smith, H.: Coccidioidomycosis in animals with a report of a new case in a dog. Am. J. Path. **24** (1948) 223.

PHYCOMYCOSIS

A phycomycosis is a localized systemic infection caused by several fungi in the class, *Phycomycetes.* For many years such infections in man and animals have been referred to as "mucormycosis" inasmuch as the fungi causing the infections belonged either to the genus, *Mucor,* or to the family, *Mucoraceae.* However, in recent years it has become obvious that fungi other than those of the family, *Mucoraceae,* are the etiologic agents of many of these infections. This is especially true in the case of equine lesions since only one report of infection with a fungus of the family, *Mucoraceae,* has been found while other fungi have been isolated numerous times.

These, like most other systemic mycoses, are quite important in each individual case because they usually lead to permanent disability or less often to death in the absence of early and radical treatment. The phycomycoses appear to be the most frequent type of internal mycotic infections of horses in many parts of the world.

Two organisms, *Hyphomyces destruens*[2] and *Entomophthora coronata*[3] are the most commonly recognized etiologic agents, although *Mucor pusillus*[12] and *Basidiobolus ranarum*[13] have been isolated from single localized lesions of the leg and lung of 2 horses.

The historical background concerning the development of knowledge of these mycoses is quite interesting. Theobald Smith reported a disease of horses in Florida during the early 1890's which the horsemen of the area called "leeches" because they thought that the elongated masses of necrotic tissue within the chronic granulomatous lesions were leeches *(Hirudinea)* which had entered the tissues while the horses were standing in water. A similar clinical disease was known in India at the same time as "bursattee" (also spelled "bursautee" and "bursati") in which the masses of necrotic tissue were called "Kunkers."[11]

In 1903, a disease of similar nature called "hyphomycosis destruens" was described in Indonesia and a nonsporulating phycomycete was isolated from the lesions and named *Hyphomyces destruens.*[5] In 1925, *Basidiobolus ranarum,* a fungus which commonly is found in the digestive tract of certain frogs, lizards and in

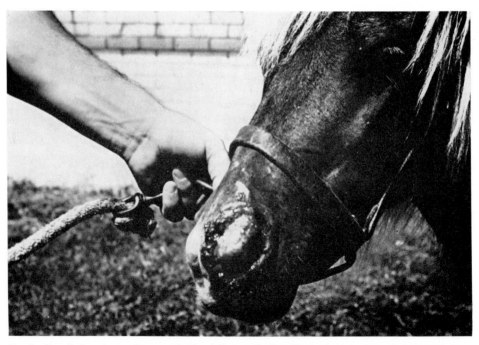

Fig. 2. Granulation tissue almost occluding left nostril of a Shetland pony. Typical lesion of *Entomophthora coronata* infection.

beetles which feed upon the excrement of equines, was isolated from a typical lesion on the leg of an Indonesian mare.[13] A similar lesion has been described on a horse in France.[6] More recently, a condition identical to hyphomycosis destruens has been described in horses in Texas and Florida, and the causative organism, *Hyphomyces destruens*, was described in detail.[2]

A clinical entity caused by *Entomophthora coronata* which produces lesions similar to those of *Hyphomycosis destruens* but has a predilection for the skin around the nostrils and mucosa of the nasal cavity has been described in Texas.[3] These mycoses were confused with the lesions of cutaneous habronemiasis for many years because of the intense local eosinophilia produced and the presence of necrotic blood vessels which simulated degenerating larvae. However, larvae have not been found in lesions with fungi, and vice versa, although such a condition should not be impossible.

Of interest is the occurrence of *Basidiobolus ranarum* and a nonsporulating phycomycete in cutaneous lesions of Indonesian children.[10] *Entomophthora coronata* has been recognized as a parasite of certain insects.[8]

Occurrence: The report of Theobald Smith[1] stressed the observation of the horse owners that the condition, called leeches, occurred most often in those animals which were in pastures containing many shallow lakes and muck ponds in which the horses waded to eat grass. Certain pastures have been recognized by the horse owners to be associated with a higher incidence of infection.[7]

The majority of the horses affected with phycomycosis caused by *Hyphomyces destruens*, as described by Bridges and Emmons,[2] are found on the flat prairies bordering the Gulf of Mexico. However, a few cases occur in the river valleys and hill lands hundreds of miles from the Gulf. Even in the latter area, small impoundments and creeks are accessible to horses. The cases with lesions caused by *Entomophthora coronata* have not had such a definite geographic distribution.[3]

Cases of phycomycosis are presented to veterinarians throughout the year. The infectious processes take the basic forms of localized granulomatous lesions, or systemic infections usually with a recognized primary lesion.

Clinical Signs: The majority of the animals are presented with one or more masses of exuberant granulation tissue on various parts of the body which have been present for a few weeks or many months (Fig. 2, 3). Simultaneous involvement of opposite limbs is not unusual. Most frequently, the lesions are reported to have developed at the site of a known injury, such as a wire cut. Occasionally, they are first recognized as focal swellings with serum exuding from small sinuses in the skin. Although the lesions occur most frequently on the legs from the hock or knee to the hoof, they are not uncommon on the abdomen, neck and lips or the skin surrounding the nostril. The mucosa of the nasal cavity, lips, trachea, or stomach may be affected occasionally.

The animals bite or lick the lesions when possible, as though there is an intense pruritus, and they may destroy portions of the granulation tissue. Lameness develops as lesions on the legs enlarge and involve functional structures. Lesions in the nasal cavity or nostril cause respiratory embarrassment, or in later

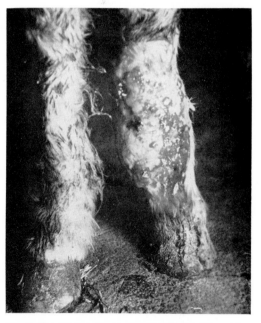

Fig. 3. Granulation tissue covered with exudate on leg of horse caused by *Hyphomyces destruens*.

stages may extend to the upper lip and thus affect prehension of food. The lesions expand peripherally in all directions. Those about the fetlock may encircle it and extend dorsally and ventrally even to the hoof. Those on the ventral abdomen form an expanding saucer-shaped mass up to 10 or 12 inches in diameter. The overlying and adjacent skin is destroyed both by the inflammatory reaction and self-mutilation by the horse.

Systemic infection is manifested by signs referable to the affected organs or may be found incidentally at the necropsy of an animal with a peripheral lesion. Metastases from gastric and cutaneous lesions have been seen.

Lesions: The superficial surface of the granulation tissue frequently is hemorrhagic due to trauma inflicted by the horse. Although the ulcerated tissue occasionally may extend some distance above the edge of the skin, it usually remains reasonably flush with it. There is sufficient, peripheral subcutaneous extension of the lesion to raise the skin which, along with trauma of the new tissue by the horse, keeps them at similar levels. In more advanced lesions, small sinuses drain pus from the deeper

foci of infection and hard, yellow, irregular masses of necrotic tissue may be expressed from them. These frequently are found on a medicated bandage when it is removed. Occasionally, one of these pieces of necrotic tissue may be found anchored firmly in the tissue but protruding slightly on the ulcerated surface.

Incision of the lesions reveals firm, fibrous tissue with cross sections of the sinuses and necrotic masses which vary from less than ½ mm. to several mm. in diameter and up to 6 cm. long (Fig. 4). These smaller ones are difficult to see with the unaided eye. The pieces of necrotic tissue from the more fulminant lesions frequently branch and rebranch in a form suggestive of blood vessels (Fig. 5). The tendons and bones ordinarily are not invaded, but the tendon sheaths may be.

Histologically, in the more advanced lesions there is granulation tissue of varying maturity surrounding a sinus in which a cross section of the necrotic tissue is embedded in purulent exudate containing numerous macrophages and occasional giant cells. Eosinophils are extremely numerous, especially in the superficial parts of the lesions, and in and about the

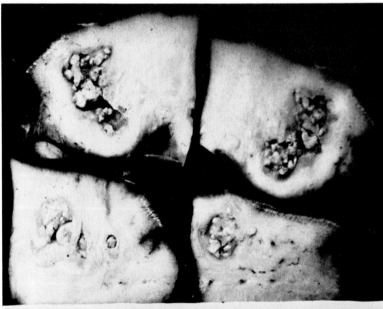

Fig. 4. Cross sections of necrotic tissue in sinuses of granulation tissue. Caused by *Hyphomyces destruens.*

sinuses. Fungi are found within the necrotic tissue.

Studies of the early foci of necrosis reveal that they begin as areas of coagulative necrosis surrounding the hyphae. Necrotic eosinophils also are numerous. Many of the larger masses, when examined at the proper time, will be found to contain blood vessels in their centers, thus explaining the branching patterns seen. The fungus can be seen as branching, occasionally septate hyphae which are scattered throughout the larger foci of necrosis and in the centers of the smaller ones (Fig. 6). The hyphae frequently are numerous in the necrotic blood vessels.

The lesions of systemic infections consist of acute purulent to chronic granulomatous inflammatory foci in which the hyphae may be demonstrated. Metastasis has been found to occur in infections with *Hyphomyces destruens* but not with *Entomophthora coronata*.[4] However, fewer of the latter have been studied.

Mycology: The hyphae of *Hyphomyces destruens* appear on all sides of the inoculum after only 24 to 36 hours' incubation. *Entomoph-*

thora coronata requires even less time to do so. The nonsporulating and nonpigmented mycelium of *H. destruens* spreads radially from the center and remains close to the agar with only short aerial hyphae. Only a few septa may be seen in the coenocytic hyphae. The organism is identified through its association with characteristic lesions and the characteristic hyphal morphology which consistently fails to sporulate.[2]

E. coronata begins to discharge, within a few hours, its characteristic conidia toward any light source from its phototrophic conidiophores, and the opposite side of the test tube or petri dish will be covered with so many conidia that a powdery deposit is present. The conidia, varying from 36 to 44 μ in diameter and having a prominent basal papilla by which they have been attached to the conidiophore, frequently are shaped somewhat like an incandescent light bulb. Aerial mycelia are minimal. These conidia may germinate on the glass surface, forming a short conidiosphore on which a secondary, smaller conidium is formed and discharged. The conidia frequently have

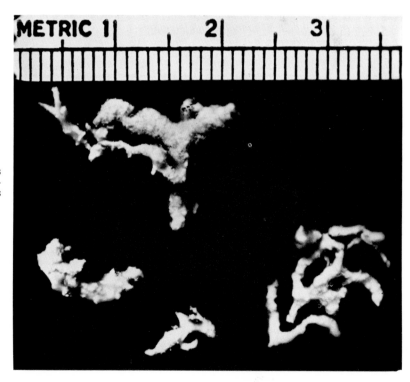

Fig. 5. Branching masses of necrotic tissue dissected from the lesions shown in Fig. 2.

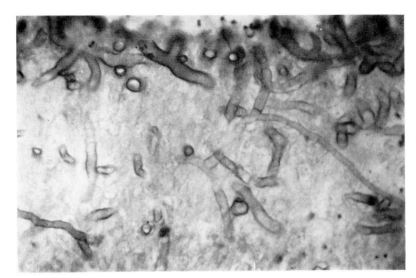

Fig. 6. Branching hyphae of *Hyphomyces destruens* in necrotic tissue. Gridley fungus stain. x950

many hair-like appendages radiating from their surfaces.[8]

Diagnosis: The presence of the large irregular, usually enlongate, gray to yellow masses of hard necrotic tissue in sinuses permeating granulation tissue is a characteristic feature. Early and slowly progressing lesions may have minute foci of necrosis with less purulent exudate and may be confused with invasive squamous cell carcinoma or cutaneous habronemiasis. In cutaneous habronemiasis, the yellow foci of necrosis and inflammation seldom are larger than a grain of rice, and they tend to regress spontaneously in the absence of repeated infection which usually stops during the colder weather.

The hyphae may be found in the necrotic tissue by microscopic examination of the sediment left after it has been treated with 10 to 20% potassium or sodium hydroxide. Care must be taken not to confuse persisting, branching elastic fibers with fungus hyphae. Histopathologic examination is preferable where possible, especially with the inclusion of special technics which stain the fungal hyphae. The necrotic masses must be included in the sections. Occasionally, the foci of infection are separated by several centimeters of granulation tissue, and a small biopsy may miss the diagnostic areas.

The fungi may be cultured with ease on ordinary media with the inclusion of antibac-terial but not fungistatic compounds (actidione). Aseptic technic is simple when a generous biopsy is made. Pieces of the necrotic tissue should be placed on agar slants.

Treatment: Because the fungus most frequently is embedded in hard, dense masses of necrotic tissue and these permeate the exuberant granulation tissue, surgical extirpation of all of the foci of infection appears essential for effective treatment. Recurrences are frequent following excision of the lesions, however, and most lesions have advanced to a stage in which surgery is impractical when the animals are submitted for treatment. The necrotic masses alone would present a formidable barrier to quick healing. The value of the antibiotics for treatment remains to be determined. Their use, however, should be complemented with surgery.

C. H. BRIDGES

REFERENCES

1. Annual report of the Bureau of Animal Industry, 1893-1894. U. S. Government Printing Office, Washington, D. C. (1896) 97-98.
2. Bridges, Charles H. and Emmons, Chester W.: A phycomycosis of horses caused by *Hyphomyces destruens*. J.A.V.M.A. **138** 1 (1961) 579-589.
3. Bridges, Charles H., Romane, William M., and Emmons, Chester W.: Phycomycosis of horses caused by *Entomophthora coronata*. J.A.V.M.A. **140** (1962) 672-677.
4. Bridges, Charles H.: Unpublished data, 1961.
5. de Haan, J. and Hoogkamer, L. J.: *Hyphomycosis destruens equi*, bosartige Schimmelkrankheit des Pferdes. Arch. f. wissensch. u. prakt. Tierheilk., Berl. **29** (1903) 395-410.
6. Drouin, V.: Sur une nouvelle mycose du cheval. Rec. med. vet. **3** (1896) 337-344.
7. Emmel, M. W.: Leeches in horses. Proc. 1st ann. conf. for veterinarians, University of Florida, Gainesville, **1** (1958) 18-19.

8. Emmons, Chester W. and Bridges, Charles H.: *Entomophthora coronata*. The etiologic agent of a Phycomycosis of horses. Mycoologia. In press.

9. Lie-Kian-Joe, Njo-Injo Tjoei Eng, Pohan, A., van der Meulen, H., and Emmons, Chester W.: *Basidiobolus ranarum* as a cause of subcutaneous mycoses in Indonesia. A.M.A. Arch. Dermat. **74** (1956) 378-383.

10. Lie-Kian-Joe, Njo-Injo Tjoei Eng, Sutomo Tjokronegoro, Emmons, Chester W.: Phycomycosis (mucormycosis) in Indonesia—description of a case affecting subcutaneous tissue. Am. J. Trop. Med. and Hyg. **9** (1960) 143-148.

11. Smith, F.: The pathology of Bursattee. Vet. J. **19** (1884) 16-17.

12. Tscherniak, W. S.: Zur Lehre von den bronchound pheumonomykosen der pferde. Arch. wiss. prakt. Tierheilk, **57** (1928) 417-444.

13. Van Overeem, C.: Beiträge zur Pilzflora von Niederlandisch Indien. 10. Ueber ein merkwurdiges Vorkommen von *Basidiobolus ranarum* Eidam. Bull. Jardin Bot. **7** (1925) 423-431.

ASPERGILLOSIS (MYCOTIC DIARRHEA)

Clinical Signs: A persistent diarrhea of foals and young horses has been observed following oral medication with antibiotics and sulfanomides. Usually, it is associated with a heavy parasitic infection. The affected animals are in fair condition, alert, have a good appetite and temperatures within normal range. The diarrheic eliminations have no characteristic odor and do not respond to conventional treatment. Often no specific pathogens other than *Aspergillus fumigatus* can be isolated from the feces on culture. Since this organism commonly is present in moldy hay it is readily understandable that it can enter the intestinal tract.

Aspergillus has also been incriminated in a few cases of equine abortion. The abortions occur during the seventh to tenth month of gestation, and the mare shows no evidence of illness. Cultures of fetal tissues reveal pure colonies of *Aspergillus fumigatus*. In 3 reported cases of mycotic abortion, 2 feti had lesions in the lungs, intestines, and skin. Fungi were isolated from each area. In the third case only pulmonary lesions were observed, from which *Aspergillus* was cultured.

Morphology of Organism: In culture, *Aspergillus* produces blue-green spores which give a typical color to the colony. A portion of a mold colony placed on a glass slide beneath a coverslip will reveal interlacing hyphae and numerous conidiophores. The conidia shatter easily and usually are seen scattered throughout the field. They are detected readily in infected tissue or in culture.

Treatment: Symptomatic treatment with astringents and intestinal emulcents will not control this cause of diarrhea, and failure of such treatment to produce at least a temporary remission should prompt suspicion of a mycotic infection.

The treatment of intestinal mycosis involves the administration of 20,000-unit nystatin boluses twice a day for a period of 10 days, and the inclusion of acidophilus milk via drench or stomach tube. Attempts should be made to prevent reinfection by changing the feed and cleaning the animal's quarters. The bedding should be removed, burned and replaced by fresh material. Although these attempts, due to the ubiquitous nature of *Aspergillus*, probably will be unsuccessful, the reduction of a good percentage of infective spores should aid in preventing reinfection.

J. F. BONE

REFERENCES

1. Carll, Forgacs, Herring, and Mahlandt: Vet. Med. **50** (1955) 210.

2. Hensel, L., *et al.*. Berl. und Munch. Tierarzl. Wchr. **74** (15) (1961) 290-293.

3. Lundvall, R. L., and Romberg, P. F.: J.A.V.M.A. **137** (8) (1960) 481-483.

4. Ticehurst, R. L., and Cameron, J. S.: Allied Vet. **30** (1959) 132.

DERMATOMYCOSES

Occurrence: In recent years there has been greater recognition of dermatophytic infections not only in small animals but also in horses. These fungi affect only the superficial keratinized areas of the body, particularly skin, hair, and hooves. There are numerous species of dermatophytes which may cause ringworm lesions in horses. The most frequently isolated dermatophytes in horses are: *Microsporum canis, M. gypseum, Trichophyton mentagrophytes,* and *T. equinum. T. verrucosum* and *T. schoenleini* have been isolated in horses relatively very rarely.

Etiology: Natural infection results from direct contact with affected animals or even with infected human beings. Indirect infection may be acquired from infected material or articles used for grooming, from harnesses, blankets or from infected clothing of man. Ringworm in horses also has been transmitted by diseased rats. Warm, damp, and dirty stables encourage mycotic infection. Conversely, sufficient sun

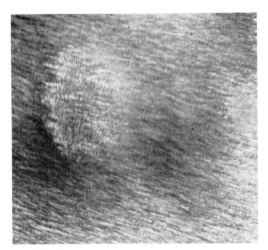

Fig. 7. Ringworm lesions caused by *Microsporum canis*.

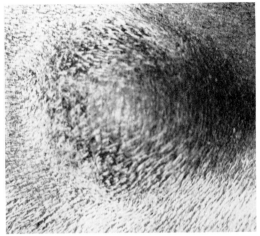

Fig. 8. Ringworm lesions caused by *Microsporum gypseum*.

and fresh air attenuate the growth of dermatophytes.

Thin-skinned horses are particularly prone to ringworm attacks. The incubation period after a natural infection is generally from a week to a month. When conditions are particularly favorable for the fungi, the incubation period may be shortened to 4 to 6 days. Minor trauma of the skin is a prerequisite for the introduction of infective spores into the horny layer or hair follicles.

Animals which are treated excessively with antibiotics may lose their previous resistance for fungus infection. Also dietary inadequacies are essential predisposing conditions for ringworm infection.[1]

The ringworm fungus lives only in the superkeratinized skin areas which are dead structures and does not penetrate the deeper living skin layers. It is most abundant in the hair follicles. The presence of the fungus causes inflammation of the skin followed by loss of hair. When the hair shafts themselves are penetrated, they become brittle and break or split, leaving short stumps. Dermatophytic lesions spread in a characteristic circular fashion. The region on the periphery of the lesions is the youngest while there may be healing in the center, even without treatment. Rieth, *et al.*[2] found that the fungus spores in skin scrapings remained infectious for longer than one year.

Identification of Dermatophytes: The diagnosis of dermatomycosis can be accomplished

in different ways. The use of a Wood's light is a valuable aid in the diagnosis of ringworm in horses only when the infection is caused by *Microsporum canis*. The ultraviolet rays transmitted through a Wood's filter cause a greenish-blue fluorescence of the affected hair. Other equine dermatophytes, such as *Microsporum gypseum*, *Trichophyton mentagrophytes*, *T. equinum*, and *T. verrucosum*, do not show fluorescence to ultraviolet radiation.

A microscopic examination of scrapings taken from suspected skin lesions or of hairs in the lesions, may be helpful in the clinical diagnosis of dermatomycoses. The material is placed on a slide and mixed with a few drops of a 10 to 15% solution of potassium hydroxide or a solution of lactophenol-cotton blue, and covered with a cover glass. Although the finding of fungus elements (spores and mycelia) indicates presence of a fungus, it does not identify the species.

The accurate differentiation of fungus species can be made only by culturing material obtained from skin lesions. Various media can be used for culturing. The standard medium used for the isolation of ringworm fungi is Sabouraud's dextrose agar. With heavily contaminated hair and skin, better culture results are obtained by the use of media to which antibiotics have been added.[3] Incubation should be done at room temperature (77 to 86 F.) for 2 to 4 weeks.

In positive cultures, the fungus colonies are differentiated macroscopically according to their characteristic shape and color, and microscopically according to the shape and size of macro- or microconidia, their walls, septation, and other morphologic characteristics.

Clinical Signs: Microsporum canis has been isolated from horses by Ainsworth, *et al.,*[4] and others. The skin lesions are characterized by rounded, hairless lesions covered with tiny scales and located mainly in the harnessed regions (Fig. 7). This ringworm is quite contagious not only to other horses but to humans as well.

Microsporum gypseum is essentially a soil-inhabiting fungus which under appropriate conditions, produces ringworm lesions in animals.[5] In horses, the lesions are characterized by multiple circular areas on various parts of the body. The affected skin is either hairless, or hairs protrude through the crusts covering the lesions (Fig. 8). The crusts are relatively thick and adherent to the base of the lesion. When removed forcibly, a moist, reddish area appears. In comparison with the lesions produced by *M. canis*, the lesions caused by *M. gypseum* are larger, more inflamed, and covered with thick crusts.

Trichophyton mentagrophytes has been isolated from horses and various animal species. Georg *et al.*[6] consider that rodents play an important role in the transmission of this infection, especially in rural areas. In horses, skin lesions caused by this fungus are located mostly on the head, neck, at the base of the tail, and on the extremities. In advanced cases, lesions occur anywhere on the body. They are either rounded or irregular in shape, of various sizes, hairless, and covered with heavy, grayish crusts with short stumps of hair. Initially, the lesions are small, then they gradually enlarge, forming round spots which may fuse into irregularly shaped areas (Fig. 9). At the onset, there may be papules, vesicles, and pustules especially at the periphery of the lesions. These lesions soon rupture and their contents dry and form crusts. When the crusts are removed, suppuration may be discovered beneath. Healing of the untreated lesions starts at the center where new hair grows surrounded by scales and crusts. There may be some evidence of pruritus during this infection.

Trichophyton equinum originally was considered to be identical to *T. mentagrophytes*. Later, it was accepted as a distinct species.[7] This fungus frequently has been the cause of ringworm in the United States, Europe, and South America. Young animals especially are susceptible to this infection, and its spread among horses is rapid. The fungi attached to hair are highly resistant to destruction. Some have been found to remain viable for a period of a year and a half when kept in a dry tube in the laboratory. Therefore, contaminated brushes, saddles, blankets, and of course, sta-

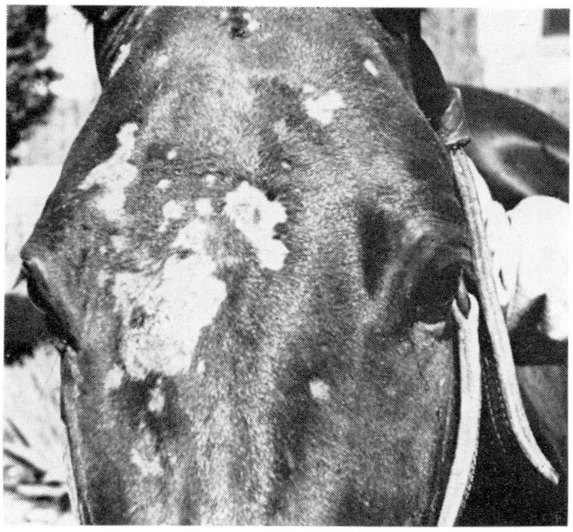

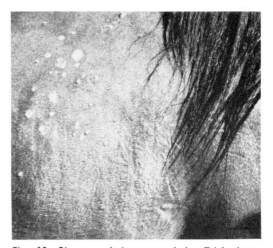

Fig. 9. Ringworm lesions caused by *Trichophyton mentagrophytes.*

Fig. 10. Ringworm lesions caused by *Trichophyton equinum.*

bles may be a source of the infection for a long period of time.

The cutaneous lesions are characterized by the development of small, rounded spots, the diameter ranging in size from 1/4 to 1 inch. They are hairless and covered with tiny scales (Fig. 10). These spots gradually enlarge and small vesicles may be palpated on their surface. The vesicles soon rupture, and their contents, together with the scales, form crusts. Healing starts at the center, where new hair grows. This type of ringworm in horses in very itchy, therefore it has been termed "girt itch." It is transmissible to humans.[8]

Trichophyton verrucosum, which is the common dermatophyte of cattle and goats, has been found in a horse which had been grazing with heavily infected cattle.[4]

Trichophyton schoenleini, the cause of favus in man, has also been isolated from horses, but relatively very rarely. The skin lesions described by Manninger, *et al.*[9] were irregularly shaped, covered with thick crusts, and located on various areas of the body surface. A characteristic odor, suggesting mold mingled with mouse urine, emanated from the crusts.

Treatment: Good nutrition and proper hygienic conditions are the essential factors of supportive therapy. Feeds rich in protein and exposure to sunshine will be helpful. The topical treatment with fungicidal preparations is, as a rule, satisfactory. Severe cases, especially in generalized ringworm, should be treated systemically with oral and intravenous administration of iodides and, in valuable horses, fulvicin could be given orally.

For effective topical treatment of ringworm in horses the following fungicidal preparations may be used:

1. Mercuric iodide in soft paraffin (1:50).
2. Salicylic acid 1.5 Gm. and chloroform 30 ml.

3. Salicylic acid 5.0 Gm., tannic acid 5.0 Gm., and alcohol (70%) 80 ml.

4. Carbolic acid 15.0 Gm., tincture of iodine 25 ml., and chloral hydrate 10.0 Gm.

The following commercial preparations are available: 2% Weladol cream; Furaspor; Fongeryl; Led-O-San; Vangard (Ortho-Tack-Wash); Chlordane; Lindane; Odylen; Mulzyl; Chlorox (10%).

In the topical treatment of equine dermatomycoses involving large areas of the body surface, it is important not to limit the therapy to affected areas only, but to treat the entire body surface by spraying or sponging with reliable fungicides.

F. KRAL

REFERENCES

1. Sellers, K. C., Sinclair, W. B., and LaTouche, C. J.: Vet. Rec. **68** (1956) **729.**
2. Rieth, H., and El-Fiki, A. V.: Berl. u. Munch. tieräztl. Wchr. **72** (1959) 201.
3. Georg, L. K.: Vet. Med. 49 (1954) 157.
4. Ainsworth, G. C., and Austwick, P. K. C.: Vet. Rec. 67 (1955) 88.
5. Ajello, L. J.: Invest. Dermat. **21** (1953) 157.
6. Georg, L. K., Roberts, C. S., Menges, R. W., and Kaplan, V.: J.A.V.M.A. **130** (1954) 427.
7. Georg, L. K., Kaplan, W., and LaVerne, B. C.: Am. J. Vet. Res. **18** (1957) 798.
8. Batte, E. G., and Miller, W. S.: J.A.V.M.A. 123 (1953) 111.
9. Manninger, R., and Mócsy, J.: Spez. Pathol. u. Therap. d. Haustiere, 11th Ed., Vol. 2, p. 887, Fischer, Jena, 1959.

KERATINOMYCES AJELLOI

This organism is a dermatophyte which has been incriminated as a cause for dermatitis in horses. The disease is rare and is characterized by a circumscribed loss of hair with an associated scaly skin surface. The underlying skin apparently is not affected. Treatment is the same as for other dermatomycoses.

J. F. BONE

REFERENCE

1. Pier, A. C., *et al.*: J.A.V.M.A. **138** (1961) 484-486.

CHAPTER 7

PROTOZOAL DISEASES

DOURINE

Dourine is one of the venereal diseases of equines and the only one due to trypanosomes. As long as it possibly exists in the United States (in the State of Arizona) or persists in the Republic of Mexico it constitutes a threat to susceptible animals in this country.

Synonyms: The synonyms used for this disease have been varied. Some of them are: equine syphilis, breeding disease, breeding paralysis, covering disease, chancrous epizootic, epizootic paraplegia, genital glanders, *maladie du coit, mal du coit, el dourine, Beschälkrankheit, Beschälseuche, slapsiekte, morbo coitale maligno,* polyneuritis infection, and *exanthema coitale paralyticum.*

Definition: Dourine is a specific, usually chronic, contagious, infectious disease of the horse and ass caused by *Trypanosoma equiperdum,* transmitted chiefly by sexual contact. It is characterized clinically by inflammation of the genitalia, followed by transitory edema of the subcutis (urticarial or dollar plaques) and paralysis.

History: As with many diseases, the origin of dourine is lost in antiquity. Apparently the original home of this disease was Asia and Northern Africa. Ammon and Dickhäuser in 1796, as reported by Zwick and Knuth,[1] described their experiences with the disease in the royal stud at Trakehnen in Northern Prussia. Since the beginning of the past century, dourine has been reported in Austria, Switzerland, France, Poland, Russia, Italy, and Spain. Reports also have been made from time to time of its occurrence in different parts of Asia and Asia Minor, Syria, Persia, India, Java, North and South Africa, Australia, Brazil, Chile, and Mexico.

In the United States, dourine was first recognized in 1886, at Wapella (in DeWitt County), Illinois, by Williams,[2] a practitioner at Bloomington. This outbreak apparently was introduced by Percheron stallions imported from France. Grade draft stallions and mares shipped from this affected area probably were the source of infection in others parts of the West and Northwest.

In 1892, the disease was recognized among breeding horses in Nebraska and, in 1893, its presence was noted in South Dakota. The reappearance of dourine in Nebraska and South Dakota caused a thorough investigation of the latent qualities of the disease and, in 1903, of 16,287 horses, 511 were found to be diseased and were destroyed; 1,899 stallions were castrated.[3]

Etiology: The protozoan *Trypanosoma equiperdum* was reported as the causal agent of dourine by Rouget,[4] in 1896, and by the French army officers, Schneider and Buffard,[5] in 1899. This monomorphic trypanosome resembles *T. evansi,* the cause of surra. It varies from 25 to 35 microns in length and 1.5 to 2.5 microns in width.[6] The large nucleus is located centrally; near the blunt end a parabasal body and a blepharoplast (basal granule) are located from which a fine flagellum runs along the free border of the undulating membrane attached to the side of the body and extends beyond the pointed end of the spindle-shaped body. Motion occurs by lashing movements of the flagellum, undulating membrane and contraction of the protoplasm. Division occurs by longitudinal fission (Fig. 1).

The virulence of the organism varies in different countries; the European strain reportedly is much more virulent than the South African and Canadian strains. Serial passage of *T. equiperdum* through equines or mice may increase its virulence. Mohler[3] was the first to be successful in growing *T. equiperdum* on blood agar. The pattern of antigenic variation in *T. equiperdum* was reported in 1960 by Cantrell.[7] Successful cultivation in developing chick embryos has been reported by Craige.[8] Electron microscopic observations also have been reported.[9]

Distribution: The trypanosomoses are diseases usually found in tropical and subtropical regions; dourine, however, is more cosmopolitan in distribution, and under natural conditions is not vector-borne.

In the United States the disease has been encountered most often in states west of the Mississippi, with the exception of Illinois, in 1886, and Virginia, in 1953. An interesting account of eradication procedures used on the Navajo Indian Reservation in Arizona has been reported by Crump.[10] The last known area of infection was in Arizona on the Papago Indian Reservation which borders the Republic of Mexico.

Transmission: The disease usually is transmitted by copulation, when the healthy genital organs are infected by the secretions from the vagina or urethral mucous membranes. A stallion may transmit dourine from an infected mare to a healthy mare without contracting the disease. The trypanosomes are not present consistently, and infection does not take place with each copulation.

The organisms usually are very scarce in the blood, and this may account for the lack of vector-borne transmission. Trypanosomes have been detected in the mammary gland and milk of infected mares and thus foals may be infected. Infection through the conjunctiva is possible if foals contact infective vaginal discharges. Occasionally, geldings are affected and this suggests the possibility of transmission by sponges or the hands of attendants and by biting flies. Mechanical transmission has been demonstrated by means of *Stomoxys calcitrans* and *Tabanus nemoralis.*

Susceptibility: The susceptibility to infection is variable with the individual animal and the virulence of the parasite. In addition to solipeds, *T. equiperdum* can be transmitted experimentally to mice, rats, cavies, rabbits, cats, dogs, monkeys, sheep, goats, and occasionally to cattle and fowls. More recently, Seager[11] reported the successful transmission to week-old ducklings.

Reservoir Hosts: There is no known reservoir other than naturally infected equines.

Clinical Signs: The period of incubation in the horse, as reported by different investigators, is indefinite and varies within the range of 1 to 8 weeks.

The signs are quite variable and some infected animals never show any clinical manifestations. In general, rather typical local and systemic manifestations are observed although no 2 cases are exactly alike. The temperature may fluctuate and seldom rises to 102 F. The red blood cells frequently are diminished in

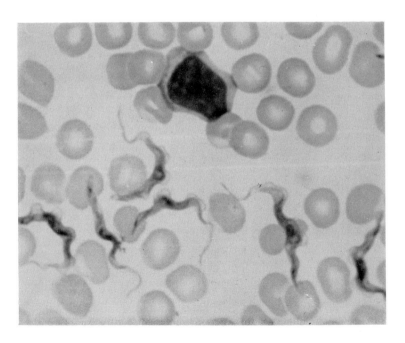

Fig. 1. *Trypanosoma equiperdum* in mouse blood. Giemsa stain. X 2395. Courtesy of Dr. William Lindquist, College of Veterinary Medicine, Michigan State University.

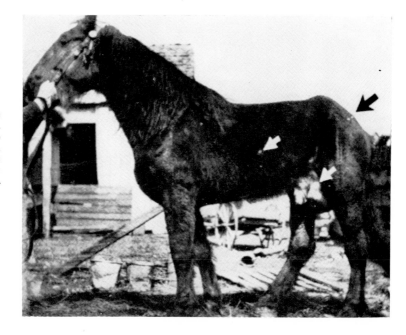

Fig. 2. Percheron stallion affected with dourine. Spots on side and croup show location of plaques. Note also the weight loss and swelling of the sheath and scrotum. From U. S. D. A. Bulletin 142 (1911).

number and there is a decided leukocytosis with a marked increase in the quantity of lymphocytic cells.

In the stallion, the first sign noticed usually is a variable swelling involving the glans penis and prepuce. The edematous process extends backward along the sheath to the scrotum, inguinal lymph nodes, and perineum with a forward extension along the lower abdomen and chest. Frequent micturition, priapism, and increased sexual desire have been observed. The penis may protrude, nodules and ulcers may form leaving white scars (leukoderma), and in some animals a discharge from a swollen, reddened urethral meatus is noted (Fig. 2).

The first signs in the mare, as in the stallion, may be so slight as to be unnoticed. The vulva, vagina, and clitoris are swollen and inflamed, with a variable amount of vaginal discharge noted. The mucous follicles may undergo nodular and pustular formation followed by ulceration. Frequent urination, switching of the tail, opening and closing of the vulvar lips, and stamping of the feet are indications of the inflammatory state of the vulvovaginal mucosa. The extent and degree of the edematous swelling, which may fluctuate by disappearing and reappearing, vary in the region of the perineum and may involve the mammary gland,

the lower abdomen, and thighs. Depigmentation (leukoderma) of portions of the genital organs, perineum, and udder may take place in several weeks (Fig. 3).

In both stallions and mares, swellings of the skin may appear on different parts of the body after a variable time. These urticarial wheals or plaques ("talerfleche") are sharply defined, round, oblong, or irregular and vary in size up to a diameter of 6 inches; they vary in number, even exceeding one hundred. The hair in these areas is harsh, erect, matted, and the swollen skin (up to 1/4 to 1/2 inch above the general level) is soft with no evidence of irritation. The eruptions may persist for days or weeks. After the edema subsides, the skin may be depigmented or covered with white hair (Fig. 4).

Advanced severe cases of dourine are characterized by emaciation and nervous signs which may occur months after the appearance of the local lesions. The weight loss is marked despite a good appetite. The most common nervous manifestations involve one or both hindquarters. Staggering, interfering, stumbling or straddling gait, partial dragging or knuckling of a hindfoot occur, all of which may be intermittent or persistent, and finally the animal is unable to stand or rise. Occasionally the fore-

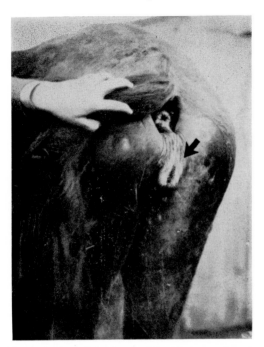

Fig. 3. Lesions of dourine involving the external genitalia and perineum of mare 47. Note the areas of depigmentation. From U.S.D.A. Bulletin 142 (1911).

limbs are involved, and the paralysis may affect the lip, nostril, eyelid or ear. Recurring swelling may appear in the joints and tendon sheaths of the fore- and hindlimbs. Mares which have been infected and conceive may abort at any time during pregnancy or carry the fetus to full term. Death of animals affected with dourine usually is due to hypostatic pneumonia or septicemia following decubital gangrene.

Lesions: Mohler[3] has described lesions as observed at necropsy. In the male, the sheath is enlarged and the skin thickened. The testicles may be enlarged and hard, or soft and atrophied. The scrotum is edematous and the tunica vaginalis may be adherent to the tunica propria. In mares, the tissues of vulva and vagina are indurated or edematous. The uterine mucosa resembles the mucous membrane of the large intestine in Johne's disease as it is thickened, infiltrated and corrugated. The ovaries may be hemorrhagic.

The lymphatic tissues in the inguinal region are inflamed. Depigmentation is noted in various affected areas of the genitals. The

bone marrow is congested and erosions and hemorrhages may be seen on the articular cartilages of joints. Ulcers may be found in the mucosa of the intestines and the mesenteric lymph nodes may be enlarged and softened or small and firm. The peritoneum is hypertrophied and edematous. The liver may be congested and it contains areas of fatty degeneration. The spleen usually is enlarged and soft but it may be normal in size and appearance. The kidneys are enlarged and soft in consistency. The lungs are very congested; suppurative foci may be present. The blood is watery and forms imperfect soft clots.

The meninges, especially the pia mater, are markedly congested and in some places adhesions have taken place between the pia and the cord. On section, softened areas and hemorrhages may be found in the cord substance. The ventricles of brain contain an excessive amount of fluid. Schoening and Formad,[12] in supplementing their spinal fluid studies, reported that degenerative changes were confined largely to the dorsal and lateral tracts of the cord.

Diagnosis: A definitive diagnosis of dourine depends upon the recognition of the clinical signs and the demonstration of the parasite in a blood film. Since *T. equiperdum* is present in the blood of horses in small numbers, attempts should be made to demonstrate the parasite in the mucoid discharge during the acute stage of the genital swelling or in serum of the edematous swellings of the genitalia or urticarial plaques. Occasionally, they may be demonstrated in milk of infected mares. The use of laboratory animals to isolate the organisms from blood or genital washing is not satisfactory.

In 1912, the use of the complement fixation test for the diagnosis of dourine was reported by Watson[13] of Canada. Mohler, Eichhorn, and Buck[14] reported on the satisfactory results of this test in the United States. Prior to this, diagnoses were based solely on physical examinations. Parkin[15] of the Union of South Africa has reported nonspecific reactions to the test in a variable number of noninfected equines, particularly donkeys and mules.

As reported in the U.S. Department of Agriculture Farmers' Bulletin No. 1146:[16]

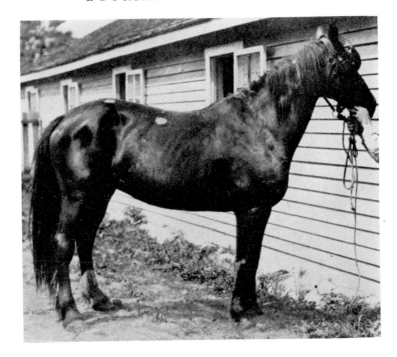

Fig. 4. Mare bred to an imported stallion March 7, 1911, and developed evidence of dourine 15 days later. Note the plaques on the croup, back, shoulder, and abdomen from which the first trypanosomes were obtained. From U.S. D.A. Bulletin 142 (1911)

The Animal Disease Eradication Regulatory Laboratories will apply the test for dourine when samples of blood serum from animals suspected of being affected with or exposed to the disease are submitted for examination. As considerable skill and experience are required in properly preparing serum samples, this work should be done by a qualified veterinarian. The samples, prepared according to the directions which follow, should be forwarded to the ADE Regulatory Laboratories, Sero-Diagnostic Center, Beltsville, Maryland. The samples should be accompanied by three copies of a letter denoting the identification of each animal (tattoo, hoof band, paint marking, or other satisfactory means), and state whether the animal is a horse, mule or burro and that dourine is suspected. The owner's name and address along with the date that the sample was collected must be clearly indicated.

Direction for the Collection of Blood Serum for Laboratory Diagnosis: As the serum is the constituent of the blood which is utilized in applying the complement fixation test, it is extremely important to send good specimens to the laboratory in order that a conclusive and reliable diagnosis may be made. To obtain a good, clear specimen of serum the following procedure is recommended:

Draw 4 ounces or more of blood from the jugular vein of the suspected animal into a dry, clean, preferably sterile, wide-mouth bottle. The blood should not be collected until a steady stream flows from the cannula of the trocar. After the bottle is filled set it carefully to one side and allow it to stand for at least 30 minutes, or until complete coagulation has taken place. It is important to see that the blood is not disturbed until complete coagulation has occurred, as the serum will not separate so readily if agitated before coagulation takes place. The sample may then be moved if desired. The clotted blood should be allowed to stand for 6 hours longer, or until the clear yellow serum separates from the clot.

When a sufficient quantity of serum has separated from the clot, pour off from 2 to 4 drams into a small vial, being very careful not to allow the entrance of any red cells. If after 6 hours the clot fails to contract sufficiently to allow the yellow serum to separate from it, the process may be accomplished by carefully loosening the clotted blood from the sides of the bottle by means of a sterile wire. The sample is then permitted to stand long enough for the clot to contract, leaving the clear yellow serum above, which should then be poured off.

If the sample is to be shipped a considerable distance or in warm weather, the serum should be carbolized 0.5% by adding 1 part of a 5% solution of carbolic acid to 9 parts of serum. It is important not to exceed these proportions of carbolic acid and serum.

The vial in which the serum is to be forwarded should be properly labeled, giving (a) description of the animal from which the sample was obtained—whether a horse, mule or burro, (b) owner's name and address, and (c) names of persons sending the sample.

Treatment:[16] Little benefit can be obtained from the medicinal treatment of dourine, nor is such treatment desirable in this country where the disease has existed only in restricted areas and where sanitary considerations demand its prompt extirpation.

The United States Department of Agriculture nevertheless has conducted experiments along lines of treatment in animals affected with the disease. Various drugs likely to be most useful in combating trypanosome infection were used, but the results were unsatisfactory. The very high cost of these drugs, together with the expense of handling the animals, would make such treatment impracticable even though beneficial results had been obtained.

Method of Eradication:[16] Sanitary measures looking to the eradication of dourine must depend on the principle that horses infected with the disease should be prevented from breeding. This conclusion is well-founded, for in spite of the possibility of recovery there are, as a matter of fact, frequent relapses, and trypanosomes may exist for many months in the sexual organs of animals apparently recovered. Therefore it is very essential to destroy diseased animals as soon as possible. The objections to spaying the mares and castrating the stallions is that such mares on the open range may be covered by stallions and that infected stallions even after castration may cover healthy mares.

Dourine, being conveyed under natural conditions solely by the act of coition, is not a difficult disease to stamp out in a farming community, but eradication is a more difficult task on the open range. It has been demonstrated, however, that with good cooperation among federal government officials, state authorities, and horse owners, these difficulties can be overcome.

The practice of the United States Department of Agriculture has been to have veterinary inspectors cooperate with the state veterinarian and his deputies in dealing with dourine where its existence is known or suspected within the state. In the spring of the year, before the animals are bred, samples of blood serum are drawn from all breeding animals in districts where dourine exists or is suspected. These samples of serum are properly identified and forwarded to the ADE Regulatory Sero-Diagnostic Center, Beltsville, Maryland and are subjected to the complement fixation test for dourine. The animals are held in virtual quarantine until the results of the test are received. Animals whose serums give positive results are destroyed. It has been customary to reimburse the owner for the value of the animal, the state and federal government usually sharing the expense equally. On Indian reservations the entire expense is borne by the federal government. Animals whose serums give negative results are considered to be free of infection and are released for breeding.

R. D. BARNER

The following data pertain to the test program described in the author's text. They were obtained by Dr. Barner through correspondence with officials of the Animal Inspection and Quarantine Division, Agricultural Research Service, U.S. Department of Agriculture. The data were contained in the Division's monthly reports. As animals may be retested when they show suspicious results to the dourine test, the total number of tests does not necessarily reflect the total number of individual animals involved. The figures refer to the dourine complement fixation tests performed on serum samples from equines offered for importation into this country from Mexico.

For the fiscal year ending June 30, 1961:

190 burro samples tested—2 dourine reactions (positive).

19 mule samples tested—all negative.

2,957 horse samples tested—10 suspicious, 36 positive reactions.

For the fiscal year ending June 30, 1960:

1,411 burro samples tested—1 suspicious, 2 positive reactions.

33 mule samples tested—all negative.

8,672 horse samples tested—11 suspicious, 176 positive reactions.—EDITOR.

REFERENCES

1. Zwick, W. and Knuth, P.: Beschälseuche oder dourine. Handbuch der Pathog. Mikro-org. 7(2) (1930) 1434-1476.
2. Williams, W. L.: Maladie du coit. Am. Vet. Rev. 12 (1888) 295-303, 341-349, 402-410, 445-450.
3. Mohler, John R.: Dourine of horses: Its cause and suppression. Bull. 142, U.S.D.A. (1911) pp. 38.
4. Rouget, J.: Contribution à l'etude du trypanosome des mammifères. Ann. Pasteur, 10 (1896) 716-728.
5. Schneider, M. and Buffard, G. E.: Transmission experimentale du trypanosome de la dourine par le coit. Bull. Acad. de Med. 42 (1899) 498-499.
6. Hutyra, F., Marek, J. and Manninger, R.: Special Pathology and Therapeutics of the Diseases of Domestic Animals. 5th Eng. ed. Alexander Eger Inc. Chicago, Ill., 1949. pp. 908-929.
7. Cantrell, William: The pattern of antigenic variation in *Trypanosoma equiperdum*. J. Inf. Dis. 107 (1960) 29-33.
8. Craige, J. E.: Infection of chick embryos and chicks with *Trypanosoma equiperdum* by the intravenous route. U. S. Army Vet. Bull. 35 (1941) 38-45.
9. Anderson, Everett, Saxe, L. H. and Beams, H. W.: Electron microscope observations of *Trypanosoma equiperdum*. J. Parasitology. 42 (1956) 11-16.
10. Crump, T. W.: Eradicating dourine in Arizona. Vet. Med. 24 (1929) 503-507.
11. Seager, L. D.: Transmission of *Trypanosoma equiperdum* to the duck. Science 100 (1944) 428.
12. Schoening, Harry W. and Formad, Robert J.: A study of the serology, the cerebrospinal fluid, and the pathological changes in the spinal cord in dourine. J. Agr. Research 26 (1923) 497-505.
13. Watson, E. A.: The serum reactions and serum diagnosis of dourine. Proc. A.V.M.A. (1912) 411-420.
14. Mohler, J. R., Eichhorn, A. and Buck, J. M.: The diagnosis of dourine by complement-fixation. Am. Vet. Rev. 45 (1914) 44-55.
15. Parkin, B. S.: The demonstration and transmission of the South African strain of *Trypanosoma equiperdum* of horses. Onderstepoort J. 23 (1947) 41-58.
16. Mohler, J. R. and Schoening, H. W.: Dourine of horses. U.S.D.A. Farmers' Bull. 1146 (1935) pp. 9-10.

BABESIASIS

Definition: Equine babesiasis is an acute, peracute, subacute or chronic tick-borne protozoal disease of solipeds characterized by fever, anemia, icterus, and by clinical signs arising from the hemolytic anemia caused by the parasites.

Etiology: Babesia equi, one of the causative organisms, is a protozoan parasite of the suborder, *Piroplasmidae.* Its synonyms are *Piroplasma equi, Nuttalia equi,* and *Nuttalia asini.*

B. equi is a small member of the genus, *Babesia,* but may attain a size of 1.5 by 4 microns. The shape varies from spherical to ovoid to pear-shaped. In blood films, the parasites are found in the erythrocytes usually singly and rarely quadrupled, when they may be seen in the classic form of a Maltese cross. The majority of parasites in a blood film are less than half the diameter of the red cell in size, and where they are scarce in blood films (which is often), the most rewarding field is at the edge of the film. Spherical and ovoid forms are seen more frequently than pear-shaped ones. Extracellular parasites occasionally are seen if there is gross infection of the erythrocytes. The small forms are actively motile.

Reproduction of *Babesia equi* in the blood of horses, takes place by division of the nucleus into four. Budding of the cytoplasm then takes place resulting in the classic Maltese cross form, which is, however, not often seen in routine clinical practice since the majority of cases are treated at an early stage. They are more numerous in smears of splenic tissue or in blood films made from the cut surface of the liver. The 4 parasites so-formed escape from the red blood cell and re-enter new erythrocytes to appear as tiny oat-shaped forms.[27] The life cycle of *B. equi* in the tick is unknown. In citrated blood at room temperature, *B. equi* can survive for 4 days.

For the clinician, the best stain is Giemsa, although parasites can be identified with methylene blue preparations. Blood films should be carefully prepared and meticulously stained, so as to be free of stain deposit or artifacts. With Giemsa stain, the parasites appear with a pale blue cytoplasm, edged by dark nuclear material of varying thickness at, or close to, the periphery.

For models of descriptive morphologic detail, readers are referred to the original papers of early workers on the subject. In countries where African horsesickness, trypanosomiasis, infectious anemia or equine influenza also occur, blood film examination is a most important diagnostic technic.

Babesia caballi (Piroplasma caballi) is the second species related to this equine disease.

This parasite differs from the preceding in being a much larger member of the genus, attaining a length of 6 microns. The majority of parasites seen in a blood film are larger than half the diameter of the red cells, and most forms are pear-shaped. They usually are more numerous and found more easily than are *B. equi.* Giemsa stain is preferred to show this organism. Their multiplication in the blood takes place by binary fission. Two pear-shaped parasites often are seen paired in erythrocytes. Extracellular parasites are occasionally seen. The life cycle of *B. caballi* in the tick is unknown. Their maximum survival time in citrated blood at room temperature is 4 days.

Transmission: Two species of *Dermacentor,* 3 species of *Rhipicephalus,* and 4 species of *Hyalomma* are known vectors of *B. equi.* Hereditary transmission has been demonstrated in *H. anatolicum,* and stage-to-stage transmission in the remaining 8 vectors.[8] Three species of *Dermacentor,* 2 species of *Rhipicephalus,* and 4 species of *Hyalomma* are known vectors of *B. caballi.* Hereditary transmission has been demonstrated in 6 of these 9 species, the exceptions being *D. pictus, H. anatolicum,* and *Rh. bursa,* and stage-to-stage transmission in all except *H. anatolicum* and *H. volgense.* It has been shown that *B. caballi* can be retained by *Rh. sanguineus* through 4 generations. Enigk considered that ticks of related species may be vectors. Adult ticks ordinarily are the important infective agents.[6, 7]

Intra-uterine transmission of both *B. equi* and *B. caballi* has been recorded quite frequently.[3,4,14,17,19,23] Aborted feti have shown varying degrees of infected erythrocytes. In feti which show gross pathologic changes plus a high percentage of infected erythrocytes, babesiasis presumably is the cause of intra-uterine death and consequent abortion.

Mechanical transmission by biting flies has not been recorded, but both *B. equi* and *B. caballi* can be transmitted readily to susceptible animals by parenteral injection of blood, or of organ emulsions. Cross-transmission also can be carried out in this way from one species of solipeds to another.

Distribution and Epizootiology: Any area where the known vectors occur concurrently with horses, donkeys, mules or zebras can be regarded either as enzootic biliary fever areas, or as potential ones. The disease has been recorded in France, Spain, Portugal, Italy, Hungary, Yugoslavia, Albania, Greece, Bulgaria, Rumania, the Middle East, the U.S.S.R., India, Indo-China, Manchuria, Central and South America, the whole of the African continent, and Madagascar. The United Kingdom, Eire, Australia, and New Zealand are free of the disease.

The seasonal and geographic incidence is related to the biology of the vectors concerned.[6,7] For example, *D. pictus,* a cold-resistant tick, has been suggested as the vector in central Russia.[8] In Europe, *B. caballi* has a more northerly distribution than *B. equi,* and is found as far north as Moscow. *B. equi* generally is regarded as the more widespread parasite. In South Africa, *B. equi* accounts for more than 99% of naturally occurring babesiasis in horses.[17]

In European countries, biliary fever occurs mainly during the spring and summer.[12,15] In Africa, it occurs at any time of the year.

In enzootic areas foals acquire the infection at an early age, unless kept free of ticks from birth; and even this precaution cannot prevent occasional intra-uterine infection, the mechanism of which is not fully understood. After early infection, foals maintain resistance by means of a premunity, *i.e.,* an immunity which is effective only so long as the animal is a carrier of the parasite. Relapses are common with *B. equi* (less frequent with *B. caballi*), particularly if the animal suffers malnutrition, overwork, change of environment, or intercurrent disease, *e.g.,* African horsesickness. Adverse conditions, such as a protracted journey, may cause a breakdown in premunity.

The state of premunity may persist for years; consequently the movement of solipeds from enzootic into nonenzootic areas may establish new foci of infection. Semenov[33] has pointed out that 30% of healthy foals may be infected with *B. caballi.*

Horses reared in enzootic areas and running on free range remain remarkably free of clinical signs unless the environment (external or internal) changes drastically. Thus, horses which have been clinically free of the disease since birth may succumb either to a relapse

DIFFERENCE IN SUSCEPTIBILITY BY SEX & AGE

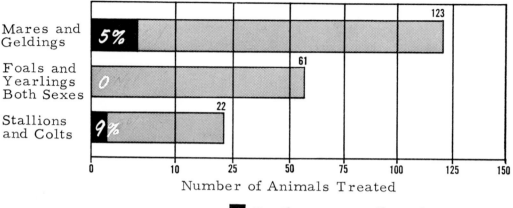

Fig. 5. Susceptibility to Babesiasis.

or to a fresh infection soon after being moved to a different province or district within the same enzootic area. Similarly on stud farms, a batch of yearlings which are brought in from range and stable-fed may develop clinical signs of babesiasis within a few weeks. There can be little doubt that stress factors play a large role in the epizootiology of equine babesiasis as in other protozoal diseases of animals. Although foals are more resistant than mature horses, many cases are seen in highly-bred foals of all ages, from birth onward. Mares and geldings have less resistance than foals, and noncastrates have least resistance of all. The most severe cases which the clinician encounters are in well-bred noncastrates and mares imported from nonenzootic countries (Fig. 5).

Donkeys have greater resistance to babesiasis (icterus is not a feature of the disease in this species), and mules have greater resistance than donkeys.[37] The susceptibility of zebras to *B. caballi* has not been established, but they are highly resistant to *B. equi*, which has been demonstrated in a series of blood smears taken from zebras in South Africa and East Africa.[21]

Pathogenesis: Invasion of erythrocytes and multiplication therein are followed by a progressively massive destruction of these cells. Hypochromasia, poikilocytosis and anisocytosis are constant findings in acute cases, and the erythrocyte count drops rapidly. A count of under 2 million is not uncommon. A clinically apparent anemia develops early in the course of the disease, usually within 24 hours of the earliest signs. A monocytosis is present, and phagocytosis of parasitized erythrocytes takes place. Hemoglobinemia and icterus develop, occasionally hemoglobinuria. The massive breakdown of erythrocytes imposes a tremendous strain on the liver, kidneys, and heart, and it is possible that the parasites themselves exude a toxin which contributes to the degeneration of these organs so regularly observed at necropsies. The presence of such a toxin has not yet been demonstrated conclusively. Quantitative spectrophotometric determinations of serum bilirubin levels in Thoroughbreds showed a variable increase of bilirubin in acute cases, but not in chronic ones.[25] There is a marked increase in blood urea.[31]

Clinical Signs: Acute, peracute, subacute, and chronic forms of the disease are recognized. The incubation period following the bite from an infected tick varies from 10 to 21 days. In an acute case of babesiasis, which is the type most frequently encountered by the clinician, the first signs noted are loss of appetite and apathy. There is a disinclination to move, and a horse on free range lags behind the rest of the group or stands alone. If stabled, a horse stands slackly inside, often with the head held lower than usual and directed toward a corner of the box. Feed is left in the manger and the hair coat loses its sheen. If walked outside, the patient moves with a swaying, weak gait.

The feces are drier and scantier than normal, and covered thinly with an orange-tinged mucus. The urine has a pungent odor and may be discolored to the extent of being port wine-colored, although in the great majority of cases the urine is either a normal color or somewhat orange.

The temperature is raised to between 102 and 106 F. In *B. equi* infection, fever is irregularly intermittent, rising to a peak every 24 to 72 hours, though with *B. caballi* the fever is more continuous. The breathing rate is increased; often there is an audible expiration. The pulse invariably is faster. In the first stages, it is strong and full, though fast, then becomes weaker, irregular and faster as the disease progresses. If the pulse rate is more than 80, the prognosis is grave. On auscultation, the second heart sound often is accentuated.

Petechial hemorrhages are present on the mucous membranes of the membrana nictitans and the conjunctivae, which are paler than normal and icteric. The buccal mucosa also is pale and yellow, but not petechiated. In mares and fillies, the best site to examine for anemia and icterus is the vaginal mucosa adjacent to the clitoris. Reddish streaks and petechial hemorrhages also may be seen on the vaginal or nasal mucosae.

Though the foregoing can be regarded as typical of the acute case, clinical signs occasionally may be absent or atypical. For example, signs of colic are noted in 4% of all cases of biliary fever. These are the usual signs of abdominal pain—pawing the ground, looking at the flank, sweating, and even lying down and rolling. Practitioners may be called to treat cases of colic which on examination are found to be babesiasis. In this connection, it is of interest to record that whenever I have done rectal examinations on such cases, the turgid and thickened posterior border of the spleen could be palpated. Whether it can be palpated in all acute cases is not known. Knuth, Behn, and Schulze considered that splenic enlargement is a contributory cause of the colic in such cases.[15] Sometimes the only definite signs are a rise in pulse rate and fever, with dyspnea. Petechial hemorrhages may be absent, and anemia and icterus may not be clinically evident in the early stages.

In subacute cases, the signs generally are milder. The appetite may be quite good and the temperature close to normal. Cases may be encountered in which the only signs are slight anemia and icterus; appetite, pulse, temperature, and respirations remain normal. In such instances, if blood films are examined daily, a rise in temperature and pulse rate coincides with the appearance of parasites in the red blood cells of the peripheral circulation. The subacute case may become acute at any stage without warning, and due cognizance must be given this possibility when instituting treatment. If an acute case is left untreated, the anemia and icterus quickly assume disastrous proportions. There is total disinterest in moving or in eating or grazing. The limbs, particularly the fetlock and cannon regions, become swollen and edematous, and pit easily on pressure. The abdominal and pectoral regions, and the head also may become edematous. Even in cases which are treated successfully at an early stage, swelling of the hind fetlocks and cannons persists for days, testifying to the derangement of the circulation caused by the disease. There also may be a marked jugular pulse.

In general, the more severe the anemia and icterus, the more difficult is the treatment and the more prolonged the convalescence. Untreated acute cases may live about 2 weeks. Subacute cases often recover without treatment.

The chronic form of babesiasis, which may follow an acute or subacute attack, or which may take an insidious course without any previously apparent signs, is characterized by a slow, progressive loss of condition in spite of a high level of nutrition. Indeed, the only complaint from an owner may be that the animal is a "poor doer." On examination, the temperature is slightly elevated, or normal. The appetite is capricious, and there is a definite loss of alertness and willingness to exercise. Icterus is absent, and anemia may be detectable only by red cell count and in hematocrit values. Careful examination of blood films, particularly if there is slight fever when the sample is taken, often reveals the parasite. However, in enzootic biliary fever areas, if presented with such a syndrome in which no parasites can be demonstrated, and if hematocrit values remain consistently low in spite of anthelminthic and symptomatic treatment (tonics, vitamins, iron, etc.), then specific treatment for babesiasis should be considered.

In general, *B. caballi* infection follows a milder course than *B. equi,* although Russian workers have recorded a mortality rate as high as 85% in untreated cases.[44]

Relapses are particularly common with *B. equi* infection, and the most common period for a relapse is 5 to 9 days after treatment of, and recovery from, the initial reaction. However, relapses can be expected any time up to 14 days afterward, and in Thoroughbreds often occur if exercise is allowed within that period. For this reason, patients recovering from biliary fever must be stabled for a minimum period of 2 weeks. After then, the danger of a relapse is small.

Peracute cases of biliary fever fortunately are rare. They provide no chance for treatment since the victims are found either dead or moribund. The clinical signs are suggestive of an acute abdominal catastrophe—sweating, trembling, and dyspnea. Soon the animal goes down, kicking and rolling violently. Closer examination reveals an elevated temperature (although this falls below normal just before death), and a pulse of more than 80. The mucous membranes show petechial hemorrhages and icterus, and may be intensely injected. Anemia is not marked. Death follows within 24 hours of the onset of signs.

Diagnosis: A diagnosis based on clinical signs can be made in about 80% of acute cases. It should always be confirmed by blood film examination, and this cannot be stressed too strongly. In enzootic areas it is usual to administer treatment first and to confirm diagnosis by blood film examination later. In view of the speed with which babesiasis can cause severe lesions or even death, treatment should not be delayed any longer than necessary. In a smaller percentage of cases when it is not possible to make a definite diagnosis on the basis of clinical signs alone, it often is advisable to administer treatment before examination of blood smears. In this connection, it should be noted that parasites begin to disappear from the peripheral circulation after the fifth day of reaction.

In differential diagnosis the following diseases must be considered:

1. Trypanosomiasis caused by these species:

T. hippicum (Murrina—Central America).

T. equinum (Mal de Caderas—tropical South America).

T. evansi (Surra—Asia, and Africa north of Sahara).

T. brucei (Nagana—tropical Africa south of Sahara).

T. equiperdum (Dourine).

Examination of blood films and hanging drop preparations help to make the diagnosis. In the final analysis, complement fixation tests or biological tests on laboratory animals may be carried out.

2. African horsesickness. In the "dikkop" or "dunkop" forms of this disease there is no difficulty. However, the "horsesickness fever" syndrome may present a clinical picture similar to the early stages of babesiasis. Careful examination of blood films is the most rewarding technic for differentiation.

3. Equine influenza. It sometimes is difficult to differentiate these infections from the early stages of biliary fever. Critical examination of the respiratory system and of blood films is of greatest value.

4. Equine infectious anemia.

5. Purpura hemorrhagica.

6. Senecio poisoning.

Gross Pathology: At necropsy, the following lesions commonly are present:

1. Generalized anemia and icterus.

2. Edema of subcutaneous and subserous tissues, and gelatinous infiltration of fatty tissues.

3. Emaciation (depending on the course).

4. Hepatomegaly and splenomegaly. The liver is a dark orange-brown color and greatly

Comparison of Treatment Results over 4-Year Periods

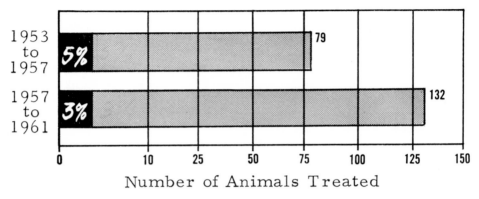

Number of Animals Treated

■ Deaths among treated animals

Fig. 6. Results of treatment for Babesiasis.

enlarged. Examination of the cut surface shows degenerative changes in the lobules.

5. The kidneys are pale, enlarged, and have small subcapsular and cortical hemorrhages.

6. Hydrothorax and hydropericardium. Subepicardial and subendocardial hemorrhages.

7. Hyperemia and edema of the lungs.

8. Marked enlargement of the lymph glands of spleen, liver, and kidneys.

In addition, the following lesions also may be found:

1. Catarrhal enteritis—usually associated with marked degeneration of liver and kidneys.

2. Myocardial degeneration—as evidenced by a "boiled" appearance.

3. Pericarditis or epicarditis may be found.[35]

4. Pneumonia also has been recorded as a complication.

Treatment: The therapy of babesiasis is aimed at elimination or suppression of the parasite, combating the effects on vital organs, and providing good nursing and environment.

Although the reports in the literature of the past 50 years point to a wide variation in the results obtained from the use of specific drugs for equine babesiasis[2,10,11,41,43] particularly in the case of *B. equi,* euflavine (gonacrine) has been widely accepted as a reliable remedy.[11,18] Of recent years, berenil (a quinaldine derivative) has come into prominence as a specific remedy for babesiasis in domestic animals. Both in laboratory trials and in clinical cases, berenil has given good results in equine babesiasis.[24,29]

Owing to an increasing number of cases of no response or relapse to gonacrine and to other drugs, even with repeated injections, in 1957 I adopted the routine use of a combination of 2 drugs, administered as follows: the initial injection of gonacrine (in the majority of cases, gonacrine was used as the first injection) is followed 16 to 24 hours later by injection of one of the following specific drugs: phenamidine, acaprin, babesan, pirevan, trypan blue, or quinine dihydrochloride. If the response to the injection of gonacrine is good and, on examination, the appetite is improved, and the pulse, temperature and respiration are within normal range, then the second injection is not administered. In the majority of cases, the second injection is indicated.

In cases of no response in which the condition of the patient has markedly deteriorated, and particularly in patients with enteritis, repeated injections of gonacrine are contraindicated. The development of enteritis appears to be associated with severe liver and/or kidney damage, and drugs other than gonacrine are advised. Occasionally, clinical assessment and blood examination indicate yet a third and even fourth treatment by different drugs in approximately 48 to 72 hours. Such refractory cases fortunately are uncommon, but they require constant and careful supervision, including daily examination of blood smears and full supportive and prophylactic treatment including antibiotics (see Theiler, 1903).[36] Relapses often are best controlled by different drugs from those used initially, and supportive therapy is fully as important as specific medicaments in the management of relapses.

Small fluctuations in temperature may occur in horses during the first 2 to 3 weeks after successful treatment, but such fluctuations are of no importance provided the appetite is good and the pulse is normal. The results obtained by the aforementioned routine are compared in Fig. 6 with the results over the preceding 4-year period, in a total series of 211 patients, of which 208 were Thoroughbreds.

Although trypan blue is regarded as ineffective against *B. equi*, I have used it with success in stables where gonacrine has given disappointing results. It cannot be recommended for routine use as a sole specific against *B. equi* in adult Thoroughbreds. The posology of specific drugs used in the treatment of babesiasis in equines is given in Table 1.

Failures of euflavine or quinuronium sulphate or their derivatives suggest the evolution of drug-resistant strains of the parasites, and this may be the case particularly in studs or stables which have occupied the same premises for many decades. As shown in Table 2, the sequelae of the disease can be a major cause of mortality. It appears that there are local variations both in virulence and in response to specific drugs, and local veterinarians in any enzootic area usually are the best judges of what remedial measures are likely to prove efficient. Early diagnosis and treatment are of prime importance.

Gilbert and Avelange (1947) reported the use of the dichlorhydrate of diamidine and the dimethane sulfonate of diamidine intravenously in a dosage of 1 Gm. in 20 ml. water.[9]

The following supportive measures are preferred by the writer:

1. Two to 3 liters of 10% dextrose-saline solution are administered during the first 24 hours. The first liter is given immediately following the gonacrine. This is repeated every day until the appetite returns; thereafter, up to 1 pound of glucose is mixed with the daily feed.

2. Vitamin therapy is administered from the start in the form of total B complex (including B_{12} and folic acid) in maximal dosage. Vitamin A also is injected intramuscularly in doses of 1 million units daily for 3 days, for its detoxifying and mucosal-protecting affects.[20]

3. Prednisolone is injected intramuscularly at the same time as the initial injection of gonacrine.

4. Arsenic therapy is instituted only after the disappearance of icterus; intramuscular injection of acetylarsan is preferred every 48 hours. Other supportive medicaments include: methionine (dosage 5 Gm. dissolved in 1 liter of dextrose-saline solution once daily), iron preparations via parenteral injection, nonirritating diuretics, and a constant supply of fresh water. Blood transfusion is a measure which should be undertaken with caution, and only if the anemia is severe and likely per se to cause collapse. Any anaphylactic reaction which results from the transfusion may be followed quickly by a relapse, and there is a danger of infecting the recipient with a labile infection of another parasite or virus. There also is danger of causing fatal pulmonary edema, by increasing the blood volume of a patient whose lungs are already stressed.

Although the value of the broad spectrum antibiotics in high dosage rates as specifics in clinical cases is unknown, they are indicated as prophylactics in severe cases, and in treating sequelae, particularly enteritis.

It should be strongly emphasized that the patient must remain in a stall for a minimum period of 14 days. The appetite of a horse suffering from babesiasis is capricious. Light, high-quality hay should be provided, plus green feed if possible. Small feedings should be provided at least 3 times daily. As a rule, only hay or green feed will be eaten during periods of fever, and the patient may even ignore good feed and concentrate on bedding. Since thirst is increased, clean fresh water always must be available. Provided it does not prevent the patient from drinking, 1

Table 1.—Drugs Used in Treatment of Babesiasis

DRUG	DOSAGE	ADMINISTRATION	RATE OF INJECTION AND REMARKS
Euflavine	Adults 20 ml./1000 lb. Foals 3 ml./50 kg. 5% aqueous solution.	Intravenous Intravenous	Causes slight depression, and orange discoloration of mucous membranes. Avoid perivascular injection. Allow 4 minutes for injection.
Quinuronium sulphate	5% aqueous solution. 1 ml./100 lbs. Maximum 6 ml.	Subcutaneous	Best given in divided doses if alarming reactions are to be avoided, especially in severely ill patients. Divide total dose into 3 or 4 and administer each portion at 30-minute intervals. Causes sweating, evacuation of fluid feces, and obvious discomfort. Avoid use in pregnant mares.
Phenamidine isethionate	5% w/v aqueous solution. 12 ml./50 kg.	Subcutaneous	Administer total dose in 6 different subcutaneous sites. Advisable to give half the total dose, then wait 10 to 15 minutes before administering remaining half. Sensitive, edematous swellings develop at sites of injection which gradually disappear. In higher concentrations, necrosis of tissue and a slough may develop. Avoid use in pregnant mares.
Berenil	2 to 3 mg./kg. in aqueous solution. Max., 10 mg./kg.	Intramuscular	No marked side effects recorded.
Trypan blue	1% aqueous solution. 20 ml./50 kg.	Intravenous	Allow 20 minutes for injection to avoid alarming reactions. Solution should be freshly prepared and filtered. Causes bluish-gray discoloration of mucous membranes.
Quinine hydro-bromide and stovarsol	5% aqueous solution. 20 ml./1000 lbs. 0.5 Gm. (Oral)	Intravenous	Repeat daily for 3 consecutive days.
Neoarsphenamine	10% w/v aqueous solution. 30 ml./1000 lbs.	Intravenous	Repeat once weekly for 3 weeks.[41]
T. 21	1.5 Gm. in 100 ml. saline.	Intravenous	Parkin (1931).[28]
Aureomycin	15.6 mg./lb.	Intravenous	Reported by Jansen (1953) in splenectomized donkey foals.[13] Value in clinical cases in horses not confirmed.
Quinine dihydro-chloride	1 Gm./100 kg. dissolved in 1 liter dextrose-saline.	Intravenous	Allow 20 minutes for injection. If given too rapidly, plunging and staggering may result.

Table 2.—Mortality Records, 1953 to 1961

Sex	Period Between First Treatment and Death	Course and Lesions	B. EQUI in Blood at Necropsy
Gelding	4 days	No response to gonacrine (twice) and trypan blue. Very anemic and icteric. Typical lesions at necropsy.	Scarce
Stallion	2 hours	*In extremis* when examined. Apparently normal and eating 14 hours previously. Typical lesions at necropsy.	Numerous
Gelding	1 week	Fibrinous epicarditis. Degeneration of liver and kidneys.	None
Mare	2 weeks	Apparent recovery followed by enteritis. Degeneration of liver, kidneys, and myocardium at necropsy.	None
Colt	68 hours	No response to trypan blue, gonacrine, phenamidine. Typical lesions at autopsy.	Numerous
Mare	2 weeks	Several relapses followed by enteritis and laminitis. Degeneration of liver, kidneys, and myocardium.	None
Gelding	6 months	Several relapses from which horse recovered, but obstinate chronic enteritis remained for months, and caused steady deterioration. No necropsy.	
Mare	1 month	Apparently successful recovery. Found dead in stall. No necropsy.	

ounce of Epsom or Glauber's salt is added per 12 pints of the water. Other purgatives should not be given. If signs of colic or laminitis are present, a mild laxative should be administered by stomach tube. A rug is provided, and the legs are bandaged if necessary.

A long convalescence—3 to 6 months—is recommended before working. The same period of sexual rest also is necessary for studs.

Some of the common sequelae to babesiasis are:

1. Mares in foal may abort as a result of an attack of biliary fever. Thus, babesiasis may cause abortion in 2 ways—by intrauterine infection of the fetus, and as a result of biliary fever in the mare. A third possibility also exists—as a result of treatment.

2. Stallions may become infertile following an attack of babesiasis. The loss of fertility may be partial or total, temporary or permanent.

3. Enteritis is one of the commonest sequelae of biliary fever. It may be acute or chronic. The exact etiology of its development remains obscure. In enteritis, laminitis is a bad prognostic sign.

4. Tissue necrosis and jugular phlebitis result from the deposition of drugs, particularly gonacrine, outside the jugular vein.

5. It can be stated with certainty that the racing potential of 90% of the horses who respond to treatment within 48 hours after the first signs is not affected.

Immunity: The immunity in equine babesiasis is not absolute. In common with that of babesiases of other animals, it is referred to as a premunity or labile infection, which may persist for many years after recovery from clinical signs.

Parasites may disappear completely as a result of autosterilization or treatment. When this occurs, the animal again is fully susceptible.[22] Animals harboring a labile infection have a fairly strong resistance to subsequent infection, but as pointed out, stress factors or reinfection with a different strain may cause a breakdown in the premunity. There is no cross-immunity in equine babesiasis; a labile infection of one parasite does not induce resistance to the other.[5] Splenectomy of premune animals is followed by a relapse.[30]

Prophylaxis: Although Theiler showed that horses could be immunized by inoculation of infected blood after passage through donkeys for 4 generations, the immunization of horses by this method is not being practiced generally.[39] The incidence of babesiasis in equines can be reduced by keeping individual animals as free of ticks as possible. In stabled horses, the use of shavings or sawdust instead of hay, for bedding, meticulous daily grooming, and regular weekly dressings with acaricide suspensions are of value in this respect. Obviously any large-scale control program must include tick eradication.

In the U.S.S.R., the prophylactic use of the urea derivative, hemosporidin, for *B. caballi* has been reported.[40] Alexandrov concluded that the duration of resistance of horses to reinfection with *B. equi* after trypaflavine therapy, was 1 year.[1] Such observations may have a wider application in future control projects.

A. LITTLEJOHN

The author gratefully acknowledges the generous advice and encouragement given by Prof. W. O. Neitz, Onderstepoort, in the preparation of this article.

REFERENCES

1. Alexandrov, N. A.: Duration of resistance of horses to repeated infection with N. equi after trypaflavine therapy. Veterinariya, Moscow, **35** (5), (1958) 49. Vet. Bull. **29** (1959) 11.
2. de Kock, G.v.d.W.: Drug treatment in Nuttalliosis. 7th and 8th Report of Director of Vet. Services, Union of South Africa, 1918, 637.
3. Donatien, A., Lestoquard, F. and Bouguet, A.: Bull. Soc. Path. Exotique, **28** (1935) 422.
4. Donatien, A., Lestoquard, F. and Sausseau, L.: Compt. Rend. Soc. Biol., **90** (1924) 1308.
5. du Toit, P. J.: Experimentelle studien über die Pferdepiroplasmose. I.Mitteilung. Trop. Hyg. **23** (1919) 121. Trop. Vet. Bull. 7 (1919) 140.
6. Enigk, K.: Die Überträger der Pferdepiroplasmose, ihre Verbreitung und Biologie. Arch. wiss. prakt. Tierheilk. **78** (1943) 209. The vectors of equine piroplasmosis; their geographical incidence and biology. Vet. Bull. **14** (1944) 85.
7. Enigk, K.: Zur Epidemiologie der Pferdepiroplasmosis Dtsch. tropenmed. Z **47** (1943) 333. Vet. Bull. **15** (1945) 42.
8. Enigk, K.: Weitere Untersuchungen zur Überträgerfrage der Pferdepiroplasmose. Arch. wiss. prakt. Tierheilk. **79** (1944) 58. Vet. Bull. **16** (1944) 218.
9. Gilbert et Avelange: La diamidine dans le traitement de la piroplasmose du cheval. Rec. Méd. Vét. **123** (1947) 226.
10. Goodall, A.: The trypan blue treatment of piroplasmosis of the domestic animals in South Africa. Parasit. (1914) 62.
11. Henning, M. W.: Animal Diseases in South Africa. C.N.A. Johannesburg. 1956.
12. Hutyra, Marek and Manninger. Special Pathology and Therapeutics of the Diseases of the Domestic Animals. Baillière, Tindall and Cox, London. 1949.
13. Jansen, B. C.: The parasiticidal effect of aureomycin on B. equi in splenectomised donkeys. Ond. J. Vet. Res. **26** (1953) 175.
14. Konstantinow, A. G.: Sovet. Vet. **13** (1936) 83. Vet. Bull. 7 (1937) 68.
15. Knuth, P., Behn, P. und Schulze, P.: Untersuchungen über die Piroplasmose der Pferde in Jahre. 1917. Ztschr. f. Veterinärk. 6 (1918) 241.
16. Laveran, A.: Contribution à l'étude de P. equi. C. R. Soc. Biol. **53** (1901) 385.
17. Littlejohn, A.: Unpublished observations. Mooi River, S. Africa, 1961.
18. Loge, G. et Guilhon, J.: Traitement de la piroplasma équine vrai par la gonacrine. Bull. Acad. vet. Fr. 8 (1935) 172.
19. Meynard, J-A.: Rec. Méd. Vét. **127** (1951) 340.
20. Moore, T.: Vitamin A. Elsevier Pub. Co. 1957.
21. Neitz, W. O.: Blood parasites of game in Zululand: a further report. Ond. J. Vet. Sci. and An. Ind. **1** (1933) 411.
22. Neitz, W. O.: Classification, transmission and biology of piroplasms of domestic animals. Ann. N.Y. Acad. Sci. **64** (1956) 56.
23. Neitz, W. O.: Personal communication 1959.
24. Neitz, W. O.: Personal communication 1961.
25. Netto, A. R. and Lima, F. S. P.: Serum bilirubin content in thoroughbred horses with specific reference to variations due to piroplasmosis. Rev. Fac. Med. Vet. S. Paulo **5** (1956) 567.
26. Neveu-Lemaire, M.: Traité de protozoologie, médicale et vétérinaire. Vigot Frères, Paris. 1943.

27. Nuttall, G. H. F. and Strickland, C.: On the occurrence of two species of parasites in equine piroplasmosis. Parasit. **5** (1912) 65.
28. Parkin, B.: Treatment of piroplasmosis with T. 21. 17th Report of Director of Vet. Serv. and An. Ind., Union of South Africa (1931) 27.
29. Quinlan, J. B.: Personal communication. 1961.
30. Quinlan, J. B., de Kock, G.v.d.W., Marais, I. P.: The operation of splenectomy in horses, cattle, sheep, goats, pigs, dogs, and some South African antelopes: a summary of the results of 98 splenectomies. Ond. J. Vet. Sci. and An. Ind. **5** (1935) 273.
31. Rossi, P.: Urée sanguine, et piroplasmose équine vraie (P. caballi). C.R. Soc. Biol. **119** (1935) 847.
32. Sebrell, W. H. Jr., and Harris, R. S.: The Vitamins. Acad. Press. Inc. N.Y. 1954.
33. Semenov, P. V.: Veterinariya, Moscow **32** (4) (1955) 49. Vet. Bull. **26** (1956) 324.
34. Simpson, L.: A note on the effect of B_{12} on the haematological picture of the racehorse. J. S. African vet. med. Assn. **32** (1961) 95.
35. Theiler, A.: Equine malaria, J. Comp. Path. and Therap. **15** (1902) 40.
36. Theiler, A. Equine malaria and its sequelae. J. Comp. Path. and Therap. **16** (1903) 97.
37. Theiler, A.: Further notes on piroplasmosis of the horse, mule and donkey. J. Comp. Path. and Therap. **18** (1905) **229.**
38. Theiler, A.: Transmission of equine piroplasmosis by ticks in South Africa. J. Comp. Path. and Therap. 19 (1906) 283.
39. Theiler, A.: Continuation of experiments on protective inoculation against equine piroplasmosis. J. Comp. Path. and Therap. **21** (1908) 97.
40. Vishker, A. S.: Chemoprophylactic action of hemosporidin in equine piroplasmosis. Veterinariya, Moscow **33** (3) (1956) 34. Vet. Bull. **26** (1956), 426.
41. Weisman, L. G.: Comments and field observations. Vet. Bull. U.S. Army **27** (1933) 167. Quoted by Udall, D. H. The Practice of Veterinary Medicine. George Banta Pub. Co., Menasha, Wisconsin. 1943.
42. Wenyon, C. M.: Protozoology. Baillière, Tindall and Cox, London. 1926.
43. Williams, A. J. Report of the treatment of Nuttalliosis in army horses. Trop. Vet. Bull. 4 (1916) 3.
44. Yakimoff, W. L. and Jodorsky: Quoted by Hutyra, Marek and Manninger. 1949. Special Pathology and Therapeutics of the Diseases of the Domestic Animals. Baillière, Tindall and Cox, London, 1935.

GLOBIDIOSIS

Globidiosis is an acute, subacute or chronic febrile disease caused by species of the protozoan genus, Globidium or Besnoitia, and affecting cattle, sheep, horses, and occasionally marsupials. It is characterized by some systemic reaction and local signs such as lacrimation, anasarca, alopecia, scleroderma, rhinitis, laryngotracheitis, enteritis, and, in bulls, sterility.

Distribution: In cattle, the disease has a wide distribution throughout Europe and large portions of Africa. Reports of equine globidiosis have been limited to Europe and Africa, and the only recorded instance of the disease in the United States has been in the white-footed mouse in Montana.[1]

The equine disease was described late in the nineteenth century in Europe as being caused by the first member of this group of organisms, *Globidium leuckarti*.[2,3] It was found in the intestinal mucosa. Subsequent descriptions of this disease in horses, involving the skin prominently and caused by *Globidium (Besnoitia) besnoiti* (the main parasite in the bovine form of globidiosis, or one indistinguishable from it) came from the Sudan and from South Africa.[4,5]

Etiology: There is considerable confusion as to the exact identity and taxonomy of the globidial parasites generally. The present concept seems to be that the intestinal parasite is *Globidium leuckarti* whereas the cutaneous pathogen is *Globidium besnoiti* or, more correctly, *Besnoitia besnoiti*.[1,6]

The latter organism multiplies by binary fission, mostly within monocytes and histiocytes, and is morphologically indistinguishable from *Toxoplasma gondii*.[1] The crescent, oval, or banana-shaped spores are found in the blood stream early in the infection. They parasitize macrophages and within them propagate by longitudinal binary fission, while the host cell enlarges until a cyst is formed consisting of a narrow rim of host cell material containing thousands of spores. The cysts as found in the skin and other locations vary in size up to 0.5 mm. wide and the spores are about 7 microns long by 2 microns wide.

In the case of the intestinal Globidium it appears that there is an Eimeria-like type of development: oocysts, sporoblasts, sporocysts, and sporozoites. The situation at the present time is not at all clear.[1]

Transmission: Cutaneous globidiosis has been transmitted fairly readily by injecting blood from an infected into a susceptible animal. The natural mode of transmission, however, is still obscure. Close physical contact between animals has not been observed to result in spread of infection.[1] Mechanical transmission is a distinct possibility as it has been shown that infection can be transferred by means of a prick with a hypodermic needle.[1] Tabanid flies have the right equipment for this type of transmission. Biologic transmission by arthropods still is an entirely open question.

Clinical Signs: Globidiosis follows, more or less, the pattern of many infectious diseases: an acute phase with parasitemia, fever, and malaise followed by a chronic phase with localization of lesions in particular tissues. In the case of horses, localization is either in the skin, subcutis, connective tissue of the scleral conjunctiva, and in the nose and pharynx in one form, and in the intestinal mucosa in another.

The incubation period in nature is unknown but that resulting from experimental injection of infected blood from the cutaneous form in cattle varies from 6 to 16 days.

During the acute stage of the intestinal form there is a hemorrhagic enteritis with dysentery developing immediately or after a few days. The animal looks very dull and depressed, and loses condition rapidly. If it recovers, convalescence is very slow.

The cutaneous form has been documented more fully in horses in the Sudan.[4] General signs of the infection include irregularly elevated temperature, marked muscular weakness, and dejection. The conjunctiva usually is reddened, often with petechiation, and the eyelids are swollen. The skin, to a variable degree, is thickened and swollen, irregularly depilated, scurfy and rough. In the relatively hairless skin of the scrotum, inner thighs, and perineum there may be blotchy areas of depigmentation where repeated bursting of cysts has caused damage. The entire skin and subcutis of the horse may be heavily parasitized as may be the nasal, pharyngeal and laryngeal mucosas, where the cysts are visible as white, spherical granules or spots up to ½ mm. wide.

Diagnosis: In the intestinal form, the diagnosis can be made by staining fecal smears with Giemsa or Wright's stain; the banana-shaped spores are about 10 by 4 microns, and are fairly regularly demonstrable.

Skin scrapings, similarly stained, or skin biopsy from thickened areas when cut and stained for histologic examination, provide suitable material for diagnosis of the cutaneous form. Recently it has been shown in bovine besnoitiosis that even in clinically inapparent cases the diagnosis may be made by visual examination of the scleral conjunctiva.[7] The diagnosis may be confirmed by biopsy and the referred report describes the technic in detail.

Treatment: There is no specific treatment known at this time, although a number of the more modern drugs have been tried.[1] Therapy consists of nursing, providing easily digestible food, plenty of water and shade where needed, and controlling the inevitable secondary infections. It has been noticed that cattle tend to improve when removed to a higher altitude and a more temperate climate.

REFERENCES

1. Pols, J. W.: Studies on bovine besnoitiosis with special reference to the aetiology. Thesis, Univ. of Pretoria. (1960) Onderstepoort J. Vet. Research **28** (1960) 265.
2. Flesch, M.: (1883) Über ein Sporozoon beim Pferde. Zool Anzeiger **6** (1960) 396. Cit. Pols.
3. Kupke, A.: Untersuchungen über *Globidium leuckarti* Flesch. Inaug. Dissertation, Tierärtzliche Hochsch., Berlin. Cit. Pols, 1960.
4. Bennett, S. C. J.: *Globidium* infection in the Sudan. J. Comp. Path. Ther. **46** (1933) 1.
5. Schulz, K. C. A. and Thorburn, J. A.: Globidiosis a cause of dermatitis in the horse. J. So. Afr. Vet. Med. Assn. **26** (1955) 39.
6. Enigk, K.: Zur Kenntnis des *Globidium cameli* and der *Eimeria cameli*. Arch. Protistenk. **83** (1934) 371.
7. Bigalke, R. D. and Naude, T. W.: The diagnostic value of cysts in the scleral conjunctiva in bovine besnoitiosis. J. So. Afr. Vet. Med. Assn. **33** (1962) 21.

NAGANA

Nagana is the name given in South Africa to an acute or chronic infectious disease of domestic animals, characterized by anemia, intermittent fever, and edema. It is caused by one or more of the following trypanosomes: *Trypanosoma congolense, T. brucei, or T. vivax.*[1] They are transmitted in nature by the so-called tsetse flies (*Glossina* spp.), but mechanical transfer of infection by biting flies is possible.

Distribution: For all practical purposes the incidence of nagana is limited to areas in Africa where the vector tsetse flies occur. The Republic of South Africa, where much of the early work was done, has been entirely free of the disease for about 10 years. The campaign to eradicate nagana from Zululand, the last remaining infected territory, by means of aerial spraying with DDT and BHC to eradicate tsetse flies was a model of modern disease control.[2] This territory is now excellent ranch country.

Much of the more recent research concerning nagana has been carried out in Central and East Africa.

Etiology: Horses exhibit considerable resistance to *T. congolense* and *T. vivax* but are highly susceptible to *T. brucei* which is a pleomorphic trypanosome varying from a short, stumpy shape without a flagellum to a longer one with a long, free flagellum. The length varies from 12 to 18 microns. It closely resembles *T. rhodesiense,* one of the causes of sleeping sickness in man, but it is antigenically different.

Transmission: The tsetse flies (*Glossina* spp.) are the most important intermediate hosts. The trypanosomes have a well-documented developmental cycle within their bodies.[3]

Clinical Signs: The incubation period in equine nagana caused by *T. brucei* depends on the degree of exposure to infection. It may be as short as 4 days. Trypanosomes appear in blood smears and progressive weakness with swaying of the hindquarters becomes apparent early. There is marked and increasing reluctance to move at a faster than slow-walking pace.

Intermittent bouts of fever are characteristic and are accompanied by loss of appetite and condition. The animals become hidebound and edema frequently is seen in the dependent parts, notably the scrotum, sheath, and lower abdominal wall. On clinical examination, anemia, a weak rapid pulse, palpitation of the heart, and accelerated respirations become increasingly evident. Icterus may be seen when the liver is damaged. Conjunctivitis and keratitis accompanied by photophobia may, in some cases, become very evident. If untreated, the disease causes heavy mortality.

Diagnosis: The parasites appear in the peripheral blood about the time of the first temperature rise. At times, they are very numerous and between these periods they may be difficult to find. Lymph node smears sometimes are better than blood smears for demonstration of the organisms, but they are not so easily made. The clinical signs and the epizootiology of the disease should prompt examination of blood smears. It has been shown that complement fixation is a good screening test in *T. brucei* infection.[4] Inoculation of laboratory animals also may be done.

Treatment: Although potassium antimony tartrate is a valuable trypanocide in other types of infection it has been shown to be virtually ineffective in the case of *T. brucei.*[5]

The Bayer 205 group of drugs was shown to have a 2-month prophylactic effect. When used in treatment these agents cleared the blood of parasites but there was survival of infection in the cerebrospinal fluid.[6] The dosage used was about 5 Gm. per 1,000 lb. of a 10% solution administered intravenously, coupled with injection of 20 ml. of a 0.1% aqueous solution given intrathecally.

Antimosan was found to be fairly effective in *T. brucei* infection at a dose rate of 3 to 6 Gm. per 300 to 400 kg. given subcutaneously at 3 weekly intervals.[7]

Of the more modern drugs, Antrycide was considered "moderately" effective against this parasite.[8]

Any drug therapy should be supplemented by good nursing care, treatment for anemia, and for liver and kidney damage when indicated.

REFERENCES

1. Henning, M. W.: Diseases of Animals in South Africa. 3rd ed. Central News Agency, Ltd., Johannesburg, 1956.
2. du Toit, R. M.: Trypanosomiasis in Zululand and the control of tsetse flies by chemical means. Onderstepoort J. Vet. Research, 26 (1952) 317.
3. Wenyon, C. M.: Protozoology. William Wood & Co., New York, N. Y., 1926.
4. Robinson, E. M.: Serological investigations into some diseases of domestic animals in South Africa caused by Trypanosomes. 11th & 12th Rep. Dir. Educ. Research, Union of So. Africa (1926) p. 9.
5. Curson, H. H.: Nagana in Zululand. 13th & 14th Rep. Dir. Vet. Educ. Research, Union of So. Africa (1928) p. 309.
6. Findlay, G. M.: Recent Advances in Chemotherapy. 1st ed. Churchill, London, England, 1930.
7. Parkin, B. S.: Antimony therapy in *Trypanosoma brucei* infection of horses. 17th Rep. Dir. Vet. Serv. & An. Husb. (1931) 67-76.
8. Richardson, U. F. and Kendall, S. B.: Veterinary Protozoology. 2nd ed. Edit. Oliver & Boyd, London, England, 1957.

SURRA

Surra is a disease primarily of horses and camels, but also affects other animals such as cattle, elephants, sheep and goats, and, occasionally, dogs. It is caused by *Trypanosoma evansi* and the symptomatology resembles that of most other trypanosomal infections.

Distribution: Surra was first detected and described in India, and is known to occur in most of the Far East, the Middle East, the North African Mediterranean littoral, the islands of Mauritius and Madagascar, and in South and Central America.[1]

Importations of the disease have occurred in the past into Australia and the United States. In both instances the disease was eradicated successfully. The exact distribution of surra has been obscured by the fact that a number of trypanosomes have been given different, locally orientated names, but are morphologically very similar to *T. evansi*. The probability exists that there are some local strain variations which have occurred in the course of time as mutants of the original organism.

Etiology: The disease is caused by the first trypanosome which was shown to be pathogenic to animals, viz. *Trypanosoma evansi*. This flagellated organism closely resembles *T. brucei*, differing mainly in that it is found to be nearly always in the "long" form, with only rare "stumpy" forms, thus being virtually monomorphic. The size is given by Wenyon as 18 to 34 microns long by 1.5 to 2.5 microns wide.[2] It has a subterminal kinetoplast and a well-developed undulating membrane usually with a long, free flagellum.

Transmission: Unlike most African trypanosomes, *T. evansi* is transmitted only by mechanical transfer of infected blood from a diseased or carrier animal to a susceptible one. The major vectors are tabanid biting flies. Others of the genera, Stomoxys, Haematopota and Lyperosia have a similar potential. Mechanical transmission by means of infected surgical instruments also is possible. Other potential vectors which have been mentioned include vampire bats and ticks.

Clinical Signs: The disease in horses, if untreated, is attended by high mortality, death supervening within 1 week to 6 months after parasites are first found in the peripheral blood. The signs are similar to those of most trypanosomal diseases: fever of an intermittent nature, anorexia, and loss of condition progressing (if the animal lives long enough) to emaciation. Edema of the dependent parts and of the serous cavities may become prominent in chronic cases, and intermittent attacks of urticaria are not uncommon. The basic lesions are anemia and liver damage, which are due largely to anoxia. This, in turn, may be responsible for some degree of icterus and for hypoalbuminemia.

Diagnosis: Diagnosis is made from the symptomatology, epizootiology, and the demonstration of parasites in smears of peripheral blood. Complement fixation tests are used. A mercuric chloride test has been described as giving good results.[3]

Treatment: Intravenous injection of sodium or potassium antimony tartrate in repeated doses of 1 Gm. in a 1% solution has been used in the past with a fair degree of success.

Later, the Antrypol-Bayer 205 group of drugs was regarded as of particular value in the treatment of *T. evansi* infection.[3] A single dose of 4 Gm. for a 1,000-lb. horse was found to be curative, but, on occasion, patients thus treated have manifested toxicity.[4]

Otherwise excellent trypanocidal drugs of the phenanthridinium group were found ineffective, but Antrycide, introduced in about 1949, is considered a most efficacious drug. About 1 Gm. is given subcutaneously in a 10% solution.

Suitable nursing and supportive treatment will improve the rate of recovery, as mentioned for nagana.

Sarcocystis

This organism as a general rule does not cause overt disease in horses or the other herbivores infected by it. It is a parasite found mainly in striated muscle, including the myocardium. Its taxonomic position and the validity of species differences described for different animals are by no means settled.

In equine infection the parasite has been named *Sarcocystis bertrami* (Doflein 1901). The "cysts" typical of the condition are microscopic in size (in horses) and are found in the diaphragm and other muscles as elliptical or fusiform bodies lying between muscle fibers. Almost invariably they are detected only by histologic examination.

The "cysts" are separated into membranous compartments which on maturation of the bodies become filled with numerous crescentic or banana-shaped "spores" about 10 to 12 microns long by 4 to 9 microns wide.

Infection is believed to be by ingestion but there is a notable lack of information about the organism's transmission and life history. As the parasite is found mainly in herbivores the ingestion of infected muscle is hardly a likely mechanism.

Murrina

Murrina is a local name for a disease of horses in Panama, caused by *Trypanosoma hippicum,* which is considered either identical to, or a strain variant of, *T. evansi,* which is described in the discussion of surra. The pathogenesis of the disease is for all practical purposes the same as that for surra.

W. D. Malherbe

REFERENCES

1. Richardson, U. F. and Kendall, S. B.: Veterinary Protozoology. 2nd ed. Oliver and Boyd, London, England, 1957.
2. Wenyon, C. M.: Protozoology. William Wood and Co., New York, N. Y., 1926.
3. Bennett, S. C. J.: The control of camel trypanosomiasis. J. Comp. Path. Ther. 46 (1933) 67.
4. Bennett, S. C. J.: Toleration of Naganol (Bayer 205) by horses. J. Comp. Path. Ther. 49 (1936) 304.
5. Davey, D. G.: Trypanocidal drugs with special reference to animal trypanosomiasis. Rept. of 14th Intern. Vet. Congr., London 2, (1949) 25.
6. Curd, F. H. S. and Davey, D. G.: Antrycide, a new trypanocidal drug. Brit. J. Pharm. 5 (1950) 25.

PROTOZOAL DIARRHEA

Occurrence: Protozoal diarrhea is an infectious disease of horses of all ages which is caused by a flagellated protozoan. The condition may vary in nature from a severe, peracute indigestion to a mild, chronic enteritis, or even an asymptomatic state. Yearlings, 2, and 3-year-old horses are the most seriously affected as a rule. A high level of nutrition (mixed sweet feed and alfalfa hay), and stress (as from overexertion or shipping) commonly are associated with the development of the disease.

Treatment with antibiotics (penicillin and dihydrostreptomycin) or use of anthelmintics (phenothiazine and carbon disulfide, or phenothiazine and piperazine) may serve as inciting factors if other factors are suitable for the development of the disease. The effect of the antibiotics and the anthelmintics may be explained by the fact that they both reduce bacteria in the digestive tract which may exist in competition with protozoa.

Poor hygiene and confinement to dirty stalls and lots foster the development and spread of this condition. The mortality rate is high in inadequately treated, acute cases, but it is low in chronically involved individuals.

Etiology: The etiologic agent is a motile flagellated protozoan that appears on direct microscopic examination to be ⅓ to ⅔ the size of a strongyle egg. This organism has been tentatively identified as *Trichomonas fecalis*.[1] The best material for microscopic examination is the fluid which has been expressed from feces collected from the rectum. A simple method of obtaining a fecal sample is directly from the rectum while wearing a plastic glove and then inverting the glove as it is taken off, leaving the feces in the inverted glove. The liquid portion can be expressed easily through a small hole made in one of the fingers of the glove.

The protozoan can often be found in large numbers in early cases even before diarrhea is evident. This organism apparently is destroyed by flotation solutions, tap water, temperature changes, dehydration, etc. It has not been possible to demonstrate it in the feces from all horses examined; however, it has been found in relatively low numbers in feces obtained from asymptomatic horses. It therefore appears that the protozoan's pathogenicity is facultative and dependent upon a number of other factors.

Spread of the infection from one horse to another, as indicated by clinical experience, may be erratic, presumably because of variations in resistance, stress, nutrition, pathogenicity, and other factors.

Clinical Signs: The acute condition is characterized by a temperature of 104 to 108 F., rapid pulse, red (sometimes extremely so) conjunctival and oral mucosas, dryness of the mouth, varying degrees of dehydration, and abdominal pain at the outset with lack of borborygmi. Later there are increased sounds of intestinal liquid as the diarrhea develops. The facial expression may be anxious, and the nostrils slightly flared in severe cases. Sweating and weakness are prominent as the climax is reached in severe cases. Laminitis, varying from mild to extremely severe manifestations, and peripheral edema occur in a portion of cases. The odor from the mouth and from the feces is characteristic.

Chronic syndromes will vary in appearance from those which are nearly asymptomatic to those patients with a severe and protracted diarrhea. The body temperature in these cases is normal, or nearly normal, and the appetite will vary from fair to good. The chronic cases with severe and protracted diarrhea are unique in that, as a rule, after the initial illness (which may go unrecognized by the horseman), the horse is bright and active and has a fair to good appetite even though it scours profusely. If the diarrhea persists, young horses may become stunted and appear to be malnourished or severely parasitized.

Laminitis varying from fairly severe to mild, or even occult, may be the only general sign in some chronic cases. There are asymptomatic carriers, and there are patients which show clinical signs limited to thinness, reduced ability to work, mild anemia, and general unthriftiness. This is true, at least to the extent that the condition of these horses is less than that expected normally of healthy animals under the level of nutrition and husbandry existing. Frequently, the feces are softer than would be expected from horses on dry feed. The excreta will form either in loose balls, or piles like cow manure.

Treatment: Treatment of the infection leaves considerable to be desired, although most acute cases may be saved and chronic cases eventually salvaged. Treatment of acute cases is to a large degree symptomatic and involves the use of intravenous fluids and electrolytes in quantities sufficient to combat the degree of dehydration existing. Erythromycin is given intramuscularly in peracute cases if for no other reason than to combat secondary invaders. Protectives such as kaolin, pectin, and bismuth subnitrate via stomach tube are indicated. Copious quantities of mineral oil, repeated frequently, are of particular value in the treatment of acute cases and seem to have some specific effect on the protozoa. Smooth muscle antispasmodics are of value in relieving pain, and reducing spasms and hyperactivity of the bowel. Belladonna is a choice additive to the kaolin mixtures for this purpose.

Spectacular results may be obtained if treatment is instituted early and is vigorous. Some acute cases may become chronic with remission of the systemic signs and establishment of a protracted diarrhea if therapy is not vigorous, or if the condition is well-established before treatment is started.

Treatment of chronic cases is more difficult than is that of acute cases. Liquamycin (2.5 Gm. terramycin) given once or twice daily via the stomach tube for several days has been successful in controlling the infection on several occasions. The condition of the feces, though improved, has not returned entirely to normal in a number of chronically involved patients so treated. The best management of chronic cases at this time seems to be turning them out in a large pasture and feeding limited amounts of grass hay and oats only as needed. Mineral and vitamin supplementation should be given. Experience has shown that it is more desirable for the pasture to be large rather than good and for the horse to be fed in a different part of the pasture every day so as to reduce the possibility of self-reinfestation.

W. H. WOHLER, JR.

REFERENCE

1. Andujar, John J.: Personal communication. 1961.

CHAPTER 8

METAZOAL DISEASES

INTERNAL PARASITES OF HORSES

INTRODUCTION

The horse harbors a wide variety of parasites. A diversity of genera and species is to be found and the individual parasites are often present in very large numbers. The endoparasites may be differentiated into nematodes, cestodes, trematodes, and insects. It is the nematodes which pose the most serious problem, and consequently it is with this group that this discussion will be largely concerned.

THE NEMATODES

The common nematode parasites of the horse are usually referred to as strongyles. They are, for convenience, divided into 2 groups, the large strongyles (sclerostomes) of the genus *Strongylus* and the small strongyles (cylicostomes). Other nematode parasites commonly found are *Parascaris equorum*, *Oxyuris equi* (the pinworm), and the stomach worms of the genus, *Habronema*. The intestinal threadworm *Strongyloides westeri* is a common parasite of foals. *Thelazia lacrimalis* (the eyeworm) also occurs as does *Dictyocaulus arnfieldi* (the lungworm); however, these species are rare.

THE LARGE STRONGYLES

The large strongyles are recognized as being the most dangerous to the horse. They belong to the genus, *Strongylus*, and comprise 3 species: *S. equinus*, *S. edentatus*, and *S. vulgaris*.

STRONGYLUS VULGARIS

Without doubt the most dangerous parasite of the horse is *Strongylus vulgaris*. The examination of feces from 1,833 horses of various ages showed 1,284 (70%) to be infected (Poynter 1958). The larvae of this worm undergo extensive migrations in the arteries, where their presence provokes a fibrous thickening of the vessel wall culminating in the typical "verminous aneurysm"; cases of coronary thrombosis are also on record.

The adults of *S. vulgaris* live mainly in the cecum of the horse, although some are found in the colon. They are equipped with well-developed buccal capsules into which they draw and erode portions of alimentary mucosa. The adult worms are about one inch in length and although often referred to as red worms, they are in fact usually a slate gray color. They are frequently found attached to the mucosa and they may be plucked away from the mucosal plugs which they hold in their mouths. Pairs of worms are often found. The female lays eggs which are passed through the horse's gut and onto the pasture with its dung. Free living development is essentially similar in all strongyles, the eggs hatching to give first stage larvae which then develop to second and then to the third stage infective larvae; the process takes about 10 days. After ingestion, the infective larvae undergo an ecdysis and penetrate the gut wall. As yet, no general agreement has been reached about the migratory route of the parasite in its host but four different theories have been advanced.

Olt (1932) was interested in the relationship between *S. vulgaris* and certain forms of colic. He thought that the development of an aneurysm of the cranial mesenteric artery was due to erratic larvae. He believed that the normal route taken was from the intestine to the liver via the blood stream, and thence to the heart and lungs, where the larvae entered the air spaces, passing up the trachea and down the esophagus to the secum. The erratic larvae, he believed, penetrated the intestinal wall and wandered between the mesenteric folds until they reached the origin of the mesentery which is around the cranial mesenteric artery. Here they either penetrated the arterial wall and initiated the development of a lesion, or they penetrated into the portal vein and were car-

Table 1.—The Distribution of Lesions in the Arterial System Due to *Strongylus vulgaris* as Found During 43 Postmorten Examinations

SITE OF DAMAGE	NO. OF POSITIVE CASES	PERCENT OF CASES AFFECTED
Arterial system (any region)	40	93.0
Origin of aorta	9	20.9
Celiac axis	12	27.9
Cranial mesenteric artery	37	86.0
Renal arteries	10	23.2
Caudal mesenteric artery	2	4.6

ried to the liver and then to the heart and lungs. Those which entered the cranial mesenteric artery were believed not to be dispersed in the blood stream.

Wetzel and Enigk (1938) did not agree with Olt, for they infected 5 foals with *Strongylus spp.* larvae and failed subsequently to find parasites in the trachea or esophagus. Enigk (1950) later studied the early phases of the migration of *S. vulgaris* by infecting 5 foals, all of which died from "haemorrhagic or anaemic infarction of the small and large intestines." He stated that larvae penetrated the mucous membranes of the cecum and colon and here shed the third cuticle, after which they entered the submucous arterioles and migrated in the intima of the intestinal arteries. No evidence was found of larvae piercing the arterial internal elastic membrane and they were therefore restricted to the intima along which they migrated to the cranial mesenteric artery.

Arterioles have a well-developed internal elastic membrane but as they become smaller this becomes thinner and then disappears. In Enigk's view, larvae could enter only small arterioles lacking the internal elastic membrane.

In a later paper, Enigk (1951) described further experiments on 4 foals in which he observed the subsequent behavior of *S. vulgaris* in the arteries. He believed that larvae could bore from the intima to the lumen of the cranial mesenteric artery and then be carried to the intestinal wall by the blood stream.

In 1941, Ottaway and Bingham reported details of the postmortem examination of 10 ponies, all of which were naturally infected with *S. vulgaris*. In their view, it seemed unlikely that development of the larvae in an aneurysm was usual, and since the larvae were so deeply embedded in the thrombus and arterial wall, and many were almost the size of adult worms, it seemed impossible for them to leave the aneurysm and migrate back to the intestine. However, these authors felt it unwise to draw conclusions concerning the normal route of migration from the material examined in their few cases. In 1941, Ottaway and Bingham were tending, with a reservation, to support Olt's hypothesis. It is interesting, therefore, to note that having dissected an additional 77 horses and carefully examined the arteries, they (1946) produced evidence suggesting that an intra-arterial migration of *S. vulgaris* larvae was part of the normal life cycle of the parasite.

Ershov (1949) also advanced views based on postmortem examinations conducted on adult horses and on foals. He considered that ingested larvae penetrated the mucous membrane of the large intestine and migrated between the muscular and serous layers of this part of the alimentary tract. Further migration then occurred and the larvae moved between the laminae of the mesentery to the cranial mesenteric artery, the wall of which they penetrated, and in the lumen of which, covered by thrombi, they developed until they were eventually carried with the blood stream to the wall of the large intestine. This view differs from that of Enigk concerning the route taken by larvae on their way to the cranial mesenteric artery.

Further thoughts on the migration of *S. vulgaris* were presented by Farrelly (1954) who described lesions of the aorta as far forward as its origin in the region of the semilunar valves. The lesions had the form of thrombi and in many of them *S. vulgaris* was found. To explain the presence of the parasite in such a situation, Farrelly extended Olt's hypothesis. He postulated that larvae did not always leave the circulation in the lung but that some of them continued to the left side of the heart and thus gained entrance to the aorta. They then entered the cranial mesenteric artery, pro-

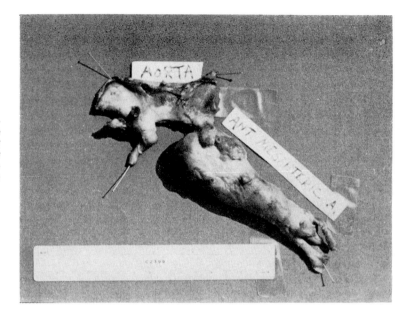

Fig. 1. Verminous aneurysm in a branch of the anterior mesenteric artery showing the bulbous type of swelling produced. Courtesy of J. H. Drudge, D.V.M.

gressed along the cecal arteries and eventually entered the lumen of the alimentary tract.

In a recent paper, Poynter (1960) presented the results obtained in 43 postmortem examinations on horses naturally infected with *Strongylus vulgaris*. A consideration of the incidence and pathogenesis of the lesions led him to support the intra-arterial hypothesis. It was shown that the lesions originated on the endothelium and gradually were incorporated into the intima. In any event, it is certain that the presence of these larval and adult nematodes in the arterial system of the horse produces an extensive endarteritis. Data are available on the incidence of these arterial lesions, and those published by Poynter (1960) who examined 43 cases are shown in Table 1.

There is no doubt that the cranial mesenteric artery is the most commonly affected vessel but other parts of the arterial system also are damaged. In Fig. 1 a typical verminous aneurysm is shown but it also must be realized that the lesion shown in Fig. 2, where a thrombus is present in the aorta, is by no means rare. Thrombi also have been found in the apex of the left ventricle. This complete or partial blockage of arteries produces a variety of signs depending on the individual vessel affected. Fortunately, the dorsal and ventral colic arter-

ies anastomose so that blockage of one does not necessarily produce death. However, occlusions of branches do occur and areas of the colon become deprived of blood, and necrosis and peritonitis result. Cronin and Leader (1952) reported a case of sudden death in a 2-year-old due to coronary thrombosis of parasitic origin.

Migrating larvae often are found in the arteries either free or within the intima (Fig. 3). They may become young adults in this situation.

STRONGYLUS EDENTATUS

Strongylus edentatus lives as an adult in the colon where it sucks mucosal tissue in a similar way to *S. vulgaris*. It may become 1¼″ in length and is a slate gray color. *S. edentatus* is a common parasite. Russell (1948) found it to be present in every one of 26 brood mares she examined in British studs. Poynter (1958), using fecal examinations, demonstrated its presence in 1317 of 1833 horses (71%). *S. edentatus* follows a complicated migratory route. Westzel and Kersten (1956) stated that the third stage larvae burrows into the wall of the gut and reaches the liver via the portal vessels. They form nodules in the liver parenchyma, and undergo the

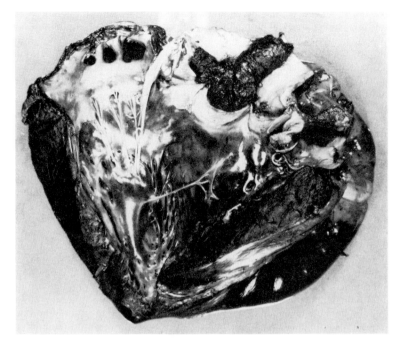

Fig. 2. Thrombus in aorta near its origin at the heart caused by migrating *Strongylus vulgaris* larvae. Courtesy of J. H. Drudge, D.V.M.

third molt. The young, fourth stage larvae wander in the liver parenchyma and increase in size, moving to the hepatic ligaments where they reach the tissues underlying the peritoneal lining of the abdominal cavity. The authors mentioned regard the liver stage as highly pathogenic. Young adults often are present in the parietal peritoneum and they frequently are found in the perinephric connective tissue and fat. Poynter (1957) has observed them penetrating the diaphragm with the anterior part of the worm present in the thorax, and the posterior present in the peritoneal cavity. This finding is, however, unusual. The young adult worms are capable of direct penetration back into the colon (Fig. 4).

STRONGYLUS EQUINUS

This parasite is the type species of its genus, and its name frequently appears in the older literature. However, it is now generally agreed

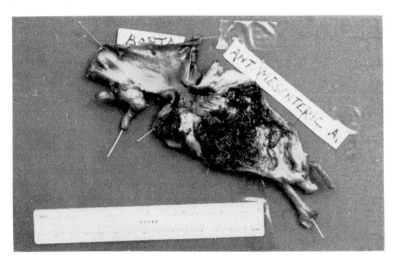

Fig. 3. Verminous aneurysm opened to show the thrombus containing immature *Strongylus vulgaris*. Courtesy of J. H. Drudge, D.V.M.

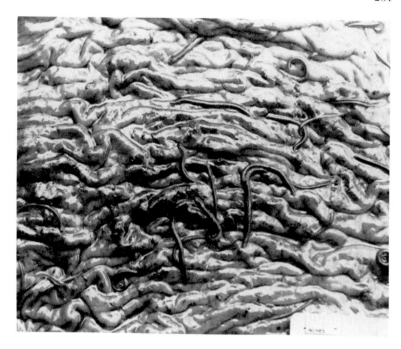

Fig. 4. *Strongylus eden-tatus* adults attached to wall of the ventral colon. Courtesy of J. H. Drudge, D.V.M.

that this is a rare parasite. Poynter (1958), in Great Britain, was able to find it only in 21 of 1833 horses (1%). Drudge (1956) attests to its rarity in Kentucky. Earlier workers often reported the finding of *S. equinus*. The apparent decline in the incidence of the parasite may not, however, be real. It seems likely that the older workers were inclined to call any strongyle nematode found in horses by this name. Since it is rare, it is difficult to judge the effects it has on a horse and little or no direct work has been done with it.

SMALL STRONGYLES

Under this title are included many small nematode parasites of the horse. The most common generally are referred to as members of the genus Trichonema. The genus contains about 40 different species. Other worms included in the group are *Poteriostomum spp.*, *Triodontophorus spp.*, *Gyalocephalus capitatus* and *Oesophagodontus robustus*. The small strongyles, which often are bright red in color, live in the large intestine. Members of the genus Trichonema penetrate as larvae into the mucosa, where they form small cysts. As the larval worm grows, the size of the cyst in-

creases until eventually it ruptures to release a young worm, which then escapes into the intestine. In a heavily infected animal, the encysted worms may be seen as numerous tiny bright red circles in the mucosa of the cecum and colon (Fig. 5). When the larval worms leave their cysts a marked inflammatory response may occur, and the cellular exudate produced is particularly rich in eosinophils. No really critical trial has been performed to show exactly how pathogenic the members of the genus Trichonema are.

As in other parasitic diseases, the relationship between nutrition and parasitism is particularly well-developed. Horses may harbor large quantities of Trichonema without showing any obvious ill effects, providing they are receiving enough to eat. However, considering the damage caused to the large intestine it is apparent that disruption of so much mucosal tissue must have an adverse effect upon the horse.

The genera: Poteriostomum, Gyalocephalus and Triodontophorus are not as common as Trichonema. The pathogenesis of the first 2 is by no means resolved, but *Triodontophorus tenuicollis* has been incriminated as causing large ulcers in the colon.

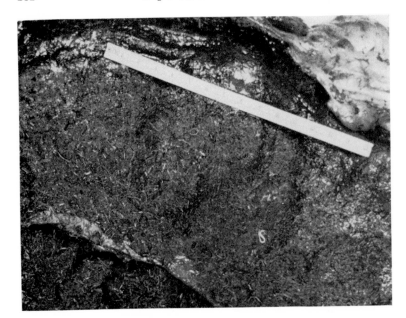

Fig. 5. Mass of small strongyles on mucosa of dorsal colon. Courtesy of J. D. Drudge, D.V.M.

TRICHOSTRONGYLUS AXEI

This is a cosmopolitan parasite that occurs in cattle, sheep, and horses; cross transmission between these animals has been demonstrated. It lives in the stomach and is common in horses when these animals share paddocks with cattle. Mild infections are usually tolerated but heavy infections cause gastritis, and long-standing ones may result in chronic inflammatory changes.

OXYURIS EQUI

Oxyuris equi is a common parasite of horses. Its eggs often are found in fecal examinations but the egg-laying habits of the female worm are sporadic. The eggs are operculated. The worms live in the posterior part of the alimentary tract, and the gravid females move to the anus to deposit their eggs. They also penetrate to the exterior where they may be found as collapsed, dead or dying forms which have voided their ova. The eggs are passed to the pasture and infection is established by ingestion of the embryonated egg.

The worms do not cause any dramatic damage, but their presence around the perineal region of the horse sometimes produces marked irritation causing the animal to rub itself on any convenient object, thereby lacerating its skin, and possibly introducing secondary bacterial invaders. The fourth stage larvae have well-developed buccal capsules with which they bite into the gut mucosa.

PARASCARIS EQUORUM

The large, white roundworm of the horse lives in the small intestine and is usually about 6 to 9″ in length (Fig. 6). It is primarily a parasite of the young foal, and horses quickly develop an immunity to it. Poynter (1958), by fecal examination, found the incidence in foals to be 58.3%, that in yearlings—36.8%, 2-year-olds—20.3%, 3-year-olds—19.8%, and 4-year-olds and upward—10.4%. The adult worm lays eggs at the rate of about 200,000 per day. These are passed on the pasture where they embryonate and become infective. The eggs are particularly resistant to climatic conditions. Infection occurs by ingestion of the infective egg and once in the alimentary tract of the horse, the egg hatches a larva. The larva migrates through the liver and lungs, where it enters the air spaces. It then travels up the trachea and down the esophagus to return to the gut.

Many foals can tolerate ascarids without any obvious ill effects, but if present in large num-

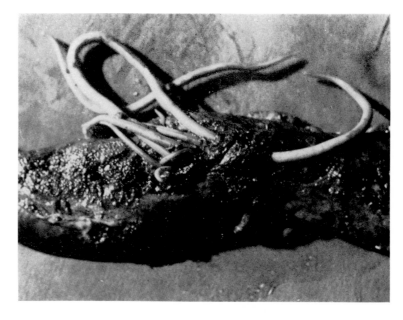

Fig. 6. Section of small intestine showing several *Parascaris equorum* protruding through a perforation located along the mesenteric attachment. Courtesy of J. H. Drudge, D.V.M.

bers they have been known to cause perforation of the small intestine with consequent peritonitis (Fig. 6). The lung migration is said by some workers to cause damage that may result in pneumonia. It has been suggested that nasal discharge in young foals may be related to ascarid migration and in this connection, the presence of viral or bacterial agents may be important.

Miller (1953) regards ascarids to be of considerable pathogenic significance and speaks of infected foals, about 3 to 5 months of age, failing to thrive in spite of good feeding. He mentions that an obvious improvement in condition occurs after treatment.

Strongyloides Westeri

This parasite normally is found in appreciable quantities only in the young foal. Horses develop an immunity to it, and it is not usually seen in older animals. Wetzel (1956) stated that the worm may remain dormant in the mare and commence egg production at the time that the mare gives birth to her foal. The parasite is very small and lives embedded in the mucosa of the small intestine. The small eggs hatch on the pasture to produce larvae which are capable of penetrating the skin.

This parasite is said to be a cause of scouring in infected animals (Davidson 1943 and Collins 1955). However, a survey conducted by Poynter (1958) revealed that only 13 (9½%) of 143 infected animals were scouring, and of 564 foals not showing S. *westeri* eggs in their feces, 18 (3.1%) were scouring. It is, therefore, obvious that there is no simple relationship between natural infections of *Strongyloides westeri* and scouring. The finding of S. *westeri* eggs in the feces of scouring foals may be incidental.

The eggs of the parasite initially are found in the feces at about 1 to 4 weeks of age and reach high figures, up to 24,000 e.p.g. (eggs per gram), during the first 3 months of life after which a sharp drop occurs so that the prevalence rate in yearlings is a mere 0 to 4%.

Thelazia Lacrimalis

This worm lives in the lacrimal duct of the eye. It can produce laceration, keratitis, ulceration of the cornea, and corneal opacities. Reactions of the nictitating membrane, superficially resembling neoplasms, also have been observed. It is a rare worm in Great Britain, but it has been found at Newmarket. Judging from the published accounts it also seems to be rare in the United States. Schebitz (1960) of Germany has recently described a case which displayed a typical parasitic granuloma and circumscribed ulcerations produced by secondary infection.

The worms are seen easily with the naked eye and at present the only logical form of treatment is their removal with forceps, and prior to doing this it is wise to tranquilize or anesthetize the horse. The adult female is viviparous and the larvae are ingested by flies, probably of the genera *Musca* or *Stomoxys*. Within the insect, the larvae develop to the third infective stage. The infective larvae are interesting in that they retain the original egg

DICTYOCAULUS ARNFIELDI

The equine lungworm is very rare in both Great Britain and the U.S.A. It is about 1 to 2″ in length and lives as an adult in the air passages of the lung. Baker and Güralp (1957) recently published an account of a donkey which died with large masses of these worms in its lungs. Lapage (1956) regards the donkey as the usual host and points out that it may serve as a reservoir of infection for horses.

There is no doubt that lungworms can produce a severe, and often fatal, pneumonia in cattle, but fortunately, there does not seem to

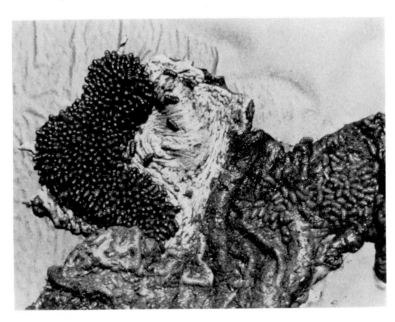

Fig. 7. Typical "clusters" of bots in the stomach. The larger "cluster" is the common bot, *Gasterophilus intestinalis*, and the smaller "cluster" is the throat bot, *G. nasalis*. Courtesy of J. H. Drudge, D.V.M.

membrane as a sheath having a characteristic end swelling.

HABRONEMA SPP.

The horse may be the host to 3 species of *Habronema*. The worms live in intimate association with the gastric mucosa where they may produce a severe gastritis and one species initiates tumor-like abscesses. The eggs rarely are seen in fecal examination since they are not usually detected by normal flotation technics. The parasite is spread by flies of the genera *Musca* or *Stomoxys* which may deposit larvae in skin wounds to produce "summer sores."

be a similar problem in horses. The parasite has a direct life cycle. The eggs are laid in the lungs and passed out via the gut by which time they have hatched to give first stage larvae which develop eventually to the third infective stage. The infective larvae upon ingestion travel in the lymph vessels to the thoracic duct and then to the heart and eventually to the lungs.

GASTEROPHILUS SPP.

The adult fly deposits eggs on the hairs of the horse. The ensuing larvae are ingested and eventually reach the stomach. The most com-

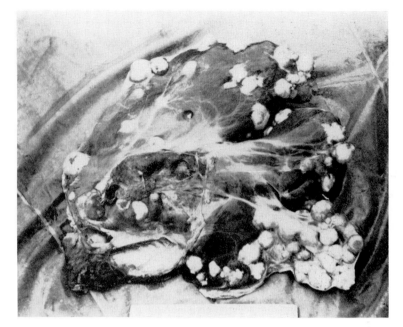

Fig. 8. Hydatid cysts in the liver.

mon species in both America and Great Britain is *G. intestinalis*. Bot larvae have well-developed biting mouth parts, and attach themselves to the mucosa of the stomach where they produce deep pits (Fig. 7). There is no doubt that horses may harbor an appreciable number of these insect larvae in their stomachs without suffering any pronounced ill effects but it is also known that the larvae are capable of perforating the gastric wall and thereby producing peritonitis. Experienced clinicians also speak of a marked improvement in the general condition of horses after treatment for bots. Some even refer to a "bot colic" which also responds to treatment.

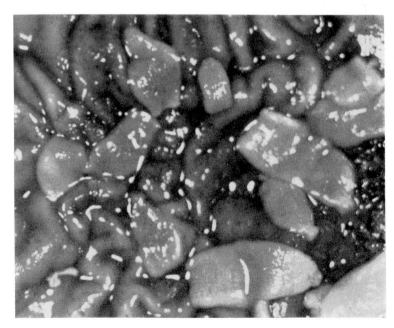

Fig. 9. Portion of cecal wall at ileocecal valve showing a cluster of tapeworms, *Anoplocephala perfoliata*. Courtesy of J. H. Drudge, D.V.M.

The pale yellow larvae of *G. nasalis,* a not uncommon bot, reside near the pyloric junction whereas the red larvae of *G. intestinalis* are found on the mucosa of the cardiac region. *G. haemorrhoidalis* also lives in the stomach but attaches itself to the rectum during its passage to the exterior. Two other species are known—*G. pecorum* and *G. inermis*—but these are comparatively rare in the U.S.A. and Britain.

A case also has been recorded by Drudge, Leland, and Behlow (1956) in which an aberrant larva was recovered from the ovary of a mare. Other aberrant wanderings have been noted and the larva also has been recovered from the brain.

Fasciola Hepatica

The liver fluke does occur in the horse but in Thoroughbred breeding regions it is rare. Diagnosis is made by demonstration of the characteristic fluke eggs in the feces.

Hydatid Disease

The incidence of hydatid disease in the horses of Great Britain is not as low as once supposed. Miller and Poynter (1956) reported a case of a mare having at least 112 cysts in the liver and 15 in the lungs (Fig. 8). This case showed that a horse can tolerate many cysts without any apparent ill effects. However, the danger of feeding the liver or lungs of such horses to dogs cannot be overemphasized since hydatid disease continues to be a serious health hazard to man.

Tapeworms

The most common species of tapeworm in horses in Great Britain and America is *Anoplocephala perfoliata* (Fig. 9). This species is the most dangerous to the horse since it lives at the junction of the ileum and the cecum. Here it produces ulcerative lesions; degeneration of the mucosa occurs and this layer may be covered with a yellow diphtheritic-like membrane. Figure 10 shows a section of small intestine with several large tapeworms (Anoplocephala magna).

Helminthiasis of the Horse

Although some indication of the effects of given parasites on the horse has been mentioned previously, it must be realized that equine helminthiasis is a complex disease. Horses harbor a variety of parasites and the effects of the individual species have not been fully evaluated due to the fact that little direct work has been carried out on them. Indeed, the effects of helminthiasis often are insidious and long term. Archer and Poynter (1957) studied some of these effects with particular reference to blood pictures and weight gains in 2 groups of foals, 1 of which grazed on an infested pasture and received no treatment while the other grazed on clean pasture and was treated regularly. They found that there was an anemia in the untreated group which correlated with the seasonal rise and fall of parasitism. The rate of growth of the parasitized animals, as measured by body weight, showed a reduction of about 30% when compared with the controls.

As in many diseases it is the young growing animal which is more susceptible, but it always must be realized that the source of infection is the older animal.

Although the acquisition of a large intestinal burden of parasites is prejudicial to health, such populations may be removed with anthelmintics. The migrating stages of the parasites are of considerable pathogenic importance, particularly in the case of *Strongylus vulgaris,* and the only way to prevent such damage is to prevent infection. The ideal management of equine helminthiasis is not treatment and control, but efficient control so that treatment is unnecessary.

The Diagnosis of Helminthiasis: The laboratory can help in the diagnosis of helminthiasis by the performance of fecal examinations for enumerating of the eggs or larvae of parasites. The strongyle eggs essentially are similar to one another. Consequently, they cannot be used to determine the species present in a given horse. This may, however, be achieved by hatching the eggs and examining the third stage infective larvae, which can be differ-

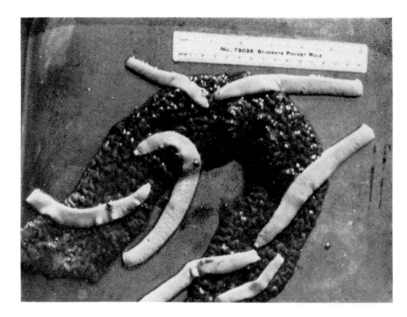

Fig. 10. Portion of small intestine opened to show several large tapeworms, *Anoplocephala magna.* Courtesy of J. H. Drudge, D.V.M.

entiated. The features used in differentiation are based on the original descriptions by Russell (1948). The other eggs are characteristic.

No great significance may be attached to the numbers of oxyurid or tapeworm eggs found. The chances of finding these depend upon whether or not the parasites concerned are reproducing at the time that the fecal sample was obtained. A sample may contain a gravid tapeworm proglottid or even an adult female *Oxyuris equi,* in which case an exaggerated count of the corresponding eggs will occur.

The strongyle egg count is more significant. It is known that a seasonal fluctuation occurs in the numbers of strongyle eggs passed by horses (Poynter 1954). In adult horses, the numbers are high in the summer and low in the winter. No hard and fast criteria may be used and individual low counts are best evaluated on a purely qualitative basis. Any single high count warrants treatment. Counts performed at regular intervals of 2-4 weeks enable one to detect whether or not the parasitism is increasing. Further, it must be realized that the worm population is dynamic, consequently as soon as the adult population is removed by anthelmintics, young strongyles will leave their histotrophic environment, attain the gut, and commence reproduction

(Gibson 1953). The result is a rise in egg count.

In general, counts below 100 e.p.g. are low, those up to 500 e.p.g. are marginal, and those more than 500 e.p.g. are high. Counts much higher are seen, and often adult horses with high counts seem to be in good condition. These obviously have reached a balance with their strongyle burdens, but it is important to realize that it is a delicate balance easily upset, to the detriment of the horse. The only safe procedure is to keep all worm burdens at a minimum. This is true particularly for the younger horses.

The routine culturing of strongyle eggs for species identification is not a step to be undertaken lightly by the busy practicing veterinarian, but it can be useful to have some sort of assessment of the species make-up of a parasitic burden. At present, we have drugs which will kill the vast majority of mature strongyles, but high percentages of S. *vulgaris* larvae in samples having high egg counts give reason to suppose that a high degree of arterial damage has taken place.

Ascarid eggs often are found in the feces of foals and the numbers may be very high, *e.g.,* 20,000 e.p.g. The finding of even 1 egg in a gram of feces indicates that, as yet, the foal or yearling has not become completely resistant to the parasite, and treatment is indicated until such time as ascarid eggs are eliminated from its feces.

Control Procedures: Having briefly reviewed the endoparasites of the horse it is necessary to consider those steps which may be taken to cure, or better to prevent parasitic diseases. The problem falls into two logical steps which are closely linked. First, the horses, and particularly foals, must be so maintained that they stand no chance of building up pathogenic parasitic populations. Second, should this build-up take place, then logical treatment must be given. The anthelmintics at our disposal are of great use in control.

Once a given pasture has been grazed by horses, it will harbor the infective stages passed by those horses. In theory, there are 4 methods by which the nematode burden on a contaminated pasture may be reduced; these include deep plowing and reseeding, not using the pasture for a period, treatment of the pasture by chemical substance, and mixed grazing. Consideration also must be given to harrowing and the manual collection of feces.

Plowing and reseeding are done when it is known that a given pasture has been grazed by horses known to be passing quantities of infective material in their dung. Any group of horses will, provided they are not under careful and consistent anthelmintic control, contaminate the pasture. The recommended procedure is to plow for a depth of at least 9 inches and then to reseed, the theory being that the parasitic eggs and larvae will be buried deeply and fail to survive. It is debatable whether even this drastic treatment is completely effective. Such a step obviously renders a paddock temporarily useless as a pasture, and although worthwhile for parasitic control it is often found to be impractical for other reasons.

Many of the recommendations for control of parasites on equine pastures are made on the basis of similar work conducted on sheep or cattle pastures and though they are probably valid, it must be borne in mind that we are dealing with different nematodes and that, in this case, extrapolation may be misleading. Work at Newmarket has led to the conclusion that if a given paddock is rested during a hot dry summer and for the next winter, it will not be heavily infested with parasitic nematodes. As a general rule, it is advisable for foals to be grazed on clean paddocks, or at least paddocks that have not been used for a season, and not to let them graze on pasture recently utilized by other horses.

There is as yet no known method for controlling the population of infective nematodes in a pasture by chemical means. Much work has been carried out on this aspect of control but no effective, inexpensive chemical has yet been found. It is likely that leads concerning this type of control may come from plant nematologists who are more actively engaged in this matter.

Cattle parasites do not infect horses, and equine parasites do not infect cattle. This fact forms the basis of control by mixed grazing. A pasture which has been used for horses is used subsequently for cattle which ingest and destroy many of the equine infective larvae and ascarid eggs. By employing this method of alternate grazing between cattle and horses, pasture infestations do not reach high figures. There is one parasite, *Trichostrongylus axei* which is unaffected by mixed grazing since it is able to infect both horses and cattle. Fortunately, this worm usually is of no pathogenic significance in horses; therefore, mixed grazing has no drawbacks and is a method to be advocated. It has been used on several Newmarket studs and a case of parasitic gastritis due to *T. axei* has not been diagnosed there yet.

It is well to mention the practice of harrowing. It often is stated that harrowing is a worthwhile part of worm control in that the dung is broken up and spread around the paddock and that nematodes are thereby exposed to adverse climatic effects. Even if this is so, it must be remembered that such a practice will spread infective material over the entire paddock. It is well-known that horses graze in a selective manner. In a paddock occupied by horses for any length of time, it readily is seen that they defecate in certain areas and graze in others. This phenomenon is well-demonstrated at times when pasture growth is at a low level. During several summers, pony mares were noticed scratching around almost barren pasture when only a few yards away were patches of luxuriant growth. On closer examination, it was seen that patches of dung were present in the long grass but that none were present where the ponies were eating. It is known that horses will not graze near their dung but away from it. Harrowing may upset selective feeding. The method is obviously inferior to the manual picking up and disposal of feces, and may in some cases actually be dangerous.

There is one simple step that is of paramount importance in any method of pasture control; this is the manual collection of feces. The dung should be removed from the pasture once or preferably twice a week. This method is rigidly employed on some well-managed studs and it is known to be effective. The strongyle eggs in the dung, under normal conditions, require about 10 days to hatch and develop to third stage infective larvae, so that if the dung is picked up before this time, pasture contamination is prevented.

Consideration has been given already to those steps which may be applied to reduce pasture contamination. Plowing and reseeding are to be recommended but they are too drastic to be employed as a routine procedure. Resting a pasture from late summer to the next spring is a convenient and practical step; allowing cattle to graze after horses so that they act as larval removers is another method of choice, together with the manual collection of feces.

Treatment: So far, consideration has been given to those methods which do not involve the actual administration of anthelmintics to horses but it must be emphasized that it is within the horse that the parasites are concentrated. Any pasture control program involves combating a dispersed population, but by treating the host horses it is possible to kill a concentration of mature worms, and thus prevent their subsequent reproduction.

The anthelmintics commonly used at present to control worms in horses are phenothiazine and piperazine. Critical tests on phenothiazine have been carried out by Habermann, Harwood, and Hunt (1941); Grahame, Sloan, and Morris (1942); Gibson (1950); and Poynter and Hughes (1958). Critical work on the

piperazine compounds was performed by Poynter (1955); Downing, Kingsbury, and Sloan (1955); Gibson (1957); Drudge, Leland, Wyant, Elam, Smith, and Dale (1957); and Campbell and Kingscote (1957). Substantial agreement has been obtained among these workers.

In general, it may be concluded that full therapeutic doses of phenothiazine (30 Gm./1000 lbs. body weight) have no effect on bots nor ascarids. The adult small strongyles are susceptible to about the 90% level but the effect on large strongyles is much less dramatic. In fact, the published figures show that the anthelmintic's efficiency against the large strongyles has gradually decreased and that although Grahame, *et al.* (1942) obtained an 85.9% kill, Gibson (1950) recorded only 31.9% and Poynter and Hughes (1958) 14.4%.

The simple salts of piperazine have no action on bots but are regularly 95-100% active against ascarids. They kill 85-95% of the small strongyles and 50-60% of *Strongylus vulgaris* but have no significant effect on *Strongylus edentatus*. The recommended dosage rate is 10 gm./100 lbs. body weight.

Recent work by Poynter and Hughes (1958) and Drudge (1960) has shown that the administration of a mixture of phenothiazine and piperazine, with both compounds present at full therapeutic levels, gives a much better kill of the large strongyles than that achieved by either anthelmintic alone. This effect is more than a purely additive one and is a case of synergism.

The best way to dose the horse is through the stomach tube. However, horses usually will consume anthelmintics in their feed. Phenothiazine usually is accepted when presented in the grain ration, but some horses must have piperazine salts mixed into a bran mash.

The chief source of infection in the foal is, without doubt, the mare. Mares and foals run together at pasture and even if the pasture is new, it will, unless the parasite population of the mare is controlled, support within a few days a larval level dangerous to foals.

Treatment of the Mare: Mares harbor in their intestines a diversity of nematode species having a tremendous reproductive potential. Egg production increases rapidly during the spring and reaches a peak in the late summer after which a drop occurs, so that egg production is again low throughout the winter. It is obvious that the number of eggs passed in the feces of the mare increases at the time she is running in pasture with her foal. Pasture infestations therefore increase at the time when the young susceptible foals are most in need of protection. It is this circumstance that leads to acute parasitism in the foal.

It is possible for mares to have egg counts as high as 2,000 to 3,000 eggs/gram of feces, and yet show no signs of parasitic disease. Provided the mare is on a high nutritional level, there is little doubt that a large intestinal burden of adult worms can be tolerated. Any treatment the mares receive will provide prophylaxis for the foal, as well as therapy for the mare.

It is important at this stage to realize that there is nothing static about a worm population. It is not merely a matter of removing the intestinal population from the host animals. Anthelmintics have no effect on worms undergoing migration. Gibson (1953) concluded that the development of large numbers of larvae is inhibited in the histotrophic stage, and that they leave the mucous membrane of the cecal wall after the adult worms in the gut lumen have been removed by an anthelmintic. There is then a store of larvae living in the tissues of the adult hosts able to enter the intestinal lumen. Thus, one dose of an anthelmintic will result only in the replacement of an existing gut population by another. Provided that mares are not subject to reinfestation, it follows that repeated anthelmintic treatment gradually will deplete the total number of worms in the body, and such was Gibson's experience in the aged horses he used for his work. As conditions exist today, however, it is likely that reinfection will occur and, consequently, additional controls must be applied.

It is necessary at this point to discuss in some detail the best practical methods which may be applied to insure that the mare is not a menace to the foal.

Full Dose Treatment: About one month prior to the expected date of foaling every mare should receive a full therapeutic dose of phenothiazine and piperazine.

It has been shown by Poynter and Hughes (1958) and Drudge (1960) that such a mixture gives a much better kill of the large strongyles than that achieved by either anthelmintic alone. Piperazine is given at the rate of 10 Gm./100 lb. body weight with a maximum dose of 80 grams, while phenothiazine is administered at the rate of 3 Gm./100 lb. body weight. Thus, a mare of 1,000 lbs. weight should receive 80 Gm. of piperazine plus 30 Gm. of phenothiazine. This combination of anthelmintics will rid a horse of the vast majority of the strongyles and ascarids in the intestinal lumen but it will not affect the histotrophic stages of these worms.

It is good practice to dose the mare again using the same anthelmintics at the same rate 10 days, or so, after the birth of the foal. The mare and her foal soon will be going to pasture and it is at this point that prophylactic treatment becomes necessary. The 2 full doses of the anthelmintic mixture will have considerably reduced the parasitic burden, but no chances must be taken that the mare will pass fertile nematode eggs in her dung.

Low Dose Treatment: Foster and Habermann (1944), Gibson (1945, 1949), Dimock (1949), and Todd, Hansen, Kelley and Wyant (1949) have all studied the effects of small, daily doses of phenothiazine on strongyles of the horse. Hansen, Todd, and Kelley (1949) have demonstrated its safety. If horses are fed 2 Gm. of phenothiazine per day then there is a significant reduction in the number of strongyle eggs passed and there also is a suppression in the fertility of such eggs.

Gibson (1960) recently reported the results of an experiment in which he fed one mare, 1 Gm. of phenothiazine daily, prior to and after she gave birth to a foal. The strongyle egg count of the mare never exceeded 2 e.p.g. and the mare and foal were on a paddock upon which horses had not grazed for several years. Despite this, the foal became infected; at its postmortem when a little more than a year old, 638 *Trichonema spp.* and 9 *S. vulgaris* worms were found. There is no doubt that after acquiring its initial infection the foal itself was responsible for pasture contamination, and its own subsequent reinfection. The experiment illustrated the fact that foals also must be administered low-level phenothiazine.

There have been many variations recommended for the low-level phenothiazine regime. On the assumption that there may be long-term toxic effects, it has been suggested that adult horses should be dosed at the rate of 2 Gm. daily for the first 20 days of any month, and that they should receive no treatment for the remaining 10 or 11 days. However, Hansen, Todd, and Kelley (1949) were unable to observe any pathologic lesions in the liver, heart, lungs, kidneys, and spleen of 4 horses which had received either 0.5, 1.0, 2.0, or 4.0 Gm. of phenothiazine every day for 14 months. Neither were there changes in the erythrocyte counts.

It has been found that 10 Gm. of phenothiazine given once a week have a similar effect in reducing the numbers and fertility of nematode eggs passed in equine dung, but that when given at this rate fertile nematode eggs reappear after about 6 months.

Enough information has been obtained to permit the recommendation of 2 Gm. doses. This regime which has been widely used in the U. S. A. and in Great Britain is satisfactory. Ten grams, or 15 Gm., once a week, also will be effective at least for the period prior to weaning.

Accounts are just beginning to appear which indicate that worms renew their reproduction in the continued presence of low-level phenothiazine administration. Drudge, Wyant, and Elam (1955) studied horses which had been treated for 4 years with small daily doses of phenothiazine and suggested that certain species of small strongyles were relatively refractory to the effects of treatment. Gibson (1960) reported that 1 mare which had daily treatment with 1 Gm. of phenothiazine still showed nematode egg counts of 200 to 400 e.p.g. He regarded this observation as unusual, but a similar case has been seen at Newmarket. It may be that this represents the emergence of equine nematodes resistant to phenothiazine.

It is wise to enlist the services of a laboratory to help with any control program. The feces of horses should be checked periodically to make sure that the control measures are proving effective; any contrary evidence should be dealt with by employing full doses of combined phenothiazine and piperazine along with any pasture changes which may be indicated. Many questions asked by stud managers can be answered only by a knowledge of the nematode picture as reflected by fecal examination.

When discussing the nematode population of the mare it is important to emphasize that any new arrivals to a stud should be isolated before being turned out to pasture. Horses must go to grass only when they have received full doses of the anthelmintic mixture, and when they are on the low-level phenothiazine regime. One horse, with a high egg count, grazing on a pasture for one day can contaminate that pasture and make it unsafe for foals, thus disrupting a control system which may have taken months to attain.

Treatment of the Foal: The foal is born free of worms, but from its first days on pasture it begins to ingest herbage and also its first parasites. These ingested forms undergo their greater or lesser migrations and return to the gut again where they commence egg-laying, and consequently are another source of pasture contamination.

The first worm to reproduce and give rise to eggs in the foal's feces is *Strongyloides westeri*. At about 8 weeks of age the first eggs denoting infection with small strongyles appear in the feces of the foal. Strongyle eggs may be seen before this time but they probably are due (Russell 1948) to the coprophagic habits of the young foal. Should egg production of the parasites within the foal remain unchecked, then a considerable degree of pasture contamination results.

The first ascarid eggs are seen in foals' feces at 9 to 11 weeks of age. The foals become infected by ingesting eggs. The prevalence of this parasite in adult horses is very low and even if mares are given 2 full doses of piperazine, which is known to be 100% efficient against this species, before foaling, their foals still become infected. There is no doubt that the chief source of pasture contamination by this species is the foal itself. Foals probably obtain their initial infection by ingesting eggs put onto the pasture by previous generations of foals or yearlings. The treatment of foals for ascarids serves a dual purpose by eliminating the ascarid population of the small intestine and also preventing pasture contamination.

Ascarids and small strongyles are both susceptible to piperazine and there is no point in treating young foals with a mixture of phenothiazine and piperazine. Piperazine is given at the rate of 10 Gm. per 100 lb. body weight; the first treatment should be given at about 8 weeks of life in order to reduce the ascarid and small strongyle burdens before they become established. Subsequent treatment will, of course, be necessary to eliminate additional worms which arrive; fecal examinations will reveal the need for this. If it is not possible to arrange for such examinations, it is still best to retreat at about 12 weeks of age.

Between the 20th and 25th weeks of life the first of the large strongyles begin to arrive in the gut; consequently, once a foal reaches this age it is necessary to employ a mixture of piperazine and phenothiazine.

It is difficult to prescribe a routine of anthelmintic treatment to suit all foals, since they apparently acquire infections at different rates. As a general guide, it is advisable to treat the animal with piperazine on the 8th, 12th, 16th and 20th week of life. Due to the presence of the large strongyles after the 25th week, any subsequent treatment should be done with the mixture. The first treatment with this mixture is required during the 25th week of life.

There, obviously, is no point in prescribing low-level daily phenothiazine treatment for foals below the age of 8 weeks since it is not until this age that they harbor egg-laying strongyles in their intestines. If the piperazine treatments mentioned before are given, there is no need for low-level phenothiazine administration for the week after each treatment with piperazine. As previously mentioned, Gibson (1960) recently demonstrated that even if the mare were given phenothiazine at the rate of 1 Gm. per day, a strongyle infection still could develop in her foal. It is a wise precaution to supplement the full doses of piperazine recommended at monthly intervals with courses of low-level phenothiazine at the rate of 1 Gm. per day. After a dose of piperazine and phenothiazine there is no need to treat for one week; after this period, low-level phenothiazine should be given daily until the next full dose is given.

Piperazine Salts: There are several piperazine salts on the market. It has been shown (Poynter 1956) that the anthelmintic properties of these compounds depend upon the piperazine content, and that the acid with which they are combined has no effect. Indeed all of the piperazine salts are efficient and suitable for horses. Piperazine has also been coupled with carbon disulfide to form a compound referred to as the piperazine-carbon disulfide complex. In general, the efficacy of the complex against small and large strongyles is comparable to the other piperazine compounds, but Drudge *el al.* (1957) have shown that lower doses, about one-half to two-thirds (piperazine base equivalent) those of other piperazine derivatives, are efficient. The complex also has been mixed with phenothiazine (Drudge 1960) to give results very close to those obtained by mixing the simple piperazine salts with phenothiazine. The chief advantage of the piperazine-carbon disulfide complex is its effect upon bot larvae.

In general, the recommendations made for treatment may include any of the piperazine salts. More work is probably required on the phenothiazine-piperazine mixture to determine whether or not the dose rates may be varied. It already has been demonstrated that the mixture is safe.

Disposal of Dung After Treatment: The proper disposal of manure from stables and yards obviously is an essential part of sound management. Fresh horse manure must never be spread on horse pasture since it will disseminate infective eggs and larvae. The manure must be stored so that it ferments. The heat generated will destroy the infective eggs and larvae. If the manure is stored in open piles, the outer 6 inches of the exposed pile must be turned over every week so that it too is heated. It has been shown that horse manure may be efficiently "sterilized" by keeping it for 2 weeks in closed boxes having double sides and double floors.

As a general rule, horse manure should be used on fields which are to be pastured by other animals, or used for crop production.

It must be remembered that after anthelmintic treatment many worms are likely to be passed in the feces of the horses and that these worms will contain eggs. If phenothiazine is being used, there seems little likelihood that such eggs will produce infective larvae, but the same may not be true with worms passed after piperazine treatment. The 2 anthelmintics act differently. Worms passed after phenothiazine are usually dead, but those passed after piperazine are narcotized and, if collected from the dung quickly, they may be revived and produce fertile eggs. It is therefore possible that a small portion of pasture could become heavily contaminated. This particularly applies to the ascarid whose body may decompose and liberate a quantity of fertile eggs. To what extent this theoretical danger is real is unknown but it does illustrate the importance of proper disposal of dung passed after treatment.

Treatment of Oxyuris equi Infection: Grahame *et al.* (1942) found phenothiazine in 30 to 35 Gm. doses for adult horses ineffective against mature *O. equi*, but 25 to 53.8% effective against the larval forms. Downing, *et al.* (1955) reported that piperazine adipate at 220 mg./kg. was 0.2% effective against larval oxyurids and estimated on the basis of subcritical tests that a similar dose removed 80% or more of the adults. Gibson (1957) also evaluated piperazine adipate at the same rate and recorded, in 2 critical tests, 0 and 28% efficiency against adults and 0.5% and 9% efficiency against the larval forms. Other critical tests have been done using the piperazine-carbon disulfide complex. Drudge, Leland, Wyant *et al.* (1957) using the drug at 75 and 100 mg./ kg., reported 64% and 75% efficiency against adults. At dose levels of 100 to 200 mg./kg. they obtained 0-28% against larvae. Campbell and Kingscote (1957) gave 60 Gm. of the complex followed by 300 ml. of 1:200 hydrochloric acid to a horse weighing 800 lbs. and recovered all of 28 mature *O. equi*. Poynter and Hughes (1958) using a mixture of phenothiazine and piperazine found practically 100% efficiency against both adult and larval stages, but only small numbers of worms were present. It appears, then, that the mixture provides the best form of treatment for infection with this parasite.

Treatment of Fluke Infection: It already has been pointed out that liver flukes do not usually pose a serious problem in horses. Farzalier (1950) reported good results in treating 13 foals with carbon tetrachloride in doses of 9 to 15 ml., the drug being given in 1 ml. capsules. No toxic effects were noticed.

Treatment for Bots: Carbon disulfide still is the most effective treatment for this condition as well as for infection with *Habronema* spp. The dose for foals is 4 to 8 ml. and for older horses 8 to 16 ml. It may be administered through a stomach tube or in gelatin capsules. Care must be taken not to break the capsule in the animal's mouth as the inhalation of the drug may produce anesthesia. Fats or oils should not be given during treatment owing to the danger of absorption of the drug; the administration of a purgative is unnecessary.

The piperazine-carbon disulfide complex has some action on bot larvae in the stomach, but most workers have found the effect to be variable. Drudge, Leland, Wyant, Elam, Smith, and Dale (1957) reported 17 to 100% efficiency against *G. intestinalis* and 63 to 100% against *G. nasalis*, using doses between 75 and 200 mg./kg. The complex is relatively nontoxic and the recommended dose level of 7.5 Gm./ cwt. is stated by Drudge (1961) to remove 80 to 85% of bots on the average.

Treatment for Tapeworms: Only slight infections with tapeworms usually are present and treatment normally is not indicated. Oil of turpentine, areca nut, Kamala, and oleoresin of male fern have been recommended.

Oil of turpentine is given in a dose of 60 ml. in capsules and continued every other day for 5 or 6 doses. The last dose is accompanied by a quart of raw linseed oil.

Freshly ground areca nut at the rate of 30 to 45 Gm. for an adult horse may be given in capsules after fasting the animal for 24 to 36 hours. If no bowel movement occurs after 6 hours, 1 or 2 pints of raw linseed oil are given.

Kamala is given in a 30-Gm. dose after fasting for 24 to 36 hours. A purgative is unnecessary.

Oleoresin of male fern is given in a dose of 10 to 20 Gm. after fasting for 24 hours. This is followed by 1 quart of raw linseed oil.

It must be remembered that the effects of these treatments have not been critically evaluated. Those given here were recommended by Morgan and Hawkins (1953).

D. POYNTER

REFERENCES

Archer, R. K. and Poynter, D. Anaemia and oesinophilia associated with helminthiasis in young horses. J. Comp. Path. 67 (1957) 196-207.

Baker, D. and Guralp, N. Lungworm disease in ponies. A case report of the respiratory worm parasitism in ponies and a donkey. Cornell Vet. 47 (1957) 456-464.

Campbell, D. J. and Kingscote, A. A. In vitro and in vivo tests of piperazine-l-carbodithoic acid as an equine boticide and anthelmintic. J.A.V.M.A. 130 (1957) 533-536.

Collins, S. In opening a discussion on "The Veterinary Surgeon and the New Born Foal," a paper by J. S. M. Cosgrove. Vet. Rec. 67 (1955) 961-969.

Cronin, M. T. and Leader, G. H. Coronary occlusion in a Thoroughbred colt. Vet. Rec. 64 (1952) 355.

Davidson, C. B. Fatal strongyloidosis in a foal. Vet. Rec. 55 (1943) 6.

Dimock, W. W. The two-gram daily dose of phenothiazine for strongylosis of the horse. Vet. Med. 44 (1949) 99-102.

Downing, W., Kingsbury, P. A. and Sloan, J. E. N. Critical tests with piperazine adipate in horses. Vet. Rec. 67 (1955) 641-644.

Drudge, J. H. Personal communication. 1956.

Drudge, J. H. Parasite control. The Blood Horse. 1960.

Drudge, J. H. Parasitic infections in horses. Vet. Scope. 6 (1961) 2-8.

Drudge, J. H., Leland, S. E. and Behlow, R. F. A bot in an equine ovary. J.A.V.M.A. 128 (1956) 72-73.

Drudge, J. H., Leland, S. E., Wyant, Z. N., Elam, G. W., Smith, C. E. and Dale, E. Critical tests with piperazine—carbon disulfide complex (Parvex) against parasites of the horse. Am. J. Vet. Res. 18 (1957) 792-797.

Drudge, J. H., Wyant, Z. N. and Elam, G. W. Continuous phenothiazine therapy for horses. II. A taxonomic study following four years of treatment. Am. J. Vet. Res. 16 (1955) 18-21.

Enigk, K. Zur Entwicklung von Strongylus vulgaris (Nematodes) im Wirstier. Z. Tropenmed, u. Parasit. 2 (1950) 287-306.

Enigk, K. Weitere Untersuchungen zur Biologie von Strongylus vulgaris im Wirstiere. Z. Tropenmed. u. Parasit. 2 (1951) 523-535.

Ershov, V. S. Development of Strongylus vulgaris in the horse. Veterinariya 26 (1949) 26-28 (in Russian).

Farrelly, B. T. The pathogenesis and significance of parasitic endarteritis and thrombosis in the ascending aorta of the horse. Vet. Rec. 66 (1954) 53-61.

Farzalier, T. A. Fascioliasis of horses and its treatment. (in Russian). Veterinariya 27 (1950) 25-26.

Foster, A. D. and Habermann, R. T. Observations on controlling horse strongyles with repeated small doses of phenothiazine. Proc. Helm. Soc. Wash. 11 (1944) 15-17.

Gibson, T. E. The effect of small repeated doses of phenothiazine on strongylid infestation in the horse. Vet. Rec. 57 (1945) 301-303.

Gibson, T. E. Further observations on the effect of small repeated doses of phenothiazine on strongylid infestation in the horse. Vet. Rec. 61 (1949) 451-453.

Gibson, T. E. Critical tests on phenothiazine as an anthelmintic for horses. Vet. Rec. 62 (1950) 341-342.

Gibson, T. E. The effect of repeated anthelmintic treatment with phenothiazine on the fecal egg counts of housed horses, with some observations on the life cycle of Trichonema spp. in the Horse. J. Helminthol. 27 (1953) 29-40.

Gibson, T. E. Critical tests of piperazine adipate as an equine anthelmintic. Brit. Vet. J. 113 (1957) 90-92.

Gibson, T. Some experiences with small daily doses of phenothiazine as a means of control of strongylid worms in the horse. Vet. Rec. 72 (1960) 37-41.

Grahame, T., Sloan, J. E. N. and Morris, P. G. D. Observations on phenothiazine as an anthelmintic in horses with reference to blood examination. Vet. Rec. 54 (1942) 213-214.

Habermann, R. T., Harwood, P. D. and Hunt, W. H. Critical tests with phenothiazine as an anthelmintic in horses. No. Am. Vet. 22 (1941) 85-92.

Hansen, M. F., Todd, A. C. and Kelley, G. W. Continuous phenothiazine therapy for horses. Part II. Haematological studies with a note on postmortem findings. Vet. Med., 44 (1949) 415-418.

Lapage, G. Veterinary Parasitology. Oliver and Boyd, Edinburgh. 1956.

Miller, W. C. The general problem of parasitic infestation in horses. Vet. Rec. 65 (1953) 213-217.

Miller, W. C. and Poynter, D. Hydatid cysts in a Thoroughbred mare. Vet. Rec. 68 (1956) 51-53.

Morgan, B. B. and Hawkins, P. A. "Veterinary Helminthology." Burgess Publishing Company, Minneapolis. 1953.

Olt, A. Das Aneurysma verminosum des Pferdes und seine unbekannten Beziehungen zur Kolik. Dtsch. tierärztl. Wschr. 40 (1932) 326-332.

Ottaway, C. W. and Bingham, M. L. Some records of parasitic aneurysm in clinically affected horses. Vet. Rec. 53 (1941) 275-282, 295-297.

Ottaway, C. W. and Bingham, M. L. Further observations on the incidence of parasitic aneurysm in the horse. Vet. Rec. 58 (1946) 155-159.

Poynter, D. Seasonal fluctuation in the number of Strongyle eggs passed by horses. Vet. Rec. 66 (1954) 74-78.

Poynter, D. Piperazine adipate as an equine anthelmintic. Vet. Rec. 67 (1955) 159-163.

Poynter, D. A comparative assessment of the anthelmintic activity in horses of four piperazine compounds. Vet. Rec. 68 (1956) 291-297.

Poynter, D. Unpublished observation. 1957.

Poynter, D. A study of certain nematode parasites of the horse in Britain. Ph. D. Thesis, University of London. 1958.

Poynter, D. The arterial lesions produced by Strongylus vulgaris and their relationship to the migratory route of the parasite in its host. Res. Vet. Sci. 1 (1960) 205-217.

Poynter, D. and Hughes, D. L. Phenothiazine and piperazine, an efficient anthelmintic mixture for horses. Vet. Rec. 70 (1958) 1183-1188.

Russell, A. F. The development of helminthiasis in Thoroughbred foals. J. Comp. Path. 58 (1948) 102-127.

Schebitz, H. von. Eine durch Thelazia lacrimalis beim Pferd verersachte conjunctivitis ukersa. Dtsch. tierärztl. Wschr. 67 (1960) 564-567.

Todd, A. C., Hansen, M. F., Kelley, G. W. and Wyant, Z. N. Continuous phenothiazine therapy for horses. Part I. Effect on the worm parasite. Vet. Med. 44 (1949) 411-414.

Wetzel, R. Personal communication. 1956.

Wetzel, R. and Enigk, K. Wandern die Larven der Palisadenwürmer (Strongylus spec). der Pferde durch die Lungen? Arch. wiss. prakt. Tierheilk. 73 (1938) 83-93.

Wetzel, R. and Kersten, W. Die leberphase der Entwicklung von Strongylus edentatus. Wien, Tierärztliche Monatsschrift., 11 (1956) 644-673.

EXTERNAL PARASITES OF HORSES

The horse may be injured in several ways by insects and related pests, the principal ones being: 1. Loss of condition caused by blood-sucking activities of mosquitoes, black flies, horseflies, stable flies, lice, and ticks. 2. Invasion of tissue by parasitic stages of screw-worms, horse botflies, and various blow flies. 3. Losses from transmission of diseases and parasites. *Habronema* spp., a roundworm, is transmitted by houseflies. The stable fly has been shown to be capable of carrying anthrax, infectious anemia, and surra.

THE HOUSEFLY, *Musca domestica*

The housefly is often a serious problem around stables as it breeds in manure. A female fly may lay as many as 2,700 eggs in 30 days. The eggs hatch into larvae within 10 to 24 hours. The larvae feed on the material in which they hatch, reaching full growth in 4 to 10 days after hatching. They then crawl to the drier surface of the breeding material and transform to pupae in a pupal case that is barrel-shaped and becomes dark brown. This stage lasts 3 to 6 days in warm weather, or a month or more in cold weather. When the pupal stage is completed, the adult fly emerges.

During the larval stage of the housefly it feeds on manure that may contain eggs of the roundworm parasite of the genus, Habronema, which lives in the stomach of horses. The roundworm eggs hatch in the intestines of fly maggots and live in the bodies of the adult fly. Horses are infected by swallowing infected flies or larvae which escape from the flies. When the worms reach the stomach of the horse, they produce tumors in which they complete their development.

Control: The most effective method of controlling houseflies is by reducing their breeding places through proper disposal of manure and garbage. Manure should be removed daily and spread thinly on fields so that the larvae will be killed. If this is impractical, manure may be stored in covered boxes or pits made of concrete which flies cannot enter.

Sprays and poison baits containing insecticides are effective in further reducing a house-fly population. Since houseflies have developed resistance to DDT and other insecticides, it has been found that chemicals used for control must be changed frequently.

THE STABLE FLY, *Stomoxys calcitrans*

The stable fly, sometimes called "biting housefly," is often noticed resting in sunny locations on the walls of stables in the summer. It is more robust than the housefly, has four dark lines on the thorax, and its abdomen is gray in color with several large, rounded, dark spots resembling a checker board. The piercing beak, or proboscis, is slender and it is held straight out in front of the face.

When horses are attacked by stable flies, they are bitten principally on the legs. If the flies are numerous, the animals get no rest from daylight until dark. They stomp their feet, run, stand in water, and crowd together trying to escape from the pain of the flies' deep piercing bites. In severe exposure an animal may lose 10 to 15% of body weight; joints may become so swollen and stiff from standing in water to avoid the flies that the animal scarcely can walk.

The life cycle and early stages in development are very similar to those of the housefly, the cycle being completed within 2 to 3 weeks. The egg, larval, and pupal stages are spent in straw stacks, wet bedding, and manure.

Control: Prompt removal and disposal of manure and straw will aid in the reduction of stable flies. This material should be scattered thinly at least once a week so that it can dry quickly.

Pyrethrum or allethrin, with added synergistric sprays, will kill all the flies on an animal and leave a residue on the coat which will kill flies alighting on it for several hours. Since stable flies bite mostly on the legs and lower parts of the body it is particularly important that these parts be completely covered by the spray. Thorough spraying of buildings with an insecticide (DDT, chlordane, lindane, or Korlan) which leaves a residual deposit also will help to control stable flies. Contamination of feed and water must be avoided.

HORSEFLY, *Tabanus* SPP., DEERFLY, *Chrysops* SPP., GREEN HEAD, *Chloratabanus* SPP.

Bites of the bloodsucking insects known as horseflies and deerflies are painful and often very troublesome to horses. These insects may transmit anthrax, surra, and other equine diseases.

Many species of horseflies and deerflies abound in marshy areas, pastures, and along streams. The eggs are laid in a compact mass on leaves of grass plants in moist areas, on aquatic plants or on rocks at the edge of streams. Hatching occurs in about a week, the young larvae dropping to the moist ground or edge of the water. After as long as a year, they pupate in the soil from which the adult fly emerges. The adults are strong, fast fliers and may range several miles from their breeding areas.

Treatment: The spraying of animals with allethrin or pyrethrum with an added synergist may give protection for short periods.

BLACKFLIES, MOSQUITOS, SAND FLIES, AND BUFFALO GNATS

These comprise a group of Dipterous insects which may cause considerable injury to horses. At least 8 species of mosquitoes have been shown to be capable of transmitting equine encephalomyelitis. Serious problems occasionally arise among highstrung animals such as race horses, due to the presence of large numbers of pests.

The immature stages of mosquitoes are found in or near water. Elimination of breeding places by drainage or landfill is the ideal method of combating these pests. Application of oil or insecticide-spray to water surfaces is effective in killing larvae or "wigglers." Well-screened stables afford protection of valuable horses against mosquitoes, but sand flies readily pass through ordinary mesh screens.

Control: Residual sprays of 5% DDT, 2% chlordane or 1% lindane on buildings and surrounding vegetation will aid in the reduction of mosquitoes. The annoyance by these pestiferous insects may be reduced by use of insecticide mists or fogs containing allethrin, pyrethrum or lindane sprays applied to the animals.

SCREWWORMS AND BLOWFLIES

In the South, the screwworm, *Callitroga hominivorax*, is a serious pest of livestock since it lives only in the living flesh of wounds of warmblooded animals. An opening in the skin of the animal is necessary for screwworm infestation. As small an opening as a tick bite will provide a starting place.

The female fly cements her eggs in shingled batches of 10 to 400 eggs on the edge or a dry portion of the wound. Once a wound is infested, it seems to become more attractive to the flies. The eggs hatch within 6 to 21 hours and the young larvae invade the wound, feeding close together and forming pockets in the flesh. They feed with the pointed end or head downward and the blunt rear end is exposed for breathing. During the larval stage, the worms shed their skins twice. Wounds infested with screwworms give off a distinctive offensive odor, and they often bleed.

When the larvae are full-grown in 5 to 8 days, they crawl out of the wound, drop to the ground, burrow into the soil, and change to the pupal stage. Adults emerge from the pupal case in 7 to 60 days. An additional 5 to 10 days are required for the female fly to become sexually mature.

Several species of blowflies invade tissue and feed on necrotic debris. Some species deposit small larvae and others place the eggs in a haphazard fashion not securely cemented together. Blowfly larvae are not embedded in live tissue but crawl about on the surface of the wound.

Control: Since the instigation of the federal-state screwworm eradication program in Florida, the Southeastern United States has not had serious outbreaks of screwworms. During this control program, screwworm flies were sterilized in the pupal stages with x-rays or gamma rays. It has been observed that male screwworm flies mated repeatedly, but that females mated only once. If a female mated with a sterilized male, only infertile eggs were laid. The release of millions of sterilized flies in the overwintering area of Florida has led to the eradication of screwworms from this area. Eradication in the Southwestern United

States by this technic has not been attempted, since insects in this area migrate from Mexico.

All wounds should be treated with a smear or spray containing diphenylamine, lindane or ronnel to prevent the invasion of tissue by fly larvae.

Face Fly, *Musca autumnalis*

A new pest, *Musca autumnalis*, commonly called "face fly," made its appearance in the United States recently. It has been reported from the states of Kansas and Nebraska, and as far south as North Carolina. Adult flies closely resemble the housefly; they usually gather in large numbers on the face of animals, especially around the eyes and nose. They suck available liquids and irritate the eyes, causing swelling and lacrimation. The nostrils, mouth, and other moist surfaces also are attractive to them.

Adult flies are found in large number on vegetation, in and around pastures. Eggs are laid on tiny stalks over patches of cow manure. The yellow larvae move into the soil to pupate. Adults are active from early spring to late autumn.

Control: Poisoned baits applied to the head of infested animals have given excellent control. An effective bait consists of a base of 75% corn syrup and 25% water mixed with 0.25% DDVP (dimethyl, dichloro, vinyl phosphate) added as a toxicant. An application of 2 to 4 ml. of the poisoned bait is applied by a paint brush to the forehead. Daily application to the infested animals during periods of heavy population has given the most relief. Provision of shelters in pastures also may be helpful.

Horselice: Biting Louse, *Bovicola equi,* Sucking Louse, *Haematopinus asini*

Infestation by lice is characterized by a dermatitis of variable intensity. The dermatitis is produced by the movement of biting lice on the animal's skin while feeding on epithelial debris and exudate, and by the puncturing of skin by sucking lice to obtain blood and lymph. In an effort to relieve this irritation, the horses rub against posts or other fixed objects. They bite or gnaw at affected areas that may be reached with their mouth. As a consequence large areas on the neck, shoulders, flanks or hips become denuded and the skin becomes susceptible to secondary infections. Infested animals often kick, paw or bite one another and may seriously injure themselves or their caretakers. Young animals which are severely infested usually fail to gain weight and, in severe cases, may lose condition rapidly. The sides of the neck, around the flanks, under the jaws, and the base of the tail are the parts of the body usually most heavily infested, but when numerous, lice may be found over the entire body.

The peak of the lice population occurs in late winter and early spring. With a temperature rise in the spring and loss of the host's heavy hair coat, there is a marked drop in number. Comparatively few lice survive the temperature of midsummer, but with the onset of cool weather the population again builds up gradually.

When an infested animal is introduced into a clean herd the infestation spreads rapidly. Direct contact is the most common method of dispersal, but lice may be transported from one animal to another on blankets, curry combs, brushes, and harnesses. Eggs attached to fallen hair may hatch under favorable conditions and young lice may live off a host for 2 or 3 days. Biting lice may live away from the host for 10 days if kept on hair. Under optimum conditions, it is possible for the premises to remain infested for 25 to 30 days.

The life history of *Bovicola equi*, the biting horselouse, may be summarized as follows: Most of the eggs, or "nits," are cemented close to the body of the animal with the end of the attachment nearest to the skin on the short fine hairs of the submaxillary space and other regions that the horse cannot reach with his lips. Eggs hatch in 5 to 10 days. The newly hatched lice resemble the adults except in size. Like adults, they feed only on particles of hair and flakes of skin. They mature in 21 to 28 days. Full-grown lice are about 1/10 inch long and are chestnut-brown in color except on the abdomen, which is yellowish with dark cross bands. The head is short, blunt, and rounded, forming a semicircle in front of the antennae (Fig. 11).

The entire life and development of the sucking louse is spent on the horse. The eggs are attached to the hair close to the skin. The incubation period is from 11 to 20 days. The young lice crawl to the skin, which they pierce, and commence feeding on blood. Feeding is done at frequent intervals and each feeding produces fresh irritation from the piercing mouth parts. A heavy infestation causes a blood loss that may seriously weaken the animal. The lice become sexually mature in 2 to 4 weeks. The full-grown lice are about 1/8 inch long, grayish to yellowish-brown in color, have a long pointed head, and short legs suited for grasping hair (Fig. 2).

Control: The application of dusting powder or spray containing one of the newer insecticides has been very effective in controlling lice. Such powders as 10% methoxychlor, 1% lindane, and 1% rotenone provide good control in cold weather. Sprays containing DDT, lindane, chlordane, toxaphene, ronnel, and methoxychlor will control both the biting and sucking lice on horses.

The stable should be sprayed with an insecticide to kill lice that have been dislodged. Hair clipped from infested animals should be collected and burned. Care should be taken not to apply sprays and dusts into the eyes, nose, mouth or into the feed of the animals.

TICKS

Several species of ticks attack horses. In the southern and western parts of the United States ticks may become a serious problem by reducing the vitality of the animals through constant irritation and the blood loss during severe infestations.

There are two families of ticks, the Ixodidae, or "hard ticks," and the Argasidae, or "soft ticks." The ixodid ticks are characterized by a dorsal scutum which covers the anterior part of the body of the adult female and immature stages, and the entire body of the adult male. As the body of the male is not capable of much expansion, it can ingest but relatively small amounts of blood. When the female is engorged with blood, the body is greatly distended and becomes ovoid. A blood meal is necessary for growth and it is obtained with

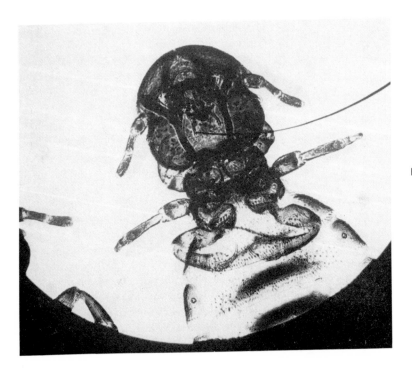

Fig. 11. The biting louse, *Bovicola equi.*

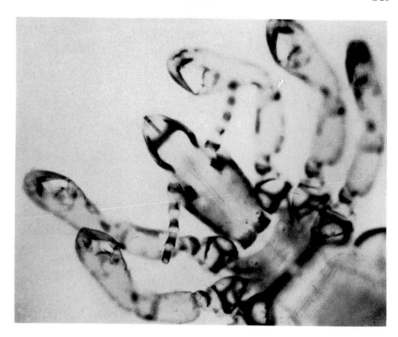

Fig. 12. The sucking louse, *Haematopinus asini.*

a barbed hypostome inserted into the skin. The argasid ticks lack a scutum and have a leathery integument. It is difficult to distinguish between the sexes of this family of ticks. The spinose ear tick is the only argasid which infests horses.

Most of the ixodid ticks mate on the host. After mating, the females continue to feed for about a week, then drop to the ground to lay eggs. If the weather is warm, the eggs hatch in 2 weeks into 6-legged larvae or "seed ticks." The larvae crawl on vegetation and when a suitable host passes, adhere to its body and crawl to a site suitable for attachment. Ticks which feed on one animal as a larva, on another animal as a nymph, and attack a third animal as adults are referred to as 3-host ticks, whether these 3 hosts are the same or different species. A few species of ticks spend all of their parasitic stages on a single individual and are referred to as a 1-host tick.

Ticks having an ornate scutum or one variegated with white or colored markings and short mouth parts belong to the genus, *Dermacentor.* The Rocky Mountain spotted fever tick, *D. venustus,* has been incriminated as a carrier of the western strain of equine encephalomyelitis. It is found in the United States between the Cascade and the Rocky

Mountains. The Pacific coast tick, *D. occidentalis,* is found in Oregon and California. The American dog tick, *D. variabilis,* while essentially a tick of dogs, has been observed on horses in the eastern United States. All of these are 3-host ticks.

A tropical horse tick, *D. nitens,* occurs in the southern tip of the United States, the West Indies, and on the eastern coast of Mexico, and is a serious problem since it invades the ears of animals. Another 1-host tick is the winter tick, *D. albipictus,* of Canada and the northern states from Maine to Oregon. Heavy infestations may result in losses through weakened condition or death.

The genus, *Amblyomma,* has the ornate scutum, long mouth parts and is a 3-host tick. The Lone Star tick, *A. americanum,* is abundant in southern United States. The Gulf Coast tick, *A. maculatum,* occurs from Texas to the Atlantic extending 200 miles inland from the Gulf of Mexico. It often is found attached to the inside of the outer ear.

Ticks belonging to the genus, *Ixodes,* have an inornate scutum, are without eyes and have 3 hosts. The black-legged tick, *I. scapularis,* and the California black-legged tick, *I. pacificus,* are found on horses in the southeastern states and on the Pacific coast (Fig. 13).

The spinose ear tick, *Otobius megnini*, is prevalent on horses in the arid and semiarid sections of the United States. They enter the animals' ears as larvae and attach themselves to the tender skin inside the external canal below the hair line where they feed for a week or two. The larval form molts to form an 8-legged nymph which continues to feed in the ear for 1 to 7 months. Upon completion of their development in the parasitic stage, they drop out of the ear to the ground where they transform into adult ticks. The adults mate, and when egg laying is completed, the female dies.

Horses infested with the spinose ear tick rub and scratch the ears while attempting to dislodge the parasite. The head is shaken and turned from side to side. Difficulty may be experienced in handling infested animals and, particularly, in bridling them. If a spinose ear tick infestation is suspected, the ear should be examined thoroughly. In a light infestation, the ticks may be in the deep folds of the ear, or down the ear canal as far as the tympanic membrane. A probe should be used to clean the ears of wax and debris while animals are restrained. The spiny appearance of the nymphs is diagnostic.

Control: Application of an insecticide as a dust, spray or dip provides effective control of ticks on horses and affords protection against reinfestation for several weeks. Sprays and dips containing 0.5% toxaphene will kill all the ticks on a horse and will reduce reinfestation by 3-host ticks for about 2 weeks and by the 1-host ticks for a month. Combinations containing 0.03% lindane and 0.5% DDT or 0.5% toxaphene give good protection. Sprays and dusts containing malathion and ronnel have proved effective. Infested animal quarters may be treated with dusts or sprays containing DDT or toxaphene.

Sprays containing lindane, DDT, toxaphene or chlordane applied at low pressure into the ear canal have provided excellent control of the spinose ear tick and prevented reinfestation for as long as a month. Hard rubber bulb syringes may be used to apply the medicament into the ear. A preparation containing 5 parts lindane, 10 parts xylene, and 85 parts pine oil may also be applied within the ear canal.

SCABIES (MANGE, ITCH)

Sarcoptes scabiei equi (SARCOPTIC MANGE), *Psoroptes equi* (SCAB MITE) AND *Chorioptes equi* (FOOT MANGE)

Three types of mange occur in horses, but the type caused by *Sarcoptes scabiei equi* is the most troublesome and injurious form. The disease commences with an intense pruritus accompanied by the development of small hairless patches and small cutaneous elevations, usually on the neck, shoulder, and head. In the early stages spread is slow, but later it is fairly rapid and occurs in irregular patches until almost the entire body surface is affected. Small vesicles are formed over and around the burrowing mite and the serous discharge forms small, dry scabs. Constant rubbing increases the size of these areas until large bloodstained scabs are formed. The skin eventually becomes dry, thickened, and wrinkled. Secondary bacterial infections often occur.

The sarcoptic mite burrows into the upper layer of the skin in areas where it is easily penetrated and the hair is thin. When the mites reach the deeper, sensitive layer of the skin, intense irritation and itching result. Mites move from the edge of the lesion to surrounding healthy skin thus spreading the condition. Each female mite may deposit 25 eggs in 2 weeks, which, in turn hatch into 6-legged larval mites that mature in about 2 weeks.

Diagnosis: Because sarcoptic mange is highly contagious, a prompt, accurate diagnosis is necessary. Microscopic examinations of skin scrapings obtained from the edge of fresh, active lesions are made to demonstrate the mite. A scalpel or knife blade may be sterilized by flaming, and after cooling it is dipped into mineral oil to moisten the skin. A fold of the skin, showing lesions, is held between the thumb and forefinger and the crest of the fold is scraped until lymph or serum begins to ooze. Since the mites may be in the deeper layers of the skin, deep scrapings must be made to find them. Several scrapings may be

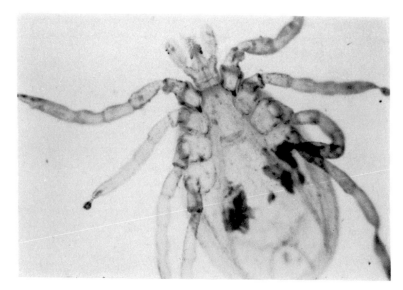

Fig. 13. The black-legged tick, *Ixodes scapularis*.

necessary before a positive diagnosis can be made, particularly when the skin has become dry and leathery.

The skin scrapings in mineral oil are transferred to a glass slide and covered with a coverglass. Examination is made with a microscope, using a low power objective and low illumination.

The mature female measures about 1/50 of an inch long and the male is a little smaller. The body is nearly round and the bluntly rounded head is as broad as it is long. There are four pair of short, thick legs; the fourth pair, and often the third pair, do not extend beyond the margin of the body. A number of short, backward projecting spines may be seen on the upper surface of the body.

Psoroptic mange, caused by *Psoroptes equi*, is more highly contagious among horses than is sarcoptic mange. It usually appears first at the base of the mane, on the head under the foretop, and at the base of the tail, but may start on any part of the body thickly covered with hair. The first noticeable sign is the rubbed or broken appearance of the hair at these sites. There is an eruption of small vesicles and papules that liberates serum which accumulates in the hair and forms crusts and scabs. These remain moist and are unlike the dry scabs found in sarcoptic mange.

As the mites multiply, they make large numbers of wounds in the skin. They live on the surface of the skin and feed on serum and lymph. As the lesions become larger, the mites migrate to the periphery of the lesions. Large areas become denuded of hair and covered with thick crusts or scabs. The skin becomes thickened and wrinkled, itching is intense, and the animal rubs and bites the affected areas.

Diagnosis: Diagnosis of psoroptic mange is made by finding the mite in skin scrapings. Superficial scrapings usually are sufficient as these mites live on the surface of the skin.

Psoroptic mites are larger than sarcoptic mites, the female being about 1/40 of an inch long, with the male slightly smaller. The head is bluntly rounded in front and is as broad as it is long. In contrast to the sarcoptic mite, all four pairs of legs of the psoroptic mite extend beyond the margin of the body.

Chorioptic, or foot mange is caused by *Chorioptes equi*, a mite which resembles the psoroptic mite by living on the surface of the skin and producing similar lesions. The lesions usually are confined to the lower parts of the limb around the foot and fetlock. These mites may spread over the legs above the hock and become established on the thighs and abdomen. The usual site, however, is the hindlegs, particularly the feet.

Infested animals stomp and rub their legs together and often try to bite the affected parts. Due to the licking and rubbing, some of the hair is removed and the skin becomes thickened and hardened.

Treatment: Mange in horses may be controlled by dipping or spraying with a suitable miticide. It is necessary that thorough coverage of the animal be provided for effective control. All horses should be treated at the same time as reinfestation may occur quickly. Two applications at a 2-week interval usually control chorioptic and psoroptic mange. Additional applications may be necessary for sarcoptic mange because of this mite's habit of burrowing into the skin.

Several products with miticidal properties are available for application to horses. They include lime sulfur, nicotine sulfate, and rotenone. Some of the newer, chlorinated hydrocarbon insecticides also are very effective in controlling mange. Benzene hexachloride and lindane have proved very effective, usually with a single application.

E. G. Batte

REFERENCES

Camin, J. H., and Rogoff, W. M., Mites Affecting Domesticated Mammals, Tech. Bull. 10, Agricultural Experiment Station, South Dakota State College, Brookings, 1952.

Dyar, H. G., The Mosquitoes of the United States, Proc. Natl. Museum, Vol. 62, Art. I, pp. 1-119, 1922.

Entomology Research Branch, Agricultural Research Service, U.S.D.A., Leaflet 338, Stable Flies—How to Control Them; Leaflet 386, Mosquitoes—How to Control Them on Your Property; Leaflet 390, The House Fly—How to Control It.

Hearle, Eric, Insects and Allied Parasites Injurious to Livestock and Poultry in Canada, Publication 604, Dominion of Canada, Dept. of Agriculture, 1938.

James, M. T., The Flies That Cause Myiasis in Man, U.S.D.A., Misc. Pub. 631, p. 175, 1947.

Schmidt, H. H., Horse Flies of Arkansas, Univ. of Arkansas, Agricultural Exper. Station, Bull. 332, p. 66, 1936.

Schwartz, B., Innes, M., and Foster, A. O., Parasites and Parasitic Diseases of Horses, U.S.D.A., Circular 148, Rev., 1948.

U.S.D.A., Animal Diseases 1956 Yearbook of Agriculture.

CHAPTER 9

DISEASES OF THE DIGESTIVE SYSTEM

ORAL AND ESOPHAGEAL CONDITIONS

LAMPAS

Lampas is not a disease entity. It is a condition which is more of the stable hand's imagination than of the horse's mouth. Lampas is a common term used in reference to the mucous membrane covering the hard palate and projecting in a prominent ridge immediately behind the upper incisors. Underlying the mucous membrane of the hard palate is a spongy tissue that fills with blood when the horse is feeding. This causes the ridges to become more prominent and helps to retain feed in the mouth. When there is some local irritation as in stomatitis, or during the eruption of the permanent incisor teeth, there may be an increased prominence of the hard palate just posterior to the dental arcade. This condition is the so-called lampas. Treatment should be directed at alleviating the stomatitis or gingivitis rather than resorting to the barbarous and injurious practice of cauterizing the area—which is sometimes done by so-called "horsemen."

R. S. JACKSON

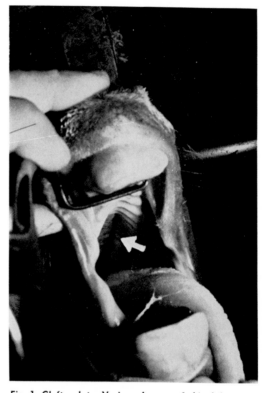

Fig. 1. Cleft palate. Various degrees of this defect may be present.

DYSPHAGIA

The inability to swallow properly is a clinical sign common to diverse etiologic factors. The difficulty may result from pain, mechanical factors, disturbed motor nerve function or brain damage.

Etiology: Difficult swallowing in the newborn may be the result of structural abnormalities such as a cleft palate. Some milk escapes through the nose during the nursing procedure. Infrequently, a foal is born that is unable to nurse. When an attempt is made to drench the foal, it seems unable to swallow the milk. The behavior of the animal is such that a defective mentality is suggested rather than a pharyngeal abnormality (Fig. 1).

Growths in the pharynx do occur but are not common. Necrotic pharyngitis similar to calf diphtheria has been found. It is not clear whether it arises as such, develops after a respiratory infection, or whether some other process has interfered with swallowing ability and allowed accumulations of irritating foodstuff to remain in the pharynx for a period of time.

Inexpert use of balling guns and long-nozzled dose syringes can injure the dorsum of the pharynx. If the animal lunges while the instrument is in the pharynx, actual penetration of the pharyngeal wall may occur. The traumatized area may react with a large edematous swelling or phlegmon.

In eclampsia of mares there may be difficult swallowing. The mare may be observed with the nose submerged in the water pail while showing persistent masticatory action. One of the early responses to calcium gluconate may be the ejection of accumulated saliva and food from the pharynx and mouth.

Strangles is a frequent cause of, at least, partial dysphagia. The mechanical pressure of the swollen adjacent lymph glands is responsible. Dysphagia may be a manifestation of an infectious disease such as rabies or viral encephalomyelitis. It may be associated with intoxications such as moldy corn poisoning and botulism. Difficult swallowing is an infrequent finding in laryngeal hemiplegia caused by granulation tissue formation on the paralyzed vocal cord, or on the epiglottis. The lesion may be seen by use of a laryngoscope. A similar problem has been encountered infrequently following the roaring operation if the cartilage of the vocal cord has been injured. Granulation tissue develops at the injured site and may extend forward.

Fracture of the hyoid bone does occur and presents a difficult diagnostic problem. X-rays are needed for confirmation of this diagnosis.

Poisoning by yellow star thistle may cause paralysis characterized by inability to prehend or swallow food.

In the Midwest, a corncob wedged between the upper arcades of teeth is a common problem.

Clinical Signs: There may be partial or complete inability to swallow. In either case, the common feature is the appearance of variable amounts of food, water, saliva and exudate at the nostrils. Long-standing problems result in inanition, dehydration, and aspiration pneumonia.

When associated with brain damage as in viral encephalomyelitis, the paralysis may not be readily apparent because of the concurrent depression and indifference to food. If fluids or nutrients are to be administered by stomach tube, the normal swallowing reflex is absent as the tube is passed into the pharynx. The tube may be introduced into the esophagus only after tedious manipulation. If the paralysis is complete, passage of the tube is virtually impossible. An audible rattling sound may arise from abnormal accumulations of fluid in the pharynx.

The animal that has been completely unable to swallow for more than a day usually spends more time at the water supply than in efforts to consume food.

Because of the long soft palate, inspection of the pharynx cannot be accomplished through the mouth without the aid of a special instrument. An endoscope may be passed through the mouth or through the nasal passage, but since only small areas can be visualized these instruments require practice for most effective usage.

Treatment: When there is paralysis of the pharynx associated with central nervous damage, the treatment is symptomatic. In viral encephalomyelitis, supportive treatment to maintain the animal's strength eventually may permit return of function. The supportive therapy consists of the intravenous administration of fluids, electrolytes, and nutrients. At times, injectable vitamin preparations are provided.

Polyps in the pharynx frequently are pedunculated and may be removed through the mouth. It is wise to precede this operation by affixing a tracheal tube. Usually, only a small hand can be introduced into the pharynx. A loop of fetatome wire is passed through a metal tube to sever the attachment of pedunculated polyps.

When surgical correction of a pharyngeal problem requires general anesthesia, it must be remembered that any mechanical pneumonia already present makes the animal a poor risk for deep anesthesia.

When the dysphagia is associated with enlarged lymph nodes, a tracheal tube may be quite helpful. Part of the difficulty in swallowing is caused by the extreme dyspnea and inability to cease the struggle for air long enough to swallow food or water.

CHOKE

Definition: Choke generally is regarded as an obstruction within the lumen of the esophagus. The obstruction may be partial or complete. It may occur in a normal esophagus or as a complication of a compressed or otherwise abnormal esophagus. Pharyngeal choke is relatively rare. It may occur in pharyngeal paralysis, or when a foreign body lodges in the pharynx.

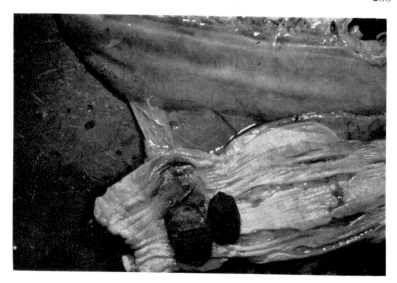

Fig. 2. Bolet in esophagus. Ulceration of the mucosa may occur both anterior and posterior to the obstruction.

Etiology: Traditionally, the majority of equine chokes have been caused by dry grain, especially oats. Older horses with faulty teeth and reduced vitality, or greedy eaters have been considered the most susceptible. In recent years, the rise in popularity of the Shetland pony has created an additional problem. The esophagus of the Shetland appears to be proportionately smaller than in the other equine breeds. A survey of the 47 most recent cases of choke presented at the Iowa State University Veterinary Clinic revealed its occurrence in 39 Shetlands, 4 Quarter Horses, 2 Palominos, 1 Thoroughbred, and 1 Hackney. Shetland colts especially are predisposed. Only 40% of the Shetlands were more than 1 year old. The majority (85%) of the chokes were caused by medicinal bolets. Dihydroxyanthraquinone (Istizen), magnesium hydroxide, anthelmintic and sulfonamide bolets were responsible most often. Foreign bodies reported in this group included several wires, one nail, and a piece of plywood (Fig. 2).

Other causes of choke include esophageal strictures, esophageal diverticula, compression of the esophagus by abscesses, and ulcers of the esophageal mucosa.

Pathogenesis: It is assumed that most food chokes develop accidentally when the esophagus is normal. It is noted, however, that certain individual animals seem especially prone to repeated or periodic chokes. Between attacks, they are asymptomatic and it has been presumed that the choke is due to greedy eating or faulty mastication. Findings at the necropsy of these individuals have been limited largely to those dying of choke, and any primary lesion is difficult to isolate from those developed during the fatal process. There does seem to be reason to suspect, however, that the choke-prone horse frequently has a congenital deformity of the esophagus, a partial stricture or other lesion, or a functional defect.

When bolets or tablets are responsible, a spasm of the esophageal musculature may contribute to the problem. There seems to be no other explanation for the difficulty in dislodging an object that has proceeded some distance down the esophagus by normal processes. Later, a local inflammatory response with associated edema aggravates the situation. The irritating property of the substance varies. Some substances cause little inflammation in several days. Others, particularly those that dissolve within an hour or so, may be sufficiently irritating to cause fatal consequences. Food chokes usually do not cause significant inflammatory reactions within 1 to 2 days. On the other hand, irregularly shaped foreign bodies may puncture or quickly necrose through the esophagus.

When choke has existed for several days other changes occur. The incidence of mechanical pneumonia is high. Ulcers develop in distant areas of the esophageal mucosa and in the gastric mucosa. These lesions are probably the result of dehydration and toxemia.

In previous years of drouth when large numbers of draft horses were wintered on low quality hay containing large amounts of weeds with beards and awns, chokes were herd problems. On postmortem, the dilated esophagus was packed with hay and the mucosa of the pharynx and esophagus was furry with the tiny vegetable fibers. The entire mucosa was devitalized and could be stripped away easily.

Clinical Signs: The early behavior is characterized by considerable distress. The horse may repeatedly arch the neck and draw the chin toward the sternum or alternately extend the head toward the ground. Periodically, the head may be shaken and, occasionally, the animal may travel around the stall in agitation. There may be an anxious facial expression. Saliva may drool from the mouth and appear at the nostrils mixed with food material. Occasional coughing may be precipitated by the accumulations of saliva and food in the pharynx.

After 18 to 36 hours, the agitation may subside. The frequent efforts to swallow disappear and the animal may stand quietly or become depressed. From this point on, the horse spends much time at the water container, frequently sloshing or sipping water which returns from the nose. Generally, the more anterior obstructions reduce the tendency to consume food more promptly than the posterior ones. When the animal is under constant attention, there may be misleading signs which indicate that the animal has recovered. Some food and water definitely are consumed without significant discomfort. Later, the material appears at the nostrils to provide evidence that the situation remains. The material had accumulated only temporarily in the esophagus.

Usually, obstructions in the cervical portion of the esophagus can be palpated. At times, the esophagus anterior to the obstruction is visibly distended with food. An inflammatory swelling or crepitation in the area is evidence of an esophageal perforation, and the prognosis is poor.

Passage of a stomach tube may confirm the diagnosis and locate the obstruction. Firm bolets are easier to identify than irregularly shaped foreign bodies which may allow the tube to slip by. These irregular objects are difficult to differentiate from strictures, diverticula, and esophageal spasms.

When choke has persisted for several days, auscultation of the lungs may reveal the noisy rales of mechanical pneumonia resulting from inspired saliva and food. Signs of dehydration become apparent.

Since many chokes are caused by medicinal preparations, it must be understood that the choke may be superimposed on a primary disease process. Most commonly, there is a history of colic, diarrhea or a respiratory infection that is being treated when the choke occurs. Thus, the signs associated with the choke may be complicated by the presence of those related to the original problem.

Treatment: The nature of the obstruction governs the urgency and selection of treatment. Grain chokes usually are the least serious. The majority recover spontaneously within several hours to 2 days. Conservative treatment usually is sufficient. A stomach tube is passed in an effort to move the mass into the stomach. The koroseal tubes commonly employed are reasonably satisfactory for this purpose. They have sufficient rigidity to apply the amount of pressure that may be employed safely. Often the results are gratifying and the mass is moved into the stomach with complete recovery. Repeated attempts with the tube at hourly intervals may be successful in removing an additional amount of feed each time as the saliva penetrates and softens the mass. After the koroseal tube is warmed by body temperature it becomes increasingly limber. The Cahill tube is more satisfactory for prolonged manipulation. If a reasonable effort is not successful, the procedure should be discontinued and more time permitted to elapse.

Carbachol, pilocarpine or arecoline may be used on the theory that increased salivary secretions assist in softening the mass. Smooth muscle relaxants also have been employed. Because of the frequent spontaneous recoveries with sufficient time, it is difficult to evaluate these treatments.

If this approach is not successful, water may be forced against the mass by use of a stomach tube and pump. The head is tied low to facilitate the escape of the return flow of fluid with less likelihood of aspiration. If these efforts are not successful, it may well be suspected that the choke is secondary to an abnormality of the esophagus. Whenever recovery is not prompt, the intravenous administration of electrolyte solutions is indicated.

Surgical invasion of the esophagus in simple food chokes seldom is necessary. Injection of water into the mass by use of a syringe and hypodermic needle has been reported to be successful although the risk of fistula formation must be considered.

The treatment of chokes caused by solid objects requires different considerations. The prospects for spontaneous recovery are somewhat less. Even if the object is passed after several days, a later stricture formation may develop in the injured area. If conservative treatment is not successful within 2 to 3 days, surgical correction should be considered. If surgery is attempted, the earlier attempts hold greater promise of success than after the esophagus has suffered some degree of necrosis.

In Shetlands, it may be simplest to perform the surgery with the animal under narcosis and lashed to a table. Other breeds require consideration of the temperament of the animal. Usually in the larger breeds it is easiest to perform surgery on the standing animal. A skin incision is made and the esophagus isolated by blunt dissection. At this point, a stomach tube may be passed against the object and a ligature of gauze or umbilical tape placed tightly around the esophagus anterior to the obstruction. Water may be injected under some pressure by means of a stomach pump in an effort to dilate the esophagus and apply pressure to the obstructing object. This is the only practical approach to surgery in thoracic chokes. After the esophagus is isolated an attempt is sometimes made to break up bolets by use of a hypodermic needle, towel clamp, dental pick or thin-bladed knife.

If the esophagus is to be incised, the opening is made only large enough to remove the foreign body. Particular care should be employed to avoid contamination of the esophageal wound. Any organisms included in the suture line greatly increase the risk of a subsequent esophageal fistula. Chromic catgut may be used to close the esophagus with care being taken not to penetrate the mucosa. Two rows of infolding sutures may be used. Additional suturing of the adjacent fascia may be done to ablate the cavity. The skin is sutured separately. If necrosis with bacterial contamination of the peri-esophageal tissue has occurred, it may be wise not to suture the skin since septic material may then follow the muscular planes to and through the thoracic aperture. Following surgery the animal should be placed in a bare stall and given only soft feeds until healing occurs.

At times, the results are completely satisfactory. Unfavorable results may be due to necrosis along the line of sutures with subsequent fistula formation, or there may be proper union of the esophageal incision but gradual formation of a stricture during the following weeks.

Prevention: Horses subject to habitual chokes may be benefited by a controlled diet. Soaked feeds may be helpful. It is surprising, however, that certain individuals show a greater tendency to choke on succulent grass than on dry hay. Possibly the necessity for more complete mastication and better lubrication of the dry roughage with saliva is a factor.

Stones may be placed in the feed boxes of greedy eaters. The purpose is to slow down the intake of feed by requiring them to nibble grain from around the stones.

It must be recognized that the problem in Shetlands is associated with lack of consideration in medication. Oral medication, especially in colts, should not be done with bolets or tablets unless this is unavoidable. A small-sized stomach tube or equine catheter should replace the balling gun whenever possible in medicating these individuals.

Differential Diagnosis: When a horse is encountered which shows inability to swallow and ejects saliva and food from the mouth, other conditions such as esophageal strictures, diverticula, esophageal spasm and pharyngeal abnormalities must be considered. In newborn foals, nursing is followed by a discharge of milk through the nostrils when a cleft palate is present. In strangles, enlarged lymph nodes in the pharyngeal area may interfere with swallowing and cause food, exudate, and saliva to appear at the nose. Pharyngeal paralysis associated with rabies and viral encephalomyelitis must be considered. Intoxications such as leukoencephalomalacia or botulism also may be manifested by dysphagia. Pharyngeal polyps and necrotic pharyngitis are infrequent causes of a similar inability to swallow properly.

Because of the possibility of human exposure to rabies as well as to identify other dysphagias associated with central nervous damage, it may be helpful to observe quietly the behavior of the animal for a time to note evidence of mental disturbance. Cerebral disturbances may not be easily differentiated from the distress associated with simple choke, but evidence of muscle spasms, incoordination, or blindness is significant.

SPASM OF THE ESOPHAGUS

The incidence of this condition is difficult to establish. The diagnosis may be justified by the clinical findings although it usually is a presumptive diagnosis since confirmatory radiologic studies have not been commonly employed. The incidence in the human is significant, and it is possible that a similar phenomenon could exist in the equine species. Postmortem findings of suspected cases do indicate that some primary lesion often is present. The incidence of esophageal spasm as a purely functional disorder is not considered common.

Generally, the diagnosis is made in foals. The nursing procedure is followed by distress and the ejection of milk through the nostrils. A stomach tube may be passed only with difficulty. No specific treatment has been suggested. When a spontaneous recovery seems to occur, the possibility of a mistaken diagnosis must be considered. When the colt first begins to supplement mother's milk with solid feed, there are certain individuals that manifest a similar distress. Eventual recovery seems to be the general rule.

In older animals, the diagnosis sometimes is made when there is a periodic inability to swallow food. A stomach tube may be passed easily at one time but is impossible to pass at another time. Probably, lesions do exist in many of these cases.

DILATION OF THE ESOPHAGUS

This term designates a cylindrical distention, or ectasia, of the esophagus. Generally, it is the result of a narrowing of the lumen at some point in the esophagus with frequent accumulations of foodstuff anterior to the obstruction. At times, the dilation seems to appear spontaneously without evidence of a stricture formation and its etiology is not clear. In such cases, neural dysfunction has been suspected.

The signs usually include frequent attacks of choke. Food may accumulate as an obvious mass in the cervical area. Radiographs outline the distended esophagus. The food accumulations eventually may be passed spontaneously; manipulations with a stomach tube may be of benefit.

Recovery from dilation is not expected. The most that can be accomplished is to adjust management procedures as indicated to reduce the incidence of choke. Softer foods generally are recommended. Usually, if the dilation is severe, even though the animal may survive indefinitely, it is difficult to maintain it in sufficient vitality for usefulness.

DIVERTICULUM OF THE ESOPHAGUS

A diverticulum is a one-sided sacculation caused by the protrusion of the mucous membrane through a defect in the wall of the esophagus. Some appear spontaneously and others develop following choke.

The clinical signs can be puzzling. The animal usually shows signs of choke. It may be possible to relieve the choke but the tendency toward repeated attacks remains. When the stomach tube is passed after the choke has been removed, an obstruction may be noted. At times, the tube will pass into the stomach, and at other times it is arrested at the lesion. To the examiner, this suggests the possibility of esophageal spasm, partial stricture or an irregularly shaped foreign body, as well as a diverticulum. When the lesion is located in the cervical esophagus, it may be possible to identify an accumulation of ingesta by palpation. Radiographs also may be used to confirm the diagnosis.

Treatment holds slight promise of success. It may be possible to control the diet and minimize the incidence of choke. Some individuals choke periodically but spontaneous emptying of the diverticulum occurs and they may remain trouble-free for a surprising period of time. More often the frequency and severity of the choke increase until eventually stricture or fistula formation causes death.

FISTULA OF THE ESOPHAGUS

Definition: Included in this designation are all esophageal defects that allow the escape of saliva or food from the esophagus. The openings may be small puncture wounds that permit the escape of small amounts of fluid into the peri-esophageal tissue or large defects that discharge a considerable flow of food to the outside through an opening in the skin. The openings may be situated in the cervical esophagus or within the thorax.

Etiology: One of the more important causes of fistula is overenergetic attempts to correct choke by use of a probang or stomach tube. This particularly is true if an area of necrosis has developed in the region of the obstruction. Strictures and diverticula can produce a local necrosis that may develop into a fistula. Careless lancing of abscessed lymph nodes also has been responsible. When draining these structures it must be remembered that an enlarged lymph node may displace the esophagus from its normal position.

Clinical Signs: The first evidence of esophageal perforation in the cervical area is the sudden appearance of a phlegmonous swelling in the left jugular furrow. Crepitation may be noted. The enlargement may develop fluctuation and eventually rupture, forming a fistulous tract to the outside. Then as the animal eats and drinks, food and water promptly are expelled through the opening.

At times, septic material that escapes from the esophagus forms a fistulous tract that empties into the thorax without creating an opening through the skin. Such fistulas cause early death.

Treatment: Surgical closure of an esophageal fistula generally is unsuccessful. Since complete asepsis cannot be established in the contaminated area, suture abscesses usually develop which result in necrosis and rupture of the line of sutures. Our attempts to join the esophageal margins over a section of plastic tube have not been successful. Surprisingly enough, some fistulas will heal spontaneously in time. Meanwhile, it is necessary to maintain the animal by providing nutrients and fluid via a stomach tube. Intravenous electrolytes also should be used. If this treatment is successful, the fistula gradually becomes smaller and heals in 10 to 21 days. Raker and Sayers collected the saliva lost from such an individual and included this in the food periodically administered through a stomach tube. As the wound closes there may or may not be stricture formation. If there is no evidence of stricture formation within the first 3 months, it probably will not occur.

STRICTURE OF THE ESOPHAGUS

Definition: Stricture of the esophagus is a narrowing of the lumen, which may affect a narrow band or a considerable length of the structure.

Etiology: Stricture is a common sequel of choke and ordinarily is produced by mechanical or chemical injury to the esophageal wall. At times, the stricture formation appears to be spontaneous although an undetected choke more probably has been responsible.

Monlux describes a peculiarity of the esophagus occasionally found at necropsy. The terminal portion of the esophagus appears to have a thickened muscularis with an accompanying decrease in the size of the lumen. The affected musculature becomes light-colored. Although this sometimes is seen in young horses it is more common in older individuals. It may be associated with an animal suffering from habitual choke, although at times the change definitely is without any history of a choke problem.

In two instances, emaciated horses were presented to our clinic with evidence of an esophageal obstruction. Both were moribund on arrival and during necropsy it was found that nearly the entire length of the cervical esophagus had slipped into the trachea through a natural defect in the tracheal rings. It was not clear whether the trachea was congenitally defective or whether inanition and loss of tone in the trachealis muscle, which stretches across the dorsal free ends of the annular cartilages, allowed the condition to develop.

Clinical Signs: Commonly, the animal shows signs of choke. The esophagus anterior to the stricture may be dilated and filled with food. If the food can be removed it is found that only the small-sized stomach tubes can be passed. If the stricture is in the cervical esophagus, barium sulfate may be administered for x-ray confirmation.

Depending upon the degree of stricture, repeated chokes may be expected. Certain individuals may remain trouble-free on a carefully controlled ration but immediately choke when fed bulky feed.

Treatment: Surgical treatment of strictures generally is unrewarding. When efforts have been made to isolate the affected portion of the esophagus and remove the connective tissue responsible for the stricture, it may be found that little of the normal esophagus remains. Surgery also may result in accidental invasion of the lumen or sufficient trauma to aggravate the stricture. In one such attempt by the authors, a stricture in the cervical esophagus finally was relieved sufficiently to pass a stomach tube, only to discover a second stricture in the thoracic esophagus.

Efforts have been made to dilate the stricture by stretching it with various sized stomach tubes and by inflating balloon-like attachments in the area. Neither approach was successful.

B. W. KINGREY
R. L. LUNDVALL

REFERENCES

Covault, C. H., Ames, Iowa. Personal communication.
Monlux, W. S., Ames, Iowa. Personal communication.
Raker, Charles W., and Sayers, Allen. Esophageal Rupture in a Standardbred Mare, J.A.V.M.A., **133** (October, 1958) pp. 371-373.
Lundvall, R. L. and Kingrey, B. W. Choke in Shetland Ponies Caused by Boluses, J.A.V.M.A. **133** (1958) 75-76.

GASTRIC DILATION

In general, the differential diagnosis between diseases of the stomach and diseases of the intestines of the horse is difficult due to the relatively small size of the stomach, its dorsal location, and the heavy abdominal musculature. The size, shape, and location of the stomach vary with the stage of digestion. The normally distended stomach of the horse after feeding lies in contact with the abdominal wall dorsally and the middle or lower third of the abdomen ventrally.[1] The long axis generally is inclined anteroventrally with the dorsal half of the anterior surface following the contour of the diaphragm. The diameter of the stomach depends on the amount of ingesta contained but usually is considered to be less than half of its length. When dilation of the stomach occurs, most of the expansion first takes place in the diameter of the organ. At this time the stomach appears globular. In the later stages of gastric dilation, expansion also occurs in length.

Etiology: Acute gastric dilation may be due to impaction, flatulence, or excessive consumption of water. The most common cause of gastric impaction is overloading it with grain when there is unrestricted access to a grain supply. Ground grains which are easily packed into a doughy mass, such as cornmeal, buckwheat, wheat, rye, and barley, especially predispose the horse to gastric impaction. Sudden changes in feed, though normal in amount, and failure to reduce the grain ration during idle periods also are factors contributing to dilation of the stomach. In addition, impaction with dilation may occur following pyloric obstruction due either to compression by a neoplastic mass or stricture of the pylorus.

Gastric dilation due to flatulence commonly follows the ingestion of succulent, easily fermentable feeds which are high in moisture content, such as oats, corn, and legumes. A more chronic type of gastric flatulence is associated with "cribbing" during which large quantities of air are swallowed.

Ingestion of excessive amounts of water, especially when the horse is still hot from work, also may cause temporary gastric dilation since motility of the intestinal tract is decreased as a consequence. Cold water also may result in pyloric spasms, thereby inhibiting the passage of water into the duodenum.

Pathogenesis: In most species, gastric dilation stimulates emesis. Because vomiting is difficult for the horse a different sequence of events occurs. Upon dilation, gastric motility is increased and strong peristaltic waves pass toward the duodenum. The peristalic action is accompanied by signs of severe pain. Dehydration tends to develop due to increase in gastric secretions and loss of body fluids through emesis and diarrhea. Increased osmotic pressure of the gastric contents aggravates the dehydration and dilation. In the early stages of the syndrome there is depression of both cardiac and respiratory functions. As toxic products develop within the stomach, however, and are absorbed into the general circulation from the devitalized gastric mucosa, cardiac and respiratory rates are increased. Laminitis is commonly associated with gastric dilation due to absorption of these toxins.

When emesis does occur in the horse, the stomach is subjected to severe pressure by strong contractions of the abdominal muscles coupled with the fact that gastric contents are not easily forced into the esophagus. Under these conditions, the possibility of gastric rupture is enhanced. Since the epiglottis of the horse lies dorsal to the extensive soft palate, vomitus usually is directed into the nasal cavity and makes its appearance at the external nares.

Clinical Signs: In acute gastric dilation, the onset of signs usually occurs 4 to 6 hours after development of the inciting cause, but it may be shorter, especially if water is given after feeding the animal. The condition may last as long as 4 days before frequently terminating in death. The affected animal exhibits depression, excessive sweating, and an anxious appearance. Initially, the temperature is normal and the pulse and respiration rates are slightly depressed. As the condition progresses, however, the temperature will range from 100.5 to 103.5 F. and becomes subnormal immediately before death. The pulse rate is rapid and the beat becomes progressively weaker until nearly imperceptible while breathing is shallow and rapid. The mucous membranes are

congested and appear reddish-blue in color, referred to as a "muddy" appearance.

The "sitting dog" position is very commonly assumed in cases of gastric dilation. The animal will sit on its haunches with forward extension of its front legs. This position tends to take some pressure off the diaphragm, thereby facilitating breathing. The animal is hesitant to move and, when forced, moves in a stiff, painful manner.

Emesis, retching, and eructation are all characteristic of gastric dilation. When emesis occurs, the vomitus is sour-smelling, red-tinged, and frothy in appearance. Small amounts of food particles adhering to the surface of the external nares are evidence of vomiting. Inhalation of vomitus may cause gangrenous pneumonia.

Retching movements are characterized by labored breathing, tenesmus, an intermittent, anterior motion of the epiglottis, and arching of the neck. Frequently, these motions are followed by eructation.

If rupture of the stomach has occurred, vomiting ceases and the animal stands quietly. Care must be taken to avoid making a favorable prognosis at this point. The animal will develop a cold sweat, tremors, a subnormal temperature, and severely congested mucous membranes. The pulse becomes very weak and has a rate of more than 120 per minute. The intestines become flaccid, and peristaltic waves are absent.

During rectal examination, the most reliable finding indicative of a dilated stomach is displacement of the spleen. In gastric dilation the spleen is displaced medially and caudally within the abdominal cavity. In severe cases its sharp, firm edge may be found in the middle of the pelvic inlet. The stomach itself may be palpated near the mesenteric root in small horses. Cases in which the stomach has ruptured present 2 characteristic signs: 1. The serosal surfaces of the intestines and other abdominal organs are roughened due to the presence of ingesta, and 2, the intestines are very flaccid due to complete absence of peristalsis.

Due to dehydration, there is a corresponding increase in the hematocrit and hemoglobin values. Evidence of shock may be seen in severe cases.[2] This syndrome is accompanied by hyperglycemia, glucosuria, and a rise of the blood urea nitrogen value.

If emesis occurs, the pH of the vomitus should be evaluated. If the ingesta has entered the stomach by reverse peristalsis, the pH usually is alkaline whereas it is acid when it comes directly from the stomach.

Diagnosis: The accurate diagnosis of acute gastric dilation hinges on a careful study of the history, clinical signs, and physical findings. An attack of colic occurring shortly after excessive amounts of food are ingested is indicative of gastric dilation. The "sitting dog" position also is quite characteristic of gastric dilation as are the signs of vomiting, eructation, and retching. Varying degrees of abdominal distention may be present. Rectal examination may be helpful in confirming the diagnosis.

Lesions: At the necropsy of a horse which has died from gastric dilation the stomach is found to be 2 to 3 times above normal in size. When dilation is due to engorgement, the stomach will contain a doughy mass of food possessing an acidic odor and a variable amount of foul-smelling gas. Petechial hemorrhages may be present in the gastric mucosa.

When gastric rupture has occurred it may be necessary to determine whether or not the rupture took place before or after death. In the case of antemortem rupture, the tear always is located along the greater curvature of the stomach. Hemorrhage is found along the edges of the tear, and ingesta mixed with blood is found throughout the abdominal cavity. Peritonitis usually is evident, but is in the early stages as death ensues shortly after rupture. When rupture has occurred post mortem, hemorrhage is limited, peritonitis is absent, and the tear may be present at any point of the stomach.

Prognosis: The prognosis in gastric dilation always is unfavorable and the owner should be informed that the animal may succumb to the condition. In spite of a good response to treatment, a favorable prognosis should not be given until at least 4 days have elapsed. It must be remembered that when rupture of the stomach occurs there appears to be an initial improvement in condition which may lead to an erroneous prognosis.

Treatment: Treatment is directed primarily toward relief of the dilation, correction of dehydration, and evacuation of ingesta. The animal should be kept walking to avoid its rolling and causing torsion of the intestines and damage to himself. If the animal is unable to rise, a large, well-bedded box stall should be provided.

When the horse is violent it is wise to sedate it immediately. Promazine hydrochloride administered intravenously at a rate of 0.4 mg. per pound usually will control the animal. Chloral hydrate also is of benefit and can be given at a rate of 30 to 40 Gm. per 1,000 lb. by means of a stomach tube, or to the desired effect intravenously. This drug has the added advantage of being an antiferment when given orally.

Passage of a stomach tube usually will provide relief when flatulence is marked or when the ingesta is still soft enough in consistency to permit siphoning of the stomach contents. In cases of engorgement in which the ingesta is firm and dry, passing the stomach tube does not provide much relief. It has been recommended that gastric lavage be performed.[2] However, this technic frequently is unsuccessful since the ingesta is too thick to return through the tube. Water should be administered in order to soften the ingesta and thereby facilitate its removal. Mineral oil also will aid in evacuation of ingesta from the stomach. The amount of water and mineral oil required will vary depending on the severity of dilation and the size of the horse. However, one gallon of water followed by one gallon of mineral oil usually is considered safe for the adult horse. The water may be repeated every hour. A saline cathartic, such as magnesium sulfate, also may be given in the water.

Carminatives such as capsicum and turpentine may be of some value in preventing further accumulation of gas when the animal is flatulent.

Fluid therapy should be instituted in cases of severe dehydration. Depending on the need, from 20 to 30 ml. of 5% dextrose per pound of body weight usually will restore the body fluid level.

The use of parasympathomimetic drugs, such as eserine salicylate, is definitely contraindicated since they may contribute to intestinal spasm and rupture of the stomach.

To avoid laminitis, antihistamines and cortisone combined with antibiotics are indicated.

Prevention: Sound animal husbandry and good feeding practices are the most important factors in prevention of acute gastric dilation. The feeding of unlimited amounts of grain, easily packed grains, and highly fermentable feeds must be avoided. In addition, abrupt changes in the type of feed should be avoided. It also is important that animals not be exercised shortly after feeding. Proper cooling after exercise likewise is necessary before the animal is allowed unlimited amounts of water.

R. C. HERSCHLER
H. E. AMSTUTZ

REFERENCES

1. Dyce, K. M.: Observations upon the gastro-intestinal tract of living foal. Brit. Vet. J. 116 (1960) 241-246.
2. Blood, D. C. and Henderson, J. A.: Veterinary Medicine. Williams and Wilkins Co., Baltimore 2, Md. 1960.

ENTERITIS

Occurrence: Enteritis refers to inflammation of the intestinal tract. It occurs commonly in the horse and is revealed in the living animal by diarrhea. Enteritis usually is accompanied by gastritis and frequently occurs secondary to infectious diseases. Since specific disease conditions which produce intestinal inflammation are discussed in other chapters, in this discussion major emphasis will be placed on feeding and management. Feeding and management errors, or other stresses, usually precede attacks of primary enteritis. Enteritis occurs in horses of all ages, but the very young and the very old are most seriously affected.

Etiology: The causes are many and varied. The foal is highly susceptible to bacterial, protozoan, mycotic, and possibly viral infections which produce intestinal inflammation. A very young foal allowed unlimited exercise after close confinement may be stressed sufficiently by compulsive running to produce a severe diarrhea.

Foal diarrhea is expected by many caretakers at approximately the ninth day of age when the mare exhibits estrus for the first time following parturition. At this time the mare often is removed from the foal for breeding, and the foal becomes unduly excited. When the mare is returned the foal rapidly engorges on the large amount of milk that has accumulated in her udder and diarrhea results. In addition to this factor, the composition of the milk may be changed at estrus and the foal is likely to ingest secretions from the mare's reproductive tract which soil the udder and teats.

Coprophagy is observed in young foals, particularly in those receiving an inadequate supply of milk, and this may be a cause of enteritis.

Intestinal parasites become a problem at a very early age and continue to plague the horse for the remainder of its life. Many cases of enteritis in horses of all ages are produced by intestinal parasites.

The quantity of feed, quality of feed, and regularity of feeding are factors in the maintenence of intestinal health from the foal's first mouthful of milk to the old horse's last mouthful of hay. The horse's digestive tract poorly tolerates moldy, frozen, or otherwise damaged feeds. The ingestion of toxic materials such as poisonous plants or nitrate fertilizers spilled in the pasture will produce enteritis.

Poor dentition which results in incomplete mastication is a potential cause of enteritis as long as the horse eats solid feed. Incomplete mastication occurs in the young horse as a result of tooth eruption and retention of caps while the major dental problems in the aged horse are enamel points, decay, overgrowth, excessive wear, and tooth loss.

Clinical Signs: The signs of enteritis are extremely variable as to severity and duration. A very young, weak foal may die from enteritis in a few hours but a mature, vigorous animal may be only mildly affected and simply have more fluid bowel movements for several days.

Diarrhea is the most constant and prominent sign of enteritis. Nearly all affected animals have a degree of diarrhea, and examination of their tails and rear parts usually reveals the evidence. The feces vary from a thin, watery fluid to a heavy "batter-like" material that has not been formed into balls. The color of the eliminations ranges from white to black.

Strands of mucus, sloughed intestinal mucosa, and blood may be included in the stool.

Affected animals exhibit evidence of pain but it usually is not as violent as that seen in intestinal obstruction. They switch their tails from side to side, draw their rear limbs up to the ventral abdominal wall, and peer anxiously at their rear flanks. Occasionally, a severely affected animal may roll and exhibit acute colicky pains. Auscultation of the abdomen reveals hypermotility of the intestines.

The appetite for solid food may be very good or totally absent dependent on the severity of the case and location of the lesions, but nearly all affected animals have an increased thirst. Dehydration usually is evident with the more severely affected animals becoming gaunt and presenting a rough, unkempt appearance. When the skin is grasped along the lateral surface of the neck and abducted, it returns very slowly to its former position. The eyes recede into the sockets as the periorbital fat is absorbed. As the condition progresses the animal becomes depressed, weak, comatose, and eventually death overtakes it.

Lesions: The intestinal lumen usually contains a thin watery fluid and an excessive amount of gas in primary enteritis. The mucosa exhibits various degrees of inflammatory changes. The lesions found in secondary enteritis are those of the primary disease.

Diagnosis: A more fluid stool is good presumptive evidence of enteritis, but it must be remembered that intense excitement may produce a temporary diarrhea without affecting appreciably the health of the intestinal wall.

Treatment: Although symptomatic treatment is necessary in some cases, every effort should be made to discover the specific cause before any treatment is attempted.

A complete history, survey of the environment, thorough physical examination, and indicated laboratory procedures often will identify the cause of enteritis. It is important to identify the cause since treatment of enteritis caused by ascarids differs widely from that caused by influenza virus. Once the cause is identified, every effort should be made to remove it. Faulty dentition should be corrected, and parasites should be removed. Stresses such as a vigorous training program for a young harness horse should be removed, or at least minimized to a practical degree. Treatment of specific diseases which include diarrhea as one of the signs is discussed in other sections of this book.

Often, the correction of feeding and management errors is all that is required to control primary enteritis. In the case of a young foal, frequent milking of a heavy producing mare and/or decreasing her feed which in turn will depress milk production, may produce a cure. In another case, prompt removal of the mare's feces from the stall or muzzling of the foal to prevent coprophagy may solve the problem. Severe or long-standing diarrhea often requires fluid therapy. Intravenous administration of approximately 1000 ml. of blood, 2.5% dextrose in Ringer's solution, or other fluids to replace lost fluids and electrolytes is indicated for the acutely ill foal. It is not necessary to determine the compatability of the first blood transfusion unless hemolytic icterus is suspected. Gram-negative and broad spectrum antibiotics administered orally and intramuscularly have produced dramatic recoveries in some foals. The specific antibiotic administered is determined by fecal culture and antibiotic sensitivity testing.

Intestinal protectants and astringents are recommended for horses of all ages. In general, the total quantity of feed and the relative amount of concentrate are reduced. If legume hay has been fed, timothy or grass hay is supplied. The horse suffering from enteritis usually is denied access to succulent pasture. Parasympatholytic drugs are of value in slowing intestinal motility where this is deemed advisable. If an excessive amount of water is consumed, the water supply should be limited and fortified with electrolytes. In some cases involving older horses, complete fasting for a week or more and intravenous feeding have been successful. Following complete fasting, the horse must be returned to full feed very slowly.

Prevention: Most enteritis can be prevented by proper feeding and management. A horse should receive a constant amount of good quality feed at regular intervals. Care should be taken that toxic substances are not ingested, and the teeth should be given proper attention to allow for satisfactory mastication. If prevention of enteritis is to be successful, enteric parasites must be controlled and infectious diseases prevented.

PERITONITIS

Peritonitis refers to inflammation of the peritoneum. This condition usually occurs secondarily to a wound or is associated with some primary disease. In the past, fear of fatal peritonitis discouraged veterinarians from attempting abdominal surgery on horses. More recently through the use of improved anesthetics, aseptic procedures, and antibiotics, equine practitioners have become convinced that their patients can and do withstand abdominal surgery.

Etiology: Penetration of the abdominal wall and peritoneum is presently the most frequent cause of peritonitis. Both accidental and intentional penetration may occur.

Accidental penetration is seen most frequently in hunters and jumpers which become impaled on fences or other barriers which they fail to clear when jumping. Harness horses become impaled on broken sulky shafts or on damaged fences in race track accidents. The abdomens of rodeo horses and cow ponies occasionally are perforated by the sharp horns of belligerent bovines. High-strung and fear-crazed animals of all classes are subject to self-inflicted abdominal perforation in the stable, at pasture, or at work.

Notwithstanding the previously mentioned improvements in the practice of abdominal surgery, intentional penetration of the abdominal wall remains a frequent cause of peritonitis. Surgical corrections of intestinal obstruction and of dystocia are 2 commonly performed operations which may lead to this condition. Trocarization of a gas-filled cecum or colon is another surgical procedure that may cause inflammation of the equine peritoneum.

Peritonitis also may develop during the course of certain infectious diseases, such as African horsesickness and equine viral arteritis.

A severe blow on the abdominal wall, such as a nonperforating kick, may cause a mild peritonitis which usually is of little clinical importance.

Fatal peritonitis usually results if the continuity of the gastrointestinal wall is interrupted for any reason and there is escape of its contents into the peritoneal cavity. This may occur as a result of gastric rupture, intestinal torsion, intussusception, parasite damage, breeding accidents, injudicious use of an enema tube, or rough palpation of the colon.

Foreign body penetration from the interior of the gastrointestinal tract rarely, if ever, occurs in the horse. This is true because the horse thoroughly masticates feed before swallowing it, and rejects foreign materials such as nails and pieces of wire.

In considering the pathogenesis of peritonitis, one must remember that it often is a secondary condition, and consideration must be given to the primary pathologic process. The signs of primary peritonitis are due to the absorption of toxins, the accumulation of fluids and gas in the peritoneal sac, intestinal stasis, and abdominal adhesions.

Clinical Signs: Acutely affected animals have an elevated temperature and exhibit marked depression. They assume a rigid stance and are reluctant to lie down. The abdominal muscles are contracted and the abdominal wall is taut. Groaning, heard at each shallow expiration, is accentuated when affected animals are forced to move. Early constipation is commonly followed by profuse diarrhea. Dehydration is evident even though animals may consume large quantities of water. Hematologic studies early in the course of the disease usually reveal the presence of a leukocytosis characterized by an increased number of neutrophilis. The pulse is accelerated and the mucous membranes are congested. Loss of body condition is marked, with death often occurring in a few days.

Mild cases exhibit the described signs to a lesser degree, and recovery is uneventful except for development of visceral adhesions, which rarely affect the animal's well-being.

Lesions: The abdominal cavity usually is distended with fluid. Since many cases of peritonitis are produced by abdominal perforation, a thorough examination of the skin may reveal a wound. When the abdomen is opened the peritoneum is found to be thickened and covered with fibrin. An excessive amount of serosanguineous fluid is observed in the peritoneal cavity. Ingesta or feces are suspended in this fluid if the gastrointestinal tract has been ruptured. The viscera is covered wtih fibrin and extensive adhesions may be observed when peritonitis has been present for some time.

Diagnosis: Since peritonitis often is a secondary condition every effort should be made to determine its origin. A complete history and thorough physical examination always are indicated, and often will reveal the cause. Peritonitis should be considered when a horse exhibits evidence of abdominal pain. A hematologic study frequently is of value in differentiating peritonitis from conditions such as cystitis and impaction of the digestive tract. In some cases, an exploratory laparotomy or paracentesis is justified in order to make a diagnosis.

Treatment: When the cause can be determined, treatment should be aimed at correcting it. If perforation of the abdomen has occurred, corrective surgery should be performed. If a specific infectious disease is identified, it should be treated accordingly. Regardless of the cause, practically all cases requiring treatment should receive broad spectrum antibiotics and/or sulfonamides systemically. If much fibrin is present and extensive adhesions are beginning to form, systemic digestive enzymes should be administered. It is essential to continue the administration of antibacterial agents for at least 2 days following enzyme therapy.

Prevention: Aseptic surgery, proper control of the animal at all times, and elimination of hazardous environmental conditions would prevent most cases of peritonitis. Nearly all of the remaining cases could be prevented by proper feeding, adequate parasite control, adequate supervision of breeding practices, exercise of care in administering enemas and doing rectal palpations, and elimination of specific infectious diseases.

H. E. AMSTUTZ
R. C. HERSCHLER

DISEASES OF THE LIVER

JAUNDICE

Jaundice, or icterus, is a staining of the tissues and fluids of the body with bile pigment. It is a clinical sign seen in many abnormal conditions and, as a primary sign, jaundice is important in the diagnosis of certain maladies. Three forms of jaundice are recognized in the horse: (1) obstructive; (2) hemolytic; and (3) hepatogenous jaundice.

Obstructive jaundice develops in horses when parasites invade the hepatic duct. Rare cases have occurred when the duct has become obstructed by a bot or roundworm. Obstructive jaundice also occurs in primary duodenitis, and also when duodenitis is secondary due to impaction of the terminal portion of the ileum, or more commonly due to impaction of the cecum or colon. A third cause, seen rarely, occurs when pressure on the bile ducts is produced by abscesses or tumors.

Hemolytic jaundice is caused by excessive destruction of red blood cells, a result of which is production of an abnormally large quantity of bile pigments. In general, it is seen in septicemic diseases and in infectious anemias. Horse and mule foals also are subject to a hemolytic anemia syndrome in which jaundice occurs. This disease is somewhat like Rh disease of human infants (erythroblastosis fetalis). This syndrome occurs when the mare becomes immunized against the red blood cells of her fetus. Hemolytic icterus of newborn foals is discussed further in Chapter 19.

Hepatogenous jaundice is caused by various chemicals and bacterial toxins which damage the parenchyma of the liver, thus preventing the normal elimination of bile pigment. Chemicals which can cause liver damage and jaundice include arsenic, lead, copper, phosphorous, soda nitrate, and carbon tetrachloride. Plants capable of producing hepatogenous jaundice are equisetum, loco weed, lupinosis, crotalaria, senechio, whitewood, and alsike clover. Icterus also is seen in many diseases in which degeneration of the liver occurs. It may occur in azoturia and cirrhosis of the liver. Infectious diseases during which jaundice frequently occurs include viral arteritis, leptospirosis, contagious pleuropneumonia and septicemias caused by hemolytic streptococci.

Jaundice is characterized by yellowish discoloration of various mucous membranes and the white parts of the skin. It is seen best in the palpebral and bulbar conjunctiva, the oral mucosa (especially of the lower lip), the nares, and the vulva of mares. In well-marked jaundice, the urine may be bright yellow, dark brown or black as in azoturia. In some cases of obstructive jaundice, the feces may be light, clay-colored and hard.

DEGENERATION OF THE LIVER

Primary degeneration of the liver probably does not occur in equines. Rarely does a horse die of fatty degeneration of the liver but cases have occurred which were presumed to be caused by a hepatotoxin, probably of plant origin. Parenchymatous and fatty degeneration of the liver usually are secondary consequences of septicemic diseases, intoxications of chemical and plant origin, infectious hepatitis, infectious anemia, azoturia, and gastrointestinal intoxications.

During the course of various diseases, hepatic involvement may be suspected when visible icterus is present. A confirmatory diagnosis can be furnished by laboratory tests including the icterus index, the Hanger flocculation test, and the bromsulphalein retention test. When liver degeneration is suspected, the treatment of the primary disease may be aided by supportive treatment consisting of 500 to 1000 ml. of 40 or 50% dextrose, injection of B-complex and cortisone, and the administration of 1 ounce of choline chloride per os daily.

SERUM HEPATITIS (X-Disease, Staggers, Liver Necrosis-Encephalosis Complex)

A highly fatal, toxic hepatitis of horses has occurred in the United States and many other countries as a sporadic or enzootic disease. Reports indicate that the majority of cases followed the use of antisera against various diseases. This form of hepatitis was quite prevalent many years ago when virus encephalomyelitis was more common and encephalomyelitis antiserum was used extensively. The syndrome, at present, is rare but occasional cases have followed the use of tetanus antitoxin and the use of pregnant mare serum in the treatment of infertility. It is characterized by icterus, signs of encephalitis, degeneration and necrosis of liver cells.

This disease was described first in 1918 by Theiler[1] in South Africa where it was termed "staggers." Its occurrence followed the use of antisera against African Horsesickness. In the United States, the disease was first described in 1933 in Utah, by Madsen,[2] following the use of encephalomyelitis antiserum. In 1937, Marsh of Montana reported losses of horses after the use of encephalomyelitis antiserum combined with virus injections.[3] Simultaneous vaccination with 2 ml. of a 1 to 10 suspension of virulent guinea pig brain tissue and 50 ml. of serum was used at that time for immunization against encephalomyelitis. The cases occurred from October 2 to November 16 and involved 89 horses of whom 79 died. Deaths occurred in 24 to 48 hours. Later, in 1939, Shahan, et al.,[4] investigated this "secondary" disease occurring subsequent to epidemics of equine encephalomyelitis. The recorded clinical signs included intense icterus, intestinal atony, and encephalitic symptoms. In the outbreaks described in the United States, demonstration of encephalomyelitis virus was impossible and inoculation of experimental and laboratory animals was not helpful.

In 1938, Slagsvold[5] described similar deaths after the use of anthrax antiserum in horses. In 1959, a similar disease in Yugoslavian horses was reported by Forenbacker et al.[6] They studied 74 cases of liver necrosis-encephalosis complex. Failure of liver function, followed by autointoxication which initiates encephalosis, appeared to be the sequence of events. These studies indicated that the hepatotoxin originated in the gastrointestinal tract and that the brain damage resulted from a noninflammatory edema. The majority of cases occurred in early summer and autumn when animals were changed to high protein feed.

The disease is manifested by an acute course ending in death in 12 to 48 hours. The reported mortality is 90%. Initial signs include depression, stupor, a vacant stare, anorexia, unsteady gait, and an absence of fever. Intense icterus, intestinal atony, and oliguria are present. The mouth may be held open. The somnolent stage usually is followed by violent nervous signs. The horse frequently adopts a spraddling stance and presses forward to balance against solid objects. Affected animals are observed to walk in circles and push against and through fences. At the terminal stages, extreme dyspnea is present and sweating is continuous. Terminal paresis is uncommon, and the horse literally dies on its feet.

At necropsy, there is generalized icterus. The liver is large, friable, paler than normal, and degenerative. The kidneys are enlarged, congested, and sometimes are petechiated. Hemorrhages of serous membranes and congestion of the stomach and small intestines usually are apparent. Microscopically, the liver contains areas of parenchymatous degeneration, central lobular necrosis, and fatty infiltration. The sinusoids frequently contain large numbers of leukocytes. Bile and iron pigments are present. The kidneys show parenchymatous degeneration. The spleen is congested. Lesions of the brain and spinal cord usually cannot be demonstrated.

Treatment usually is without effect. Shahan reported some recoveries following prompt intestinal evacuation. The Yugoslavian investigators report that "therapy with glucose, vitamins, and lipotropic substances reduced losses from 90 to 30 per cent." They also noted that the administration of antihistamines relieved the clinical signs.

REFERENCES

1. Theiler, A. Acute Liver Atrophy and Parenchymatous Hepatitis in Horses. Rep. of Director, Vet. Res. S. Afr. (quoted by Shahan). 1919.
2. Madsen, D. E. Equine Encephalomyelitis, Utah Academy of Science, Arts, and Letters, Vol. 11, p. 95. 1934.
3. Marsh, Hadleigh. Losses of Undetermined Cause Following an Outbreak of Equine Encephalomyelitis. J.A.V.M.A. 91 (1937) 88.
4. Shahan, M. S., Giltner, L. T., David C. L., and Huffman, W. T., "Secondary" Disease Occurring Subsequent to Infectious Equine Encephalomyelitis. Vet. Med. 34 (1939) 354.
5. Slagsvold, L., Ikterus hos Hester Behandlet Med. Miltbrandserum. Norsk. Veterinair. Tidskrift. Nr. 2-69, 94. 1938.
6. Forenbacher, S., Morzan, B. and Topolnik, E. Liver Necrosis in Horses and its Etiology and Therapy. Vet. Arhiv., 29 (1959) 344.

CIRRHOSIS OF THE LIVER
(WALKING DISEASE, WINTON DISEASE)

Over a number of years, a fatal disease of horses has been described as being characterized by cirrhosis of the liver. It is known to occur in certain regional areas of the United States and Canada, as well as other areas of the world.

In 1884, Bessey and Stalker[1] demonstrated that *Crotalaria sagittalis* was the cause of "Missouri River Bottom Disease," which resulted in death of horses. In 1892, Schroeder[2] described "bottom disease," cirrhosis of the liver, among horses in the same region. In 1900, Gilruth[3] of New Zealand, reported cirrhosis occurring in horses and cattle in the Winton district, and the condition was termed "Winton disease." The disease was attributed to the ingestion of *Senechio jacobeus*. In 1906, Robertson[4] reported the frequent occurrence of chronic atrophic hepatic cirrhosis, "stomach staggers," in pastured horses in Cape Colony, and he produced the disease by feeding *Senechio*. In 1929, Van Es *et al.*[5] reported on the nature and cause of "the walking disease" of northwestern Nebraska. The cause was proved to be *Senechio riddelli*.

Hepatic cirrhosis in horses also occurs in New York State and presumably is found only in horses fed alsike clover. Schofield,[6] in Canada, also described cirrhosis of the liver caused by feeding alsike clover. Murnane and Ewart[7] described "walk-about disease" of horses in Australia caused by *Atalya hemiglauca* (whitewood), in which a saponin proved to be the toxic substance. Enzootic cirrhosis of horses has been reported by McCullough[8] as due to the seeds of *Amsinckia intermedia* (yellow tarweed).

Cirrhosis of the liver in horses is diagnosed frequently and often is due to the ingestion of *Crotalaria spectabilis* or *C. sagittalis*. Gibbons[9,10] has described hepatic cirrhosis in Alabama and Mississippi caused by *Crotalaria*, the toxic species of which contain a hepatotoxin, monocrotaline ($C_{16}H_{26}O_6N$). In Czechoslovakia, Vanek[11] has made extensive studies of hepatic cirrhosis of horses, or Zdar disease, due to the ingestion of *Senecio erraticus*. He also studied the toxicity of alkaloids isolated from this plant in producing typical liver lesions. Similar hepatic diseases of horses have been reported from Bavaria, the Soviet Union, Iceland, England, and Japan.

Clinical Signs: The clinical signs encountered in cirrhosis of the liver in horses vary. A chronic progressive type and a more acute type have been identified in which striking signs of illness occur suddenly and resemble an acute central nervous disturbance. In the acute syndrome, the horse shows nervous signs characteristic of motor irritation. The signs include walking in circles, delirium, pressing forward and pushing the head against objects. The progressive, or more common form, is characterized by gradual onset, loss of condition, inability to work, and incoordination of the rear limbs. Later, the affected animal is somnolent and progresses to a stage of "dummy-like" behavior.

In some cases, both stages may appear in the same animal. Even in the patients suddenly affected with nervous signs, it may be revealed by careful questioning of the owner that loss of condition, periods of incoordination, or inability to eat or work existed previously. Fever is not present, and only one-half or so of the affected horses show visible icterus.

Diagnosis: The diagnosis of hepatic cirrhosis is based on the typical attitude, incoordination, dragging of the rear feet, nervous signs in some cases and the presence of icterus. The last sign can be demonstrated by determination of the icterus index. The icterus index in clinical cases usually is from 25 to 200, with an average of 75. In most cases, the icterus index rises as the disease progresses. In most observed cases, the icterus index has given a reading of at least 50. Cases of hepatic cirrhosis in horses frequently are mistaken for toxic encephalitis (moldy corn poisoning), encephalomyelitis (sleeping sickness), and occasionally for rabies. Toxic encephalitis has a shorter, more violent course, with pronounced signs of encephalitis. Death usually occurs in 48 to 72 hours. A history of feeding moldy corn, and characteristic lesions of brain degeneration are conclusive evidence. Brain lesions are not found in cirrhosis. Encephalomyelitis is a viral disease characterized by fever, violent nervous signs, followed by somnolence and progressive paralysis in a few days. A positive diagnosis can be made by serum-neutralization tests, guinea pig inoculation of brain tissue, and histopathologic examination of brain tissue for characteristic lesions. Rabies in horses produces nervous signs of a violent nature, and death in 2 to 5 days. The syndrome in horses generally is the furious type. Positive diagnosis

can be made by mouse-inoculation tests and by the demonstration of Negri bodies.

The treatment of hepatic cirrhosis of horses usually is hopeless. Three cases of supposed early cirrhosis characterized by slight incoordination recovered with heavy feeding, injections of B-complex, and the feeding of choline chloride, 1 ounce per day for 30 days. Many other cases with more advanced signs were treated similarly to no avail.

W. J. GIBBONS

REFERENCES

1. Bessey, C. E. and Stalker, M.: The rattle-box (Crotalaria sagittalis Linn) Iowa Agric. Col. Dept. Bot. Bull. (1884) 111-115.
2. Schroeder, E. C.: "Bottom disease" among horses in South Dakota 8th and 9th An. Rpts. U.S.B.A.I. 1891-92. p. 371.
3. Gilruth, J. R.: Cirrhosis of the liver in horses. Veterinarian, 73 (1900) 309.
4. Robertson, Wm.: Cirrhosis of the liver in stock in Cape Colony, produced by two species of senechio (Senechio burchelli and S. latifolins) J. Comp. Path and Ther. (1906) 19, 97.
5. Van Es, L., Cantwell, L. R., Martin, H. M., and Kramer, J.: On the nature and cause of "the Walking Disease" of Northwestern Nebraska. Univ. Neb. Agr. Sta. Res. Bull., 43, Lincoln, 1929.
6. Schofield, F. W., Enzootic hypertrophic cirrhosis of the liver of the horse caused by the feeding of alsike clover, Report of the Ontario Veterinary College, p. 31. 1932.
7. Murnane, D., and Ewart, A. J.: Kimberley Horse Disease (Walk-about-Disease), Commonwealth of Australia, Council for Scientific and Industrial Research, Bull. No. 36, Melbourne, 1928.
8. McCulloch, E. C.: Hepatic Cirrhosis of horses, swine and cattle due to the ingestion of seeds of the tarweed (Amsinckia intermedia), J.A.V.M.A. (1940) 96, 5.
9. Gibbons, W. J., Hokanson, J. F., Wiggins, A. M., and Schmitz, M. B. Cirrhosis of the Liver in Horses, No. Am. Vet., 31 (1950) 229-232.
10. Gibbons, W. J., Durr, E., and Cox, S. A. No. Am. Vet., 34 (1953) 556.
11. Vanek, J.: Senecio Poisoning (Senecio Erraticus SSP. Barbaracifolius) as the cause of ZDar Diseases in Horses; Toxicity of Isolated Alkaloids. Rev. Czech. Med. 1957, III-4.

INTESTINAL OBSTRUCTION

TORSION OR VOLVULUS

In this condition, a portion of the intestines becomes twisted on itself. The lesion may occur in any area of the intestinal tract.

Etiology: Volvulus usually follows an attack of colicky signs related to various etiologies. It occurs when horses roll and writhe in pain. It also may result from casting an animal.

Clinical Signs: This condition is characterized by the acute onset of severe and continuous colicky signs. Rectal palpation may or may not assist the diagnosis, depending on the location of the lesion and the degree of flatulence.

Cases of volvulus often end fatally within 8 to 24 hours after continuous manifestation of severe abdominal pain.

Diagnosis: As volvulus generally terminates fatally, the lesion is most often identified at necropsy. The history and signs should prompt suspicion of this lesion, and it occasionally can be identified by rectal palpation.

Treatment: Prompt surgical correction offers the only hope of saving an affected horse. Generally, the prognosis is poor.

Intussusception

Intussusception can occur in adult horses but more often is seen in younger animals. The lesion ordinarily is located in the ileum, near the ileocecal valve.

Etiology: This lesion is a consequence of abnormal peristalsis which forces a portion of the intestine to telescope into the bowel immediately behind it. Both ascariasis and strongylosis have been indicted as causes for intussusception.

Clinical Signs: The signs of intussusception usually are not severe at the outset, probably because the bowel is not completely occluded then. There often is a history of intermittent colic which has persisted for 2 to 3 days or longer. The horse manifests mild pain by lying on its back for prolonged periods, frequent stretching, and kicking at the abdomen. The conjunctivae are moderately congested, the abdomen may be slightly distended, the temperature is slightly elevated, and the pulse rate may be 60 to 70 per minute.

Rectal examination reveals that it is nearly empty. The few feces are covered with mucus, sometimes mixed with blood. Often a large crepitant mass can be palpated anterior to the pubis, and evidence of pain is elicited when it is touched.

The course of the disease depends on when occlusion of the bowel occurs. When this develops, there is a sudden increase in temperature and evidence of continuous pain. Untreated cases pass suddenly into a terminal phase which is characterized by signs of shock, and death usually occurs within 48 hours or less after appearance of acute signs.

Lesions: At necropsy, the stomach and intestines anterior to the lesion are found to be distended with fluid and gas. Peritonitis is usually present.

Treatment: Recovery depends on prompt surgical intervention. Sedatives, as demerol hydrochloride or chloral hydrate, and antispasmodics, as coecolysin, give temporary relief and are indicated as preoperative therapy. The condition should be corrected, if possible, without exteriorizing the bowel, and without manipulating it excessively. Postoperative therapy includes systemic antibiotics and a diet of concentrates and liquids.

The prognosis is good if the condition is diagnosed early and the surgical correction is done promptly.

IMPACTIONS OF THE COLON

Cecal Impaction

Causes and Predisposition: Impaction of the cecum is seen less often than other forms of intestinal obstruction. It still may be seen when coarse roughages, such as grain hays, straw, and chaff are fed. When treating one horse with signs of cecal impaction, rectal examination of several others in the herd may show some degree of impaction, especially when horses are being wintered on straw stacks. Similar impactions have been seen in horses grazing in prune orchards, the indigestible pits collecting in the cecum. Horses with perverted appetites may be subject to the same condition. I have seen two cecal impactions which developed secondary to aneurysm of the anterior mesenteric artery. Other coarse roughages such as coarse alfalfa, sweet clover, corn stalks and sorghum also have been implicated.

Since most impactions seem to occur between October and April, it is believed that changes from warm to cold weather, from green feed to dry hay diets, from warm to icy cold water, and changes from regular exercise or work routines to no work at all contribute heavily to their occurrence. Old age, bad dentition, and a less motile digestive tract also seem to be important. In addition, cecal impactions are thought to be associated with the continuous feeding of one particular type of feed the year around.

Generally speaking, cecal impactions are the most difficult food obstructions to treat successfully. We feel fortunate to have 50% survive. Survival rates probably are lower because of the insidious onset with relatively mild signs at first, plus the presence, in many cases, of diarrhea. The early syndrome often fails to alarm the owner enough to call for veterinary service until the trouble is well-advanced.

Clinical Signs: Cecal impaction initially produces the least painful signs of any intestinal obstruction. Dull pain is manifested by pawing and lying down for an hour or so. Between periods of such behavior, the horse may eat and drink normally for a while, and then lie down again and show mild signs of colic. Bowel movements are about half the usual amount and the feces soon lose the characteristic pellet formation, becoming more like those of a cow. The occurrence of diarrhea is no indication of improvement, as liquid intestinal contents readily pass between the entrance and exit of the cecum, despite the presence of the mass of impacted material below it. Examination of the mucous membranes often will reveal some icterus and congestion which increase later. Pulse, respirations, and temperature may be elevated slightly, but more often they will be normal. Auscultation over the abdomen will reveal normal sounds in all areas except the cecum, where there is no sound except an occasional low rumble replacing the active tinkling, bubbling sound present normally.

Rectal palpation facilitates the diagnosis if the base of the cecum is impacted. The consistency of the impaction ranges from that of a soft loaf of bread to the hardness of a board. Since cecal contents normally are fluid, any palpable mass may be considered as tending toward impaction. If the mass is low in the cecum, it may be difficult to reach. The signs, however, usually are characteristic enough to indicate treatment. This particularly is true when the feces are not formed and colic recurs after eating.

Treatment: Fatalities easily can be caused in these cases by treatment with harsh-acting drugs. The impaction must be softened before it can be removed and the atonic musculature of the bowel should be stimulated gradually and carefully to move the softened mass. First and most important is complete withholding of food. Patient, persistent massage of parts of the mass that can be reached is of considerable help. This may be done daily or every other day for 5 or 6 times. Encouraging water intake is most important. The administration of a quart of bran mixed with 1 or 2 tablespoonfuls of salt and 1 cup of mineral oil 2 or 3 times daily may encourage drinking as well as help soften the mass. Administration of 500 ml. of Lang's solution intravenously usually will cause the horse to drink large amounts of water.

The use of therapeutic doses of strong purgatives is contraindicated. I prefer initially to control pain with coecolysin (to stimulate gastrointestinal peristalsis) or Novin (an analgesic and antispasmodic) and then follow with Turcapsul (an antiferment and antispasmodic) or aromatic spirits of ammonia. I advise withholding food other than bran and oil mashes, while periodically massaging the mass. In particularly severe cases I have administered powdered nux vomica daily until the horse exhibits excitability. Recovery takes time— from 3 to 4 days at best, and sometimes as long as 3 weeks, during which period the horse must have no feed of any kind except the bran and oil mashes. In prolonged cases, the administration of vitamins, minerals, intravenous and oral dextrose and amino acids provides useful support. Intestinal antibiotics, as neomycin, bacitracin, or streptomycin, also are advisable in protracted cases to prevent colitis.

Cecal impactions secondary to aneurysms occur occasionally and recoveries are not to be expected. Other fatalities occur from pressure necrosis, and ultimate rupture, usually near the tip of the cecum, and peritonitis. It is important to continue treatment until the expected fecal content has been passed and the horse can eat a small amount of feed without recurrence of clinical signs.

IMPACTION OF THE SMALL COLON
(INCLUDES TRANVERSE COLON AND RECTUM)

Causes and Predisposition: The usual predisposing causes common to other types of feed impactions also apply to small colon impactions. Dental irregularities and certain hays probably are especially important as predisposing influences for this condition.

Most small colon impactions are seen in horses before they are full-mouthed and after they are smooth-mouthed, probably because of inadequate chewing and a tendency of horses with bad teeth to avoid drinking cold water. Reduced water intake, common during the winter months, likely plays a major role in causing small colon impactions. Most important, however, is the tendency for impaction to occur when certain types of hay (Chinese lettuce, sweet clover and alfalfa) are fed. The majority of cases seen in the Northwest occur in horses fed alfalfa. The most difficult occur in those few areas where Chinese lettuce is mixed with alfalfa. It has been suggested that tannates in these feeds help glue the material together.

It also is possible that good alfalfa hay, which is highly palatable and nutritious, with 16% or more protein, can cause mild engorgement effects similar to those caused by overeating of grain, and thereby produce a mild gastroenteritis and atony. This may reduce bowel motility sufficiently to allow masses of fibers to collect and form an impaction. Sudden changes in the ration from other hays to alfalfa, and changes from limited amounts of alfalfa to free choice, are especially dangerous. This is particularly so when combined with a change of weather from warm to cold, and reduced water intake.

Clinical Signs: Impaction of the small colon may take several days to develop and generally will produce no clinical signs until it has completely occluded the bowel, and tympany occurs. Then the onset of colic is sudden. A history of acute abdominal pain for several hours, complete inappetence, scanty evacuations, and bloat gives good reason to suspect complete obstruction of the bowel. A thorough search for a small colon impaction is advisable, especially if there is alfalfa hay in the ration. The horse rolls and tumbles, gets up and lies down, and looks at his sides. There apparently is little, if any, relief from pain. It may take only a few hours before the animal becomes so exhausted that it is difficult to get him on his feet.

Since these horses are beyond help within 24 hours, it is important to check temperature and pulse at once. Congested and icteric mucous membranes plus a rapid, thready pulse of more than 100, sweating and dyspnea indicate that death probably is imminent and a poor prognosis should be given. Such animals may die quite suddenly while straining during a rectal examination, or while resisting the introduction of a stomach tube.

Treatment: Before attempting rectal examination, coecolysin is administered to obtain maximum relief from pain and make the rectal examination safer. If a small amount of dark, dry, sticky feces is found in the rectum and the rectum itself is dry and sticky, an enema should be given to make palpation possible. In advanced cases with excessive bloat, it may be impossible to palpate beyond the pubis until gas is released by introducing a trochar into the cecum. Even after the tympany is relieved, impactions of the small colon are not always easy to find. However, thorough and persistent palpation of the entire hypogastric region usually will reveal the mass.

There are three common locations for these impactions: the left hypogastric area on the abdominal floor, the right hypogastric region, and the upper central region where the transverse colon is located. A few impactions will be found in the posterior part of the small colon where they can be palpated directly. Persistent efforts to mechanically reduce these masses, and repeated enemas usually will effect removal of this type. By pulling loops of colon posteriorly or by following tight bands of mesentery downward one may locate the impaction. Having an assistant push the horse's abdomen upward may bring the impaction within reach. If this is not successful a tranquilizer is given and the horse is cast on the left side, 3 legs are tied, and the search is continued on the ground. Usually, this will bring the impaction within easy reach. In small horses, even impactions of the transverse colon may be reached in this position.

It is important to keep in mind the possibility of detecting other obstructive conditions during the examination. One may find an aneurysm, torsion, volvulus, or intussusception. On 2 occasions while searching for impactions, I found a loop of the bowel incarcerated in a mesenteric tear, and by careful manipulation relieved the obstruction. The differentiation of impaction from other obstructive conditions depends primarily on rectal examination.

When finally located, the small colon impaction will be found to be very hard, with nearly the feel of a concretion. It may be smaller than anticipated, varying in size from a turkey egg in Shetlands to the size of a large coconut in draft animals. Except when located in the transverse colon, the mass is movable and often can be drawn back to or within the pelvic inlet. Neglected impactions may seem so hard as to defy efforts to reduce their size. In the absence of the critical signs mentioned earlier, it pays to try. In cases where much pain and tympany have occurred, only immediate surgery may offer a slight chance of recovery. In the majority of cases, however, when rectal palpation is possible, reducing the mass by hand will afford the needed relief. Massage is done much more quickly if the impaction can be withdrawn into the pelvis. In a mare, rectovaginal manipulation, using both hands, will break the hardest mass in a few minutes. In other animals, massage is more effective if the impaction is pushed against the brim of the pubis or the shaft of the ilium, and pressure applied with the tips of the fingers or the side of the hand. One should not attempt massage nor allow the hand to remain in the bowel while the horse strains because the rectal wall can be ruptured under these conditions.

Attempts should be made to divide the mass into four pieces, first by grooving it longitudinally until it divides, then by squeezing each half into two pieces. Complete reduction will prevent a re-forming of the mass in the posterior bowel. Gas usually will be expelled before the first groove is completed, providing consequent relief to the horse. Breaking of

recently formed impactions may take only a few minutes; older ones may take several hours of hard work. Since, in my experience, drug therapy gives highly variable results, I stay with the horse until manual breakup of the mass is accomplished. During extended massage, the hand occasionally should be moved to different locations in the rectum to avoid damaging the mucosa and producing edema and hemorrhage. Occasional cold water enemas may help reduce swelling of the mucosa.

After the impaction has been reduced, oral and systemic antibiotics may be administered along with injectable cascara. No hay of any kind should be fed for 24 hours, and alfalfa hay should not be fed for at least 6 weeks.

In Shetlands, colts, or other small horses, when rectal massage is impossible or ineffective, immediate surgery is indicated. Use of a tranquilizer and local anesthesia at the operative site is preferable to general anesthesia. The operation may be done standing with a flank incision or the horse may be cast and tied in dorsal recumbency. In the latter case, a midline incision is used. The impaction may be reduced with the colon in the abdomen or the colon may be brought outside. Only rarely will enterotomy be required. At least 90% of the cases caused by small colon impactions should recover, if treated promptly.

IMPACTION OF THE LARGE COLON

Causes and Predisposition: The etiology of large colon impactions is similar in most respects to that of other impactions—bad teeth, internal parasites, lowered water intake, eating coarse roughages, and lack of exercise. Of major importance in certain areas is the feeding of alfalfa or grain hays. Grain hays, especially wheat, are highly palatable because of the grain heads. Horses tend to eat them too fast and this can produce mild irritation of the digestive tract, which coupled with the long stringy hay fibers comprise the ingredients for impaction.

Although alfalfa seems good from the standpoint of nutritional value it is, in my opinion, a poor horse feed for several reasons, not the least of which is its tendency to cause impactions of the large and small colons. Impactions seldom are seen where good bright grass or timothy hays are fed, no matter how poor the other phases of management may be.

Clinical Signs: The signs of large colon impaction are more severe than those in a horse afflicted with a cecal impaction, but they are not as severe nor continuous as in a small colon impaction. Typically, the horse may have had colic intermittently for 2 or more days. He is observed to get up and down more than usual, and frequently looks around at his sides. While standing, he may strain as if to pass urine. He may do some pawing when the pain is greatest. He may for 2 or 3 days pass fairly normal looking feces, but the amounts will be smaller than usual. When signs are present the animal usually will not eat nor drink, but between periods of overt signs the appetite may be almost normal. Over a period of days the signs become more severe and the periods of relief are fewer and of shorter duration. The feces become darker, sticky, and scant. Bloat seldom is present. The temperature, pulse, and respiratory rate usually are normal in the early stages, but generally are elevated in the later stages. The presence of dyspnea and stiffness of gait may indicate the impaction of the diaphragmatic or sternal flexure.

Rectal examination usually reveals the left ventral colon to be impacted, with the hardest part of the mass located at the pelvic flexure. The impaction starts near the brim of the pubis and extends anteriorly beyond reach. In advanced cases, the pelvic flexure may be pushed posteriorly on the floor of the pelvis and it can be palpated as soon as the fingers pass the anal sphincter. A horse with such an impaction may assume peculiar positions such as kneeling, sitting like a dog, or stretching and straining apparently in an effort to expel the impaction, or to relieve pain. The consistency of the mass is harder than that of the cecal impaction; the impacted pelvic flexure often is so hard that it is difficult to dent. If there is considerable pain evinced by the horse when palpated or if there is a crepitant feel to the bowel, the prognosis is poor. Fiery red mucous membranes combined with elevated temperature, a thready pulse of more than 100, and listlessness also indicate that death is imminent.

Treatment: Withholding food and massaging the mass are most important in treating these impactions. I avoid the use of severe cathartics and attempt to promote water intake. Thirty minutes or more are often spent kneading, squeezing, and massaging mostly on the pelvic flexure, but also massaging forward as far as possible. This is followed by a cold water enema to help reduce inflammation caused by the massage, and to keep the posterior bowel well-lubricated for the fecal masses soon to be passed. An initial injection of coecolysin provides prompt relief from pain and is followed by daily injections of cascara as needed. If mineral oil is used, the initial dose should be ½ gallon or more. After 24 hours of witholding food, some bran, oil, and salt mashes are advised. The horse should not have any other food until 2 to 3 buckets of manure are passed. In an early case, this treatment usually will result in complete evacuation within 24 to 48 hours and no further treatment will be necessary. In neglected cases, it may require 10 days or more to pass the entire impaction, and in these cases especially, the use of drastic purges is to be avoided.

If there is a recurrence of signs within 24 to 48 hours, then rectal massage, plus coecolysin and cascara, are administered again. After 2 consecutive daily treatments, massaging on alternate days is preferred; 5 or more massages can be performed without damage to the rectum. The use of intestinal antibiotics is advisable if additional treatment is necessary after 2 days.

After passage of normal amounts of feces has occurred and the impaction is not palpable, the horse's regular feeding is resumed gradually. If the signs recur, treatment must be repeated. For ponies or colts which cannot be massaged, withholding food plus medicinal treatment usually will solve the problem, but more slowly. If this is not effective, then massage can be accomplished successfully via a laparotomy performed after tranquilization and local anesthesia. Use of general anesthesia is to be avoided if possible, since many of these animals are too toxic to tolerate it. Ninety percent or more can be expected to recover if treated properly.

N. Van Hoosen

CHAPTER 10

DISEASES OF THE RESPIRATORY SYSTEM

LUNGS AND AIR PASSAGES

In considering the diseases of the respiratory system it is essential to keep in mind its anatomic features and the need for examination of deformities that may be present. Perhaps of greater and more directly related importance is the physiologic function of the system and its requirements for maintenance of life. For detailed discussions of pulmonary function in health and disease the reader is referred to *The Physiological Basis of Medical Practice,* by Best and Taylor, and *A Textbook of Medicine,* by Cecil and Loeb.

Examination of the respiratory system is necessary in all routine physical examinations of the horse because of the many conditions that may influence its functions. Inspection, palpation, percussion, and auscultation are all quite readily employed and should be done with the animal at rest and following exercise. Only the more important diseases of this system will be treated in this chapter, as space does not permit an attempt to cover the numerous conditions encountered. Some of these will be discussed in other sections of the book.

RHINITIS, PHARYNGITIS, AND LARYNGITIS

This group of diseases usually appears together, but in rare instances one may be the predominant problem. They are characterized by nasal discharge with or without a cough or temperature elevation. The degree of severity depends largely on the intensity of the inflammatory agent causing the injury to the mucosa.

Etiology: The etiology may be inhalation of injurious fumes or chemicals, or infections of the mucous membrane and adjacent structures. *Streptococcus equi* or *Streptococcus equisimilis* are the most common causes of pharyngitis with extensions to the nasal and laryngeal mucosa and adjacent lymphocytic structures. Recent work suggests that *Pseudomonas aeruginosa* is also involved to some extent. Chronic inflammation of the guttural pouches also may be a source of irritant exudates or infection.

Clinical Signs: The signs observed following inhalation of injurious agents are dependent on the intensity of exposure to the irritant and the depth of penetration into the respiratory tract. The most important manifestations are a serous, serohemorrhagic, or mucoid nasal discharge, a dry, harsh cough, and moderate increase in respiratory rate. The regional lymph nodes may be hypertrophic, the conjunctiva usually is congested, and excessive lacrimation may be noted. Animals affected with these conditions usually are afebrile, and in severe cases one observes subnormal temperatures.

The infections commonly encountered involve the pharynx, and acute cases have a sudden onset with a sharp temperature rise to 103.5 to 105 F. The horse will have little or no interest in food but will show a desire for water. The inflammation, when severe, causes partial pharyngeal paralysis and fluids taken into the mouth are partially discharged through the nose. Such fluids will contain particles of feed, and may also contain exudates.

The attitude of the animal is that of marked depression. In severe cases the head is held with the neck extended to alleviate the dyspnea resulting from swelling of the pharyngeal mucosa and interference with opening of the glottis. Light palpation over the region of the pharynx will stimulate a cough response. If the stomach tube is passed for administration of medication or to rule out the possibilities of choke, a marked objection by the horse is demonstrated when the end of the tube enters the pharynx. The resistance ceases when the tube enters the esophagus.

In less acute cases or those seen at 24 to 48 hours following the initial signs, enlargement of the retropharyngeal lymph nodes with varying degrees of involvement of the anterior cervical and mandibular nodes will be observed. The nasal discharge is serous at the onset of the disease or may be serosanguineous. As the disease progresses the exudate becomes mucoid and later mucopurulent, and congestion of the nasal mucosa may be noted. An intermittent nonproductive cough develops.

Lesions: The pathologic changes noted on direct examination of the pharynx are swelling of the mucosa in its dorsal portion with redness and, in some cases, small accumulations of exudate. Few cases are fatal, so little has been reported on postmortem findings. The common changes found on terminal cases are either edema of the glottis or acute fibrinous pneumonia and pleuritis.

Diagnosis: The diagnosis of pharyngitis is based on clinical observations. At certain seasons it may be epizootic among young horses. Its association with strangles frequently is ascertained through comparison or association with other horses manifesting more marked evidence of that disease. Horses which develop an intermittent but unrelenting or unresponding cough during or after an attack of pharyngitis are thought to harbor a *Pseudomonas* species. Such cases should also be examined carefully for evidence of chronic inflammation of the guttural pouches. In our experience, acute pharyngitis usually is evident early in strangles. It must often be differentiated from cases of choke if regurgitation is noted. The response to treatment generally is favorable, with complete recovery occurring in 3 to 5 days.

Prognosis: The prognosis on acute pharyngitis is very favorable when treatment is administered without delay. The more chronic cases are prone to remissions and exacerbations. At times, they develop into a chronic bronchitis or mild bronchopneumonia which may be a factor in the induction of chronic pulmonary emphysema.

The treatment of choice is the intramuscular administration of 4000 units of aqueous procaine penicillin per pound of body weight daily. The addition of streptomycin offers some promise of enhancing recovery, but should be given twice daily in doses of 250 mgm. per pound to avoid side reactions. In most cases the response to penicillin therapy is striking. Those cases with poor response and a persisting cough usually become chronic. The administration of 100,000 units of a proteolytic enzyme, in 40 ml. of water containing 2,000,000 units of aqueous procaine penicillin, provides relief in more chronic or subacute cases. Relapses are, however, quite common.

Preventive measures in outbreaks of pharyngitis among large stables of horses or for those recently on exhibition include application of strict sanitary practices, segregating the ill, and prophylactic treatment of the healthy with one dose of benzathine penicillin of 4000 units per pound given intramuscularly.

Pneumonia

Most textbooks of veterinary medicine refer to "Equine Contagious Pleuropneumonia." Some of the early work on equine pneumonia suggested the presence of an organism resembling the pleuropneumonia group, but this soon was discounted. Schutz considered streptococci to be the primary etiology, but the studies conducted by Gaffky and Lührs demonstrated the presence of a virus during the first few days of the disease which was followed in most cases by invasion of the lungs and pleura by streptococci.[4] Many of the signs reported for equine contagious pneumonia are suggestive of viral arteritis as recognized today.[1,2] The presence of pneumonia, distribution of the virus in the host, and the reported incubation period of the viral disease reported by Lührs is quite different, however. Equine contagious pleuropneumonia as reported in the older literature does not, to my knowledge, present a problem in the United States at this time.

Pneumonia in the horse as it occurs now is principally a disease of the young, the aged, and the debilitated animal. In foals and young horses it is acute, and in aged or debilitated horses it usually is chronic and progressive.

Etiology: Streptococci and Pasteurellae are the most frequent causes of the disease. But it is also recognized that Staphylococci, Salmonellae, coliforms, Pseudomonas, Klebsiella, and other groups of bacteria also may be incriminated. Current information on bacteriologic studies of equine pneumonia is very limited because of the effective control of these infections or due to interference in bacteriologic examinations as a consequence of antibiotic therapy.

Predisposition of horses to pneumonia results from infections of the upper respiratory tract such as infectious rhinopneumonitis, influenza, strangles, and parasitism. Transport for long distances in open vans, confinement to dusty quarters, and malnutrition also contribute to the problem. The inhalation of smoke, irritant chemicals, and aspiration of fluids also enhance development of pulmonary infection.

Clinical Signs: By the time pneumonia has developed, the primary inciting condition is either obvious, has been self-limiting, or is revealed only through the history. In many instances the owner or groom has noted a serous nasal discharge a few days to a week previously, but no alarming signs. In other instances a navel infection may be noted, or complications of strangles still will be apparent. The history usually will disclose anorexia of significant degree and lethargy.

Physical examination of affected horses will disclose an elevation of temperature—seldom less than 102.5 F. and frequently 104 to 105 F. In the latter instance sweating is frequently observed. Feed generally is refused but water is taken sparingly. The horse is depressed and amenable to handling. The pulse is full and moderately accelerated in most cases. An intermittent moist cough may be noted during the course of the examination. The respirations are increased in rate and are abdominal in character.

At the onset of pneumonia percussion of the thorax is not revealing, but when the horse has been sick for 12 to 24 hours as much as the lower third of the lung field may be dull on percussion. At this stage the animal frequently resists blows to the thorax because of pleuritis. Percussion late in the course of the disease reveals areas of dullness in the lower thorax as a result of pleural effusion. At this stage thoracic breathing is restricted, dyspnea is present, and abdominal breathing is prominent.

Auscultation early in the course of pneumonia detects moist rales which may be heard on inspiration over widely spread areas of the ventral third to one-half of the thorax. Later in the disease a friction rub may be detected in the lower part of the thorax with absence of vesicular sounds. If pleural effusion develops all sounds disappear from the area, and there is a marked decrease in cardiac sounds. A succession splash seldom develops.

Most fatal cases of pneumonia become chronic and progressive prior to death. General emaciation or cachexia is commonly present. The course of acute pneumonia unless prolonged by treatment varies from 24 to 96 hours. From the onset of obvious signs until the development of frank pneumonia varies from 12 to 24 hours. The presence of extensive pulmonary consolidation and fibrinous pleuritis can be detected by 24 to 48 hours.

Lesions: At necropsy, there is extensive pleuritis with a thin fibrinous exudate over the visceral and parietal pleura, and few if any adhesions. The amount of pleural exudate present is highly variable but usually is greater in acute cases. Cases resulting from acute Pasteurella infection present extensive lung involvement with quite uniform fibrinous pneumonia of the lower one-third to one-half of the diaphragmatic lobes and most of the cardiac and apical lobes.

Streptococcal pneumonias more frequently involve only the diaphragmatic lobes and usually are bilateral, but may be unilateral. Pleural effusion and pleuritis are more intense and lung lesions show mixed areas of fibrinous pneumonia, peribronchitis, suppurative bronchitis, and, occasionally, frank pulmonary necrosis. Pulmonary abscesses surrounded by pneumonic lung also may be noted. Chronic pneumonia of the debilitated or aged animal usually is lobular with lesions of varying stages of duration. Pleuritis is present less frequently but if observed usually is fibrous and adherent in character. All cases show evidence of compensatory emphysema of the unaffected lung and also may show interlobular edema.

Prognosis: The acute pneumonias of the horse offer a favorable prognosis if treated early. When treatment is delayed or is inadequate, up to 50% die or become chronic. Chronic cases run a protracted course requiring prolonged treatment. Chronic bronchitis and emphysema are frequent sequelae.

Treatment: The treatment of pneumonia depends upon factors initiating the disease, conditions under which therapy must be conducted, and to a large extent upon personal preferences. Most of the antibacterial agents are effective. The sulfonamides, particularly triple sulfonamide mixtures at 1½ grains per pound of body weight administered intravenously, are effective. They should be continued at 1 grain per pound for 3 to 5 days. They also provide a broad spectrum of action against the potential infectious agents, and are of some value as expectorants. Fluid intake must be encouraged, particularly for young animals on sulfonamide therapy.

Cases of pneumonia resulting from streptococcal infections respond well to 4000 units of penicillin per pound given intramuscularly, but they should be treated over a period of at least 7 to 10 days. The addition of streptomycin will expand the antibacterial spectrum and should be used if Pasteurella or other gram-negative infections are suspected. Some veterinarians prefer the tetracyclines for treating pneumonia. These drugs provide a broad coverage of organisms that may be involved. They do, however, lack the direct lethal action so characteristic of penicillin and streptomycin. None of the antibiotics have been used widely enough in horses to create populations of resistant organisms.

A horse with a respiratory infection should have well-ventilated, draft-free quarters. During stages of the acute febrile reaction, blanketing is desirable to prevent discomfort and avoid chilling. Fresh water and palatable feeds should be offered frequently to encourage eating and drinking. The state of hydration is of considerable importance and balanced electrolyte solutions given intravenously help prevent serious fluid depletion. Recovery can be measured by return of the temperature to normal, improved appetite, and increased alertness. A period of 2 to 3 weeks should be allowed for convalescence. Retraining should be delayed to avoid relapses.

Pleuritis

Pleuritis in the horse is infrequent in occurrence except for its association with pneumonia. Introduction of infection into the pleural cavity usually is a result of injury or thoracic

puncture. Trauma to the thorax resulting in rib fracture may cause damage to the parietal pleura and lead to an open thorax. One such case was observed to develop a suppurative pleuritis on the affected side and to terminate fatally. It is noteworthy that only the lung on the affected side was collapsed, which is contrary to the accepted theory that the mediastinum is always fenestrated and that pneumothorax of the horse is always bilateral.[3]

The nature of the pleuritis encountered in the horse depends on the type of invading organisms. Pleuritis usually is acute, involving both parietal and visceral pleura with thickening, roughness of the surface, and a coating with a meshwork of fibrinous strands. The subacute or chronic cases develop pleural effusions. The exudate present in such cases may be voluminous and usually is cloudy. In rare instances, long-standing or recovered cases may develop adherent fibrous bands between the parietal and visceral pleura in localized areas.

Clinical Signs: The signs of primary pleuritis in the initial stages are moderate temperature rise, depression, loss of appetite, reluctance to move, and, occasionally, mild signs of colic and accompanying anxiety. On detailed examination, respirations are found to be increased in rate, with restriction of thoracic breathing and shallow abdominal excursions. The heart rate is increased. Percussion of the thorax may elicit evidence of pain and produce a painful cough. Auscultation of the thorax reveals a decrease in intensity of vesicular sounds and the presence of a friction rub. When pleural effusion has developed, the friction rub is no longer present and respirations become labored and remain abdominal in character. The animal prefers to remain standing, and edema of the pectoral region and forelimbs frequently develops. The presence of pleural effusion may be confirmed by noting an area of dullness on percussion limited dorsally by a horizontal line and exudate can be removed by thoracentesis.

Diagnosis: The diagnosis of pleuritis is dependent on clinical findings and history. The cases with pleural effusion are confirmed by thoracic puncture and visual and laboratory observation of the exudate.

Acute cases may be mild and of short duration with spontaneous recovery. Cases with pleural effusion usually terminate fatally within 2 to 3 weeks. Cases of suppurative pleuritis are unfavorable in prognosis.

Treatment: Treatment consists of good nursing care and antibacterial therapy. Combinations of penicillin and streptomycin in dosages as used for pneumonia will reduce extension and severity of the involvement. In cases with pleural effusion, the dyspnea can be alleviated by withdrawal of exudate. Thoracentesis must be done aseptically and care should be exercised in respect to the rate of fluid removal and total quantities withdrawn to avoid cardiac collapse.

HYDROTHORAX

This disease results from accumulation of transudate into the pleural cavity. The most common and singularly important cause of this condition in the horse is chronic heart disease. Hydrothorax may be associated with long-standing cases of chronic pulmonary emphysema.

The principal clinical evidence of the condition is dyspnea without fever. An area of dullness can be demonstrated by percussion of the ventral portion of the thorax.

The diagnosis is established by the physical findings and withdrawal of fluid which has a lower specific gravity and protein content than exudates.

The course is progressive and the prognosis is unfavorable. Temporary relief may be provided by thoracentesis, but this is hazardous because of the circulatory deficiency of the patient.

PNEUMOTHORAX

The presence of air in the pleural cavity may occur as a result of trauma to the thoracic wall which produces an opening into the pleural cavity, or by rupture of the lung resulting from severe coughing, or through the development of a fistula from a bronchiole through the pleura. The significance of this condition is dependent on the quantity of air that enters the pleural cavity and the persistence of the opening that admits the air.

Pneumothorax causes partial collapse of the lung, reduces the vital capacity, and affects the negative intrathoracic pressure thus causing interference with pulmonary circulation. If the opening into the pleural cavity is large, the lung on the affected side will collapse completely in a short time. Because of the thinness or fenestration of the mediastinum of the horse, it is generally accepted that the pneumothorax becomes bilateral.

Clinical Signs: A suddenly developing severe dyspnea is the most prominent sign of pneumothorax. If the point of access of air persists, the dyspnea increases in severity with the development of cyanosis and death within a few hours. Frequently, the continued introduction of air is prevented by closure of the opening by tissue swelling or fibrinous exudate. In this case the air in the thorax is absorbed, with subsequent improvement. Examination of the thorax while air is present reveals a tympanitic resonance on percussion and absence of vesicular sounds on the affected side. If the condition persists a pleuritis may develop.

Lesions: Terminal cases of pneumothorax show atelectasis of both lungs in acute cases. In more prolonged cases, partial atelectasis may persist and be complicated by pleuritis which is usually suppurative.

Diagnosis: The diagnosis of pneumothorax is established by the presenting history, rapid onset of characteristic signs, and the progressive and usually short course of the disease.

Prognosis: The prognosis is unfavorable unless the point of air access is closed promptly, either surgically or through normal healing. In the latter case, the outlook will depend on the amount of air admitted to the pleural cavity and the presence of infection in the pleura.

Treatment: Pneumothorax may be treated first by surgical closure of the site of air access followed by withdrawal of the air in the thorax. This assists in correcting the atelectasis of the lung and hastens re-establishment of normal pulmonary ventilation and intrathoracic pressure relationships. Prevention of secondary pleuritis should be attempted by maintenance of the patient on a broad spectrum antibiotic until recovery is complete. Treatment usually is fruitless if the pneumothorax cannot be corrected within 8 hours.

CHRONIC PULMONARY ALVEOLAR EMPHYSEMA

Definition: The disease of horses commonly referred to as "heaves" or "broken wind" is a chronic, progressive condition affecting respirations, circulation, stamina, and general condition. It is considered to be a disease of horses 5 years of age or older. Recently it has been noted to develop in some instances in younger horses, following acute respiratory diseases. Chronic alveolar emphysema is characterized by an expiratory dyspnea, chronic cough, intermittent nasal discharge, intestinal flatulence, unthriftiness, and lack of stamina. These signs are exaggerated by exercise, feeding of heavy roughage, and confinement to dusty stables.

Etiology: The specific etiology of chronic alveolar emphysema is a controversial subject, but there is general agreement about the factors contributing to its development following its induction. Consideration has been given to the role of legume roughage as an inciting agent because of its influences on vagal innervation as a result of digestive disease. It now is thought that the effects of infections causing chronic bronchitis are important contributors to development of emphysema. Bronchitis resulting from allergic responses to natural antigens must be considered. There is experimental evidence to indict the role of allergic reactions, but there also is a surprising absence of this disease among horses employed for production of biologics, despite their frequent challenge with antigenic substances. This may be due to the fact that the allergens must be inhaled. Remission of signs may be attributed to changes in the concentration of allergens in inspired air.

Lesions: On opening the thorax, the lungs fail to collapse and are fully distended. In severe cases the lateral surfaces of the lobes may show depressions at their points of contact with the ribs. The lungs are pale or grayish, have lost their elasticity, and are drier than normal. Alveolar and interstitial emphysema are prominent. The margins of the lobes are thickened and rounded, and local areas,

particularly at the periphery of the apical and diaphragmatic lobes, may show bulbous dilations of alveoli or confluence of alveoli forming sacs. Chronic bronchiolitis invariably is present with the bronchioles being thickened and containing focal accumulations of tenacious, mucoid exudate. In the more rapidly developing cases, the decrease in pulmonary circulation and the loss of elasticity of the lung are less prominent and the lesions of bronchitis are more obvious.

Microscopically, the normal pulmonary architecture is lost; the alveolar walls show atrophy and are much thinner than normal. Alveoli are ruptured and there is union of adjacent alveoli to form a number of large, irregular air sacs. Much of the capillary network has disappeared, resulting in a marked decrease in the vascularity of the lung parenchyma. Dilation of the bronchioles also is evident. A diffuse but irregularly distributed bronchitis, bronchiolitis, and peribronchiolitis are always prominent.

Pathogenesis: The pathogenesis of chronic alveolar emphysema emphasizes the importance of the several factors that may contribute to its development. The presence of bronchitis and exudate in the bronchial tree results in narrowing of the bronchioles. Bronchial spasm resulting from an allergic response may produce similar changes. This leads to increased inspiratory effort and hyperventilation. The constriction of the bronchioles and the presence of exudates in their lumens increase resistance to expiration and an increase in residual air. The increase in residual air, in effect, reduces vital capacity and further exaggerates the condition. Exercise increases the demand for oxygen resulting in further hyperventilation. The increase in residual air causes a thinning of the alveolar walls and reduction in size and number of the capillary vessels, causing local anoxia, rupture of the alveolar walls, and their coalescence.

Continued distention of alveoli and the development of air sacs resulting from alveolar rupture cause portions of the lung to become ineffective for exchange of gases, and in essence increases the dead air space.

Other factors that influence the degree of distention and rupture of alveoli are coughing and extreme muscular contraction of the abdomen against a closed glottis, as occurs in pulling a heavy load. The reduced ventilation and decreased perfusion with blood of local areas in the lung cause a progressive increase in the severity of the disease.

Pulmonary emphysema is further complicated by alteration of the oxygen-carbon dioxide relationship in the blood and alveolar air. The reduction in breathing capacity is marked because of the increase in dead air space and residual air and the reduction in vital capacity. The reduction in ventilation causes a decrease in oxygenation of the blood which alters the oxygen-carbon dioxide equilibrium and results in an increase in carbon dioxide in blood. This causes a diminished sensitivity of the respiratory center and further aggravates carbon dioxide retention.

In addition to the effects on ventilation, emphysema also affects circulation and the mechanics of respiration. With reduction of the capillary bed of the lungs, the work of the right heart is increased and, subsequently, pulmonary blood pressure is increased. This leads to hypertrophy of the right ventricle and, in time, congestive heart failure with hepatic enlargement and general passive congestion. A tendency to develop edema of the appendages may occur in extreme cases.

The continuous and progressive expiratory dyspnea and increased abdominal effort to forcefully empty the lung produce several changes. To increase lung volume, the diaphragm contracts and the abdomen relaxes. This leads to hypertrophy of the diaphragmatic muscles and reduction of the diaphragmatic cupola. This expands the percussible lung field. Abdominal relaxation causes a pendulous abdomen. Marked springing of the rib cage on inspiration increases the thoracic girth. Difficulty in removal of air from the emphysematous lung requires more abdominal effort on expiration so that instead of being a normal passive act there is active contraction of the abdominal muscles, producing the classic expiratory lift or double expiration. This results in hypertrophy of the external abdominal oblique muscles and formation of a ridge, "heave line," seen along the lateral side of the thorax

in the region of the costochondral junctions and extending in the direction of the hip.

Clinical Signs: Chronic alveolar emphysema is not generally accompanied by fever, but moderate temperature rises at the onset have been recorded. Such instances suggest the presence of a bronchitis as an inducing factor. At the onset, the horse is alert and active, with a normal appetite and regular eliminations. An intermittent or occasional cough or a short paroxysm of coughing may be noted in the morning, following watering or when the horse is first taken out for exercise. Some moistness of the nostrils may be noted or there may be a moderate discharge of mucoid exudate, either unilateral or bilateral. This may be observed when the head is lowered to eat or drink when the animal is first attended to in the morning. Initial concern about emphysema usually is aroused by the development of dyspnea, or in the horseman's terms when "shortness of wind" is observed following exercise. At this stage of the disease, the abdominal phase of expiration may be shown slightly, particularly after exercise.

As the disease progresses, the signs become more prominent. The cough is more marked and is observed intermittently but with less tendency to be paroxysmal. The nasal discharge may be absent or seen only occasionally as a mucoid or mucopurulent exudate in the morning. An increase in inspiratory effort is manifested by dilation of the nostrils, more springing of the ribs, and abdominal relaxation. Expiration is the most prominent phase of breathing with relaxation of the intercostals and normal contraction of the abdominal muscles followed by a marked secondary active contraction of the abdomen. At this time, the increase in abdominal pressure caused by exaggeration of dyspnea through exercise or coughing frequently is accompanied by expulsion of gas from the rectum. In extreme cases, the rectum will protrude at each expiratory effort. A horse which has been affected for an extended period will exhibit hypertrophy of the external abdominal oblique muscles by the presence of the "heave line."

On detailed examination of the thorax, palpation may disclose a prominent apical impulse of the heart on the left side and if hypertrophy of the heart is marked, it may also be palpated on the right. It is more common to find that the emphysematous lung has obscured the cardiac impulse. On percussion, the lung field is found to be expanded posteriorly due to distention of the lungs and depression of the diaphragmatic cupola. The percussible area of the heart is reduced due to an increase in the size of the adjacent apical and cardiac lobes of the lung.

On auscultation, a variety of sounds may be detected. In all stages, the vesicular murmur is increased in magnitude in proportion to the severity of involvement. In early cases, dry rales are heard frequently, and at times moist rales may be detected. As the disease progresses, the tubular sounds increase in prominence in relation to the increase in dyspnea, and most cases exhibit asthmatic wheezes. In advanced cases, the vesicular sounds in the lung periphery often are accompanied by crepitant rales. Auscultation of the heart invariably reveals an increased rate and prominent systolic sounds which are enhanced on exercise.

The heart rate is slow in returning to normal following exercise in all but very early cases. When the heartbeat is irregular following exercise and is slow in returning to the initial rate, cardiac hypertrophy and right heart failure are likely present.

Diagnosis: The diagnosis of chronic alveolar emphysema is made on the basis of the clinical signs and the history. The early stages present the greatest difficulty in diagnosis due to the confusion caused by cases of compensatory emphysema. Evidence of bronchitis manifested by dry rales or asthmatic wheezes and increased vesicular sounds is indicative of the onset of the disease but some evidence of expiratory dyspnea should be present. To obtain confirmatory evidence of the disease, the administration of atropine ⅛ to ¼ grain (8 to 16 mgm.) per 1,000 pounds subcutaneously will alleviate the dyspnea in 20 to 30 minutes and persist for 3 to 4 hours. Excessive dosage causes dryness of the mouth and may cause uneasiness in the horse. The use of atropine and other related products may be employed by unscrupulous individuals to obscure the signs of emphysema. This should be checked by inspection of the mouth for dryness and for dilation of the pupils before declaring a horse to be sound on presale examination.

The course of chronic alveolar emphysema is progressive. The reduction or removal of conditions that aggravate the disease may alleviate it, but the pathologic changes of the lung are irreversible. Cases which are reported to have recovered were in all probability, either a simple bronchitis or cases of acute or compensatory emphysema. Because of the progressive character of the disease, the prognosis is unfavorable, particularly if any demanding work is expected from the animal. In most instances, affected mares can be used for breeding for several years after the disease is initiated.

Treatment: The treatment of horses with chronic emphysema is purely palliative. It does not influence the course of the disease, but may prolong the usefulness of the horse. Most of the effort should be directed toward relieving clinical signs by removing factors conducive to their production. Legume roughage should be avoided and only limited amounts of native meadow grasses should be fed. The roughage should be moistened to reduce dustiness. Most of the ration should consist of grain, preferably whole, dust-free oats. Grain rations must be increased to maintain condition. Green pasture is the most efficacious roughage. Stables should be well-ventilated and kept dust-free. Pasturing is better than stabling to avoid dust exposure. Withholding water for a brief time (2 to 4 hours) before working often will reduce the severity of the dyspnea.

The drugs employed principally are products that cause bronchial dilation to alleviate the dyspnea. They also may increase circulation by increasing the heart action. Expectorants are helpful in early stages for removal of bronchial exudate. Most of the products used are prepared as powders and added to the grain ration.

In recent years the use of beet pulp as roughage has aided in alleviation of the signs of emphysema, and the currently available, pelleted horse rations should aid in its control.

H. H. Hoyt

REFERENCES

1. Bryans, John T. *et al.*: Cornell Vet., **47** (1957) 42-52.
2. Doll, E. R. *et al.*: Cornell Vet., **47** (1957) 3-41.
3. Hutyra, Marek, and Manniger: Special Pathology and Therapeutics of the Diseases of Domestic Animals, 4th ed. Alexander Eger, Chicago, Ill., 1938.
4. M'Fadyean, Sir John: J. of Comp. Path. and Therap., **51** (1938) 108-118.
5. Best and Taylor: Physiologic Basis of Medical Practice, 6th ed., Williams and Wilkins Co., Baltimore, Md., 1955.
6. Cecil and Loeb: A Textbook of Medicine, 9th ed., William B. Saunders Co., Philadelphia, Pa., 1955.
7. Law: Textbook of Veterinary Medicine, 2nd ed., published by the author, Ithaca, N. Y., 1905.
8. Udall: The Practice of Veterinary Medicine, 6th ed., published by The author, Ithaca, N. Y., 1954.

THE GUTTURAL POUCHES

The guttural pouches are organs peculiar to the horse and other solipeds. Varied hypotheses have arisen through the years as to their function but at this writing these organs still are involved in obscurity.

The pouches are two in number and each is suspended from a ventral slit in each Eustachian tube, forming ventral diverticuli. They are located at the base of the sphenoid and occipital bones. The sacs envelop the great cornua (stylohyoids) and extend to the sides of the pharynx and larynx ventrally. The upper margin of the posterior nares, or a point just anterior to the vertical ramus of the mandible, is the anterior limitation. Posteriorly, they extend to the atlanto-axial articulation, the occipital artery and the atlantal attachment of the longus colli muscle. Medially, they lie against each other but are partially separated by the ventral straight muscles of the head. The lateral anatomic relations are multiple. Each pouch is separated from the innerface of the parotid gland by the many muscles, nerves and vessels in the area (Fig. 1, 2, & 3).

The size and shape of the sacs are quite variable and may differ in the same individual. The capacity of each pouch usually is between 275-300 cc.[1]

In the horse, the Eustachian tubes extend for about 4 inches connecting the middle ear with the pharynx. They are composed of fibrocartilage, lined with mucous membrane, flattened on both sides, and open into the tympanic cavities by narrow orifices. The pharyngeal openings are slit-like apertures 2

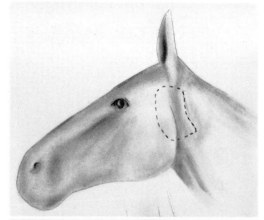

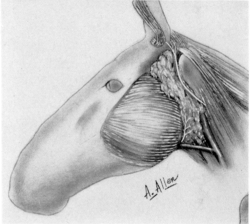

Fig. 1 and 2. Outline of the approximate position of the guttural pouch (top). Parotid region showing the posterior auricular nerve and Viborg's triangle. Parotido-auricular muscle is reflected (bottom).

inches in length, located on the postero-superior walls of the lateral pharynx. The Eustachian tubes serve to equalize the air pressure on both sides of the tympani.

The guttural pouches contain air which they receive from the pharynx through the Eustachian tubes. Warm air is thought to fill the pouches during expiration, and part of this is exchanged for cold air during inspiration.[2] The amount of air in the sacs varies with the extensibility of the mucous membrane. Their dilation is produced by the palatopharyngeus muscle fibers imbedded in the membrane. The pouches may be seen to expand and fill during expiration.

Fig. 4. Illustrated is the operative method employed in the removal of chondroids with drainage of the guttural pouch. (A) Skin incision made one inch anterior to the wing of the atlas. The skin, posterior auricular nerve and fascia reflected posteriorly. Parotid gland is freed from its attachment to the atlas and reflected forward and laterally. The hypoglossal and glossopharyngeal nerves observed crossing the protruding guttural pouch. (B) Removal of chondroids from bulging pouch showing adequate reflection of the carotid artery, parotid gland, and hypoglossal and glossopharyngeal nerves. (C) Dorsal incision closed with interrupted sutures. Ventral incision through Viborg's triangle. (D) Stab wound into protruding guttural pouch taking care to avoid the parotid duct, external maxillary vein, and parotid gland. (E) A gauze strip being inserted into the pouch to facilitate drainage.

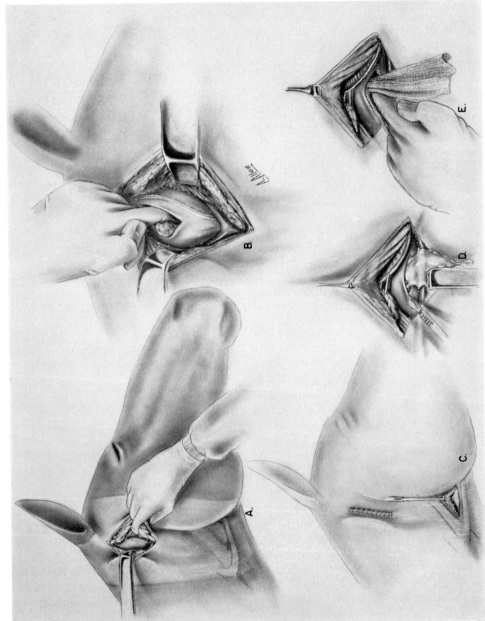

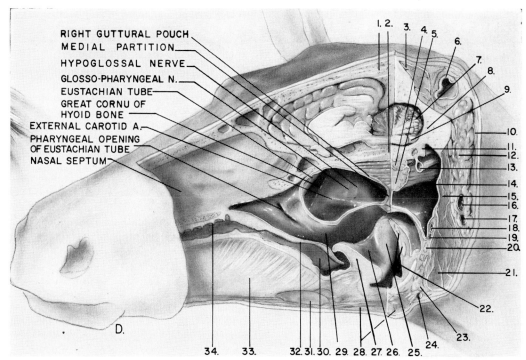

RIGHT GUTTURAL POUCH
MEDIAL PARTITION
HYPOGLOSSAL NERVE
GLOSSO-PHARYNGEAL N.
EUSTACHIAN TUBE
GREAT CORNU OF
HYOID BONE
EXTERNAL CAROTID A.
PHARYNGEAL OPENING
OF EUSTACHIAN TUBE
NASAL SEPTUM

Fig. 3. Sagittal and cross section of head showing the guttural pouches. (1) occipital bone (2) base of occipital bone (3) temporal muscle (4) rectus capitis ventralis minor (5) rectus capitis ventralis major (6) conchal cartilage (7) cerebellum (8) petrous temporal bone (9) medulla oblongata (10) parotido-auricularis muscle (11) glossopharyngeal, vagus, spinal accessory and sympathetic nerve (12) parotid gland (13) internal carotid artery (14) left guttural pouch (15) occipito-hyoideus muscle (16) jugular vein (17) maxillary vein (18) external carotid artery (19) external maxillary artery (20) pharyngeal lymph gland (21) stylo-maxillaris muscle (22) glottis (23) submaxillary salivary gland (24) submaxillary vein (25) arytenoid cartilage (26) aditus laryngis (27) epiglottis (28) omohyoideus muscle (29) pharynx (30) fauces (31) hyoglossus muscle (32) soft palate (33) genioglossus muscle (34) hard palate.

The mucous membrane lining the guttural pouches is the same as that lining the Eustachian tubes except that it is thicker and stronger. The epithelium is ciliated and pseudostratified with goblet cells. Beneath the epithelium, the propria contains smooth muscle cells, elastic fibers, lymph nodules and both serous and mucous glands. The adventitia is fibroelastic and includes vessels, nerves and adipose tissue.[3]

The guttural pouches are quite susceptible to infection introduced by way of the Eustachian tubes, usually being the aftermath of strangles or other respiratory infections. The two most important diseases of this area are empyema and tympanites.

EMPYEMA OF THE GUTTURAL POUCHES

Empyema results from an eustachitis which extends to the mucous lining of one or both of the guttural pouches. Drainage is interfered with because the orifices are situated at the upper part of the pouches and the lumina of the inflamed tubes become occluded. A mucopurulent, tenacious exudate which can develop into caseous or solid concrements, called chondroids, accumulates in the affected cavities.

A tentative diagnosis of empyema in the guttural pouch can be confirmed by passing a metal, mare catheter into the pharyngeal orifice and observing a flow of pus.

Treatment of simple empyema consists of incision and drainage in the most ventral part of Viborg's triangle, being careful not to cut into the external maxillary vein, parotid gland or its duct which parallels the ramus of the mandible. Viborg's triangle includes the area bounded by the vertical ramus of the mandible in front, the external maxillary vein below and the tendon of the sternocephalicus muscle behind and above. Another ventral approach is an incision between the sternocephalicus and the omohyoideus muscles.

If chondroids are present, a dorsal approach is necessary. Only in this manner is it possible to make a large enough incision to remove these solid concrements. This procedure requires a general anesthetic as complete relaxation is necessary to avoid injury to the auricular branch of the second cervical (posterior auricular), hypoglossal and glossopharyngeal nerves, and the carotid artery in the operative field. After the area is surgically prepared, an incision is made 3 to 4 inches in length, 1 inch anterior and parallel to the anterior border of the atlas. The posterior auricular nerve now is easily visible on the parotid gland just posterior to the parotido-auricularis muscle. It is whitish-yellow in color, ribbon-like, and the only superficial nerve in the area. The posterior border of the parotid, which is under the fascia, is freed from its attachment to the atlas, and is retracted forward and laterally. The clearly visible pouch is pierced with a blunt instrument (carefully avoiding the carotid artery which lies directly above it), opened and enlarged with the fingers and the chondroids removed. After removal of the chondroids, a ventral incision is made either through Viborg's triangle or between the sternocephalicus and the omohyoideus muscles, for drainage. The dorsal incision is closed first by suturing the guttural pouch, dropping the parotid gland into position, and then closing the fascia and skin. A gauze strip is inserted into the ventral incision to facilitate drainage, and to prevent closure of the wound. The gauze drain should be changed as often as necessary until drainage ceases (Fig. 4).

Healing will be accomplished by granulation in 2 to 4 weeks. The prognosis is favorable if the solid concrements are removed and drainage is established.

Tympanites of the Guttural Pouches

Tympanites occasionally is found in the newborn foal and in young horses up through a year of age. It is thought to result from a congenital defect or an inflammation of the Eustachian tubes. A ventral fold forming a one-way valve is the result of either disorder. Strenuous coughing and swallowing force air through the swollen tubes into the pouches from whence it cannot escape.

Respiratory difficulties usually are present a few days previous to the clinical symptoms. A unilateral or bilateral pneumatic swelling in the region of the parotids can be observed. The distended area is painless, tense, and drum-like on percussion. Stertorous breathing is characteristic and the animal may stand with its head extended, exhibiting symptoms of suffocation.

The treatment consists of opening the distended pouch ventral to the external maxillary vein. The mucous fold lying over the entrance to the Eustachian tube from the guttural pouch is located with the index finger and excised to allow the free exchange of air between the pouch and the tube. The wound is left to close by granulation.[5]

A favorable prognosis can be expected if the valve-like mucous membrane is removed successfully.

R. A. Holmes

REFERENCES

1. Sisson, S., Grossman, J. D.: The Anatomy of the Domestic Animals. 4th. ed. Philadelphia, W. B. Saunders Co. (1956).

2. Chauveau, A.: The Comparative Anatomy of the Domesticated Animals. 2nd ed. New York and London. D. Appleton and Co. (1910).

3. Trautmann, A., Fiebiger, J.: Fundamentals of the histology of domestic animals. 9th ed. Ithaca, New York, Comstock Publishing Associates. (1957).

4. Frank, E. R.: Veterinary Surgery. 6th ed. Minneapolis, Burgess Publishing Co. (1959).

5. Wirstad, H. F.: Tympanites of the guttural pouches of the horse. Nord. Vet. Med. 3 (1951) 87-101.

CHAPTER 11

DISEASES OF THE URINARY SYSTEM

URINARY CALCULI

Urinary calculi are stony precipitates found anywhere along the urinary tract. The calculi also are referred to as uroliths and the condition as urolithiasis.

Grossly, there are 2 main types of calculi which occur in the horse. One type has a rough crystalline appearance and is yellowish to brown. Its chief constituent is calcium carbonate. This type is found in horses fed largely hay or pasture grasses. The second variety is smooth and almost white. It is encountered in horses on a grain ration high in phosphorus. Calculi may vary in size from a grain of sand to the size and shape of a large cantaloupe.

VESICAL CALCULI

Although calculi may be found anywhere along the urinary tract, the bladder is the most common site in the horse. Usually only one stone is encountered (Fig. 1, 2).

Etiology: The calculi may be formed in the kidney and pass to the bladder, or they may be formed in the bladder. Several factors contribute to their formation. Smith and Jones state that "the aggregation of dispersed insoluble material into concretions depends upon the presence of particulate nuclei and upon alterations in the quantity and quality of protective colloids in the urine."[1] The aforementioned nuclei around which calculi form can be fibrin, leukocytes, whole blood, albumin, or other organic elements which are the result of infection or inflammation of some part of the urinary tract. The nucleus also may be epithelium desquamated from the urinary tract during avitaminosis A. High mineral and low water intake also play a role in urolithiasis but the conditions mentioned previously must be present before the stone will be formed.

Clinical Signs: The signs are quite variable depending on the size, nature, and location of the stone. The horse may show evidence of abdominal pain, walk with a stilted gait, trot or gallop reluctantly, and when at rest often will stand in a stretched position. Other signs include tenesmus while voiding urine, frequent attempts to urinate, and gross blood or blood clots in the urine. Blood may appear only in the last small amount of urine voided.

Diagnosis: If the clinical signs and history are indicative of a calculus, a rectal examination should be made. Intravenous promazine or epidural anesthesia often makes this examination much easier. If present, the calculus is located most easily when the bladder is empty. If the bladder is fully distended and frequent attempts at urination are being made, the neck of the bladder and urethra should be examined. In the differential diagnosis, cystitis of other origin and neoplasia of the lower urinary tract must be considered.

Treatment: Treatment consists primarily of surgical removal of the stone. In the male animal, a urethrotomy is performed with the horse preferably in a standing position after an epidural anesthetic has been administered.

The skin ventral to the anus should be thoroughly cleansed and a suitable antiseptic applied topically. A catheter is passed into the bladder so that the urethra can be located more easily. A cutaneous incision is made on the midline extending from immediately below the anal sphincter to below the ischial arch. The incision is continued through the subcutaneous tissues until the urethra is exposed. The urethra is incised sufficiently to admit a forceps for removal of the calculi. Several types of forceps are described for this operation. Frank[9] suggested the use of small animal obstetrical forceps. They are passed through the incision and into the bladder. At this point, it is best that either the surgeon or an assistant pass his hand into the rectum and guide the stone into the jaws of the forceps. After a firm grip on the stone is obtained it may be necessary to rotate it to free it from the mucous membrane. It also may be necessary to free the calculus from the mucous membrane by blunt dissection as it is brought through the urethral incision. If the calculus is large it should be crushed with a heavy forceps, and the fragments removed one at a time. When hemorrhage is profuse, the bladder should be packed with sterile gauze. This is removed in 24 hours and the bladder is irrigated with penicillin and streptomycin in normal saline. The incision in the skin and urethra is left to heal as an open wound.

In the mare, the stone often can be removed through the external urethral orifice by using suitable forceps. No incision is required.

If the calculus is extremely large or seems too deeply imbedded in the mucosa, the operator may deem it wise to perform a cystotomy. This can be done either through the flank with the horse standing or with the horse in dorsal recumbency.[8] In the latter approach, an incision is made lateral to the prepuce or mammary gland and extended obliquely toward the umbilicus. Details for laparotomy are discussed in Chapter 27. When the bladder is exposed 2 stay sutures are placed in it, and it is brought through the skin incision. An incision is made through the vertex of the bladder large enough to remove the calculus. It may be necessary to free the calculus from the mucosa by blunt dissection before it can be removed. A suction apparatus is helpful to pick up small fragments of calculi and to remove blood from the area so that the surgeon has a better view.

Following removal of the stone, 5 Gm. of dihydrostreptomycin is instilled into the lumen of the bladder. The mucosa is sutured with a single row of simple, continuous sutures using O chromic catgut, and the serosal layers are infolded with a double row of Cushing or Lembert sutures. Closure of the abdominal incision is described in Chapter 27.

Regardless of whether cystotomy or urethrotomy is performed, penicillin and streptomycin are given intramuscularly and ammonium chloride is administered orally for 4 or 5 days postoperatively.

URETHRAL CALCULUS

The signs of urethral calculi include restlessness, abdominal pain, and frequent attempts at urination. On rectal examination, the bladder is found to be distended. The stone can be located with a catheter, one made of metal being preferable. Sometimes it is possible to dislodge the calculus with the catheter, and it subsequently may be expelled. The use of smooth muscle relaxants such as Jeno-

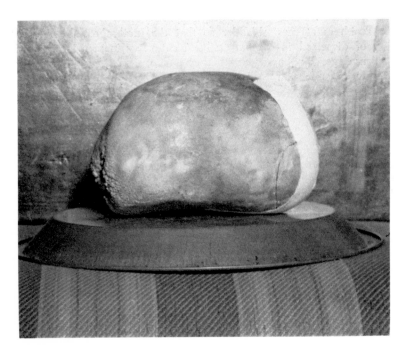

Fig. 1. Calculus removed from urinary bladder of a 17-year-old mare at necropsy. Weight — 2⅜ pounds. Size—5 x 3 x 3 inches. Courtesy of A. C. Herzberger, D.V.M.

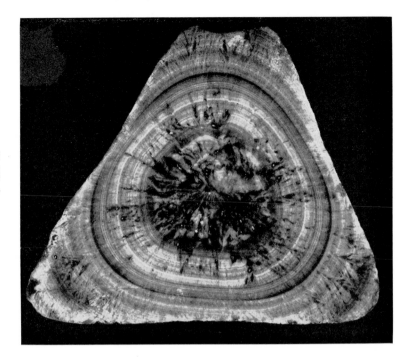

Fig. 2. Cross section of vesical calculus. Manifestation—X 1.2. Courtesy of Colorado State University.

tone (Jen-Sal) also may be helpful in allowing the stone to pass through the urethra. If these attempts fail, the horse is given an epidural anesthetic and a catheter is passed to the calculus. A midline skin incision is made directly over and down to the stone. It is removed with forceps and the incision allowed to heal as an open wound.

Nephrosis

Under the heading of nephrosis or degeneration of the kidney are included a number of pathologic processes which lead to cloudy swelling, fatty degeneration, and necrosis of the tubular epithelium. Nephrosis generally occurs secondary to a variety of disease conditions, the damage to the kidney being caused when it is exposed to toxic substances brought to it by the circulating blood.

Etiology: Chemical poisons which cause nephrosis include mercury, arsenic, copper, carbon tetrachloride, tetrachlorethylene, cantharides, iodoform, bipp, sulfas, and insecticides belonging to the chlorinated hydrocarbon group such as toxaphene. Plant poisons include those of the *Senecio* spp. Substances causing damage to the kidney and produced within the body include myoglobin liberated during the course of azoturia, products of protein destruction in extensive burns and widespread skin diseases, and toxins produced in the bowel during intestinal diseases such as impaction. The presence of icterus regardless of cause will be associated with some kidney degeneration, although there is no certainty as to whether bile pigments or other circulating agents are the cause. Bacterial toxins damage the kidneys in acute septic diseases, such as metritis.

Clinical Signs and Pathogenesis: Signs of renal disease usually are masked by those of the primary condition and treatment is directed toward the basic cause. If the patient survives, regeneration of kidney tissue is possible if necrosis has not been too extensive. In severe cases, parts of the renal parenchyma may be replaced by fibrous connective tissue, and the remaining functional tissue undergoes hypertrophy. Although there is sufficient functional tissue remaining to keep the horse alive, he will secrete large volumes of poorly concentrated urine and remain a "poor doer" for the rest of his life.

Diagnosis: Diagnosis of nephrosis often is made at necropsy but may be made on the live animal with the aid of a urinalysis. In nephrosis the albumin content of urine is increased, and hyaline or granular casts often are present. At necropsy, which should be done early to avoid postmortem autolysis, large, pale kidneys are observed. The paleness, often almost white, is caused by fat, necrotic cells, and the fact that increased internal pressure has expelled much of the blood from the renal vessels. Microscopic changes include cloudy swelling, fatty degeneration, and necrosis of the epithelial cells lining the tubules. In azoturia, some renal tubules are filled with brownish pigment.

R. G. ROLOFSON

REFERENCES

1. Smith, H. A. and Jones, T. C.: Veterinary Pathology. Lea and Febiger, Philadelphia, Pa. 793-795, 651-654. 1957.
2. Hutyra, F.; Marek, J.; and Manninger, R.: Special Pathology and Therapeutics of the Diseases of Domestic Animals. Alexander Eger, Inc., Chicago, Ill., p. 14-16, 1949.
3. Nicholson, J. A.: Lander's Veterinary Toxicology. Alexander Eger, Inc., Chicago, Ill., pp. 36, 55, 59, 153. 1947.
4. Puntriano, G. O.: Urinary calculi in livestock. J.A.V.M.A. 124 (1954) 55-61.
5. Swingle, K. F.: The chemical composition of urinary calculi from range steers. Am. J. Vet. Research 14 (1953) 493-498.
6. Marsh: The relation of limited water consumption to the incidence of urinary calculi in steers. Am. J. Vet. Research 14 (1953) 16-18.
7. Smith, H. A. and Jones, T. C.: Veterinary Pathology, Lea and Febiger, Philadelphia, Pa., p. 807-810, 1957.
8. Usenik, E. A., Larson, L. L. and Saver, F.: Cystotomy and removal of a urolith in a Shetland mare. J.A.V.M.A. 128 (1956) 453.
9. Frank, E. R.: Veterinary Surgery Notes. Burgess Publishing Co., Minneapolis, Minn., p. 240-41. 1947.
10. Law, James and Shahan, M. S.: Special Report on Diseases of the Horse. Washington, D. C., United States Government Printing Office, p. 115-143, 1942.
11. Herzberger, A. C.: Personal communication.

CHAPTER 12

DISEASES OF THE ENDOCRINE SYSTEM

INTRODUCTION

Very few records exist concerning the occurrence of organic or functional endocrine abnormalities in the horse, and the number of different endocrine conditions encountered by veterinarians of long experience in horse practice is small. They include the disorder termed "dry-coat," seen in race horses in certain tropical countries, and sexual disturbances related to ovarian disorders which are observed fairly frequently in mares. Goiter, common among human beings and many other animals throughout the world, appears to affect the horse very rarely, and pancreatic dysfunction, as evidenced by the occurrence of diabetes mellitus, does not appear to have been recorded in the horse.

Anhidrosis (Dry-coat)

This condition in horses is characterized by the loss of ability to sweat. It has been observed in horses imported to hot, humid countries from those possessing drier and more temperate climates. Anhidrosis has occurred in Australian and British Thoroughbreds, principally among those located in coastal areas of Malaya, India, Ceylon, the Philippines, the West Indies, and Indonesia. It is seen rarely in South Africa and Australia, and does not often make its appearance in horses born and reared in the countries in which "dry-coat" affects imported animals.

When anhidrotic animals are removed to cooler and drier climates they automatically recover within a few weeks. No predisposition related to sex or color has been noticed but high-strung or nervous animals appear more susceptible.

The secretion of sweat in the horse is under the control of secretory nerve fibers which leave the spinal cord as part of the sympathetic system and communicate with the sweat centers in the central nervous system. The sweat centers are stimulated by impulses transmitted from the skin during heat stimulation, by an increase in the temperature of the blood circulating through the sweat centers, by an increased carbon dioxide (hydrogen ion) concentration in the blood, or by psychic disturbances such as fear or stress. Pilocarpine, injected subcutaneously, causes sweating which is antagonized by injection of atropine. Epinephrine also is effective in producing sweating in the horse, an indication that the sympathetic fibers to the equine sweat glands are adrenergic.

In the horse, the sweat glands are tubular and their secretory portions often are coiled into spirals or balls, which lie in the dermis at the bases of hair follicles. The excretory ducts open into the orifices of the hair follicles near the skin surface. All the sweat glands of the horse are associated with hair follicles and are regarded as apocrine glands which secrete a necrobiotic discharge of secretory cytoplasm.

Etiology: In anhidrosis of horses it has been found that approximately 10% of sweat gland ducts are blocked by plugs of keratin at their orifices. The ducts also may be occluded by homogenous material derived from sweat mixed with phagocytic cells. In other instances, casts composed of desquamated epithelial cells are present in the distended ducts.

It appears unlikely, however, that occlusion of so small a percentage of ducts should bring about cessation of sweating, and it seems more likely that duct occlusion is the result of anhidrosis rather than its cause. Attention has been drawn to the part which the suprarenal glands may play in the production of "dry-coat," and the part which these glands play in the physiology of sweating. Circumscribed areas of skin may be rendered anhidrotic by repeated intradermal injections of epinephrine. The sweat glands in areas thus treated are similar histologically to those removed by skin biopsies from horses which have developed anhidrosis.

The experiments which involved repeated injections in the same area of skin with epinephrine have led to the belief that sweat glands become refractory to increases in circulating adrenalin which would be sufficient to cause profuse sweating in normal, untreated animals. This acquired tolerance may explain why most of the sweat glands appear to be morphologically normal but functionally inactive.

Clinical Signs: The condition of anhidrosis is preceded by excessive sweating, increased pulse rate, and abnormal "blowing" after exercise, although the same signs may be shown by a horse at rest in the stable. In affected horses, the nostrils may be constantly dilated. A few horses eventually become acclimatized and, after showing transient signs, recover and proceed thereafter to sweat normally. Others, however, sweat only beneath the jaws, along the neck, and at the base of the ears, between the hindlimbs, and under the saddle. It should be remembered that few horses, when normal, sweat from the skin of the limbs and certainly never below knees and hocks— the sweat seen running down the limbs comes from sweat glands higher on the body.

The onset of signs of "dry-coat" in horses in Malaya often is very gradual and the state of anhidrosis may remain only partial; the animals continue to sweat along their manes. The areas where the skin is firmly adherent to underlying tissues, such as over the rump and gluteal muscles, remain dry, giving a patchy appearance after exercise. In advanced cases, the skin becomes scurfy and there is a tendency to lose hair. Such animals are useless for racing and if subjected to severe exertion may die from cardiac failure. In these advanced cases, there is loss of condition, elevated blood pressure, and a very rapid pulse. The body temperature may be raised little while the horse is at rest but after exercise it may reach 105 to 108 F.

Polyuria always is present as compensation for lack of sweating. The urine often contains albumin and casts. After exercise, the rise in temperature may persist for several hours. Horses which fail to sweat at exercise, may break out in sweat in the stable as long as an hour later. Such horses eventually become completely anhidrotic. A similar delayed sweating is quite common in normal horses in temperate climates.

Pathogenesis: The regulation of body temperature normally is controlled by thermoregulators situated in the hypothalamus. The intravenous injection of 0.5 to 1.0 mg. of epinephrine causes profuse sweating in normal horses in temperate latitudes. Exercise and excitement liberate epinephrine from the adrenal glands and result in increased sweating along with other actions. It is probable that the heat centers in the hypothalamus are determined genetically to maintain a normal, steady temperature and that acclimatization requires a new adjustment. In certain horses, the sweat glands may accommodate to a raised epinephrine level and cease to respond unless the high level is maintained. There also may be failure of reserves in the adrenal medulla, a restriction of peripheral circulation, and degeneration of sweat glands with occlusion of some sweat ducts. It was observed in Malaya that dry-coated horses showed less response to adrenalin injection than free sweaters although none failed to show some evidence of response. The adrenalin content of equine blood in Malaya was found to be higher than that in horses during summer conditions in England.

Treatment: The only treatment of value has been removal of affected horses to a cooler climate, but good results were sometimes obtained by air conditioning and cooling of stables. This, however, is not always possible or economic. Maqsood described anhidrosis in race horses and Tonga ponies in Lahore, Pakistan, and stated that horses developed the condition during the summer but that it persisted through the winter months. It was observed that the administration of 10 to 15 Gm. of iodinated casein (Protamone) for a period of 4 to 8 days cured the affected animals. The condition was attributed to endocrine disturbance of the heat-regulating mechanism caused by overwork. This suggests that the thyroid may play some obscure part in the process.

Anhidrosis has been treated with alpha tocopherol in conjunction with other treatments.[5] Animals also have been treated under ordinary stable conditions. Alpha tocopherol administered orally at a level of between 1000 and 3000 units daily for one month has given beneficial effects. The amount required varies with the animal and the stage of the disease. The first observable effect is the absence of labored breathing and dilated nostrils. The coat is gradually replaced, the new hair is bright, and the skin becomes smooth and pliable. Sweating commences on the neck and around the anus at first, and as recovery proceeds, appears between the hindlimbs and in the flank and saddle regions. The effectiveness of alpha tocopherol is directly connected with the type of management employed. Best results are obtained when the drug is used together with air conditioning and the worst with ordinary stable conditions. The treatment has had approximately 90% success when used with all types of management.

REFERENCES

1. Dukes: The Physiology of Domestic Animals, Comstock Publishing Associates, Ithaca, N. Y., 1955.
2. Evans, C. Lovatt; Ross, K. A.; Smith, D. F. G.; and Weil-Malherbe, H.: Vet. Rec. 69 (1957) 1-9. Comp. Path. 67 (1957) 397-404.
3. Maqsood, M.: Vet. Rec. 68 (1956) 475.
4. Maqsood, M.: Proc. 9th Pakistan Sci. Conf. Peshawar, Part III, (1957) 123.
5. Marsh, J. H. Treatment of 'dry coat' in Thoroughbreds. Vet. Rec. 73 (1961) 1124.

NYMPHOMANIA IN THE MARE

Mares, unless they have become pregnant, normally come into season at regular intervals during the sunny, light months of the year and remain more or less sexually quiescent during the remaining period. Not uncommonly, however, mares remain in constant estrus throughout the year, or they may behave in this way intermittently throughout the winter. Their behavior includes flashing the clitoris, passing jets of urine, kicking, squealing, and exhibiting bad temper. Although such behavior often is ascribed to cystic ovaries, it is unusual to find these when one makes a rectal examination. An apparently normal follicle may be present, but when one follows these cases by regular examinations it usually becomes evident that the follicular rupture is not followed by the formation of a corpus luteum. The structure is not raised above the surface of the ovary, or only slightly so for 3 to 5 days, and then is replaced by a cavity, which feels like foam rubber on palpation. Another follicle will then make its appearance and rupture, and the process may be repeated indefinitely. The often described cystic ovaries of large or enormous size are rarities. The real cause appears to be absence of luteinization.

In hunters and mares used for hacking, the subcutaneous injection of gonadotrophic luteinizing hormone sometimes produces temporary amelioration of the signs, and in mild cases may be sufficient. It must be remembered however, that mares which behave in this way are never really "cured." In marked cases of persistent nymphomania, ovariectomy is the only remedy. Whether the adrenal glands also are involved, or whether the abnormal behavior once established is not easily forgotten, is uncertain, but the fact remains that some mares, especially those which for years have been the victims of their own hormones, show only temporary improvement or none at all after the ovariectomy.

INTERSEX

Von F. Freudenberg reported on the genital organs of a female foal born partner to a male twin. The defects of the female included intersexuality due to hormonal influence. The placenta could not be examined, thus the existence of vascular anastomosis was not proved.

REFERENCE

1. Von F. Freudenberg: Dtsch. tierärztl. Wschr. 67 (1960) 214-216.

ENDEMIC GOITER

Endemic goiter appears to be an exceptionally rare condition in the horse. The Handbook of the Chilean Iodine Educational Bureau lists 1,014 references to reports on goiter from all over the world, and although farm animals, dogs, and rats are mentioned several times, there is no reference to goiter in the horse. Michi described the use of insulin therapy in general unthriftiness (thought to be due to hyperthyroidism) in a race horse. Pantic and Jovanovic have described cases of chronic thyroiditis in a dog and a horse. In 50 years' experience I have met with only one case of thyroid abnormality but this was not true goiter. The horse was a gray Shire stallion and the left thyroid was invaded by a melanotic neo-plasm. During life, no signs of thyroid disturbance were manifested.

R. H. Smythe

REFERENCES

1. Michi, V.: Profilassi **28** (1955) 150-154.
2. Pantic, V. and Jovanovic, M.: Acta. vet. Belgrade **6** (1956) 101-105.

CHAPTER 13

DISEASES OF THE SKIN

NONINFECTIOUS DERMATITIS

Eczema

Dermatitis usually is defined as an inflammation of the skin affecting both the superficial and deep layers. Eczema is classified as a catarrhal dermatitis affecting the epidermis, or superficial layer of the skin. Eczema varies from dermatitis in degree of severity as well as in the parts of the skin affected. When the deeper layers are involved, the epidermis may suffer secondarily. A rigid classification of noninfectious dermatitis cannot be held because in dermatitis resulting from trauma or exposure to chemicals, heat or irradiation, both the superficial and deep structures of the skin are affected primarily. For practical purposes, equine eczema can be considered a mild form of dermatitis.

Eczema is characterized by superficial inflammation, in many cases resembling a catarrhal dermatitis. Not all cases of eczema, however, are characterized by a moist catarrhal exudation. The lesions that become subacute or chronic frequently are dry and scaly.

Etiology: The cause of eczema frequently is undetermined and may be complex. Horses fed poor diets, especially in the winter months, may develop a dry, scaly skin and loss of hair over the most seriously affected areas. These animals often are kept in dark, dirty, and damp quarters which contribute to the etiology. In some cases, itching and consequent rubbing change the appearance of the early lesions. Horses suffering from malnutrition have a dry, scaly skin that loses its elasticity. They fail to shed hair normally in the spring and present a rough, shaggy appearance. Whether equines are affected to any extent with eczema due to avitaminoses or hormonal imbalances is not clearly established. The vitamin requirements of horses are easily satisfied and when lacking, the problem is general malnutrition rather than a specific vitamin deficiency. Hormonal imbalance may cause eczema in mares but this is rare.

Eczema due to allergy is not common in equines. Horses occasionally suffer from food rashes. When pastured on clover they sometimes salivate excessively and develop eczematous lesions around the mouth, and on the skin of the neck and breast. This has occurred on red clover, *Trifolium pratense*, pasture. Horses pastured on alsike clover, *Trifolium hybridum*, have in mild cases developed redness and moderate swelling of unpigmented parts of the skin of the face and legs. This condition is a form of photosensitization and in severe cases, necrosis of the skin develops (see Chapter 19). Horses that are heavily infected with ascarids or strongyles frequently fail to shed with the advent of warm weather and are afflicted with eczema.

Leather preservatives, gasoline or raw linseed oil used on the harness or saddle may produce a harness or saddle eczema in some animals.

Other forms of equine eczema include summer eczema which disappears during the colder months but returns again during hot weather. This condition in some cases apparently is a consequence of excessive sweating and poor care of the skin. An eczema called "scratches" usually is associated with exposure to mud and filth, and involves the heels and fetlock areas. When the condition is sufficiently aggravated and becomes chronic, inflammation occurs and the condition is referred to as "grease heel."

A chronic eczema of unknown etiology characterized by a dry, scaly skin is not uncommon in horses (Fig. 1). In chronic eczema the long-haired parts—the mane and tail—are affected. Eczema at the base of the tail is manifested by a dry, rough skin and loss of hair due to rubbing. Tail rubbing has been considered a sign of rectal irritation due to oxyuriasis but it occurs independent of parasitism. Eczema of the tail is observed frequently in horses whose tails are bandaged and kept in a tail-set for long periods.

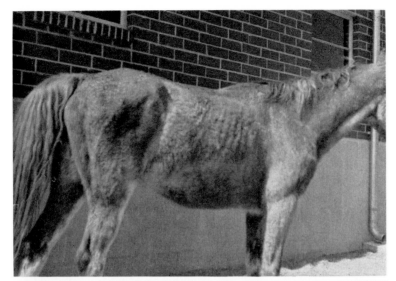

Fig. 1. Chronic eczema with lesions distributed widely over the body.

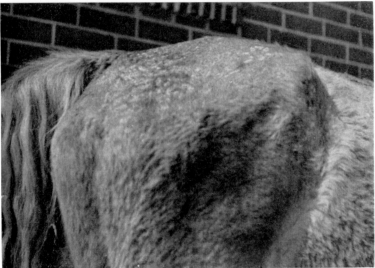

An occasional case of seborrheic eczema due to a functional disorder of the sebaceous glands is encountered. The disease usually is characterized in horses by the formation of fatty crusts over the back and sides of the body. The disease occurs most frequently in the cold months of the year when the hair is long. The skin generally is dry and is covered with excessive dandruff. The lesions are round or oval areas of crusted material and resemble a fungus infection. Microscopic examinations and cultures of material from these lesions fail to reveal a specific etiology.

Chronic eczema of equines resulting from inadequate feeding and poor care of the skin is observed in old, debilitated animals (Fig. 2). Lesions may be diffuse over the sides of the neck and chest or they may appear in patches well-distributed over the body. The affected areas are scaly, crusted, thickened, and denuded.

DERMATITIS

Dermatitis is an inflammation of both the deep and superficial cutaneous layers and is

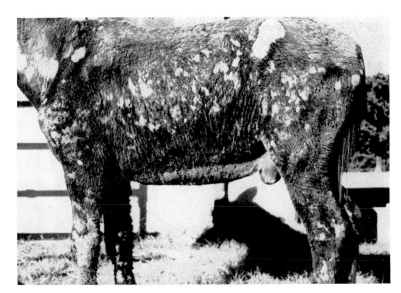

Fig. 2. Chronic eczema in a debilitated mule.

characterized by hyperemia, exudation, proliferative changes in vascular tissue, and even by necrosis in some cases. In addition to infectious causes, dermatitis may be due to trauma, chemical irritation, thermic causes, and irradiation.

Etiology: The cutaneous regions most subject to trauma are over the hip, the supraorbital region, the outer hock, and the carpal and elbow regions. Decubital injuries are included in this classification. In work horses, dermatitis is produced by harness friction or by pressure from an ill-fitting collar. A variety of lesions may be produced by collar pressure. Saddle pressure causes dermatitis and necrosis when the saddle or a saddle blanket or pad is not properly adjusted.

Dermatitis may develop subsequent to close clipping of hair of the fetlock region. A chronic dermatitis above the coronary region of the front feet may result from continued use of training chains placed around the phalangeal region to induce the horse to step higher. Dermatitis of the extremities also is caused by constant exposure to filth and mud.

A wide variety of chemical irritants is responsible for various degrees of dermatitis. Toxic dermatitis occurs more readily in fine-skinned horses. Escharotics applied on granulating wounds when carried by secretions may produce a severe dermatitis below the wound unless the skin is protected. Wound secretions themselves induce a "scalding" form of dermatitis. Hoof treatments or dressings used for the treatment of thrush or other hoof infections may cause dermatitis below the fetlock when carelessly applied. Preparations containing formalin and tar are especially dangerous. Kerosene and many oil insecticides will blister the skin of horses. A scaly dermatitis with hyperkeratosis may develop from continued contact with stall boards freshly treated with wood preservatives.

Thermic causes include freezing and burns. Though equines are not particularly subject to frostbite, dermatitis due to freezing may occur around the muzzle, the tips of the ears, and the tender cutaneous areas of animals kept in damp, unventilated stables during subzero weather. More common is dermatitis of the fetlock and coronary region in animals working or being ridden for long periods in snow and freezing weather. Such dermatitis frequently is associated with poor grooming practices.

Burns occur in horses exposed to stable or barn fires. Burns usually are found over the head, back, and rump and they are characterized by edema, blistering, exudation of serum, and subsequent necrosis.

The effects of solar irradiation would not be noticeable clinically in equines kept under normal conditions. Sunburn usually does not occur in horses due to the protection of hair and pigmented skin. In animals having white cutaneous areas, apparent sunburn almost always is due to a mild form of photosensitization.

Damage of the skin due to atomic irradiation has been produced experimentally, and it also occurred in horses exposed in Hiroshima, Japan, in 1945. Animals in the near vicinity of an atomic explosion suffer a high mortality. One-third of the deaths may be due to flash and thermal burns. Further from the explosion, animals will suffer burns that lead to depigmentation and epilation. A chronic thickening of the skin may develop.

X-ray damage to the skin of horses has been infrequent. The amount of exposure necessary for diagnostic purposes is not sufficient to produce radiodermatitis. With the probable increase in x-ray therapy of animals, the possibility of dermatitis due to overexposure likely will increase. Only the veterinarian thoroughly trained in radiology should practice x-ray therapy.

Treatment: Before therapy is attempted the diagnosis of eczema or more severe dermatitis should be confirmed. A history which reveals the etiology enables the clinician to make a positive diagnosis in many cases. In cases of traumatic injury and burns the cause often is evident. Of primary importance is the differentiation of dermatitis due to ectoparasites and bacterial or fungus infections. In all cases of dermatitis of doubtful diagnosis, skin scrapings should be submitted for laboratory examination.

The first objective in the therapy of dermatitis is removal of all known and possible causes. An adequate diet should be provided and when possible, access to good pasture is essential. The addition of vitamin and mineral preparations to diets is beneficial in the correction of skin conditions even when the ration apparently is adequate.

Arsenical solutions have long been used on an empiric basis for therapy of skin diseases. Fowler's solution, a solution of potassium arsenite, administered orally in 1-ounce doses 3 times daily, will aid in the recovery of many cases of eczema. The intravenous injection of 4.5 Gm. of neoarsphenamine well-diluted in water seems beneficial in many cases. Iodine may be prescribed for intervals of 10 days in the forms of potassium iodide or organic iodides.

When allergic dermatitis is suspected, antihistamines are indicated but the results are hard to evaluate. In all forms of dermatitis, rational treatment includes the use of cortisone or ACTH. An old remedy reported to be of value in some cases of dermatitis is the injection of 80 to 100 ml. of the patient's own blood intramuscularly.

The extent to which topical treatment is indicated depends upon the area involved and the character of the lesions. When lesions are extensive, the entire body should be clipped of hair. Even when lesions are confined to certain areas of the body, clipping may reveal them to be more extensive than realized. Areas of local dermatitis also should be clipped. Washing of the skin is indicated when there is an accumulation of scales, crusts or sebaceous material. Green soap and warm water exert a good influence on many lesions. The washing of dry, eczematous skin with a 2% creolin solution in warm water has a stimulating effect in some cases. The most reliable treatment for many cases of dermatitis is the application of a 2% aqueous solution of lime-sulphur. The chemical is dissolved in hot water and applied thoroughly with a stiff brush. When lesions are extensive only one-half of the body should be treated on alternate days. When the skin is dry and scaly, grooming with a stiff brush favors the healing process.

Treatment of certain forms of dermatitis requires more specific remedies. When areas of the skin are burned, liberal application of carron oil is indicated. Carron oil can be made by mixing linseed oil, cottonseed oil or olive oil with lime water in equal proportions. When moist lesions are present in dermatitis, the application of 5% tannic and salicylic acids in alcohol is indicated. This treatment is followed by the application of zinc oxide ointment or 10% ichthammol ointment or a combination of both. Skin lesions around the fetlock or "scratches," respond to cleaning with 70% alcohol or alcoholic sublimate solution and the subsequent application of astringent ointments or solutions. Either zinc oxide or 10% ichthammol ointments are beneficial as is lead acetate solution.

When secondary bacterial infection is present, an alcoholic sublimate pack may be indicated. A useful remedy in acute dermatitis is prepared as follows: Zinc oxide powder is added to a gallon of cottonseed oil until it is a thick, creamy mixture. Then 5% scarlet red in oil (scarlet oil) is added until the mixture has a bright pink color. This mixture promotes healing and seems to be insect-repelling. In chronic dermatitis, 1 part Lugol's solution in 3 parts glycerin is a good medicament for topical application. The use of 5% silver nitrate solution also is useful in chronic cases.

When chronic, productive lesions are present the use of a caustic such as silver nitrate, or actual cautery may be necessary. Eczematous lesions at the base of the tail are best treated with ointments that promote healing and relieve the pruritus. Bacon fat has been advocated by some horsemen and actually seems to be of benefit. Prevention of tail rubbing by the use of wall-boards may be necessary to prevent secondary lesions and loss of hair.

W. J. GIBBONS

REFERENCES

1. Fröhner, E.: Lehrbuch der Toxicologie, ed. 3, 347. (1910) 347. (quoted by Udall, 2).
2. Udall, D. H.: The Practice of Veterinary Medicine, Ithaca, N.Y. Published by the author. 1954.
3. Kral, R. and Novak, B. J.: Veterinary Dermatology, J. B. Lippincott Co., Philadelphia, Pa., 1953.

GREASE HEEL (MUD FEVER, CRACKED HEELS)

Grease heel is primarily a dermatitis of the posterior aspect of the pastern and of the heel. The hindfeet are affected most often.

Etiology: This condition usually is the result of inflammation and infection caused by constant wetting of the area, and is most common in breeds having long hair about the pastern and fetlock region. Improper shoeing which causes a folding of the skin of the posterior face of the pastern may produce sufficient irritation to allow the disease to begin. Chronic "stocking" may predispose or cause the condition. Chemical irritants such as soap, lime dust from floors or roads, salt solutions, or other substances such as irritating liniments may produce a dermatitis sufficient to begin the process. Allergic reactions, such as photosensitization caused by certain chemicals or plants, and contact dermatitis from plants such as poison ivy and certain clovers may produce the dermatitis. Secondary infection with a variety of bacteria and fungi usually occurs as the dermatitis persists.

Clinical Signs: The process often begins at the periople of the heel or in the skin of the posterior aspect of the pastern. At the outset, there is an inflammation of the superficial layers of the skin. At this stage, lameness is not exhibited. The dermatitis gradually becomes more severe, the involved area exhibits heat, swelling, and some lameness. Serum then begins to exude from the affected area. The skin becomes encrusted with dried serum, and the hair at the cleft of the heel and on the posterior aspect of the pastern becomes erect. Edema and lymphangitis may develop and extend for varying distances up the affected leg or legs. Skin fissures then appear on the posterior face of the pastern. The whole area often becomes wet and encrusted with serous exudate. Necrosis and ulceration of the skin occur and secondary bacterial and fungal infections produce a pronounced fetid odor. Proliferation of the subcutaneous connective tissue begins, and the pastern area especially is involved.

Later, granulations may appear in the skin fissures or the ulcerated areas, sometimes becoming pedunculated. The granulations bleed easily and their surface often is necrotic. The skin granulations and the subcutaneous connective tissue proliferations have a tendency to circumscribe the pastern with considerable enlargement of the part. Infection and inflammation of the hair follicles, of the entire thickness of the skin, and of the subcutaneous tissues result. The infection may extend into the cleft of the frog and may even undermine the frog and sole, occasionally with granulations being present under the horn.

Treatment: The treatment varies with the cause and the extent of the disease process. In all cases, the exciting cause should be removed. Early cases, in which only the superficial layers of the skin are affected, will respond to clipping the long hair, careful cleansing, removal of any loose periople, drying, and the application of a mildly antiseptic and astringent emollient. The area should be protected from further irritation. The use of astringent solutions for several days, followed by ointments to prevent excessive drying and further fissuring of the skin generally is preferred. Petrolatum products should be used with caution, as they may produce a dermatitis in certain animals. Zinc oxide ointment, lanolin, and scarlet oil often are used as protective ointments. Fungicidal ointments may be indicated if a mycosis is suspected.

If the infection extends into the periople of the heel, the frog or the sole, it will be necessary to remove the loose horn down to healthy tissue to permit effective treatment. An astringent pack usually is bandaged over the affected area for several days in such cases, and ½% formalin is suitable since it tends to dry and toughen tissues in addition to having bacteriostatic and fungicidal properties.

In its chronic form, grease heel is characterized by exuberant granulations. This form of the disease is treated in various ways depending upon the character and extent of the granulations. If they are not excessive in size, pressure bandages, with or without use of stronger astringents, may be effective. The larger granulations may be removed surgically, by cautery or by the application of caustics. These procedures usually are followed by the use of astringent dressings under pressure packs to prevent recurrence. Ointments should be avoided until the surface remains dry.

R. L. LUNDVALL

CHAPTER 14

DISEASES OF THE NERVOUS SYSTEM

INTRODUCTION

Paucity of knowledge of neuroanatomy and neurophysiology discourages many veterinarians in large animal practice from attempting to make specific diagnoses of the less common neurologic disturbances. With a reasonable knowledge of the anatomy and function of the central nervous system, it is often possible to locate neurologic lesions more exactly than lesions involving other systems. Probably more failures in neurologic diagnosis arise from the lack of careful clinical examination and the application of basic information than from lack of detailed knowledge.

Nervous disorders of horses are caused by a variety of conditions which include developmental defects, infectious agents, toxic disorders, trauma, deficiency diseases, disturbances in circulation, and neoplasms. In some disorders, the cause(s) have not been determined. Often neurologic manifestations are observed following the occurrence of clinical signs related to other systems. Though space does not permit a detailed discussion, some of the factors influencing the resistance or the vulnerability of the nervous system to disease will be discussed.

The brain and spinal cord are well-protected by coverings which aid in shielding them from injury. The bony calvarium and vertebral column maintain relatively constant support for the nervous tissue within their confines, and afford good protection against moderate external violence. The pia-glia membrane covering the blood vessels which supply the central nervous system provides additional protection from infection carried by the circulatory system. This blood-brain barrier also has the function of selective permeability, and it protects the nervous system from gross variations of the body environment as well as prevents access of many undesirable substances.

Defects in this protective mechanism are apparent, however. Through the upper air passages, infections may gain direct entrance through the cribriform plate, or indirect entrance by retrograde thrombosis of the cortical veins, and by direct extension from the frontal, sphenoidal or ethmoidal sinuses. Direct routes of infection also may follow the optic nerve or enter through the inner ear. Once the infection reaches the cerebrospinal fluid, it may spread very easily as one portion of the subarachnoid space communicates freely with all others.

The blood-brain barrier also poses a problem in the treatment of infections of the central nervous system since many of the drugs fail to penetrate this membrane readily. On the other hand, some toxic substances pass through the pia-glia membrane very easily and affect components of the nervous system without causing demonstrable changes in other tissues. Also, certain neurotrophic bacteria or viruses apparently have the ability to destroy this barrier by ischemic degeneration.

DEVELOPMENTAL DEFECTS OF THE NERVOUS SYSTEM

Malformations involving the nervous system are reported less frequently in horses than in other classes of livestock. In only a few instances have these defects been concluded to be hereditary in origin. More often they are the consequence of various noxious, physical, and/or chemical stimuli adversely affecting the developing embryo.

CONGENITAL HYDROCEPHALUS

Congenital hydrocephalus is characterized by an increased quantity of cerebrospinal fluid within the cranial cavity. Varying degrees of cranial distention usually are apparent at birth, and in well-marked cases the fontanelles are very large, with the skin stretched tightly over the widely separated frontal and parietal bones (Fig. 1). The degree of involvement may be so severe that destructive craniotomy or cesarean section must be performed before the foal can be delivered. In other instances, little or no enlargement of the skull is evident, and diagnosis is made on the basis of the clinical signs. Radiographs of the skull may demonstrate an increased size in the cranial vault as compared to the facial bones, and the walls of the cranium are observed to be thinner than normal.

Etiology: The pathologic changes causing hydrocephalus may be varied, and they often are difficult to demonstrate. Hydrocephalus generally is considered to result from obstruction or lack of patency of some of the small drainage structures of cerebrospinal fluid near the site of its formation by the choroid plexus in the lateral and third ventricles of the brain. The points of obstruction may be the interventricular foramen (of Monroe), the aqueduct of Sylvius, or the foramina of Magendie or Luschka. Also the septum pellucidum may be improperly formed, allowing the unsupported fornix to sag and act as a valve to obstruct the interventricular foramen. With any of these conditions, the ventricles anterior to the obstruction are greatly distended with fluid. The cerebral cortex eventually is compressed to a thin layer of nerve tissue around the ventricles.

In external or communicating hydrocephalus, increased cerebrospinal fluid results from interference of absorption somewhere along the course of subarachnoid drainage, or it may result from rupture of the thin dorsal wall of the third ventricle. In external hydrocephalus, pressure atrophy proceeds from the exterior of the brain.

The clinical signs usually progress in severity due to increase in the intracranial pressure. The brain is forced posteriorly into the foramen magnum and against the incisura cerebelli, further obstructing the flow of cerebrospinal fluid into the subarachnoid villi or the spinal canal.

Clinical Signs: Signs of hydrocephalus vary with the degree of cerebral atrophy. In advanced cases, the foal usually is stillborn or dies shortly after birth. With less severe involvement, the foal generally is unable to stand, but may nurse if given the opportunity. Since the vital centers are located in the midbrain and hindbrain, some foals may live for several days with a marked reduction of cerebral tissue. In mild cases of hydrocephalus, the foal usually appears lethargic and at times is unsteady on its feet. Sometimes while walking, the foal may suddenly appear very drowsy and begin to stagger, carry the head low to the ground, but react to external stimuli. Though most cases become progressively worse, spontaneous arrestment may occur and

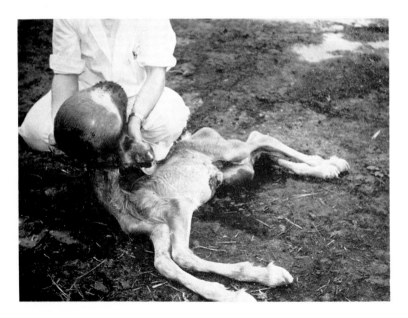

Fig. 1. Congenital hydrocephalus.

the condition may remain unchanged for some time.

No reports of effective therapy for congenital hydrocephalus have been found in the veterinary literature. Euthanasia generally is prescribed.

Cerebellar Hypoplasia

Cerebellar hypoplasia has been reported in the horse. The occurrence of bilateral symmetrical defects in the lateral hemispheres of the cerebellum has been described; this horse had fallen backward several times while being trained as a jumper. No other abnormalities of gait had been observed by the owner prior to a fatal injury incurred in a fall.

The Epilepsies

Etiology: True, or idiopathic, epilepsy occurs without a demonstrable cause and often is classified as a developmental disorder. The role of heredity in this defect has not been clarified completely. Symptomatic epilepsies are due to a demonstrable disease process. It should be emphasized that the seizures are indistinguishable from those observed in true epilepsy. The conditions causing symptomatic epilepsy may be inflammatory, traumatic, metabolic, toxic, vascular, neoplastic, or degenerative disorders of the brain.

Clinical Signs: Epilepsies generally are characterized by recurrent, sudden and usually brief disturbances of consciousness, with or without tonic-clonic convulsions. Some forms of epilepsy cause paroxysms of nonpurposive movements without loss of consciousness. Frequency and severity of attacks vary greatly from animal to animal. Classification is based on the nature of the seizures and not on the cause.

Grand mal or severe epileptic attacks are characterized by many of the following signs. The horse suddenly appears to be in great distress and has a dazed expression, the respirations increase in depth, and the nostrils are flared. The animal then becomes unsteady on its feet and falls to the ground in a state of semiconsciousness. Immediately, all the skeletal muscles are tensed in tonic spasms, and the nictitating membrane covers the eye. Breathing is arrested for a few moments due to tonic spasm of the diaphragm, and the mucous membranes become cyanotic. Peripheral veins are engorged by the severe muscular contractions. When it appears that the animal is near death from asphyxia, the tonic spasms cease and clonic movements begin as the breathing becomes deep and labored. As the tonic movements continue, the muscular contractions become stronger but less frequent, until they cease altogether. Twitching of the facial muscles and ears, masticatory movements, grinding of the teeth, and foaming of the mouth may occur during the course of the seizure. The head may be pulled to one side, and the eyes are rotated backward. The pupils are dilated, and reflexes (including the corneal) are abolished. The sphincter muscles are relaxed and involuntary elimination of urine and feces is common. The duration of the attack may vary from 1 to 30 minutes, or longer. Some horses recover immediately at the end of the seizure, but others exhibit lassitude or muscular weakness for several hours.

Petit mal or mild epileptic attacks are much less dramatic than the grand mal syndrome and may be difficult to differentiate from fainting. The horse may show a sudden impairment or loss of consciousness with little or no tonic or clonic movements. There may be immobility with a staring expression during which there seems to be a loss of contact with the environment.

Jacksonian epilepsy is characterized by a focal involvement always of the same group of muscles and a "march" of the spasms to other muscles on that side of the body. Consciousness is not impaired unless the opposite half of the body is involved. This form of epilepsy generally is associated with organic brain disease.

Treatment: Treatment of symptomatic epilepsy should be directed toward elimination of the basic disease process. During a major attack, efforts should be made to prevent the animal from injuring itself, and if the seizure is prolonged chloral hydrate or other sedatives should be administered intravenously. Bromides or barbiturates have been used to prevent recurrent attacks (20 to 50 Gm. daily of equal parts of sodium bromide, potassium bromide, and ammonium bromide). The horse should be placed in a well-bedded stall and care exercised to prevent external stimuli from precipitating a seizure. Elimination of parasites and attention to the general health of the animal must be included in the therapy. Nothing more than control of the signs can be expected in true epilepsy. Severe seizures in young animals are indicative of a hopeless condition.

TRAUMA OF THE CENTRAL NERVOUS SYSTEM

Injuries of the brain or spinal cord of the horse may accompany various accidents in which direct or indirect forces impinge on the skull or vertebral column. Kicks or blows to the head, running against solid objects, falling forward on the head or neck, and falling over backward are examples of direct forces which may cause injury to the central nervous system.

It is common for lesions of the brain or spinal cord caused by indirect forces to be located some distance from the point of impact. For example, an accident in which the horse falls forward with the chin striking the ground may transmit force through the mandible to cause fracture of the sphenoid bone. Similar fractures of the sphenoid bone have occurred when the horse fell backward. When horses rear and strike the head on a solid object, the indirect force may cause fracture of cervical vertebrae.

Concussion, contusion, laceration, or hemorrhage in the central nervous system may occur singularly or in various combinations. Severe clinical signs of the injury may be apparent immediately, or may be delayed several hours in cases of compression of the brain or cord by hemorrhage or edema. Meningitis or encephalitis also are delayed complications likely to follow certain fractures of the skull.

Traumatic lesions frequently result in death or permanent disability of the animal, and the veterinarian is helpless when confronted with these cases. However, certain therapeutic procedures are very helpful in some injuries, and their application certainly will enable practitioners to save many animals that would otherwise be lost.

SKULL FRACTURES

Skull fractures usually are not the major concern in injuries to the head. The important considerations are the extent and nature of the injury to the brain. It is possible to have a skull fracture without serious injury to the intracranial contents, just as it is possible to have serious injury to the intracranial contents without fracture of the skull. Linear fractures of the cranial vault are of little importance and require no treatment.

Fractures of the skull, however, are most important when they extend into the ear, ethmoid area, or into the paranasal sinuses. Fractures of these areas may show but mild signs of brain damage immediately following the accident, but they open avenues for infection into the intracranial cavity and subsequent meningitis or encephalitis. Basilar fractures usually are very difficult to visualize on radiographs, but they should be suspected if bleeding occurs from the nasal passages or the ear in the absence of external wounds that would account for the hemorrhage.

Compound and depressed skull fractures often cause immediate death and the veterinarian rarely is called to attend this type of injury. In compound fractures, the wound should be debrided very carefully, and all foreign material removed. Small fragments of bone should be discarded, but larger pieces which are not grossly contaminated may be saved. If the brain is exposed and contaminated, debridement should include the cerebral substance. After the wound is closed, the animal should be administered broad spectrum antibiotics to aid in control of infection. Meningitis or intracerebral abscess often is the result of failure to remove foreign material and badly contused tissue.

Depressed fractures usually do not require emergency treatment. However, if they are associated with severe hemorrhage or pressure on the cerebellum which forces it downward against the fourth ventricle (causing an acute noncommunicating hydrocephalus), prompt attention will be required.

CONCUSSION

Concussion is a term often loosely applied to all nervous disturbances resulting from a blow on the head. Most neurologists agree that this term should be reserved for injuries resulting in an instant period of unconsciousness lasting only a few minutes and followed by an apparently complete recovery. Unconsciousness or other signs of cerebral disorder lasting more than 10 minutes is indicative of brain injury more serious than concussion. The cause of the temporary unconsciousness is not understood, but it is associated with a momentary rise in intracranial pressure, a transitory ischemia, and a marked electrical discharge in the central nervous system. It is not necessarily associated with any cerebral lesion that may be apparent on gross examination of the brain.

CONTUSIONS AND LACERATIONS

Contusions and lacerations are more serious brain injuries causing generalized or focal cerebral disturbances of longer duration. The surface of the brain may be bruised or torn and the cortex may be swollen and edematous or hemorrhagic. In very severe injuries of this type, death may be instantaneous or the horse may die within a few minutes while convulsing. In moderately severe contusions or lacerations, the period of unconsciousness usually is of longer duration than in concussion, and there is a gradual recovery period. During this time the animal may have dilated pupils, slow and irregular breathing, and the pulse usually is slow and weak. Nystagmus often is observed, as are muscular twitchings which may increase to strong clonic contractions. After several unsuccessful efforts, the horse may get up but usually it will continue to manifest signs of general or focal neurologic disturbance. General disturbances may include depression or generalized muscular weakness. Focal disturbances are indicated by rolling movements or falling to one side, or by partial or complete paralysis of groups of muscles on the side of the body opposite the injury. Impairment of one or more of the cranial nerves may be evident.

Mild contusions or lacerations may occur with or without the loss of consciousness, but there may be generalized or focal nervous disturbances that are temporary or permanent.

BRAIN HEMORRHAGE

Brain hemorrhage occurs in almost every severe head injury. Trauma seldom causes bleeding within brain substance which is more extensive than numerous, discrete hemorrhages. The signs associated with these lesions are not understood. Subarachnoid hemorrhages allow blood to escape into the subarachnoid space and produce blood-tinged cerebrospinal fluid. The signs may not be evident for several hours following the injury. The products of red cell disintegration in the cerebrospinal fluid are irritating to nerve tissues and cause signs of meningitis which may vary from hyperirritability to convulsions. The first manifestations are hypertonicity of muscles, causing the horse to stand with the neck and back arched. Then movement of skeletal muscles becomes increasingly difficult. The temperature usually is slightly elevated. The signs may be arrested at this point and slowly regress, or the horse may fall and be unable to rise. Its convulsive efforts to do so may become violent in some cases. Further increase in intracranial pressure may cause lethargy or coma. The diagnosis of subarachnoid hemorrhage can be confirmed by the detection of erythrocytes or hemoglobin in the cerebrospinal fluid.

Subdural and extradural hemorrhages may or may not cause immediate clinical signs depending on the rapidity with which blood escapes into the area. Extradural hemorrhages almost always are associated with linear fractures of the skull. If an artery is injured, the pressure of the blood is sufficient to separate the dura from bone, and the hematoma develops rapidly. If bleeding is from one of the dural sinuses, the pressure of the blood is much lower and the hematoma develops slowly. Usually the animal is unconscious at the time of injury due to cerebral concussion, and as consciousness returns it may be apparently normal for a variable period of time. As pressure from the hematoma develops, signs of somnolence, stupor, and coma supervene. If there are contusions or lacerations, however, the original injury may be sufficiently severe to produce prolonged coma which merges with that resulting from the hematoma. This possibility is suggested by the progressively down-hill course evidenced by a continued slowing of breathing rate and pulse. The pupils may be of unequal size, and pupillary dilation occurs most often on the side on which the hematoma is located. The possibility of bilateral hematomas must not be overlooked.

TREATMENT OF BRAIN INJURIES

Though few reports which pertain to treatment of large animals can be found, certain recommendations for the care of horses with brain injuries should be emphasized.

The veterinarian should insist that the patient be kept as quiet and comfortable as possible for many hours following the accident. In cases of apparently simple concussion, this rule should be followed because of the possibility of hemorrhage into the cranial cavity. If this conservative advice is followed, the degree of cerebral compression will be minimized. An effort to induce the horse to stand or move may cause the effect of the trauma to be more severe. Stimulants are contraindicated for the same reason. Examinations should be conducted with the least possible disturbance of the patient. Particular attention should be given to ocular reflexes, pulse, and breathing rate. Subsequent observations will be helpful in determining changes in the patient's condition.

Active intervention will be required in some cases. Increasing the tonicity of the blood vessels may be helpful in the treatment of cerebral edema resulting from contusions or lacerations. This treatment was described by Bullock et al., and has been used by McGrath in the treatment of dogs suffering from this condition.[1,2] A solution containing 50% sucrose or 50% sorbitol is administered intravenously every 4 hours until the animal improves. Approximately 1 ml. per pound of body weight should be given slowly over a 30-minute period.

The signs related to subarachnoid hemorrhage may be relieved by the withdrawal of cerebrospinal fluid. If prompt improvement follows, it may be repeated from time to time, depending on the severity and duration of the signs.

The term "shock" sometimes is given misplaced emphasis when referring to cerebral injuries. If a condition simulating surgical shock is present, it probably is due to blood loss and should be the first concern of the attending veterinarian. It seldom is the result of cerebral trauma per se.

SPINAL CORD INJURIES

Sprains, dislocations, or fractures of the vertebral column often result in injuries to the spinal cord. Tumors, abscesses, disc herniation, foreign bodies, and subdural or epidural hemorrhages are less common causes. The lesions produced in the spinal cord are classified similarly to those of the brain.

TYPES OF INJURIES

Concussion signifies a temporary physiologic disturbance of the function of the cord manifested by paresis or paralysis of the body caudal to the lesion. Recovery usually is complete and occurs within a few minutes to a few hours.

Contusions result from more severe injuries in which there is swelling and hemorrhage into the substance of the cord. The neurologic manifestations depend on the severity of the injury, but have a longer duration than in concussion.

Lacerations cause interruption in the continuity of the cord with hemorrhages and swelling which result in spinal shock. This lesion usually is comparable in effect to transection of the cord, and the resulting paralysis is permanent.

Compression usually is the result of focal pressure on the spinal cord and may be caused by any of the factors already mentioned. The manifestations may be those of acute or subacute myelopathy. Relaxation of intervertebral ligaments with misalignment of the vertebrae may result in focal pressure on the cord. Compression of the spinal cord is considered a cause of "wobbles," or equine spinal ataxia.

Hematomyelia is hemorrhage into the substance of the cord, and this frequently occurs with contusions or lacerations. Occasionally, it may result from a fall in which there is no obvious trauma to the spinal column or spinal cord substance. The blood liquefies in time, and usually is absorbed. There is a gradual remission of signs, but the recovery period is prolonged. The onset of clinical signs may be immediate or delayed several hours following the accident.

CLINICAL SIGNS OF SPINAL CORD INJURIES

Signs of spinal cord injury vary with the severity and location of the trauma. Paresis or ataxia that is temporary or permanent may be the only sign associated with minor lesions. More often, injuries of this structure result in paralysis of the body distal to the lesion.

Spinal shock is a phenomenon frequently observed immediately following severe injury to the spinal cord. Caudal to the injury, the muscles are in a state of flaccid paralysis and the sphincters are relaxed. Sensations and reflexes are absent and vasomotor paralysis may be detected.

After a variable period of time, the shock and vascular reactions disappear and spinal cord reflexes return. If any portion of the cord remains undamaged, function is resumed in the corresponding part of the body. Anterior to the lesion, the muscle tone and reflexes are normal. In an area adjacent to but just above the lesion, the tissues are in a state of hyperesthesia, apparently caused by damaged tissue acting as an irritant. In the area supplied by the damaged portion of the spinal cord all reflexes are lost and the muscles exhibit flaccid paralysis. Caudal to the lesion the muscles are in a state of spastic paralysis (increased tone, contraction in response to local stimulus, but not under voluntary control), and the tendon reflexes are exaggerated.

The location and extent of the lesion usually can be determined by the presence or absence of reflexes. Injuries affecting the upper cervical section of the spinal cord usually result in death within a few minutes because of paralysis of all respiratory movements. Rarely, the lesion may be incomplete and the animal may live for some time with paralysis of all muscles except those of the head (quadriplegia). Lesions in the cervical enlargement behind the origin of the phrenic nerves also will cause quadriplegia, but this condition can be differentiated on the basis of flaccid paralysis and areflexia in areas of the forelimbs supplied by the injured nerve segments. Paralysis of the posterior part of the body is termed paraplegia.

Rarely, the lateral half of the spinal cord may be injured by extramedullary cord tumors, abscesses, or disc herniations. When this occurs, spastic paralysis is present on the side of the lesion and caudal to it, with pain loss on the opposite side of the body beginning 3 or 4 segments posterior to the lesion. This condition is called spinal hemiplegia.

DIAGNOSIS OF SPINAL CORD INJURIES

In severe spinal cord injuries resulting in paraplegia, diagnosis can be made easily on the basis of loss of muscle tone and sensation in the posterior parts of the body. Azoturia might be confused with paraplegia, but it can be differentiated through the history and the detection of myoglobinuria. Pelvic fractures may cause the horse to be unable to stand on the hindlimbs, but usually voluntary muscle contractions may be observed and the fracture may be detected by rectal palpation.

Mild spinal cord injuries causing paresis may be more difficult to diagnose. Iliac thrombosis may be differentiated by rectal examination as a vibrating mass with no pulsations distal to the thrombus. In foals, pyosepticemia with polyarthritis may cause difficulty in rising or posterior weakness. Depression and the general febrile reaction serve to differentiate this condition.

TREATMENT OF SPINAL CORD INJURIES

In cases known to be caused by an accident, the horse should be kept as quiet as possible until the extent of the injury can be ascertained. If it is obvious that a fracture-dislocation of the vertebral column has occurred the animal should be destroyed at once. In instances in which the extent of the injury cannot be determined, it is advisable to observe the progress of the patient for 2 or 3 days. There are no clinical means of differentiating paralysis due to physiologic block of spinal cord function with possible recovery from complete anatomic severance of the pathways which result in permanent paralysis. The rapid recovery from spinal shock may be indicative of less severe lesions.

During the observation period, the horse must be well-bedded to prevent the development of decubital ulcers. Particular attention should be given to evacuations of the bowel and bladder. Enemas or catheterization may be necessary to induce eliminations. Antibiotics should be given to prevent pneumonia and urinary tract infections. The horse should be turned twice daily to its other side even though the possibility of vertebral fracture and dislocation is suspected. In this case, movement may further injure the spinal cord, but the additional trauma is unlikely to influence the final outcome of the case. The use of a sling is helpful in some instances. If the horse is unable to stand within 3 days after the accident, recovery is unlikely.

CRANIAL NERVE INJURIES

Impairment of one or more of the cranial nerves commonly is a result of various craniocerebral injuries, meningeal infections, tumors, or the action of toxins.

OLFACTORY NERVE INJURY

Olfactory nerve injuries resulting in anosmia rarely are recognized in the horse, but anosmia may be detected by failure of the animal to show appreciation of the presence of grain in the feed box until it is actually seen. Tests for this condition are rendered useless if the horse sees or hears sounds associated with the act of providing the food. Rhinitis must be excluded before a diagnosis of olfactory nerve injury can be made.

OPTIC NERVE INJURY

Optic nerve injury can be determined by tests for visual acuity in the absence of observable ocular lesions. When conducting the test, it generally is best to stand in front of the horse and slightly to one side. Care must be exercised to identify reactions to odors or sounds. Quick movements of the hand near the eye may cause air currents that can be felt and cause the horse to close the lids or to flinch, thus creating a false impression that the hand has been seen. Failure of the pupil to react to light may be caused by impaired oculomotor nerve function as well as by injury to the optic nerve.

OCULOMOTOR NERVE INJURY

Oculomotor nerve injury causes ptosis of the eyelids, dilation of the pupil, and paralysis of all extrinsic muscles of the eye except the lateral rectus, retractor oculi, and superior oblique muscles. The resulting paralysis of the extraocular muscles causes a diverging strabismus in which the eye is rotated outward and slightly upward. (Sympathetic fibers originating in the superior cervical ganglion reach the eye through the ciliary nerves; injuries of these fibers which result in constriction of the pupil are exceedingly rare.)

TROCHLEAR AND ABDUCENT NERVE INJURIES

Trochlear and abducent nerve injuries seldom are recognized in the absence of oculomotor injury. The coordinated and combined actions of the eye muscles are complex, and the resultant paralysis following the injury of one or both of these nerves without other involvement is difficult to detect.

The motor nerves to the eye may be involved peripherally by many types of lesions. Not infrequently they are involved in multiple neuritis along with other peripheral nerves, or a basilar meningitis may extend along these nerves to cause a perineuritis. Congenital aplasia of the oculomotor nucleus is manifested by ptosis and stationary upward and outward deviation of the eyes.

TRIGEMINAL NERVE INJURY

Trigeminal nerve injuries may be associated with intracranial lesions, lesions in the area of the Gasserian ganglion, or neuritis of its branches without visible inflammatory changes. The clinical signs of this disorder are anesthesia over the area supplied by the sensory fibers and paresis or paralysis of the muscles of mastication from involvement of the motor root.

Injuries of the ophthalmic branch cause a loss of cutaneous sensation over the affected side of the forehead as far back as the ears. The conjunctiva, cornea, upper lid, and mucous membranes of the upper nasal passage also are affected. Keratitis and conjunctivitis are likely complications. Because of the absence of corneal reflex, dust and food particles may collect on the cornea and conjunctival sac without causing increased lacrimation. Injuries by foreign materials may result in erosions and serious infections of the cornea. Vision is unimpaired except as the result of keratitis or other complications. Often ophthalmic nerve paralysis is not suspected until the eye is examined and the absence of the corneal reflex is detected.

Injury to the maxillary branch causes anesthesia of skin over the lower lid, nose, cheek, nostril, upper lip, mucosa of the lower nasal passage, upper part of the mouth, and the upper teeth. Disturbances of parasympathetic fibers traversing in this nerve cause a decrease in nasal secretions and an abnormal dryness of the affected nostril.

Injuries of the mandibular branch cause anesthesia of the anterior part of the tongue, the mucosa of the lower part of the mouth, lower teeth, lower lip and chin, and paralysis of the muscles of mastication. In unilateral involvement, the lower jaw deviates toward the paralyzed side, and the lack of tone is evident in the masseter, temporal, and pterygoid muscles. The upper and lower teeth on the affected side do not come in contact, and food tends to accumulate between the cheek and the teeth. Because of the anesthesia of the tongue, it may be injured seriously by chewing movements.

Bilateral trigeminal nerve involvement causes a very disabling condition. The animal is unable to close the mouth, and it hangs open with the tip of the tongue protruding and saliva drooling from the lips. Movement of the tongue is not impaired. Corneal lesions may develop as the horse is insensitive to drying of this tissue and seldom blinks.

Differential diagnosis seldom presents a problem. Fractures or dislocation of the mandible and nigro-pallidal encephalomalacia cause no alteration of sensation. Dumb rabies has not been recognized in horses.

No effective treatment is known. Horses with a unilateral lesion will require daily care of the eye and inspection of the tongue. Cases with bilateral involvement should be fed through a stomach tube until it can be determined whether or not function will be restored.

Trigeminal neuralgia occasionally is observed in horses. The cause is unknown. It is characterized by repeated, irregular periods of discomfort or pain about the lips or face. The head is shaken violently or rubbed against accessible objects. The first evidence of signs may be mistaken for pruritus, and only after repeated attacks is the true nature of the disease recognized. No specific treatment is known but the injection of 95% alcohol into the peripheral branches of the nerve may be used in severe cases.

FACIAL NERVE INJURY

Facial paralysis occurs frequently in horses. The clinical manifestations vary depending on the severity of the lesion and the portion of the nerve that is injured. The sensory fibers of this nerve are unimportant; the principal function is motor innervation of the lips, nostrils, cheek, eyelids, and ear.

Etiology: The common cause of facial paralysis is trauma of the nerve as it rounds the posterior border of the mandible approximately 1½ inches below the articulation of the jaw. At this superficial point, it is easily crushed against the bone by a variety of injuries such as blows, or the pressure of a buckle or a cheek strap of a halter while the horse is lying down. The incidence is increased following such disorders as colic or chronic lameness which causes the horse to lie down much of the time.

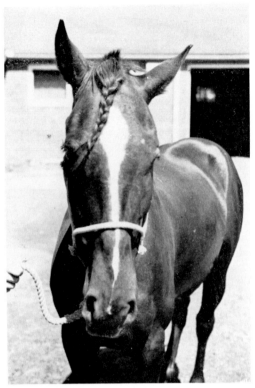

Fig. 2. Paralysis of left facial nerve causing drooping of ear, ptosis of eyelid, and deviation of lips to right side.

Other causes of facial paralysis include neuritis following exposure to cold or drafts, neuritis resulting from such infections as influenza or pneumonia, and inflammations in the parotid area such as abscesses of the parotid lymph node. Intracranial pathology as trauma, meningoencephalitis, or brain tumor may cause unilateral or bilateral injuries of this nerve.

Clinical Signs: Unilateral lesions involving the entire nerve cause a characteristic paralysis which is particularly evident by its effect on the ear, upper eyelid, nostril, and lips (Fig. 2). The paralyzed ear hangs laterally in an oblique or horizontal position, and cutaneous sensation may be lost on the convex and concave surfaces. The upper eyelid droops due to paralysis of the corrugator supercilii muscle, but this is in part compensated by the action of the levator palpebrae superioris muscle supplied by the oculomotor nerve. The horse is unable to completely close the eyelids on the affected side because of paralysis of the orbicularis oculi muscle. The accumulation of foreign material consequently may cause keratitis and increased lacrimation. Corneal sensation is not impaired.

The nostril of the paralyzed side is partially collapsed and hangs lower than the other; on inspiration it tends to fall inward. The upper lip on the affected side often sags and is drawn medially, causing the muzzle to deviate toward the normal side. On lateral view, the lower lip on the paralyzed side will hang loosely from its attachments.

Other indications of facial nerve injury include interference with prehension of food because of the unilateral lip paralysis, and a tendency for food to collect between the cheek and molar teeth. Impaired inspiration seldom is evident except after strenuous exertion.

Unilateral nerve injuries involving only the dorsal and ventral buccal branches of this nerve are common and cause the clinical signs described previously, except those involving the ear and eyelid.

Bilateral facial paralysis is a very disabling condition primarily because of its effect on prehension of food and interference with inspiration. Good nursing is necessary to prevent the horse from losing condition rapidly. Since the paralyzed lips cannot be used to move food into the mouth, eating becomes difficult. Food and saliva drool from the mouth when the horse attempts to eat. Drinking is also difficult. The corners of the mouth must be immersed in order to prevent the water from flowing back.

Equally serious in bilateral facial nerve injuries is the interference with breathing due to paralysis of the muscles which dilate the nostrils. Since the horse breathes only through the nose, failure to dilate the nostrils seriously interfers with inspiration. While the breathing is quiet an affected nostril will fall inward on inspiration and the false nostril collapses, but a sufficient opening generally remains and dyspnea is not evident. There is no interference with expiration of air. Following mild exertion or excitement which causes an increased breathing rate, the nostril collapses on inspiration, and a snoring sound is heard. In bilateral paralysis, inspiratory snoring sounds may be noticeable while the animal is at rest, and if forced to exercise the horse may collapse due to the inspiratory dyspnea.

Prognosis: The outcome of facial nerve paralysis depends upon the cause. Cases caused by trauma generally recover in 4 to 8 weeks. If no improvement is apparent within 2 or 3 months, the chances of recovery are not good. Cases in which the ear and eyelid are involved indicate more serious conditions.

Treatment: Treatment should be directed toward prevention of additional irritation to the nerve, and good nursing. If the condition is the result of trauma, the horse should be placed in a well-bedded stall and the halter removed. If caused by abscesses or tumors, appropriate measures should be taken. Medicaments such as cortisone, B-complex vitamins, and nerve tonics containing strychnine are of questionable value. Mild counterirritants applied to the skin over the mandibular ramus may be helpful, and such measures serve to satisfy the owner.

A soft, easily masticated ration should be offered, and in the case of bilateral paralysis, should be placed in a deep receptacle so that the food can be worked into the mouth. Water must also be available from a deep container. Food which collects between the teeth and the cheeks should be removed after each meal. If the horse is unable to close the eye on the affected side, dust or debris should be washed from the eye frequently and secondary infections controlled.

Cases in which inspiratory dyspnea is evident should not be exercised until the condition has improved. In some cases, it is necessary to place a wire suture through each nostril and tie the ends together over the nose. In cases of permanent damage to the nerves it is advisable to remove a portion of the external wall of the nostril. In some instances, tracheotomy may be indicated.

ACOUSTIC NERVE INJURY

Acoustic nerve injury may involve either or both the cochlear branch related to hearing and the vestibular branch concerned with balance.

Dysfunction of the cochlear branch is only one of the causes of deafness. It also may result from lesions in the external ear, middle ear, or cochlea. Unilateral involvement seldom is recognized; bilateral involvement is easily detected by observing the movements of the ears. If hearing is normal, the horse will turn the ears toward the direction from which the sounds originated.

Trigeminal nerve injury may cause temporarily reduced auditory acuity due to paralysis of the tensor tympani muscle which is supplied by a branch of this nerve. Inherited deafness occurs in horses of various breeds and colors, and is associated with degeneration of the organ of Corti. (Hypersensitivity to sound is occasionally observed in a facial nerve paralysis that includes the branch of this nerve which supplies the stapedius muscle.)

The vestibular portion of the eighth nerve is physiologically and anatomically distinct from the cochlear nerve and is concerned with maintenance of posture and equilibrium during motion. Lesions of the vestibular apparatus cause the animal to hold the head obliquely so that the affected side is downward, and there is a tendency for the horse to fall to that side. If recumbent, the animal may be uncomfortable when made to lie on the sound side. Bilateral lesions cause signs comparable to cerebellar ataxia. The most common cause of vestibular involvement is trauma with hemorrhage into the internal ear, although infections or neoplasms occasionally are responsible.

Treatment of deafness can be successful only when it is caused by lesions in the external ear. Vestibular involvement due to trauma generally improves spontaneously within a few weeks; when caused by infection, antibiotics may be effective in treatment. Paracentesis of the tympanic membrane may be attempted in severe cases.

GLOSSOPHARYNGEAL NERVE INJURY

Glossopharyngeal nerve injuries seldom are detected in the horse. They cause loss of sensation in the nasopharynx and pharynx with loss of palatal and pharyngeal reflexes; other structures innervated by the nerve have obscure clinical manifestations. Motor fibers supply the stylopharyngeus muscle. The glossopharyngeal nerve is so closely associated with the vagus nerve that both are often involved simultaneously, and motor paralysis of the palate and posterior pharyngeal wall formerly attributed to glossopharyngeal nerve injury is known to be the result of damage to the vagus nerve.

VAGUS NERVE INJURY

The vagal paralysis most commonly encountered in the horse involves one of its branches, the recurrent nerve. This condition is discussed separately under the title of "roaring."

Lesions involving the pharyngeal branches are much less common and cause partial or complete paralysis of the palate and pharynx. Difficulty in swallowing is evidenced by regurgitation of food or water through the nose while attempting to eat. Material often is aspirated into the respiratory tract, resulting in gangrenous pneumonia. Stertorous breathing may be caused by vibration of the paralyzed soft palate. In unilateral paralysis, the free border of the soft palate is pulled toward the healthy side.

Disturbances of visceral function may be evidenced by tachycardia which is caused by the functional loss of inhibitory fibers of the vagus nerve to the heart. Alterations in gastric motility and secretions also occur.

The cause of vagus nerve injury often is obscure. The pharyngeal branches may be damaged by severe inflammatory processes in the area. Causes of central lesions include trauma, infections and neoplasms involving the brain stem, toxins of *Cl. botulinum* and of plants of the *Lathyrus* spp., and chemical poisons such as lead and arsenic.

Treatment depends on the cause. Spontaneous recovery often occurs in cases when the paralytic signs are caused by local inflammation. In cases resulting from chemical or plant poisons, the source of the noxious agent should be removed and the known antidotes administered (E.D.T.A. for lead, and BAL for arsenic). The horse should be fed by stomach tube as long as there is danger of aspiration pneumonia.

LARYNGEAL HEMIPLEGIA (ROARING)

Introduction: This condition is characterized by a whistling or roaring that can be heard when the horse is breathing deeply from exertion. The noise is made only during inspiration and is accompanied by inspiratory dyspnea in severe cases. Due to impaired function of one or both recurrent nerves the intrinsic laryngeal muscles are unable to draw the arytenoid cartilage and vocal fold laterally, in the normal manner, during inspiration. Instead, these enfeebled structures are drawn medially, and caused to vibrate by the inrushing air, thus producing the whistling or roaring sound and inspiratory dyspnea. During exhalation they are pushed harmlessly aside, offering no resistance to the outflowing air.

Occurrence: Only the left recurrent nerve is affected in most cases. Of the roarers examined by Kral, laryngeal paralysis was restricted to the left side in 92%, on the right in 6%, and was bilateral in only 2% of the recorded cases.[2] All breeds of horses may be affected. Though laryngeal hemiplegia is more often recognized in animals used at a fast gait, it is not uncommon in draft horses. Apparently, it is rare in Shetland ponies and mules. The incidence is greatest in animals 3 to 6 years old, and the condition is more frequent in geldings than in mares.

Etiology: Impaired function of the recurrent nerve(s) is the basic cause. This results in paresis or paralysis of the intrinsic laryngeal muscles. On occasions, the impaired function can be associated with mechanical injury to the nerve or with the ingestion of certain poisons. In the great majority of cases, however, roaring is related to a recent, prolonged respiratory infection. In many instances, the antecedent disease is thought to be a form of strangles; roaring also follows rhinitis, pharyngitis, bronchitis, pneumonia, or influenza in which *Streptococcus equi* may have been a complicating agent. It is thought that an allergic response in previously sensitized horses results in injury of the affected nerve.

Maguire presented serologic evidence that *Bacterium viscosum equi* may be the cause of laryngeal hemiplegia.[6] He suggested that strains of this organism have a predilection for the recurrent nerve, and other strains cause neuritis in other parts of the body. Beta-hemolytic streptococci were isolated from some of his cases.

The predominance of left recurrent nerve paralysis has been attributed to the unique course of this structure. After branching from the vagus nerve opposite the aortic arch, it passes backward and medially around the concavity of the aorta and turns anteriorly on the left ventral surface of the trachea. In passing around the aorta, this nerve lies beneath the bronchial lymph nodes and passes between the aorta and trachea. It has been suggested that constant pulsations of the aorta predispose the nerve to injury by toxins, or that it is traumatized by pressure between the aorta and enlarged bronchial lymph nodes associated with respiratory infections. The report by Cole does not support this theory because he found that marked degeneration was confined to the distal portion of the recurrent nerve, with little or no neuropathology found in the region of the aortic arch.[4]

Roaring has been produced experimentally by neurotomy. Occasionally, comparable lesions are caused by abscesses, tumors, or granulomatous masses along the course of the recurrent nerve. Esophageal diverticulum or aortic aneurysm may cause similar damage.

Other known etiologic factors include poisoning by lead or certain plant toxins. In lead poisoning, other clinical signs often are present. Recurrent nerve paralysis has been observed in about a third of the horses which ingested rations containing plants of the genus, Lathyrus, *Cicer arietinum* (chick pea), or lucerne. According to Kral, the roaring caused by these toxins is temporary if the offending feed is withdrawn.[5]

Clinical Signs: In cases in which paresis is slight, signs are evident only while the horse is breathing deeply from strenous exercise. Often the first sign is a high-pitched whistling sound that is called "high breathing" by trainers. In show horses, this noise may be heard only when the neck is arched and the head is flexed. In other cases these sounds may be detected only when the horse is eating grain. During this stage of the disease the inspiratory dyspnea is slight. Occasionally, the condition

remains static for some time, but more often the signs increase in severity within a few weeks.

In other cases, the onset of the disease appears to be sudden. Well-defined signs may develop suddenly; inspiratory stertor is heard easily after mild exercise and inspiratory dyspnea is evident. In moderate cases, the signs subside after a short period of rest. In severe cases or in those with bilateral recurrent nerve paralysis, sounds may be clearly audible during quiet respiration. If cases of this type are forced to exercise, dyspnea may be so acute that the horse becomes unsteady on its feet.

Lesions: Pathologic changes consist of atrophy of the intrinsic muscles of the larynx and degeneration of the recurrent nerve on the affected side. Calcification of the laryngeal cartilages often is present in chronic cases. The first 2 lesions are restricted to the left side of the larynx in more than 90% of the cases, but calcification often is bilateral.

Most of the crico-arytenoideus dorsalis, crico-arytenoideus lateralis, and arytenoideus transversus muscles on the affected side are replaced by connective tissue. The ventricularis and vocalis muscles generally are involved to a lesser extent. The crico-thyroideus dorsalis and extrinsic muscles are normal since they are not supplied by the recurrent nerve.

Cole reported interesting observations on the larynges of 174 horses that were examined post mortem. Varying degrees of laryngeal muscle degeneration were found in 47 (27%) of these animals. Many of the horses were exercised and examined for roaring before euthanasia, but signs were not detected in those found to have less than 50% atrophy of the laryngeal muscles. In fact, signs were detected in only a third of those with more than 50% atrophy. This study indicates that there is a wide variation of laryngeal muscle degeneration in horses that roar, and that recurrent nerve injury is more common than was previously recognized. Bilateral calcification of the laryngeal cartilages was present in approximately half of the animals with marked atrophy of the intrinsic muscles, but the importance of this lesion in roaring was not discussed.

Marked decrease in the size of the left recurrent nerve near its termination is a constant finding. Though the left nerve normally is slightly smaller than the right, the terminal portion of this structure in horses with laryngeal hemiplegia is only half the size of the right recurrent nerve. Wallerian degeneration usually is found on histopathologic examination.

Diagnosis: In well-developed cases, this disease can be recognized from the clinical signs alone. In mild cases of laryngeal hemiplegia, the use of an endoscope as described by Kral may be helpful. When the larynx is observed through this instrument, the arytenoid cartilage on the affected side has little or no lateral movement during inspiration. The vocal cord on that side appears shorter, has a steeper angle than its partner, and is set in vibration during forced inspiration (Fig. 3). The opening into the ventricle of Morgagni is larger on the affected side, and in advanced cases, the epiglottis may be shifted from its central position toward the paralyzed side.

Occasionally, intermittent roarers are encountered in which it is difficult or impossible to evoke signs at the time of the examination.

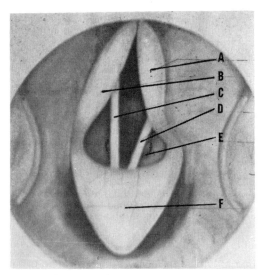

Fig. 3. Endoscopic view of the larynx of a horse with left recurrent nerve paralysis (schematic). The left arytenoid cartilage (A) projects farther into the lumen than does the right arytenoid cartilage (B), The right vocal fold (C) is longer than the left vocal fold (D) which may be seen vibrating during forced inspiration. The opening of the left ventricle of Morgagni (E) is larger than that of the right side. The epiglottis (F) may be shifted toward the paralyzed side in some cases. Courtesy of Dr. F. Kral.

Many practitioners place emphasis on the palpation of a pit between the arytenoid and thyroid cartilages. This depression results from atrophy of underlying muscles. Many horses with laryngeal hemiplegia make a peculiar grunting sound when a sudden motion is made as though to strike it in the ribs after it has been hit once or twice. This sound apparently is caused by the escape of air through the partially paralyzed larynx when intrathoracic pressure is increased.

Edematous folds of pharyngeal mucosa may cause upper respiratory sounds by partially blocking the rima glottidis (Fig. 4). Tumors such as lipomas, papillomas, or carcinomas may cause similar interference with respiration. Pedunculated retention cysts located near the epiglottis are occasionally found (Fig. 5). Deformed tracheal rings sometimes are confused with roaring. As a general rule, differential diagnosis can be made by careful consideration of the respiratory sounds. With pharyngeal edema, tumors, or cysts the adventitious sounds are heard during both inhalation and exhalation. Endoscopic examination may be necessary to further identify the lesion that is present.

Treatment: Surgical removal of the mucous membrane from the laryngeal saccules (William's operation) is the safest and most effective method of relieving the signs of roaring. In the healing process, firm adhesions form between the lateral surface of the vocal cord and the arytenoid cartilage. They prevent these structures from being drawn medially during inspiration. Most equine practitioners share the opinion that the condition is likely to recur unless the saccule is removed from both sides. Tetanus antitoxin and a broad spectrum antibiotic should be administered following surgery. See technic in Chapter 22.

Aftercare is very important. The horse should be tied in a stall to restrict movement of the head. During the first few postoperative days, the horse should be observed at frequent intervals for signs of dyspnea caused by swelling of the tissues. Should this occur, an ice pack applied over the incision is very helpful in preventing additional swelling. Tracheal intubation should be employed if the dyspnea becomes acute. In all cases, the margins of the incision should be cleaned twice daily with a

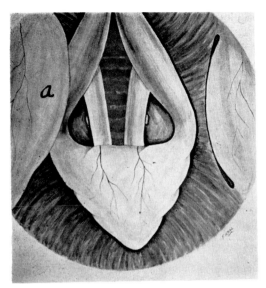

Fig. 4. Endoscopic view of a "false roarer" caused by edematous fold of pharyngeal mucosa (a) partially covering the entrance of the larynx (schematic). Courtesy of Dr. F. Kral.

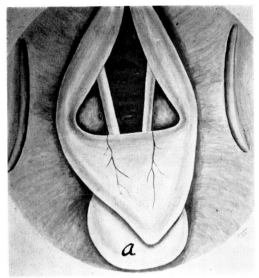

Fig. 5. Endoscopic view of the larynx of a horse with a retention cyst (a) located under the epiglottis and causing respiratory sounds that were confused with roaring (schematic). Courtesy of Dr. F. Kral.

cool water compress. Generally, it is not advisable to apply antiseptics or antibiotics into the incision.

Healing usually is complete in about 3 weeks, but exercise should be restricted for at least 2 months following the surgery.

Relief from roaring is not instantaneous. Gradual improvement during the first 30 days is the rule, but complete recovery may require several months. The prognosis is most favorable in the heavier breeds that are used at a slower gait. It is least favorable in the saddle breeds that are shown under tight rein.

SPINAL ACCESSORY NERVE INJURY

Spinal accessory nerve injury causes paralysis of the trapezius and/or the sternocephalicus muscles only if the cervical segments contributing to this nerve are also involved. This condition rarely is recognized.

HYPOGLOSSAL NERVE INJURY

Hypoglossal nerve injuries occur infrequently in horses. The resulting paresis or paralysis of the tongue may be uni- or bilateral. In bilateral paralysis, the tongue hangs from the partly opened mouth and cannot be retracted. Eating and drinking are difficult. Pain sensation to the tongue and ability to close the jaws are not affected unless fibers of the trigeminal nerve are also involved.

Unilateral paralysis causes a deviation of the tongue toward the affected side when it is voluntarily extended from the mouth. This deviation is caused by the posterior fibers of the genioglossus muscle on the unaffected side which pull the base of the tongue forward. Their unopposed action allows the tip of the tongue to be carried toward the paralyzed side. If the tongue is retracted, its tip deviates similarly toward the unaffected side because of the unopposed action of the styloglossus muscle. Interference with eating and drinking is less evident in unilateral paralysis.

Lesions more often are located along the hypoglossal nerve or in its nucleus, causing flaccid paralysis followed by atrophy. The affected side of the tongue becomes wrinkled, furrowed, and wasted. Inflammation of the nerve or the nucleus may cause paresis. Occasionally, coarse muscular fasciculations are observed on the affected side. Lesions above the hypoglossal nucleus may cause spastic paralysis with weakness and deviation of the tongue without atrophy or fasciculations.

Etiology: Causes of unilateral glossoplegia

include trauma, tumors, or neuritis following such infections as influenza and strangles. Central lesions, such as meningoencephalitis, aneurysms of the vertebral artery, or tumors of the brain stem usually result in bilateral paralysis, and often involve other bulbar nerves.

Excessive traction of the tongue or constriction of the upper neck by ropes drawn too tightly may cause glossoplegia, but more often impaired mobility of the tongue is the result of hemorrhage or edema into the tissues. In this case, recovery usually occurs within a few days.

Diagnosis: Differential diagnosis seldom is difficult. "Tongue-lolling" is a vice of horses in which the tongue is allowed to hang from the mouth while resting or working, but they have no detectable impairment of muscular activity of the tongue. Some trainers have shown horses successfully only after the tongue was tied to the mandible by some material such as a shoestring that was dyed to blend with the color of the horse.

The tendency to expose the tip of the tongue in trigeminal or facial paralysis seldom is confused with glossoplegia. Inflammation of the tongue caused by penetration of a foreign body or infections can be distinguished by the presence of swelling or local tenderness.

Treatment: Treatment of unilateral lesions may only require the provision of a moistened ration which can be moved easily into position for mastication. Hot compresses applied to the skin over the pharyngeal area several times daily may be helpful in cases caused by trauma or inflammation of the nerve. If the horse is unable to eat, it must be fed by stomach tube. Unless improvement is evident within a few weeks, the paralysis is likely to be permanent.

REFERENCES

1. Wheat, J. D., and Kenny, P. C.: Cerebellar hypoplasia and its sequela in a horse. J.A.V.M.A. **131** (1957) 291-293.
2. Bullock, L. T., Gregeson, M. T., and Kinney, J.: The use of hypertonic sucrose solution intravenously to reduce cerebrospinal fluid pressure without a secondary rise. Amer. J. Physiol. **112** (1935) 82-86.
3. McGrath, J. T.: Neurological Examination of the Dog. 2nd ed., p. 216. Lea & Febiger, Philadelphia, Pa., 1960.
4. Cole, C. R.: Changes in the equine larynx associated with laryngeal hemiplegia. Amer. J. Vet. Research **7** (1946) 69-77.
5. Kral, F.: Examination by endoscope. N. Amer. Vet. **32** (1951) 91-95.
6. Maguire, L. C.: The role of *Bacterium viscosum equi* in the causation of equine disease. Vet. Rec. **70** (1958) 989-991.

MENINGITIS

Inflammation of the meninges may be caused by various factors. Bacteria, fungi, nematode larvae, and larvae of the bovine warble fly are etiologic agents of this disease in the horse. The distinction made here between meningitis and encephalitis or myelitis is more convenient than it is real, but it serves to separate the etiologies mentioned from the nonsuppurative encephalomyelitides caused by viruses (equine encephalomyelitis, Borna disease), by protozoa (mal de caderas, surra, dourine), and by toxins (leukoencephalomalacia) that will be discussed elsewhere. Seldom does the causal agent of meningitis remain localized in the meninges; in the majority of cases it spreads to the neural tissue, resulting in meningeoencephalitis or meningomyelitis.

Etiology: Animals have no primary meningitis comparable to that caused by the meningococci in man. Except for those organisms gaining entrance through penetrating wounds involving the coverings of the brain or spinal cord, meningitis almost always is the result of extension of infection to the central nervous system from other parts of the body.

Bacterial meningitis in horses is caused most often by *Streptococcus equi.* This organism gains entrance through the blood stream, or by extension of a contiguous abscess. Jones and Maurer after a study of equine influenza reported that hemolytic streptococci were present in the lungs of most of the horses that died from complicated influenza, and that this organism caused purulent meningoencephalitis in some of the cases.[3] In a few instances the infection had produced brain abscesses.

Mixed infections of the meninges may follow an acute bacteremia associated with navel ill. Staphylococcal infections occasionally are found. In countries where glanders or tuberculosis is still a problem the etiologic agents occasionally extend into the meninges of the horse. Fungus infection of the central nervous system of horses was reported by McGrath and by Irwin and Rac.[1,4] Blindness and incoordination were the predominant neurologic signs in this disease caused by *Cryptococcus* spp.

Parasitic lesions of the brain or spinal cord of horses have been reported. The *Setaria* spp.

which cause neurologic disorders in Asian horses will be discussed with "wobbles." It also is known that Strongyle larvae migrate through tissues and occasionally reach the brain or spinal cord. Partial paraplegia in a mare caused by a hydatid cyst was described by Miller.[5] The brief mention of these few reported cases of mechanical injury to the central nervous system by parasites belies the importance of this problem. Innes and Saunders point to many references which indicate that parasites become located in the brain or spinal cord much more commonly than generally is realized and that their presence may not produce clinical signs or be associated with non-specific neurologic reactions.[2] They also refer to evidence that nematode infections may facilitate viral invasion of the nervous system.

In passing, it seems advisable to review observations made by Radeleff on the use of systemic parasiticides in cattle infected with *Hypoderma bovis*.[6] If treatment was delayed until early winter, the disturbed or killed grubs contiguous to the spinal cord often caused transitory or prolonged paralysis. The mechanism of this "side reaction" could not be determined, but it is possible that anaphylaxis or mechanical damage to the spinal cord were caused by the disturbed grub, or that myelitis may be due to metabolites from the decomposing grub. It may be that other comparable effects caused by other parasites in the nervous system of horses will be recognized some day.

Clinical Signs: The signs of meningoencephalitis and meningomyelitis vary greatly, depending on the portion of the central nervous system that is affected and the severity of the inflammatory reaction. Except for focal lesions, the manifestations seldom remain static but change daily as the disease progresses. A description of the many possible combinations of signs is not within the scope of this chapter or the ability of the authors. The following observations, however, should help the interpretation of neurologic manifestations.

Meningitis results in varying degrees of hyperesthesia and excitement. If the spinal meninges are affected, the body is held rigid, and any attempt to flex the head will elicit pain. The muscles innervated by nerves passing through affected meninges have increased tone, often with muscle spasms or cramps. Later the inflammatory reaction may cause paresis or paralysis by pressure on the nerve.

As the inflammation extends to the neural tissue, signs of encephalitis or myelitis develop. Disturbances of consciousness that vary from dullness to coma are caused by encephalitis. Abnormal movements are common and ataxia, compulsive movements (circling or pushing against objects), or convulsions are observed. Myelitis interferes with impulse conduction and causes signs that vary from incoordination to paralysis.

Fever usually is present and remains high, but occasionally it follows a fluctuating pattern. If the infection tends to localize, the febrile reaction may diminish. Disturbances of pulse and respiration are grave signs.

Brain abscesses of the cerebrum caused by *S. equi* simulate the signs caused by viral encephalitis. The horse is drowsy and the lack of coordination causes an unsteady gait. It may fall and have difficulty in rising to its feet. While standing, the legs may be placed in an unnatural position, and one or more of the joints tends to collapse repeatedly. Focal disturbances may include twitching of an ear, nystagmus, trismus, or inability to swallow. Diminished appetite, urine retention, and constipation may occur.

Treatment: Supportive measures and the use of antibiotics may save some cases. It is imperative that treatment be initiated early in the course of the disease; if it is delayed the horse may die or become permanently affected because of neural damage even though the infectious agent is eliminated by the antibiotic.

The intravenous administration of large quantities of electrolyte solutions appears to be helpful. Sedation may be required to control convulsions. A sample of cerebrospinal fluid may furnish information about the causal agent when it is stained or cultured. Antibiotic sensitivity tests should aid in the selection of the effective therapeutic agents. The intrathecal injection of antibiotics or antiserum is often followed by arachnoiditis, and should not be used except as a last resort.

REFERENCES

1. Irwin, D. F. P., and Rac, R.: Cryptococcosis infection in a horse. Austral. Vet. J. **33** (1957) 97-98.
2. Innes, J. R. M., and Saunders, L. Z.: Comparative Neuropathology 560. Academic Press, New York and London, 1962.
3. Jones, T. C., and Maurer, F. D.: The pathology of equine influenza. Am. J. Vet. Research **4** (1943) 15-31.
4. McGrath, J. T.: Cryptococcosis of the central nervous system in domestic animals. (Abstract). Amer. J. Path. **30** (1954) 561.
5. Miller, W. C., and Poynter, D.: Hydatid cysts in a Thoroughbred mare. Vet. Rec. **68** (1956) 51-53.
6. Radeleff, R. D.: Problems associated with the use of the newer insecticides for livestock pests. J.A.V.M.A. **136** (1960) 529-537.

"Wobbles"

Although the syndrome described as "wobbles" in the United States is fairly well-defined, certain etiologic aspects of this disease have not been determined. Other conditions causing similar clinical signs in horses of various ages have been reported in this and other parts of the world, but their relationship to "wobbles" in this country has not been established. Until such points are clarified by further investigation, these various conditions will be discussed separately.

Equine Incoordination (Equine Spinal Ataxia, Ataxia of Foals)

This sporadic, nonparalytic disease of young horses is characterized by an awkward, incoordinated gait. In addition to the name "wobbles," other common terms as "weak loin" and "jinxed back" are sometimes used because of the swaying or lurching of the pelvic limbs as the animal walks. The incidence of this disease is low, with rarely more than a few cases occurring each year in large breeding establishments. Apparently all breeds are susceptible, but it is less common in draft horses and mules.

This disease usually develops before the horse is 2 years of age. Signs may be apparent in sucklings as young as 3 months, but more often they are recognized in weanlings or yearlings. Well-nourished and heavily muscled individuals are affected most often. Definite signs may be delayed until after the horse is 2 years or older, but in many of these cases occasional movements suggestive of incoordination had been observed at an earlier age. It rarely develops in horses older than 4 years.

Etiology: The pathologic changes associated with equine incoordination (*i.e.*, osteoarthritis of the vertebrae and lesions of the spinal cord) are well-documented, but the underlying cause has not been definitely established. In all probability diverse etiologic factors will be found.

This disease has long been known to equine practitioners in the United States, and for many years it was thought that the disorder was caused by a fall or similar accident. Dimock and Errington first reported the changes in the cervical vertebrae and spinal cord.[2] They suggested that the condition was inherited, but the genetic nature has never been defined. Olafson compared equine incoordination to "swingback" in lambs (congenital demyelination caused by prenatal copper deficiency), and indicated that the conditions may have common etiology.[2]

Cerebrospinal nematodosis (discussed later) is the cause of comparable clinical signs in horses in the Far East, but differences in the age incidence and the asymmetric arrangement of lesions within the spinal cord indicate different etiology. This factor warrants further investigation.

Clinical Signs: The salient feature of this disease is incoordination which is characterized by a wobbling gait. This locomotor disturbance is bilateral and varies from slight ataxia that is detectable in the movements of the hindlimbs only when the horse is turning or backing to marked wobbling in all directions as if inebriated. When standing quietly, the attitude is normal except in the terminal stages of the disease. The onset may be insidious or sudden. In some cases, the condition is not recognized until the horse is ridden for the first time, when it appears to sway from the weight of the rider. In other instances, a horse that appeared normal in the morning may exhibit typical or extreme ataxia by evening.

In mild cases, the wobbling gait is not apparent when the horse is walking straightaway. However, it tends to overreach occasionally, and there may be intermittent dragging of the toes on forward movement. The signs usually are exaggerated by turning the horse from side to side; incoordination is evidenced by swaying or lurching of the posterior part of the body, and the horse frequently knuckles over in the fetlocks. Steel *et al.* reported that blindfolding an affected horse exaggerated the signs.[7] Mildly affected animals may be able to trot or gallop surprisingly well without showing definite signs until turned or stopped. During these movements swaying of the hindquarters or knuckling of the fetlocks may be noted. Backing usually is difficult for affected animals.

Though the striking feature of this disease is ataxia of the hindquarters, the forelimbs are affected as well. If the development of the disease is slow, ataxia in the posterior parts may be detected several days or weeks before involvement of the forelimbs becomes apparent. Often the peculiar gait makes it difficult to determine that the forelimbs are affected except in extreme cases.

As the condition progresses the horse loses condition. It moves with the forelimbs abducted in an effort to maintain balance. When galloping, it overextends the hindlimbs, and they appear to swing forward from momentum rather than from muscular effort. In many cases, the horse tends to cross the hindlimbs at the faster gaits. It is surprising how seldom severely affected animals fall, and generally they are able to get up and down until the terminal stages of the disease develop.

Lesions: Detailed studies of the lesions found in 30 cases of equine incoordination were reported by Jones *et al.*[4] The only consistent lesions were restricted to myelinated tracts in the spinal cord. The changes were most severe in the cervical region, usually at the junction of C3 and C4, C5 and C6, or C6 and C7. In some cases primary lesions of severe malacia were found in the ventral, lateral, and dorsal funiculi. In all cases, secondary (Wallerian) degeneration was present. Mild lesions of this type were present in the dorsal funiculi cephalad to the primary focus; more severe degeneration was found in the ventral (and to a lesser extent in the lateral) funiculi caudad to the primary lesion. A particular feature of the lesions was their bilateral symmetry, with the most severe malacia concentrated on both sides of the median fissure in the ventral funiculi caudad to the primary foci.

Osteoarthritis involving the articular processes of the cervical and thoracic vertebrae appear to be the important lesions of the spinal column. It has been suggested that these changes permit increased movement of the vertebral articulations, and injury to the spinal cord results from impingement or stretching. Arthritic changes occasionally are found between the bodies of the cervical vertebrae, and are most frequent at the junction of C3 and C4.

Constrictions of the spinal canal by projections of the vertebrae or intervertebral discs were found in 14 of 30 cases studied by Jones *et al.*[4] They reported that bony changes of this type were seldom present in horses killed earlier than 30 days after the onset of signs. In many cases, the constrictions were not related anatomically to the malacic foci found in the spinal cord. Steel *et al.* found stenosis of the spinal canal in 2 of 11 cases studied and in old fracture of the arches of C6 and C7 in 1 horse.[7] In the 2 studies just mentioned, the authors were unable to find parasitic larvae in the central nervous system.

Jones *et al.* reported an interesting lesion that warrants further study.[4] A rather severe epineuritis in which there was a large accumulation of lymphoid cells was present in both spinal and peripheral nerves of horses killed early in the course of the disease (10 and 12 days after the onset of signs). The significance of these changes has not been determined, but it may be an early manifestation of the disease.

Prognosis: The course is unpredictable, but it always is unfavorable and insurance companies recognize this disease as an acceptable reason for euthanasia. The extent to which the signs will develop cannot be determined in the early stages. Any change for the better or worse, however, is likely to occur within the first week after the onset of signs. Recovery is very rare, but individuals with mild incoordination may survive for some time, or without warning, they may be found dead in a pasture field. At necropsy, subarachnoid hemorrhages may be found. Mares or stallions with mild ataxia have been used for breeding purposes for years, and the progeny seldom are affected.

Treatment: No therapeutic measure has proved effective. Cortisone and related products may cause temporary remission of signs, but almost invariably they return after treatment is discontinued. Possible nutritional deficiencies should be corrected in an effort to prevent or alleviate this disease. The use of antifilarial drugs will be discussed with cerebrospinal nematodosis, but, as stated before, these parasites have not been proved to be a cause of equine incoordination in this country. It appears that "wobbles" in Brazil may have a different etiology, as it has been reported that cases in that country often make uncomplicated recoveries when given unlimited access to pasture.

CEREBROSPINAL NEMATODOSIS (KUMRI)

Etiology: In the Far East, a nervous disorder of horses comparable in many respects to equine incoordination is caused by larvae of *Setaria* spp. (the peritoneal worm of cattle). Arthropod vectors serve as intermediate hosts of this parasite and can pass infective larvae into horses, sheep, or goats. In these unnatural hosts, the larvae can penetrate the central nervous system and cause varying degrees of incoordination, imbalance, and motor weakness. Since these filarids are widely distributed in cattle it has been suggested that their larvae may occasionally cause similar signs in horses in this and other areas, as well as in the Orient.

Clinical Signs: In some cases, the clinical manifestations are similar to those of equine incoordination. The onset may be insidious or sudden. Often only the pelvic limbs are affected, causing marked swaying in the posterior parts of the body, and the horse tends to drag the toes on forward movement. In other cases, all 4 limbs are involved, and ataxia may be severe.

Several differences in the signs of cerebrospinal nematodosis and equine incoordination are often observed. In the former condition, the clinical manifestations depend on the random location and extent of injury to the nervous system that is caused by the burrowing larvae. Muscular weakness is associated with imbalance in the majority of cases. Monoplegia, hemiplegia, paraplegia, or quadriplegia sometimes are seen. Spontaneous recovery occurs occasionally with little or no residual neurologic effects, which is very unlikely in equine incoordination. Also of differential significance is the age incidence and seasonal occurrence of the 2 diseases. This parasitic invasion of the nervous system very rarely occurs in foals; it usually is found in horses older than 2 years. Cerebrospinal nematodosis occurs most often in late summer or fall, when the arthropod vectors are most numerous. There may be a latent period of 15 to 60 days following entrance of the larvae into the horse before signs are detected.

Lesions: Scattered malacic lesions are found in the spinal cord and/or brain. Varying degrees of cellular infiltrations are present in subdural, epidural, leptomeningeal tissues, and spinal nerve roots. Hemorrhages may occur if the migrating larvae penetrate blood vessels in the central nervous system. Secondary degeneration of the tracts may be found anterior and posterior to the primary foci.

The important difference in these lesions, as compared to those of equine incoordination, is the random arrangement. Bilateral symmetry is not found in cerebrospinal nematodosis. Portions of parasitic larvae may be recognized in stained sections of the nervous system in some cases of this disease, but osteoarthritic lesions in cervical and thoracic vertebrae have not been reported.

Treatment: Shoho treated and prevented the disease successfully with a product known as caricide (American Cyanamid Company, Princeton, New Jersey).[6] The treatment was effective in horses with minor neurologic signs of motor weakness and wobbling.

"WOBBLES" IN BRAZIL

Bardwell studied a form of "wobbles" in horses in Brazil that differs in several respects from equine incoordination in this country.[1] Its cause was thought to be a nutritional deficiency. Histopathologic studies were not described.

Clinical Signs: Broodmares more than 6 years old developed typical signs of wobbles during the last quarter of gestation. They became progressively ataxic until parturition. After foaling, the condition improved and by the time the mare weaned the foal, incoordination often was hardly detectable. With subsequent pregnancies, however, impairment of gait again would increase in severity and duration until the mare either died or was destroyed. Foals from these mares apparently were normal, but they had a marked tendency to become unsound while racing.

A condition described as incoordination or "sloppy coordination" was present in as many as 3 to 10% of the yearlings. After lying in the stall during the night, the affected horses were unable to rise to more than a "dog sitting" position unless assisted to their feet. Normal, playful movements were suppressed when the yearlings were on pasture, and affected individuals stood in one place for many hours, frequently shifting the weight on the hindlimbs. Gradual improvement followed by complete recovery within several months was the rule.

Treatment: No specific treatment was suggested, but yearlings allowed to run on pasture for 24 hours each day seemed to respond much better than those confined in lots or stalls for all or part of the time. Many of these horses later raced successfully.

"Pseudo-Amyloid" Multiradicular Degeneration of Spinal Nerve Roots

Innes and Saunders described a condition that has long been recognized in newborn Shetland ponies in Maryland and Virginia.[3] From birth, the foals resemble "wobblers" in that they are ataxic. Motor weakness is apparent and the foals are not inclined to move. Eating is impaired, and the animals remain in good flesh. Necropsy of one case revealed lesions described as ill-defined "pseudo-amyloid" or "pseudo-mucoid" degeneration of spinal nerve roots at many segmental levels. The lesions were comparable to an inherited disorder of children. Although the condition is congenital in ponies, no genetic relationship has been proved.

REFERENCES

1. Bardwell, R. E.: Osteomalacia in horses. II. Nutrition as an etiologic factor. J.A.V.M.A., **138**: (1961) 159-162.

2. Dimock, W. W., and Errington, E. J.: Incoordination of equidae: "Wobblers". J.A.V.M.A., **95**: (1939) 261-267.
3. Innes, J. M. R., and Saunders, L. Z.: Comparative Neuropathology. Academic Press, New York and London, 1962.
4. Jones, T. C., Doll, E. R., and Brown, R. G.: The pathology of equine incoordination (Ataxia or "Wobbles" of Foals) Proc. A.V.M.A. 91st. Annual Meeting, (1954) 139-149.
5. Olafson, P.: "Wobblers" compared with ataxic (swingback) lambs. Cornell Vet. **32** (1942) 301-314.
6. Shoho, C.: Prophylaxis and therapy in enzootic cerebrospinal nematodiasis of animals by 1-diethylcarbamyl-4-methylpiperazine dihydrogen citrate. Report of a second field trial. Vet. Med. **49** (1954) 459-464.
7. Steel, J. D., Whittem, J. H., and Hutchins, D. R.: Equine sensory ataxia ("Wobbles"). Clinical and pathological observations on Australian cases. Austral. Vet. J. **35** (1959) 442-449.

Suprascapular Nerve Injury (Sweeny)

The suprascapular nerve is an important branch of the brachial plexus. It innervates muscles that serve as lateral collateral ligaments of the shoulder joint. After passing between the supraspinatus and subscapularis muscles, this nerve passes over the coracoid border of the scapula, where it is exposed to trauma or may be overstretched. Severe injury results in flaccid paralysis followed by neurotrophic atrophy of the supraspinatus and infraspinatus muscles. Horsemen refer to these changes as sweeny, or swinny (also spelled sweeney and swinney).

Etiology: Various forms of trauma to the suprascapular nerve cause sweeny. Lunging against a post or other fixed object, kicks on the shoulder, or the collision of horses in sports such as polo may result in bruising or severing of the suprascapular nerve. Pulling the forelimbs backward violently may cause injury by overstretching the nerve. This is encountered sometimes when horses are cast by roping the forefeet. In draft horses, pressure from ill-fitting collars is a common cause of suprascapular nerve injury and this is particularly common in young horses that are forced to walk in the furrow or on the ridge while plowing.

Clinical Signs: Atrophy of the supraspinatus and infraspinatus muscles leaves a depressed surface on either side of the scapular spine and this may be the only detectable change in some cases. Lameness may not be apparent unless bruising of other tissues accompanies the nerve injury. In other cases, abduction of the scapulohumeral articulation occurs when weight is placed on the affected leg. By walking the animal slowly toward the observer, he will see that the shoulder joint is suddenly abducted from the thorax the moment the affected limb is bearing weight and is perpendicular to the body. If the degree of nerve injury is slight, winging of the shoulder may be missed if viewed from the side. In marked cases, the lateral excursion of the shoulder may lead the inexperienced horseman to suspect dislocation, or "slipped shoulder."

Prognosis: The prognosis varies with the rapidity and degree of atrophy. Complete atrophy within 7 to 10 days following trauma often indicates permanent nerve paralysis, but with proper care the horse may serve many useful years. If the atrophy is incomplete, the horse may recover full use of these muscles in 4 to 8 weeks.

Treatment: Cold compresses should be applied to the area at frequent intervals during the first 24 hours following the trauma. After this, hot packs are beneficial, and later counterirritation may help to hasten recovery. When it is apparent that the nerve injury is permanent, irritants should be injected into the atrophied muscle tissue.

Several preparations have been used for this purpose; they include equal parts of turpentine and chloroform, equal parts of turpentine and alcohol, a 2% solution of silver nitrate, tincture of iodine, or Dondren (Knoll Pharmaceutical Company). In our experience, the turpentine and chloroform mixture has given the best results. After disinfection of the site, 1 milliliter injections spaced 2 inches apart are injected into the atrophied muscle. From 5 to 15 ml. are used, depending on the size of the horse. Following the injections, the site should be massaged thoroughly. The owner should be informed that this agent causes a painful reaction, and the horse may be reluctant to use the leg for several days. If the area does not fill in completely, more injections should be given.

OBTURATOR PARALYSIS

Etiology: Injuries to the obturator nerve occur infrequently in horses. It rarely is associated with parturition. In fractures of the pelvis, this nerve may be crushed between bony fragments or compressed by callus formation during the healing process. Abscesses or tumors (usually melanomas) which occur along the course of the nerve occasionally cause obturator paralysis.

Clinical Signs: Clinical signs result from impaired ability to adduct the leg. While the 4 muscles of the pelvic limb most important in this function are paralyzed (obturator externus, pectineus, adductor, and gracilis muscles), slight adduction is possible through action of the sartorius muscle supplied by the saphenous nerve, and by the semimembraneous muscle supplied by the sciatic nerve. In unilateral involvement, no signs may be apparent while the horse is standing, other than slight abduction of the affected limb, but when walking or trotting the effect is more conspicious. The limb is moved forward with an outward sweep of the femur so that only the inside of the hoof touches the ground. The stride is shortened on the affected limbs and the horse moves obliquely toward the sound side.

In unilateral involvement the horse may have difficulty in rising when it is lying on the sound side, or with bilateral involvement it may be unable to gain its feet without assistance. Sprains of muscles or ligaments are complications of obturator paralysis that may increase the severity of the disability. The limb may be held in abduction, and while attempting to walk the hoof is dragged along the ground, or the horse may hop on the unaffected limb and tend to fall toward the sound side. In other cases, the stifle is drawn upward and outward as in stringhalt. In long-standing cases, atrophy of the adductor muscles may be marked.

Prognosis: Prognosis varies with the cause. Injuries from parturition usually repair quickly. Paralysis caused by abscesses or tumors along the course of the nerve, or by callus formation following fractures, is likely to be permanent.

Treatment: Treatment should be directed toward the prevention of injuries that may follow the occurrence of obturator paralysis. Less seriously affected horses only require comfortable quarters but may be allowed restricted exercise. Stimulating embrocations applied to the adductor muscles may be of some value.

Recovery usually follows in uncomplicated cases within 2 or 3 weeks.

The more seriously affected cases require the use of a sling. If the hindlimbs tend to straddle, they should be loosely hobbled to prevent overabduction of the hip joint that may result in myorrhexis of the adductor muscles or injuries to the ligaments of the coxa-femoral joint.

Pudic Nerve Injury:

Etiology and Clinical Signs: The pudic nerves supply motor fibers to the retractor penis muscle and sensory fibers to the penis. In rare cases, injuries of these nerves occur and result in paraphimosis and loss of sensation in the glans penis. This condition infrequently follows castration. Pudic nerve paralysis can be differentiated from the more common paraphimosis resulting from swelling of the prepuce, penis, or inguinal region by the absence of pain sensation in the glans penis.

Other causes of pudic nerve injury are trauma to the nerve in the perineal region where it may be crushed against the bone as it passes over the ischial arch, contiguous abscesses, tumors, or neuritis following respiratory infections as influenza or strangles. In these instances, the paraphimosis develops without detectable abnormalities of the penis or prepuce in the early stages, except for the impaired sensitivity of the glans. The penis hangs limply from the sheath. Since there is no swelling, it can be pushed into the sheath but immediately prolapses again.

Prognosis: The prognosis generally is unfavorable. If swelling is present for several days and becomes firm, it is unlikely that the tissues will be restored to normal even if function of the nerve is restored. Surgical intervention (amputation of the penis) should be reserved for those cases considered incurable by more conventional methods.

Treatment: Treatment should be directed toward the protection of the penis from trauma. A suspensory apparatus or other device should be employed to hold the penis in the sheath or to protect it from injury until the nerve is again functional. Unless constant care is given, swelling or ulceration of the penis is a likely sequel to paralysis of the retractor muscles.

Cauda Equina Paralysis

Postinfectious neuritis of the cauda equina may not occur in this country. The only reports are from northern Europe. Observations on the pathogenesis of this disorder, however, warrant its inclusion with the other neuropathies.

Etiology: Fractures of the sacrum or injuries of the coccygeal vertebrae from pulling on the tail or forceful bending of it during copulation have been reported but usually cause only tail paralysis. Reports of neuritis of the cauda equina following infectious diseases have originated from Germany,[1] Holland, and Denmark.[2] Innes and Saunders[3] refer to these reports in which roaring, neuritis of the cauda equina, or other neurologic complications followed recovery from infections (usually respiratory) that were caused or complicated by streptococci. In addition to the nerve involvement, myocarditis, glomerulonephritis, and internal hydrocephalus were seen. The cause of the lesions was thought to be an allergic response evoked by streptococci in horses sensitized by previous infection. Other causes may be tumors, abscesses, or parasitic larvae which invade the cauda equina.

Clinical Signs: The salient features of this condition are paralysis of the tail and cutaneous anesthesia of the perineum and posterior gluteal region. Tone of the anal and urinary sphincters is decreased and the area of anesthesia often includes the rectal and vaginal mucosa. The tail hangs limply and is not raised during defecation or micturition. Feces accumulate in the rectum causing constipation, and in the mare, the tail and perineum become soiled with urine. Cystitis is a frequent complication.

Treatment: No specific treatment is known, but with proper care the horse may live many useful years. Manual evacuation of the rectum may be necessary, and prevention of urinary infections by frequent cleaning of the vulva and protection of the skin from infection is indicated.

REFERENCES

1. Beijers, J. A.: Enkele ervaringen omtrent de aandoeningen der luchtwegen en longen bij het paard, gedurende het laatste jaar. Tijdschr. Diergeneesk. 69 (1942) 141-159.
2. Eberbeck, E. and Hemmert-Holswick, A.: Zur pathogenese der spatschaden des ansteckenden datarrhs der luftwege bzw. der druse des pferdes. Arch. Tierheilk, 78 (1943) 334-351.
3. Innes, J. R. M., and Saunders, L. Z.: Comparative Neuropathology. P. 794 Academic Press, New York and London, 1962.

Convulsive Syndrome of Newborn Foals (Barkers, Dummies, and Wanderers)

A nervous disorder of newborn foals characterized by convulsions and/or blindness has been recognized in Thoroughbred breeding centers in England, Ireland, France, and Italy for many years.[1] The terms, "barker," "dummy," or "wanderer," are descriptive of the signs of this disease which is caused by cerebral anoxia. Premonitory signs develop within a few minutes to hours after birth, and generally consist of jerking the head up and down in a strange fashion, aimless leg movements, and clonic spasms of muscles of the limbs, body, neck, and head. The "barker" syndrome is followed by marked convulsions, during which the foal may make a peculiar noise resembling the bark of a small dog. "Dummies" and "wanderers" generally have less severe convulsions and are so-called because of apparent blindness and failure to respond to external stimuli. The "dummy" tends to stand or lie quietly in one place with a more or less drowsy attitude. The "wanderer" moves about aimlessly showing no fear of man or other animals. If the "barker" survives the convulsion, it passes into the "dummy" or "wanderer" stage. Affected foals will not nurse, but with forced feeding many make complete recovery.

Mahaffey and Rossdale state that this disease apparently is restricted to Thoroughbred foals born indoors under human supervision, and the incidence has been as high as 2% of the foals born on some farms.[3] Millar and Bailey reported a convulsive syndrome in a newborn foal in which human intervention was not a factor. They noted that this condition has been more common in Australia than was previously recognized.[5] No reports of this disease were found in the American literature.

Etiology: Mahaffey and Rossdale report that loss of placental blood is the underlying cause.[4]

This deficit reduces blood pressure in the capillaries of the lungs and results in its improper inflation. Cerebral hypoxia is suggested as the cause of nervous derangement. Since this condition has not been observed in foals born outdoors without human intervention, it is thought that the cause in some way is related to the events at parturition.

When the mare is allowed to foal unattended, both mare and foal rest for a time after parturition. During this period, virtually all the blood from the placenta passes into the circulatory system of the foal, and it is difficult to collect even 50 ml. of blood from the placenta when the cord is ruptured at this stage. When an attendant is present, it is a common practice to apply traction to the forelimbs of the foal as they emerge from the vulva. Also the foal may be dragged to the mare's head almost immediately after birth. This unwarranted assistance causes premature rupture of the umbilical cord, and in such cases from 1000 to 1500 ml. of blood may be recovered from the placenta. This quantity amounts to approximately 30% of the foal's potential blood volume. It has been shown that blood pressure causing capillary erection is very important in effecting expansion and aeration of the lung in the newborn infant, and fluid pressure is necessary to produce proper aeration of the lung. The patent ductus arteriosus was larger than normal in convulsive foals, and it was suggested that this may be a contributing factor.

Another possible cause is proposed by Millar and Bailey.[5] At the necropsy of an Australian case, contusion of the right ventricle of the heart, fractures of the second, third, and fourth ribs, marked bruising of the pectoral muscles, and edema of the subcutaneous tissue were found. In this instance, it appeared that circulatory dysfunction and anoxia were caused by injury to the thorax and heart during the birth process. References are cited in which other investigators found similar lesions associated with a convulsive syndrome.

Clinical Signs: Mahaffey and Rossdale have described the clinical signs in comprehensive studies of this disease.[3,4] Following delivery, the foal may appear normal for a time, and the first respiratory movements occur without noticeable difficulty. The onset of signs often is detected within minutes after birth, but they may be delayed as long as 12 hours.

The "barker" syndrome usually is preceded by a period of restlessness and irritability, followed by a rapid onset of signs. While trying to get on its feet for the first time or while standing, the affected foal may suddenly begin jerking its head up and down. If standing, it becomes unsteady on its feet, and usually falls. Respiratory distress is pronounced in severe cases, with marked pallor of the mucous membranes. Clonic movements follow, and during this time the foal may emit a sound resembling the yapping of a dog. While in lateral recumbency, the foal paddles wildly with the forefeet, and this stage is followed by violent convulsions in which galloping movements and powerful contractions of the jaw, neck, and back muscles are seen. Nystagmus often is present, pulse and respiratory rates are greatly increased, and sweating may be profuse. Occasionally, the foal is able to maintain its feet, and it may exhibit acute mania by charging blindly into walls or other obstacles in its path. When convulsions subside or are controlled by sedation the foal lapses into semicoma, but convulsive movements are easily provoked by various stimuli. This stage of the disease may last several days, but with proper care about half of the foals survive but pass through the "dummy" or "wanderer" stage before recovery.

"Dummies" and "wanderers" represent less severe manifestations of this syndrome. They appear to be blind, fail to respond to most external stimuli, and are without inclination or ability to nurse. These signs may be apparent at birth, delayed several hours or, as previously stated, follow the "barker" stage of this disease. The "wanderer" is able to walk, wanders about aimlessly bumping into objects, and shows no fear or recognition of man or other animals. It seldom lies down voluntarily. If laid down, the affected animal may remain in the same position for several hours. With proper care, improvement may be seen in 36 to 48 hours and this is first evidenced by weak sucking movements. Recovery by the fifth day is the rule, with visual function being the last faculty to return.

Lesions: The lesions support the theory that anoxia causes the syndrome. In normal foals lung expansion is very rapid and is probably complete within 10 minutes following birth. By this time the lungs are pale and feathery. By contrast, most of the lung tissue of convulsive foals is dark purple and has almost no aerated areas. Pieces of lung tissue from affected foals sink rapidly in water.

Microscopically, the outstanding and constant lesion is resorption atelectasis. Normal alveolar patterns completely disappear and patency seems to end at the bronchioles. Another lesion involves the spleen. In foals living more than 24 hours, the Malpighian corpuscles are markedly depleted of cells, and may appear as hyaline masses in animals living as long as 4 days. This change is not specific as it may occur in foals dying from hemolytic diseases of the newborn or from neonatal pneumonia. Lesions in the central nervous system have not been described.

Diagnosis: Prenatal and postnatal infections by *Actinobacillus equuli* cause somewhat similar signs in foals in this country. Dimock *et al.* reported that foals were in a semicomatose condition at birth but later were stricken suddenly and lived but a short time.[2] In those animals which die within the first 24 hours after birth the only lesion is severe enteritis. These authors also mentioned that 2 foals were destroyed because of blindness, but the lesions were not described.

Treatment: No specific treatment has been described. With proper care, many foals recover without residual effects. The barker syndrome may require sedation to control convulsions. Since the sucking reflex is absent, foals must be fed by stomach tube several times daily until they are able to drink from a pan. It has been estimated that about 50% of convulsive foals given proper care make complete recoveries, and the prognosis for "wanderers" and "dummies" is even more favorable.

REFERENCES

1. Cosgrove, J. S. M.: The veterinary surgeon and the newborn foal. Vet. Rec. 67 (1955) 961-969.
2. Dimock, W. W., Edwards, P. R., and Bruner, D. W.: Infections observed in equine fetuses and foals. Cornell Vet. 37 (1947) 89-99.
3. Mahaffey, L. W., and Rossdale, P. D.: Convulsive syndromes in new-born foals. Vet. Rec. 69 (1957) 1277-1288.

4. Mahaffey, L. W. I., and Rossdale, P. D.: A convulsive syndrome in newborn foals resembling pulmonary syndrome in the newborn infant. Lancet (1959) 1223-1225.

5. Millar, R., and Bailey, K. C.: A clinical case of convulsive syndrome in a newborn foal. Aust. Vet. J. 35 (1959) 489-492.

Shivering

Shivering is a chronic neuromuscular disorder primarily affecting the heavier breeds that are used for hard work regularly. Since the few remaining draft horses in this country seldom are used extensively, shivering is very rare today in the United States. This disease is still encountered, however, in some European countries where draft horses are worked regularly. Shivering has been occasionally observed in lighter breeds of horses.

Etiology: The etiology of shivering has not been determined. Hereditary influence has been suggested but not proved. In some countries, it is recommended that stallions with this disease not be used for breeding purposes. Other workers believe that shivering may be a result of neuropathic lesions caused by such diseases as influenza, strangles, or other systemic infections. It also has been attributed to accidental injuries, as might be incurred from a fall.

Clinical Signs: The signs are variable. The most commonly recognized form of shivering involves muscles of the hindlimbs and tail. When the horse is moved backward, the tail is elevated in a series of spasmodic jerks and the muscles of the hindlimbs are tensed and trembling. The farther the horse is moved backward, the more difficult this movement becomes and in advanced cases the affected animal may be unable to move backward more than a few paces. Some affected horses will lift one hindlimb from the ground and hold it away from the body in a rigid, semiflexed position. During this spasm, the limb and superficial thigh muscles often quiver or shake violently, and the tail is elevated and tremulous. After a few moments the spasm ceases, and the tail and limb are returned slowly to their normal position, but signs may reappear when the horse is again forced to move backward.

Other horses evidence shivering during the first few steps forward with movements that could be mistaken for stringhalt. In shivering, however, the limb is abducted and poised for a few moments in a spastic state and is not returned to the ground in the quick motion characteristic of stringhalt. An occasional horse will exhibit signs when made to move laterally in a tie stall. Here the movements are awkward and spasmodic, with the tail moving up and down in a pumping motion.

Involvement of the muscles of the forelimb, neck, or face is seen occasionally. When the horse lifts the forefoot, the limb may be thrust forward in full extension and held with the foot barely touching the ground, or it may be flexed and abducted with quivering in the extensor muscles above the elbow. When muscles of the head or neck are involved, they contract spasmodically.

Diagnosis: The diagnosis of well-developed shivering seldom presents a problem. In advanced cases the signs may be apparent when the horse is backed, moved sideways, or turned. Severely affected animals may be hesitant to lie down, and recumbent horses may be unable to rise without assistance.

Slight or intermittent shivering often requires careful observation before it can be diagnosed. Repeated tests under various conditions may be necessary before an opinion can be formed in doubtful cases. In mild cases the horses may appear normal until exercised for some time. Rest for several weeks may mitigate signs, so horses which have shown marked shivering may pass tests for soundness.

Prognosis: The prognosis generally is unfavorable. The condition may remain unchanged for some time but as a rule shivering is a chronic, debilitating disease, and with regular work the muscle spasms will increase in severity and frequency until the hindlimbs become stiff and the horse no longer can be used. Signs tend to subside when long periods of rest are allowed. Some jumping or hunting horses known to be occasional shiverers may be used for several seasons, but gradually they lose their ability to clear obstacles.

Treatment: No specific treatment for shivering is known.

F. C. Neal
F. K. Ramsey

CHAPTER 15

DISEASES OF THE EYE

INTRODUCTION

The procedure employed during examination of the eye has been described in Chapter I. The parts now to be considered are the: 1. Eyelids. 2. Conjunctiva. 3. Cornea. 4. Aqueous and Vitreous Humors. 5. Lens and Retina.

SUPERFICIAL OCULAR LESIONS

THE EYELIDS

The eyelids of the horse may be torn by contact with nails, hooks, thorns, or barbed wire. The tear may be at right angles to the lids, longitudinal, or a piece of lid may have been removed. The condition is marked by epiphora and frequently is attended by closure of the lids (blepharospasm). The puncta may be torn away, or the lacrimal duct may be occluded or partially missing. Healing may result in deformity due to cicatricial contraction, persistent epiphora, and sometimes with development of entropion or ectropion (Fig. 1).

Lacerations of the lids are difficult to manage because most cases are not presented for veterinary care until several days after the injury occurred. During the very early stages it is possible to suture the edges of lacerations with some possibility of union resulting. Often, the lacerated edges must be debrided before it is possible to suture them. If the animal is docile it may be possible to do this after administration of a tranquilizer and a local anesthetic. In many cases, however, much better surgical technic can be employed if the patient is under general anesthesia.

If the laceration is deep, extending entirely through the lid, the muscular layers should be sutured with interrupted No. 0 or 00 catgut sutures; the skin should be approximated with tension sutures of a nonabsorbable material. The skin sutures should be removed in about 7 days. The horse should be crosstied or a cradle should be applied to prevent its rubbing the sutured site.

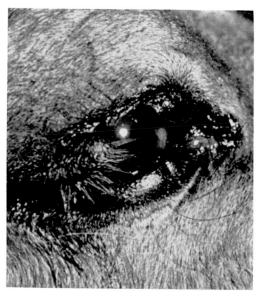

Fig. 1. Laceration of upper lid.

If the injury is old, the prospect of obtaining primary union after suturing is not good. In most of these cases, the sutures will slough in 3 or 4 days. Often, irregular edges are observed after healing of such lesions by second intention. These uneven tags of tissue should be excised flush with the edges of the eyelids.

When suturing eyelids one should never attempt to close obvious gaps; also avoid penetrating the tarsal cartilage or the conjunctiva. Any tissue gaps remaining after healing may be closed later by plastic surgery.

The daily application of penicillin ointment may be preferable to suturing. The occasional instillation of a solution of tetracaine hydrochloride, or other topical anesthetic, relieves pain and permits the eyelids to be stretched. This lessens the risk of lid contraction during the healing process.

BLEPHAROSPASM (Spasmodic Closure of the Lids)

This condition is encountered when a foreign body irritates the cornea or conjunctiva,

327

or when there is abrasion or a puncture wound of the cornea. It also is present in periodic ophthalmia. It is a dangerous condition in the horse as friction of the cornea by hair often produces more trouble than the inciting cause. Prolonged spasm of the orbicularis muscle may give rise to a chronic condition resembling entropion, accompanied by contraction of the lid, which then turns inward. This causes a keratitis and sets a vicious cycle into operation. A congenital blepharospasm may be encountered in foals; this is usually accompanied by entropion.

Treatment: One should endeavor to find and remove the cause. The use of a local anesthetic, such as a solution of Pontocaine, produces temporary relief and frequently enables the cause, such as a foreign body, to be discovered and removed. Corneal lesions must be treated topically and entropion corrected by surgery.

In foals, the lids may be everted by skin sutures applied below the lower lid without skin incision. This produces the necessary dilation of the palpebral orifice. When the blepharospasm is congenital but the degree of entropion is slight, the injection of a few drops of warm, sterile, liquid paraffin beneath the skin of the eyelid along the free edge and a quarter of an inch below it, often is corrective.

Some practitioners first inject procaine with a very fine needle, then introduce a thicker needle parallel with the palpebral margin and withdraw it slowly as the paraffin is being introduced beneath the skin. The puncture is sealed by application of petroleum jelly.

Foreign Bodies

Horses do not frequently suffer from the introduction of plant material into the conjunctival sacs, but not infrequently mud or grit enters the sacs during racing. Rarely, an awn of wild barley grass may enter the conjunctival sac of colts in pasture. The parasite, *Thelazia lacrimalis*, also has been found in both the conjunctival sacs and in the anterior chamber of horses' eyes.

Occlusion of the Naso-Lacrimal Duct

In the horse the puncta lacrimalia, the ducts through which the tears escape from the conjunctival sac into the nasal chambers, lie close to the caruncle on the margins of both the upper and lower lids near the nasal commissure. The caruncle may be oversized and as it carries a number of short hairs it may form an obstacle to the passage of tears.

The lower punctum is more apparent than the upper in the horse. In this species, the first portion of the duct consists of a bony canal occupying a third of its total length. At the middle of its length, overlying the first premolar, a marked dilation occurs. The lower orifice takes the form of well-defined puncta on the lower floor of the nostril. There may be 1 to 3 such puncta. When the lacrimal duct is patent, a few drops of fluorescein instilled into the lacrimal sac can be seen coming through the nasal puncta.

Occlusion of the lacrimal duct may be the result of its obstruction with a foreign object such as a weed seed, or inspissated exudate following conjunctivitis or strangles, or due to injury of the bony lacrimal canal. It is nearly impossible to probe or flush the canal or duct from the punctum lacrimalis at the palpebral orifice due to the small orifice and the resistance usually shown by the animal when this is attempted.

Retrograde flushing from the nasal opening of the lacrimal duct is relatively simple. The nasal orifice is rather large, and is easily entered. Nervous animals must be twitched before the canal can be flushed. A blunt-pointed 12- or 14-gauge hypodermic needle or a larger tomcat catheter can be passed into the nasal orifice. Physiologic saline alone or combined with an aqueous antibiotic solution may be used to flush the duct. If there is evidence of infectious exudate the procedure should be repeated daily until the flushed solution is free of exudate.

Conjunctivitis

Etiology: Conjunctivitis may be regarded as the most common of all conditions affecting the eye of the horse. The causes for conjunctivitis include: 1. Bacterial or viral infection, 2, presence of foreign bodies or finely divided solids, 3, trauma, 4, allergy. Normally, the tears which bathe the conjunctival surface possess a lubricating, flushing and antiseptic action. The conjunctiva withstands low-grade infection better than the presence of a chemical or mechanical irritant.

Clinical Signs: An attack of conjunctivitis is initiated with engorgement of the superficial vessels, which are extendable as they are arranged more or less spirally in the loose membrane. The deeper vessels are straight and appear only at the corneoscleral margin. When these are inflamed and form a visible circle at the limbus, it is an indication that the cornea also is injured.

A slight scratch or introduction of a foreign body will produce simple catarrhal conjunctivitis. There will be excessive tearing which will spill over the lower lid and soil the face of the animal. Later, the discharge becomes mucoid and glutinous, and that which collects on the face will contain leukocytes. The eyelids become swollen and inflamed. Their edges may become adherent, but usually the condition is not as painful as in keratitis. Blepharospasm, a spasmodic closure of the eyelids, seldom is seen in uncomplicated conjunctivitis.

When the infection is not quickly overcome the conjunctival discharge becomes purulent. Pus exudes from the conjunctival sacs and usually causes adherence of the lids. Purulent conjunctivitis almost invariably is associated with subsequent involvement of the cornea.

Treatment: Frequent flushing of the conjunctival sac with normal saline should be the foundation of treatment. Apart from the application of penicillin ointment, the frequent instillation of liquid paraffin, castor oil or cod-liver oil usually will prevent damage to the cornea. When corneal damage appears likely to occur due to the animal's rubbing the eye, a topical anesthetic may be indicated. (Cocaine has a damaging effect on the cornea and should be avoided.) If penicillin solution is used instead of the ointment, it should be at a strength of 1500 to 3000 units per ml. of normal saline solution.

KERATITIS

Etiology: Inflammation of the cornea is not as commonly encountered in the horse as in most other animals. Its causes include trauma, foreign bodies, entropion, dermoid cyst, and parasitic invasion of the eyelids, conjunctival sacs or of the anterior chamber. The cornea also manifests inflammatory changes during periodic ophthalmia.

Clinical Signs: In the very early stages of keratitis, minute bullae appear as dark, clear spots on the cornea against a surrounding haziness. This appearance resembles that caused by a few drops of paraffin on the surface of a clear pool and it is accentuated by oblique lighting. The substantia propria then is invaded by leukocytes and other blood elements which produce a corneal haziness. The lids probably will be tightly closed in blepharospasm. The conjunctival vessels will extend from the corneoscleral junction and branch over the corneal surface which normally is nonvascular. When the cornea becomes invaded in its depth, the vessels proceed from the ciliary arteries and travel across the cornea in straight lines to coalesce in a circle or in concentric circles.

Despite the great number of new vessels and the dense opacity which thereby is produced, the neovascularization starts to disappear as soon as the irritation causing the condition is removed. The vessels arising from the early inflammation disappear rapidly, but when new fibrous interstitial tissue has been laid down with the appearance of blood vessels, the prognosis, so far as complete resolution is concerned, must be very guarded.

When cellular precipitates appear in the anterior chamber of the eye below the pupil, this indicates that extension of the inflammation to the ciliary body has taken place.

Pus in the anterior chamber of the eyeball (hypopyon) can result from extension of infectious keratitis or corneal perforation. It is seen most frequently as a complication of strangles (Fig. 2). If the infection can be controlled, the exudate will gravitate to the ventral portion of the chamber within a few days.

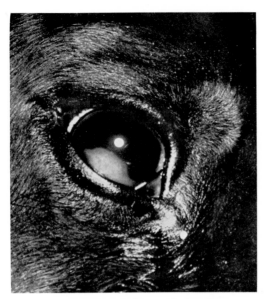

Fig. 2. Hypopyon in horse with strangles.

In most cases, the exudate will gradually be resorbed, but in a few the fibrin and debris will form a permanent adherent band at the lower rim of the cornea.

Treatment: Early identification of the cause and its prompt removal or correction are the objectives of therapy for keratitis. When the cause is not apparent, the corneal inflammation frequently is related to an external source of irritation or injury and subsequent bacterial, mycotic, or viral infection.

During the early stages of superficial keratitis, a beneficial therapeutic regimen includes the application of hot packs to the involved eye 3 or 4 times daily, keeping the animal in a darkened stall, instillation of an antibiotic ointment after each application of the hot pack, and twice daily application of atropine ointment if miosis is observed. Superficial corneal lesions generally will heal within 7 to 10 days if this therapy is followed. If the corneal erosions are deeper and accompanied by extensive neovascularization the healing process will require 3 to 4 weeks.

If healing is prolonged or an ulcerative process becomes chronic, cauterization of the invasive corneal vessels at the limbus is indicated. Cauterization is performed most easily by the cautious use of 90% phenol which may be ap-plied to the edges of the ulcer as well as to the vessels at the corneoscleral junction. Intramuscular injections of a foreign protein, such as sterile milk or hog cholera serum, may be given at 5- to 7-day intervals to stimulate the healing process. Cortisone preparations should be used with caution and preferably not in the early stages of corneal ulceration. When applied they should be used in combination with a broad spectrum antibiotic or after the infectious process is controlled.

The frequent administration (4 to 6 times daily) of 30% sulamyd sodium (sodium sulfacetamide) solution also is recommended for treatment of infectious keratitis.

CORNEAL PERFORATION

On occasion, a foreign object will completely penetrate the cornea, allowing escape of aqueous humor. If the iris, lens, or other structures inside the eyeball are not injured and the corneal wound is small, sealing of the perforation occurs in a short time. Aqueous humor regenerates promptly and healing will be uneventful if intraocular or corneal infection can be controlled. The application of hot packs and instillation of an antibiotic ointment are indicated for this purpose. Corneal scarring and corneo-iris adhesion (anterior synechia) are common sequelae of corneal perforation.

If the perforation is sufficiently large to permit the iris to prolapse through it, there is greater danger of intraocular infection and subsequent panophthalmitis. Treatment of this lesion for the first several days is aimed at preventing infection. The protruding iris will form granulation tissue rapidly and after several days the protruding tissue may be removed by excision flush with the corneal surface. Removal of prolapsed iris also may be accomplished by cauterization with a hyfrecator or by the repeated use of 90% phenol. The use of phenol is quite satisfactory. It is applied only to the granulating portion of the protruding iris with a metal or wooden rod at 24- to 48-hour intervals until the cornea has healed. When healing occurs, anterior synechia and a corneal scar are usual sequelae but some visual function and a nearly normal appearance are regained.

If penetration of the cornea results in luxation of lens, loss of vitreous, and/or infection of iris, the eyeball should be enucleated immediately. Extirpation of the eyeball and surrounding tissues in the horse is not a difficult procedure. The most common indications are panophthalmitis, collapse of the eyeball following corneal perforation, and the occurrence of malignant neoplasms which cannot be removed otherwise.

DERMOID CYST

This lesion of the cornea is by no means rare in horses. It usually appears as a raised, flat area, or as a rounded, wart-like growth, usually at the junction of sclera and cornea, and extending a bit over the corneal surface. The dermoid invariably carries a number of fairly stiff hairs which may be an inch in length and cause a great deal of local irritation. Surgical removal is corrective.

DISEASES ASSOCIATED WITH FILTRATION OF THE ANTERIOR CHAMBER

In the horse, the filtration of fluid from the anterior chamber into the suprachoroidal space is remarkably efficient so that true glaucoma is a rarity except during an attack of periodic ophthalmia in which hypertension of the eyeball may appear transiently during the acute stage. The hypertension disappears when the acute inflammatory signs subside, and usually is followed by intraocular hypotension.

Hydrophthalmos also is rare and when it occurs the lesion usually is due to intraocular neoplasms.

ABNORMALITIES OF THE LENS

LUXATION

There are few records of this condition in the horse. It has been mentioned on several occasions in connection with periodic ophthalmia, and it possibly occurs occasionally as the result of trauma. I (R.H.S.) have encountered only one case of anterior lens luxation in a horse and this resulted from contusion. In this case the degree of damage caused to the eye-lids and supraorbital structures prevented close examination of the eyeball and the luxation was not observed until 2 weeks later when local swelling, accompanied by edema of the eyelids, had lessened. Hydrophthalmos resulted and it would have been difficult to say whether the luxation occurred as the result of the contusion or was secondary to the hydrophthalmos.

CATARACT

This condition is present when an opacity, partial or complete, of the lens substance or its capsule interferes with the passage of light to the ocular fundus.

Etiology: As in other animals, cataract in the horse may be congenital or acquired. In the latter case, it may result from trauma, or it may arise as a degenerative process during the animal's lifetime. Congenital cataracts are regarded by some as hereditary. Cataract has been known to horse owners as a serious defect but probably only a minor percentage of congenital cataracts ever cause complete loss of vision unless they were already diffuse at the time of birth.

A cataract in a horse of any age may be only of pinpoint size even if it has been in existence for some time. On the other hand, it may partly occlude the lens, or less commonly the lens may become completely opaque.

The smaller cataracts may cause very little interference with vision. Anyone sufficiently interested to paint dots or streaks on the lens of his camera before taking some photographs may be surprised at the little difference they make to the image on the prints.

In spite of these remarks, cataract, in whatever stage or form it may exist, must be regarded as an unsoundness. Some small opacities remain quiescent throughout the horse's life while others, of similar size, tend to spread. Their importance and the prognosis must depend considerably upon their cause and their position in the lens. Cataract may arise in some cases from trauma, but years ago, when periodic ophthalmia was rampant, cataract was a very frequent complication.

Those cases which develop following trauma show little or no tendency to spread after the effects of contusion have subsided. A small cataract, occurring as a sequel to periodic ophthalmia, is more likely to increase in size especially when attacks of this disease recur. This lesion may result when nourishment of the lens is inadequate due to disease of the uveal tract. Frequently after an attack of ophthalmia, the passage of light to the fundus is interfered with by a deposition of fibrinous exudate on the rim of the iris, or suspended in the aqueous, or attached to the anterior capsule of the lens. (Called a spurious cataract.) In the course of time such deposits tend to shrink but they may continue to interfere with the clarity of vision.

In aged horses, some apparent grayness or blueness may be observed when one attempts to look through the pupil into the depths of the eye. This may have no connection with cataract and it causes no loss of vision. It is due to the fact that the deeper layers of the aging lens no longer refract all the rays of light but tend to reflect them. Occasionally, a sclerosis of the lens nucleus may produce a similar appearance. This may be a little more serious but at the same time a moderate degree of sclerosis, enough to cause an appearance of grayness, may have no apparent effect on vision.

The opacity of a true cataract may result from an abnormal arrangement of the lens fibers, or to the irregular or abnormal distribution of the fluid content of the lens. Excess fluid may collect in the spaces between the cortical and nuclear layers and thus impair translucence. This is a common occurrence in congenital cataract.

Very few lenses affected with cataract appear white when removed from the eyeball, except in those rare instances when they are wholly calcareous. The apparent opacity, when viewed through the pupil, results from impaired translucence which may not be evident when the lens is removed and viewed from outside the eyeball.

Types of Cataract: According to their position, cataracts may be nuclear when centrally placed in the lens, or capsular when they involve the capsule of the lens rather than its substance. A cataract is said to be polar when it affects the most prominent part of the cortex beneath the capsule, either at the front or back of the lens.

Anterior cortical cataract may follow corneal ulceration and perforation. It is known as pyramidal cataract. Diffuse cataract spreads evenly throughout the whole lens substance. True lamellar cataract is rare in the horse and is associated usually with maternal malnutrition during pregnancy, particularly when there is a deficiency of vitamin D in the mare's diet. When this type of cataract does appear in the horse, it is usually perinuclear in location. It begins as an opaque ring surrounding the lens nucleus. The outermost portion of the lens remains clear, and through the ophthalmoscope the surface of the lens beneath the capsule shows crenation or a series of denser dots which may appear gray with oblique illumination.

Cortical cataract involves the outer layers of the lens which lie beneath the capsule, and generally it is more diffuse than polar cataract. One may distinguish between the two by the use of the ophthalmoscope. Such opacities are usually progressive in nature and sooner or later the nucleus generally becomes involved.

Quite frequently, cataracts at birth are minute in size and may easily be missed. They may remain completely static, or may extend with age. Congenital cataracts of the foal are more commonly bilateral.

Diagnosis: Demonstration of the 3 light images formerly were used to ascertain the transparency of ocular media. The 3 images represent reflections of a light source held in front of the eye. An erect image can be seen on the cornea itself. A second erect image appears on the anterior capsule of the lens. An inverted image is seen on the posterior surface of the lens capsule. The corneal reflection is small and bright. That from the anterior capsule is smaller, erect, and not so bright. The image on the posterior surface of the lens capsule often is difficult to locate even in the normal eye. It not only is inverted but it also is very much smaller than the second image, and not at all bright. By manipulating the light source slightly it should be possible in a normal eye to see all 3 stages at the same time and from all reflective surfaces. This method of determining the translucency of the lens requires a patient horse and a good deal of practice on the part of the examiner.

Today, the electric ophthalmoscope is used more often and is far more reliable. Some practitioners still employ the indirect method of ophthalmoscopy by which a light is introduced into an eye from a distance. This method may have some advantages in the case of an unruly stallion as the operator need not come within reach of the teeth or forefeet of the horse.

For ophthalmic examination, a darkened stall is sufficient and instillation of a mydriatic is unnecessary. Opacities in the refractive media of the eye, the cornea, lens, and vitreous fluid can be recognized as black specks or as dark gray or blackish areas when viewed against the greenish-blue and gold tapetum lucidum of the horse.

The optic papilla, the point at which the optic nerve enters the eyeball, lies a little laterally, on the temporal side of the fundus. It is pinkish-white in color. In the absence of any opacity this structure can be seen clearly when the viewer looks slightly downward through the pupil. Any opacity of the lens, even when small, can produce obliteration of some part of the fundus of the eye. In normal eyes, the lens is translucent throughout its whole substance. By watching the passage of light through the lens and noting particularly the parts which impede it, one endeavors to identify the portions of the lens which are opaque.

One can do little for cataract in the horse when it is present but the importance of being able to recognize it cannot be overestimated.

ABNORMALITIES OF THE VITREOUS

Hyalitis

Inflammation of the vitreous is a rare condition in the horse except as a complication of periodic ophthalmia. It may be caused occasionally by contusion, and is accompanied sometimes by detachment of the retina. It may also be caused by perforating foreign bodies which produce damage to other ocular structures at the same time. Although in small animals gunshot injuries frequently are responsible, it is seldom that the horse is exposed to this kind of accident.

In a few horses, incomplete absorption of the hyaloid artery may leave minute fragments which move freely in the vitreous. Such bodies also may originate from the remains of the original covering of the embryonic lens. It is thought by some veterinarians that these may give rise to shying or headshaking, but there is no real proof of this.

In periodic ophthalmia, when liquefaction of the vitreous (synchisis) occurs, portions of membrane may be seen floating across the ophthalmoscopic field. In some cases, crystals of tyrosine or cholestrol appear in the vitreous and can readily be seen, producing the appearance of the sky on a starry night.

ABNORMALITIES OF THE RETINA

Retinitis

In the horse, this condition may be associated with periodic ophthalmia, or it may follow influenza or purpura hemorrhagica. Hemorrhages are present in the vitreous and possibly beneath the retina, and its detachment probably will ensue.

Papilledema with constriction of the central vessels and blanching of the optic papilla may accompany an increase in intracranial pressure. In cases of psammoma and after cranial concussion, there may be swelling and congestion of the optic papilla and it may protrude into the vitreous. Venous engorgement of the retinal vessels also may occur. When verminous aneurysm involves the aortic arch, congestion of the optic disc may become evident on ophthalmic examination following a gallop. The vessels appear to be purple or dark blue.

Posterior staphyloma has been reported to occur in the horse. This condition has been diagnosed clinically in the horse and confirmed by postmortem examination.

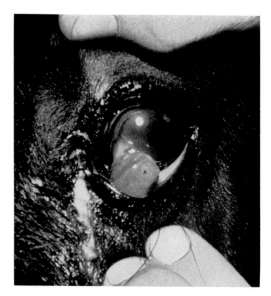

Fig. 3. Sarcoma extending from conjunctiva to invade the cornea.

NEOPLASMS INVOLVING THE ORBIT AND EYEBALL

A granulomatous condition of the caruncle which may be confused with a neoplasm is due to the presence of parasitic embryos of *Habronema* spp. Hydatid cysts have been encountered in the orbit of the horse and botryomycosis may produce lesions of the eyelids which resemble tumors. Neoplasms may range from simple lipoma to various benign and malignant types.

Lipomata may vary from small to very large in size. They appear as lobulated, fatty tumors of soft consistency, filling the spaces between the oculomotor muscles. They may be present in a lean animal and give rise to exophthalmos and strabismus. Other benign tumors include fibromata, papillomata, and dermoids. Along the malignant tumors, epithelioma, sarcoma, melanosarcoma, osteosarcoma, and lymphosarcoma may be encountered. True sarcoma usually starts in the conjunctiva. The neoplasm generally is covered with epithelium and is smooth and pigmented (Fig. 3). Melanotic sarcoma originates in the choroid or uveal tract. Endothelioma usually is encapsulated, slow growing, and seldom recurs following its sur-

gical excision. Epithelioma, or squamous-cell carcinoma, may occur in the membrana nictitans or in the conjunctiva. Such growths always recur after incision; in fact the wounds seldom heal but granulate and become neoplastic at once. This tumor may eventually involve the bony orbit and adjoining lymph nodes (Fig. 4).

AMAUROSIS

Blindness resulting from failure of the retina to convey impressions to the occipital lobes of the brain, may occur after excessive hemorrhage, cranial trauma, lightning shock, and certain encephalitides. Blindness, without visible change in the ocular structure (apart from constant dilation of the pupils), has been known to appear suddenly in a previously normal horse. It is accompanied by rapid ear movements and high-stepping, cautious movements of the forelimbs. Horses which are partially blind move in this way when coming out of a dark stable into daylight.

R. H. SMYTHE
R. L. LUNDVALL

Acknowledgement: The text of this chapter contains portions of an article written by Dr. R. L. Lundvall. It originally appeared in *Biochemic Review* (Fort Dodge Laboratories), Vol. 31, No. 1, 1961. The illustrations were contributed by Dr. Lundvall and several of them appeared in the original article in *Biochemic Review*.

PERIODIC OPHTHALMIA

Inflammation of the ciliary body and iris (iridocyclitis) and sequelae to this reaction are the most common cause of defective vision in the horse. Periodic ophthalmia is a recurrent iridocyclitis that produces alterations in the ocular structures as a result of reaction to the acute inflammatory process. It occurs in horses of all ages, usually resulting in blindness.

Etiology: A reasonable assessment of the available information relating to the cause of equine periodic ophthalmia leads one to the conclusion that this disease must be regarded

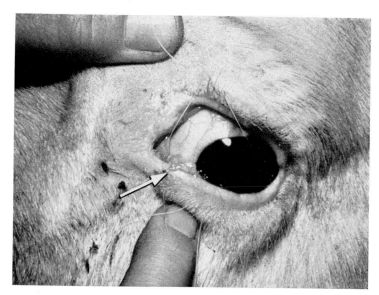

Fig. 4. Epithelioma extending from the membrana nictitans.

as idiopathic. A critical consideration of the many unconfirmed theories of infectious, hereditary or nutritional causation will serve no useful purpose here.

It is pertinent to discuss the evidence for a leptospiral etiology because this is the most recent in a line of suspected causes for the disease. Leptospiral infection is suspected to be the cause of equine periodic ophthalmia for 2 principal reasons: that uveitis is a rather common sequel to leptospiral infection in man, and that leptospiral agglutinins are demonstrable in the serum and aqueous humor of a majority of horses with periodic ophthalmia.

Two hypotheses have been advanced to explain the pathogenesis of periodic ophthalmia as a recurrent leptospiral uveitis. One of these holds that periodic ophthalmia occurs as a result of localization and persistence of leptospira in the uveal tissues. There is no good evidence in support of this concept. Leptospira have neither been demonstrated to be routinely recoverable nor histologically identifiable in affected eyes. Further, recurrent iridocyclitis has not been shown to be reproducible by inoculation of horses with cultures or other infectious material containing leptospira.

The second hypothesis is based on sensitization of the eye during the bacteremic stage of leptospirosis. Recurrent attacks of iridocyclitis would then be provoked by leptospiral antigens originating from a chronic extraocular focus of infection. If this hypothesis is valid, then injection of an affected horse with either live or killed leptospires should produce such an attack. I have attempted to provoke such an attack by this method in several horses with naturally occurring periodic ophthalmia. The results were negative. A second factor for establishment of this mechanism must be either the presence of a chronic focus of infection or demonstration of repeated infection of the horse. It has been our experience that chronic leptospiral infection does not occur in the horse and that horses having experienced a leptospiral infection are quite solidly immune.

A reasonable hypothesis for explanation of the cause of equine recurrent iridocyclitis is that this disease is a hypersensitivity reaction of the bacterial type. Recurrent iridocyclitis may be provoked in the previously sensitized eye of animals by using a variety of antigenic substances. This has been repeatedly demonstrated in experimental animals, including the horse. The inflammatory reaction in an affected equine eye is characterized by the presence of cellular elements that would be expected to be present in a lesion produced by this type of hypersensitivity.

Recurrent uveitis of equally obscure etiology occurs in humans, and surgical manipulation of focal infectious processes in certain of these patients has been associated with acute exacerbations of uveitis. The vascularity of the uveal tract, especially that in a previously affected eye, seems to render this structure quite accessible to circulating antigenic material arising from extraocular focal lesions. The common occurrence of localized streptococcal infections in the horse or the constant presence of parasitic nematodes with their attendant tissue damage might well satisfy the requirements for initiating and maintaining this type of tissue hypersensitivity. *Strongylus vulgaris* infestation and the resultant verminous arteritis could be considered a prime suspect.

Treatment: Because no specific therapy is available, treatment of acute iridocyclitis should be directed toward prevention of the intraocular lesions secondary to the inflammatory process.

The horse should be stabled in a darkened stall. An effort should be made to prevent the formation of synechia by achieving maximal pupillary dilation. This usually requires repeated instillation of atropine at short intervals to achieve initial dilation. Mydriasis should be maintained by repeated instillation of atropine until the acute inflammation has subsided. Pain may be relieved by use of a topical anesthetic. Corticosteroid therapy may be of value for controlling the inflammatory reaction. Cortisone or hydrocortisone ophthalmic ointments should be used locally. These ointments should be applied every 4 to 6 hours. Cortisone or corticotropin may be given parenterally.

Antibiotic or foreign protein therapy is of no proven value. Foreign protein therapy may produce serious reactions in the horse. There is no form of therapy that is known to prevent recurrent attacks in equine periodic ophthalmia.

Clinical Signs and Diagnosis: Diagnosis of periodic ophthalmia depends upon observation of repeated attacks of iridocyclitis or upon a history of such attacks coupled with demonstration of residual ocular lesions attributable to iridocyclitis.

Horses afflicted with periodic ophthalmia may exhibit a transient (1- to 2-degree) rise in body temperature without other extraocular signs of disease. Nonrecurrent attacks of iridocyclitis occur as sequelae to or during the acute stage of other equine diseases. Affected animals present all of the ocular signs occurring in acute attacks of periodic ophthalmia. Iridocyclitis with hypopyon may occur as a sequel to equine arteritis virus infection or as a result of trauma. Nonrecurrent intraocular inflammation may produce residual damage comparable to that resulting from periodic ophthalmia. Many horses without history of periodic ophthalmia have defective vision due to lesions similar or identical to those produced by that disease.

The clinical signs of acute iridocyclitis are detectable by examination with the naked eye. The earliest signs consist of catarrhal conjunctivitis, marked photophobia, miosis, and epiphora. These signs become more marked with time. Conjunctival and pericorneal congestion, cloudiness of the cornea, and the presence of a diffusely distributed or precipitated exudate in the anterior chamber usually are apparent by the second or third day. The normally avascular cornea usually shows peripheral vascularization and the narrowed pupil responds only after repeated instillation of a mydriatic. The intraocular tension is decreased and pain is evident upon palpation. The acute phase may last for periods as long as a month. The inflammation may be present in only one eye, in both eyes, or may occur unilaterally in opposite eyes during repeated attacks. The interval between attacks varies greatly; no distinct periodicity is apparent in most cases, and the quiescent period may be more than a year. The quiescent period seems to be more prolonged in horses that have experienced several recurrences.

Diagnosis during the quiescent period depends upon history of recurrent attacks and detection of resultant residual lesions. These lesions are produced mainly by organization of the inflammatory exudate formed during the acute stage. The pupillary response to light commonly is affected by adhesions limiting the movement of the iris. The iris may therefore have irregular margins. Bits of the pigmented iris may be seen adherent to the anterior lens capsule as a result of torn adhesions. The adhesions formed between the iris and the anterior lens capsule (posterior synechia) may be so complete as to cause obliteration of the pupil (total posterior synechia). Interference with fluid exchange caused by adhesions leads to accumulation of aqueous humor in the posterior chamber which causes the iris to balloon, and adhesions between the iris and cornea (anterior synechia) may form. Ophthalmoscopic examination usually reveals dark bodies in the vitreous humor which represent exudate formed during the acute stage. The presence of exudate in the vitreous may preclude satisfactory visualization of the fundus.

Cataract is a usual finding in horses experiencing repeated attacks. Cataract may be partial in these cases but usually is complete. Retinitis and detachment of the retina may occur as a sequel to recurrent iridocyclitis.

It should be realized that the degree of alteration of ocular structure depends on the number and severity of acute attacks. The lesions detected in a horse having experienced only a few attacks may consist of no more than opacities in the vitreous body. Errington has observed that estimation of the intraocular tension is an important prognostic sign in periodic ophthalmia, loss of tension being indicative of an unfavorable prognosis. He also has emphasized that vitreous opacities are very commonly seen in horses with no history of ophthalmitis.

J. T. BRYANS

REFERENCES

Bryans, J. T.: Studies on equine leptospirosis. Cornell Vet. 45 (1955) 16.

Errington, B. J.: Equine ophthalmology. Vet. Med. 37 (1942) 16.

Foss, B.: Experimental anaphylactic iridocyclitis. Acta. Path. et. Microbiol. Scand., Supp. 81, (1949).

Gordon, D. M.: The clinical use of corticotropin, cortisone and hydrocortisone in eye disease. Pub. No. 162, Amer. Lect. Series. Chas. C Thomas, Springfield, Illinois, (1954).

Jones, T. C.: Equine periodic ophthalmia. Am. J. Vet. Res. 3 (1942) 45.

Manninger, R.: Untersuchungen uber die Atiologie der mondblindheit. Arch. fur Wiss. u. Prakt. Turheilk. 61 (1930) 144.

Woods, Alan C.: Endogenous Uveitis. Williams & Wilkins Co., Baltimore, Md. 1956.

CHAPTER 16

DISEASES OF THE BLOOD AND CARDIOVASCULAR SYSTEM

THE HEART

INTRODUCTION

Cardiovascular disease in the horse requires further study to provide an adequate basis for clinical purposes. Most of the knowledge available is based on postmortem observations of animals which were not examined by modern cardiological methods prior to death.

Cardiac arrhythmias and murmurs are more frequent in horses than in other domestic mammals, but the significance of many of these clinical signs has not been established for this species. The prevalence of heart disease in horses has not been determined. Sudden death attributable to myocarditis or rupture of the great vessels is not rare, and occasional horses with congestive heart failure are encountered.

EXAMINATION OF THE HEART

Inspection: Before centering attention on the cardiac region, the animal should be examined as a whole. Particular attention should be paid to the color of the visible mucous membranes, the degree of filling of peripheral veins, the jugular pulse, and the presence or absence of edema in dependent areas.

In subjects with a thin thoracic wall, the apex beat may be visible at the fifth left intercostal space about the middle of the lower third of the thorax.

Palpation: To palpate the cardiac region (the lower third of the thorax on each side between the third and fifth intercostal spaces), use the left hand on the left side and the right hand on the right side, with the palm at the fifth intercostal space and the fingers extending forward under the shoulder musculature over the third intercostal space and downward toward the sternal margin.

The cardiac impulse is felt between the third and fifth left intercostal spaces in the lower third of the thorax, being strongest at the fifth left intercostal space, about the middle of the lower third of the thorax, and on the right side between the third and fourth intercostal spaces above the right sternal border.

Cardiac murmurs which are sufficiently intense are accompanied by palpable thrills. Detection of a thrill establishes the location of the point of maximum intensity of a murmur and usually indicates heart disease. Thrills may be felt over large arteriovenous fistulas and aneurysms and may be present over the cardiac region in severe anemia in the absence of valvular disease or other cardiac defects.

Forward shift of the caudal limit of the palpable cardiac impulse may occur owing to marked ascites or excessive tympany. Abnormal masses within the thoracic cavity (large abscesses, tumors) may shift the heart position. Relative weakness of the cardiac impulse occurs when the thoracic walls are thick, in the presence of pleural or pericardial effusions, or when any abnormal mass is interposed between the heart and the chest wall. The cardiac impulse is increased in strength under conditions of exercise and excitement, febrile diseases, and in postblock or postextrasystolic beats.

Percussion: Gross cardiac enlargement may be demonstrated by delineation of the areas of cardiac dullness. The area of absolute cardiac dullness is bounded on the left side of the thorax by the edge of the sternum ventrally, and the third left intercostal space anteriorly. Dorsally and caudally it is bounded by an arc passing from a point on the fourth rib about 5 or 6 inches above the sternal border, through the fifth left intercostal space at a distance of 1 or 2 inches above the sternal border to reach the sternal border in the sixth left intercostal space. On the right side of the thorax, the area of cardiac dullness extends from the third to the fourth right intercostal space and to a distance of 1 to 2 inches above the sternal border. To expose these areas for percussion, it is necessary to pull the foreleg far forward.

These limits of the area of cardiac dullness are only approximations which vary from individual to individual, depending on the shape of the thorax and thickness of the chest wall. When the heart is markedly enlarged or the pericardial sac is greatly distended with fluid, the area of cardiac dullness may be extended in a dorsal direction and caudally to the sixth left intercostal space with corresponding, but lesser, enlargement on the right side.

In the presence of marked pulmonary emphysema, the area of cardiac dullness disappears first in the fifth left intercostal space, is lower in the fourth left intercostal space and may disappear entirely on the right side of the thorax.

Auscultation: This is the most important part of the physical examination of the heart. It requires time, patience, adequate control of the subject, and absence of external noise.

The Auscultation Areas: Sounds associated with the various valves of the heart are best heard in different locations and these areas are correspondingly named. The mitral area is located at the caudal border of the area of cardiac dullness at the fifth left intercostal space just below the level of a horizontal line drawn halfway between the point of the shoulder and the edge of the sternum; the aortic area is at the fourth left intercostal space about one inch below the level of the point of the shoulder; the pulmonic area is at the third left intercostal space or fourth rib below a line drawn through the middle of the lower third of the thorax; the right atrioventricular valve area is located at the third or fourth intercostal space in the lower half of the ventral third of the thorax. The characteristics of the heart sounds will be described in a later section (see p. 347 *et seq.*).

Examination of the Arterial Pulse

The arteries ordinarily palpated are the submaxillary, coccygeal, and the transverse facial. When investigating cardiac rate and rhythm alterations, auscultation of the heart or palpation of the cardiac impulse should be combined with simultaneous palpation of the pulse. For this purpose the common digital artery, when palpable, is within easy reach while auscultating the cardiac region.

The volume and contour of the arterial pulse depend upon the cardiac output (stroke volume) and the contractile tone of the arteries and arterioles (peripheral resistance). The volume or "strength" of the pulse is dependent on the pulse pressure (*i.e.* difference between systolic and diastolic pressure) and its duration. Marked variations may occur from cycle to cycle in various arrhythmias since the pulse volume ordinarily will increase with increased stroke volume following relatively prolonged diastolic periods. The average pulse volume is increased relatively when there is central regurgitation of blood (*e.g.* aortic insufficiency), decrease in peripheral resistance (*e.g.* arteriovenous anastomosis, vasomotor relaxation), and increased stroke volume (*e.g.* bradycardia). The average pulse volume is decreased relatively in conditions which result in diminished forward stroke volume such as aortic stenosis, mitral insufficiency, myocardial decompensation, and tachycardia above a critical rate (usually 90 per minute or more).

The contour of the pulse may be roughly determined by palpation. An anacrotic pulse has 2 summits, the second higher than the first, and may occur in aortic regurgitation. A dicrotic pulse also has 2 summits, the second lower than the first. This type of pulse is a normal finding at slow pulse rate in the horse, and may be exaggerated in arterial hypotension. In aortic regurgitation, the pulse may have 2 summits of approximately equal height (pulsus bisferiens). A bounding or collapsing pulse (celer pulse) characterized by a sharp rise and fall, may be found in aortic regurgitation and patent ductus arteriosus. Tardus pulse or plateau pulse occurs when the volume of the pulse is diminished as in aortic stensis. There is a gradual rise and fall of the pulse wave separated by a plateau. Pulsus alternans, alternate strong and weak pulsations, occurs rarely in the presence of severe myocardial disease. Paradoxical pulse decreases in volume during inspiration and is expected in pericarditis with effusion. (We have not, as yet, observed this condition in horses although traumatic pericarditis has been reported.)

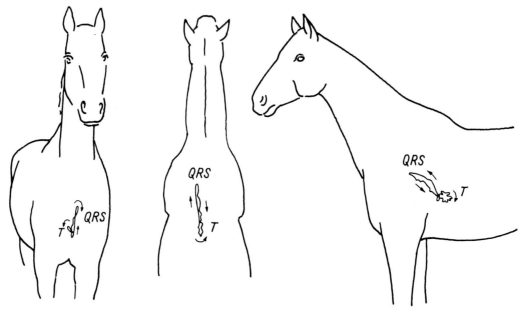

Fig. 1. Vectorcardiogram of a horse. From left to right: transverse projection, dorsal projection, and saggital projection. The cube technic of electrode placement was used. In this animal the QRS spatial loop is directed dorsally and cranially.

EXAMINATION OF THE JUGULAR PULSE

The jugular veins and their contained blood act like an elastic fluid manometer, reflecting pressure changes occurring in the right atrium and in the thoracic cavity. The extent to which pulsation in these veins is visible depends upon the mean pressure within the atrium, the amount of tissue overlying the veins, the height of the veins with respect to the level of the right atrium (this varies with the height at which head and neck are held), and the amplitude of the pulse pressure. Obviously many of these factors are variable under normal circumstances. Consequently, the interpretation of visible pulsation in the jugular veins must be made with due regard to normal variations.

The normal jugular pulse consists of several waves during each cardiac cycle (see p. 347 *et seq.*) When the right atrium contracts, a pulse wave (A wave) is transmitted to the jugular veins. This wave is followed by a second wave due to bulging of the right atrioventricular valve into the right atrium during early ventricular systole and to transmission of the pulse from the adjacent carotid artery (C wave). As the base of the heart moves downward and the papillary muscles shorten and move the atrioventricular valves downward in systole, a negative wave occurs (X wave). This is followed by a positive wave as the atrium and veins fill with blood during ventricular systole (V wave). When the atrioventricular valves open, the blood flows rapidly into the ventricles and another negative wave (Y wave) is seen. These waves occur in sequence during each cardiac cycle and are further complicated by pressure changes in the thorax and modifications of the wave form resulting from the elasticity of the veins and surrounding tissues and pressure effects from contiguous muscles and organs.

Pulsations and undulations of the jugular veins usually are visible at the thoracic inlet and often for a variable distance along the veins above the level of the heart base. A rhythmic swelling and collapsing of the veins may be seen with respiration, the veins filling somewhat during expiration and emptying partially during inspiration. This effect is exaggerated by factors increasing expiratory intrapleural pressure (expiratory dyspnea). If the head is lowered and the veins reach a level below that of the heart, they are seen to fill with blood. In the commonly occurring incomplete heart block with dropped beats, the veins may be seen to fill during the doubled diastolic interval.

The atrial wave occurs just before the end of ventricular diastole. It often can be identified by visual inspection and its time in the cardiac cycle verified by palpating the apex beat of the heart simultaneously. It precedes the palpable apex beat by a brief interval.

Insufficiency of the tricuspid valve is accompanied by regurgitation of blood which, when the volume is great enough, produces strong systolic pulsation in the jugular veins. It is distinguished from the atrial pulse since it occurs later in the cycle (*i.e.* during ventricular systole).

ELECTROCARDIOGRAPHY

Readers unfamiliar with the basic principles of electrocardiography will find the introductory texts of Schamroth[1] and Burch and Winsor[2] and the books by Lepeschkin,[3] Sodi-Pallares[4] and Grant[5] useful since space limitation does not permit a discussion of them here.

The form of electrocardiographic waves in various leads depends on the direction and relative magnitude of electrical forces from moment to moment during the cardiac cycle. The direction of these electrical forces is determined by the anatomic position of the heart and the course taken by the spread of excitation throughout the myocardium. These factors vary in different species. For example, in horses the pathway followed by the excitation wave over the atria is in general the same as that in the dog, though the course of the excitation over the ventricles differs from that of the dog.[6] Consequently, the form of the ventricular complex in comparable leads in these 2 species is not the same but the direction of the P waves is similar.

The electrical forces determining the form of the QRS complex in various leads can be represented as a spatial vector loop. This loop in the dog is directed approximately along the long axis of the body; in the horse it is directed at approximately a right angle to that of the dog, *i.e.* generally from the sternum toward the vertebral column. It is for this reason that the directions of the major deflec-

tions of QRS in certain leads in the horse differ from those in the dog. A QRS spatial vector loop is depicted in Fig. 1. Figure 2 is a map of isopotential lines determined during the peak of the R wave in lead II and Fig. 3a, 3b, and 3c illustrate the forms of QRS complexes in unipolar leads taken over the body surface of a horse. These records, based on detailed observations on a few normal animals, give a general idea of the form of QRS complexes which can be anticipated in various leads. Marked departures from the general ventrodorsal orientation of the spatial vector loop of QRS indicate that the process of ventricular excitation is following an abnormal pathway

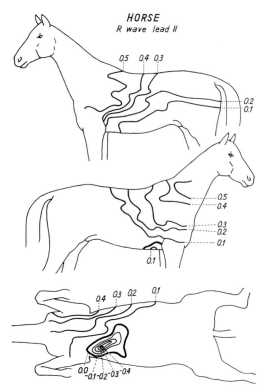

Fig. 2. Isopotential lines mapped on the body surface of a horse during the peak of R wave in lead II. The values are in millivolts and represent the potentials recorded against the Wilson central terminal. The area of greatest negativity (−0.4 mV.) was located on the ventral thorax to the right of the sternum and the area of greatest positivity (+0.5 mV.) toward the head. A line connecting these two areas has approximately the same direction as that of the QRS spatial vector loop shown in Fig. 1. The isopotential lines were determined using the method of Mauro et al., Am. J. Physiol., 168 (1952) 584–591.

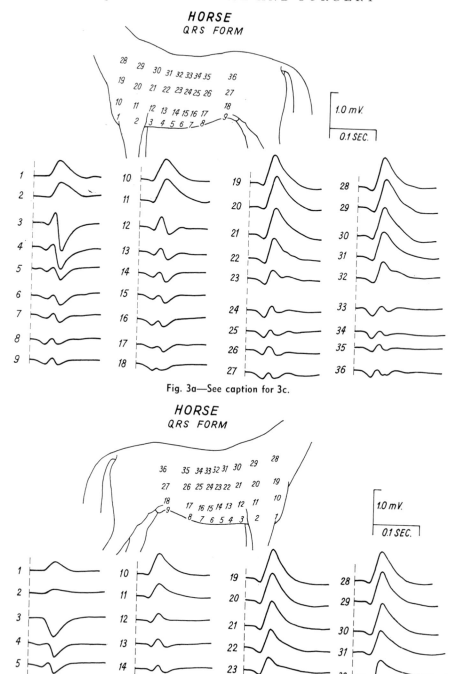

Fig. 3a—See caption for 3c.

Fig. 3b—See caption for 3c.

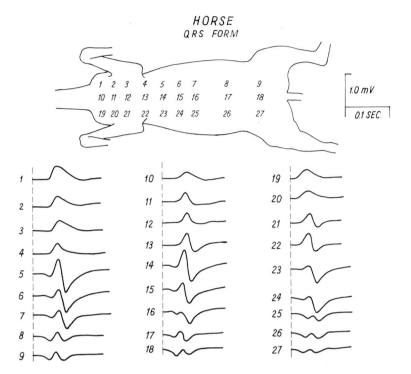

HORSE
QRS FORM

1.0 mV.

0.1 SEC.

Fig. 3c. Form of the QRS complex on the body surface of a horse. Unipolar leads against the Wilson central terminal were taken at the anatomic points indicated by the numbers. The QRS complexes recorded at each point are shown below each diagram. The paper speed employed was 260 mm. per second. These maps show the form of QRS over various points on the body surface.

and this can be recognized from scalar body surface electrocardiograms. Detailed knowledge of normal electrocardiographic variations and changes characteristic of cardiac disease is still inadequate for most diagnostic purposes in the horse. Based on present knowledge, however, major QRS vector changes, conduction disturbances, and arrhythmias can be recognized.

The chief waves of the electrocardiogram are labeled P, Q, R, S, and T. The P wave represents the process of excitation (depolarization) as it spreads from the sinu-atrial node through both atria. In the horse the repolarization wave following atrial excitation often produces a visible deflection in body surface leads which is frequently opposite in direction from the P wave and is termed the atrial T or Ta wave. The P-R interval is measured from the beginning of P to the beginning of the QRS complex. It represents the time required for the passage of the excitatory process from the sinu-atrial node through the atria to the atrioventricular node, through the atrioventricular node and bundle of His and into the ventricular musculature. The QRS complex is

inscribed during depolarization of the ventricular musculature. This complex may consist of from one to several waves which are labeled in accordance with their direction and relative position. Any upward deflection is labeled R. If there are several upward deflections, the additional ones are labeled R′,R″, etc. A downward deflection is termed Q if it precedes R and S if it follows R. A single downward deflection unaccompanied by other waves is labeled QS. The S-T segment designates that part of the tracing between the end of the QRS complex and the beginning of the T wave. The S-T junction (ST_J) is the point where the QRS complex joins the S-T segment. The T wave represents the ventricular recovery process (repolarization), which occurs as ventricular systole subsides. The Q-T interval, which represents the period of ventricular excitation and recovery, is measured from the beginning of QRS to the end of T. The durations of these various electrocardiographic intervals are given in Table I.[7]

Electrocardiographic Leads: Standard bipolar limb leads, unipolar and augmented unipolar limb leads, and precordial leads have

Table 1.—Duration of Electrocardiographic Intervals (in Seconds) in Horses, Lead II

	P	P-R	QRS	Q-T	HR/MIN.
Warm-blooded horses					
Upper probable abnormal limit................	0.175	0.429	0.155	0.625	79.3
Upper normal limit..........................	0.155	0.382	0.140	0.575	70.2
Mean.......................................	0.117	0.286	0.111	0.475	42.6
Lower normal limit..........................	0.079	0.190	0.082	0.376	24.2
Lower probable abnormal limit................	0.059	0.143	0.068	0.326	19.6
Cold-blooded horses					
Upper probable abnormal limit...............	0.172	0.465	0.139	0.589	96.8
Upper normal limit..........................	0.154	0.410	0.126	0.567	86.1
Mean.......................................	0.120	0.298	0.100	0.475	43.6
Lower normal limit..........................	0.085	0.187	0.074	0.339	27.7
Lower probable abnormal limit................	0.067	0.131	0.061	0.293	22.4

Source: From Lannek and Rutqvist (1951).[7]

been employed for clinical purposes in horses. Various electrode positions have been proposed for precordial leads, but no given system is in general use.[7,8,9,10,11,12]

Standard Bipolar Limb Leads: These are counterparts of the three leads Einthoven originally used in man. They are right foreleg and left foreleg (lead I), right foreleg and left hindleg (lead II), and left foreleg and left hindleg (lead III).

Augmented Unipolar Limb Leads: In these leads 2 of the 3 limbs used in the standard bipolar limb leads are paired against the third limb. Records are taken from each limb in sequence and are labeled in accordance with current terminology aVR, aVL, aVF; R designates right foreleg, L left foreleg, and F left hindleg. In each lead the limb designated by the letter is connected with one pole of the galvanometer and the remaining 2 limbs connected together with the opposite pole. The less commonly employed unipolar limb leads (labeled VR, VL, VF, respectively) are taken by connecting all 3 limbs with one pole of the galvanometer and the limb designated by the letter with the opposite pole. The unipolar limb lead records are of the same form as the corresponding augmented unipolar records, but are of lower amplitude.

Chest Leads: In these leads an exploring electrode is placed on various locations on the chest and paired with an electrode or group of electrodes located at a distance from the heart.

A precordial lead with the exploring electrode over the cardiac apex, paired with a relatively indifferent electrode at the base of the neck on the right side was introduced by Lautenschlager in 1928.[13] This is often referred to as a base-apex bipolar lead because the electrodes are placed on the body surface where an extension of the anatomic longitudinal axis of the heart would meet the skin.

Electrocardiographic data from 212 horses for standard bipolar limb leads and three precordial leads are given in Table 2.[7] The locations of the three precordial leads used were as follows: CV_6RL on the right side of the thorax, 3 to 5 cm. above a horizontal line drawn through the highest point of the olecranon behind the triceps brachii at the sixth rib (*i.e.* over the free wall of the right ventricle); CV_6LL on the left side of the thorax at the same height as a horizontal line through the highest point of the olecranon behind the triceps brachii at the sixth rib (thus over the left ventricular apex); CV_6LU on the left side of the thorax about 8 cm. above CV_6LL (thus over the free wall of the left ventricle). In lead V10, the exploring electrode is placed over the vertebral column vertically above CV_6LL.

Table 2.—Amplitudes of Electrocardiographic Waves in Various Leads in Horses*

LEAD	P	Q	R	S	S-T	T
I	0.07 ± 0.07 0.06 ± 0.04	0.10 ± 0.07 0.10 ± 0.10	0.42 ± 0.22 0.28 ± 0.15	0.11 ± 0.04 0.14 ± 0.17	-0.01 ± 0.02 -0.01 ± 0.02	-0.18 ± 0.22 -0.12 ± 0.16
II	0.23 ± 0.09 0.18 ± 0.07	0.18 ± 0.10 0.12 ± 0.07	0.80 ± 0.47 0.49 ± 0.29	0.21 ± 0.17 0.21 ± 0.18	-0.02 ± 0.04 -0.02 ± 0.03	0.20 ± 0.39 0.05 ± 0.26
III	0.17 ± 0.11 0.14 ± 0.06	0.17 ± 0.14 0.17 ± 0.16	0.60 ± 0.37 0.38 ± 0.27	0.34 ± 0.22 0.28 ± 0.18	0.00 ± 0.02 0.00 ± 0.01	0.41 ± 0.25 0.22 ± 0.21
VR	-0.09(0/-0.2)	0(0/0.20)	0.10(0.02/0.20)	0.36(0.20/1.00)	....	(-0.30/0.60)
VL	-0.03(-0.20/0.08)	0(0/0.10)	0.19(0.02/1.00)	0.21(0/0.60)	....	(-0.60/0.25)
VF	0.10(-0.05/0.20)	0.06(0/0.20)	0.34(0.02/1.00)	0.09(0/0.40)	....	(0.05/0.60)
CV₆RL	-0.004 ± 0.10 -0.002 ± 0.05	0.10 ± 0.05 0.10 ± 0.04	0.27 ± 0.23 0.19 ± 0.14	0.45 ± 0.30 0.18 ± 0.11	0.02 ± 0.03 0.00 ± 0.01	0.16 ± 0.29 0.03 ± 0.15
CV₆LL	0.25 ± 0.10 0.12 ± 0.09	0.13 ± 0.08 0.09 ± 0.04	0.44 ± 0.34 0.19 ± 0.12	0.84 ± 0.54 0.34 ± 0.23	0.02 ± 0.04 0.00 ± 0.02	-0.16 ± 0.41 -0.09 ± 0.23
CV₆LU	0.31 ± 0.13 0.17 ± 0.09	0.15 ± 0.10 0.11 ± 0.05	0.66 ± 0.44 0.42 ± 0.24	0.36 ± 0.33 0.19 ± 0.15	-0.01 ± 0.03 0.00 ± 0.01	-0.05 ± 0.29 -0.03 ± 0.17

*Mean and standard deviation or mean and range (in parentheses) given in millivolts. Where two values are given, the upper values are for warm-blooded and the lower for cold-blooded horses.
Source: From Lannek and Rutqvist (1951) and van Zijl.[7,10]

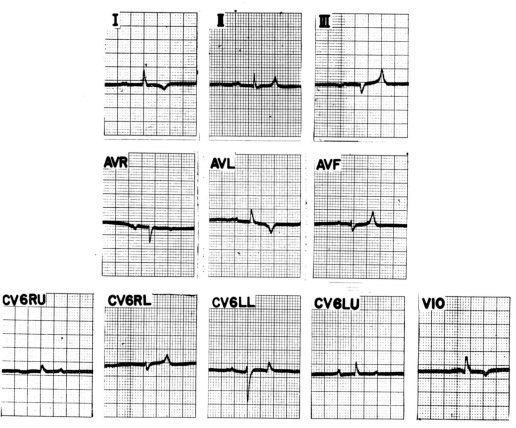

Fig. 4. Electrocardiogram from a 3-year-old Thoroughbred stallion in a standing position. Standard limb leads I, II, III. Augmented unipolar leads AVR, AVL, AVF. For the precordial leads, Wilson's central terminal is paired with the exploring electrode in the following positions: CV_6RU, right side of thorax at the sixth rib at the level of a horizontal line drawn through the point of the shoulder; CV_6RL, right side of thorax, just above the highest point of the olecranon, behind the triceps brachii at the sixth rib; CV_6LL, left side of thorax at the same height as a horizontal line drawn through the highest point of the olecranon behind the triceps brachii at the sixth rib; CV_6LU, left side thorax directly above CV_6LL, at the level of a horizontal line drawn through the point of the shoulder; V_{10}, over the vertebral column vertically above CV_6LU.

Van Zijl has provided values from a few horses for the unipolar limb leads.[10] Electrocardiographic data are given in Tables 1 and 2 and a representative electrocardiogram in Fig. 4. In this figure, the electrode position for lead CV_6LU is slightly higher than that employed by Lannek and Rutqvist, since it is positioned at the level of a horizontal line drawn through the point of the shoulder, and that for lead CV_6RL is lower, since it is positioned on a level with the olecranon.

The P wave usually is positive, most often notched, sometimes diphasic in the standard limb leads. These variations are considered normal by most workers, although Brooijmans, on the basis of vector analysis and the well-known variation in P wave form seen in equine electrocardiograms, regards only positive P waves normal in leads I, II, and III.[9] P is negative in lead aVR.[14] The QRS complex is variable in form and amplitude in the standard limb leads. Although a prominent R wave is usually present, the amplitudes are frequently small and the entire complex may possess a complicated configuration with slurring and notching of the various waves. The QRS in aVR is usually negative (deep S or QS) and in aVL and aVF usually predominantly positive or diphasic.

The heart rate, determined in the electrocardiogram, averaged 35 per minute (range: 27 to 47) in a series of 49 horses.[15] Lannek

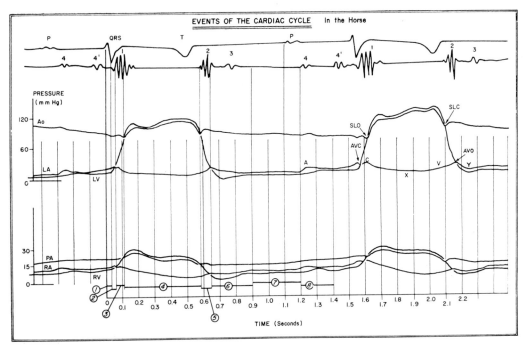

Fig. 5. The cardiac cycle of the horse. From the top: electrocardiogram, phonocardiogram, pressure tracings from the various chambers of the heart and great vessels in a normal 5-year-old horse. This diagram was constructed from a series of recordings in which the electrocardiogram, phonocardiogram, and 2 pressure curves were recorded simultaneously. Pressure recordings were obtained by using 2 micromanometers mounted on the tips of cardiac catheters (Telco Inc., Paris, France). Simultaneous pressure recordings from the various chambers and vessels were then superimposed, and the composite diagram constructed. The left atrial pressure curve was not recorded, but was approximated from records obtained in open chest experiments on horses, and from the right atrial pressure curve. (1) Electropressor latent period—.035 second, (2) Entrant phase—.025 second, (3) Isometric contraction phase—.05 second, (4) Ejection phase—0.47 second, (5) Isometric relaxation phase—.065 second, (6) and (7) Ventricular filling phase—0.55 second, (8) Atrial systole (duration of A wave)—approximately 0.20 second. 4, early atrial sound; 4', late atrial sound; 1, first heart sound; 2, second heart sound; 3, third heart sound; Ao, aorta; LA, left atrium; LV, left ventricle; PA, pulmonary artery; RA, right atrium; RV, right ventricle; AVC, atrioventricular valve closure; SLO, semilunar valve opening; SLC, semilunar valve closure; AVO, atrioventricular valve opening; A, A wave; C, C wave; X, X wave; V, V wave; Y, Y wave.

and Rutqvist found the average to be 43.6 per minute for cold-blooded horses[7] and 42.6 per minute for warm-blooded horses. This disparity in average heart rates may be accounted for by the fact that in the first series the total number of animals was much smaller than the group studied by Lannek and Rutqvist, and many of the records were taken without removing the horses from their accustomed stalls.

EVENTS OF THE CARDIAC CYCLE. THE HEART SOUNDS

More information concerning the functional status of the heart can be obtained through careful auscultation and thoughtful interpretation of the heart sounds, than by any other routine method of clinical examination.

Because of the relatively great intensity of the low frequency sounds and the slow heart rate, 4 heart sounds often are readily heard in the horse during routine auscultation. An understanding of the relationship between various electric, hemodynamic, and acoustic events which accompany the heartbeat is essential for correct interpretation of cardiovascular sounds. A diagram showing the relationship of various events of the cardiac cycle in the horse is presented in Fig. 5.

EVENTS OF THE CARDIAC CYCLE

The cardiac cycle may be divided into 2 phases, ventricular systole and ventricular diastole. Electrical systole begins with the onset of the QRS complex of the electrocardiogram, and ends at the end of the T wave. The beginning of mechanical systole lags somewhat behind electrical systole, starting with the onset of the pressure rise in the ventricles, and ending with closure of the semilunar valves. The duration of mechanical systole is roughly determined by the time interval between the onset of the first heart sound, and the onset of the second heart sound. Mechanical ventricular diastole extends from the closure of the semilunar valves to the onset of the next ventricular systolic pressure rise, or roughly, from the beginning of the second heart sound to the beginning of the first heart sound of the succeeding beat. At normal resting heart rates in the horse, ventricular diastole comprises about 70% of the cardiac cycle. It is this long diastolic interval which the examiner often uses intuitively to identify the heart sounds (the first heart sound is heard after a long diastolic interval). In tachycardia, the diastolic interval shortens, making identification of the first and second heart sounds difficult solely on the basis of timing.

For a more detailed understanding of the events of the cardiac cycle, systole and diastole can be further subdivided into a number of phases (Fig. 5). The *electropressor latent period* is defined as the period from the onset of the QRS complex to the initial pressure rise in the ventricles. The *entrant phase* extends from the onset of ventricular pressure rise to closure of the atrioventricular valves. The *isometric contraction phase* is a period of rapidly rising ventricular pressure which begins with the closure of the atrioventricular valves and extends to the opening of the semilunar valves. During this period, the atrioventricular and semilunar valves are closed, so that no blood is ejected from the heart. The volume of blood in the ventricles remains constant until the rising ventricular pressure exceeds that in the aorta and pulmonary arteries, and the semilunar valves open. The *ejection phase* begins with the opening of the semilunar valves and ends with their closure. The *period of maximum ejection* extends from the onset of the ejection phase to the peak of the aortic and pulmonary artery pressure curves. The *period of reduced ejection* extends from this point to the dicrotic notch in the aortic and pulmonary artery pressure curves (closure of the semilunar valves). The latter period represents the time of subsiding ventricular contraction. When the pressure in the corresponding ventricle falls below that in the aorta or pulmonary artery, the pulmonary and aortic semilunar valves close and ventricular systole is ended.

Diastole begins with a phase of rapidly decreasing intraventricular pressure, the *period of isometric relaxation*, which starts with closure of the semilunar valves and extends to the opening of the atrioventricular valves. As in the case of isometric contraction, both the atrioventricular and semilunar valves are closed, so that no blood enters or leaves the ventricle during this period. When the intraventricular pressure falls below that in the corresponding atrium, the atrioventricular valves open, and the *filling phase* begins. It extends to the onset of the next ventricular contraction, and begins with a *period of rapid filling* during which there is a sudden inflow of the blood which has accumulated in the atrium during ventricular systole. Following the period of rapid filling, the ventricles fill at a slower rate until the beginning of atrial systole. Our records did not make it possible to determine when rapid filling ends and slow filling begins. These periods are arbitrarily labeled 6 and 7 in Fig. 5 without trying to designate the actual point of separation.

Atrial systole occurs at a variable time just prior to the onset of ventricular systole, adding an additional complement of blood to the ventricle. If atrioventricular conduction is relatively slow (P-R interval of the electrocardiogram is long) atrial contraction may occur well before ventricular systole begins. In the horse, the onset of the atrial systolic wave as recorded in the atrium (A wave) follows the onset of the P wave by about 0.10 to 0.13 second.

Other Atrial Waves: Other passive waves are recognized in the pressure recording from the atrium. The C wave is a sharp positive wave which occurs at the time of closure of the atrioventricular valves, presumably owing to the bulging of the valves into the atrium. The X wave is a negative wave following the C wave, and is ascribed to the lengthening of the atrium as the ventricle moves downward during ventricular systole. The V *wave* is a slowly rising positive wave due to gradual filling of the atrium by the return of blood from the great veins. The Y *wave* is a negative wave which begins at the time of atrioventricular valve opening. It represents a decrease in intra-atrial pressure which occurs as the atrial blood drains into the corresponding ventricle during the period of rapid filling. The pressure waves of the right atrium are transmitted to the great veins and may be visible in the jugular pulse (see jugular pulse, p. 340).

Vibrational Characteristics of Cardiovascular Sound

The major part of cardiovascular vibrations is not audible, being either two low in frequency, or too feeble in intensity to be detected by the human hearing mechanism. The ear is able to perceive sounds below 30 cycles per second only if they are of great intensity. Much of the sound associated with cardiac activity is in this low frequency range. Although the human hearing mechanism tends to accentuate sounds of increasing frequency so that they are subjectively louder than sounds of the same intensity but of lower frequency, cardiovascular sounds of more than 500 cycles per second usually are of such low energy that they are inaudible. The audible range of cardiovascular sound vibrations is thus between 30 and 500 cycles per second. In the horse, low frequency components of certain sounds are heard at the thoracic wall because of their relatively high intensity, whereas they seldom are detected in smaller animals.

Cardiovascular sounds may be described as transients (sounds of short duration, usually referred to as heart sounds) or murmurs (groups of sound vibrations of longer duration). Friction sounds usually are distinguished from murmurs, but likewise are of long duration. The transients include the 4 normal heart sounds as well as abnormalities such as gallop sounds and clicks. Murmurs have a wide variety of distinguishing characteristics.

Characteristics of heart sounds and murmurs which are important in their interpreta-

tion are: 1. Time of occurrence in the cardiac cycle and duration, 2, frequency, 3, intensity, 4, quality. The time of occurrence in the cardiac cycle and the duration of transients and murmurs often furnish important clues as to the underlying hemodynamic lesion. Such descriptive terms as early diastolic, holosystolic, and mid-systolic are used in this regard. The frequency of pitch of a transient or murmur may be low, medium, or high. The intensity of cardiovascular sound may be described as soft or loud; however, several more quantitative systems for grading the intensity of murmurs have been suggested and, though arbitrary, form a better basis for exchange of information concerning intensity. One classification in common use grades murmurs from 1 to 5: a Grade 1 murmur is the softest audible murmur; Grade 5 remains audible with the stethoscope chest-piece just removed from the thoracic wall; Grade 2 is a faint murmur, clearly heard after a few seconds' auscultation; Grade 4 is the loudest murmur which is still inaudible when the chest-piece is just removed from the chest wall; and a Grade 3 murmur is immediately audible after auscultation begins and is heard over a fairly large area.

The term, quality of sound, refers to a subjective impression which is best described through the use of words such as snapping, clicking, and thudding in the case of transients; blowing, harsh, or musical in the case of murmurs. The arrangement and the intensity of the various frequency components of a sound or murmur determine its quality. Transients and murmurs rarely consist of vibrations of homogeneous frequency, and thus are usually not pure tones. Occasionally, murmurs may have a definitely musical quality and when examined graphically are seen to consist primarily of sound vibrations of a single frequency and its harmonics (Fig. 6).

Murmurs may exhibit another distinguishing characteristic often described as "shape." This is best demonstrated in phonocardiograms, but may be evident on auscultation as well. Systolic murmurs which result from the obstruction of outflow of blood from either of the ventricles, for example, tend to have a crescendo-decrescendo or diamond shape. That is, their amplitude is small early in systole, builds to a maximum at about mid-systole, then falls off again in late systole before the second heart sound. As will be discussed in the section on cardiac murmurs, the "shape" of a murmur is often useful in determining its underlying hemodynamic cause.

PHONOCARDIOGRAPHY

The graphic recording of heart sounds is a useful adjunct to auscultation and often is essential to the correct interpretation of auscultatory phenomena. It provides a lasting record which can be studied objectively without the biases inherent in human hearing. A phonocardiograph consists basically of a microphone, audio-amplifier, and recording galvanometer together with a second system for recording an electrocardiogram or pulse curve for timing purposes. Most phonocardiographs incorporate one or more filters which allow certain areas of the vibratory spectrum to be amplified, while others are attenuated. The lower frequency components of cardiovascular sounds are generally of much greater amplitude than the higher ones, though not as well heard. If a linear phonocardiogram is recorded, in which all frequency components are equally presented in their true amplitude proportions, the lower frequency components deflect full scale, and the higher frequency vibrations are barely visible. The main purpose of most filter systems used in phonocardiography is to attenuate the lower frequency components so that the higher ones can be amplified to the point of easy visibility. Various filter systems have been advocated, but there is no uniform agreement as to which should be adopted as a standard. A logical system advocated by Luisada and Zalter is the recording of 6 bands consisting of one octave each.[16] This is accomplished through the use of band-pass filters which attenuate vibrations both above and below the desired ranges.

Most of the phonocardiographic illustrations in this chapter were recorded by a 2-channel, photographic, portable phonocardiograph (Sanborn Twin-Beam, Sanborn Instrument Co., Waltham, Mass.) which incorporates 2 filter systems (equalizers). Tracings obtained are termed either stethoscopic or logarithmic. Stethoscopic recordings represent the frequency characteristics of sound vibrations as they arrive at the ear through an average acoustic stethoscope. Logarithmic tracings simulate the approximate logarithmic response of human hearing, and represent the sound as heard by the ear through an acoustic stethoscope. The stethoscopic system, hence, tends to accentuate sounds in the lower frequency range, and the logarithmic response accentuates higher frequency vibrations. A phonocardiogram recorded from the 4 valve areas of a normal horse is shown in Fig. 7.

Some phonocardiographic values from 25 normal horses are shown in Table 3.[17] Only values obtained from stethoscopic phonocardiograms recorded in the mitral area are presented in this table.

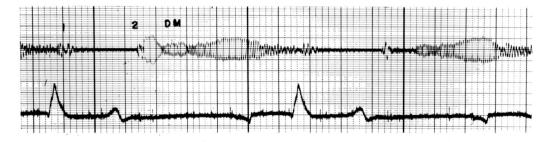

Fig. 6. Logarithmic phonocardiogram (top) from the aortic area, and electrocardiogram (thoracic unipolar lead V10, with the exploring electrode on the dorsal spine of the 7th thoracic vertebra) from an 11-year-old Thoroughbred gelding with signs of aortic insufficiency due to bacterial endocarditis. An intense diastolic murmur (DM) begins with the second heart sound and lasts throughout diastole. On auscultation, the murmur had a peculiar musical quality and varied in intensity, being at first loud, then soft, then loud again, finally decreasing in intensity just before the first heart sound. Most of the vibrations of the murmur in the phonocardiogram are of the same frequency.

Table 3.—Some Phonocardiographic Values in 25 Normal Horses*

	Frequency** (CPS)		Duration (sec.)		Intervals (sec.)		
	S_1	S_2	S_1	S_2	$P-S_4$	$P-S_4'$	S_2-S_3
Number of Observations	25	25	25	25	4	11	12
Mean	37	58	0.20	0.09	0.12	0.31	0.19
Range	21–53	31–91	0.16–0.28	0.08–0.13	0.06–0.16	0.24–0.36	0.15–0.26

*Obtained from stethoscopic phonocardiograms recorded only in the mitral area (atrial and third heart sounds were not observed in all horses).

$$**\text{Frequency} = \frac{\text{no. of vibrations observed}}{1 \text{ sec.}}$$

The Normal Heart Sounds of the Horse

The First Heart Sound: The first heart sound is usually a low-pitched sound of longer duration than the second and is best heard at the mitral and tricuspid areas. It occurs at the onset of ventricular systole, and is therefore associated with the onset of the apex beat and is heard just before the rise of the arterial pulse. The major audible portion of the first heart sound is attributed primarily to closure of the atrioventricular valves, but other events probably contribute to its production. Three groups of vibrations are often visible in the graphic tracings of the first heart sound (Fig. 5, 7, and 8). An early, low amplitude, low frequency portion apparently is associated with the initial movement of the ventricles during the entrant phase, preceding closure of the atrioventricular valves. The possibility that this component is the result of atrial contraction is ruled out by its persistence in atrial fibrillation (Fig. 9). A central, higher amplitude, higher frequency component occurs at the time of closure of the atrioventricular valves, and is probably related to the abrupt deceleration of the moving blood column at this time.

The fact that at the onset of systole, left ventricular pressure rises before the right has been presented as evidence in man[18] and the dog[19] that the mitral valve closes slightly before the tricuspid, and that the initial vibration of the main component of the first sound is mitral in origin. Spörri notes that the onset of pressure rise in the ventricles in the horse and cow likewise occurs first in the left ventricle.[20] This agrees with observations in our laboratory, but it is doubtful on the basis of present information that one can identify the mitral and tricuspid components of the first heart sound in the phonocardiogram of the horse.

The terminal vibrations of the first heart sound are low in amplitude and frequency, and occur at the time of initial ejection of blood from the ventricles. Presumably these vibrations are associated with the opening of the semilunar valves, and the initial acceleration of blood in the aorta and pulmonary artery.[19,21]

The Second Heart Sound: The second heart sound is of higher pitch (frequency) and shorter duration than the first heart sound (Fig. 5, 7, and 8). It occurs on the descending limb of the central arterial pulse, and ordinarily is best heard in the pulmonic area. The second heart sound is attributed primarily to closure of the semilunar valves. Opening of the atrioventricular valves may contribute to the second heart sound, but these events are normally inaudible. Littlewort suggests that the opening sound of the mitral valve may be a separately identifiable component of the equine phonocardiogram.[22] In normal horses, in which phonocardiograms are recorded simultaneously from the surface of the aorta and pulmonary artery near the semilunar valves, separate aortic and pulmonic components of the second heart sound can be distinguished.[17] At the thoracic wall, these two components usually are not heard separately nor recorded phonocardiographically, the second heart sound being a single series of vibrations.

In man and the dog, aortic valve closure normally precedes pulmonic valve closure by a brief interval. On inspiration, when pul-

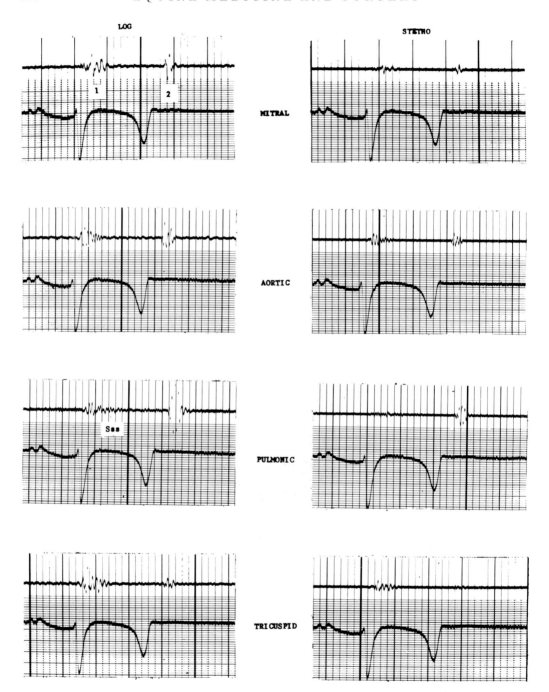

Fig. 7. Phonogram from a normal horse. Base-apex electrocardiogram and complete phonocardiogram of a 7-year-old, 960 pound, gelding Hunter with no clinical or gross postmortem evidence of cardiac disease. The P-R interval is 0.28 second. The first heart sound begins at the nadir of the S-wave. Atrial and third heart sounds cannot be identified. An early systolic murmur (Sss) is present in the pulmonic area (See Fig. 8). The second heart sound in the mitral area is short in duration, consisting of only 2 to 3 vibrations. In the aortic area, the second sound is slightly longer in duration and more complex. It is of maximum duration and amplitude in the pulmonic area.

monic valve closure is delayed because of the increased right ventricular stroke output engendered by the augmentation of venous return to the right heart, separation of the aortic and pulmonic components of the second heart sound may be great enough to be detected as slight splitting of the second heart sound. The question of sequence of closure of the aortic and pulmonic valves in the horse has not been adequately studied. Spörri indicates that there is some evidence that pulmonic closure precedes aortic closure, the reverse of that in man and the dog.[20] Our observations on this point are not conclusive. If this is true, one would expect inspiration to have the reverse effect on splitting of the second sound, the 2 components coming closer together during inspiration, and separating on expiration. We have occasionally observed this so-called reversed splitting in horses with no apparent heart disease (Fig. 10). Pathologic splitting of the second heart sound occurs in horses as well as other species (see splitting of the heart sounds p. 359, and Fig. 15).

The Third Heart Sound: The third sound is a short, low-pitched one of low intensity which occurs in early diastole, closely following the second heart sound (Fig. 5 and 11). It usually has a dull, thudding quality and is best heard in the mitral area. Charton, Minot, and Bressou detected a third heart sound in phonocardiograms from 8% of the normal horses they examined, but in our experience it is more common.[23] A third heart sound was detected in stethoscopic phonocardiograms from 12 of a group of 25 normal horses examined in our clinic when recordings from all of the 4 areas of auscultation were examined.

The third heart sound occurs during the period of rapid ventricular filling (Fig. 5), 0.14 to 0.28 second after the onset of the second heart sound. The precise mechanism involved in its production has not been established, but most evidence indicates that it results from sudden distention of the ventricular walls by the in-rushing blood from the atrium at the time of rapid filling. It has been suggested that transient closure of the atrioventricular valves also may be involved.

Phonocardiographically, the third heart sound in the horse is usually a mono- or di-phasic vibration of low amplitude and low frequency, but may consist of a series of vibrations or may appear to be split into 2 components (Fig. 11). The significance of these

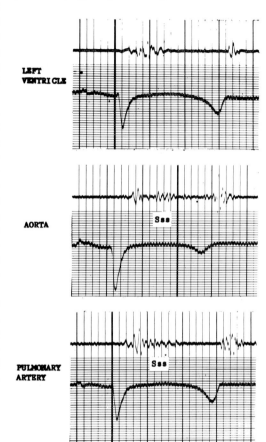

Fig. 8. Stethoscopic phonocardiograms recorded directly from the left ventricular surface, over the aortic base, and the pulmonary artery base. Recordings from the thoracic wall of the same horse are shown in Fig. 7. The left ventricular phonocardiogram closely resembles that taken from the mitral area. The first heart sound begins at the nadir of the S-wave. It consists of 3 groups of vibrations: initial medium-low frequency, low-amplitude vibrations; a central series of deflections of higher frequency and amplitude; and a terminal group of vibrations of medium-low frequency and low amplitude. The onset of the second heart sound in the left ventricular phonocardiogram coincides with the onset in the aortic and pulmonary artery tracings, but the sound is shorter in duration over the left ventricle.
An early decrescendo systolic murmur, similar to the one recorded over the surface of the thorax in the pulmonic area (see Fig. 7) is seen in the pulmonary artery and aortic recordings.
Gross postmortem examination of the heart and great vessels in this animal revealed no evidence of cardiac disease. The erythrocyte count was within normal limits.

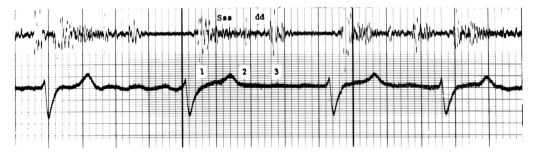

Fig. 9. Mitral regurgitation and congestive heart failure. Base-apex electrocardiogram and stethoscopic phonocardiogram from the mitral area of a 3-year-old Thoroughbred filly which had subacute endocarditis and myocarditis. On postmortem examination, there was extensive cardiac dilation and thickening and deformity of the mitral valve.
Atrial fibrillation is present. The first heart sound (1) begins at the nadir of the S-wave with a diphasic low amplitude, medium-low frequency wave similar to that seen in normal horses. A decrescendo, holosystolic murmur (Sss) begins with the high-amplitude, high-frequency vibrations of the first heart sound. A series of medium-low frequency, low-amplitude vibrations (dd) begin with the end of the second heart sound and terminate in a third heart sound (3) which is interpreted as a protodiastolic gallop sound because of its high amplitude. The gallop sound begins 0.16 second after the onset of the second heart sound.

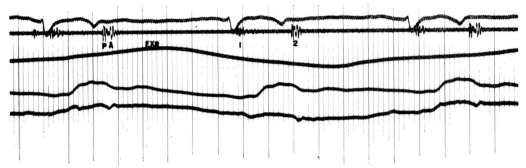

Fig. 10. Expiratory splitting of the second heart sound. From the top: base-apex electrocardiogram, phonocardiogram from the pulmonic area, pneumogram, aortic pressure tracing, and pulmonary artery pressure tracing from a 2-year-old Standardbred filly with no other clinical evidence of cardiac abnormality. Cardiac catheterization demonstrated unusually marked respiratory variations of intracardiac pressure, but no other hemodynamic abnormalities.
Splitting of the second heart sound occurs on expiration (exp.). The second sound becomes single on inspiration (downward slope of the pneumograph curve). The horse was moderately anemic. Postmortem examination revealed recent focal hemorrhages in the lungs and minimal endocardial thickening of the right atrium.

variations of the third heart sound is not clear, but the occurrence of multiple vibrations during the period of rapid filling is not surprising since ventricular filling is not a discrete event, but continues for a variable period of time during ventricular diastole. The possibility that separate third heart sounds may be produced in the right and left ventricles is supported by evidence in the dog that rapid filling occurs asynchronously in the 2 ventricles.[19]

Although the inital impact of the filling wave on the ventricle appears to be most effective in producing audible sound, other factors such as flow through the atrioventricular valve

orifice may produce sound vibrations as well. Though audible diastolic vibrations due to atrioventricular flow in man are considered evidence of relative or absolute mitral stenosis, the greater volume involved in the horse may make normal atrioventricular flow an audible phenomenon at times.

The third heart sound may change or disappear in the same normal animal in association with changes in the heart rate and other factors which alter ventricular filling (Fig. 12).

During tachycardia, in normal horses, if atrial contraction occurs at the time of the period of rapid ventricular filling of the previ-

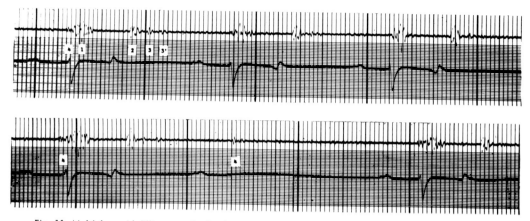

Fig. 11. Multiple rapid filling sounds. Stethoscopic phonocardiogram from the mitral area of a normal 3-year-old Thoroughbred gelding. The 2 strips are continuous. Incomplete atrioventricular block with dropped beats is present. The P-R interval varies from 0.32 second to 0.40 second. The longest P-R interval occurs in the first beat of the lower record, just prior to the blocked atrial beat (second beat in the lower record). The P-4 interval is consistently 0.36 second in all beats including the blocked beat. When the P-R interval is shortest, as in the third beat of the upper tracing (P-R .32 second), no atrial vibrations are visible preceding the first heart sound. In beats with longer P-R intervals, atrial vibrations can be seen before the nadir of the S-wave and, in most instances, before the onset of the QRS complex.
Two low-frequency vibrations are consistently present following the second heart sound. The first (3) occurs 0.16 second after the onset of the second heart sound. The second is recorded 0.12 second later (3'). Both of these vibrations probably are associated with the period of rapid ventricular filling.

ous beat, a summation sound is produced which may be of great intensity (see Tachycardia, p. 357 and Fig. 13). Cardiac disease may result in accentuation of the third heart sound, yielding with the first and second heart sound a triple rhythm resembling the cadence of a galloping horse (see Gallop rhythms, p. 359 and Fig. 9).

Atrial Sounds: The sound vibrations associated with contraction of the atria are often referred to in the singular as the fourth heart sound. There is evidence, however, that atrial activity gives rise to two groups of vibrations which are produced by different mechanisms. An early group of vibrations begins during or at the end of the P wave of the electrocardiogram, presumably as a direct result of atrial contraction (Fig. 5, 12 and 14). A later series of vibrations apparently results from the impact of the blood ejected from the atria on the standing column of blood in the ventricles (Fig. 5, 12, 13 and 14). The latter mechanism resembles that which is thought to be responsible for the third heart sound. In man and in most other species, atrial sounds are seldom heard during auscultation in normal individu-

als, although they can be recorded from the thoracic surface using phonocardiographic equipment with an appropriate low-frequency response. In most species, the atrial sounds detected at the thoracic surface by either phonocardiography or auscultation usually are of the second group, which presumably originate in the ventricle. The early atrial sound, attributed to atrial contraction, is seldom detected on the thoracic surface in man and in other animals, but can be consistently recorded from the esophagus.[24]

In horses, both early and late atrial sounds often may be recorded and late atrial sounds heard at the thoracic wall. In a series of 25 healthy horses, atrial vibrations were present in at least 1 auscultatory area in phonocardiograms from 16. Late atrial vibrations were most common and of highest amplitude, beginning 0.24 to 0.38 second after the onset of the P wave (Fig. 5, 12, 13 and 14). Early atrial vibrations also were present in 7 of 16 horses, beginning 0.04 to 0.16 second after the onset of the P wave. Early atrial vibrations were observed only in horses in which late atrial vibrations also were recorded.

On auscultation, atrial sounds are best heard in the mitral area, just prior to the onset of the first heart sound. The atrial sound as heard by the ear is usually only the late atrial sound. It is a low-pitched, low intensity sound similar in quality to the third heart sound. In phonocardiograms the early and late atrial vibrations may be continuous, a series of low amplitude vibrations extending between the two. If of long duration, a series of atrial vibrations may be heard as a low, short, presystolic rumble which often fuses with the first heart sound (Fig. 12). If slightly separated from the first heart sound, a discrete late atrial sound may give the impression that the first heart sound is split. The audibility of the atrial sounds depends somewhat upon the time of occurrence of atrial systole with respect to ventricular systole, and is thus related to the PR interval of the electrocardiogram. If atrioventricular conduction time is relatively long (PR interval exceeds 0.32 second), the late atrial sound may be heard as a separate sound just preceding the first heart sound (Fig. 11 and 13). As the PR interval lengthens, the late atrial sounds are separated from the first heart sound by a greater interval.

Isolated atrial sounds may be heard under certain circumstances. In incomplete atrioventricular block with dropped beats, in which some atrial contractions are not followed by a ventricular response, isolated atrial sounds may be heard and recorded during the ventricular pause (Fig. 11 and 13). Regular atrial sounds at a rate of 3 to 4 times the ventricular rate may be heard in complete atrioventricular block and are helpful in the diagnosis of this condition. In complete atrioventricular block there is no consistent relationship between the atrial sounds and the first heart sounds. The first heart sound may change in intensity as the preceding atrial contraction varies in its time of occurrence with respect to the onset of ventricular contraction (see Variations in intensity of the first heart sound, p. 358 and Fig. 14).

The presence of an atrial sound is clinical evidence that organized atrial contraction is occurring. The atrial sound is absent in atrial fibrillation (Fig. 9).

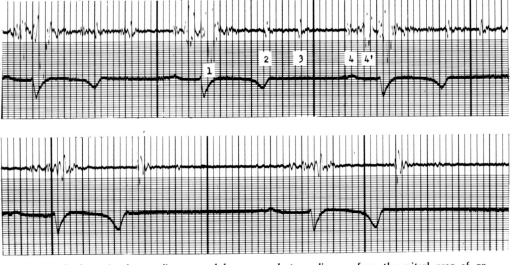

Fig. 12. Stethoscopic phonocardiogram and base-apex electrocardiogram from the mitral area of an 8-year-old Quarter Horse gelding with no evidence of cardiac disease. Multiple atrial vibrations and a third heart sound are present. In the upper recording, the heart rate is approximately 50 beats per minute. Early, low amplitude atrial sounds (4) occur at the middle of the P-wave. Higher amplitude, later atrial vibrations (4') occur .08 second later following the end of the P-wave. A third heart sound is seen 0.24 second following the onset of the second heart sound. In the lower tracing the heart rate is 37, and the character of the atrial and third heart sounds has changed. The atrial vibrations are much lower in amplitude and consist of a continuous series which merges with the first heart sound. The third heart sound is reduced in amplitude and is preceded by a series of low amplitude vibrations which follow the second heart sound.

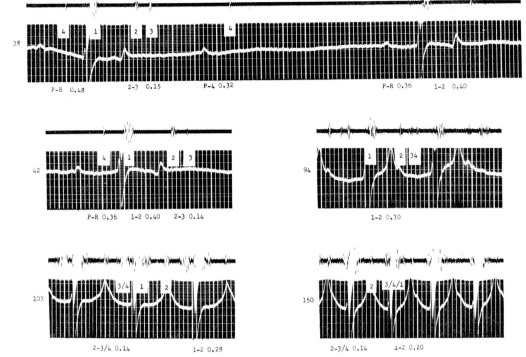

Fig. 13. Effects of changes in heart rate on the phonocardiogram. Base-apex electrocardiogram and phonocardiogram from the mitral valve area of a normal 6-year-old Thoroughbred mare.
A. The resting heart rate is approximately 38 beats per minute. Incomplete atrioventricular block with dropped beats of the Wenckebach type is present. The PR interval prior to the dropped ventricular beat is 0.48 second, but the PR interval of the post-block beat is shorter (0.36 second). Four heart sounds are recorded. An atrial sound (4) consistently occurs 0.32 second following the onset of the P-wave and is well-demonstrated in the dropped beat. The third heart sound follows the onset of the second heart sound by 0.15 second. The first heart sound (1) is diminished in amplitude following the post-block beat.
B. Heart rate-42. Essentially the same as A.
C. Heart rate-94. The PR interval has not shortened appreciably. The P-wave occurs during the descending limb of the preceding T-wave. The third heart sound follows the P-wave and occurs just before the fourth heart sound.
D. Heart rate-103. The P-wave is buried in the preceding T-wave. The third and fourth heart sounds summate (3/4), producing a sound which equals the first heart sound in amplitude. The second heart sound (2) is relatively low in amplitude, and occurs before the end of the QT interval (here at the peak of the T-wave).
E. Heart rate-150. The PR interval has shortened slightly. The summation sound approaches and fuses with the first heart sound (3/4/1), giving the appearance of a high amplitude murmur which begins prior to and ends after the QRS complex. The second heart sound is lower in amplitude. Note that acoustic systole (1-2 interval) shortens progressively as the heart rate increases.

NORMAL VARIATIONS OF THE HEART SOUNDS

All of the 4 heart sounds may be audible (Fig. 11, 12, and 13) but often only the first and second; the first, second, and third; or the fourth, first, and second are heard in a given horse. If all 4 sounds are heard, they resemble the syllables: Ba Lub - Dup Bup (S_4 S_1–S_2 S_3).

Tachycardia: In tachycardia the heart sounds may change markedly. If the rate increases to

the point that atrial contraction occurs during the period of rapid filling of the previous beat, summation of the third and fourth heart sounds occurs (Fig. 13), producing a loud, diastolic sound which may exceed the first and second heart sounds in intensity. This gives rise to a triple rhythm resembling the cadence of a galloping horse. In some horses the second heart sound decreases in intensity during tachycardia so that the summation sound and

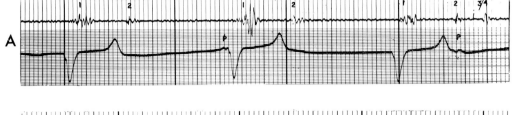

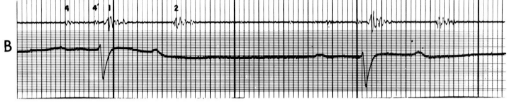

Fig. 14. Atrioventricular dissociation.

A. Bottom, base-apex electrocardiogram. Top, stethoscopic phonocardiogram from the tricuspid area of a 4-year-old Thoroughbred stallion suspected of having myocarditis. Atrioventricular dissociation resulted from an ectopic ventricular pacemaker having a rate slightly faster than the atrial rate. The ventricular complex is a QS deflection beginning with a slurred downstroke (compare with B below). There is no consistent relationship between the P-waves and ventricular complexes. In the center, a P-wave coincides with onset of the ventricular complex. The first heart sound is markedly accentuated in this beat (*bruit de canon*). The next P-wave occurs immediately following the T-wave of the previous beat (in early diastole, during the period of rapid filling). A low-frequency vibration (3/4) occurs 0.24 second after the onset of the second heart sound, owing to summation of the events responsible for the third and fourth heart sounds.

B. Base-apex electrocardiogram from the same horse, recorded one hour after the tracing in A. Normal sinus rhythm is present. The ventricular complex is normal in configuration, beginning with a small R-wave and ending in a large S-wave. Early (4) and late (4') atrial sounds are present.

the first heart sound are the only clearly audible sounds. As summation of the atrial and rapid filling sounds occurs in normal horses with marked tachycardia, either artificially induced with an electronic pacemaker or following exercise or excitement, it must be considered a normal phenomenon.[17,25] Summation also has been observed in isolated beats (atrial premature beats, atrioventricular dissociation) when atrial contraction closely follows the previous ventricular contraction (Fig. 14).

Variations in the Intensity of the First Heart Sound: Variations in the intensity of the first heart sound may occur in normal horses in association with variations in the P-R interval. In man and in other animals, the first heart sound tends to increase in intensity as the P-R interval shortens. The generally accepted explanation of this phenomenon is that the intensity of the first heart sound depends, at least in part, on the position of the atrioventricular valves at the time of ventricular contraction. If atrial contraction occurs well before the onset of ventricular systole, filling of the ventricles allows the valves to float upward into a nearly closed position. The excursion of

the valve leaflets at the time of full closure is then slight and the resulting sound is low. Conversely, if atrial contraction occurs late, just before ventricular systole, the valves are in a more widely open position at the time of ventricular contraction. The degree of valve excursion at closure is thus greater and the resulting sound is more intense. In the horse as in other species, the first heart sound tends to become louder as the P-R interval shortens. This phenomenon often is audible in incomplete atrioventricular block in the horse in which spontaneous variations in the P-R interval occur from beat to beat.

Our experimental observations in intact horses in which the atrium was driven by an electronic pacemaker indicate that if the P-R interval lengthens beyond a certain point, the first heart sound again begins to increase rather than becoming lower in intensity. Further study is required to explain this phenomenon.

In certain abnormal arrhythmias and conduction disturbances in which there is atrioventricular dissociation, atrial contraction may nearly coincide at times with the onset of ventricular systole. If atrial contraction is superimposed on the onset of ventricular contraction, the first heart sound suddenly increases in intensity (*bruit de canon*) for that beat (Fig. 14).

Splitting of the Heart Sounds: Splitting of the first heart sound was reported frequently in early studies of the horse, but in most instances this phenomenon was actually produced by the occurrence of an atrial sound just before the true first heart sound.[26] True splitting of the first heart sound in man and in the dog presumably results from asynchronous closure of the mitral and tricuspid valves. Splitting of a minor degree may occur normally, but is exaggerated in intraventricular conduction disturbances. Early systolic clicks (ejection sounds) have often been confused with splitting of the first heart sound in man, but they have not been described in the horse.

Splitting of the second heart sound is uncommon in the horse and results from asynchronous closure of the aortic and pulmonary valves. It is best heard in the aortic and pulmonary areas. Splitting of the second heart sound is a well-documented physical sign in man[24,27] and also has been reported in the dog. As stated in the foregoing, the sequence of aortic and pulmonary valve closure in the horse has not been established. Available evidence indicates that pulmonary valve closure precedes aortic valve closure, the reverse of the sequence in man and the dog.[20] The asynchronous closure in the horse, if present, usually is so slight that it does not result in separate aortic and pulmonary components of the second heart sound at the thoracic wall. We have observed splitting of the second heart sound in 2 horses in which the splitting became evident on expiration. This implies that the pulmonary valve closes prior to aortic closure. The expected increase in right ventricular ejection time, which occurs on inspiration secondary to the increased venous filling of the right heart, would delay pulmonary valve closure and tend to decrease the splitting interval during inspiration and increase it during expiration (Fig. 10). One of the horses in question suffered from a chronic anemia of undetermined cause. It was studied by cardiac catheterization and at postmortem examination. The only demonstrable hemodynamic abnormality was an unusually large respiratory fluctuation of intracardiac pressures. On postmortem examination a few recent, focal pulmonary hemorrhages and minimal endocardial thickening of the right atrium were the only gross or microscopic lesions in the heart or lungs. Splitting of the second heart sound on expiration also was observed in a 4-month-old Welsh pony with no clinical evidence of cardiac disease.

Corticelli reports splitting of the second heart sound in a horse with advanced chronic pulmonary emphysema.[29] We have observed a similar case (Fig. 15). Although pulmonary arterial blood pressures were not recorded in either case, splitting of the second heart sound presumably was associated with pulmonary hypertension due to chronic pulmonary disease. In such instances, an increase in right ventricular ejection time is required to eject the right ventricular volume against an increased pulmonary vascular resistance. Delay in closure of the pulmonary valve results in splitting of the second heart sound.

Gallop Rhythms: The term, gallop rhythm, refers to a 3-beat or triple rhythm which resembles the cadence of a galloping horse. In other species, they are classified as protodiastolic (ventricular), presystolic (atrial), or summation gallops.

Protodiastolic or ventricular gallop rhythms are produced by abnormal accentuation of the third heart sound. In man, dog, and ox they are usually associated with advanced myocardial disease and congestive heart failure. As the third heart sound may be of relatively great intensity in normal horses, the question of when a normal third heart sound becomes a pathologic gallop has not been resolved. We have observed marked accentuation of the third heart sound in a horse with myocarditis, endocarditis, mitral valve insufficiency, and congestive heart failure (Fig. 9).

In man and the dog, presystolic or atrial gallop rhythms result when atrial sounds become audible. They usually are associated with prolongation of the PR interval. As rather loud atrial sounds often are present in normal horses, the question of differentiating pathologic accentuation from the normal range of variation is difficult, as in the case of the ventricular gallop. We have not observed what could be described as a true atrial gallop rhythm in the horse.

A summation gallop rhythm results from the fusion of atrial and ventricular gallop sounds. Its significance is similar to either atrial or ventricular gallop rhythms in man and the dog. We have not observed this phenomenon in cardiac disease in the horse and since a summation gallop is readily produced at rapid heart rates in normal horses (Fig. 13), its significance in the presence of cardiac disease is equivocal.

CARDIOVASCULAR MURMURS

Mechanism of Production of Murmurs: Cardiovascular murmurs are series of sound vibrations produced by disruption of laminar flow in the heart or vessels. If as a result of the disturbance, sufficient energy of fluid motion is transferred into acoustical energy, a murmur becomes audible at the thoracic wall.

The concept of turbulent flow has been used for many years to explain the occurrence of cardiovascular murmurs. It is based on the work of Reynolds, who showed that turbulence develops at a certain critical flow velocity depending on the caliber of the tube and the viscosity and density of the fluid. The critical velocity is defined as the velocity at which laminar flow becomes turbulent. In a given tube the critical velocity (Vc) is determined by the formula:

$$Vc = \frac{Kn}{pR}$$

where K is Reynolds' number (about 1,000 for blood), n is the viscosity of the blood in poises, p is the density in grams per milliliter, and R is the radius of the tube. When laminar flow changes to turbulent flow, eddies and whirlpools occur, presumably giving rise to noise.

More recently, Bruns has advanced the hypothesis that cardiovascular murmurs are not simply the result of random turbulence as predicted in the foregoing concept, but are caused by vortex shedding downstream from an obstruction, resulting in periodic wake fluctuations in the stream.[30] On a physical and mathematical basis, periodic wake fluctuations as described by Bruns appear to be a more sound explanation for the production of murmurs in the cardiovascular system than that of random turbulence. The obstruction to blood flow responsible for vortex shedding need not be severe. Minor deformities or even natural irregularities in various orifices of the heart could be expected to produce periodic wake fluctuations, if the velocity of flow is relatively great.

As in other species, the mere presence of a murmur is not definite evidence of cardiovascular abnormality. The interpretation of cardiac murmurs is rendered somewhat more difficult in the horse, than in man and the dog, owing to the prevalence of both systolic and diastolic murmurs in normal horses. This fact, plus the lack of adequate clinical data concerning the heart sounds in disease states, necessitates caution in the interpretation of all cardiovascular sound, including murmurs, when dealing with the horse.

Functional Systolic Murmurs: The occurrence of systolic murmurs in horses without other evidence of organic heart disease is well-known.[31-36] Such murmurs usually are heard over the heart base (aortic and pulmonic valve areas), and have been reported in as many as 66% of normal horses.[32] In a sample of 25 normal horses examined in our clinic, early systolic murmurs were recorded in phonocardiograms over the heart base in 15 (Fig. 7, 8).

Although references to functional heart murmurs in horses are common, most of the published observations have not been documented through the use of phonocardiography. Their description, however, and our phonocardiographic observations of these murmurs, resem-

Fig. 15. Phonocardiogram of an 8-year-old Thoroughbred gelding with chronic pulmonary emphysema. Splitting of the second heart sound was consistently present in the aortic and pulmonic areas. The degree of splitting increased slightly during inspiration. The second component of the second heart sound presumably represents closure of the pulmonic valve. It is equal in amplitude to the first component in the stethoscopic recording at the pulmonic area, and exceeds it in the logarithmic tracing. The initial (aortic) component of the second heart sound is seen well in the records from the mitral and tricuspid areas, but in these areas the second component appears only as a series of low amplitude vibrations not definitely separated from the initial component.

STETHO

LOG

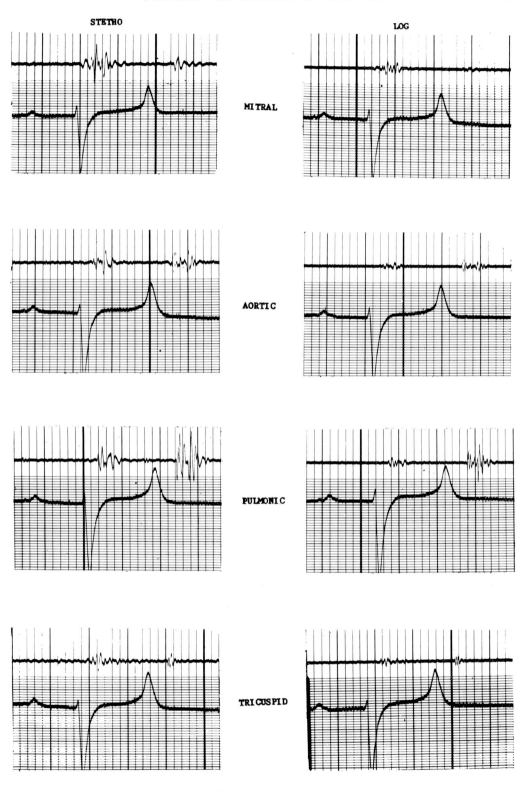

MITRAL

AORTIC

PULMONIC

TRICUSPID

ble the "normal flow murmurs" which can be recorded from the thoracic surface in the pulmonary area in man, and from the surface of the pulmonary artery in the dog.[24,37] A number of theories have been advanced to explain this "normal flow murmur." Some authors attribute the murmur to turbulent flow in the aorta and pulmonary artery during the phase of rapid ejection.[38] A calculation of the blood velocity in the pulmonary artery and aorta in the horse based on knowledge of the cardiac output, diameter of the great vessels, and the viscosity of blood, reveals that the critical velocity is exceeded under normal physiologic conditions, particularly during the early phase of rapid ventricular ejection.

Another mechanism postulated is that the retracted edges of the pulmonic and the aortic semilunar valve cusps may offer some obstruction to flow.[39] In support of this view, one investigator removed the pulmonary valve leaflets in the dog and found that the systolic murmur disappeared.[37]

The functional systolic murmur heard in normal horses usually is a soft, high-pitched decrescendo, early systolic murmur which tends to die out before the end of systole (before the second heart sound) (Fig. 7). A similar murmur to that recorded on the thorax has been recorded from the surface of the pulmonary artery and aorta in a number of horses in which open-chest experiments have been performed (Fig. 8).[17]

Systolic murmurs heard in anemia without organic heart disease in the horse and in other species probably are produced by a similar mechanism. Because of the increased velocity of blood flow and a decreased blood viscosity, either mechanism of murmur production is favored.

Functional Diastolic Murmurs: Diastolic murmurs are considered reliable evidence of cardiac disease in dog and man, but groups of diastolic vibrations of sufficient duration to be considered murmurs are found in normal horses. These murmurs tend to occur in presystole, between the onset of atrial contraction and the first heart sound, and in early diastole.

A continuous series of atrial vibrations beginning at about the end of the P-wave of the electrocardiogram and lasting 0.32 to 0.40 second may be observed in sound horses (Fig. 12). These atrial vibrations are occasionally detected by auscultation as a low-pitched, rumbling murmur just preceding the first heart sound (see Atrial sounds, p. 355).

Series of early diastolic vibrations which occur closely following the second heart sound can be recorded phonocardiographically (Fig. 11, 12), and may be heard in some normal horses. As discussed in the section on the third heart sound, these vibrations probably are associated with rapid ventricular filling.

The presystolic and diastolic murmurs which occur in mitral insufficiency and ventricular septal defect in man and the dog are ample evidence that murmurs can be produced by increased flow through the mitral valve ring during diastole without the presence of anatomic mitral stenosis. In the horse, the amount of potential acoustic energy which may result from minor disruptions of laminar flow is great enough that audible sound may be generated during normal flow through the atrioventricular valves.

Atrioventricular Valve Regurgitation: Deformity of the mitral or tricuspid valve cusps, or dilation of the valve ring may result in regurgitation of blood into the atrium during ventricular systole. Atrioventricular regurgitation gives rise to a pansystolic (throughout systole) murmur, which begins with the first heart sound and extends to the second heart sound. The murmur is best heard in the mitral and tricuspid valve areas. A systolic murmur from a horse with mitral insufficiency associated with endocarditis and cardiac dilation is shown in Fig. 9. When loud, the pansystolic murmur of atrioventricular valve insufficiency may mask the first and second heart sounds, so that only the murmur is heard.

Atrioventricular Valve Stenosis: This condition is rare in the horse and has not been observed in our clinic. In mitral or tricuspid stenosis there is obstruction to ventricular filling during diastole, thus yielding a decrescendo diastolic murmur beginning after the second heart sound. If organized atrial contraction is occurring, a presystolic accentuation of the diastolic murmur occurs due to the increased velocity of flow through the stenotic orifice during atrial systole.

Semilunar Valve Regurgitation: Insufficiency of the aortic or pulmonic valve allows regurgitation of blood into the corresponding ventricle during diastole. We have observed aortic insufficiency owing to bacterial endocarditis, chronic valvular fibrosis, and, in one horse, it apparently was the result of dilation of the valve ring. A calcified nodule in one aortic semilunar valve cusp, probably associated with strongyle infection, was the cause of mild aortic insufficiency in another case. Fenestration of the semilunar valve cusps, which apparently is a congenital anomaly, has been described as an incidental postmortem finding in horses, but clinical evidence of aortic insufficiency from this cause has not been reported.[40] We have not observed pulmonary valve insufficiency in the horse.

The decrescendo diastolic murmur of aortic insufficiency begins with the second heart sound. It is best heard over the heart base (aortic and pulmonic valve areas), and usually is transmitted well to the cardiac apex. Significant degrees of aortic insufficiency are associated with a bounding pulse (waterhammer pulse; Corrigan pulse), owing to the high pulse pressure and rapid fall in pressure resulting from regurgitation during diastole. In some horses with proven aortic insufficiency, the diastolic murmur is not a classic decrescendo murmur, but displays a series of rising and falling intensities (Fig. 6). These diastolic murmurs, of high intensity in the horse, often are mistaken for systolic murmurs by the inexperienced, particularly at rapid heart rates.

Semilunar Valve Stenosis: Stenosis of the aortic or pulmonic valves is usually of congenital origin in the dog. Except in the tetralogy of Fallot we have not seen pulmonic stenosis in the horse, nor have we observed aortic stenosis. Semilunar valve stenosis results in obstruction to the outflow of blood from the ventricle during systole, causing a crescendo-decrescendo (diamond-shaped) systolic murmur, which usually begins after the first heart sound and ends before the second. Based on observations in other species, the murmurs of aortic or pulmonic stenosis are best heard over

the aortic and pulmonic areas respectively. The murmur of aortic stenosis in man and the dog often is transmitted cephalically, and is easily heard in the second to third right intercostal space and at the thoracic inlet.

Interventricular Septal Defect: Defects in the interventricular septum characteristically produce harsh murmurs which result from the rapid flow of blood from left to right through the defect during systole. The murmur is usually pansystolic in time since a pressure gradient between the 2 ventricles exists throughout systole.

In 2 horses in which clinical studies were performed, the murmur was most intense in the second and third right intercostal spaces at the level of the olecranon, and also was heard well in the mitral area.

The systolic murmur of interventricular septal defect is accentuated by vasopressor agents and lessens in intensity if the systemic blood pressure is lowered with vasodilators.[41,42] This phenomenon is related to the velocity of flow across the defect, and is a useful diagnostic aid in differentiating interventricular septal defect from certain other lesions. The murmur of mitral regurgitation is similarly affected by these agents.

Figure 16 illustrates an increase in the systolic murmur following administration of l-arterenol (Levophed bitartrate, Winthrop Laboratories, New York, N. Y). to a Welsh pony with an interventricular septal defect.

Patent Ductus Arteriosus: The ductus arteriosus normally closes within the first 24 hours after birth. Amoroso *et el.* noted continuous murmurs in newborn foals which disappeared shortly after birth.[43] The murmurs were typical of those in patent ductus arteriosis of other species, and were best heard in the left third intercostal space.

The murmur of uncomplicated patent ductus arteriosus often is described as a machinery murmur because of its continuous nature and alternating periods of increasing and decreasing intensity. It resembles the murmur of other types of arteriovenous fistulas (Fig. 17a). The continuous nature of the murmur is explained by the fact that aortic pressure exceeds pulmonary artery pressure throughout the cardiac

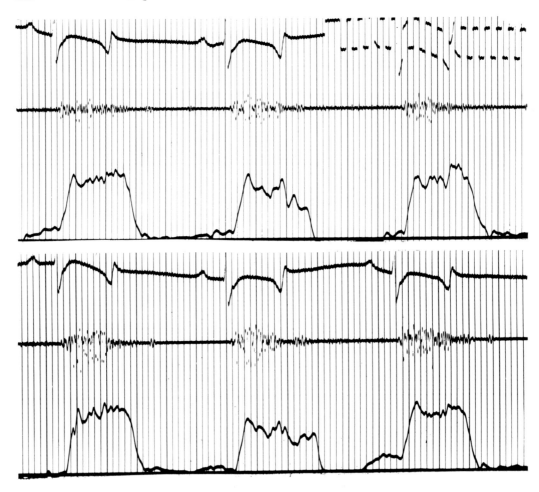

Fig. 16. Base-apex electrocardiogram (top), phonocardiogram from the right third intercostal space at the level of the olecranon (middle), and right ventricular pressure tracing (bottom) of a 1-year-old Welsh pony stallion with an interventricular septal defect. The upper and lower series are portions of a continuous recording made to show the effect of a vasopressor on the intensity of the murmur. The control tracing is shown at top. The standardization signal in the electrocardiographic tracing marks the intravenous injection of ½ ml. of a 0.2% solution of l-arterenol bitartrate. At the bottom is a portion of the record made 8 seconds after injection. The murmur is noticeably accentuated. A third heart sound is seen clearly in the first and third beats, lower series.

cycle, resulting in continuous blood flow through the ductus. The gradient between the aorta and pulmonary artery is greatest at the time of the rise of the aortic systolic pulse curve, resulting in accentuation of the murmur during late systole and early diastole. If pulmonary hypertension is present, the murmur may not be continuous, or may disappear entirely.

Venous Hum: A continuous murmur may be heard over the jugular veins and at the thoracic inlet in horses with accelerated blood flow such as occurs in anemic states. This murmur may be transmitted to the thoracic wall and interpreted as a murmur of cardiac origin. If the jugular veins are occluded, the murmur ceases (Fig. 17B).

Peripheral Arterial Murmurs: Peripheral arteriovenous fistulas may be of congenital or traumatic origin. They give rise to continuous murmurs which are heard over the site of the fistula (Fig. 17A) and often are transmitted

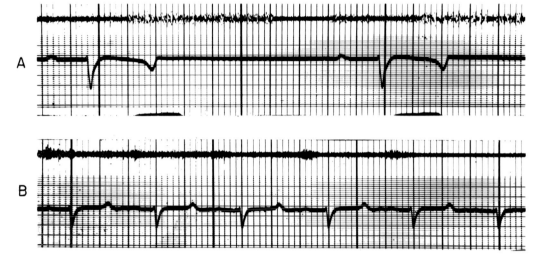

Fig. 17. Vascular murmurs.
A. Arteriovenous fistula. Base-apex electrocardiogram (bottom). Phonocardiogram (top) of a continuous murmur recorded from a swelling on the right front fetlock of a 7-year-old Thoroughbred gelding. A continuous thrill could be palpated over the area. Multiple arteriovenous anastomoses, found at surgery, were believed to be congenital in origin. The murmur reaches maximum intensity late in ventricular systole (around the onset of the T-wave) owing to the delay of the systolic pulse wave at the site of the fistula.
B. Venous hum. Base-apex electrocardiogram (bottom). Phonocardiogram (top) recorded over the thoracic inlet near the left external jugular vein in a 1 year-old Thoroughbred filly with equine infectious anemia. The murmur is continuous, but is accentuated in mid-diastole (midway between the end of the T-wave and succeeding QRS complex). The velocity of flow in the jugular vein would be expected to increase during ventricular diastole due to the decrease in right atrial pressure at that time. At the right of the record, the murmur is abolished by occluding the jugular veins.

well along the veins leading from the site. Occlusion of the artery obliterates the murmur.

Pericardial Friction Rub: Pericardial friction rubs have a "leathery" or "scratchy" quality. They often occur in more than one phase of the cardiac cycle. A short friction rub may be associated with atrial systole and another with ventricular contraction, producing a "to and fro" sound. A third component may occur at the onset of diastole. The multiple timing of pericardial friction rubs is explained by the fact that roughened epicardial and pericardial surfaces can rub together and produce sound during any movement of the heart.

OTHER DIAGNOSTIC AND TECHNICAL METHODS

Circulation time is the time interval between the injection of a substance into a vein and its arrival at some distant part of the body. It represents the approximate reciprocal of the average blood velocity between the two points and is related to the cardiac output and the volume of circulating blood. The determination of circulation time is of value to confirm the clinical diagnosis of congestive heart failure and to demonstrate other interferences with circulation between the points of injection and detection. The relationship between circulation time (CT), cardiac output (CO), and blood volume (BV) can be expressed as follows:

$$CT = K\frac{BV}{CO}$$

in which K represents a constant that may vary in different individuals or in the same individual under changing conditions. If blood volume and cardiac output increase together and to the same relative extent, the circulation time will not change. If the blood volume increases and the cardiac output decreases, as occurs in congestive heart failure, the circulation time will be increased. An increase in cardiac output with no change or a decrease in blood volume will result in shortening of the circulation time. Thus, circulation time is reduced when the cardiac output is increased in exercise, excitement, anemia, and febrile states.

Three substances for determining the circulation time under clinical conditions have been used in horses: lobeline,[44,45] ether,[46] and fluorescein sodium.[17] In experimental animals, lobeline reflexly stimulates the respiratory center through its action on the carotid body and aortic body. In the horse, the hyperpnea following its injection is presumed to occur when the drug reaches these chemoreceptors. Thus, when it is injected into the jugular vein, the circulation time from the jugular vein through the right heart, pulmonary circulation, left heart and to the chemoreceptors is determined. In healthy horses, this time interval was 15 to 35 seconds (average 25 seconds) but in those with cardiac decompensation, it exceeded 35 seconds (36 to 51 seconds). The dose employed was 15 mg. per 100 kg. body weight in a solution containing 10 mg. per ml. Because of the possibility of dangerous side effects in animals with heart disease, this drug is not recommended for routine clinical use.

Ether, when injected into the jugular vein, reaches the pulmonary capillaries and can be detected in the expired air. Thus the circulation time through the jugular vein, right heart, and pulmonary arterial tree to the pulmonary capillary bed, plus the time required for diffusion and expiration are measured. In healthy horses, this time ranged from 9 to 14 seconds (mean, 11 seconds). In horses with heaves, the range was 8 to 23 seconds, with a mean of 15.4 seconds in moderately severe cases and 20.2 seconds in severe cases. The dose used was 2 ml. of ether combined with 2 ml. of physiologic saline solution.

Fluorescein sodium, when injected into the jugular vein, can be detected on arrival at visible mucous membranes by viewing the area under an ultraviolet lamp (maximal emission at 3,600 A° units). A Wood's lamp is suitable for this purpose. The tongue is most convenient for observation; the yellow-green fluorescence often is first visible in the papillae. The course over which the circulation time is measured is about the same as with the lobeline method. Values ranging between 20 and 35 seconds have been observed in healthy horses and in one horse with congestive heart failure (q.v.), the circulation time was 48 seconds.

The determination of cardiac output is a more direct measure of cardiac function, but this will not be discussed in detail here. Values for healthy horses determined by the use of T.1824 dye ranged from 62 to 94 (mean 74 ± 9) ml./kg./min.[47]

Postexercise Electrocardiographic Abnormalities: Horses with inflammatory and degenerative myocardial lesions may show electrocardiographic alterations associated with myocardial damage (S-T segment shifts, abnormal arrythmias, and conduction disturbances) at rest. Exercise may elicit electrocardiographic abnormalities in horses with myocardial disease and in conditions in which hypoxia develops (pulmonary disease, laryngeal hemiplegia). Defining coronary insufficiency as any condition causing inadequacy of the coronary circulation to meet the metabolic needs of the myocardium, Brooijmans lists the following postexercise electrocardiographic changes as characteristic:[9]

1. Elevation of the S-T segment in leads II, III and aVF; depression of S-T in lead aVR.
2. The occurrence of arrhythmias of all types.
3. The occurrence of conduction disturbances.
4. Elevation or depression of T waves beyond normal limits.

Changes in the electrocardiogram observed after exercise in normal horses are described by Landgren and Rutqvist.[48] With increased heart rate there is shortening of all electrocardiographic intervals (*e.g.*, PR, QRS, QT, etc.) and characteristic T wave changes (*e.g.*, elevation of the T wave in lead I or CV_6LL).

In carrying out an exercise test, control limb lead and precordial lead electrocardiograms are taken with a direct writing apparatus. The animal is exercised sufficiently to produce tachycardia and hyperpnea, but within the limits of its tolerance as indicated by previous training history and the ability of the subject to perform work. As soon as possible after exercise, the electrodes are applied and records of the

Table 4.—Blood Pressure Values in 7 Normal Horses

Site	Pressure (mm. of Hg)		
	Systolic	Diastolic	Mean
Right atrium	20 (16 to 28)	0 (−2 to +1)	6 (4 to 8)
Right ventricle	46 (30 to 53)	1 (−4 to +7)	11 (9 to 12)
Pulmonary artery	39 (34 to 48)	16 (14 to 19)	22 (16 to 24)
Brachial artery	166 (144 to 187)	105 (82 to 125)	106 (94 to 113)

various leads taken continuously for 2 minutes and then at intervals of 3,4,5,10,15,20, and 30 minutes following cessation of exercise.

Arterial and Venous Blood Pressure: Values for arterial blood pressure obtained by direct needle puncture of an artery are presented below. The indirect method employing a Riva-Rocci cuff applied to the tail or foreleg is suitable for clinical purposes.[49,50,51] The cuff is applied over the median artery in the foreleg, using this artery or its continuation (the common digital artery) 1 or 2 inches above the carpus for palpation or auscultation. The middle coccygeal artery is employed in the tail. Values obtained at these points in standing horses will differ from the arterial pressure at the base of the heart because the weight of the column of blood above or below the heart base will be added to or subtracted from the pressure obtained. The specific gravity of blood is about 1.050 to 1.060 and that of mercury about 13.6, so that for every 13 mm. above or below the heart a pressure of 1 mm. Hg is added or subtracted by the weight of the blood. Absolute pressures obtained at the tail range from 86 to 133 mm. Hg systolic and from 40 to 72 mm. Hg diastolic.[50,51] Those obtained at the foreleg range from 144 to 194 mm. Hg systolic and 108 to 150 diastolic.[49]

Venous pressure determined by direct puncture of the cephalic humeral continuation of the cephalic vein ranged from 8 to 24 cm. of water in a series of healthy horses.[52]

Cardiac Catheterization: Catheterization of the heart and great vessels can be performed in unanesthetized horses with comparative ease and is a useful diagnostic procedure where derangement of normal hemodynamics is suspected. In routine catheterization, pressure pulse curves in the various chambers of the heart are recorded and compared with normal values. Determination of the oxygen saturation of blood samples from each vessel and chamber also may yield information of diagnostic value if intracardiac or intravascular shunts are present (see interventricular septal defect, p. 363).

Recording of intracardiac pressures is best accomplished through the use of a physiologic pressure transducer connected to a suitable catheter. To enter the right heart and pulmonary artery the catheter is passed through a needle inserted in the jugular vein. It is advanced successively to the right atrium, right ventricle, and pulmonary artery. If a flexible catheter is used, the normal flow of blood carries it to the pulmonary artery with little difficulty. The aorta and left ventricle are entered by performing a carotid artery cut-down under local anesthesia and passing the catheter in a retrograde fashion to the aortic root, and through the aortic valve. A uniformly successful method of catheterizing the left atrium has not been devised in the intact horse. A technic of puncturing the brachial artery for the collection of arterial blood samples and recording of arterial pressures has been devised by Fisher.[53]

In a series of 7 normal horses, right heart catheterization and brachial artery puncture yielded the data in Table 4.[54]

Catheterization data from 2 horses with interventricular septal defects are shown in the section on congenital heart disease (p. 385). In both cases a left-to-right shunt at the level of the right ventricle is indicated by an increase in oxygen saturation in blood samples from that chamber. In case two, pulmonary hypertension and congestive heart failure had developed secondary to the large left-to-right shunt. Pressures in the right heart and pulmonary arteries were 3 to 4 times above the normal values, and end-diastolic pressure in the right ventricle was elevated.

CARDIAC ARRHYTHMIAS AND CONDUCTION DISTURBANCES

INTRODUCTION

Cardiac arrhythmias are ordinarily classified in accordance with the location of the pacemaker or pacemakers involved. Under such a classification there are 4 possible types: sinuatrial node irregularities and irregularities owing to ectopic pacemakers located in either the atria, atrioventricular node, or ventricles.

Conduction delays usually are classified in accordance with the anatomic location of the interference with conduction. The following types are recognized: sinuatrial, atrioventricular, blocking of the branches of the bundle of His, and parietal blocks occurring peripherally in the ventricular myocardium.

Studies of the electrical activity of single cardiac fibers indicate that disturbances of rhythm owing to ectopic pacemaker activity are most likely to have their origin in the specialized conducting tissues rather than in the ordinary muscle fibers of the atria or the ventricles. Further, many conduction disturbances are known to result from disordered function of the specialized conduction tissue.

NORMAL RATE AND RHYTHM

Under usual conditions the heart rate of the horse ordinarily is from 32 to 45 beats per minute. This range includes the rates often seen at rest, but it is obvious that horses usually are neither at complete rest nor in a basal state when examined. Heart rates in the horse as low as 22 per minute occur, but the lower limit usually is about 26 or 27 per minute. Though the cardiac rhythm is approximately regular in horses, it is not uncommon to find individuals with sinus arrhythmia, i.e., they skip beats from time to time owing to atrioventricular or sinuatrial block.

TACHYCARDIA AND BRADYCARDIA

These are relative terms and, because of the wide variations in heart rate encountered clinically, they are difficult to define with precision. The significance attached to a given heart rate depends on a number of factors, including the age and temperament of the animal, the presence or absence of exciting influences and diseases, and whether the cardiac rhythm is irregular or regular.

Sinus Tachycardia: This is a term reserved for rapid heart rates in which the sinuatrial node is the pacemaker. When tachycardia occurs in abruptly initiated bursts, the term paroxysmal tachycardia is used. Sinus tachycardia which persists when the animal is quiet and at rest occurs in fever, in anemia, following hemorrhage, in shock, and in congestive heart failure.

Sinus Bradycardia: This is an abnormally slow heart rate owing to infrequent discharge of the sinus node. It must be distinguished from bradycardia which occurs in atrioventricular block and atrioventricular nodal rhythm. In sinus bradycardia the heart rate should increase as usual with exercise, excitement, or following administration of atropine. It may result from stimulation of the vagal nerve anywhere along its course (e.g., intracranial tumors, increased intracranial pressure, meningitis, or inflammatory or neoplastic processes along the path of the nerve). Sinus bradycardia also occurs in jaundice and may accompany malnutrition.

ATRIAL ARRHYTHMIAS AND CONDUCTION DISTURBANCES

The arrhythmias which fall under this heading have their origin either in the irregular activity of the normal sinus pacemaker or in the establishment of an ectopic pacemaker located somewhere in the atria (see p. 375 for a discussion of the role specialized fibers are thought to play as ectopic pacemakers). Although it is apparent that atrial conduction disturbances occur, it rarely is possible to establish their presence beyond noting abnormalities in the form of the P wave or in excessive increase in its duration (widening of the P wave). Under certain circumstances shortening of the PR interval may be taken as evidence that the pacemaker has moved closer to the A-V node.

The term, sinus arrhythmia, is applied to the periodic increase and decrease of the heart rate governed by variations in frequency of the sinuatrial node pacemaker owing to waxing and waning of vagal activity. When this has a fixed relationship to the respiratory cycle, it is called respiratory sinus arrhythmia. Sinus arrhythmia, both respiratory and nonrespiratory, is not rare in horses and always is present in incomplete atrioventricular block with dropped beats. Anything which reduces vagal tone, *i.e.*, adequate exercise, excitement or atropine, ordinarily will reduce the degree of the arrhythmia or result in its disappearance. Except that marked sinus arrhythmia suggests abnormal fluctuations in vagal tone, this arrhythmia has no important clinical significance.

Atrial Premature Systoles (Fig. 18): These are heartbeats which occur early in time and have their origin in an ectopic pacemaker located in the atria. Although premature beats presumably can occur in the sinus node, it is difficult to establish their location here unequivocally. In the electrocardiogram, premature atrial systoles are characterized by the early occurrence and bizarre configuration of the atrial wave (P wave). The P wave must be premature and of a different configuration from the dominant P waves. The change in shape may be distinct or almost imperceptible. When the P wave is inverted in leads in which it ordinarily is upright, or vice versa, it is called retrograde. Such P waves often are caused by the reversed conduction of an impulse arising in the atrioventricular node. If the dominant rhythm is regular, the arrhythmia resulting from premature contractions may be recognized because of the characteristic short diastolic pause preceding the premature systole and long compensatory pause which follows. In this arrhythmia the basic sinus rhythm is disturbed so that the contraction following the compensatory pause occurs somewhat earlier than expected, whereas in the case of ventricular premature contractions the basic sinus rhythm is preserved. This difference can be detected by tapping out the dom-

inant cardiac rhythm while listening to the heart sounds. In the case of premature ventricular contractions, the beat following the compensatory pause will be synchronous with the tapping, whereas with the premature atrial contractions this beat will appear earlier. If sinus arrhythmia also is present, the basic dominant rhythm itself is irregular and this criterion is useless. The clinical significance of atrial premature systoles in horses has not been well-established. Atrial myocardial damage should be suspected when they are present.

Paroxysmal Atrial Tachycardia: This is characterized by periods of rapid, usually regular, contractions which start suddenly and stop abruptly. The tachycardia may last for only a few heartbeats or persist for a long period. To be classified as atrial tachycardia the pacemaker must be located ectopically in the atria; *i.e.*, this is an ectopic rhythm which actually can be looked upon as a series of premature atrial systoles. Abrupt onset and termination of rapid heart action establish the diagnosis of paroxysmal tachycardia and can be diagnosed by auscultation. That the pacemaker is located in the atria can be determined by an electrocardiogram. In paroxysmal atrial tachycardia, the electrocardiogram is characterized by the sudden onset of rapid heart action accompanied by deformation of the P waves. If the rate is fast enough, it is difficult to find the P waves since they may be hidden in the T wave of the preceding complex. Under these circumstances, since the P wave is inevitably somewhat distorted owing to its occurring simultaneously with the T wave, it is difficult to establish the fact that the P waves are bizarre. In general, however, when such rapid rates are encountered and are not related to exercise, excitement, or drugs, and it can be established that P waves are occurring (*i. e.* that the rhythm is supraventricular), then the diagnosis of paroxysmal atrial tachycardia is not infrequently used. The term, supraventricular tachycardia, is preferable under these circumstances. Paroxysmal atrial tachycardia in man and the dog usually indicates disease of the atrial myocardium, and presumably this is true in horses and other mammals.

Atrial Flutter: This term is employed for rapid, regular atrial tachycardia characterized

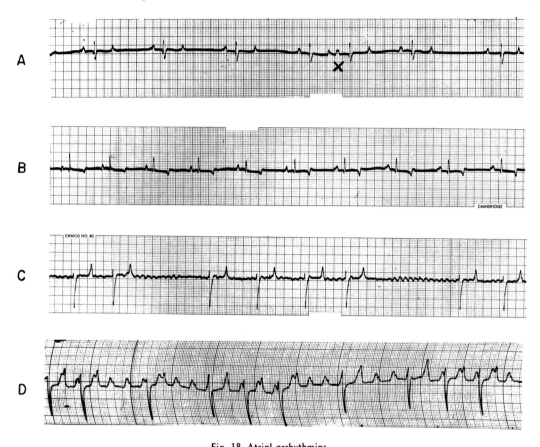

Fig. 18. Atrial arrhythmias.

A. Atrial premature beat (**X**). Lead CV$_6$LU from an 8-year-old Thoroughbred gelding. Note the P-wave in the fifth PQRST complex from the left. It occurs early and is changed in form, indicating a shift in the site of the pacemaker. The P-wave in the following complex is similar in form. The last P-wave has returned to the original configuration.

B. Wandering pacemaker: Lead II from a 2-year-old Thoroughbred mare with no evidence of heart disease. Note the change in shape of the P-wave beginning with the sixth complex from the left.

C. Atrial fibrillation. Base-apex lead from an 8-year-old Thoroughbred gelding with a grade 3 late diastolic murmur in the tricuspid area.

D. Atrial tachycardia with varying atrioventricular block in a 3-year-old Thoroughbred mare with mitral insufficiency.

in the electrocardiogram by atrial oscillations (flutter waves) which are regular in rhythm and form. Whether or not atrial flutter has been identified in horses depends on the criteria accepted for the electrocardiographic diagnosis. Brooijmans,[9] accepting the criteria of Holzmann[55] which required a regular and constant relationship between the flutter waves and ventricular complexes and perfectly regular flutter waves, could find no instances of this arrhythmia in his collection nor in the literature. At present, the diagnosis of atrial flutter and its distinction from rapid atrial tachycardia in horses must be based on criteria which are open to question owing to inadequate data.[56] It is questionable whether such a distinction is of clinical importance. The electrocardiogram in atrial flutter is characterized by the absence of P waves and the presence of flutter (F) waves which are uniform in amplitude, contour, and spacing except where distorted by the ventricular QRST complex. F wave rates reported for the horse by van Zijl were 220 to 350 per minute,[57] which correspond to rates reported for man and are slower than those found in the dog.[56] In man, atrial flutter ordinarily is a sign of serious cardiac disease. Not infrequently this arrhythmia appears during the treatment of atrial fibrillation with quinidine in the horse. No recommendations regarding treatment can be offered for the horse owing to absence of experience in managing this disturbance.

Atrial Fibrillation: (Fig. 18, 19): This dysfunction has been reported frequently in horses,[9,56-79] and clinical experience indicates that it occurs in this species with less severe underlying heart disease than in the dog. Moreover, the arrhythmia usually responds to quinidine therapy in the horse, whereas, in the dog quinidine ordinarily is ineffective. Numerous impulses arise in the atria, producing localized, incoordinated contractions of the atrial myocardium. Consequently, the atria fail to contract as a whole and lose their pumping action. The ventricular rate is variable and the rhythm and force of ventricular contractions are absolutely irregular. This characteristic is reflected in the names previously applied to the condition: delirium cordis; absolute, gross, or total irregularity of the heart; and perpetual or permanent arrhythmia. The horse played an interesting role in the early studies on atrial fibrillation. Sir Thomas Lewis, having shown the similarity between experimental atrial fibrillation in dogs and clinical atrial fibrillation in man, sought visual proof that the atrial activity seen in the experimental dog occurred spontaneously in disease. A veterinarian obtained 5 horses with atrial fibrillation, in 2 of which he was able to directly observe atrial activity following thoracotomy.[77,78] Thus, the first direct visual proof that spontaneous atrial fibrillation occurs in disease was obtained from horses.

The clinical diagnosis of atrial fibrillation, without the aid of an electrocardiogram, may be based on the following signs: 1. An absolutely irregular ventricular rhythm, 2, an elevated heart rate (between 50 and 90 per minute, although bradycardia, normal rate, and rates exceeding 100 per minute sometimes are found), 3, a "pulse deficit", *i.e.*, pulse rate less than the audible heartbeat rate, some contractions having occurred before the left ventricle has filled with sufficient blood to produce a palpable pulse (this is decreased or absent when the ventricular rate is relatively slow), 4, in some instances, absence of the second heart sound when, following a short diastolic period, the ventricles fail to fill sufficiently with blood to permit opening of the semilunar valves, 5, a variation in the strength of the peripheral pulse, 6, variation in intensity of heart sounds and murmurs, and 7, absence of an audible atrial sound. Although the atrial sound is not necessarily audible in normal horses, when it is heard then organized atrial contractions must be occurring. The first 6 signs listed result from rapid and irregular ventricular action. Electrocardiographic diagnosis is based on the absence of P waves, the presence of rapid atrial oscillations (fibrillation or f waves), which are irregular in form and frequency and have a frequency range of 300 to 500 per minute, and an irregular ventricular rhythm. In man and the dog the absence of P waves and the presence of grossly irregular ventricular rhythm are usually accepted as diagnostic even though characteristic f waves cannot be seen. In the horse, f waves usually are present in limb and precordial leads. Their amplitude is variable (up to 0.3 mV. in lead II in typical cases) and stretches with very low amplitude may alternate with runs of large, distinct f waves. They often are largest in lead II, base-apex bipolar lead, and lead CV₆LL. The QT intervals often vary, being shortened after prolonged RR intervals. The T wave may be altered in form when the QT interval is shortened.

Some horses with atrial fibrillation may show little evidence of cardiac disability if the heart rate is slow at rest. Stamina is invariably reduced, however, and the ability to perform strenuous work is limited. In individuals with a slow resting ventricular rate, the heart rate increases excessively and the rhythm becomes more irregular as vagal tone is reduced during and following exercise. Evidently, the ability of some horses to carry out mild activity despite the presence of this arrhythmia depends upon the presence of high resting vagal tone, characteristic of the species, which produces sufficient atrioventricular block to protect the ventricles and maintain a relatively slow rate and fairly regular rhythm. In other horses, the

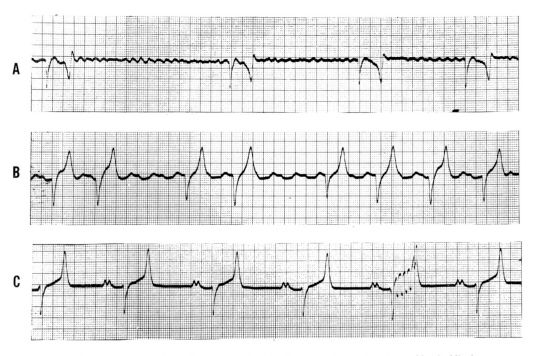

Fig. 19. The effect of quinidine sulfate on atrial fibrillation in a 4-year-old Thoroughbred. All electro-cardiograms are base-apex lead.

A. On the previous day, a 5 Gm. test dose of quinidine sulfate had been given. This record was taken 24 hours later when the quinidine blood level was 0.8 mg./liter.

B. Record taken on the fourth day of treatment. The quinidine level in the morning of this day was 8.0 mg./liter. Forty Gm. of quinidine were given in 2 divided doses 3 hours apart, and this record was taken 6 hours after the last dose. The quinidine blood level was 13.8 mg./liter. Note the rapidly occurring P-waves (atrial tachycardia) with variable ventricular response.

An additional 20 Gm. dose of quinidine sulfate was given at the time of the tracing in B, and 4 hours later the blood level reached 16 mg./liter. This had fallen to 8.4 mg./liter 12 hours later on the morning of the fifth day. Forty five Gm. of quinidine sulfate in 2 divided doses, 3 hours apart were given on this day, and the blood level reached 15.8 mg./liter.

C. During the evening of the fifth day the rhythm returned to normal, and this record was taken on the sixth day after the initiation of treatment, when the blood level had dropped to 7.3 mg./liter.

rate is high and the rhythm quite irregular. These subjects show considerable reduction in stamina and may develop a state of frank congestive heart failure. Rarely, syncope may occur but this has never been reported to be a major problem in the horse. The available postmortem reports indicate that degenerative or inflammatory myocardial changes usually are found in horses with atrial fibrillation. Chronic valvular endocarditis with resultant valvular damage is sometimes found. In a few cases, postmortem findings have been negative. In general, the clinical course in horses with persistent atrial fibrillation has been unfavorable. This is to be expected since many have

serious heart lesions. Only a few instances of paroxysmal atrial fibrillation have been reported in the horse. A few individuals, however, have continued to work up to 5 years despite the presence of the arrhythmia.[79]

Recently the use of quinidine sulfate treatment (Fig. 19) has been found to be effective in the horse[25,58] and several race horses in which the arrhythmia has been abolished with quinidine have returned to work and performed as well as they did before the arrhythmia developed.[80] These early experiences with therapy support the impression that atrial fibrillation occurs in horses more readily than in the dog and with less severe underlying cardiac disease. The following dose schedule for oral administration is the one used:

1st day	5 Gm. (test dose)
2nd day	10 Gm., 2 x daily
3rd and 4th days	10 Gm., 3 x daily
5th and 6th days	10 Gm., 4 x daily
7th and 8th days	10 Gm., 5 x daily

Only in exceptional cases has it been necessary to give higher doses as follows:

9th and 10th days	15 Gm., 4 x daily
11th and 12th days	20 Gm., 4 x daily
13th day	22 Gm., 4 x daily

These doses should be given at 4-hour intervals. In most of our cases it has not been necessary to exceed a dose of 40 Gm. daily, but one animal required 90 Gm. Doses at these higher levels are dangerous and extreme care must be taken to avoid serious toxic effects. A common complication is marked swelling of the nasal mucosa. In one case the nostrils were nearly occluded. This is a reaction that has usually occurred to a greater or lesser extent in all treated animals. As horses ordinarily cannot breathe through the mouth, the danger is obvious. This reaction is related to dosage and usually subsides if the drug is stopped or the dose reduced to the level tolerated on previous days. Urticarial wheals have been seen, and 2 horses among 14 treated developed severe laminitis following treatment, which in 1 animal caused permanent damage to the feet.

Wandering Pacemaker (Fig. 18): This is a term applied to certain P wave changes (and in some instances PR interval changes) which are attributed to shifts in the position of the pacemaker. In man and dog at least, this shift may be from one part of the sinuatrial node to another or from the sinus node to the atrioventricular node and back again. It is apparent from experimental work that the pacemaker may move out of the sinuatrial node into surrounding atrial tissue, although how often this occurs spontaneously in clinical cases is not known.

Experimental work in the dog has shown that the location of the pacemaker may shift from the head to the tail of the sinuatrial node as a result of vagal stimulation[81,82] and that in a rabbit it probably could shift out of the sinuatrial node into the sinuatrial ring bundle in the region of the cranial vena cava[83] (pp. 371). Such changes in position of the pacemaker would alter the course of the spread of excitation with resultant changes in the form of the P wave. The P wave in the dog may even become inverted in limb leads, and the PR interval may be shortened. Similar alterations in the form of the P wave have been produced experimentally in the dog by placing ligatures a few millimeters apart, starting at the head end of the sinuatrial node and progressing toward the tail.[84] Vagal stimulation also can shift the location of the pacemaker from the sinuatrial node to the atrioventricular node.[85] In man, both types of pacemaker shifts are described (*i.e.*, shifts within the sinuatrial node and shifts to the atrioventricular node).

The electrocardiographic criteria suggested for wandering of the pacemaker within the sinus node are: 1. P waves varying in contour without becoming retrograde, 2, only minor variations in the duration of PR interval (in man PR does not become shorter than 0.12 second). The electrocardiographic criteria for wandering of the pacemaker from the SA node to the AV node are: 1. P waves vary in form and size and may even become retrograde simultaneously with slowing of the heart rate, 2, changes in the PR interval, the PR interval becoming abnormally short (in man less than 0.12 second).

In the horse electrocardiogram, the form of the P wave may change abruptly with the new configuration persisting for several heartbeats, and then returning to the original form. Usually some variation in the PR interval occurs.

Wandering pacemaker has been correlated with heart disease in horses by some investigators. There is reason to think that this is not a valid conclusion, however. Presumably, the reason for the occurrence of marked changes in the form of the P wave in horses is that the distance of the pacemaker shifts within the SA node may be rather large. The sinus node in the horse is extensive and horseshoe-shaped, curving around the opening of the cranial vena cava and extending a lateral branch to a point midway between the opening of the 2 venae cavae and a medial branch through the medial groove for ⅔ of its length.[86] Shifting of the pacemaker within such an extensive sinuatrial node could result in marked alterations in the P wave form. In the horse, the characteristic P wave changes do not necessarily occur when other effects of increased vagal tone appear, such as atrioventricular block and sinus arrhythmia. Thus, such a pacemaker shift could not be attributed to vagal stimulation alone. In 2 horses with wandering pacemaker, startling the animals was sufficient to produce changes in the form of the P wave. Whether or not this can be considered a characteristic reaction must be determined by further trials. That vagal action may play a role is suggested by the fact that in our series wandering pacemaker has never been seen when tachycardia was present nor in horses given atropine.

Brooijmans considers wandering pacemaker in the horse to be an abnormal mechanism in which the pacemaker shifts "from the sinus node to a focus in the auricular walls and back."[9] To explain the frequency of this phenomenon in the horse, as contrasted with man and the dog, he points to the presence in horse atria of Purkinje fibers which might have a higher degree of automatism than the atrioventricular node. Such fibers are found in the atria of other hooved mammals which are not known to show P wave changes as frequently as the horse. No evidence is at hand which definitely shows that the pacemaker shifts entirely out of the SA node.

In a series of 48 horses examined in our clinic which were selected as having no clinical evidence of cardiovascular disease, wandering pacemaker was observed 16 times.[15] Brooijmans found such P wave changes in 53 horses, in about half of which cardiac failure was present.[9]

Because of its common occurrence in apparently healthy horses and lack of evidence that it is caused by cardiac disease, this phenomenon should be considered a normal variant. It is probable that P wave changes are more common in diseased hearts. As they also occur in the absence of other signs of heart disease, the diagnosis of cardiac disease should be based on other signs in the horse.

Atrioventricular (AV) Nodal Rhythm and AV Nodal Premature Beats: These are forms of ectopic impulse formation in which the pacemaker is located in the atrioventricular node. Because these arrhythmias have not been described in horses nor seen in our series, they will not be discussed further.[9]

Sinus Arrest or Sinus Standstill: This is a disturbance of rhythm in which the sinuatrial node fails to initiate an impulse for a period of time. If the standstill persists long enough, an ectopic pacemaker in the AV node or in the ventricle takes over and maintains the heartbeat. The arrhythmia has not been described in horses and is mentioned only because a distinction is made between it and sinuatrial block which is described next.

In *sinuatrial block*, both the atria and the ventricles are not activated by the sinus node pacemaker for one or a series of beats (Fig. 20). Theoretically, this can be accounted for by the assumption that the impulse is initiated in the sinuatrial (SA) node but not conducted to the rest of the heart. Such a condition can be produced experimentally by isolation of the SA node by ligation. Since activity in the pacemaker is not registered on the electrocardiogram, the condition is diagnosed clinically by inference. Actually, sinuatrial block cannot be distinguished from sinus arrest. When both the atria and the ventricles fail to contract with fairly regular periodicity or every so often as an isolated event, the electrocardiographic diagnosis usually is sinuatrial block.

An electrocardiogram is required for certain diagnosis. Pauses equal to one or several PP intervals (or a little less) are found. In the absence of any P waves during the pause, SA block must be distinguished from sinus arrhyth-

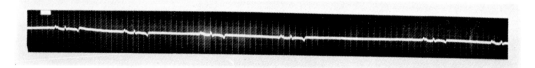

Fig. 20. Sinuatrial block. Lead I. This record was taken from a 4-year-old Thoroughbred stallion, which exhibited no evidence of heart disease.

mia in which, as a rule, the approximate doubling of the PP interval is lacking and the change from rapid to slower rate and vice versa ordinarily is more gradual. Actually, a certain diagnosis of sinuatrial block usually cannot be made if marked sinus arrhythmia is present. A type of SA block is described in which the PP intervals become progressively shorter until the missed beat and the PP interval following the missed beat is longer than all of the others. This corresponds to the arrhythmia of the ventricles described as Wenckebach periods which is seen in incomplete atrioventricular block with dropped beats (to be described later). Although this form of SA block resembles sinus arrhythmia, it can be distinguished on the basis of finding the phasic shortening of PP intervals followed by a pause, since this particular PP spacing is not expected in sinus arrhythmia.

In the horse, sinuatrial block occurs as an apparently normal phenomenon owing to elevated vagal tone at rest. This arrhythmia is much less frequent than atrioventricular block with dropped beats in horses. For example, in a series of 82 horses there were 10 instances of second-degree atrioventricular block and 3 of sinuatrial block in 12 animals (in 1 of the animals both types of block occurred).[87] In Brooijmans' series, there were 46 horses with second-degree AV block as against 2 with SA block.[9] Though there is some belief that SA block in horses should be considered a sign of heart disease,[9,88] the evidence is not convincing. As its occurrence is rare, it seems most reasonable to classify SA block as an unusual expression of either increased vagal activity or increased sensitivity of the SA node to vagal effects, which may or may not be related to primary heart disease. (See also the following section.)

ATRIOVENTRICULAR CONDUCTION DISTURBANCES, INTRAVENTRICULAR CONDUCTION DISTURBANCES, AND VENTRICULAR ARRHYTHMIAS

These arrhythmias and conduction disturbances involve primarily the specialized conduction tissues of the heart, i.e., the atrioventricular (AV) node, the bundle of His, the bundle branches, and the Purkinje fibers. The cardiac impulse arising in the sinuatrial node is conducted from the atria to the ventricles through these tissues. Interference with or interruption of conduction in the AV node or bundle of His will slow or stop conduction to the ventricles. Intraventricular conduction will be altered if the bundle branches are impaired functionally. When this occurs, impulses reaching the ventricular myocardium will be conducted in part through the ordinary cardiac muscle fibers. This results in slower conduction and an alteration in the pattern of spread of excitation because the usual specialized pathways are not followed. Although it has been assumed that any myocardial fiber is a potential pacemaker, when ectopic foci have been located, they have been found only in specialized conduction fibers.[83]

Thus, these specialized tissues currently are considered the seat of both arrhythmias and conduction disturbances. Even in the atria, specialized fibers are found which could be the site of ectopic impulse formation.

Atrioventricular Block: The term, heart block, is used to indicate delay or interruption in conduction of the impulse somewhere in its course from the pacemaker to the ventricles. There are 3 types: sinuatrial (SA) block, atrioventricular (AV) block, and bundle branch block (BBB). SA block has been discussed previously.

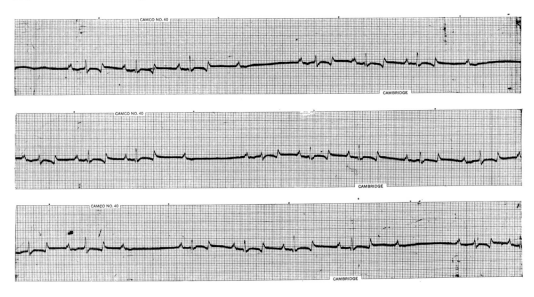

Fig. 21. Incomplete atrioventricular block with dropped beats. A continuous record, lead II from a 5-year-old Thoroughbred gelding which had no evidence of heart disease.

In *atrioventricular block,* the conduction between the atria and the ventricles is impaired. In incomplete AV block (first-degree AV block), the conduction is merely delayed. In incomplete AV block with dropped beats (partial heart block; second-degree AV block), conduction is interrupted at intervals so that the ventricles fail to contract periodically (Fig. 21). In complete AV block (third-degree AV block), none of the impulses arising in the atria are conducted to the ventricles (Fig. 22). In complete AV block, the atria and ventricles beat independently—the ventricles in response to an ectopic pacemaker in the nodal or ventricular tissue, and the pulse rate is usually slow. Incomplete AV block can be diagnosed with certainty only by electrocardiography.

In horses, the fourth or atrial heart sound often becomes audible preceding the first sound when the PR interval is long enough (*i.e.* exceeds 0.18 sec.).[26] When the interval between this sound and the first sound is greatly prolonged, the diagnosis of incomplete AV block should be considered. In incomplete AV block with dropped beats, the ventricles fail to contract periodically as in sinuatrial

block. If during the pause an atrial sound is heard, the presence of incomplete AV block with dropped beats is demonstrated. In the absence of this sign, an electrocardiogram is required for diagnosis. In complete AV block, the ventricular rate is slow (10 to 20 per minute or slower in some cases) and the rhythm is regular as long as the ventricles respond to a single pacemaker.* Regular atrial sounds (systoles en echo) may be heard during diastole, often occurring at a rate 2 to 3 times those of the ventricular beats. If the atria and ventricles contract simultaneously, the first sound is increased in intensity (*bruit de canon,* see p. 359 and Fig. 14).

Electrocardiographically, incomplete AV block is present when the PR intervals are prolonged abnormally. The upper limit of normal PR interval in horses may be arbitrarily placed at 0.47 second.[7] The validity of this value remains to be shown. The PR interval frequently is variable even when AV block with

---

*In the cases found in the literature, irregular ventricular activity has been reported frequently, presumably owing to occasional conducted beats or participation of additional ventricular ectopic pacemakers.

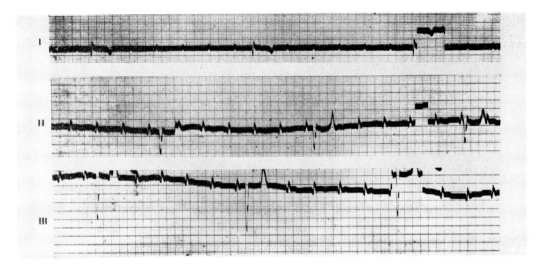

Fig. 22. Complete atrioventricular block. Leads I, II, III from a 10-year-old Thoroughbred-cross gelding. From thesis by A. W. M. Brooijmans.[9]

dropped beats does not occur. The length of the PR interval increases to a maximum and then decreases to a minimum periodically. There are 2 types of incomplete AV block with dropped beats recognized; in Type 1, which is most commonly observed, there is progressive lengthening of the PR interval starting with the first complex after the missed beat and continuing until the first complex preceding the missed beat. This is called the Wenckebach phenomenon, and the entire sequence from one missed beat to the next is referred to as a Wenckebach period. In a completely characteristic example of this phenomenon, the PR interval progressively lengthens but the increment is greatest at the second postblock beat and this increment of lengthening diminishes in ensuing beats. Owing to this peculiar relationship, the ventricular rate actually accelerates so that while the PR interval is increasing, the interval between beats (RR interval) decreases. Wenckebach periods can also occur in SA conduction.

In Type II AV block with dropped beats, which seldom is seen, the ventricular beats are dropped out periodically without any progressive change in the PR duration. Under clinical conditions, the characteristic or ideal

Wenckebach phenomenon may be distorted by other influences such as variations in the atrial rhythm and other, possibly reflex, effects which may change the conduction time between the atria and the ventricles from beat to beat. In the horse, changes in the PR interval do not always follow the classic Wenckebach pattern although, in general, the tendency is clear. The PR interval just preceding a missed beat may actually be shorter than the maximum PR interval in a given series.

In complete AV block (Fig. 22), the ventricular complexes occur regularly at a slow rate and the atrial complexes (P waves and Ta waves) occur usually at a rate 2 to 3 times faster than the ventricular rate.

In the horse, the Wenckebach type of AV block is the most common. For example, in a series of 46 cases, only one was Type II AV block.[9] In about 1 of 5 of these cases some paired blocked beats were found and in about 1 in 23 only paired blocked beats occurred. The postblock PR interval frequently is not the shortest, although it usually is shorter than the preblock interval and, as mentioned before, the preblock PR interval is not necessarily the longest. Sinus arrhythmia always accompanies incomplete AV block with dropped beats in the horse. The PP interval, which begins with the blocked P wave, usually is the longest. The PP intervals increase gradually to a maximum and decrease following the postblock beat.

Characteristic features of the postblock beat in incomplete block with dropped beats in the horse are shortening of the QT interval and reduction in T wave amplitude (or change in form, *e.g.*, from diphasic to positive). These changes are invariably present in our records. They also may occur following prolonged diastolic pauses in other arrhythmias (atrial fibrillation, premature ventricular systoles) in horse electrocardiograms. In the horses thus far studied phonocardiographically, it was found that the interval between the first and second heart sound was not shortened despite the shortening of the QT interval in the postblock beats. This suggests, but does not prove, that although electrical systole is shortened, mechanical systole remains unchanged. Adrenergic blockade can abolish these postblock effects or at least reduce them.[89]

Spörri observed that the dropped beats coincided with the longest PP intervals in records from 33 horses and he concluded that the slowing of AV conduction and block is due to respiratory variations in tone of the efferent nerves, especially the vagus.[90,91,92] He did not record a simultaneous pneumogram, and in a series of records (simultaneous electrocardiograms and pneumograms) taken on 10 horses, no simple relationship between the phases of the breathing cycle and atrioventricular block was observed.[93] Although the phase of the respiratory cycle may influence atrioventricular conduction through reflex effects, this is not the only influence involved, and a more detailed study of reflex and hemodynamic factors is required to understand the genesis of this conduction disturbance in horses.

The PR interval in horses frequently is variable even when incomplete atrioventricular block with dropped beats does not occur. The length of the PR interval periodically increases to a maximum and then decreases to a mini-

mum. Brooijmans recorded 28 instances of this variation in AV conduction, of which 20 were associated with incomplete atrioventricular block with dropped beats.[9] Presumably, these variations in AV block are the result of changes in vagal tone and represent a lesser degree of the vagal effect which causes incomplete block with dropped beats.

There is divided opinion about the significance of incomplete AV block with dropped beats in horses. A widely held view is that in most cases this is a functional phenomenon resulting from the action of the vagus at rest. Generally when the block disappears following excitement or exercise, it is considered benign. Spörri states that in only about ⅕ of the horses exhibiting this arrhythmia is it associated with disease.[90] On the other hand, Brooijmans feels that functional incomplete AV block with dropped beats is rare and that conclusive evidence of its occurrence has never been presented.[9] Though this lack of conclusive evidence cannot be denied, the common occurrence of this arrhythmia in horses supports the view that it ordinarily should not be considered of pathologic significance. For example, in electrocardiographic studies on supposedly normal horses it has been found to occur in from 12 to 18% of the individuals studied.[90,94,95] Further, it is well-known that somewhere between 10 and 15% of horses which show no other signs of heart disease have this arrhythmia and continue to work for years with no other evidence of heart disease. As it is a vagal phenomenon and the vagal tone may be increased under certain pathologic conditions, it would not be surprising if this arrhythmia were more frequent among horses with heart disease. Sound evidence to support this conclusion is not available, however.

In the horse, the action of the vagus at rest apparently produces AV block more often than SA block, but in a small percentage of individuals the relationship is reversed. The early effect of atropine sulfate is of interest in this regard.[96] Before the peripheral parasympathetic blocking action of atropine develops, its central vagal stimulant effect may be seen. In 6 trials in 2 horses, it was found that incomplete AV block with dropped beats was induced initially. As the peripheral effect developed, acceleration of the heart rate occurred first while the AV block persisted at rates exceeding those at which it ordinarily is observed. Finally, with further cardio-acceleration, normal AV conduction appeared. Thus, it seems that the effect of vagal stimulation on the rate of SA node pacemaker activity is more readily blocked than its effect on AV conduction. A similar phenomenon has been observed in experimental dogs.

Complete AV block is a definite pathologic sign in the horse as are the more severe grades of incomplete block with dropped beats. A frequently reported phenomenon in horses with these marked degrees of AV block is fainting (Adams-Stokes syndrome).[97-108]

The pulse rate in these cases usually was quite slow (10 to 20 per minute) and often irregular, with intervals of 10, 20, 40, and even 60 seconds between beats. The long pauses lead to cerebral anemia and fainting. Since a single ectopic ventricular pacemaker usually is quite regular, the characteristic irregularity reported may be the result of irregularly conducted atrial beats or participation of additional ventricular pacemakers. As many as 100 attacks per day have been reported and one horse had several hundred fainting spells on its last day of life.[98,99] One horse had severe attacks over a period of 8 to 9 months but still performed heavy work.[97]

The relationship between atrial and ventricular activity may be established without an electrocardiogram by counting the arterial pulse (ventricular systoles) and jugular pulsations (atrial systoles) between ventricular beats. For example, Krinizen counted an arterial pulse of 24 per minute and a venous pulse rate of 48 per minute.[103] Three days later the arterial pulse was 22 to 24, but the venous pulse had increased to 86 per minute. In some cases the atrial sounds can be heard and counted between ventricular systoles.

Although specific pathologic lesions accounting for this conduction disturbance cannot always be found, histologic studies in some cases have revealed chronic inflammatory changes involving the AV node and bundle of His.[97,99,101]

Decreasing vagal tone with atropine sulfate (30 mg. subcutaneously) may increase ventricular rate when AV block is not complete, and result in increased pulse rate. Drugs which increase the irritability of the heart have been recommended in man, but in general are not too effective, and in many cases the use of electronic pacemakers is necessary. Digitalis preparations are contraindicated owing to their effect of elevating vagal tone with consequent increase in the degree of AV block.[103]

Bundle Branch Block (BBB): This is a conduction disturbance in which the impulse is delayed or blocked in either the right or left branch of the bundle of His. The ventricular muscle supplied by the blocked branch contracts later than the remaining ventricular myocardium and the pattern of depolarization of the ventricular mass is abnormal. In the dog, right or left BBB can be produced by sectioning the appropriate bundle branch, and dogs with similar electrocardiographic patterns have been observed.[109] Surgical section of the bundle branches in calf hearts produces relatively little change in the duration and form of QRS when contrasted with that produced in the dog.[110,111] Presumably, this is accounted for by the characteristically rich Purkinje network in ungulates. An instance of intraventricular conduction disturbance interpreted as right bundle branch block has been reported in the horse.[112] Whether or not this is an example of true BBB is conjectural.

The large variation in the electrocardiogram of normal horses, the relatively small effect of experimental section of the bundle of His in other ungulates (calves), and the lack of information on experimental BBB in horses make an electrocardiographic interpretation unreliable because similar prolongation of the QRS interval and alterations in the QRS axis can be caused by a variety of other factors, such as

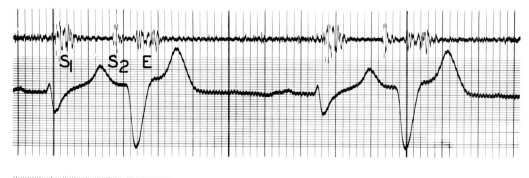

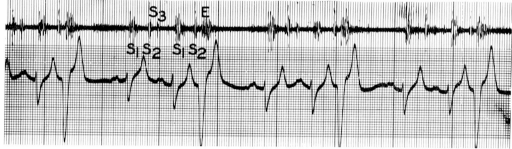

Fig. 23. Ventricular premature beats. Lead CV₀LL and phonocardiogram with the microphone at the cardiac apex of 10 year-old Thoroughbred stallion with chronic alveolar emphysema and pneumonia. Note the coupled ventricular premature beats which produce only the first heart sound. A physiologic third heart sound is present when the coupled premature ventricular systoles are absent (lower record). The sound associated with the premature beats is longer than the third heart sound and extends throughout much of systole.

unilateral ventricular enlargement and widespread myocardial disease affecting intramural conduction.

Ventricular Premature Beats: These are contractions which arise in an ectopic pacemaker in the ventricles and appear early in time (Fig. 23). The term, ventricular extrasystole, frequently is used for these premature ectopic systoles but has been rejected by some authorities on the grounds that the ectopic beats seldom are "extra," as they ordinarily replace the normal beat rather than occur in addition to the regular sequence of beats. Rarely, a ventricular ectopic beat may be interpolated exactly between two normal beats occurring at the dominant rate. In this case, a true "extra" systole has occurred.

Ventricular premature beats often can be diagnosed by auscultation and palpation of the pulse. The beats occur early and are followed by a compensatory pause. The second heart sound and the peripheral pulse may be absent during the premature beat (Fig. 23). Electrocardiographically, ventricular premature systoles are characterized by the presence of bizarre QRST complexes which are not preceded by a true premature P wave, and there is prolongation of the QRS complex beyond that of those occurring in the dominant beats. The normal P wave will occur at its expected time but may be invisible if it is buried within the QRS complex of the premature systole. The most frequent type of premature ventricular systole shows complexes which are identical in contour and coupling. Their form remains the same and the interval between the end of the previous T wave and the beginning of the premature QRS complex is constant (constant coupling). Premature systoles which have identical form but varying coupling usually are instances of parasystole. This arrhythmia will be discussed later. Premature ventricular systoles with constant coupling but variable contour may occur, apparently owing to varying degrees of interference with conduction of impulses originating in the same ectopic focus. Two or more types of premature systoles with respect to the coupling interval and form of QRST complexes may occur in the same record. In such cases, presumably more than one ectopic focus exists. If the ventricular ectopic pacemaker initiates an impulse after the impulse from the normal pacemaker has already entered ventricular tissue, then the ventricles will be excited from 2 sources and the QRST complex will be found intermediate in form between that of the premature systoles and of the dominant beats. These are called ventricular fusion beats.

Coupled ventricular extrasystoles, occurring after each normotopic beat early enough in the diastolic period following the normal beat so that only one heart sound is heard, may be confusing on auscultation. The horse often has an audible third heart sound normally, and such premature systoles causing a single sound early in diastole may be confused with this physiologic third heart sound (Fig. 23). The single sound produced by premature systoles early in diastole usually is louder and more prolonged than a physiologic third heart sound.

Ventricular premature beats cannot be said to be common in the horse, although a number of investigators have reported their occurrence in the presence of recognizable heart disease and in animals in which other signs of heart disease were absent.[9,62,65,113,114,115] Certainly, heart disease should be suspected when ventricular premature beats are present, as there is no question that they are more common in the presence of myocardial damage. On the basis of present information, it is advisable to regard ventricular premature systoles as evidence of cardiac lesions, especially when induced following exercise. If these ectopic ventricular systoles are frequent and if they arise from two or more foci within the heart (i.e., have differing electrocardiographic configuration), the degree of cardiac damage may be considered greater than when they are infrequent and arise from a single focus. Various drugs, toxins, and electrolyte disturbances increase myocardial irritability and this fact must be kept in mind in judging the significance of ectopic pacemaker activity in a given case.

Paroxysmal Ventricular Tachycardia: A rapidly-firing ectopic pacemaker assumes control of the heart beat in this condition. Actually, the resulting systoles may be looked upon as a series of rapidly recurring ventricular premature beats. The heart rate is rapid and regular; the periods of tachycardia start suddenly and stop abruptly, and may last for only a series of several heartbeats or persist for hours or days or weeks. Electrocardiographically, a series of QRST complexes of bizarre contour are seen. Sometimes P waves can be identified as occurring independently and at a slower rate than the ventricular complexes. Occasionally, initiated by an impulse arriving from the atria and conducted normally, ventricular complexes may be seen with shorter QRST complexes than in the beats of the tachycardia. Ventricular fusion beats may occur. These assume a form intermediate between the normotopic beats and the ectopic beats. In most instances, this arrhythmia has been associated with inflammatory or degenerative myocardial lesions. The underlying cardiac condition is usually more severe when several ectopic pacemakers cause the ventricular paroxysmal tachycardia (polymorphic ventricular complexes). So-called bidirectional ventricular tachycardia, characterized by alternate QRS complexes which occur in opposite directions, also is taken as a grave prognostic sign in man, since it frequently precedes fatal ventricular fibrillation.

In man, paroxysmal ventricular tachycardia may occur in the absence of organic heart disease, frequently in association with gastrointestinal disturbances, excessive fatigue, overindulgence in tobacco, alcohol, or coffee, especially when associated with emotional stress, and sometimes following the effect of certain drugs, including aspirin and digitalis. It also may accompany thyrotoxicosis. When it does occur in association with organic heart disease, it has the same serious significance usually associated with the condition in animals.

In the horse, of a total of 11 cases reported in the literature, the etiology was not established in 2, 5 were attributed to septicemia or toxemia, in 3 the paroxysms occurred during severe digestive disturbances, and only 1 was attributed to primary heart disease.[9] The ventricular rates reported by Brooijmans varied from 80 to 140 per minute.[9] Both bidirectional ventricular tachycardia and polymorphic ventricular complexes occurred in some cases. Noerr described a case in a 15-year-old riding horse with rates up to 240 per minute.[116] Despite the presence of heart disease, the work-capacity of the animal was not reduced. It was destroyed 6 years later owing to lameness, and was found to have a grossly enlarged heart.

Ventricular Fibrillation: Coordinated contraction of the ventricles ceases in this condition, and continuous chaotic activity replaces the alternate systole and diastole. The heart ceases to function as a pump and death follows immediately. Transient ventricular fibrillation, as has been reported in man, is not known to occur in horses.

In ventricular fibrillation, there is sudden cessation of the pulse and heart sounds, and a precipitous fall in blood pressure. Unless the heart can be viewed directly or an electrocardiogram is made, the condition cannot be distinguished from simple cardiac standstill. The conventional electrocardiogram shows bizarre, irregular oscillations without any normal QRST complexes. This arrhythmia is so rapidly fatal that it is rarely detected clinically, except in animals under anesthesia. It probably is frequently the immediate cause of death in moribund animals.

Idioventricular Rhythm: This term may be applied to any response of the ventricles to an ectopic ventricular pacemaker. Thus, it could include ventricular tachycardia (*i.e.,* rapid idioventricular rhythm). Whenever the supraventricular pacemakers fail or their rate is excessively slow, a ventricular pacemaker will take over and maintain the heartbeat. Thus, idioventricular rhythm is seen in complete atrioventricular heart block and not infrequently is observed during the final activity in a dying heart. Since experimental work indicates that it probably is specialized conduction tissue (*e.g.,* Purkinje fibers) which usually initiates ectopic rhythms, and since the site of impulse formation in idioventricular rhythms often appears to be in the septum, it is probable that AV nodal tissue, the bundle of His, or the bundle branches are the most common sites of impulse formation.[83]

The Pararrhythmias

In this group of arrhythmias, two or sometimes more pacemakers act independently to produce contractions of the heart (or parts of the heart) in the absence of primary disturbances of atrioventricular conduction. The 2 independent pacemakers coexist, because the one with the lower rate of impulse formation is protected from becoming depolarized by the impulses initiated by the center with the fastest rate.

Two groups of pararrhythmias are distinguished: 1. Parasystole, in which an automatic center is located usually in a ventricle and may produce impulses interfering with those of the normal pacemaker, 2, dissociation with interference, in which a faster atrioventricular rate coexists with a slower sinuatrial rate.

There are 2 varieties of parasystole: 1. Parasystole with simple interference, and 2, parasystole with exit block.

In *parasystole with simple interference,* the impulses from a slower ectopic center interfere with those of the faster sinuatrial node, so that either pacemaker may govern contraction of the heart when it falls outside of the refractory period of the preceding beat. Electrocardiographically, the following characteristics are found: 1. The ectopic beats show varying coupling with the preceding sinuatrial beat, 2, the intervals between consecutive ectopic beats separated by one or more sinuatrial beats (interectopic intervals) are divisible by some common denominator, which is assumed to be the basic interval between discharges of the ectopic pacemaker (ectopic cycle length, which may be directly measurable when 2 ectopic beats occur in succession), 3, the occurrence of fusion beats, intermediate in configuration between those of the sinuatrial beats and those of the ectopic beats.

Parasystole with exit block differs from the foregoing in that the rate of impulse formation in the ectopic center exceeds that of the SA pacemaker, and some of these ectopic impulses are prevented from spreading to the remainder of the heart by a mechanism, which has been termed exit block. Were it not for such exit blocks, an ectopic tachycardia would be present.

In *dissociation with interference* a faster ventricular or atrioventricular nodal (or rarely ventricular) pacemaker exists simultaneously with a slower sinuatrial pacemaker, and the SA nodal rhythm interferes at times by conducted beats with the faster AV rhythm. Like parasystole, the slower center of impulse formation must be protected in some way from the impulses arising in the faster center, but this condition differs from parasystole with simple interference in that here the faster center is located in the AV node or ventricle, and the normal pacemaker is the slower center. It differs from parasystole with exit block in that the ectopic impulses fail to excite the ventricles only during the refractory period of conducted sinuatrial beats. If in beats arising from either of the 2 pacemakers the ventricles are depolarized along the usual pathways, the configuration of the QRST complexes is identical and normal in the 2 types of beats. If the ectopic pacemaker is located below the atrioventricular node or bundle of His, these ventricular complexes will be bizarre in configuration. Simple atrioventricular dissociation is illustrated in Fig. 14. In this record interference did not occur.

Parasystole may occur spontaneously in organic heart disease, and it is a not infrequent arrhythmia in digitalis toxicity. Dissociation with interference may also occur in organically diseased hearts, as well as with digitalis toxicity. Parasystole has been reported in horses.[9]

Accelerated Conduction (Wolff-Parkinson-White Syndrome, WPW, Pre-excitation Syndrome): In this conduction abnormality, the interval between atrial and ventricular contraction (or excitation) is shortened. Thus, in a record showing normal sinus rhythm, a short PR interval is found. The latter is associated with a ventricular complex of abnormal configuration in that the QRS complex is of bizarre shape and is widened, especially in its initial portion. In appropriate leads, the QRS complex may show a very slow rising, slurred deflection, called the delta wave. The T wave ordinarily is more or less in an opposite direction from this delta wave. In man, this arrhythmia often is associated with rapid ectopic supraventricular rhythms. The diagnosis is based on the finding of short PR intervals, prolonged QRS intervals, and QRS complexes of abnormal contour.

It seems that this conduction disturbance is a variant of AV conduction, rather than an accompaniment of some disease. It is not infrequent in man, occurring at a rate of about 2 per 1,000 of routine electrocardiograms in a hospital series,[117] and has been reported in the horse,[48,118,119,120] ox,[121] and dog.[109] The occurrence of accelerated conduction in several species suggests that the phenomenon might be found in mammals generally if other species were studied as extensively as these.

Examples of the changes in duration of PR and QRS intervals, in the same horse, from normal complexes to complexes showing accelerated conduction are as follows: PR shortened from 0.27 to 0.10 second and, simultaneously, QRS lengthened from 0.12 to 0.16 second; PR from 0.26 to 0.14 second and QRS from 0.10 to 0.12 second.[119,120]

During the shortened PR intervals the intensity of the first heart sound may be increased,[120] a finding characteristic of short PR intervals but, surprisingly, not ordinarily detected in the WPW syndrome in man.[38]

Accelerated conduction in horses has been observed after strenuous work,[48] in the presence of heart disease,[118] in a horse which fell while racing,[119] during cardiac catheterization,[122] and in a 3-year-old filly which continued to race and win.[120]

THE PREVALENCE AND TYPES OF VARIOUS ARRHYTHMIAS IN HORSES

As is well-known, cardiac irregularities are fairly common in horses. Most of these are the result of incomplete atrioventricular block with dropped beats. Estimates of the prevalence of this arrhythmia based on electrocardiographic studies vary from 12 to 18%.[90,94,95] Earlier observations on the prevalence of cardiac irregularities in the horse are in the same range. Sixty-two of 200 (31%) military horses (average age of 12.5 years) examined by Pietzsch had irregularities of the rhythm and quality of the pulse and heartbeat.[123] Dreyer similarly investigated 272 military horses, finding an overall prevalence of 15.5% (42 horses) with an age distribution as follows: 15 to 18 years, 36%; 10 to 14 years, 27%; 7 to 10 years, 14%; 4 to 6 years, 6%.[124] Undoubtedly, in these last cited reports, most of the arrhythmias resulted from atrioventricular block with dropped beats. The mere presence of a pulse irregularity obviously may be of little clinical significance. It is important, however, to distinguish the benign arrhythmias (sinus arrhythmia and incomplete atrioventricular block with dropped beats) from those often associated with heart disease (e.g., atrial fibrillation, ventricular premature beats, paroxysmal ventricular tachycardia, etc.).

In a series of 100 horses with arrhythmias and conduction disturbances, 60 had atrioventricular conduction disturbances; 15 had ectopic premature systoles; 9 had sinus arrhythmias; 6 had atrial fibrillation; 4 had sinuatrial block, and the remainder had various combination of these arrhythmias, bradycardia, and tachycardia.[62] Included was one instance of pulsus alternans. In another series of arrhythmias and conduction disturbances in horses, the distribution was as follows: atrial fibrillation, 89; wandering pacemaker, 53; incomplete atrioventricular block, 7; paroxysmal ventricu-

lar tachycardia, 5; sinuatrial block, 2; sinus tachycardia, 2; complete atrioventricular block, 1; accelerated conduction, 1; right bundle branch (or parietal) block, 1; and sinus premature beats, 1.[9]

THE FETAL ELECTROCARDIOGRAM

Deflections caused by the fetal heart appear in maternal limb lead electrocardiograms in advanced pregnancy and through the use of abdominal leads[125,126] with or without special amplifiers.[125] The fetal electrocardiogram may be detected as early as the sixth or seventh month of gestation. In one instance, the cardiac frequency of a 7-month fetus was 130 per minute and that of a fetus at the end of the tenth month was 100 per minute.[126] Although fectal electrocardiography in horses was introduced many years ago, the method has been used little and is not generally practiced.[127,128,129] In our clinic, it has been used on rare occasions to establish fetal viability when this was in question.

CONGENITAL HEART DISEASE

The prevalence of congenital heart disease among horses has never been determined and cannot be assessed from the literature. Lilleengen surveyed the reported cases of congenital heart disease in animals up to 1934, adding 37 cases of his own.[130] Among the 166 cases in various species, cattle were represented most frequently (91 cases) and horses next (28 malformations in 26 horses). The congenital cardiac lesions which have been reported in the horse include the following: various valvular malformations, patent ductus arteriosus,[131] cor triloculare biatriatum,[132] interventricular septal defects,[133] persistent foramen ovale,[134] tetralogy of Fallot,[135] persistent foramen primum,[130] persistent truncus arteriosus,[130] atresia of the right atrioventricular ostium,[130] and various malformations of the great vessels. The 28 malformations surveyed by Lilleengen were distributed as follows:

DEFECT	CASES
Interventricular septal defect	13
Semilunar valvular defects of various sorts	4
Persistent truncus arteriosus	3
Atrioventricular valvular defects	3
Atresia of the right atrioventricular ostium	1
Hematocysts on mitral valve	1
Persistent foramen primum	1
Cor triloculare biatriatum	1
Duplicated cranial venae cavae	1

Clearly, subaortic interventricular septal defects and valvular anomalies are the most frequently reported malformations (Fig. 24).[130]

As most reports on cases of congenital heart disease in the horse are limited primarily to a description of the necropsy findings, the clinical signs of the various conditions are not known in detail.

The valve of the foramen ovale in the horse consists of a dilated membranous tube which is divided into a fenestrated apical region and a nonfenestrated area.[136] Patency of the foramen ovale varies at birth. Not infrequently some of the fenestrations remain unoccluded and this situation may persist into adult life. The time of anatomic closure may be as early as 15 days postpartum, although earlier reports indicate closure occurs at least as late as the ninth week after birth.[136] Persistence of the foramen ovale has rarely been reported in the horse and seldom has been considered a lesion of clinical significance.[134,136] Presumably, as in other species, an open foramen ovale, when the aperture is functionally small, may persist into adult life and remain of little consequence.

Patent ductus arteriosus is likewise apparently uncommon in the horse.[131] Presumably, a typical machinery murmur would be audible in the pulmonic auscultatory area. One case reported had reached advanced age (more than 20 years) before being used as an anatomic subject, although it was suffering from dyspnea and the right atrium and ventricle were hypertrophied. In 3 foals examined, 7 to 7½ hours after birth, the machinery murmur of an open ductus arteriosus was heard over the third, left intercostal space.[43] The area over which the murmur was audible was not extensive. A case of pentalogy of Fallot in which patent ductus arteriosus is one of the anomalies is described in the following.

In *interventricular septal defects* (Fig. 16, 24) the location of the point of maximum intensity and the configuration of the systolic murmur are variable from case to case. The results of cardiac catheterization in 2 cases were:

SITE	PRESSURE SYSTOLIC/DIASTOLIC (MM. HG)	PERCENT OXYGEN SATURATION
Case 1: Welsh pony, male, 1 year old		
Jugular vein	—	55
Right atrium	7/−7	51
Right ventricle	35/0	70
Pulmonary artery	35/11	68
Case 2: Thoroughbred, gelding, 3 years old.		
Cranial vena cava	—	58
Right atrium	60/22	72
Right ventricle	170/−4 to 30	87
Pulmonary artery	130/60 to 80	87

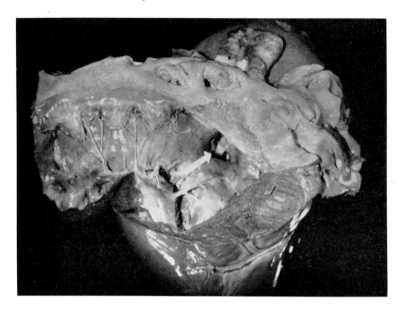

Fig. 24. Opened left ventricle of a 3-year-old Thoroughbred gelding, showing a large interventricular septal defect (arrow). The septal cusp of the mitral valve has been reflected to show the defect, which is high in the interventricular septum just below the aortic valve. The left ventricular wall is markedly hypertrophied.

A presumptive diagnostic test, useful in suspected cases of interventricular septal defect, involves the accentuation of the systolic murmur by the injection of vasopressor agents (see p. 363 and Fig. 16).

The *tetralogy of Fallot*, a complex anomaly consisting of pulmonic stenosis, high interventricular septal defect, dextroposition and consequent over-riding of the aorta, and right ventricular hypertrophy has been described in a Shetland pony.[135] In this condition, cyanosis is present, but may not be pronounced, and a systolic murmur is audible. We have observed a 2-month-old Thoroughbred foal with a *pentalogy of Fallot*. In this anomaly the features of the tetralogy of Fallot are complicated by the presence of a patent ductus arteriosus.

The presence of a patent ductus arteriosus in the pentalogy of Fallot permits more blood to reach the lungs than in the tetralogy and thus is of some benefit to the afflicted animal.

DISEASES OF THE PERICARDIUM

Pericarditis

Pericarditis occurs most often secondary to pneumonia and pleuritis and has been reported in various respiratory infections of horses.[137] Distention of the pericardial sac with excess pericardial fluid sometimes occurs in horses with respiratory infections described as influenza (equine respiratory disease complex).[138] Of the virus diseases which produce clinical signs corresponding to those classically described as equine influenza, equine viral arteritis is known to be accompanied occasionally by distention of the pericardial sac with excess fluid.[139] A specific arthritis with pericarditis, thought possibly to be caused by a virus with secondary streptococcal invasion, has been described in horses in Tasmania.[140,141]

Rare instances of fatal traumatic pericarditis caused when a hard alfalfa stem, horseshoe nail, or similar object pierced the lower esophagus, stomach, or upper duodenum and the pericardium have been reported.[137,142]

The clinical sign of diagnostic significance in acute pericarditis is a scratching or grating sound which may occur during both systole and diastole (pericardial friction rub). When excessive pericardial fluid accumulates, the heart sounds are muffled and if the intrapericardial pressure is great enough to interfere with venous return to the heart, chronic passive congestion and venous engorgement will develop owing to cardiac tamponade. Amounts of pericardial fluid as great as 35 to 40 liters have been reported.[137]

Rupture of the pericardium in horses, associated with violent activity, occurs occasionally.[143,144,145] In the cases described, death occurred suddenly and in at least one horse the immediate cause of death appeared to be an associated rupture of the aorta at its root.[144] Since it is unlikely that rupture of the pericardial sac, in itself, would be fatal, associated or subsequent damage to the heart presumably was the cause of death in the rapidly fatal cases. In one animal, death occurred 30 days following a collision with another horse.[145] Serofibrinous pericarditis, hydropericardium, and parenchymal myocarditis were observed at necropsy.

DISEASES OF THE MYOCARDIUM

Myocarditis

Inflammatory lesions of the myocardium are not rare in horses, but since they have not been well-characterized, classification is difficult. Myocarditis occurs in various infectious diseases and may develop as the result of metastasis or extension from primary endocardial or pericardial lesions.[137,146,147] Acute and chronic interstitial myocarditis, often associated with endocarditis, are described in horses having a locus of infection elsewhere in the body. Rubarth described 5 cases of sudden death in horses following exercise.[148] A chronic pharyngitis and infection of the retropharyngeal lymph nodes were found. On histologic examination, changes were seen in the myocardial parenchyma or conduction system. Positive bacterial cultures were obtained in 3 cases (*Streptococcus equi* in 2 and streptococcus type Schuetz in 1). Myocarditis of allergic origin is considered especially common in streptococcal infections in horses, and sudden death has been associated with myocarditis in horses recently recovered from either strangles or influenza.[146,149] Apparently, these lesions often do not produce clinical evidence

of disease, although in certain cases clinical signs of cardiac insufficiency develop and death may follow.[150,151]

Ossification of the right atrium, especially the auricular appendix, has been reported frequently in the European literature.[137,146, 152-162]

One view of the pathogenesis of this lesion has been that it is secondary to dilation of the right atrium with resultant damage to muscle fibers and proliferation of the intermuscular tissue, followed by ossification.[152] Cohrs and Streich found this lesion in 5 horses with tuberculosis.[152] Tuberculous lesions were found in the affected atrial wall in 4 of these and it was concluded that the lesion was an allergic myositis caused by localization of the tuberculous process in the wall of the right atrium in a sensitized animal. From the literature it appears that from 50 to 80% of the horses with this lesion have had tuberculosis.[146,152] The lesion also is found in horses in which tuberculosis has not been diagnosed.[153] Farrelly has suggested that infarction in the atrium resulting from thrombotic lesions in the aorta caused by strongyle larvae may have etiologic significance because in his 3 cases with such infarctions the right atrium was involved.[163] This condition has not been described as a clinical entity and has been recognized only at necropsy, although in some cases it has been associated with sudden illness and death.[152]

Other Myocardial Lesions

Fatty degeneration and hemorrhage of the myocardium are not infrequent in purpura hemorrhagica of horses. Cardiac lesions are often prominent and extensive in horses which have died from equine infectious anemia.[164] In acute cases, hemorrhages and areas of necrosis occur and, in some, extensive induration and small areas of infarction may be found.

In aged horses, especially draft horses, small or large indurations are sometimes seen in the myocardium. These consist of collagenous connective tissue poor in nucleated cells, sometimes hyalinized, and not infrequently containing fatty tissue. The origin of these lesions is obscure. Although they have been attributed to coronary circulatory disturbances, it is difficult to trace or establish their pathogenesis.[146]

Horses with paralytic myoglobinuria may develop myocardial lesions similar to those found in the skeletal muscle. These may be extensive enough to produce clinical signs of myocardial damage.

Spontaneous rupture of the heart is an occasional cause of death in horses. The sudden death and dramatic nature of postmortem findings account in part for the frequency with which this fatal event has been reported. Leonhardt assembled 34 cases; the rupture occurred in the right ventricular wall in 15, in the right atrium in 7, in the left atrium in 8, in the left ventricle in 3, and in the interventricular septum in 1. The usual cause is underlying myocardial disease, such as infarction or other myocardial lesion with loss of substance. Primary disease of the coronary arteries has not been recognized often and coronary atherosclerosis does not appear to occur as a primary lesion in horses. Myocardial infarcts owing to embolism or thrombosis are encountered occasionally. Bacterial emboli arising from vegetative lesions of bacterial endocarditis account for some of these. Farrelly described 4 cases of parasitic endarteritis and thrombosis at the origin of the aorta caused by larvae of *Strongylus vulgaris*.[163] In 2 cases, thrombo-embolism of the right atrial branches of the right coronary artery had caused infarction of the right atrium. In a third case, previously reported by Cronin and Leader, occlusion of the right coronary artery was caused by a vegetation located in the aortic bulb.[166] A fourth horse died owing to thrombo-embolism of the common brachiocephalic trunk.

Farrelly points out that myocardial infarction is not a common lesion in the equine heart and that, when found, the right atrium is usually involved. The anterior and ventral location of the orifice of the right coronary artery

in the aortic bulb favors entrance of particulate matter, facing as it does the oncoming flow of blood. This is in contrast to the left coronary orifice direction which is almost opposite to that of the right. It is not clear why the atrial branches of the right coronary should be more commonly affected than the other branches. Farrelly describes a fifth case in which a healed infarct in the right atrial myocardium was found and suggests that this lesion was probably the result of parasitic thrombosis of the aortic sinuses. It appears that parasitic arteritis at the origin of the aorta is fairly common in horses since Poynter found an incidence of 20.9% in a series of 43 horses examined as part of a study of the migratory route of *Strongylus vulgaris*.[167]

Clinical Signs: The clinical features of myocarditis and other myocardial lesions are quite variable. Ordinarily, one cannot distinguish inflammatory myocardial changes from other types of myocardial damage under clinical circumstances. Thus the term, myocarditis, as used by the clinician often refers to inflammatory, degenerative, or other pathologic processes affecting the myocardium. There are no pathognomonic signs of myocardial involvement. Very often myocardial disease goes undetected clinically and is found only on postmortem examination. Myocarditis, secondary to an infectious process, often may fail to produce clinical signs until one to several weeks after the infection is recognized clinically.

The clinical signs which are associated with myocarditis include: 1. Tachycardia disproportionate to any fever present, 2, murmurs and gallop sounds, 3, various cardiac arrhythmias (atrial or ventricular premature systoles, paroxysmal ventricular tachycardia, atrial fibrillation), 4, certain abnormalities of the electrocardiogram, such as S-T segment deviation, prolongation and slurring of the QRS complex, and prolongation of the Q-T interval, 5, signs of congestive heart failure, 6, acute circulatory collapse, and 7, sudden death attributable to a fatal arrhythmia.

DISEASES OF THE ENDOCARDIUM

ENDOCARDITIS

Inflammatory lesions affecting the cardiac valves or mural endocardium are of relatively frequent occurrence in the horse. From a clinical point of view, it is the valvular lesions which are of greater importance owing to the occurrence of valvular malfunction and thrombo-embolic phenomena which may accompany these lesions.

Etiology: Allergic tissue reaction and bacterial infection have been the etiologic factors most commonly incriminated in endocarditis of horses. In bacterial endocarditis, streptococci have been most commonly isolated, although other organisms such as *Shigella equirulis* may be found.[168,169,170] The occurrence of arterial and venous thrombi and of secondary embolism is not rare in horses with verrucous valvular endocarditis, and visceral infarction in lungs, liver, kidneys, and brain with or without accompanying signs may be expected.[171-174] Endocarditis may result as part of an antigen-antibody reaction in previously sensitized animals.[175-177]

Clinical Signs: Animals with bacterial endocarditis present a difficult diagnostic problem. There may be a history of a recent infection, followed by continued fever associated with weakness, weight loss, and possibly the development of a cardiac murmur. A positive blood culture may be found but often the blood cultures are negative. The other signs of disease which develop are associated with septicemia and the amount and character of valvular damage which has occurred. Other organs, such as the brain and kidneys, may be affected as the result of arterial embolism originating from the primary lesions in the heart.

Lesions: Endocarditic lesions are located most often in the left atrium and left ventricle.[168] The aortic valves are most frequently affected followed by the mitral, tricuspid, and pulmonary valves, in that order.[168,171,178] In 14 serum production horses which developed valvular endocarditis while under immuniza-

tion with meningococci, all had only left heart lesions and the aortic valves were more frequently involved than the mitral.[171] Although stenotic lesions occur, usually due to large verrucae obstructing a valve orifice, aortic or mitral insufficiency has been the most common valvular impairment observed in our clinic.

Valvular Fenestration: Fenestration of the free edge of the cusps of the aortic and pulmonic valves is a common finding in horses of all ages.[40] Such lesions were found in 22 of 27 horses of various ages from an 8-month fetus to a 20-year-old stallion and were present in all horses examined which were more than 2 years old. The aortic valves were most often involved, although large fenestrations also occurred in some pulmonic semilunar cusps. Dysfunction is likely only when the lacunae happen to coincide if they are limited to the overlapping edges of the cusps, or when they extend into the body of the cusp beyond the line of overlap. Ordinarily, these lesions are of no clinical significance.

BLOOD CYSTS OF VALVES

Blood cysts or telangiectases of the valves are not infrequent in horses. For example, in one series 22 cases were found in 251 necropsied horses (8.76%).[179] The mitral valve is involved most often. Ordinarily, these so-called valvular hematomas do not interfere with the function of the valves and are of no clinical importance.

DISEASES OF THE ARTERIES AND VEINS

The aorta of horses increases in thickness to varying degrees with aging, through intimal proliferation, and medial alteration.[146] The latter consists of primary medial necrosis with replacement later by connective tissue. Medial calcification is common in horses 14 to 16 years of age or older, occurring initially in the thoracic aorta. In advanced cases, the inner surface of the thoracic aorta may be markedly roughened by ridges and indentations. Primary intimal calcification is sometimes observed in the thoracic aorta and may appear in young as well as in older animals.

ARTERIAL LESIONS

Etiology and Lesions: Arterial lesions caused by migrating *Strongylus vulgaris* larvae are the basis of the most commonly recognized and clinically important vascular disease of horses.[179a] These lesions consist of fibrin tracks on the intimal surface, arteritis, thrombosis, embolism, and aneurysm formation. The incidence of these arterial lesions is said to be from 90 to 95% by various investigators.[167,180] As a result of the inflammatory and thrombotic arterial changes, secondary arteriosclerosis and atherosclerosis occur.[167] The cranial mesenteric artery is the usual site of the most severe lesions and was found to be affected in from 86 to 95% and more of horses examined.[167] Other enteric vessels are also commonly involved. Nine of 43 horses (20.9%) had developed parasitic arteritis at the root of the aorta,[167] and thrombotic and embolic lesions have been reported in the coronary and cerebral arteries, and the more posterior branches of the aorta.[146,163,166] To account for the distribution of these lesions, it appears that the migratory pathway of larvae from the gut must include the outflow tract of the left heart, although the classic view of retrograde travel from the gut up into the mesenteric arteries and aorta also may occur.[146,147]

In the aorta, the earliest lesions seen are fibrin tracks produced by the larvae.[167] Small thrombi form at places where these fibrin tracks cross. Similar changes also occur in other affected areas and lead to thromboendarteritis. For example, in the cranial mesenteric artery and for a considerable distance in the aorta above and below the origin of the mesenteric artery, the intima may be covered with parietal thrombotic masses containing strongyle larvae. The induced inflammatory infiltration reaches deep into the media. In larger vessels, the intima, thickened with fibrin, may be separated from the media by a space filled with debris, producing an atherosclerotic lesion.[167]

Aneurysms are frequently found in horses and are almost always the result of arterial disease caused by strongyle larvae. An incidence of 90 to 95% has been reported.[146,180] Newborn foals have no aneurysms, but these lesions have been found as early as the 10th and 38th day of life.[146,180] The most frequent site of development is the cranial mesenteric artery, and other arteries supplying abdominal viscera are commonly affected. Rarely, other regions (*e.g.,* carotid and femoral arteries) may develop aneurysms. These lesions may lead to thromboembolic colic, rupture with fatal hemorrhage, or infection and subsequent pyemia.

Clinical Signs: Considering the extremely high prevalence of these mesenteric artery lesions, the occurrence of thromboembolic colic is relatively rare. Clinically, it is difficult to distinguish this type of colic from other types, and the cause usually is discovered at necropsy. It should be suspected in cases of colic which appear without evident cause (often during or shortly after work) and recur. Thrombosis of arteries supplying the posterior limbs may lead to intermittent lameness. In records assembled some years ago by a Swiss insurance firm 0.1% of all insured horses and 1.5% of horses for which damages were claimed were afflicted with this condition.[180] Rectal palpation of the aorta and its major branches may be of value in diagnosing aneurysms of arteries which can be reached.

OTHER LESIONS

Viral arteritis of horses results in necrosis of smooth muscle cells of the arterial media with disappearance of nuclei and replacement of the cytoplasm by homogeneous, eosinophilic or fibrinoid material. These arterial lesions appear to be the underlying cause of the edema and hemorrhages in many organs and of the infarctions in the intestine and lungs.[181] The abortion produced by this virus in pregnant mares is attributed to infection of the fetus rather than a consequence of disease in the mare.[182]

Obliterating endarteritis has been reported in such diseases as infectious anemia and as an isolated finding affecting the digital arteries. Dahme's view is that the latter lesions result from trauma and that true Buerger's disease (endarteritis obliterans) has not been observed in domestic animals.[183]

Three types of *noninflammatory thickening of the pulmonary arteries* have been distinguished: 1. Intimal hyperplasia of the pulmonary artery and its larger branches, 2, sclerosis of the arteries, arterioles, and capillaries resulting from mitral insufficiency, which has led to pulmonary hypertension and hypertrophy of the right ventricle, and 3, arteriosclerosis and arteriolosclerosis in chronic alveolar emphysema.[184]

Rupture of veins, although of rare occurrence, has been reported more frequently in horses than in other species. The caudal vena cava has been most commonly involved, the cranial vena cava next, followed by the jugular, portal and femoral veins.[146,188] For the most part, these appear to have been traumatic in origin, although local disease of the veins (varices, extension of a neoplastic process) was responsible in some cases. Varices also have been found in horses more frequently than other domestic species. They usually involve the cutaneous veins. *Venous thrombosis* is encountered most commonly in the jugular vein as the result of faulty intravenous injection of irritant substances with consequent periphlebitis. *Phlebitis* is not common in horses and generally results from local infections (*e.g.*, subcutaneous or intramuscular phlegmon) extending along the vessels.

A variety of vascular anomalies have been reported in horses such as double jugular veins, double cranial venae cavae, absence of the bicarotid trunk, absence of the internal iliac artery, and arteriovenous anastomoses of the carotid and jugular vein.[188] Multiple congenital anastomoses of the small arteries and veins in the region of the fetlock were corrected surgically in a horse in our clinic (Fig. 17a).[189] Wherever possible, arteriovenous anastomoses should be corrected because the accompanying loss of peripheral resistance increases the cardiac output and may impose a harmful workload on the heart.

Rupture of the Aorta and Other Arteries: Aortic rupture, although rare, has been reported more frequently in horses than in other domestic animals. The usual site of rupture is at the root of the aorta between the aortic valves and the ligamentum arteriosum. In this region the aortic wall is thinner than at the aortic arch. Winterhalter investigated 7 cases of spontaneous aortic rupture in horses.[185] The site of rupture in each case was just above the semilunar valves. Histologic sections revealed fine medial necrosis in the region of the rupture. Except for the tear in the aortic wall, macroscopic alterations were not visible. Atheromatous degeneration, arteriosclerosis, and parasitic (*S. vulgaris*) arteritis are among the lesions described in other cases.

Rare instances of fatal hemorrhage owing to rupture of other arteries (*e.g.*, the cranial mesenteric artery and the renal artery) have been described also.[186,187]

CLINICAL SYNDROMES

The cardiovascular syndromes recognized clinically in the horse are chronic cor pulmonale, congestive heart failure, and Adams-Stokes disease. In addition, sudden death associated with cardiovascular disease may be included under this heading. The convulsive syndrome of newborn foals, which has been described by English workers, though not fully understood, possibly is related to the hemodynamic effects of depriving the foal of placental blood.

Chronic Cor Pulmonale

Chronic cor pulmonale or pulmonary heart disease refers to pathologic cardiac changes secondary to chronic disease of the lungs or pulmonary circulation. In horses, hypertrophy and dilation of the right heart, secondary to chronic alveolar emphysema (heaves) occur. The pulmonary arterial pressure and pulse pressure are increased.[190,191,192] In advanced cases, right ventricular dilation may progress until the tricuspid valve becomes incompetent. A systolic murmur is then audible at the tricuspid area, and right heart failure with dependent edema may supervene, leading to death from congestive heart failure.

CONGESTIVE HEART FAILURE

This syndrome develops when the cardiac output no longer meets body needs, and there is resultant retention and accumulation of sodium and water. Diagnosis is based on the presence of clinical signs of passive venous congestion and edema attributable to heart disease. The congestion involves the venous bed behind either the right side of the heart ("right heart" failure), the left side of the heart ("left heart" failure), or both ("generalized" failure).

The clinical signs of right-sided heart failure, which result from congestion involving predominantly the systemic veins, include dependent edema, ascites, and generalized venous engorgement. The liver is enlarged, but this is difficult to diagnose in the horse. In left-sided heart failure, the signs are referable to congestion in the pulmonary venous bed and include coughing, dyspnea, and pulmonary rales. Fatigability is common in both types of failure. In generalized heart failure, both groups of signs are present. The circulation time is increased and one would expect reduced cardiac output when resting values can be obtained. The presence of moderate ascites sometimes is difficult to detect in the horse by observation or palpation, and abdominal paracentesis may be required to confirm its presence. In contrast to the dog, in which ascites often precedes dependent edema, edema of the limbs and ventral surface of the body usually is evident before ascites is marked.

The mechanism of sodium and water retention in congestive heart failure has not been studied in horses, and current concepts are based on work carried out on man and experimental dogs.[193-197] Presumably, these mechanisms are common to all mammals. There is general agreement that the inciting cause of disturbed renal function in congestive heart failure is a reduction in cardiac output below that required to meet bodily needs, at first during exercise and finally even at rest, and the associated venous congestion. Antidiuretic hormone and aldosterone have been implicated as the humoral agents responsible for water and sodium retention, although the former does not appear to be essential. The factors responsible for the release of aldosterone in congestive heart failure remain controversial and will not be discussed here.[196]

Horses which develop congestive heart failure seldom are treated for long periods of time, and experience with therapy is meager. As in the dog, the general principle of giving a digitalization dose followed by a maintenance dose should be followed. The digitalization dose may be administered in 6 divided doses, distributed over 48 hours. The following digitalization doses for various preparations are recommended with the caution that we have had only limited experience in treating congestive heart failure in the horse:

Preparation	Digitalization dose
Digitalis (powder, tablets)	1.5 to 3.0 Gm./100 lb. body weight (0.03 to 0.06 Gm./kg.)
Digitalis tincture	15 to 30 ml./100 lb. body weight (0.3 to 0.6 ml./kg.)
Digitoxin	1.5 to 3.0 mg./100 lb. body weight (0.03 to 0.06 mg./kg.)
Digoxin	3.0 mg./100 lb. body weight (0.06 mg./kg.)

Signs of effective digitalization include cardiac slowing (especially marked if atrial fibrillation with rapid ventricular rate is present), relief of dyspnea, coughing, pulmonary rales, fatigability, and reduction in edema through diuresis. If no effect is observed by the third day, more digitalis may be given, using as the daily dose ⅓ of the calculated digitalization dose. This dose may be continued until a therapeutic effect is produced, or signs of digitalis toxicity occur (ventricular premature beats, atrioventricular block, marked depression, inappetence). Diarrhea may develop and, unless severe, is not considered a contraindication to continued therapy. The daily maintenance dose selected following digitalization should be from ⅙ to ⅕ of the originally calculated digitalization dose. This may have to be increased or decreased, using clinical response as a guide.

Ouabain may be employed for intravenous digitalization. The dose required for a 1,000-pound horse may be determined by injecting 3 mg. intravenously at 2-hour intervals until cardiac slowing or other signs of effective digitalization appear or a total dose of 9 mg. has been given. The dose required can then be given daily for several days to maintain digitalization, provided the animal can be carefully observed for evidence of toxicity.

Other therapeutic measures include limitation of exercise and a light, palatable diet without the addition of salt.

MORGAGNI-ADAMS-STOKES SYNDROME

This, or simply Adams-Stokes syndrome, is the term applied to the condition in man characterized by syncope and epileptiform convulsions caused by cerebral anemia resulting from marked slowing of the heart. The cardiac slowing usually is the result of complete atrioventricular block, although similar fainting spells can occur with cerebral anemia due to extreme tachycardia or cardiac (atrial and ventricular) standstill. In horses, syncope associated with advanced degrees of atrioventricular block occasionally occurs. For further discussion of this syndrome and for references, see the section on complete atrioventricular block on page 379.

SUDDEN DEATH

Sudden death in horses, attributable to cardiovascular disease, has been reported in ani-

mals with myocarditis,[148,149] rupture of the heart,[165] rupture of great veins,[146,188] and rupture of the aorta or other large arteries.[185,186,187] These conditions have been discussed previously (see page 387ff).

In addition, several instances of sudden death in young horses have been encountered which were caused by coronary embolism or massive thrombosis in other vital organs resulting from emboli originating from friable parasitic thrombi in the aorta.[166,179a]

CONVULSIVE SYNDROME IN FOALS

In England and Ireland a convulsive syndrome is described which occurs in about 2% of newborn Thoroughbred foals. In many respects it resembles pulmonary hyaline membrane syndrome of newborn infants.[198,199,200] Clinical signs of this condition usually appear within an hour or so after birth, although they may be delayed 12 or more hours, but never longer than 24 hours. The affected foal becomes incoordinated; violent clonic convulsions appear accompanied by a "barking" sound. About 50% of the foals die, and the remainder recover. Full recovery often is preceded by a period during which there is apparent blindness and failure to respond normally to environmental stimuli. Such foals are called wanderers or dummies. This syndrome is not described as occurring in other regions nor in births unattended by man. There is extensive atelectasis of the lungs. In the foals developing this syndrome, the umbilical cord has been cut early by attendants. Early severance of the umbilical cord results in a blood loss of from 500 to 1500 ml. (i.e., up to 25% of the foal's blood volume). This has led to the suggestion that initial expansion of the lungs fails secondary to the hemodynamic effects of this blood deprivation.[198,199,200] The mechanism responsible for this condition is not understood, although too early ligation of the umbilical cord is thought to be a significant factor in its etiology. Other factors may produce similar clinical signs. For example, the same syndrome has been reported in a foal with fracture of the ribs and contusion of the right ventricle in which birth was presumably normal and humans were not present to sever the umbilical cord.[201]

D. K. DETWEILER

D. F. PATTERSON

REFERENCES

1. Schamroth, L.: An Introduction to Electrocardiography. Charles C Thomas, Springfield, Ill., 1956.

2. Burch, G. E. and Winsor, T.: A Primer of Electrocardiography. 4th ed., Lea and Febiger, Philadelphia, Pa., 1960.

3. Lepeschkin, E.: Modern Electrocardiography. Vol. 1, Williams and Wilkins Co., Baltimore, Md., 1951.

4. Sodi-Pallares, D. and Calder, R. M.: New Bases of Electrocardiography. Mosby, St. Louis, Mo., 1956.

5. Grant, R. P.: Clinical Electrocardiography. McGraw-Hill, New York, N. Y., 1957.

6. Spörri, H. and Detweiler, D. K.: Ueber die Ausbreitung der Erregungswelle in Pferde- und Rinderherzen. Helv. Physiol. Pharmacol. Acta, 14 (1956) 79-81.

7. Lannek, N. and Rutqvist, L.: Normal area variation for the electrocardiogram of horses. Nord. Vet.-Med. 3 (1951) 1094-1117.

8. Brooijmans, A. W. M.: Standardization of leads in veterinary clinical electrocardiography. Tijdschr. Diergeneesk. 79 (1954) 801-811.

9. Brooijmans, A. W. M.: Electrocardiography in Normal Horses and Cattle. Laboratory of Veterinary Physiology, State University, Utrecht, 1957.

10. van Zijl, W. J.: The electrocardiogram of the normal horse using the techniques of Einthoven and Wilson. Tijdschr. Diergeneesk. 76 (1951) 85-96.

11. Nakamura, R. K., Too, K., and Matsuhashi, A.: Studies on applications of electrocardiograms in horses; I, II, and III. Jap. J. Vet. Research 3 (1955) 24-32; 3 171-180; and 4 (1956) 33-43.

12. Kusachi, R.: Fundamental studies on electrocardiograms of the horse. I. Unipolar semidirect lead. Jap. J. Vet. Research 3 (1955) 120-135.

13. Lautenschlager, O.: Grundlagen der Aufnahmetechnik des Elektrokardiogrammes von Pferd und Rind und ihre Ergebnisse. Dissertation, Giessen, 1928.

14. Steel, J. D.: Electrocardiogram of racehorses: A preliminary communication. Med. J. Austral. 1 (1957) 78-79.

15. Detweiler, D. K.: Electrocardiogram of the horse. Fed. Proc. 11 (1952) 34.

16. Luisada, A. A. and Zalter, R.: Phonocardiography. III. Design of the ideal phonocardiograph. Amer. J. Cardiol. 4 (1959) 24-39.

17. Patterson, D. F., Cooper, S. H., and Detweiler, D. K.: Unpublished observations, 1961.

18. Braunwald, E., Fishman, A. P. and Cournand, A.: Time relationship of dynamic events in the cardiac chambers, pulmonary artery and aorta in man. Circulation, 4 (1956) 100-107.

19. Luisada, A. A., Liu, C. K., Aravanis, C., Testelli, M., and Morris, J.: On the mechanism of production of heart sounds. Amer. Heart J. 55 (1958) 383-399.

20. Spörri, H.: The study of cardiac dynamics and their clinical significance. Advances in Vet. Sci. 7 (1962) 1-41.

21. Orias, O.: Genesis of heart sounds. New Eng. J. Med. 241 (1949) 762-769.

22. Littlewort, M. G. C.: Certain extra sounds associated with the equine heart beat. From a Seminar-Conference of Veterinary Surgeons of Europe; Cambridge, April, 1961. (Abstr.: Schw. Arch. Tierheilk. 103 (1961) 623.)

23. Charton, A., Minot, G., and Bressou, M.: Les bruits normaux de coeur du cheval: Étude phonocardiographique. Bull. Acad. Vét. France 16 (1943) 218-224.

24. McKusick, V. A.: Cardiovascular Sound in Health and Disease. Williams and Wilkins Co., Baltimore, 1958.

25. Detweiler, D. K.: Examination of the equine heart. Univ. Pennsylvania Vet. Extension Quart. 40 (1958) 14-33.

26. Corticelli, B.: Sull'origine e sulla natura dello sdoppiamento del primo tono cardiaco del cavallo. Arch. Vet. Ital. 2 (1951) 257-261.

27. Leatham, A.: Splitting of the first and second heart sounds. Lancet 2 (1954) 607-614.

28. Patterson, D. F. and Detweiler, D. K.: The diagnostic significance of splitting of the second heart sound in the dog. (Zbl. Vet.-Med., 1962—in press.)

29. Corticelli, B.: La fonocardiografia in clinica veterinaria. Nuova Vet. 30 (1954) 218-239.

30. Bruns, D. L.: A general theory of the causes of murmurs in the cardio-vascular system. Amer. J. Med. 27 (1959) 360-374.

31. Reisinger, L.: Physiologische funktionelle Störungen am Pferdeherzen. Berl. Münch. tierärztl. Wschr. 12 (1949) 181-182.

32. Niemetz, E.: Ueber das funktionelle systolische Geräusch an der Pulmonalis bei Pferden. Wien. tierärztl. Mschr., 1924. (Cited by Reisinger—#31.)

33. Papadaniel, S., and Matthaiaki, E.: Souffles cardiaques provoquées chez le cheval par le réflexe "oto-cardiaque". Ann. Méd. Vét. 81 (1936) 49-55.

34. Perevezentsev, V. V.: Diagnosis of the functional heart murmurs in horses. Trudy Troitsk. Vet. Inst. 3 (1940) 135-140. (Abst.: Vet. Bull. 14 1944.)

35. Alatorzeff, A. P.: Zur Frage der funktionellen Diagnostik des Herzens. Arch. wiss. Tierheilk. 65 (1932) 272-278.

36. Sudakov, N. A.: Functional heart murmurs in thoroughbreds and trotters. (In Russian.) Trudy Mosk. Vet. Akad. 24 (1959) 171-177.

37. Rogers, W. M., Simandl, E., Bhonslay, S. B., and Deterling, R. A., Jr.: The pulmonary valve in direct phonocardiography. Circulation, 18 (1958) 992-996.

38. Levine, S. A. and Harvey, W. P.: Clinical Auscultation of the Heart. 2nd Ed., W. B. Saunders Co., Philadelphia, Pa., 1959.

39. Chrisholm, D. R.: Trigoniadation of the semilunar valves and its relation to certain basal systolic murmurs. Amer. Heart J. 13 (1937) 362-372.

40. Mahaffey, L. W.: Fenestration of the aortic and pulmonary semilunar valves in the horse. Vet. Rec. 70 (1958) 415-418.

41. Crevasse, L.: The use of a vasopressor agent as a diagnostic aid in auscultation. Amer. Heart J., 58 (1959) 821-826.

42. Vogelpoel, L. M.: The use of amyl nitrite in the diagnosis of systolic murmurs. Lancet 2 (1959) 810.

43. Amoroso, E. C., Dawes, G. S., and Mott, J. C.: Patency of the ductus arteriosus in the new-born calf and foal. Brit. Heart J., 20 (1958) 92-96.

44. Louf, R. and Bouchard, N.: Mésure du temps de circulation avec la lobeline chez les chevaux sains. Rev. Corps Vét. Armée, 3 (1954) 102-105.

45. Louf, R. and Bouchard, N.: Mésure du temps de circulation chez les chevaux cardiaques. Ibid, 106-111.

46. Romagnoli, A. and Salutini, E.: La velocità del circolo polmonare negli equini affeti della sindrome bolsaggine. Ann. Fac. Med. Vet. Univ. Pisa, 3 (1950) (15 pp.).

47. Fisher, E. W. and Dalton, R. G.: Cardiac output in horses. Nature, 184 (1959) 2020.

48. Landgren, S. and Rutqvist, L.: Electrocardiogram of normal cold-blooded horses after work. Nord. Vet.-Med. 5 (1953) 905-914.

49. Chowdhury, A. K. and Banerjee, A. K.: Blood pressure in horse. Indian Vet. J., 37 (1960) 341-348.

50. Covington, N. G. and McNutt, G. W.: Studies of normal blood pressure in animals. I. Blood pressure in the horse with a brief note on the ox. J.A.V.M.A. 79 (1931) 603-624.

51. Grauweiler, J., Spörri, H. and Wegmann, H.: Zur graphischen Ermittlung des systolischen und diastolischen Blutdruckes bei Haustieren mittels des Infratonmikrophons und Druckmarkengebers von Brecht und Boucke. Schw. Arch. Tierheilk. 100 (1958) 297-318.

52. Dohmen, E. S.: Determinación de la presión venosa en el caballo. Rev. Fac. Ciencias Vet.La Plata 1 (1959) 51-55.

53. Fisher, E. W.: Arterial puncture in horses. Vet. Rec. **71** (1959) 514-515.

54. Fisher, E. W., Detweiler, D. K., and Patterson, D. F.: Unpublished observations.

55. Holzmann, M.: Klinische Elektrokardiographie. 2nd ed., Thieme, Stuttgart, 1952.

56. Detweiler, D. K.: Electrocardiographic and clinical features of spontaneous auricular fibrillation and flutter (tachycardia) in dogs. Zbl. Vet.-Med., **4** (1957) 509-556.

57. van Zijl, W. J.: Electrocardiografische opmerkingen over het boezemfibrilleren bij het paard. Tijdschr. Diergeneesk., **76** (1951) 553-555.

58. Detweiler, D. K.: Experimental and clinical observations on auricular fibrillation in horses. Proc. Book, Amer. Vet. Med. Assoc., 89th Ann. Mtg., 1952, 119-129.

59. Detweiler, D. K.: Auricular fibrillation in horses. J.A.V.M.A. **126** (1955) 47-50.

60. Roos, J.: Auricular fibrillation in domestic animals. Heart, **11** (1924) 1-7.

61. Roos, J.: Vorhofflimmern bei den Haustieren. Arch. wiss. Tierheilk., **51** (1924) 280 (Abst.: Deut. tierärztl. Wschr. **33** (1925) 408.)

62. Nörr, J.: 100 klinische Fälle von Herz- und Pulsarrhythmien beim Pferde. Monatshf. prakt. Tierheilk. **34** (1924) 177-232.

63. Krupski, A.: Ueber Vorhofflimmern, Arrhythmia perpetua sive completa beim Pferd. Schw. Arch. Tierheilk. **73** (1931) 51-55.

64. Fodroczy, E.: Elektrokardiographische Untersuchungen bei Rhythmus- und Reizleitungsstörungen beim Pferde. Dissertation, Budapest, 1938. (Abst.: Jahresber. Vet.-Med. **66** (1939) 94.)

65. Szakmary, G.: Formveränderungen der Herzstromkurve beim Pferde. Auszug aus der Dissertation, Budapest, 1940.

66. Batt, H.: Three cases of heart disease in horses. Cornell Vet. **31** (1941) 71-76.

67. Dukes, H. H. and Batt, H.: Studies on the electrocardiogram of the horse. Amer. J. Physiol. **133** (1941) P265-P266.

68. Wirth, D.: Vorhofflimmern und -flattern beim Pferd. Wien. tierärztl. Mschr. **29** (1942) 241-251.

69. Spörri, H.: Ueber das Wesen und die Bedeutung der Reizleitungs- und Reizbildungsstörungen im Herzen. Festschrift für Dr. O. Bürgi, Zürich, 1943. 21 pp.

70. Spörri, H. and Leeman, W.: Die Beurteilung der Herzkraft bei kranken Tieren durch das Elektrokardiogramm. Schw. Arch. Tierheilk. **88** (1946) 113-133.

71. Donald, D. E. and Elliot, F. J.: Auricular fibrillation in horses. Vet. Rec. **60** (1949) 473-474.

72. Corticelli, B.: Fibrillazione e flutter atriale nel cavallo. Arch. Vet. Ital. **1** (1950) 177-196.

73. Corticelli, B.: Fibrillation auriculaire chez le cheval et le bovin. Atti XV Cong. Intern. Vet., Stockholm, **7** (1953) 220.

74. Domracev, G.: An unusual case of tricuspid insufficiency accompanied by marked sinus arrhythmia and cardiac fibrillation in the horse. (In Russian.) Uchen. Zap. Kazanskovo gosudarst. Vet. Inst. **38** (1928) 100-110. (Abst.: Jahresber. Vet.-Med. **48** (1928) 538.)

75. Monti, F. and Regni, M.: La fibrillazione atriale bradicardiaca nel cavallo. Clinica Vet. **81** (1958) 289-299.

76. Glazier, D. B., Nicholson, J. A. and Kelly, W. R.: Atrial fibrillation in the horse. Irish Vet. J. **13** (1959) 47-53.

77. Lewis, T.: Irregularity of the heart's action in horses and its relation to fibrillation of the auricles in experiment and to complete irregularity of the human heart. Heart **3** (1911-1912) 161-171.

78. Lewis, T.: Auricular fibrillation and its relationship to clinical irregularity of the heart. Heart **1** (1909-1910) 306-372.

79. Beijers, J. A.: Klinische waarnemingen over het boezemfibrilleren bij paard en rund. Tijdschr. Diergeneesk. **76** (1951) 540-552.

80. Detweiler, D. K. and Patterson, D. F.: Unpublished observations, 1962.

81. Lewis, T., Meakins, J. and White, P. D.: The excitatory process in the dog's heart. Part I. The Auricles. Philosoph. Trans. Roy. Soc., Ser. B, **205** (1914) 375-420.

82. Meek, W. J. and Eyster, J. A. E.: Experiments on the origin and propagation of the impulse in the heart. IV. The effect of vagal stimulation and of cooling on the location of the pacemaker within the sino-auricular node. Amer. J. Physiol. **34** (1914) 368-383.

83. Hoffman, B. and Cranefield, P. F.: Electrophysiology of the Heart. McGraw-Hill, New York, 1960.

84. Schütz, E.: Physiologie des Herzens. Springer, Berlin, 1958; p. 17.

85. Lewis, T.: The Mechanism and Graphic Registration of the Heart Beat. Shaw and Sons, London, 1925; p. 193.

86. Meyling, H. A. and TerBorg, N.: The conducting system of the heart in hoofed animals. Cornell Vet. **47** (1957) 419-455.

87. Detweiler, D. K.: Unpublished observations.

88. Nicholson, J. A., Glazier, D. B., and Heffernan, M.: Sino-atrial heart block in the horse. Irish Vet. J. **13** (1959) 168-172.

89. Lannek, N.: The terminal ventricular complex of the post-block beat in the horse's electrocardiogram. Nord. Vet.-Med. **3** (1951) 425-434.

90. Spörri, H.: Ueber die Genese und klinische Bedeutung des partiellen Herzblockes beim Pferd. Schw. Arch. Tierheilk. **94** (1952) 337-346.

91. Spörri, H.: Ueber den atmungsgesteuerten reflektorischen Herzblock des Pferdes. Tierärztl. Umschau, **6** (1951) 419-431.

92. Spörri, H.: Der respiratorisch induzierte Herzblock des Pferdes. Cardiologia, **20** (1952) 180-187.

93. Detweiler, D. K.: Unpublished observations, 1959.

94. Detweiler, D. K.: Unpublished observations on 82 horses.

95. Nörr, J.: Das Elektrokardiogramm des Pferdes. Seine Aufnahme und Form. Ztschr. Biol. **61** (1913) 197-229.

96. Detweiler, D. K.: Physiological effects of atropine on military animals: horse and mule. Chem. Corps Med. Lab. Contract Rept., 1955, 1-64.

97. Bosnić, L. and Rapić, S.: Two further cases of Adams-Stokes syndrome in horses. Vet. Arkhiv, **11** (1941) 166-179. (Abst.: Vet. Bull **18** [1948] #548.)

98. Desliens, L.: Les arhythmies cardiaques du cheval. (Anémie cérébrale et syndrome d'Adams-Stokes). Bull. Acad. Med., Paris **133** (1949) 327-330. (Abstr.: Vet. Bull. **22** [1952] #1449.)

99. Bosnić, L. and Rapić, S.: Adams-Stokesov sindrom kod parcialnoga srcanoga bloka konja. Vet. Arkhiv **11** (1941) 1-17. (Abst.: Vet. Bull. **17** [1947] #2586.)

100. Wirth, D.: Adams-Stokes'sche Krankheit bei zwei Pferden, bedingt durch Herzblock. Wien. tierärztl. Mschr. **14** (1927) 1-8. (Abst.: Jahresber Vet.-Med. **47** [1927] 556.)

101. Martincic, M.: (Pathology of changes in the atrioventricular system of the horse with Adams-Stokes syndrome). Vet. Arkhiv. **11** (1941) 76-99. (Abst.: Vet. Bull. **18** [1948] #574.)

102. Marek, J. and Mócsy, J.: Zwei Fälle von Adams-Stokes'scher Krankheit infolge von Herzdissoziation beim Pferd. Prag. Arch. Tiermed. vergl. Path., **6** (1926) (A) (1), 43-54.

103. Krinizin, D. J.: Adams-Stokes'scher Symptomenkomplex bei partiellen Herzblock bei Pferde. Arch. Tierheilk. **60** (1929) 444-463. (Abst., Jahresber. Vet.-Med. **49** [1929] 519.)

104. Kozma, I. and Szekely, E. G.: Ein Fall von Adams-Stokes'scher Krankheit beim Pferd. Állatorvosi Lapok, **50** (1927) 299-300. (Abst.: Jahresber. Vet.-Med. **47** [1927] 557.)

105. Bang, O., Peterson, G., and Petersen, O.: Bradykardie bei Pferden. Herzblock und Sinusbradykardie. Vet. og. L. Aarsskr., 1920. p. 180. (Abst.: Jahresber. Vet.-Med. **39-40** [1919-1920] 145).

106. Domracev, G.: (A case of Adams-Stokes disease in horse). Učenye Zap. Kazan. Vet. Inst. **37**(1) (1926) 154-165. (Abst.: Jahresber. Vet.-Med. **47** [1927] 557).

107. Moretti, B.: Sindrome di Morgagni-Adams-Stokes in un cavallo determinata da blocco totale del cuore. Atti Soc. Ital. Sci. Vet., **2** (1948) 1-19.

108. Dukes, H. H.: A case of heart-block in a horse. Cornell Vet., **30** (1940) 248-251.

109. Patterson, D. F., Detweiler, D. K., Hubben, K., and Botts, R. P.: Spontaneous abnormal cardiac arrhythmias and conduction disturbances in the dog. Amer. J. Vet. Research **22** (1961) 355-369.

110. Alfredson, B. V. and Sykes, J. F.: Studies of the bovine electrocardiogram: II. Bundle branch block. Proc. Soc. Exp. Biol. Med. **43** (1940) 580-584.

111. Pruitt, R. D.: Electrocardiogram of bundle-branch block in the bovine heart. Circ. Research **10** (1962) 593-597.

112. van Zijl, W. J.: Een geval van rechten bundeltak-block bij het paard. Tijdschr. Diergeneesk. 77 (1952) 417-422.

113. Glazier, D. B. and Nicholson, J. A.: Premature ventricular beats. Irish Vet. J. 13 (1959) 82-86.

114. Krinitzen, J. and Philippoff, J. J.: Die kombinierte Form der extrasystolischen ventrikulären Arrhythmie und der sinus Arrhythmia beim Pferde. Arch. wiss. prakt. Tierheilk. 64 (1931) 281-289.

115. Nörr, J.: Hochgradige Herzhypertrophie, Erweiterung des Arteriellensystems und Extrasystolen bei einem Pferde. Berl. tierärztl. Wschr., 1922, 393. (Abst.: Jahresber. Vet.-Med 41-42 [1921-1922] 208).

116. Nörr, J.: Paroxysmale Tachykardie und partielle Vorhof-Kammerblock bei einem Reitpferd mit Aortenin-suffizienz. Arch. Tierheilk. 63 (1931) 104-119.

117. Katz, L. N. and Pick, A.: Clinical Electrocardiography. Part I. The Arrhythmias. Lea and Febiger, Philadelphia, Pa., 1956.

118. Brooijmans, A. W. M.: Syndrome of Wolff-Parkinson-White in a horse. Acta Physiol. Pharmacol. neerland. 5 (1956) 112-113.

119. Delhanty, D. D. and Glazier, D. B.: The Wolff-Parkinson-White (atrioventricular conduction) syndrome. Irish Vet. J., 13 (1959) 205-207.

120. Cooper, S. A.: Ventricular pre-excitation (Wolff-Parkinson-White syndrome) in a horse. Vet. Rec. 74 (1962) 527-530.

121. Spörri, H.: Die ersten Fälle von sog. Wolff-Parkinson-White Syndrom, einer eigenartigen Herzanomalie, bei Tieren. Schweiz. Arch. Tierheilk. 95 (1953) 13-22.

122. Detweiler, D. K., Fisher, E. W., and Patterson, D. F.: Unpublished observations.

123. Pietzsch: Untersuchungen über das Vorkommen von Arrhythmien der Herztätigkeit bei unseren Truppenpferden. Ztschr. Veterinärk. 38 (1926) 239-244. (Abst.: Jahresber. Vet.-Med. 46 [1926] 638).

124. Dreyer, W.: Untersuchungen über des Vorkommen von Arrhythmien der Herztätigkeit bei unseren Dienstpferden. Ztschr. Veterinärk., 1912, 276 (Abst.: Jahresber. Vet-Med., 32 [1912] 157).

125. Larks, S. D., Holm, L. W., and Parker, H. R.: A new technic for the demonstration of the fetal electrocardiogram in the large domestic animal (cattle, sheep, horse). Cornell Vet. 50 (1960) 459-468.

126. Rehmet, L.: Versuche über Altersbestimmung der Föten durch die fötale Elektrokardiographie. Dissertation, Berlin, 1939.

127. Nörr, J.: Fötale Elektrokardiogramme vom Pferd. Ztschr. Biol. 73 (1921) 123-128.

128. Nörr, J.: Ein neuer Trächtigkeitsnachweis durch galvanometrische Aufnahme der Aktionsströme des fötalen Herzens. Berl. tierärztl. Wschr., 1921 (1 and 2).

129. Glazier, D. B., Nicholson, J. A., and Hyde, D.: A preliminary report on the appearance of waves in the maternal electrocardiogram due to activity of the foetal heart. Irish Vet. J. 13 (1959) 87.

130. Lilleengen, K.: Hjärtmissbildningar hos djuren. Skand. Vet.-Tijdskr. 24 (1934) 493-555.

131. Hare, T.: Patent ductus arteriosus in an aged horse. J. Path. 34 (1931) 124. (Abst.: Jahresber. Vet.-Med. 51 [1931] 566).

132. Avtokratov, D.: Cor triloculare biatriatum equi. Izv. Donsk. Vet. Inst. 4 (1928) 62-64. (Abst.: Jahresber. Vet.-Med. 49 [1929] 519).

133. Aellig, A.: Das Foramen interventriculare persistens cordis bei den Haustieren. Schw. Arch. Tierheilk. 72 (1929) 509-525 and 73 (1930) 10-29. (Abst.: Jahresber. Vet.-Med., 50 [1930] 562).

134. Wilson, A. P.: Persistent foramen ovale in a foal. Vet. Med. 38 (1943) 491-492.

135. Wensvoort, P.: De Tetralogie van Fallot, met atresie van de arteria pulmonalis, bij het hart van een Shetland pony. Tijdschr. Diergeneesk. 84 (1959) 939-942.

136. Ottaway, C. W.: The anatomical closure of the foramen ovale in the equine and bovine heart: A comparative study with observations on the foetal and adult states. Vet. J. 100 (1944) 111-118 and 130-134.

137. Ackerknecht, E.: Kreislauforgane. In: Joest, E.: Spezielle pathologische Anatomie der Haustiere. Band IV, Schoetz, Berlin, 1925.

138. Manninger, R. and Mócsy, J.: Spezielle Pathologie und Therapie der Haustiere. Band I., Fisher, Jena, 1954.

139. Doll, E. R., Bryans, J. T., McCollum, W. H., and Crowe, M. E. W.: Isolation of a filterable agent causing arteritis of horses and abortion by mares. Its differentiation from equine abortion (influenza) virus. Cornell Vet. 47 (1957) 3-41.

140. Ramey, J. W.: A specific arthritis with pericarditis affecting young horses in Tasmania. Austral. Vet. J. 20 (1944) 204-206.

141. Ryan, A. F. and Ramey, J. W.: A specific arthritis with pericarditis affecting horses in Tasmania. Austral Vet. J. 21 (1945) 146-148.

142. Jaehnke, H.: Traumatische Pericarditis bei einem Pferd. Ztschr. Veterinärk. 3 (1918). (Abst.: Jahresber. Vet.-Med. 38 [1918] 71).

143. Hughes, W.: Rupture of the pericardium in a horse. Vet. J. 79 (1923) 266.

144. Wilson, A. C.: Rupture of the pericardium in the horse due to fright. Vet. Rec. n.s. 5 (1925) 173.

145. Anon.: Statistischer Veterinärbericht über das deutsche Reichsheer für das Jahr 1923. Jahresber. Vet.-Met. 43 (1923) 317.

146. Cohrs, P.: Nieberle und Cohrs Lehrbuch der speziellen pathologischen Anatomie der Haustiere. 4th ed., Fischer, Stuttgart, 1962.

147. Smith, H. A. and Jones, T. C.: Veterinary Pathology, Lea and Febiger, Philadelphia, Pa., 1957.

148. Rubarth, S.: Plötsliga dödsfall hos häst och derar samband med fokalinfektioner. Svensk. Militärvet.-sallskap. Kvartalskr. 30(4) (1943) 1-16.

149. Monlux, W. S.: Sudden death in the horse due to myocarditis. Iowa State Univ. Vet. 29 (1961-1962) 40-41.

150. Lorscheid: Herzkrankheiten bei Truppenpferden. Deut. tierärztl. Wschr., 1918, 136. (Abst.: Jahresber. Vet.-Med. 38 (1918) 71).

151. Petersen, G.: Einige Fälle von Herzleiden bei Pferden. Maanedsskr. Dyrlaeger 39 (1928) 579-585. (Abst.: Jahresber. Vet.-Med.48 (1928) 538).

152. Cohrs, P. and Streich, W.: Verknöcherung der rechten Herzvorkammer beim Pferde, die Folge einer tuberculösen hyperergischen Myositis. Deut. tierärztl. Wschr., 51 (1943) 92-95. (Abstr.: Vet. Bull. 16 (1946) 133, #776).

153. Garbers, H.: Verknöcherung der rechten Herzvorkammer beim Pferd. Dissertation, Hannover, 1949.

154. Viebrock, A.: Ein weiterer Fall von Herzvorhof-verknöcherung beim Pferd. Münch. tierärztl. Wschr. I (1929) 310-313.

155. Pallaske, G.: Totale Herzvorhofverknöcherung mit Verkalkung beim Pferd. Deut. tierärztl. Wschr. II (1928) 523-527.

156. Nienhaus, H.: Verknöcherung der rechten Herzvorkammerwand eines Pferdes. Deut. tierärztl. Wschr. 33 (1925) 854-855.

157. Morpurgo, E.: Di un caso di ossificazione del miocardio nel cavallo. Nuova Vet., 7(3) (1929) 13-19.

158. Land, N.: Zur Frage über Verknöcherung des Herzens beim Pferde. Arch. Vet.-Wiss. 44 (1917) 1333.

159. Joest, E. and Schieback, P.: Ueber Herzwandver-knöcherung. Virchows Arch. 253 (1924) 472-504.

160. de Graaf, C.: Verknöcherung der Herzmuskel bei einem Pferde. Tijdschr. Diergeneesk. 49 (1922) 340.

161. Cisowski, A.: Przypadek skostnienia uszka i ściany przedsionka w sercu u konia. Przegl. Wet. 48 (1935) 724-733.

162. Altmann, L.: Ueber die Verknöcherung der rechten Herzvorhofwand beim Pferde an der Hand von zwei Fällen. Állatorvosi Lapok 49 (1926) 259-261. (Abst.: Jahresber. Vet.-Med. 48 (1926) 637).

163. Farrelly, B. T.: The pathogenesis and significance of parasitic endarteritis and thrombosis in the ascending aorta of the horse. Vet. Rec. 66 (1954) 53-62.

164. Detweiler, D. K.: Personal observations.

165. Leonhardt: (Cited by Ackerknecht-#137).

166. Cronin, M. T. I. and Leader, G. H.: Coronary occlusion in a Thoroughbred colt. Vet. Rec. 64 (1952) 8.

167. Poynter, D.: The arterial lesions produced by Strongylus vulgaris and their relationship to the migratory route of the parasite in its host. Res. Vet. Sci. 1 (1960) 205-217.

168. Winqvist, G.: Topografisk och etiologisk sammanställning av de fibrinösa och ulcerösa endokarditerna hos en del av vara hujsdur. Skand. Vet. Tidskr. 35 (1945) 575-585.

169. Innes, J. R. M., Berger, J. and Francis, J.: Subacute bacterial endocarditis with pulmonary embolism in a horse associated with Shigella equirulis. Brit. Vet. J. 106 (1950) 245-250.

170. Svenkernd, R. R. and Iversen, L.: Shigella equirulus (S. viscosum equi) som arsak til klappeendocarditis hos häst. Nord. Vet.-Med. 1 (1949) 227-232.

171. Miller, J. K.: Meningococcal endocarditis in immunized horses. Amer. J. Path. 20 (1944) 269-276.

172. Middeldorf, R.: Gehirnembolie eines an Endocarditis verrucosa chronica erkrankten Pferdes. Berl. tierärztl. Wschr. 35 (1919) 111.

173. Aston, W. F.: Endocarditis with secondary embolism and infarct in a shire. Vet. Rec. II (1929) 610.

174. Danelius, G.: Endocarditis verrucosa mit Metastasen bei Pferde. Svensk. Vet. Tidskr., 1923, 183.

175. Klein, P.: Bakteriologie und Immunologie der Endokarditis. Verhandl. Deut. Ges. Kreislaufforsch. **20** (1954) 176-191.

176. Weidlich, N.: Beitrag zur Biologie des Rotlaufserumtieres. Berl. Münch. tierärztl. Wschr., 1943, (10/20), 135-140.

177. Richter, W.: Immunobiologische und klinische Beobachtungen bei Rotlauf-serumpferde. Monatshefte Vet.-Med. **5** (1950) 85-91.

178. Engström, K.: Zwei Fälle von Endokarditis rheumatica. Svensk. Vet. Tidskr., 1918, 352.

179. Kowanz, R.: Beitrag zum Vorkommen von Blutzysten, sog. Klappenhämatomen an den AV Klappen beim Pferd und Hund. Deut.-Oesterreich. tierärztl. Wschr. **3** (1921) 153.

179a. Miller, W. C.: Cardiovascular disease in horses. Vet. Rec. 74 (1962) 825-828.

180. Ris, H.: Untersuchungen über Erkrankungen des arteriellen Gefässsystems des Pferdes. Schw. Arch. Tierheilk. **66** (1924), 1-14 and 34-47.

181. Jones, T. C., Doll, E. R., and Bryans, J. T.: The lesions of equine viral arteritis. Cornell Vet., **47** (1957) 52-68.

182. Doll, E. R., Knappenberger, R. E., and Bryans, J. T.: An outbreak of abortion caused by equine arteritis virus. Cornell Vet. 47 (1957) 69-75.

183. Dahme, E.: Personal communication.

184. Dahme, E.: Der Gestaltwandel der Lunge und arteriellen Lungenstrombahn bei Störungen des kleinen Kreislaufs. Berl. Münch. tierärztl. Wschr. **73** (1960) 333-336.

185. Winterhalter, M.: Uebe spontane Aortenrupturen bei Pferden. *Medianecrosis aoratae.* Vet. Arkhiv, **8** (1938) 471-497. (Abst.: Jahresber. Vet.-Med., **65** (1939) 203-204).

186. Danelius, G.: Fatal hemorrhage caused by rupture of the anterior mesenteric artery due to excessive aneurysm, thrombi, and abscesses of the mesenteric trunk in a colt. Cornell Vet. **31** (1941) 307.

187. Huber: Seltener Fall einer Blutgefässruptur. Mitt. Ver. bad. Tierärzte, **27** (1927) 70. (Abst.: Jahresber. Vet.-Med. 47 (1927) 561).

188. Ackerknecht, E. and Krause, C.: Kreislauforgane; Gefässe. In: Joest, E.: Handbuch der speziellen pathologischen Anatomie der Haustiere. Band V., Schoetz, Berlin, 1929.

189. Raker, C., Detweiler, D. K., and Patterson, D. F.: Unpublished observations.

190. Spörri, H. and Schlatter, Ch.: Blutdruckerhöhungen im Lungenkreislauf. Schw. Arch. Tierheilk. **101** (1959) 525-541.

191. Spörri, H.: Ueber die Untersuchung der Herzdynamik und ihre diagnostische Bedeutung. Wien. tierärztl. Monatsschr. 47 (1960) 251-268.

192. Fisher, E. W. and Patterson, D. F.: Unpublished observations.

193. Thompson, D. D.: Salt and water retention in heart failure. Progr. Cardiovasc. Dis. 3 (1961) 520-536.

194. Gauer, O. H., Henry, J. P., and Sieker, H. O.: Cardiac receptors and fluid volume control. Progr. Cardiovasc. Dis. 4 (1961) 1-26.

195. Davis, J. O.: A critical evaluation of the role of receptors in the control of aldosterone secretion and sodium excretion. Progr. Cardiovasc. Dis. 4 (1961) 27-46.

196. Davis, J. O.: Adrenocortical and renal hormonal function in experimental cardiac failure. Circulation **25** (1962) 1002-1014.

197. Laragh, J. H.: Hormones and the pathogenesis of congestive heart failure. Circulation 25 (1962) 1015-1023.

198. Mahaffey, L. W. and Rossdale, P. D.: Convulsive and allied syndromes in new-born foals. Vet. Rec. 69 (1957) 1277-1286.

199. Burch, G. E. and Pasquale, N. D.: Diffuse hyaline pulmonary disease of foals and infants. Amer. Heart J. 63 (1962) 428-429.

200. Tizard, J. P. M.: The pulmonary hyaline membrane syndrome of the newborn. In: Waley, R., Goodwin, J. F. and Steiner, R. E.: Clinical Disorders of the Pulmonary Circulation. Little, Brown and Co., Boston, 1960. pp. 288-297.

201. Millar, R. and Bailey, K. C.: A clinical case of convulsive syndrome in a new-born foal. Austral. Vet. J. **35** (1959) 489-492.

HEMORRHAGIC DISEASES

Hemorrhagic diseases are defined as conditions due to vascular weakness, defective number or function of blood platelets, or faulty coagulation of the blood. In the horse we have only two diseases generally classified as hemorrhagic diseases. These are purpura hemorrhagica and primary idiopathic thrombocytopenic purpura. The rest of the hemorrhagic diseases are ill-defined in the horse or not well-documented. Only the two types of purpura will be discussed in this section.

Purpura Hemorrhagica

This disease is a nonthrombocytopenic purpura of horses usually occurring secondary to strangles or equine influenza and characterized by a generalized edema of the subcutaneous tissues. Synonyms of the disease as reported in the older literature are petechial fever and morbus maculosus.

Purpura hemorrhagica is an old disease of horses and the first accurate description of the disease according to Biggers and Ingram was written by Field in 1839.[1] The disease apparently was present for a considerable time prior to this description but documentary proof is missing. Since this time, the disease has been recognized in many parts of the world with most reports of the disease coming from Europe and the United States.

There are no accurate data on the prevalence of the disease. It occurs primarily following an outbreak of either strangles or influenza in horses. For this reason, it occurred most frequently in army remount stations or in stockyards where horses are assembled for sale. Following most outbreaks of these diseases purpura hemorrhagica does not occur, but in certain outbreaks a number of horses will develop purpura. From the author's experience, the percentage of animals developing purpura will range from approximately 1 to 10% in a severe outbreak. On occasion, an animal will develop purpura hemorrhagica without a history of any previous respiratory infection. The reason why purpura occurs subsequent to some outbreaks of strangles or influenza and not

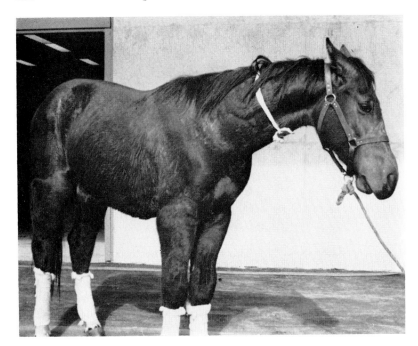

Fig. 25. Edema of face and limbs.

others is not known. Results of a survey of 339 veterinarians in Minnesota and part of Wisconsin revealed that 100 cases of purpura hemorrhagica were diagnosed by them in the past 10 years. Since the disease in its more severe form is reasonably easy to recognize, it probably reflects the general prevalence of the disease at the present time in this area.

Etiology: The cause of the disease is not known. There are several theories about the etiology, and the most generally accepted theory today is that it is a result of a hypersensitive reaction. The theory was first advanced by Marek when he apparently produced a case of the disease by sensitizing a horse with extracts of streptococci and challenged it a month later. Seven days later the animal developed purpura and died. Kramer has described a case that developed 20 days after a second injection of tetanus antitoxin which further suggests the relationship to anaphylaxis.[2] The frequent history of a strangles infection also suggests that *Streptococci equi* or *equisimilus* are concerned in the pathogenesis and the possibility that streptococcal antigens are the sensitizing agents. The occasional occurrence of urticarial wheals on the body of

the horse also suggests a relationship to a hypersensitive reaction.

Clinical Signs: The onset of clinical signs usually occurs within 2 to 4 weeks after a respiratory disease. There is considerable variation in the severity of the disease, and though the severe form is most easily recognized and described, mild forms of the disease also occur. The less severe form of the disease will be considered first.

The mild form is characterized clinically by muscle soreness, stiffness, and the animal's reluctance to move its neck or to walk. There is difficulty in walking and the animal has the clinical attitude of a horse with acute laminitis. Upon clinical examination, the temperature is normal, the pulse rate is in the normal range, and the respiratory rate is either normal or high-normal. The appetite usually remains good, and urine and fecal eliminations are normal. Urticarial lesions may appear on various parts of the body. They usually do not involve the extremities. The lesions vary in size, usually are circumscribed, raised, and will pit on pressure. Palpation of the muscles reveals them to be tense and harder than normal. Slight to moderate edema of one or more legs, the prepuce, or ventral abdomen may develop. The disease may become more severe at this time, or the signs may regress with complete recovery occurring within 3 to 7 days.

The severe form of the disease is characterized by the appearance of pronounced edema. The animal usually goes through an initial period of muscle soreness and stiffness before the appearance of edema. The edema usually is slight initially and may be observed first in the intermandibular area, the anterior pectoral region, or as "stocking" of the limbs. The edema usually becomes progressively more severe. Its development may be gradual, changing little from day to day, or it may become rather marked within 2 to 3 days. As the edema develops the head also becomes involved, starting first in the lips and ventral aspects of the head and progressing dorsally above the eyes. At the same time the edema is developing the nasal mucosa usually is congested. Petechial or ecchymotic hemorrhages may or may not be present (Fig. 25, 26).

The edema may become so severe that several complications occur. Edema of the head, face, upper respiratory passages, and larynx may lead to moderate to severe inspiratory dyspnea. This may become more severe and result in edema of the lungs, and death may result from asphyxiation. A nasal discharge may develop in some animals; it may be serosanguineous in nature or it may progress to a purulent exudate if necrosis of the upper respiratory passages occurs. The edema of the legs and ventral abdomen frequently is well-defined and sharply delineated from the non-edematous area dorsally. If the edema becomes severe, serum may ooze from the skin and areas of skin necrosis may develop. This particularly is true in areas over the joints. The eyes also may become involved, with the lids and periorbital tissues becoming so edematous that the lids will be forced together to completely obstruct vision.[3]

During this time the animal has difficulty walking and is reluctant to lie down, or it may go down and have difficulty in rising. The appetite diminishes as the disease becomes more severe. Urination may be difficult due to the edema of the prepuce. The temperature usually

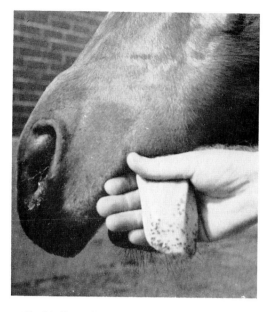

Fig. 26. Hemorrhages on ventral surface of tongue.

is normal or high-normal. It may become elevated, up to 105 F. for several days. This may be associated with secondary infection. The pulse usually is normal or slightly elevated, and the respiratory rate usually is normal unless edema of the upper respiratory passages causes some occlusion.

The hematologic findings in purpura hemorrhagica are rather consistent, although in the past there has been some confusion about them. In the mild or moderate forms of the disease there is no alteration in the number of red blood cells. In the severe form there is a gradual progressive decrease in the hemoglobin from normal to about 7 to 8 Gm. %. The total red blood cells may decrease to between 3 and 4 million cells.

A leukocytosis with a neutrophilia usually is found in purpura hemorrhagica. This occurs quite early in the disease, frequently on the second or third day after its onset. There is a tendency for the total leukocytes to increase in proportion to the severity of the disease, although total leukocytes counts of 15,000 to 18,000 per cmm. also have been recorded in mild cases. In most cases, the total leukocyte count increases to approximately 15,000 to 20,000 per cmm. withm the first week of the disease, and remains elevated until the clinical signs regress. White blood counts of 40,000 to 50,000 per cmm. have been recorded. A neutrophilia and a shift to the left with more immature forms usually accompanies the leukocytosis. An absolute eosinopenia and lymphopenia may be present, although on some occasions it may be only relative.[4]

Whether or not a thrombocytopenia is present has caused some confusion in the past. Total platelet counts on 6 horses studied by the author and his colleagues have revealed normal platelet values. The platelet values ranged from 135,000 to 300,000 per cubic millimeter. The disease therefore is classified as a nonthrombocytopenic purpura. Studies on blood coagulation also have revealed no alterations in prothrombin time, clot retraction time, and clotting time.

Blood biochemical values in cases of purpura hemorrhagica, with the exception of the albumin-globulin ratios, are within the normal ranges. Total protein values usually are in the normal range of 6.0 to 9.0 Gm. %, but in some cases there is a decrease of albumin causing a lower A/G ratio. The normal A/G ratio usually is between 0.5 to 0.8, and in purpura hemorrhagica the ratio may decrease to 0.3.

Blood glucose, calcium, phosphorus, chloride, and blood urea nitrogen values appear to be normal. Total bilirubin values on occasion may be slightly elevated.

Course of the Disease: The course of the disease is variable with mild cases recovering in 7 to 10 days, and severe cases taking 4 weeks to several months to recover. Usually the edema recedes and disappears in 2 to 4 weeks, but in cases with considerable skin necrosis the convalescent period can extend 2 to 3 months.

The mortality rate is variable and the usual estimate is approximately 50%. It appears that this rate can be reduced by good treatment and care. The mortality rate also varies from one outbreak to the next and is dependent on the severity of the cases.

Diagnosis: The diagnosis of severe cases usually is not difficult and a clinical diagnosis based on the history and clinical signs can generally be made. The milder form of the disease can be confused with laminitis, and viral arteritis may be difficult to differentiate in some cases. Total leukocyte counts may be helpful as a laboratory aid in diagnosis.

Lesions: The most characteristic gross lesions are subcutaneous edema and fluid in the peritoneal cavity. Edema also can be found in the intermuscular fascia. The presence of hemorrhages is variable; some degree of hemorrhage may be found in the subcutaneous tissues, viscera, or muscles in some cases.[5] The severity of the gross lesions corresponds to the severity of the clinical disease. The histologic changes are primarily confined to the muscles and consist of hemorrhages, hyaline changes, necrosis of the muscle fibers, and inflammatory cellular infiltration.

Treatment: Many therapeutic agents have been advocated as beneficial for the treatment of purpura hemorrhagica. Some of these are blood transfusions, calcium gluconate, formalin, potassium dichromate, adrenalin, caffeine sodium benzoate, and antibiotics. It appears that none of them are specific although some are helpful. Blood transfusions were recommended to correct the anemia and thrombocytopenia but since neither sign is critical in this disease, it is difficult to recommend it. It is equally as difficult to see the rationale of the other recommended treatments.

Good nursing care which includes deep bedding, restricted activity, fresh water, palatable feed, and daily grooming is perhaps the most essential. The use of corticosteroids or ACTH may be beneficial since there is evidence that purpura hemorrhagica of horses possibly is a hypersensitive reaction, and that it is a vascular purpura associated with increased capillary permeability. There is evidence that these steroid products will decrease capillary permeability on sustained administration. Unfortunately, this therapy has not been evaluated adequately in horses.

Tracheotomies may have to be done in cases when breathing is obstructed. Antibiotics may be indicated with a rise in temperature or in cases with skin necrosis. Massage of the legs and bandaging plus mild exercise also may be helpful in reducing the edema.

PRIMARY IDIOPATHIC THROMBOCYTOPENIC PURPURA

Primary idiopathic thrombocytopenic purpura in the horse has not previously been reported. This discussion is based on one case diagnosed and studied in the Veterinary Clinic at the College of Veterinary Medicine, The University of Minnesota. This disease has been diagnosed in the dog and is well-documented in man. The disease in the horse is similar to the disease in dogs and man.

Thrombocytopenic purpura in the horse is characterized by hemorrhage in the skin and other tissues, from the nose or intestinal tract, and a thrombocytopenia.

Etiology: The cause of the disease is not understood clearly. It has been conjectured that an autoimmunologic state is present.[6] The thrombocytopenia is usually accepted as the cause of hemorrhage. The cause of the decrease in platelets is not known. It is thought to be due either to their excessive destruction or inhibition of platelet production through depression of megakaryocyte maturation.[7]

Since splenectomy usually is effective in correcting the condition, it is obvious that the spleen plays an important role in the pathogenesis. It has been postulated that the spleen either removes platelets which have been sensitized or produces humoral factors which influence the platelet production through depression of megakaryocyte maturation.[8] This disease may be one manifestation of hypersplenism as this appears to be true in man and in dogs. Other manifestations of this syndrome are pancytopenia, hemolytic anemia, and neutropenia.

Clinical Signs: Physical examination of the animal being reported disclosed the occurrence of hemorrhage from both nostrils. Petechial hemorrhages of mucous membranes of the tongue, mouth, and nose were observed. There were petechial or ecchymotic hemorrhages of the skin on the prepuce, the inguinal region, and on the muzzle. Considerable bleeding from the prepuce had occurred as evidenced by the amount of dried blood on the tail and hair in this region. A small localized area of edema was present on the ventral aspect of the thorax. The appetite and eliminations were normal and the horse was in good condition. Other than the hemorrhages the animal appeared to be in good health.

Hematologic studies initially revealed a normal hemoglobin level (11.4 Gm. %), a normal hematocrit (35%), and a leukocytosis (18,100 per cmm.) with a neutrophilia. The platelets were decreased to 33,000 per cmm. The prothrombin time, total protein level, albumin-globulin ratio, serum bilirubin, blood glucose, and blood urea nitrogen values all were normal. On the basis of the clinical signs and thrombocytopenia a diagnosis of primary idiopathic thrombocytopenic purpura was made. Subsequent blood studies during the next 4 days revealed that the platelet count remained depressed and there was a decrease in hemoglobin values. Five days later the hemoglobin had dropped to 6 Gm. %. This decrease was found to be due largely to gastrointestinal bleeding.

Treatment: At present there are 3 courses of therapy available for treatment of this condition in man. These include corticosteroid products, platelet or blood transfusion, and splenectomy. Cortisone was used in this case as the therapeutic agent, and with good success. The animal was maintained on cortisone for 10 days and the platelet count increased to a normal value by the fifth day of treatment. There was cessation of hemorrhage as the thrombocytopenia was corrected and the horse made an uneventful and complete recovery. Six months later the animal was still in good health and had a normal platelet count.

Such marked success with corticosteroids is not always the case in this disease. In man, permanent results are not invariably affected by cortisone therapy. In some cases there is little response, or there may be good response initially but remissions occur and a splenectomy must be performed.[9,10]

D. K. SORENSEN

REFERENCES

1. Biggers, J. D. and Ingram, P. L.: Studies on equine purpura hemorrhagica. Review of the literature article No. 1, Vet. J. **104** (1948) 214.
2. Udall. D. H.: The Practice of Veterinary Medicine. 5th Ed. Published by the Author, Ithaca, N.Y. p. 435, 1947.

3. Bennett, P. M. and King, A. S.: Studies on equine purpura hemorrhagica, Article No. 2. Symptomatology, Vet. J. **104** (1948) 414.

4. Biggers, J. D., Ingram, P. L. and Murray, C. B.: Studies on equine purpura hemorrhagica. Article No. 4. Hematology. Vet. J. **105** (1949) 191.

5. King, A. S.: Studies on equine purpura hemorrhagica. Article No. 3. Morbid anatomy and histology. Vet. J. **105** (1949) 35.

6. Harrington, W. J. et al.: Immunologic mechanisms in idiopathic neonatal thrombocytopenic purpura. Ann. Int. Med. **38** (1953) 433.

7. Dameshek, William and Estren, Solomon. The Spleen and Hypersplenism. Grune and Stratton, New York, N.Y., 1947.

8. Robson, H. N.: Idiopathic thrombocytopenic purpura. Quart. J. Med. **18** (1949) 279.

9. Steffon, M., and Dameshek, W.: The Hemorrhagic Disorders. Grune and Stratton, New York, N.Y., 1955.

10. Quick, A. J.: Hemorrhagic Diseases, pp. 197-254. Lea & Febiger, Philadelphia, Pa., 1957.

HEMATOLOGY AND ITS RELATIONSHIP TO TRACK PERFORMANCE

INTRODUCTION

Race horse trainers are constantly concerned with the question of whether the animals in their care are responding well to their training program and reaching the "peak of fitness" which will enable them to win races. As a result of a long and close association with horses, many trainers assess the fitness of their charges by a series of more or less empiric observations that are given different emphasis by different trainers and often are of uncertain significance to their veterinary advisers.

The more common guides to lack or loss of fitness used by trainers include loss of appetite, loss of weight, excessive "blowing" after work, the development of a dry, harsh coat, profuse watery as opposed to beady sweating, and "blowing up" over the loins. Since most of these signs are nonspecific and some may be figments of the imagination, veterinarians attending racing stables have used various blood examinations in the hope that such objective assessments will assist their understanding the physical state which lies between disease and peak fitness. This general idea has provided motivation for the more recent hematologic studies of horses in training and racing by Brenon, Irvine, and Steel and Whitlock.[1,2,3,4] Since the original observation by Neser[5] that race horses had higher red cell counts than other horses, a number of valuable contributions to our knowledge of the equine blood picture have been made by MacLeod and Pon-

der, MacLeod et al., Hansen et al., Archer and Miller and Archer.[6,7,8,9,10] The excellent book, *Veterinary Hematology,* by Schalm describes and compares with great care the various technics for estimating blood values and reviews the literature on equine hematology in detail.[11] Because of this valuable source of information it seems best to concentrate here on the interpretation of blood counts in relation to track performance.

It should be emphasized that accurate interpretation depends on good technic and if significance is to be attributed to relatively small changes in the range of blood values, great care must be taken during the collection, preservation, and analysis of the blood samples. The various tests performed during a routine blood count are not of equal value. Some, such as the packed cell volume, provide considerable information and others, such as the mean corpuscular hemoglobin, are of minor clinical importance. For accuracy in interpretation, all the factors in the blood picture need consideration and while short-cut procedures relying on 2 or 3 of the main tests are of some value, they often fail to indicate some of the possible causes for loss of racing form.

Slight variations in the technic of performing blood counts in different laboratories make it certain that no single set of blood values, purporting to describe the normal range of values, will have absolute accuracy. Because of this, the individual veterinarian must select a technic, follow it carefully, and use the published values as a guide for his own accuracy in estimation and interpretation.

Blood values that are applicable for Thoroughbreds and Standardbreds and form a useful basis for interpretation are presented in Table 5. These values indicate that the hemoglobin level, red cell count, and packed cell volume are significantly higher in the Thoroughbred than in the Standardbred. The white cell count is slightly higher in the Thoroughbred, and the mean corpuscular volume and mean corpuscular hemoglobin are higher in the Standardbred.[4] Although these differences make it possible to adopt separate standards of interpretation for each breed, it seems more convenient to adopt a single standard which

Table 5.—Blood Values

	Thoroughbreds					Standardbreds				
	Mean Values		Range		S.D.	Mean Values		Range		S.D.
Hemoglobin	13.44 Gm./100 ml.		9.1-21.3		1.88	12.4		7.7-17.8		1.86
Red Blood Corpuscles	9.66 million		6.72-13.6		1.29	8.66		5.42-13.5		1.35
White Blood Corpuscles	10,428		6,350-20,000		2,568	9,763		5,000-17,500		2,475
Packed Cell Volume	41.7		31-55		4.5	39.4		26-58		4.4
Erythrocyte Sedimentation Rate	36.3		2-62		15.7	44.0		5-67		14.3
Mean Corpuscular Hemoglobin	13.8		10.9-18.7		1.76	14.3		11-18.4		1.33
Mean Corpuscular Volume	43.8		30.7-58.1		4.62	45.5		36.2-61.6		4.12
Mean Corpuscular Hemoglobin Concentration	31.5		25.8-37.4		1.99	31.4		26.5-37		2.4
	Relative	Absolute	Relative	Absolute		Relative	Absolute	Relative	Absolute	
Differential White Cell Count										
Neutrophils Segmented	53.57	5,586	15.5-77	985-15,400	10.14	59.9	5,848	31.5-82	1,575-14,350	10.1
Neutrophils Band	0.09	9	0-3	0-600	0.4	0.2	19.5	0-8	0-1,400	0.96
Lymphocytes	40.11	4,183	16-80	1,016-16,000	10.61	32.8	3,203	6-62	300-10,850	10.63
Monocytes	3.63	378	0.5-14	2-2,800	2.08	3.4	332	1-9	50-1,575	1.7
Eosinophils	2.28	237	0-7.0	0-1,400	1.47	3.1	303	0.5-9	25-1,575	2.45
Basophils	0.32	33	0-3.0	0-600	0.49	0.6	59	0-4	0-700	0.35

Reprinted from Aust. Vet. J., April 1960.

Table 6.—Thoroughbred and Standardbred Groupings Based on Certain Hemogram Values

	HEMOGLOBIN GM./100 ML.	RED BLOOD CELLS MILL./CMM.	PACKED CELL VOLUME %
Group 1	> 16	> 11.0	> 45
Group 2	14–16	9–11	40–45
Group 3	12–14	8–9	35–40
Group 4	< 12	< 8	< 35

can be modified by the individual veterinarian according to his circumstances and experience.

INTERPRETATION OF BLOOD COUNTS

By using the homoglobin level, red cell count, and packed cell volume, the blood values encountered during routine hematologic work can be divided into the 4 groups shown in Table 6. When a Thoroughbred or Standardbred horse is found with a hemoglobin level of less than 12.0 Gm. per 100 ml., a red cell count of less than 8.0 million per cmm., or a packed cell volume of less than 35%, it is regarded as being anemic. Blood counts of this type (Group 4) are found in about 18% of horses. Clinically, they show the following signs in variable degree, depending on the severity of their anemia. There may be slight to marked pallor of the visible mucous membranes, lethargy, and failure to maintain body condition. They tend to stop badly in races and show a decrease in tolerance to exercise which is evidenced by excessive "blowing," or dyspnea that is disproportionate to the work done. Vascular, or hemic, murmurs may be heard on auscultation of the heart. These murmurs are difficult to time but mostly systolic and usually are heard best when auscultating over the base of the heart. In severe cases during which the hemoglobin and/or red cell levels have fallen 50% or less below mean values there is tachycardia at rest, increased cardiac impulse on palpation, increased intensity of the heart sounds, and a greater than normal audibility of the heart sounds over a wider area of the thorax.

About 5% of horses have blood counts in which the hemoglobin level exceeds 16.0 Gm. per 100 ml., the red cell count exceeds 11.0 million per cmm., and the packed cell volume exceeds 45%. These horses (Group 1) are regarded as having a polycythemia. The term, polycythemia, is used to indicate an increase above the normal in the number of circulating erythrocytes. There usually is an accompanying increase in the amount of hemoglobin and of the packed cell volume. Polycythemia may be transient, relative, or absolute. The transient form which occurs in response to excitement or exercise has been observed by a number of authors.[1,2,3,5,12,13,14] Apart from being a source of diagnostic error, transient polycythemia seems unlikely to be of clinical significance.

Relative polycythemia occurs as a result of reduced fluid intake or marked loss of body fluids which cause a decrease in plasma volume. Unless plasma volume estimations are performed it is a difficult condition to diagnose. An elevated red cell count found in association with severe diarrhea, polyuria, profuse sweating or refusal to drink, and other signs of dehydration such as rapid loss of weight, dry buccal mucosa, dry conjunctiva, sunken eyes, and loss of skin elasticity may indicate a relative polycythemia.

Absolute polycythemia occurs when oxygen tension is reduced at high altitudes or in conditions interfering with gaseous exchange, such as emphysema or fibrosis of the lungs. It also occurs in congenital or acquired heart disease.

Horses with relative or absolute polycythemia race unsatisfactorily and fail to thrive in the stable. Their appetite frequently is poor and they may show transient cyanosis after training or racing.

Most horses which show consistent, good racing form have hemoglobin levels between 14 to 16 Gm. per 100 ml., red cell counts between 9 to 11 million per cmm., and packed cell volumes between 40 to 45%. Although about 17% of horses fall into this Group 2 category, it must not be inferred that they will necessarily be good performers or that any horse with a blood picture outside this range is going to be incapable of winning races. Many factors affect racing form and the blood picture is only one factor in a complex biologic situation.

Nearly 60% of the horses examined have hemoglobin levels between 12 to 14 Gm. per 100 ml., red cell counts between 8 to 9 million per cmm., and packed cell volumes between 35 to 40%. These horses (Group 3) have blood pictures which are difficult to interpret. Some are undoubtedly progressing toward anemia and others are recovering from a depression of hematopoiesis. Many horses with such a blood picture are capable of winning races but, in general, they fall short of being top-class performers. When values of this type are encountered there is a strong temptation to suggest that if the blood picture could be improved to the Group 2 level, the racing performance would be better. Some of these horses do respond to hematinics but in most the response to such therapy is disappointing. One possible explanation for this is that most of the Group 3 horses are carrying all the red cells and hemoglobin they are capable of developing and, as such, have less potential for good racing performance than the horses in Group 2. The other possibility is that there is still insufficient knowledge regarding the etiology of equine anemia and the ways of stimulating hematopoiesis.

Additional information can be obtained by calculating the mean corpuscular volume and the mean corpuscular hemoglobin concentration. If the mean corpuscular volume is less than 36 cubic microns the red cells are microcytic and if the volume is greater than 50 cubic microns they are macrocytic. If the mean corpuscular hemoglobin concentration is less than 30% the red cells are hypochromic. Although a low mean corpuscular hemoglobin concentration can be regarded as the strongest single indication of an iron deficiency anemia, many horses with mean corpuscular hemoglobin concentrations of more than 30% respond to iron therapy by an increase in red cell numbers and hemoglobin.

The sedimentation rate in horses is quite variable and difficult to interpret. Neumann-Kleinpaul observed in young trotters that the sedimentation rate became slower as peak of fitness was reached after training, and it increased again when the horses became "stale" due to overtraining.[15] Although these observations can be confirmed in a general way it seems unlikely that they have an overriding significance in relation to whether a horse is ready to win races.[4] Good horses, at the peak of their racing form, usually have sedimentation rates of less than 30 mm. per hour. Very slow sedimentation rates (8 mm. per hour or less) often are found in horses with polycythemia. If the sedimentation rate exceeds 55 mm. per hour it is abnormal. High sedimentation rates are commonly, but not invariably, associated with an anemia.

The white cell count and differential count are just as important as the red cell count and hemoglobin estimation. Variations in white cell count are not likely to be specifically related to physical fitness. They are, however, important indicators of disease processes which may make it difficult for a horse to become or remain fit. It should be remembered that 23.5% of the horses with anemia have a leukocytosis and unless an effort is made to deal with the cause of the leukocytosis the results of attempting to treat the anemia are likely to be disappointing. If the total white cell count is in excess of 12,000 per cmm., it is abnormal. Counts as low as 10,000 per cmm. are regarded as abnormal if the differential count shows more than 67% neutrophils, more than 50% lymphocytes or more than 10% monocytes. If the eosinophil count is in excess of 7%, it probably is abnormal. The possible causes of a leukocytosis in the race horse are too numerous to be discussed here.

THERAPY FOR ANEMIA

In practice, the treatment of anemia in race horses is of the empiric, "shot-gun" variety. This does not imply that treatment is frequently ineffective. It does, however, mean that much more precise information is required before what is being done is truly understood. The usual method of treating horses with anemia is to administer iron and cyanocobalamine (vitamin B_{12}). Theoretically, it should be possible to treat properly selected cases with one or the other agent but in practice the common procedure is to use both substances. A wide variety of iron preparations, suitable for oral or parenteral administration, are available. One of the cheapest, effective preparations is ferrous sulfate ($FeSO_4.7H_2O$) which is given orally in doses of 2 to 4 Gm. daily for about 2 weeks. Ferrous sulfate is not ingested readily if it is added directly to the horse's feed. If 30 Gm. of ferrous sulfate are dissolved in 500 ml. water and 30 ml. of the solution is added to the food or drinking water, most horses ingest it readily. More palatable and expensive preparations, such as ferrous gluconate, are available. They are added to the feed to provide a daily intake of 1.5 to 3.0 Gm. per animal.

Preparations of ferrous gluconate, iron adenylate, and saccharated iron oxide, which are suitable for intramuscular or intravenous injection, also are available. They usually are given in doses of 500 mg. at intervals of one week. Although iron given parenterally is utilized efficiently, severe local reactions at the site of intramuscular injection may occur, and there is an occasional death following intravenous use. In general, there seems to be reason for avoiding the administration of iron parenterally unless the animal is suffering an alimentary tract disturbance likely to interfere with the absorption of iron given by mouth.

Wide variations in the method of giving cyanocobalamine exist. Some veterinarians give an intramuscular injection of 1000 mcg. daily for 7 to 10 days. Others give from 2000 to 5000 mcg. twice a week for 3 to 4 weeks. Cyanocobalamine zinc tannate (repository vitamin B_{12}) may be given in a dose of 2500 mcg. once a week. Sometimes folic acid is given at the rate of 60 to 120 mg. 2 or 3 times a week. There is no critical evidence that the addition of folic acid to the commonly used iron and vitamin B_{12} therapy is of distinct benefit although, on theoretical grounds, it should be possible to establish a place for folic acid in the rational treatment of some equine anemias.

Ascorbic acid and members of the vitamin B-complex often are added to complete the "shot-gun" nature of current therapy but apart from adding to expense and satisfying the client that the animal "has got the lot," their true role in the therapy, if any, remains to be determined.

J. D. STEEL

REFERENCES

1. Brenon, H. C.: J.A.V.M.A., **128** (1956) 343.
2. Brenon, H. C.: J.A.V.M.A., **133** (1958) 102.
3. Irvine, C. H. G.: J.A.V.M.A., **133** (1958) 97.
4. Steel, J. D. and Whitlock, L. E.: Aust. Vet. J. 36 (1960) 136.
5. Neser, C. P.: Ninth and Tenth Report. Div. Vet. Ed. and Research, Union of South Africa (1923), Gov't. Printing Office, Pretoria.
6. MacLeod, J. and Ponder, E.: Science **103** (1946) 73.
7. MacLeod, J., Ponder, E., Aitken, G. J. and Brown, R. B.: Cornell Vet. **37** (1947) 305.
8. Hansen, M. F., Todd, A. C., Kelley, G. W. and Cawein, M.: Bull. 555, p. 19, Kentucky Agric. Exper. Sta. (1950).
9. Archer, R. K., and Miller, W. C.: Vet. Rec. **71** (1959) 278.
10. Archer, R. K.: J. Comp. Path. 69 (1959) 390.
11. Schalm, O. W.: Veterinary Hematology, 1st ed., Lea and Febiger, Philadelphia, Pa., 1961.
12. Scheunert, A. and Krzywanek, F. W.: Pflügers Arch. **213** (1926) 198.
13. Holman, H. H.: Proc. Roy. Soc. Med., **40** (1947) 185.
14. Sreter, F. A.: Canad. J. Biochem. Physiol. 37 (1959) 273.
15. Neumann-Kleinpaul, K.: Berl. Tierärztl. Wchschr. **65** (1952) 175.

CHAPTER 17

DISEASES OF THE LOCOMOTOR SYSTEM

DISEASE OF BONE

INTRODUCTION

A review of bone disease in the horse must, of necessity, deal in generalities with occasional reference to specific entities known to occur in the horse. Despite the many years during which the horse has been studied, examined, and worked for man's benefit and pleasure, specific basic knowledge of the normal and pathologic characteristics of equine bone is extremely meager.

The available literature contains many theories and speculations largely derived, it appears, from clinical and experimental work on species other than the horse. Only a few reports, for example, are available on the nutritional aspects of equine bone, but many reports speculate on the possible importance of nutrition and bone disease.

The major aims of this review will be to provide:

1. An outline of the normal structure and development of bone.
2. A discussion of specific bone disease entities which occur or which may occur in the horse.

NORMAL BONE STRUCTURE

It is not appropriate to enter into a detailed discussion of bone structure. Rather, certain salient features will be presented with appropriate introductory references for those wishing to probe deeper.

Bone, as a tissue, is composed of an organized organic matrix-collagen and an unorganized or homogenous organic matrix (ground substance), in which are imbedded bone cells, osteocytes. Osteoblasts, bone-forming cells, lie on the surface of the bone. The organic matrix, with the exception of the osteocytes, is ossified—impregnated with a calcium-phosphate crystal complex generally considered to be of the hydroxyapatite type. A number of other inorganic elements are included in or on the basic calcium-phosphate crystal. Under certain conditions, in young, rapidly growing animals and in rickets-osteomalacia, the organic matrix may be present in a nonossified state known as osteoid.

Bones, as organs, are composed of compact (cortical) bone tissue and cancellous (spongy, medullary) bone tissue. The relative proportions of compact and cancellous bone vary in different bones and different parts of the same bone. The mechanical properties of bones are, to a large measure, related to these proportions and the orientations of the osteones and cancellous bone trabeculae. The proper study of the biomechanic properties of bones must include consideration of:

1. Mechanics of bone strength, orientation and load.
2. Vascular, neural supply.
3. Nutrition and chemical composition.
4. Endocrine mediation and control.
5. Early growth and development.

These factors are closely interwoven, and adequate understanding of both normal and abnormal bone must be based on a consideration of all of them.

Although cognizant of the objections which have been raised, I, feel that the trajectorial theory of bone architecture offers a fruitful approach to many of the problems of equine bone disease. Koch's classic analysis of the human femur led to a clear exposition of the trajectorial theory:[26]

". . . it has been shown that in every part of the femur there is a remarkable adaptation of the inner structure of the bone to the mechanical requirements due to the load on the femur-head. The various parts of the femur taken together form a single mechanical structure wonderfully well-adapted for the efficient, economical transmission of loads from the acetabulum to the tibia; a structure in which every element contributes its modicum of

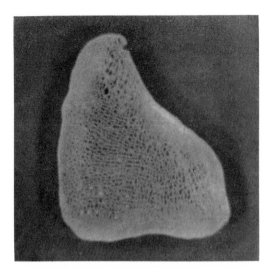

Fig. 1. Normal bone structure. Proximal sesamoid from 2-year-old Thoroughbred.

strength in the manner required by theoretical mechanics for maximum efficiency. . . . the internal structure is everywhere so formed as to provide in an efficient manner for all the internal stresses which occur due to the load on the femur-head. . . . the bony material is arranged in the paths of the maximum internal stresses, which are thereby resisted with the greatest efficiency, and hence with the maximum economy of material."

It may be of interest at this point to illustrate the pattern of bone structure in a proximal sesamoid from the foreleg of a 2-year-old Thoroughbred (Fig. 1).

The vascular supply of a bone is an important determinant of the strength and quality of that bone. In general, the diaphysis is supplied by major nutrient arteries entering the middle third of the shaft, while the epiphyses and metaphyses are supplied by a number of smaller vessels located near the margins of the articular surfaces. Small numbers of periosteal vessels penetrate the cortex and may reach the marrow cavity. Before epiphysial closure the blood supplies of the diaphysis and epiphysis are said to be separate, but after closure, they unite.

Variations in the pattern of blood supply in different bones and under different conditions can be of considerable pathologic significance: aseptic necrosis of carpal navicular bone (human).[27]

The nerves entering bones probably are exclusively vasomotor in nature and the effects of neural lesions undoubtedly are mediated through the vessels.

The chemical composition of bone has been considered previously. Some aspects of nutrition in relation to bone will be considered later as will the endocrine relationships.

The bones are first formed as condensations of mesenchyme, which subsequently are converted to cartilage and invaded by blood vessels followed by calcification and ossification. This process of endochondral ossification is complete in some bones before or at the time of birth, but others continue to grow for several years postpartum. Certain bones, of course, develop directly by calcification and ossification of the mesenchymal condensation without an intermediate cartilaginous stage (intramembranous ossification).

There is very little detailed information on the time of appearance of ossification centers in the several bones of the horse. The following information has been abstracted from Zietzschmann and Krölling, and Sisson and Grossman.[28,29]

Ossification centers in the bones of the appendicular skeleton:

Scapula: 4 or 5 centers. 1, Main center for body and spine, 2, center for tuber scapulae and coracoid process, 3, distal epiphysial center for articular cavity (glenoid cavity), 4, center for tuber spinae and cranial part of glenoid cavity. The proximal border of the cartilage model remains as the scapular cartilage which may ossify partially later in life. The tuber scapulae fuses with the body at about 3 years of age and the tuber spinae still later.

Humerus: 6 centers. 1, Diaphysis, 2, head and medial tuberosity, 3, lateral tuberosity, 4, distal epiphysis (condyles), 5, lateral and medial epicondyles, 6, deltoid tuberosity.

Radius: 3 centers. Proximal and distal epiphyses and diaphysis.

Ulna: 3 centers. Olecranon, shaft and distal end. The cartilaginous embryonic ulna extends as far distad as the radius but the distal part of the shaft usually is reduced and disappears, or a part may ossify. The distal tip fuses with the radius before birth.

Carpus: 1 center for each bone.

Metacarpal: 2 centers (Sisson and Grossman, 3 centers). Diaphysis and distal epiphysis. According to Zietzschmann and Krölling, a proximal epiphyseal center is very rare in the 70 cm. fetus and already is closing at birth. The small metacarpal bones ossify from 2 centers. The distal end is cartilaginous at birth and the center does not appear until 3 months after birth and fuses with the diaphysis of the small metacarpal at the beginning of the second year.

First Phalanx: 3 centers. Diaphysis, proximal, and distal epiphysis. The last fuses just before or after birth.

Second Phalanx: 3 centers. Same as first phalanx. Proximal epiphysis fuses somewhat earlier than in the first phalanx.

Third Phalanx: 1 center. A thick perichondral end cap of bone forms in relation to the hoof while the proximal part of bone still is cartilaginous.

Femur: 4 or 5 centers. Diaphysis, head, trochanter major and eventually trochanter minor, distal epiphysis, and third trochanter.

Tibia: 4 centers. Diaphysis, proximal and distal epiphyses, and tibial tuberosity. Lateral malleolus—see fibula.

Fibula: 3 centers. The fibula is, like the ulna, fully developed in the cartilaginous model (3.2 mm. embryo). The distal fibular epiphysis separates in the 7.4 cm. embryo from the regressing diaphysial part and is joined to the tibia in the 15.5 cm. embryo by connective tissue. At birth, the diaphysis of the fibula is ossified, while the proximal and distal epiphyses ossify after birth. The distal epiphysis (lateral malleolus of tibia) is separate at birth, completely uniting with the tibia during the second year of life.

Tarsus: 1 center for each bone. The fibular tarsal bone has 2 centers—one for the main mass of bone and an apophysial center for the tuber calcis which appears shortly before or after birth and fuses at about 3 years of age. The metatarsus and rear phalanges essentially are identical to the metacarpus and fore phalanges.

The patella and other sesamoid bones each have one center which, in general, appears after birth. In my experience, the proximal sesamoids of Thoroughbreds and Standardbreds always are well-ossified before birth.

The following table (from Zietzschmann and Krölling) lists the times of anatomic closure of the various epiphysial plates. As is well-known, roentgenologic evidence of epiphysial closure may be some months earlier than actual anatomic fusion.

Vertebra	4 to 5 years
Scapula-Coracoid . . .	10 months to 1 year
Humerus: proximal . .	About 3.5 years
distal	15 to 18 months
Radius: proximal . . .	15 to 18 months
distal	About 3.5 years
Ulna: proximal	About 3.5 years
distal	?
Ilium-Pubis-Ischium .	10 to 12 months
Femur: proximal	3 to 3.5 years
distal	3.5 years
Fibula: proximal	?
distal	2 years
Metacarpus-Metatarsus	10 to 12 months
1st Phalanx: proximal	12 to 15 months
distal	1 week postpartum
2nd Phalanx: proximal	10 to 12 months
distal	1 week postpartum
3rd Phalanx: proximal	Last part of pregnancy
Tuber Calcis (fibular tarsal bone)	3 years

CONGENITAL DEFECTS

Congenital defects of bone may be conveniently discussed as: 1. Generalized developmental disturbances. 2. Localized developmental disturbances.

GENERALIZED DEVELOPMENTAL DISTURBANCES

There appears to be little information available on generalized congenital defects in the horse. A brief discussion of several more common conditions in man and other animals, however, may be pertinent for purposes of future recognition.

Osteogenesis Imperfecta: This is a hereditary fragility of bones in man. The bones grow normally in length since epiphysial cartilage

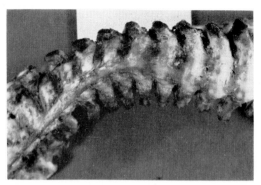

Fig. 2. Scoliosis involving thoracic vertebrae of foal.

growth and calcification are normal.[30] Ossification of the calcified trabeculae and transverse growth of cortical bone are retarded, however, apparently because of a primary defect in the osteoblasts. The end result is bone markedly deficient in bone tissues with thin cortices and trabeculae which are liable to fracture from mild trauma or normal functioning.

A similar condition has been observed in cats, in which it appears to be dietary in origin (low calcium diet).

Osteogenesis imperfecta has not been described in the horse, but should it appear, one might expect marked deficiency of bone tissue on radiographs and multiple fractures of the limb bones in young foals.

Osteopetrosis (Marble Bone Disease): This condition has not been recorded in horses. In man the condition is characterized by severe osteosclerosis, thickening of the ends of the bones, and increased bone fragility (poor quality in spite of increased quantity). The primary defect is hereditary and is related to disharmony of bone formation and resorption—the former greatly exceeding the latter.

Chondrodystrophia Fetalis (Achondroplasia): This is a hereditary dwarfism of man and animals related to failure of growth of epiphysial and articular cartilage. Although such dwarfism apparently has not been recorded in the horse, there may be manifestations of localized or restricted chondrodystrophy escaping detection. Such restricted manifestations are seen in a number of breeds of dogs.

The so-called *enchondroses* will be discussed later.

"Contracted Foal" (Ankylosed foals): This condition does not appear to be primarily a congenital defect of bones. The basic neuromuscular disorder seems, however, to result in widespread bony malformations. The articular ends of the limb bones may be distorted by the severely shortened muscle-tendons. Varying degrees of vertebral scoliosis and distortion of the cranial skeleton are found (Fig. 2). Although they undoubtedly are secondary lesions, failure of performance in a foal contracted at birth and straightened by surgical means, may be related to persistent scoliosis. It is noteworthy that moderate scoliosis involving the last portion of the thoracic region (a favored site) cannot always be detected by external examination.

Hereditary Multiple Exostoses: This is a hereditary disease of man characterized by multiple exostoses related to and apparently derived from epiphysial cartilages. The exostoses consist of cartilage which gradually is replaced by bone. Carlson described 2 cases in horses, sire and colt, of a condition radiologically similar to the disease in man.[31] It was stated that other animals of the same blood lines were involved as well. Necropsy studies would be of great interest.

LOCALIZED DEVELOPMENTAL DISTURBANCES

Localized disturbances of skeletal development, in contrast to generalized, are seen with some frequency in horses.

Vertebral Column: Stecher and Goss have described the frequent occurrence of a variety of ankylosing lesions of the equine vertebral column.[32] The lesions which they considered to be developmental in origin included:

1. Fusion of caudal vertebrae to sacrum.
2. Fusion of lateral facets with ankylosis of lateral transverse joints (lumbar vertebrae).

In addition, they described ankylosis of intervertebral joints and spinous processes which they did not necessarily consider as being developmental. In my experience many of these latter lesions probably are developmental since no gross nor microscopic evidence of arthritis or other pathologic changes can be detected.

Kyphosis, lordosis, and scoliosis are not uncommon in the horse. Though kyphosis and lordosis may be acquired, I know of one normal appearing mare that has produced 2 successive lordotic foals. Scoliosis has been seen, by the writer, only in contracted foals.

The perplexing "wobbler" (equine incoordination) appears to be an example of cervical retrolisthesis. The asymmetrical, improper orientation of the intervertebral articulations of the cervical region allows upward slipping or displacement of one vertebra on another with consequent spinal cord pressure, spinal tract degeneration, and clinical signs of incoordination.

Appendicular Skeleton: Fractured splint bones may be related to their mode of development. The late appearance of the distal epiphysial center and the fusion with the shaft of the bone during the second year may predispose the distal epiphysis to epiphysial fracture.

So-called fibular fractures have been shown to be, in reality, congenital defects occurring in a rudimentary organ.

Minor variations may occur, without apparent significance, in the carpus and tarsus. The first carpal bone may or may not be present. Although usually fused, the first and second tarsal bones may remain separate.

In man, sesamoid bones frequently are double as a result, possibly, of 2 ossification centers. I have seen several proximal sesamoids in horses that may have developed from 2 ossification centers though no examples of double bones have been encountered. Carlson presents a radiograph which is suggestive of a bipartite sesamoid.

James described a case of supernumerary bone in a horse's foot, but the description is too brief to allow any decision concerning the congenital or acquired nature of the bone.[19]

An interesting aspect of localized developmental disturbance of bone is the angulation of joints. Improper joint angle may well be related to development of osteoarthritis and fractures, also spavin and curb in certain lines of horses.

DEFECTS IN THE IMMATURE ANIMAL

In this section we shall be concerned primarily with localized skeletal lesions appearing in the immature animal. Metabolic and/or nutritional and endocrine bone diseases will be considered later under the appropriate headings.

I have adapted as a matter of practical convenience the classification of Mau to a variety of localized skeletal lesions in the horse.[20] Whether such lumping, with the implied interrelationship of such varied conditions as "wobbler" and epiphysial fractures is justified, only time, research, and the discerning reader can decide.

Even the selection of the title, enchondrosis, for the following grouping is fraught with difficulty. With the clear understanding that the definition of the word, as here used, is coined by the writer, it may serve to enlighten the reader. Enchondrosis may be defined as any one of a variety of pathologic conditions affecting epiphyses or epiphysial cartilages and bone immediately related to them. The conditions may be grouped as follows:

1. Enchondrosis on the predominantly endogenous, dysostotic basis (dysostosis—defect in the normal ossification of fetal cartilages). This group is characterized by a malformation or malfunctioning of cartilage—bone transformation (ossification) on a congenital and/or hereditary basis.

2. Enchondrosis related to mechanical influences applied to already dysostotic cartilage—bone tissue.

3. Enchondrosis related to mechanical effects on cartilage—bone tissue affected by aseptic bone necrosis. This group corresponds to those conditions in man known as: osteochondritis juvenilis, idiopathic osteosis, Osgood-Schlatter, Legg-Calvé-Perthes, Köhlers, etc.

4. Enchondrosis on purely mechanical grounds.

In man, this variety is characterized by symmetrical disturbance of cartilaginous growth. Syndromes are known as Leri, Morquiro, and Pfaundler-Hurler. I am not aware of an example of this "pure" hereditary or congenital group in the horse. The charac-

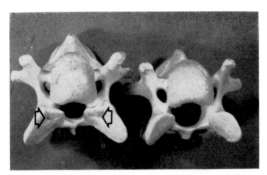

Fig. 3. Abnormal development of articular surfaces of cervical vertebra from a "wobbler." Abnormal vertebra on left. Normal on right.

teristics of the group are familial incidence and multiple, bilateral lesions which appear soon after birth.

One entity which may belong in this group is "wobbles." As discussed earlier, the evidence now indicates that malformation of the intervertebral joints of the cervical vertebrae is the major gross anatomic defect. Asymmetric articular facets, with or without over- or undergrowth and with altered planes of articular surfaces are characteristic (Fig. 3). Preliminary studies indicate that morphologically recognizable disturbances of cartilage growth and ossification cause the gross anatomic changes. Although definitive genetic studies are not available, there is a considerable body of "opinion" in support of a familial basis for equine incoordination. The condition usually appears in weanlings, yearlings, less frequently in 2-year-olds, and rarely in older animals.

A history of trauma sometimes is related to the onset of incoordination. In such cases of a predisposition being manifested as a result of superimposed mechanical factors we must consider Group 2.

This second group—with the exception, perhaps, of some wobblers—has no well-defined equine examples. Some cases which now are included in Groups 3 or 4, however, may eventually be shown to belong in Group 2.

With reference to Group 3, some radiologic evidence is available to indicate that true aseptic necrosis of bone does occur in the horse as in man.[31] There has been considerable speculation on this point with little basis in fact. It is certain that only adequate pathologic studies can provide the information necessary to decide whether avulsions, "collapses" and fractures involving epiphyses and epiphysial cartilages have aseptic bone necrosis as their basis.

In man, the picture is not much clearer than in the horse. Though radiologic evidence is convincing and some pathologic data are available, there still appears to be considerable confusion as to the cause and precise nature of aseptic necrosis of bone.[21] Some hypotheses which have been proposed as the pathogenesis are:

1. Minute bone fractures as a result of compression or other repeated trauma (stress or fatigue fracture).

2. As 1 plus cartilaginous callus formation and refracturing of the callus.

3. Hypermia and hemorrhage in the bone.

4. Angioneurotic imbalances or instabilities.

5. Embolic phenomena.

With Group 4 the footing becomes somewhat less treacherous. Here we are dealing with purely mechanical trauma producing damage to epiphysial cartilage and associated bone. It may be well to immediately cast some doubts, however, as far as the horse is concerned. Rather than categorically accepting all members of this group as purely mechanical, adequate studies are needed to prove that some, any or all of the factors discussed in 1 and 3 are or are not operating.

A condition known as "epiphysitis" appears rather commonly in young, light horses. Similar conditions have been observed in man and the dog. Clinically, the condition is characterized by a firm swelling on the medial side at the level of the distal epiphysial cartilage of certain long bones, principally the radius and cannon bone. Pathologically, the epiphysial cartilage appears crushed and thinned on the involved sides and new bone formation is apparent (Fig. 4). Microscopic findings are compatible with the later stages of experimental compression of epiphysial cartilage as reported by Trueta and Trias.[33]

Clinical observations support the concept of epiphysitis as a compression lesion of the epiphysial cartilage. Rapidly growing, fattening animals, particularly those tending to stand base-narrow in front, are prone to develop

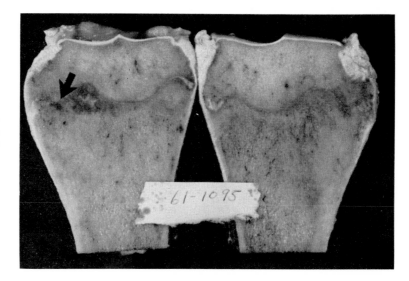

Fig. 4. Epiphysitis at distal epiphysis of radius. Note thinning of epiphysial cartilage.

medial, distal radial epiphysitis. One instructive case involved intractable, nonweight-bearing lameness of the right foreleg. A short time after the onset of lameness, epiphysitis appeared on the distal end of the medial side of the left radius.

Frank fractures involving the epiphysial cartilages of the femoral neck, olecranon process of the ulna and other bones are not uncommon in foals. At the present time these fractures are considered purely mechanical in nature. The presence or absence of predisposing factors, mentioned earlier, must be considered and investigated. Stress and fatigue fractures will be considered later.

Finally, a consideration of osteochondritis dissecans should be included in this section. "Loose bodies" in joints as a result of direct needle trauma, arthritis, infection, etc., are considered elsewhere.

I consider osteochondritis dissecans in the narrow sense of a partial or complete splitting of a piece of articular cartilage and underlying bone into a joint cavity. The evidence for man, and in a very few necropsy cases for the horse, is that osteochondritis dissecans is simply a form of enchondrosis (as herein defined) and may occur in association with any of the 4 groups presented before. Nagura's concept of stress fracturing of cancellous bone, cartilaginous callus formation, fracturing of the callus, etc., is attractive

(Group 4).[22] There is a rather striking incidence of loose joint bodies in the cervical intervertebral joints of wobblers even prior to the onset of recognizable osteoarthritis.

ROLE OF THE ENDOCRINE SYSTEM

The endocrine system exerts profound effects on the skeletal system. We shall review briefly those abnormalities related to endocrine hyper- and hypofunction. Details of the normal role of hormones in bone growth and maintenance must be left to the pertinent literature.

PITUITARY GLAND

Five anterior pituitary lobe hormones have significant effects on bone: 1. Growth hormone, 2, follicle-stimulating hormone, 3, luteinizing hormone, 4, thyrotropic hormone, and 5, adrenocorticotropic hormone.

In brief, growth hormone acts directly, and thyroid hormone acts indirectly to stimulate bone growth. The ultimate effect of the gonadotropic and adrenocorticotropic hormones is inhibition of growth.

Gigantism caused by overproduction of growth hormone (eosinophilic adenoma) is a result of excessive stimulation of endochondral ossification, continued over a longer period of time than normal. This condition has not been reported in the horse. Indeed, most, if not all, pituitary adenomas of horses arise from the pars intermedia, while growth hormone probably is elaborated by the eosinophilic cells of the pars anterior.[24]

Acromegaly is the adult (after epiphysial closure) form of excessive growth hormone production.

Hypopituitarism, as might be expected, is a result of deficient growth hormone production with proportionate dwarfism. (In man, this usually is related to destruction of the anterior lobe.) Acromicria is the adult form of hypopituitarism and is rare in man. Neither condition has been defined in the horse.

THYROID GLAND

The thyroid and pituitary glands are, as is well-known, interdependent levels of thyrotropic hormone determining thyroid growth and activity, while thyroxin regulates, in part, the production of thyrotropic hormone.

Low levels of thyroxin appear to exert at least 3 effects on growing bone:

1. Since the metabolic rate of bone tissue, as other tissues, is dependent in part on thyroxin, the effect may be inability of slowly

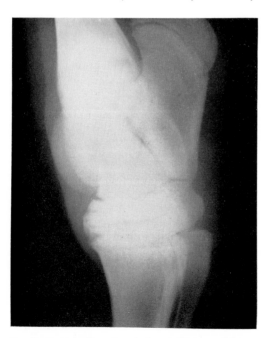

Fig. 5. Comminution of central and third tarsal bones in foal with hypothyroidism.

metabolizing bone to react to pituitary growth hormone.

2. On the other hand, the general depression of metabolic rate influences the pituitary as well as other organs and may result in decreased growth hormone production.

3. The most direct action of thyroxin on bone appears to be on maturation instead of growth of bone.

In general, hypothyroidism causes slowing and eventual cessation of skeletal growth as a result of cessation of epiphysial cartilage growth and ossification. As a corollary, certain bones may remain cartilaginous for a long period as a result of failure of ossification.

The writer has had the opportunity to examine 2 cases (and radiographs of a third) of apparent hypothyroidism in foals. Since no reports of this condition in foals have been found, a brief discussion is included here.

Two suckling foals, a colt and a filly, of quite different bloodlines but on the same farm, developed bilateral rear leg lameness with firm swelling of the distal parts of the hocks. Both animals had dry haircoats and loose, flabby-appearing muscles. There was bilateral, visible, and palpable enlargement of the thyroid glands. The animals were not growing at a normal rate. Radiographs revealed collapse and crushing of the central and third tarsal bones with increased density and mushrooming (Fig. 5).

The colt was destroyed and the macerated hock specimen is shown in Fig. 6. Microscopic sections revealed persistence of cartilage as described by Looser.[23] Sections of the thyroid revealed only a tendency of the acinar epithelial cells to be columnar (evidence of activity). Protein-bound iodine determinations were performed on serum from the affected colt and one normal colt. The affected colt had 2.0 mcg.% and the normal 4.2 mcg.% (normal for man is 4.0-8.0 mcg.%; no normal values could be found for the horse).

The filly seemed to be recovering slowly. A course of thyroid hormone therapy appeared to accelerate her growth and general condition. Radiographs indicated that the bone lesions were resolving slowly. Although these studies hardly are extensive enough to be definitive, the evidence strongly suggests that hypothyroidism does occur in foals and may be related to localized bone lesions.

Hyperthyroidism in man may cause acceleration of bone growth in the young and osteoporosis in adults. Four cases of hyperthyroidism have been recorded in the horse, but no mention was made of skeletal lesions.

SEX HORMONES

Hypogonadism, as a result of spaying or castration of young animals, causes delay of skeletal maturation and suppression of secondary sex characteristics. In effect, removal of the sex organs causes a form of gigantism with the limbs being relatively long in comparison to the body. It would be interesting to validate this observation in geldings.

Hypergonadism probably is rare in animals except in cases of cryptorchidism and prolonged therapeutic use of hormone preparations. Excessive amounts of sex hormones lead, in general, to accelerated growth and maturation of the skeleton. The skeletal status of ridglings would provide a most interesting study.

The effect of estrogen on storage of calcium and phosphorus, as bone, in the medullary cavities of bones of female animals probably represents an adaptation for providing large amounts of minerals for the developing fetus. Such an estrogenic action has not been reported in mares.

ADRENAL GLAND

There appears to be little evidence that adrenal hormones play a significant role in normal bone metabolism. It is known that hypercorticalism (Cushing's disease) causes osteoporosis. In this connection, work with rabbits and rats has shown that under certain conditions osteoporosis can be induced by administration of cortisone. In view of the extensive local and systemic use of cortisone-type compounds in equine lameness, the possibility of localized or generalized osteoporosis should be borne in mind.

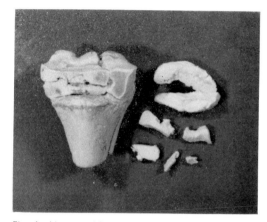

Fig. 6. Macerated bones from hock illustrated in Fig. 5.

PARATHYROID GLAND

Of all the endocrine glands, the parathyroid is most directly concerned with bone metabolism, and it is here that there is, if possible, the least amount of information for the horse. Some of this paucity of information may be related to the difficulty of finding the parathyroid glands during routine necropsies. The following information concerning the parathyroids is derived from Vermeulen:[8]

Gross structure: lobated, fine capsule with finely granular surface; 5 to 6 mm. long and weighing up to 45 milligrams.

Position:

1. Lying on or near the cranial thyroid artery.

2. Lying on the upper, medial border of the thyroid.

3. In the connective tissue lateral to the thyroid.

4. On the upper, tracheal surface of the thyroid (2).

5. May be imbedded in the thyroid.

Hypotheses relating to parathyroid function are legion. The best evidence, at the present time, suggests that the parathyroid hormone (parathormone) acts to:

1. Raise the blood level of calcium by inducing osteoclastic bone resorption.

2. Increase renal excretion of phosphorus.

3. Inhibit calcification of newly formed osteoid.

The important stimulators of parathormone production are hypocalcemia and, perhaps, hyperphosphatemia.

Hyperparathyroidism (osteitis fibrosa): Primary hyperparathyroidism caused by a tumor or tumors of the parathyroid glands is not uncommon in man but appears to be rare in animals. Krook could not accept any of the canine cases reported in the literature and described 3 definite ones of his own.[9] I am not aware of any definite cases in the horse.

The condition is characterized by: 1. A chronic, progressive course with loss of bone strength, deformities, and spontaneous fractures, 2, loss of compact bone which is replaced by poor quality spongy bone and fibrous tissue, 3, bone swellings or "cysts" of fibrous tissue and giant cells, 4, widespread metastatic calcification of kidneys, lungs, stomach, arteries, and pleura, 5, hypercalcemia, hypophosphatemia, hyperphosphatasemia, calciuria, and phosphaturia.

Hyperparathyroidism may develop as a result of extraparathyroidal factors. As indicated previously these must involve either low blood calcium or high blood phosphorus. Secondary hyperparathyroidism, then, could be expected as a result of:

1. Low calcium diet.
2. Failure to absorb calcium from intestine.
3. Pregnancy and lactation (heavy drain on maternal blood calcium).
4. Rickets, osteomalacia.
5. Chronic renal insufficiency.
6. High phosphate intake.

One reasonable hypothesis concerning the pathogenesis of secondary hyperparathyroidism is that as a result of low serum calcium the glands enlarge and release parathormone which, in turn, causes resorption of bone and elevation of serum calcium and phosphorus. If the hypocalcemia is prolonged, the bones lose structural elements which are replaced by fibrous tissue (osteitis fibrosa). Metastatic calcification is common. The elevation of serum phosphorus, of course, constitutes further stimulation for parathormone production in order to eliminate the excess phosphates. Obviously, correction of the calcium deficiency will break the cycle.

High phosphate intake may initiate the same cycle of events by causing parathormone hypersecretion in order to eliminate the excess phosphate. Unfortunately, the hormone is non-discriminatory and will resorb bone as well as induce renal phosphate excretion. The bone resorption, in turn, serves to increase blood phosphate levels. The vicious cycle may be broken by reducing phosphate intake.

In chronic renal insufficiency, there generally is retention of phosphate. Whether the retention of phosphate alone is sufficient for parathormone release, or whether the relative hypocalcemia caused by hyperphosphatemia causes its release has been long debated. Here we shall adopt the middle road, considering both hypocalcemia and hyperphosphatemia as stimulators of parathormone release. In any event, hyperphosphatemia leads to parathormone release, and osteitis fibrosa and metastatic calcification result. The renal insufficiency will eventually be aggravated by metastatic calcification in the kidneys.

Fortunately, the horse is relatively free of renal disease.

The hyperparathyroidism of rickets and osteomalacia will be discussed later.

Biochemic findings in secondary hyperparathyroidism are: 1. Hyperphosphatemia, 2, hypo- or normocalcemia, and 3, hyperphosphatasemia.

Hypoparathyroidism: As might be anticipated osteosclerosis, increased bone deposition, occurs in hypoparathyroidism. Uncontrolled hypocalcemic tetany would, under most conditions, be expected to far overshadow such bone effects.

NUTRITIONAL DISEASES OF BONE

Since basic information on the nutrient requirements of horses is meager, nutrition has become a favorite field for theorizing on the causes of equine lameness. There is no question that various nutritional deficiencies, or excesses, are related to the development of frank bone lesions in horses. It is unfortunate that these gross syndromes have been used as a basis for postulating nutritional bases for localized bone lesions. Facts are needed to demonstrate that certain bone lesions are nutritionally related, and that many are not.

A discussion of nutritional diseases of bone must begin with inanition. Inadequate intake of total nutrients or any given nutrient may cause nonspecific slowing of both cartilage proliferation and new bone formation in the young animal, and rarefaction of bone in the adult (inability of new bone formation to keep pace with resorption).

VITAMIN A

Hypovitaminosis A causes, in skeletal tissues, a nonspecific slowing and, eventually, cessation of bone growth. In some species, at least, neurologic manifestations are related to cessation of growth of the skull, while the nervous tissues continue growing at a normal rate.

Dimock recorded the occurrence of night blindness in 2 of 4 horses on a vitamin A-deficient diet for 1 year.[10] The 2 animals, both pregnant mares, foaled at term. One foal, normal at birth, died 2 months later of pneumonia. The second foal was small, thin, light-boned, and never grew well.

Howell, Hart, and Ittner studied the effect of vitamin A deficiency in horses.[5] Although their observations on joint erosions are incorrect—to judge from the illustrations—a definite osteoporotic bone effect was observed.

Sandstedt et al. in an excellent, thorough study on causes of death in young foals, found vitamin A deficiency of varying degrees to be an important factor.[11] They described bone lesions similar, in many respects, to scurvy in other species, and unlike those seen in laboratory animals on vitamin A-deficient diets. Whether horse bone responds to vitamin A deficiency in a manner different from other species, or whether the observations of Sandstedt et al. were misinterpreted requires further study.

Hypervitaminosis A may be more of a threat to the horse with an overzealous handler than hypovitaminosis. Toxic amounts of A in experimental animals cause marked acceleration of bone growth and remodeling, with fragile, osteoporotic bone resulting.

VITAMIN B GROUP

Vitamin B-complex deficiency apparently exerts little or no specific bone effect. An interesting aspect of some B-vitamin deficiencies (riboflavin, folic acid) concerns development of congenital skeletal defects in offspring of deficient mothers. Carroll et al. reported the production of thiamine deficiency signs in horses on low B-complex diets.[25]

VITAMIN C

Avitaminosis C has not been defined in the horse. As mentioned in the discussion of hypovitaminosis A some bone lesions in foals appear to resemble scurvy, and it may be well to describe the characteristic lesions.

Characteristic skeletal changes include enlargement of the ends of the long bones and costochondral junctions. The basic defect is a failure of osteoblast formation of bone, so that a broad, calcified cartilage lattice develops beneath the epiphysial cartilage.[12] With weight-bearing the lattice collapses, crushes and fractures, producing a "trummerfeld" or zone of calcified debris. Bone lesions are most significant during the growing period.

VITAMIN D (RICKETS AND OSTEOMALACIA)

There appears to be no reliable information available on the effects of vitamin D deficiency in the horse. Many investigators in the past have denied the existence of true rickets (as seen in man and some animals) in the horse.[13] More recent authors apparently assume that rickets occurs in completely comparable form in animals and man.[2]

One essential difficulty may be a lack of understanding of the several and interrelated effects of vitamin D, calcium, phosphorus, bone tissue, and the parathyroid glands. These factors will be considered as they have been elucidated in work with man and experimental animals. The application of these studies to the horse remains to be done.

The effects of vitamin D-deficiency include the following:[30]

"1. The absorption of calcium, and secondarily of phosphorus, from the gastrointestinal tract is diminished.

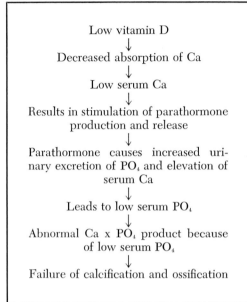

Low vitamin D
↓
Decreased absorption of Ca
↓
Low serum Ca
↓
Results in stimulation of parathormone production and release
↓
Parathormone causes increased urinary excretion of PO_4 and elevation of serum Ca
↓
Leads to low serum PO_4
↓
Abnormal Ca x PO_4 product because of low serum PO_4
↓
Failure of calcification and ossification

Fig. 7.

"2. The calcium blood level remains normal or nearly normal. The phosphorus level is depressed.

"3. The excretion of phosphorus in the urine is increased.

"4. The parathyroid glands are enlarged.

"5. Calcification of cartilage, osteoid and cementoid tissue, and predentin is prevented."

The development of rickets or osteomalacia as a result of vitamin D deficiency may then be visualized (Fig. 7, after Nordin).[14]

The discerning reader now will see the complexity of the interrelationships of the Ca-P controlling mechanisms. The role of the parathyroids in vitamin D deficiency is significant.

Vitamin D-resistant rickets, apparently hereditary, has been recorded in man.[15] The outstanding characteristic of this type of rickets is resistance to treatment with usual doses of vitamin D. Resistant rickets appears to be based on a congenital defect of the renal tubular reabsorption mechanism for phosphorus. Failure of reabsorption causes serum phosphate to be permanently low. Therefore, the Ca x P product will be low and rickets results (Fig. 7).

Hypervitaminosis D: Undoubtedly vitamin D, vaguely understood by many laymen to be concerned with bone, is fed promiscuously or injected into horses with some hope that "better" bone will result and all forms of unsoundness disappear. The writer has necropsied several young horses with lesions highly suggestive of hypervitaminosis D. In one case a feed supplement containing massive amounts of vitamin D was being fed. In hypervitaminosis D without severe renal damage there will be increased calcium-phosphorus absorption, formation of new bone (osteosclerosis) and metastatic calcification. With the onset of renal damage from metastatic calcification in the renal tubules, secondary hyperparathyroidism would be expected along with the bone changes of osteitis fibrosa.

OSTEOMALACIA

This specific disease of Equidae has been described by Theiler[16] and Kintner and Holt,[17] among others. It has been variously known as: osteomalacia, osteoporosis, osteitis fibrosa, big head, bran disease, etc.

According to Kintner and Holt[17] this is a deficiency disease related to inadequate intake of calcium or excessive intake of phosphorus. With a diet low in calcium and high in phosphorus, the previous discussion reveals clearly that either 1 or both of 2 mechanisms may be set in motion:

1. Rickets-osteomalacia will appear as a result of low calcium, high phosphorus serum levels with disturbance of the Ca x P product.

2. Secondary hyperparathyroidism will appear as a result of low serum Ca and elevated serum P.

With mechanism 1, histologic examination of the bones should show impaired calcification with the appearance of osteoid borders. With 2, the microscopic picture should be dominated by bone destruction, osteoclasis, fibrosis, and osteoid borders only as part of abortive repair phenomena. According to the descriptions and illustrations of Kintner and Holt,[17] and Theiler,[16] this second picture—osteitis fibrosa—is, indeed, what is seen in so-called equine osteomalacia. Theiler preferred to call the condition osteodystrophia fibrosa—a synonym for osteitis fibrosa.

A comparison of the characteristic blood findings in various conditions strongly indicates that so-called equine osteomalacia is, indeed, osteitis fibrosa as a result of secondary hyperparathyroidism.*

| | Blood Serum Levels | |
Condition	Calcium	Phosphorus
Rickets-osteo-malacia	Normal or low	Low
Primary hyper-parathyroidism	High	Low
Secondary hyper-parathyroidism	Normal or low	High
Equine osteo-malacia	Normal or low	High

(Kintner & Holt's data)

Although variations from these findings are to be expected and do occur, the weight of evidence appears in favor of secondary hyperparathyroidism as the cause of the bone lesions in horses on high phosphorus, low calcium diets.

The several points remaining for elucidation are:

1. Does metastatic calcification, a hallmark of hyperparathyroidism, occur?

2. What is the status of the parathyroid gland?

3. Would serial studies reveal that osteomalacia (in the true sense) occurs early in the course of the disease, to be superceded by hyperparathyroidism-osteitis fibrosa?

MINERALS

Most of the pertinent information on minerals in relation to bone metabolism already has been presented. Only those points not previously discussed will be mentioned here.

Calcium: It appears at the present time that simple calcium deficiency uncomplicated by other factors can, at least in the cat, cause osteoporosis. Nordin indicates simple calcium deficiency can result from: 1. Low dietary intake, 2 malabsorption, and 3 hypercalciuria.[14]

At this point it may be well to discuss osteoporosis as an entity and place it in proper relation to the several bone diseases already discussed.

OSTEOPOROSIS

The term, osteoporosis, often is used in a general way to describe absence of normal quantities of bone whatever the cause. It might be well, however, to restrict the term to atrophy (inability of new bone formation to keep pace with resorption) or failure of new bone formation without signs of specific entities such as rickets, osteitis fibrosa, etc. Frost's definition is apropos: "In osteoporotic bone the bone substance is of normal quality with respect to the properties of organic and inorganic material, the strength, the hardness and the rigidity. The quantity of bone, however, is diminished because of thinning of the cortices and trabeculae, the presence of fewer trabeculae and the enlargement of Haversian canals and marrow spaces. The total mass and volume of bone substance (marrow excluded) are thus reduced, rendering the bone less dense on the roentgenogram."[18]

Osteoporosis may be either generalized or localized. The generalized form affects virtually every bone in the body and may result from inanition, calcium deficiency, various vitamin deficiencies, old age (senile osteoporosis), hyperthyroidism, copper deficiency, and lead poisoning in lambs.[1] (Osteosclerosis is reported in human lead poisoning.)

Localized osteoporosis may result from disuse, diminished vascular supply, nerve lesions, and internal or external pressure.

Generalized osteoporosis apparently is not common in the horse. Howell *et al.* presented a picture of a cannon bone of a vitamin A-deficient horse which appeared osteoporotic.[5] In a large series of necropsies on old mares (10 to 30 years of age) I have seen no examples of generalized osteoporosis.

Localized osteoporosis undoubtedly is more common. The crushing of the coffin bone following bilateral neurectomy may be an example of a neurovascular, localized osteoporosis.

Phosphorus: Aphosphorosis is discussed in Chapter 22. Suffice it to note here that dietary phosphate deficiency should lead to the development of rickets—osteomalacia in essentially

*Lowe (Thesis, Cornell, 1962) has recently demonstrated that so-called equine osteomalacia is, indeed, secondary hyperparathyroidism.

the same fashion as phosphate deficiency conditioned by vitamin D-deficiency (Fig. 7). The difference would be that low serum phosphorus would upset the Ca x P product directly and parathyroid participation would not be anticipated.

Other Minerals: No definitive work is available on the skeletal effects of various other mineral deficiencies in the horse. Work with other species indicates that copper and manganese deficiencies lead to osteoporosis.

Excessive chronic ingestion of fluorine and selenium exerts significant effects on the skeletal system of horses as well as other animals. These have been described elsewhere.

Conclusion: Experimental work is urgently needed to define the clinical, radiologic, biochemic, and pathologic features of simple calcium deficiency, simple phosphorus deficiency, hyperphosphorosis, vitamin D deficiency, hyperparathyroidism, etc., as related to equines.

FRACTURES

In this section, consideration is given to the problem of why and how fractures occur. There are at least 4 factors involved:

1. Predisposing factors.
2. Mechanical factors.
3. Stress or fatigue fractures.
4. Enchondrosis.

Fractures related to enchondrosis have been discussed previously. The many facets of track condition, cushion, etc., must be omitted. We shall limit ourselves to a consideration of those factors and inferences which can be developed by examination of the horse alone. Healing of fractures is adequately covered in a number of textbooks.

Predisposing Factors

Studies, presently in progress, have revealed that some spontaneous fractures of long bones may be related to pre-existing lesions. To date, precise correlation of the predisposing lesion and the acute fracture has been difficult. It is hoped that increasing comprehension of the dynamic and mechanical aspects of horse

movement may allow more precise correlations to be established.

One case of fracture of the humerus is illustrative. An older mare was running in a paddock when the humerus fractured. Necropsy revealed severe degeneration of the lower cervical intervertebral disks with greatly increased mobility of adjacent vertebrae. Fresh hemorrhage, originating in the vicinity of the dorsal part of the annular ligaments of 2 of these disks, pressed against the ventral surface of the spinal cord.

In a second case, fracture of the tibia was associated with a pedunculated joint mouse (osteochondritis dissecans) on the distal articular surface of the tibia.

Mechanical Factors

Mechanical factors have already been discussed. Koch's study of the human femur revealed that the sites for the most common femoral fractures (other than neck) could be predicted by application of mathematical principles and the laws of probability. Such studies on horse bones, though tedious, might be highly rewarding.

Stress or fatigue fractures bear certain affinities to the Type 3 enchondroses discussed earlier. Since these fractures are not confined to young bone, however, they constitute a separate group for consideration.

The essential features of stress or fatigue fractures appear to be:

1. Localized lameness.
2. Variable degree of loss of continuity of cancellous and/or compact bone.
3. Late appearance of radiologic signs. The loss of continuity may be apparent only as the development and recession of internal or external callus; the actual fracture line may never be visualized.
4. Causally related to repeated, subthreshold, mechanical insults leading by summation to changes in structure and loss of continuity (weakness of the basic architecture of the bone may predispose).

The reason for loss of continuity as a result of repeated trauma or insult is not clear.

Devas' discussion of navicular fractures in Greyhounds is thought-provoking:[3]

"Although many theories on the fatigue of bone have been advanced, it must also be considered that a stress fracture may, in fact, be a pathologic fracture occurring in bone in which the soft-tissue elements, either within the bone or on its surface, have been damaged, with impairment of the blood supply to a certain part of the bone. Thus, in that part, the bone is deprived of its ability to undergo continuous reconstitution and it remains no longer healthy, and perhaps, in fact, no longer living. Under these circumstances fatigue, in the metallurgical sense, would set in, a small break would appear, and this would cause further pathologic changes with further oedema of the soft tissues to compress the blood supply and a vicious circle would soon be in operation. It must, however, be emphasized that it is extremely unlikely that there be but one cause for all forms of stress fractures."

In the horse, chip fractures of the radial carpal bone may well be stress fractures. The radial carpal is subject to a number of mechanical factors:

1. It is on the medial side of the limb where compression forces are greatest.
2. The radial carpal moves or "flips" up and down in relation to the intermediate carpal as the carpus is flexed and extended (readily demonstrated on the postmortem specimen).
3. Many animals, when reaching, or extending the forelimb, overextend the carpus at the moment of contact with the ground, thus putting extreme compressive force on the front portion of the radial carpal. This seems to be particularly true when the animal is tiring.

In the few pathologic specimens I have had an opportunity to examine, the radial carpal has shown severe bruising of the soft tissues within the bone. The forces acting on this bone may lead to stress fracturing and/or arthritic changes with osteosclerosis.

Fractures of the proximal sesamoid bones also may represent stress or fatigue fracturing. Fresh fractures, removed surgically, should be examined by a pathologist for evidence of predisposing conditions.

So-called "bucked shins" in young horses may be yet another example of stress fracturing of the compression type, involving small cortical cracks on the dorsal aspect of the cannon bone.

As a corollary, perhaps, of these forms of fracturing, nonunion is a frequent complicating factor. Proximal sesamoid fractures are notorious in this respect, undoubtedly as a result of the near impossibility of immobilizing the fragments. Preliminary studies on the vascular supply of these bones do not indicate that loss of blood supply should be a significant factor. Vascular interruption as a cause of nonunion is well-recognized in man. The blood supply of the radial carpal bone should be investigated in this regard.

OTHER DISEASES OF BONE

Pulmonary osteoarthropathy has been seen in the horse. The characteristic features of the condition are acute vascular disturbances of the limbs succeeded by chronic formation of osteophytic new bone. There usually is an associated chronic pulmonary or cardiac lesion. An extended discussion of the causes of this condition is beyond the scope of this chapter. Perhaps it is sufficient to note that ringbones, osselets, and sesamoiditis have not been related to pulmonary osteoarthropathy.

INFLAMMATION AND NEOPLASIA OF BONE

As with fracture healing, inflammation of bone (osteitis, osteomyelitis) is well-described elsewhere and need not be considered in detail here. Several points might, however, be mentioned:

1. Abscesses, solitary or multiple, are not uncommon in the bones as well as joints of foals with navel ill.

2. Persistent proud flesh may, at least on occasion, be related to sequestering of underlying bone.

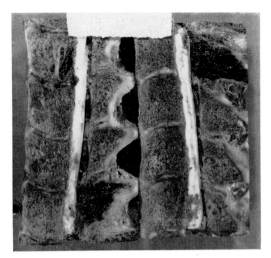

Fig. 8. Metastatic melanoma in vertebra of horse.

3. Metastatic tumors and abscessing processes may involve long bones and vertebrae (Fig. 8).

4. Primary bone tumors are rare in horses with most reported cases involving the head.[4]

J. R. ROONEY

REFERENCES

1. Butter, E. J., Nisbet, D. I., and Robertson, J. M.: J. Comp. Path. & Therap. **67** 378-396.
2. Smith, H. A. and Jones, T. C.: Veterinary Pathology, Lea & Febiger, Philadelphia, Pa., 1957.
3. Devas, M. B. J.: Bone and Joint. Surg., **43-B** (1961) 540-551.
4. Cotchin, E.: Neoplasms of the Domesticated Mammals. Commonwealth Agricultural Bureaux. England, 1956.
5. Howell, C. E., Hart, G. H., and Ittner, N. R.: Am. J. Vet. Research, **2** (1941) 60-74.
6. Sattler, H.: Basedow's Disease. Grune and Stratton, New York, N. Y., 1952.
7. Storey, E.: Brit. J. Exp. Path. **XLI** (1960) 16-213.
8. Vermuelen, H. A.: Berl. tierräztl Wchr. **33** 1-4, 13-17.
9. Krook, L.: Acta Path. et Microbiol., Scand. Suppl. **122** (1957) 41.
10. Dimock, W. W.: Incoordination of Horses (Wobbles). Kentucky Agric. Exp. Sta. Bull. **553** (1950).
11. Sandstedt, H., Obel, A-L., Sjöberg, K., and Karlsson, K.-F.: Skand. Veterinärtidsk. **21** (1946) 321-351.
12. Follis, R. H., Jr.: Deficiency Disease. Charles C Thomas, Springfield, Ill., 1958.
13. Nieberle and Cohrs. Lehrbuch der Speziellen Pathologischen Anatomie der Haustiere. Gustav Fischer, Jena, E. Germany, 1954.
14. Nordin, B. E. C.: Clin. Orthopaed. **17** (1960) 235-258.
15. Hsia, D.: Inborn Errors of Metabolism. Year Book Publishers, Chicago, Ill., 1959.
16. Theiler, A.: Vet. J. **90** (1934) 143-175, 183-206.
17. Kintner, J. H. and Holt, R. L.: Philippine J. Sci. **49** (1932) 1-89.
18. Frost, H. M.: J. Bone and Joint Surg. **42-A** (1960) 447-456.
19. James, N. V.: Canad. J. Comp. Med. **15** (1951) 94-95.
20. Mau, H.: Clin. Orthopaed. **11** 154-167.
21. Axhausen, G. in Henke and Luharsch: Handbuch der speziellen pathologischen Anatomie und Histologie 7, Vol. 9. Julius Springer, Berlin, Germany, (1937).
22. Nagura, S.: Clin. Orthopaed. **18** (1960) 100-122.
23. Looser: Verhandl. I. Deutsch. Pathol. Ges. **24** (1929) 352-360.
24. Brandt, A. J.: Skand. Veterinärtidsk. **59** (1940) 881-917.
25. Carroll, F. D., Goss, H. and Howell, C. E.: J. An. Sci. **8** (1949) 290-299.
26. Koch, J. C.: Am. J. Anat. **21** (1917) 177-298.
27. Obletz, B. E.: J. Bone & Joint. Surg. **20** (1938) 424-428.
28. Zietzschmann, O., and Krölling, O.: Lehrbuch der Entwicklungsgeschichte der Haustiere. Paul Parey, Berlin, Germany, 1955.
29. Sisson, S., and Grossman, J. D.: The Anatomy of the Domestic Animals. W. B. Saunders, Philadelphia, Pa., 1953.
30. Weinmann, J. P., and Sicher, H.: Bone and Bones, C. V. Mosby, St. Louis, Mo., 1955.
31. Carlson, W. D.: Veterinary Radiology. Lea and Febiger, Philadelphia, Pa., 1961.
32. Stecher, R. M., and Goss, L. J.: J.A.V.M.A. **138** (1961) 248-255.
33. Trueta, J., and Frias, A. J.: Bone & Joint Surg. **43B** (1961) 800-813.

DISEASES OF JOINTS, TENDONS, LIGAMENTS AND BURSAE

INTRODUCTION

Arthritis, bursitis, synovitis, and tendinitis can logically be discussed together because all these disorders cause some alteration in the animal's ability to move and perform as its owner desires. Further, it has been pointed out elsewhere in this volume that the musculoskeletal system represents a mechanical system of levers to provide the power for locomotion. The joints are the fulcrums and the tendons are the means of applying muscular power to the levers, which are the bones. The bursae and tendon sheaths serve to cushion and lubricate their associated structures so that power may be applied without damage to them.

ANATOMY

In order to understand the abnormal and to be able to plan rational therapy, it is necessary to fully understand the normal. With this in mind, a brief review of the normal structure of bursae, joints, tendon sheaths, and tendons is provided. The chapter on the locomotor system in Sodeman's *Pathologic Physiology* is recommended for a more complete discussion of this subject.

The joints are composed of a layer of hyaline cartilage covering the opposing ends of the bones. A joint is surrounded by a fibrous capsule lined with specialized cells, the synovium, which secrete synovial fluid. This capsule is reinforced by ligaments. Strictly speaking, the joint cavity is a tissue space, and the normal amount of synovial fluid is very small. The cohesive force of the synovial fluid as well as the strength of the joint capsule and its reinforcing ligaments serve to maintain joint stability and proper alignment.

Bursae and tendon sheaths are connective tissue structures lined with synovium and containing a small amount of synovial fluid. Bursae may be found where tendons or muscles lie upon bones, and at other points of stress, such as where the extensor tendons lie next to the skin at the fetlocks. Tendon sheaths surround the tendon where they pass around joints or where they are bound down at the joints by the annular ligaments. The tendons themselves are composed of bundles of collagenous fibers with fibroblasts between them, bound together in varying-sized structures. The ligaments are different from the tendons only in that their structure is less regular.

PHYSIOLOGY

A brief word also is in order as to the physiology of these structures. The articular cartilage is nourished by the synovial fluid, from subsynovial vessels lying at the junction of the joint capsule and the cartilage, and from the bone beneath the cartilage. Of these 3, the synovial fluid is the most important. Therefore, injuries to joint cartilage are slow to heal if they heal at all. The synovial membranes of the joint capsules, bursae, and tendon sheaths are relatively inelastic and highly resistant to tearing. These tissues are well-supplied with blood and have considerable regenerative capacity. The tendons are poorly supplied with blood, and their healing is a slow process.

PATHOGENESIS

Arthritis, bursitis, and tendovaginitis can all occur as septic processes, either as the result of localized infections of the structures themselves or as an extension of infections elsewhere in the body. Navel ill or joint ill in foals illustrates the latter, and poll evil and fistulous withers are examples of the former. These entities will be dealt with at appropriate places in this volume. It is sufficient to emphasize here that prompt removal of pus and control of infection are vital if damage to the affected structures is to be held to a minimum.

Our chief interest in this discussion is directed to the damage caused by stress and mechanical factors to the structures under consideration, in other words to aseptic inflammations of the joints, joint capsules, bursae, tendon sheaths, tendons, and ligaments. It is well to note here that severe, long-standing, untreated rickets also will produce degenerative joint damage. Proper and adequate nutrition from the time of conception is extremely important. However, it is of interest to note that exostoses and spur formation can occur at the joint margins in young horses fed heavily supplemented rations, particularly when nutritional imbalances are created.

CLINICAL ENTITIES

Arthropathies can be classified on the basis of their severity; the mildest condition is a strain. A strain is excessive stretching of the joint capsule ligaments which produces some edema and congestion around the joint. It usually occurs as an isolated traumatic incident. Greater trauma will produce synovitis of the joint capsule with an increase in joint fluid. These conditions respond well to topical therapy and heal quickly. A more severe trauma, or trauma repeated over a period of time, will affect the joint cartilage. If the injury to the cartilage is in the center of the joint, little or no healing will take place, and an irregular joint surface with consequent interference of movement will occur. Injuries at the junction of the cartilage and the capsule will result in proliferative and degenerative changes. Further injuries to weight-bearing joints that cause central damage and irregular joint surfaces will result in joint dysfunction and pathology at the joint margin. Thus, the consequences of trauma to weight-bearing joints at early ages will plague the animal later in life.

The pathologic result of severe joint trauma is osteoarthritis and this involves destruction of the joint cartilage, roughening of the joint surfaces, and bony spur formation at the margins of the joint. Ankylosis of the joint can occur when the degenerative changes of the joint surface are accompanied by prolonged synovitis.

Bursitis and tendosynovitis are inflammations of the synovial lining of these structures as a result of trauma, usually a strain. Prolonged inflammation of these structures leads to the deposition of calcium in the synovial membrane. The tendinitis usually seen in horses is the result of a strain in which there has been rupture of varying numbers of tendon fibers. An exception to the statement is the condition known as contracted tendons which will be discussed later.

DIAGNOSIS

A few general remarks on diagnosis will save repetition later. An effort should be made to acquire a thorough knowledge of the normal gaits of a horse. Variations from the normal can then be attributed to appropriate structures by an exercise of logic. This is particularly true when, as is often the case, more than one cause may be responsible for dysfunction in movement. When in doubt you can use diagnostic nerve blocks, but first keep moving the horse until you feel that you can spot the site of the trouble. Frequently, continued movement will help by making the site of the lameness more apparent. Conversely, it is important if the horse warms into or out of the lameness. Radiographs are in many cases a vital necessity in diagnosis, and they also serve in the planning of therapy by providing an accurate estimate of the extent of the damage. In brief, to diagnose the site of a lameness use your eyes and your head, and take your time.

THERAPEUTIC PROCEDURES

Let us now consider methods of therapy and the therapeutic agents used for disorders of the locomotor system. Primary considera-

tion is the presence or absence of heat in the affected part. If heat is present it should be removed. Heat is a sign of inflammation and the greater the inflammation and the longer it is present, the more severe the pathologic changes in the structures will be. Cold water is an efficient agent to counteract acute inflammation. I prefer using a hose, but a tub of water or ice boots will do. A point to remember in the use of a hose is that the flow of water should be slow and the nozzle of the hose should be laid against the part so that the water flows down the part as a sheet. Cooling, astringent lotions, such as white lotion or Burow's solution, applied liberally to cotton bandages also are good. Such soaked bandages or foot swabs should never be allowed to dry because when they do they become hot.

The corticosteroids and phenylbutazone can play an extremely useful part in reducing inflammation. They may be injected either parenterally or directly into the affected joint, bursa or tendon sheath. Extreme care is indicated when injecting into a joint as to both aseptic technic and the avoidance of further damage to articular cartilage. One undesirable consequence related to the use of corticosteroids is that by the reduction of inflammation and pain, the horse can be returned to work long before adequate time for repair has passed. As a consequence, the trauma is repeated and frequently magnified, to the detriment of the animal. The owner's efforts to use corticosteroids for this reason must be resisted at all times although it often will be a losing battle.

Rest is of prime importance. It frequently is difficult, especially in race horse practice, to adequately rest the injured animal. The owner will not permit complete rest of the animal for the necessary time and some compromise must be made about limited exercise to keep the horse fit. On occasion, the use of the firing iron, although not strictly warranted by the case in question, will make imperative a decent interval of rest.

Externally applied counterirritant preparations vary in severity of the reaction they produce. Further variation in effect can be achieved by bandaging the part, by using waxed paper or oilcloth under the bandage, and by the vigor with which they are applied, *e.g.*, steaming them in, scrubbing with stiff brush, etc. Various counterirritants are available commercially but many practitioners prefer to make their own favorite prescriptions. In order of severity from mild to strong, they are termed sweats, liniments, paints, and blisters. Sweats are used primarily under bandage to prevent filling (edema) of the legs after work. The astringent lotions are used this way also, and their use is a matter of personal preference. Liniments usually are used to prevent muscle soreness and to remove tissue fluid accumulations that sweats cannot. They usually are not used under bandage.

Paints are made in all strengths and are a compromise between more rigorous therapy which will confine the horse, and keeping him in full training. Blisters, or vesicants, are used in conjunction with the firing iron or by themselves in radical treatment of joint and tendon disorders. Some iodine preparations are injected subcutaneously or intramuscularly as internal blisters. There is some controversy regarding the relative efficiency of external and internal blisters, and there is little scientifically derived evidence on either side. Most practitioners use both methods on occasion. Perhaps the best approach until more accurate evidence is available, is to select the method which personal experience proves best for the case in question.

The third line of attack in the therapy of locomotor disorders is the procedure known as "firing." This ordinarily is accomplished with a hot iron. Acids have been used as a method of firing; however, I have never seen this. Firing with an iron is done either as point firing or line firing. In point firing, as the name implies, a round tip of varying sharpness and diameter is used. Line firing is done with a point shaped like a short, dull, knife blade. Point firing is by far the more common procedure, line firing usually being reserved for a second treatment when necessary. Combinations of the 2 allow the practitioner to indulge his artistic bent in the patterns created. As a matter of personal preference, I use small,

relatively sharp points, but whatever the size and shape preferred, the objective usually is to barely pierce the skin with the tip of the point. Some veterinarians make an exception to this rule when firing jack spavins and actually fire into the bone itself. A light touch is indicated, or an unsightly degree of scarring will result. Particular care is necessary when firing joints to avoid penetrating the joint capsule. The severity of this treatment is determined partly by varying the distance between the fired points. When line firing, considerable care must be exercised not to cut the skin. It should be understood that nerve blocks are applied to the part to be fired. In addition to creating an increased blood supply resulting from the subsequent inflammation, the purpose of firing is to promote the development of fibrous tissue to add strength to the part under treatment.

A fourth method of therapy is diathermy, the application of which is determined by the type of equipment being used. Diathermy devices are expensive but, in my opinion, well worth the price. Diathermy is useful in the treatment of all the conditions under consideration here and is most useful when the injury is of recent origin. A word of caution—do not use diathermy on a lesion which has been blistered within one month at the least, and vice versa. This warning also applies to paints and liniments, although the time limits are less restrictive. Reactions caused by such a procedure can be alarmingly severe.

As a fifth form of therapy, ultrasonic rays are used. The use of ultrasonic devices is attended with some difficulty in that the part being treated must be either under water or liberally greased. In human therapy, these machines are used to a considerable degree in the treatment of bursitis as well as arthritis. A limited number of personal observations has caused some question in my mind concerning the possibility of damaging sound bone if this therapy is not used with extreme care.

A sixth therapeutic method involves the application of x-rays or their components. The use of radiation therapy equipment is beyond the physical and financial reach of most practitioners. However, with the advent of the radioisotopes and with the aid of a special boot, methods presently are being developed to deliver measured doses of radiation to selected areas of a horse's leg. My understanding from personal contact with men who have used this treatment is that it is most effective when the pathology is of recent origin.

Lastly, whirlpool baths have become very popular in recent years. This is, of course, a variation on the tried and true method of standing the horse in a creek. Both warm and cold water are used as well as many different chemical solutions. This form of treatment can be as varied as the indications of the individual case and the practitioner's imagination dictate. The standard approach in physical therapy, however, is to use plain water moving at considerable velocity, the temperature of the water being cold on a newly inflamed part, and warm (100 to 105 F.) when the acute inflammatory changes have subsided.

In summary, the treatment used can and should be varied to suit the case in question. There are, however, several important considerations that always should be kept in mind. First, inflammation following the injury should be reduced as promptly and completely as possible. Second, rest always is indicated to give the injured parts time to heal. Third, in view of the fact that many of the injured structures have a poor blood supply, any increase that can be produced will aid in healing.

POLL EVIL AND FISTULOUS WITHERS

Poll evil is an infection of the occipital bursa. In fistulous withers the supraspinous bursa is involved. They once were considered to result from mechanical trauma with the resulting collection of serosanguineous fluid serving as an excellent culture medium for subsequent bacterial infection. However, there is every indication that trauma is not necessary to initiate the infection. *Brucella abortus*, or occasionally *B. suis*, regularly can be cultured from these lesions. Also, it has been demonstrated that the prevalence of these entities in a given area closely parallels the prevalence of *B. abortus* infection in the cattle population. *Actinomyces bovis* also is frequently cultured

from these lesions. The practitioner usually will have to rely on clinical impressions to judge the presence or absence of infection.

If infection is present, the object is to get it under control, and, if necessary, to establish surgical drainage as quickly as possible. Parenteral antibiotics and fibrinolytic products usually will control infections, and hot water application will aid in promoting drainage by localizing the purulent process. The intravenous use of sodium iodide is of benefit in many cases.

Surgical drainage often is necessary when treating poll evil and fistulous withers. When the lesion is incised all the fistulous tracts should be explored with a probe and if they extend a distance below the level of the opening originally made, these tracts should be opened at their lowest point. Fluid from these lesions should be cultured and sensitivity tests made so that the most effective antibiotic therapy can be administered. The fistulous tracts should be flushed daily until the infection has been controlled. I favor packing the infected tracts daily with sterile gauze soaked with Lugol's solution and one of the enzyme preparations. If packing is impossible, setons with the same medication should be used. The indicated antibiotics are administered parenterally. As the infection is controlled and healing commences, the routine of packing should be adjusted to allow the formation of granulation tissue from the bottoms of the tracts so that the wound is filled solidly with granulation tissue. In both poll evil and fistulous withers it is important to place water buckets, feed tubs, and hay at a height from the floor that is convenient for the animal. Horses with these conditions frequently will be unwilling to alter the position of the head or neck even to eat or drink.

The practitioner occasionally will see a sterile inflammation of the supraspinous bursa. Such lesions will be sharply defined, fluctuating masses with little or no heat present. In determining the cause the saddle and, if a stock saddle is used, the saddling procedure always should be checked. My experience is that regardless of claims to the contrary, 99% of these lesions are caused by an improperly fitting English saddle or by not pulling up the front of the saddle blanket after the saddle is put on when western tack is used. Therapy starts with pointed advice on this subject. Usually the practitioner will see these swellings several days after they occur. If one is fortunate enough to be called immediately, an ice bag applied for 20 minutes twice a day will usually be effective. The ice bag treatment is less effective the longer the condition has existed. The application of a liniment for 4 or 5 days is the next line of attack. If this is ineffective, the swelling should be incised at its most ventral site. I have found that unresponsive lesions in this area contain chicken fat clots, despite their feeling like fluid on palpation. Removal of clots, application of Lugol's solution to the interior of the sac, and the continued external application of liniment generally will alleviate this condition.

H. CRESSWELL

INTRODUCTION TO SECTION ON LAMENESSES

Special consideration is given in this section to the clinical syndromes which are characterized by lameness. The grouping of these syndromes seems warranted in view of their importance in the practice of equine medicine. These conditions compose a large number of equine ailments for which veterinary care is solicited. Their significance is intimately related to the economic value of most equines and, consequently, lameness syndromes are regarded with considerable concern by horse owners.

It has been difficult to assemble this section without introducing some repetition of other parts of the book. This generally has been avoided, however, and the advantage of having the discussions of lamenesses grouped for convenient reference easily justifies the repetition which does occur.

The contributions of two outstanding equine practitioners have been combined in the lameness section. By so doing, the range of syndromes covered is more extensive and the individual discussions are more comprehensive. This section, likewise, has benefitted from the

merger of experience obtained over a period of years in both the United States and Great Britain.—Editor.

FOOT LAMENESSES

INTRODUCTION

Foot lameness, insofar as this text is concerned, involves the structures distal to the fetlock joint. Before discussing the various forms of lameness which may occur in, or in connection with, the foot of the horse, it may be helpful to refer to some features which are peculiar to the soliped, and which have a considerable bearing upon lameness, its prognosis, and treatment.

Let us regard the visible differences which exist when we compare the fore- and hindfeet. While doing this we must remember that although lameness in a forefoot is common, it is far less common in a hindfoot, except when it arises from a nail badly driven during shoeing, or from a punctured sole. The hindfoot is well-protected against concussion. The fetlock, hock, and stifle all work in unison, each joint with its attached muscles acting as an efficient shock absorber.

The forefoot, when it exerts pressure upon the ground, forms the extremity of a solid bony column, and the concussion sustained when the forefoot strikes the ground is transmitted through the whole limb. The ability of the forelimb to absorb the effects of concussion depends not only upon the structure of the foot but also upon its individual peculiarities and, not least, upon the part which man has played in reshaping and providing it with a metal shoe. This is why navicular disease, laminitis, fractures, corns, and even injuries arising from sole puncture are more common in the forefoot than in the hind.

CHANGES IN THE SHAPE OF THE FOOT

Apart from keratoma which causes the hoof to bulge, a foot may carry a "false quarter" or have one side of the hoof flattened or even concave instead of being rounded. This usually is the result of an injury to the coronary band immediately above the false quarter, and the scar resulting from this injury may often be evident. The condition may or may not give rise to lameness.

Horses occasionally have "odd feet," one of which does not quite match the other. There may be no lameness in such instances, but one must not be led to believe that such feet are not usually a result of unnatural causes. One may be assured by the owner, particularly if he is also offering the horse for sale, that the horse cast a shoe and either wore the wall away, or broke the wall before the loss of the shoe was noticed. It is true that this occasionally may be the case but one must always examine odd feet very carefully and try to discover the reason for their existence.

Lameness, of some duration, almost always causes contraction of the foot of the involved limb, even though the seat of the lameness was not located in the foot. A lessening of weight-bearing diminishes the blood pumping action that occurs within every sound foot and lessens the degree of spreading of the sole and heel of the hoof on the lame side.

Such a foot always grows longer (higher) and narrower than its fellow; in fact the latter may appear the smaller and flatter of the two. The difference is obvious when one picks up each foot in turn and looks at their sole surfaces. The heels of the contracted foot will be narrower; the sole may be a little longer but not so wide as in the sound foot, and the wall may be a little higher. In most cases, the sole of the contracted foot will be more concave, and the frog will be smaller and will show less sign of wear (Fig. 9).

A contracted foot is not necessarily a cause of lameness but it is an indication that lameness has existed, or does exist, in that particular limb. Contraction almost invariably is present in cases of navicular disease and in horses lame from chronic or suppurating corns. It is nearly a constant feature in lameness from ringbone, and in lameness associated with any part of the limb if it exists for more than a few days.

Odd feet, which occur naturally, will have normally rounded soles and wide-open heels, and frogs which make contact with the ground.

LAMINITIS

Etiology: Inflammation of the sensitive laminae occurs in all classes of horses, but it is seen more commonly in overfed and underworked ponies which are confined, and in mares after foaling. It is accompanied by general circulatory congestion within the feet together with venous stagnation. It usually affects the forefeet only, although occasionally, the hindfeet also may become involved. A great many own-

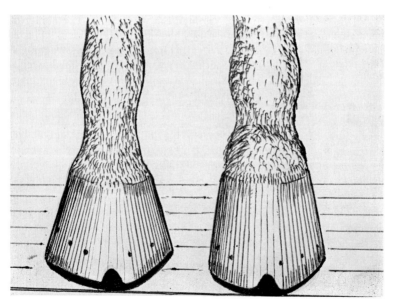

Fig. 9. Contracted foot with ringbone on right.

ers imagine that lameness exists in the hind-feet when only the front ones actually are involved because, in acute laminitis of the fore-feet, the horse flexes the hocks and carries the 2 hindfeet beneath the center of the body in order to remove the weight from the front soles. If, for any reason, the 2 forefeet are rendered insensitive by plantar nerve block, the horse temporarily will walk sound on all 4 feet.

Clinical Signs: In acute cases, the 2 forefeet are extended in front of the body in an attempt to take weight on the heels, and the 2 hind-feet are placed in the manner just indicated. In the rare cases in which all the feet are involved, the horse, if it is able to stand at all, places all its feet beneath the body. The position assumed has been described as appearing as though the animal were attempting to balance itself on the lid of a barrel.

In cases of laminitis affecting the forefeet, the movement, when forced, is typical. One forefoot is advanced a few inches, then the other. When both are side by side, the back is arched and one hindfoot brought as far under the belly as possible. The second hind-foot then is advanced beside the first. The horse flexes the hocks, lowers the quarters, emits a groan, and holds the weight of the body on the 2 hindfeet, while the forefeet again advance in turn. Once recumbent, the horse lies flat and has great difficulty in rising.

One form of acute laminitis is accompanied by systemic signs: some elevation of the temperature, rather labored breathing, loss of appetite, and marked depression. This form is not uncommonly encountered after a protracted or difficult foaling, particularly if the fetal membranes are retained for 48 hours or longer.

Chronic laminitis is encountered in fat horses receiving limited exercise. It occasionally may be encountered in ponies kept on good quality pasture, which results in their being overweight. The clinical signs are much milder but the forefeet are still advanced even when standing and the hindfeet carried well beneath the body. The complications of laminitis are dropped soles and, in some instances, perforation of the horny sole by the rim of the pedal bone (Fig. 10).

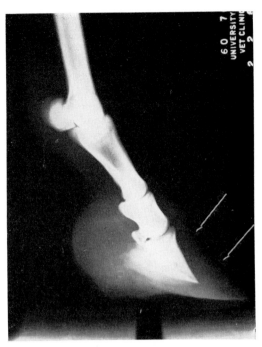

Fig. 10. Rotation of third phalanx in horse with laminitis. Radiograph by J. P. Manning, D.V.M.

The local signs are similar to those associated with acute inflammation. The feet feel hot, and the animal experiences difficulty in lifting one as the other is unable to carry the weight due to severe pain. Pulsation in the digital arteries may be marked.

Inflammatory exudate weakens the attachment existing between the horny and sensitive laminae, causing the front edge of the pedal bone to drop on the upper surface of the sole, which it may eventually penetrate. When this does not happen, the pressure of exudate and the weight of the pedal bone combined cause the normal arching of the foot to disappear until the sole viewed from below becomes convex instead of concave. This distortion of the sole apparently is an irreversible process. After the acute signs have abated, and the horse is again able to walk, a well-seated shoe will be necessary in order to avoid undue pressure on the sole.

Treatment: Rapid recovery from severe attacks of acute laminitis has been observed following the administration of antihistamines. Previous to the use of these agents, laminitis was a very damaging condition, and apt to recur. Purging, poulticing, enforced rest, bleeding, hoof incising, and even trephining the sole have been employed with little or no benefit.

Laminitis is encountered less frequently today. Antihistamines, combined with keeping the feet cold and moist, restricting the diet, use of diuretics, and anti-inflammatory agents such as corticosteroids or phenylbutazone produce more rapid recovery with less serious aftereffects. Chronic laminitis in ponies may be treated similarly, paying special attention to diet restriction, regular exercise, and avoiding constipation. The practice of administering from 1 to 2 ounces of magnesium sulfate daily in a small feed of bran is of value in the prevention of further exacerbations.

NAVICULAR DISEASE AND NAVICULAR FRACTURE

Anatomy: The navicular bone is a small, flat bone which lies behind the articulation of the second and third phalanges, to form the "coffin joint." The bone is elongated from side to side and has 2 surfaces, 2 edges, and 2 ends. Its articular surface is smooth, but its opposite tendinous surface is rougher and broader.

The tendinous surface is covered by fibrocartilage over which the tendon of the deep flexor tendon passes, and it carries the synovial membrane which lies between the bone and tendon—the navicular sheath.

The upper edge of the navicular bone is wide and grooved in its middle portion, becoming narrower toward the extremities. The groove gives attachment to the postero-lateral ligaments of the coffin joint and they anchor the upper edge of the navicular bone to the side of the second phalanx and to the os pedis behind its articular surface, as well as to the lateral ligaments of the pastern joint with which the postero-lateral ligaments are continuous. The ends of the navicular bone also are attached by small fibers to the wings of the os pedis, and to the inner surface of the lateral cartilages.

The navicular bone is anchored firmly at both ends, above and below. It is supported by the plantar aponeurosis and its reinforcing sheath.

When the foot lands from a jump with the coronary band upright, the tendons tensed, and weight falling on the frog, the navicular bone is tightly squeezed. It is even more tightly squeezed when the second forefoot lands in front of the first in the position in which the heel is being used as a brake, the toe advanced to its limit, and the tendon pulled to its most taut position. The fact that the navicular bone is attached firmly at either end would tend to fracture it where such fractures usually occur, at ⅓ of the length of the bone taken from each terminal point.

Pathogenesis: It has been pointed out that sudden violent pressure on the navicular bone exerted, perhaps, via the second phalanx, might cause the body of the bone potentially to have a greater backward displacement than its extremities. This might produce sufficient leverage to cause fracture at the usual sites, which are the weakest parts of the normal bone. This appears to be 10 to 15 mm. from the extremities.

Navicular disease may be regarded as a chronic osteitis with roughening of the articular cartilage, production of osteophytes or proliferating calcium deposits, and bony rarefaction which occasionally terminates in fracture. In most cases, the disease begins as a bursitis affecting the navicular bursa, followed by adhesions between the bone and the deep flexor tendon and its aponeurosis. Sometimes calcification appears in the ligaments of the navicular bone, especially in those connected with its pointed ends. More often both forefeet become affected, rather than a single foot. Ulcers appear on the tendinous surface of the bone, and these may invade and weaken its substance (Fig. 11).

Etiology: The etiology is uncertain, but heredity and concussion are major influences. The conformation of the horse, particularly upright shoulders and upright pasterns, increases the risks from concussion. Other possible causes include penetrating wounds of the frog, contracted heels, and extension of the ossifying process of sidebone to the suspensory ligaments of the navicular. The condition is seen more commonly in upright, narrow, and contracted feet but whether the type of foot is important is difficult to determine since many cases occur in the best-looking feet. Horses which possess weak, flat heels often are affected, although this may be the result of the disease rather than its cause.

Clinical Signs: The clinical signs make their appearance very gradually and consequently the condition may be already well-advanced when the attention of the owner is first attracted. At first, the horse points his feet a good deal, *i.e.* advances them to relieve weight and pressure, first one, then the other. Pointing seems to be widely regarded as pathognomonic of navicular disease, but this is a fallacy. A horse will point with any painful disorder involving the leg below the fetlock. When led from the stable, the animal fails to stride out, but shuffles and takes short steps. The condition is more noticeable when only one foot is affected—when both are involved the lameness may be partially disguised. The lameness is more marked on hard ground and it is particularly evident when the horse is turned in a short circle. The horse rotates on the lame leg instead of lifting the foot from the ground, and he frequently stumbles. Pressure applied to the frog produces pain. As the disease progresses, the hoof becomes narrow and high in its walls, and the shoulder muscles and those of the forearm atrophy. Heat is present in the heels only when there is acute lameness in the later stages.

Diagnosis: Diagnosis often may be confirmed by x-ray examination, but when rarefaction of the bone is present interpretation may be difficult and a fracture may be invisible. The upright pedal position for radiographing the navicular bone still is the best. It has been noted that a widening of the foramina which carry the blood vessels of the bone is the first radiographic evidence of the disease. Often a rarefaction of the central portion of the bone is seen, with osteophytes at its ends and at the center of its upper edge, most of which point upward. Since the diagnosis of navicular disease often is considered to be a death sentence or an indication of a drastic reduction in the useful life of the animal, radiographs should be obtained of all suspected cases.

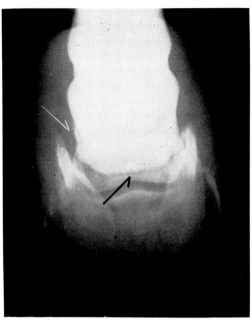

Fig. 11. Pitting of navicular bone. Top arrow indicates fracture of second phalanx. Radiograph by J. P. Manning, D.V.M.

Treatment: No treatment is of permanent value although it may temporarily provide relief on some occasions. Most so-called cures probably are the result of mistaken diagnosis. Treatment is palliative and symptomatic, and will not result in a cure. The horse should be shod with a rolled toe or half-round shoes and heel caulks. The foot should be trimmed with as short a toe and as much heel as possible. If a bar shoe can be applied without touching the frog, this will help. It will make things worse, however, if the bar transmits pressure to the frog. Aspirin and ice boots will serve to get the horse through a race on a day-to-day basis. Posterior digital nerve blocks and/or phenylbutazone are used similarly for show horses.

Digital neurectomy has been practiced, but its effect is only temporary and rupture of the deep flexor tendon is a common sequel. Denerved horses are barred from racing and are unsafe for jumping or anything but the slowest hacking.

CORNS

A corn is a contusion arising from pressure from the heel of a shoe, usually the inner branch. The origin is at the angle of the sole between the main wall of the foot and the portion of the wall which turns in to form the bar of the foot.

Clinical Signs: The appearance of corns, after the shoe has been removed and the foot scrubbed, is not always the same. It depends considerably upon how long the corn has been in existence and whether the shoe still is causing pressure on the spot indicated. In an early case, one sees evidence of a localized inflammation. There is heat and pain in the heel, together with signs of serum extravasation. To see this, it may be necessary to trim a little of the sole within the angle between bar and wall. The trimming should be as superficial as possible, otherwise infection may be introduced and a simple bruise may then develop into a serious, suppurating corn.

There will have been an escape of blood from the injured vessels with staining of the underlying horn, visible through the surface in many instances. In a recent bruise, the color may be red or bluish. Later the bruise takes on a liver color, and finally it becomes yellow or copper-colored.

Treatment: While the corn remains aseptic it is possible to remedy it by removing the cause of pressure. The shoe is removed and the foot soaked in warm water which softens the horn. A kaolin poultice is even more effective. The horse is reshod, using a ¾-shoe, until the pain has disappeared, and then the shoe is replaced by one made a little wide at the heels, or with a feather-edged shoe which causes no pressure on the bar.

If the corn has been excised and has become infected, the foot will require drainage, an antibiotic dressing, and a ¾-shoe. In very lame horses suffering from a purulent corn, a ¾-bar shoe may be used, with exercise restricted to walking. The etiology of corns includes faulty conformation of the foot. Narrow, boxy feet are particularly susceptible and so are the direct opposites, flat, shallow feet which lack heels. Such feet, when viewed from the side, show no depth of heel whatever. Close shoeing which keeps the inner branch of the shoe well in from the wall to avoid brushing, is also a common cause of corns. Another cause is the wedging of a stone between the shoe and the base of the frog near the heel.

Chronic corns, when undiagnosed, often produce signs which may be attributed to navicular diseases, low ringbone, or sidebone. The lameness may be mild and intermittent, or it may be severe and continuous. An untreated suppurating corn has been regarded as the cause of quittor. Marked pain usually is evinced when the heel of the affected foot is gently squeezed.

Corns may be prevented by allowing the frog to make slight contact with the ground and thus take some of the weight off the foot. Heels should be allowed to grow down instead of being trimmed away. The toe should be kept short to avoid weight being thrown upon the heels, and a ¾- or feather-edged shoe may be worn. Many horses suffering from corns are inclined to turn in the toe of the affected foot, and thus throw more weight upon the inside heel. Any measures which lessen this tendency will be helpful. Sometimes a little more depth of shoe on the inner branch may help to correct this. An inch of the ground surface at the heel of the inner branch may be recessed.

SANDCRACK

This is characterized by a fissure in the horny wall of the foot which commences immediately below the coronary band and extends part way down the wall. Although cracks occur which appear to commence below the level of the coronary band and extend to the ground surface of the wall, these may be accounted for in 1 of 2 ways. The first explanation may be that the original sandcrack has commenced to undergo repair and the new wall has already grown some way down from the coronary band. If all goes well, complete recovery will be only a matter of time. It takes 8 to 10 months for a sandcrack to grow out after sound horn has started to develop from the coronary band. The second explanation is that a shoe has been cast or not used and the horse has split the hoof wall from the bottom edge upward.

True sandcracks appear more often at the quarters of a forefoot, and at the toe of the hindfoot, although they may make their appearance in other positions in either foot. Some cracks are simple and occur at right angles to the wall of the foot; others are set obliquely so that one thin layer of horn overlaps the other. The crack usually extends vertically down the foot and includes the whole thickness of the horny wall. It opens when weight is put upon the sole and the foot spreads; it closes when the foot is raised from the ground. According to the shape of the foot and the nature of the sandcrack, it may behave in the opposite fashion, opening when the foot is raised. The opening and closing of the crack pinch the sensitive laminae, producing pain and promoting the onset of a localized laminitis.

Etiology: The predisposing causes include complete drying of the foot which often may be attributed to routine rasping of the periople. Feet differ in texture. Some are dry and brittle, others more moist, plastic, and also more elastic, in much the same way that human fingernails vary. A lack of thyroid secretion may be responsible for sandcrack and broken hoofs. Many neglected sandcracks become infected and then they cause extreme lameness. Very frequently, the infection produces a painful enlargement of the coronet above the crack, and this may suppurate and rupture.

Clinical Signs: In hindlimb lameness related to an anteriorly situated sandcrack, the foot is lifted high, carried far forward, and brought to the ground heel first. This mode of progression is characteristic when lesions occur in the front of the coronet, including pyramidal disease and treads in this region. It is seen in both the fore- and hindfeet in these same circumstances.

Horse dealers once filled the cracks with pitch, wax, or gutta percha, polished the foot, and sold the animals as sound. Perhaps the vendors of horses today are more honorable men, but when examining a horse for soundness it always is well to look at the foot and make certain that a crack is not present.

Treatment: The wall should be completely divided transversely, through the crack, immediately below the coronary band, to prevent further opening and closing of the fissure which prevents the closing of the crack as new horn is secreted. The division may be be made with a hoof groover, a hoof saw, or better still with a flat, firing iron at a red heat. The foot may be rendered insensitive by a plantar nerve block. Movement of the wall at the cleft is then brought to a stop by the insertion of one or more soft iron clamps, made for the purpose. These are inserted in slots made with a special iron at a red heat, and they are closed by means of special forceps. For sandcrack at the hind toe a special shoe is worn, carrying 2 quarter-clips, one on either side of the fissure. This greatly helps to arrest its movement.

To hasten the growth of horn mild but repeated counterirritation applied over the coronary band is useful. An application of a biniodide of mercury blister every tenth day is sufficient.

KERATOMA

This is a growth of horn from the coronary band which extends gradually down the foot, causing pressure upon the sensitive laminae and the os pedis, in which it may produce a localized atrophy and grooving.

The growth nearly always appears at the toe of the foot although a few cases have been recorded in which it was situated at the quarter. These unusual positions usually are associated with damage to the coronary band. Cases have been seen in mules in which extensive growth of horn not only caused pressure within the foot but also extended down the external surface at the outer quarter (Fig. 12).

Etiology: The etiology of the ordinary type of keratoma which extends down the anterior surface of the foot is obscure. It is not always associated with apparent injury to, or irritation of, the coronary band but appears to arise from abnormal secretion of horn, and when the growth of horn is removed surgically there is no guarantee that it will not continue to be produced.

Clinical Signs: The onset of lameness is gradual, and in the early stages before bulging of the horn becomes apparent it may be considered to be the result of an injury to the anterior coronary region. There usually is no evidence that any trauma has occurred.

The presence of keratoma can be confirmed by removing the shoe, scrubbing the foot, and, if necessary, by paring away a thin wafer of horn from around the toe where the horny growth may be seen. This will be the case only when the condition has been present for at least 8 months. Sometimes the tumor does not grow down so far but may appear to be arrested when only part way down the wall. In a few cases, a sinus may be present at the toe through which a probe can be passed to encounter the more solid horny growth higher up inside the wall. Infection of the growth is rare.

Treatment: Treatment consists of removing the wall over the keratoma and extirpating it. The foot then is bound with an adhesive plaster bandage, the orifice at the toe of the sole may be covered by a piece of metal plate, and the shoe replaced. The horse rapidly improves in some cases, but in others the tumor continues to grow downward.

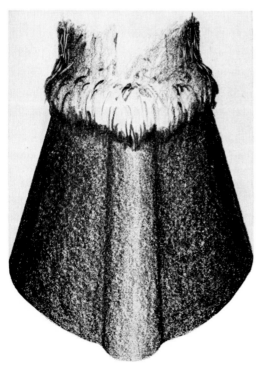

Fig. 12. An advanced keratoma.

SEEDY TOE

This condition should be mentioned although it does not frequently give rise to lameness. It is characterized by a separation at the toe of the foot between the wall and the sensitive laminae. The space becomes partly filled with degenerated, crumbly horn so that a hollow cavity exists which becomes visible when the sole is pared at the toe after removal of the shoe. Sometimes infection by various fungi may be suspected as the cause, but these usually are secondary invaders.

The cavity may be packed with cotton wool and tar, and the shoe replaced. There are more modern preparations which may be employed, but with no considerable prospect of greater success.

QUITTOR

Quittor is a sinus which connects the coronet with a suppurating or necrotic lateral cartilage. It was more common in draft horses and frequently arose from treads when horses were worked in pairs. It also can result from a suppurating corn. Like canker, quittor may be almost disregarded today as a cause of equine lameness.

SIDEBONE

A lateral cartilage of a foot which has undergone partial or complete ossification is identified as a sidebone. This ossification appears to be a physiologic process in the horse, especially in certain breeds, but there are a great many horses and ponies in which any degree of conversion of the cartilage into bone is a rare occurrence. The change occurs more commonly in heavy draft horses and in heavyweight hunters. Sidebones are seen far less commonly in the light breeds, although in advanced age a degree of ossification is frequently palpable. The occurrence of sidebones usually is bilateral and they are rarely found in the hindfeet (Fig. 13).

Etiology: Although heredity undoubtedly plays a part in the development of sidebone, there can be little doubt that the process of ossification is excited and accelerated by the effect of concussion upon the pedal bone, with which the cartilage is continuous. Faulty shoeing, leading to contracted heels, as well as laminitis can also result in sidebone. Any palpable degree of ossification of the lateral cartilage must be considered an unsoundness and animals showing the condition should not be bred.

Clinical Signs: In heavy breeds, the cartilage commences to harden at its anterior end, starting at its junction with the wing of the third phalanx at about the seventh year. This process continues until the 12th to 15th year when ossification may be complete.

The rate at which the cartilage becomes converted into bone is not constant in all 4 cartilages of the forefeet. Usually the lateral cartilage ossifies sooner than the medial, and in some instances one cartilage will change more markedly. Sidebone development may become so excessive that the entire lateral cartilage becomes ossified. When this happens, it is quite usual to find that the production of new bone is not confined to the lateral cartilage and there may be evidence that a concurrent ringbone is affecting the articulation between the second and third phalanges. This frequently starts in the pyramidal process and extends around the joint margins often with erosion of the articular surface. The accompanying lameness then is partly due to the low ringbone rather than to the sidebone.

Interference with the free movement of the foot arising from complete ossification of both lateral cartilages, in the absence of ringbone, is due to the fact that the alternate expansion and contraction of the foot normally produced by pressure upon the frog and plantar cushion are restricted because the lateral cartilages have become unyielding. The pumping action which maintains the pedal circulation of blood is thus impeded.

The spurs of bone which on rare occasions develop upon an ossified cartilage undoubtedly cause lameness whether or not ringbone is present, but these are encountered infrequently. It is likely that their origin is trauma such as a tread from another horse. When lameness is present and the horse is moved in a circle, the greatest pain is shown when the affected leg is on the inside. On inspecting the

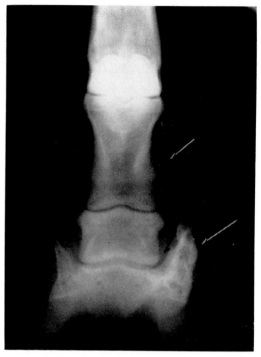

Fig. 13. Sidebones, navicular periligamentitis, and periostitis of first phalanx. Radiograph by J. P. Manning, D.V.M.

shoe of such a horse, it will be noted by the character of wear that the foot is breaking over at the outside of the toe. Close inspection will show that when the horse puts the affected foot down, the outside wall strikes first and then the foot rocks to the inside wall. When the ossification process is somewhat advanced, pressure on the cartilage above the coronet almost always will produce pain.

Diagnosis: The diagnosis of sidebone is easy when the cartilages have ossified throughout a considerable part of their length but it may be quite difficult to diagnose by palpation early changes in the cartilages. To do so, one must be familiar with the feel of a healthy lateral cartilage. Even with horse's foot firmly planted on the ground, it is easy to depress the cartilage with one's thumb. To make quite certain a sidebone is present or not, the foot should be lifted from the ground and supported by one hand while the thumb and fingers of the free hand follow the cartilage from back to front and test its flexibility. The free edge of each cartilage should be palpated and its resistance compared with the opposite foot, noting the degree and extent of the flexibility. It never is wise to conclude that one cartilage is normal and the other abnormal, since some degree of abnormality may be present in both cartilages.

Perhaps the best way to distinguish sidebone from navicular disorders is by observing that in navicular disease the horse is lame when going either way in a circle. Differentiating sidebone from other foot lameness occasionally can be difficult. Bruised soles will react to hoof testers and can be demonstrated with a hoof knife. Gravel or penetrating foreign bodies show more inflammation and a fuller pulse as well as localized tenderness. There is more heat and pulse pressure associated with laminitis. Fractures of the os pedis produce more heat, pulse pressure, and lameness and also are characterized by sudden onset.

Radiographs taken to confirm a diagnosis of sidebone will, in a considerable number of cases, present difficulties of interpretation. It must be kept in mind that replacement of cartilage by bone is part of the normal aging process. Consequently, one cannot decide whether or not a horse is lame simply by examining a radiograph.

Treatment: Surgical treatment will produce excellent results if the inflammation and ossification of the cartilages have stopped. The surgical procedures include posterior digital neurectomy and operations designed to increase the width of the foot. A more conservative therapeutic approach is to soak the feet or use ice boots to reduce inflammation. Having the foot balanced properly is helpful and if difficulty is encountered here, removing the shoes and pasturing the horse for a month often will accomplish this. The use of full leathers under the shoes will help reduce pain and lameness, and aspirin will provide relief for short periods. The corticosteroids or phenylbutazone will be helpful in acute cases.

PUNCTURE WOUNDS

A longitudinal section of a horse's foot will show that the navicular bone with its synovial attachments lies above the frog approximately an inch behind its terminal point. The pedal bone does not lie flat upon the sole of the foot for its hind part is raised as it rests upon the plantar cushion. Thus, the sharp outer rim of the floor of the pedal bone is directed downward and its toe rests upon the sensitive sole close to its periphery where sole and wall meet.

The os pedis is anchored in place by the sensitive laminae which are attached to the periosteum of the bone over its anterior and lateral aspects. These laminae mesh with those of the horny wall and sole. The sensitive laminae become shorter as they are traced backward and end in a number of short laminae which unite with the horny laminae of the bars of the foot.

When looking at this section of the foot, it is apparent that a nail which penetrates and enters the lateral lacuna of the frog at any point between its extremity and halfway up its length may enter the navicular synovial sheath and reach the navicular bone itself. Fortunately, it would require a nail of 1½ to 2 inches in length to reach the navicular bone, and it is not very often that a nail penetrates the foot for such a distance. Deep penetration is not necessary for a nail to cause serious damage since feet, as well as nails, are never sterile and when infection is carried into the plantar cushion it may easily spread in an upward direction, especially if bottom drainage is not provided. Punctures of the sole of the hindfoot are more likely to terminate at or in the plantar cushion owing to the distance between the ground and the lateral lacuna of the frog when the foot rests on the ground. However, a nail entering the lateral lacuna of the frog, close to the heel, might well puncture the synovial membrane of the coffin joint near the anterior end of the lateral cartilage (Fig. 14).

In either a fore- or hindfoot, a nail more than 1 inch in length, which enters the horny sole between the toe and a circle of a ½ inch radius, having the point of the frog as its center, will in all probability puncture the pedal bone. It may chip small fragments from its surface, or cause a fracture through the body of the bone.

A nail which enters the lateral lacuna of the frog may, by repeated blows as the foot strikes the ground, be driven out of sight and its presence may be detected only by trimming the area and by careful inspection. When a small-headed nail enters the sole of the foot, its presence may be made apparent only by scrubbing the foot and trimming away thin layers of the sole with a hoof knife.

Horses and cattle differ a good deal with regard to the type of foreign bodies which they collect in their feet. Cattle pick up short objects, though horses which possess slightly concave hoofs raised from the ground level by shoes, collect nails which are seldom less than an inch in length. Most of these are found in the forefeet, but the shoe of a forefoot of a trotting horse sometimes may land upon a nail lying flat on the ground and set it spinning on its own axis. It may then be picked up by the descending hindfoot.

A blacksmith occasionally may injure a foot by driving the nail through the horny wall into the junction of the horny and sensitive laminae. On other occasions, a nail may bend very slightly beneath the hammer and if this is not noticed, the curved nail will exert undue pressure upon the sensitive laminae even if it does not actually puncture them. This is termed "nail-binding." The offending nail usually can be detected by gentle blows from a light hammer applied over each nail. Special testing pincers may be used to accomplish the same thing.

Before removing the shoe, the foot should be brushed clean with soap and water. After the shoe has been removed the nails should be examined to determine whether they are blood-stained, or are damp and black in color due to the action of purulent exudate. Frequently, the nail will show no sign of anything unusual. The foot should again be subjected to gentle pinching with a forceps to observe if any blackened pus emerges from a nail hole. If the foot has been shod for 8 to 10 days, this may be observed. Usually, however, pain and lameness are manifested from 3 to 5 days after shoeing and by this time little pus will have developed.

Treatment: The suspected nail hole should be enlarged with a suitable knife, at the same

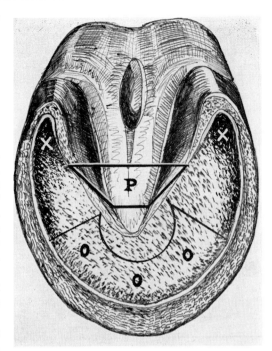

Fig. 14. Ground surface of hoof. The X's mark common sites for occurrence of corns. Punctures in this area may reach the joint capsule of the pedal joint. Punctures in area labeled P may reach the navicular bone or bursa. Nail punctures at sites labeled 0 may reach the third phalanx.

time thinning the horn of the sole in close proximity to the nail hole to relieve pressure and pain. After drainage of entrapped pus, the whole foot should be immersed in warm water to which 2 to 3 tablespoons of salt are added. The horse should be given an injection of tetanus antitoxin at once. An antibiotic may be injected parenterally and a dressing of an antibiotic applied to the infected area. The antibiotic may be administered topically by use of tubes prepared for intramammary infusion. A warm kaolin poultice applied to the sole and wall and covered with a thick layer of cotton wool will ease pain, keep the part clean, and provide a comfortable surface on which the foot may rest. When the shoe is replaced, the infected nail hole should be left empty.

Quite frequently, the owner does not suspect the foot to be the origin of lameness and fails to solicit veterinary care. In this instance, an abscess may develop within the foot, commencing at the puncture site and continuing upward between the sensitive laminae. The abscess eventually ruptures and discharges above the coronary band, usually at the quarters of the foot. This gives the horse a little relief but still does not provide sufficient drainage, and the offending nail remains. These coronary abscesses often have been confused with a quittor, but they usually do not involve necrosis of the lateral cartilage, nor do they persist after drainage has been obtained at the sole of the foot.

One of the common objects which may puncture the sole of the foot, and not infrequently cause damage to the pedal bone, is the toe clip of the horse's own shoe. A partly cast shoe is the basic cause of this injury. This dangerous accident has caused the death or destruction of a great many horses. Sometimes, a horse treads not on his own toe clip, but upon that of a discarded shoe.

Pyramidal Disease

Pyramidal disease is a periostitis of the extensor process of the third phalanx with resultant exostosis. Frequently, there will be an avulsion fracture of the extensor process

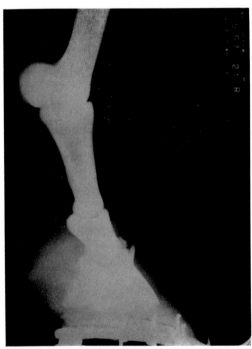

Fig. 15. Pyramidal disease.

or of the exostosis. In many cases there will be some development of low ringbone. A differentiation between pyramidal disease and low ringbone by palpation is impossible. The bump on the hoof resulting from an exostosis may appear to be somewhat lower in pyramidal disease than in low ringbone. This enlargement will grow down to the ground, producing a foot which is longer and less round than before. Cold applications are useful if inflammation is present and analgesics are about the only medicaments regularly indicated. In the radiograph, the animal shown with this condition has been used in hunting for 2 seasons with nothing but daily applications of vaseline to the coronary band. (Fig. 15).

Lameness Originating in the Second Phalanx

Acute inflammation of the second phalanx may be caused by treads from other horses, and some animals tread on their own coronets when turning while in harness. Horses which work in pairs frequently sustain treads on the outer aspect of the coronet, from the feet of their partners. Light horses not infrequently rap the coronet on the top rail of a gate or fence, and kicking bouts between 2 horses also may give rise to injuries of the second phalanx.

Sometimes dermatitis occurs over the coronets of heavy draft horses, particularly of those with a good deal of feather. This usually involves the heels and the posterior aspect of the fetlocks, and may cause serious cracks or fissures of the heels and hind part of the pasterns, resulting in severe lameness.

Swelling of a coronet's anterior surface may be associated with pyramidal disease. This disease, like all other lesions which affect this part of the coronet, produces a characteristic type of lameness in which the foot is advanced a little farther than its fellow, with the toe of the foot slightly elevated. The foot comes to ground heel first and toe last. Once seen, this type of lameness never can be mistaken for any other, and always will be related to its correct source.

The diagnosis of coronitis is easy and in most cases, apart from those associated with ringbone or with disease of the pyramidal process of the pedal bone, the prognosis is good.

The possible complications include the formation of an exostosis on the second phalanx and its extension to the third; also damage to the coronary band which may give rise to false quarters, a sandcrack, or in rare instances to a keratome. If the lateral cartilage is extensively bruised, a quittor may develop subsequently.

The treatment is enforced rest with intermittent, light exercise and the application of warm (not hot) fomentations, or a kaolin poultice. In some cases, antibiotics are indicated.

Sesamoiditis

Inflammation at the sesamoid region is encountered more frequently in the lighter breeds, being particularly common among hunters and steeplechasers. There is an associated lameness that is either constant or increases with work. Years ago it was seen rather frequently in Shires that were worked on hard roads but the importance of this occurrence is now mainly historical. Most of the cases encountered today occur in steeplechasers and to a slightly less degree in horses raced on the flat.

Etiology: The etiology is either trauma or tearing of the attachments of the suspensory ligament to the sesamoid bones by strain or concussion. Sesamoiditis usually is associated with inflammation and distention of the metacarpophalangeal sheath. The synovial membrane of this sheath lubricates the intersesamoid ligament which forms a pulley-like surface for the passage of the deep flexor tendon.

The inflammatory changes usually occur first in the substance of the sesamoid bones with necrotic changes in their articular surfaces resulting in ulceration. Both the anterior and posterior surfaces often are involved. Not infrequently, fusion occurs between the anterior surface of the sesamoids and the posterior surface of the lower end of the metacarpal bone. In advanced cases, the articulation between the lower end of the third metacarpal (or metatarsal) and the upper end of the proximal phalanx may become involved, and not infrequently ulcerated. Sesamoiditis affects both fore- and hindlimbs but as the forelimbs suffer most from concussion, the condition is more prevalent in front than behind. Suspected cases should always be x-rayed, because a distinct possibility exists that a fracture is present.

Clinical Signs: Swelling at the back of the fetlock joint with distention of the metacarpophalangeal sheath characterizes sesamoiditis. The affected area is painful and the horse resists gentle squeezing of the hind part of the fetlock between fingers and thumb. In the standing position, the fetlock is held in flexion with the heel of the shoe raised slightly from the ground. When walked and trotted, the horse shows difficulty in starting and makes several rather ineffectual steps, using the toe of the foot without placing a great deal of weight on the foot or heel. By careful palpation, the diseased sesamoids can be distinguished and usually some degree of thickening of the flexor tendons also is distinguishable, especially in the region of the intersesamoidean ligament. This usually leads to some shortening of the tendons with moderate knuckling at the fetlock. In advanced cases, adhesions may occur between the bones of the fetlock and the sesamoids with fixation of the fetlock joint (Fig. 16, 17, 18).

The prognosis never is good, although if the condition is diagnosed early, it can sometimes be arrested.

Treatment: Shoeing with heels or with a bar welded across the 2 heels of the shoe, to raise these ½ inch from the ground, relieves pressure on the intersesamoidean ligament and the underlying sesamoid bones.

Cold water, diathermy, blistering, astringents, and sedative applications have all been employed. Probably the most effective treatment is the application of an elastic adhesive bandage over a thick layer of cotton wool, the bandage extending from halfway up the hoof to within a few inches of the lower limit of the knee or hock. In the early stages, corticosteroid therapy may be instituted. If improvement is manifested, the heels of the shoe should be gradually reduced to normal. When the acute stages have subsided, line firing and

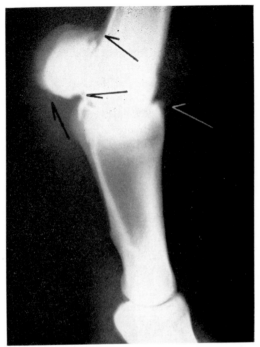

Fig. 16. Sesamoiditis and exostosis at anterior surface of proximal end of first phalanx. Radiograph by J. P. Manning, D.V.M.

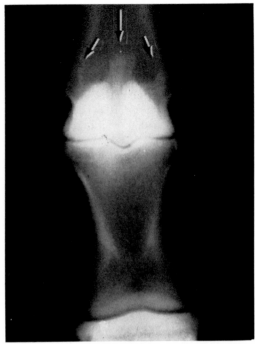

Fig. 17. Calcification of abaxial attachments of the suspensory ligament to the proximal sesamoids. Calcification of the intersesamoidean ligament. Radiograph by J. P. Manning, D.V.M.

blistering followed by 3 months at pasture without shoes are advisable.

FRACTURE OF THE SESAMOID

Horses which have developed an ostitis of the sesamoid with rarefaction of the bone, are likely to sustain fracture of one or both sesamoid bones when galloping.

Each sesamoid bone is subjected to the opposing pull of the suspensory ligament above and the ventral sesmoidean ligaments below at the moment when the full weight of the front end of the body is thrown upon the fetlock joint. In the normal course of events, the attachments of the superficial digital flexor tendon behind the intermediate phalanx, and of the deep digital flexor tendon into the distal phalanx, provide a margin of safety and prevent overextension of the fetlock. This margin, however, is dependent entirely upon perfect synchronization between the flexor and extensor muscles. If the flexors fail to contract at the proper time, the extensor muscles will pull the toe of the foot forward, overextending the

fetlock joint. As a result, the proximal phalanx stands in danger of being broken in half.

Clinical Signs: Fracture of the sesamoids may occur in either of 2 directions, longitudinally or transversely. The latter direction is by far the more common. When both sesamoids fracture transversely the fetlock naturally sinks toward the ground. If the flexor muscles function in time, however, the fetlock will not contact the ground and the foot will retain its normal position with the sole flat and without upward tilting. This will not be so if the deep digital flexor tendon ruptures simultaneously with the occurrence of fracture.

Following fracture or fissure of a sesamoid, marked inflammatory changes will occur in the sesamoid region with evidence of severe pain on palpation. The degree of swelling usually will make palpation difficult, although immediately following the accident and before the swelling becomes tense, it may be possible to detect the separation between the broken portions of the bone. X-ray examination will verify the diagnosis (Fig. 19).

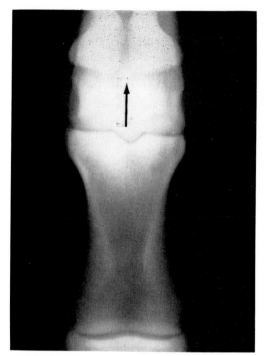

Fig. 18. Rupture of sesamoidean ligaments and upward displacement of the proximal sesamoids. Radiograph by J. P. Manning, D.V.M.

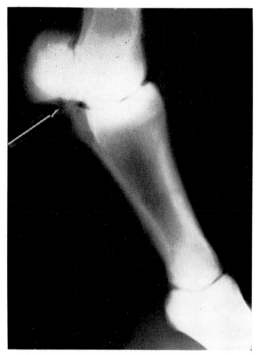

Fig. 19. Fracture of proximal sesamoid. Arrow indicates fragment. Radiograph by J. P. Manning, D.V.M.

When the fracture occurs longitudinally, which is not common, dropping of the fetlock will not be observed.

Treatment: Maintaining reduction of a transverse fracture of the sesamoid bones is quite hopeless, especially when it is the culmination of previous ostitis. If after prolonged treatment some degree of fibrous union should result, the horse probably will be of little use.

When the fracture is longitudinal, with no sinking of the fetlock, the horse should be confined to a stall and the heel raised by means of a special shoe. The fetlock may be supported additionally by plaster bandages. After 2 to 3 months, the horse should be shod with wedge heels, the height of which is reduced at each successive shoeing.

The prognosis is never good even in this type of fracture, and few horses recover sufficiently to run again.

When union between the fractured portions occurs, it is only fibrous and may break down again later. Another 6 to 12 months' rest is needed after the horse is fit to wear a normal shoe, and during this period one may line-fire and blister to provide further support. American veterinarians experience good results following surgical removal of the smaller fragments of the fractured bone. See Chapter 26.

OSTEOPERIOSTITIS OF THE FIRST PHALANX

An osteoperiostitis affecting the medial head of the proximal phalanx where it articulates with the lower end of the metacarpal bone once was extremely common in horses employed for pulling carriages. When horses turned sharply, they frequently would injure the inner side of a fetlock with the inside of the opposite foot. This produced an inflammation and eventual production of a ring of osteophytes surrounding the medial articular surface of the joint. In a certain percentage of cases, small erosions appeared on the articular surface and caused even more marked lameness (Fig. 20).

The prognosis was not good in these cases and although some horses returned to work it was never long before they were lame again.

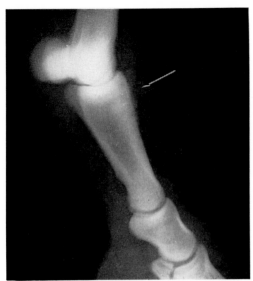

Fig. 20. Chronic, calcifying periostitis of anterior surface of first phalanx. Radiograph by J. P. Manning, D.V.M.

This condition is by no means uncommon in race horses and particularly in polo ponies. The painful enlargement on the medial head of the proximal phalanx and the continuous lameness are sufficiently diagnostic. Prevention is easier than cure, and in polo ponies brushing pads are recommended where practicable. In the treatment of fetlock injuries, a crepe bandage covered by an adhesive, elastic bandage, not too tightly applied, will produce good results when recovery is possible. As in all lamenesses, resting the animal in a level field is one of the best treatments.

Osselets

Osselets occur at the fetlocks along the anterior margin of the articular cartilage of the large metacarpal bone. When they appear they are hot, painful, and comparatively soft swellings. The horse travels with a choppy, stilted gait, and the lameness is constant. Flexion of the fetlock joint often will produce pain. Radiographs will show a rarefaction of the bone where the joint capsule is attached. Later, calcium will be deposited and an exostosis will form in the area. The degree of lameness will depend on the distance the lesion invades the joint and the articular cartilage.

Treatment includes rest, reduction of inflammation with cold water and astringents, and firing when the inflammation is gone. The firing pattern generally includes the whole ankle and both sides of the joint. Radiation therapy for new osselets has proved quite successful. Diathermy also is useful when these lesions are starting.

Ringbone

Probably more disagreement has resulted concerning the diagnosis of ringbone than about any other form of equine unsoundness.

There are 2 main reasons. The first is that no one definition of ringbone has ever been universally agreed upon. The second is that it is difficult to determine the nature of the changes taking place in bones and articulations while the horse is still alive. Radiographs provide some information concerning the extent and development of the process.

The term, ringbone, applies whenever the articular surfaces of one or more joints from the fetlock down are diseased and eroded. Arthritis of any of these joints usually is attended, sooner or later, by the development of osteophytes surrounding the edges of the articular surfaces.

The bones below the fetlock, however, also may develop an osteoperiostitis which produces swelling of the phalangeal region and the production of exostoses, even larger sometimes than those present in "true ringbone." The only difference between the 2 conditions is that in true ringbone the presence of exostoses is complicated by erosive arthritis. In "false ringbone" the exostoses are present, but the joint surfaces are normal. In either condition, the bony outgrowths from the 2 bones which contribute to the joint may become ankylosed, and immobilize the joint. Even if the pain is lessened, or ceases altogether, the horse still will show some impairment of gait owing to an inability to make further use of the articulation. If the limb from the fetlock down is anesthetized, the restriction in gait will persist.

It is not easy for the most experienced observer to run his fingers and thumb over a pronounced bony swelling in the phalangeal region and decide without a doubt that the enlargement represents a true articular ringbone with surrounding exostoses, and is not the result of an osteoperiostitis involving the shaft of the bone and its periosteum with no actual invasion of the joint cavity.

The degree of lameness sometimes may be of assistance in making a diagnosis. If the lameness has appeared within the past few weeks, is severe, and is accompanied by a swelling, still compressible, which can be traced around the articular edges, one may be justified in suspecting the presence of ringbone. At this stage, a radiograph likely will not reveal significant changes.

In false ringbone, the exostosis tends to form first around the shaft of the bone and extend to the articular edges. The rate of growth of the exostosis usually is considerably faster (and more extensive) than in early cases of true ringbone.

Although these statements are based on experience, too much value must not be placed upon them since a great deal of variation exists in the nature and position of the lesions, and the rate of growth of exostoses in both true and false ringbone.

Etiology: True ringbone is believed to have a genetic influence, or a susceptibility for arthritis. What happened during the life of the horse will be influenced by the nature of the work and its amount, the surface on which the work is performed, and the sensitivity of the particular animal to the influences of concussion.

False ringbone also appears to have a familial incidence. It certainly occurs far more commonly in some breeds than in others, and more frequently in the progeny of certain stallions.

Ringbone may result from traumatic injury, especially from blows upon the coronet, faulty shoeing, wirecuts, or rope burns. Such cases may remain lame for many months but the prognosis is hopeful. However, the prognosis in articular ringbone, if it can be diagnosed, always is poor. Ringbone also may appear as a sequel to degenerative bony diseases such as osteomalacia and rickets.

A great deal of the difference in incidence of ringbone may be attributed to the degree of concussion transmitted to the coronets and pasterns in different breeds. Thoroughbreds advance the limbs and land upon their heels rather than upon a flat sole. Most ponies do the same. The larger draft breeds possess large, flat feet and considerable knee action, which cause them to hammer their feet upon the ground.

An inflamed bone, such as the first phalanx when exposed to the effects of concussion, loses its pinkish-grayness and changes to a livid or dark blue color, and this is more obvious when one views the bone through its articular cartilage. This cartilage contains no lymphatics, blood vessels or nerves, but is surrounded by a highly vascular layer which nourishes it. The inflammatory changes travel down the long axis of the bone to the perichondrium. Exudates form there and isolate areas of articular cartilage from the perichondrium with the result that necrosis occurs, followed by ulceration. This happens more readily on a concave surface than on a convex one since the articular concavity lies nearer the center of the inflammatory area.

Clinical Signs: Ringbones occur in 2 locations, high and low. A high ringbone involves the distal end of the first phalanx and the pastern joint. A low ringbone involves the distal end of the second phalanx and the coffin joint. The first points of inflammation and ossification in ringbone are at the attachments of the collateral ligaments of the involved joint. In high ringbone, this point also is the insertion of the superficial digital flexor tendon. From these points, the inflammation and proliferative changes proceed around the bone passing to the dorsal, but possibly to the volar surface. The amount of lameness is in direct relation to the extent that proliferative changes invade areas under the extensor tendon above or the deep digital flexor tendon below. The proliferating bone also invades the surfaces of the involved joint and ankylosis is possible. High ringbones are somewhat more common than low. They occur in all 4 feet impartially.

There is a possibility of error if one concludes that all cases of lameness in which there is marked pain and formation of bony exostoses surrounding the pastern are due to either true or false ringbone. In light horses, especially in race horses, steeplechasers, and hunters, such signs often accompany split pastern.

Peculiarities in the gait may help locate the exact site of the ringbone. When it occurs in front, the heel often strikes on the ground first, and when the lesion is behind, the toe strikes first. The fetlock of the affected leg often is held rigid and this produces a hitch in the flight of the foot when moving. These clues are a help only in well-developed cases. They do not appear when the trouble is starting.

A well-developed high ringbone will show a convex bulge in the upper surface of the pastern and a low ringbone will, for a time, create a bulge just below the coronet at the toe. Little heat is present with this condition and swelling is the result of underlying calcium deposits.

When a ringbone is starting the horse will warm out of the lameness. Later, the lameness will be constant and may increase with exercise, depending on the position of the lesion. It is only in the later stages when calcium deposits have formed, that the lesion can be palpated.

Radiographs will demonstrate the lesions before they can be felt. Anteroposterior and lateral views should be taken. On occasion, oblique views will show the lesions when the other views are negative (Fig. 21, 22, 23).

Treatment: Treatment of true ringbone always is unrewarding. When one appears to have attained some measure of success, he may conclude that the diagnosis was at fault. A good many cases of lameness arising from false ringbone recover in time, with or without treatment. Most of these are fired and blistered or treated by short-wave therapy.

Two granulating articular surfaces given rest and freedom from concussion sometimes unite, and a deposit of bony material around their articular margins may assist in producing fixation of the joint. This is the way in which cure may, in theory, be brought about. In practice, too often the healing of one joint causes undue strain upon another, and the process may commence again at a new site.

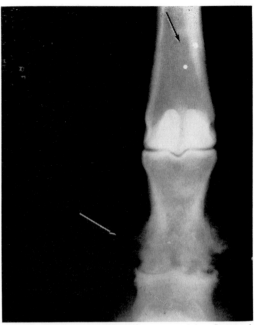

Fig. 21. Ringbone involving the pastern joint. Proximal arrow indicates gunshot. Radiograph by J. P. Manning, D.V.M.

The only real hope in ringbone therapy lies in prolonged rest, preferably in a level field, and where grass is not too plentiful so that the horse will have to move about to keep fed. The horse should be unshod and should not be worked until some months after the lameness has disappeared. When put to work, attention must be paid to the shoeing and the feet must be kept perfectly level. Whether a light or a heavy shoe gives the better result has been a debatable point through several generations. In any case a stout leather, a rubber sheet, or a bar pad between foot and shoe diminish concussion. Sectioning the horn may relieve the pain in low ringbone when the pyramidal process is involved and when exostoses are present on the lower half of the intermediate phalanx, but it can do nothing to relieve pain caused by ulceration of the articular surfaces. Point firing combined with blistering has been used for many years, but whether this has any salutary effect apart from insuring rest is doubtful.

Once the lesion has ankylosed, affected horses can be worked to a limited extent.

The economic consideration often is the primary one, and one must consider whether

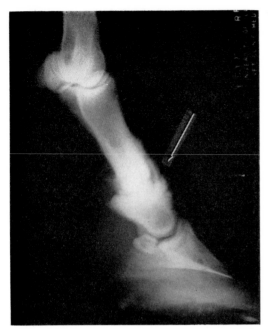

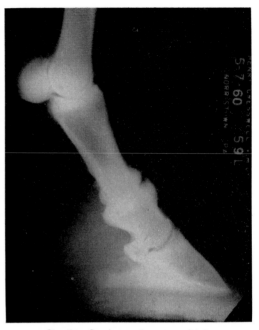

Fig. 22. Ringbone at pastern joint. Radiograph by J. P. Manning, D.V.M.

Fig. 23. Ringbone at pastern joint.

the expense of an idle horse is justifiable when the prospects are small for the animal's regaining permanent usefulness.

SPLIT PASTERN

The bony injuries arising in cases of split pastern range from comminuted fractures in which the bones have broken into a number of pieces, to cases in which both the shaft of a bone and one of its articular surfaces are included, down to bony fissures. When the fissure does not include an articulation (a rather rare event) recovery usually follows, with some permanent enlargement. Cases in which an articular surface is involved hardly ever become free from lameness.

KNUCKLING AT THE FETLOCK

Etiology: This condition, together with bowing of the knees, may be congenital in foals. With manipulation and patient treatment quite a large proportion of such newborn which can receive milk from the mother and survive the first week or two, grow into normal foals. The tendons appear to withstand

a great deal of stretching provided the plantar surface of the foot reaches the ground. When the deep digital flexor tendon is included the prospects are not so good. One may wonder sometimes whether the condition is wholly one of shortened tendons or if a great deal of the apparent contraction may not be due to a too firm and close connection between the various tendinous and ligamentous structures behind the knee and cannon, and the peritendinous aponeurosis.

In adult horses, knuckling at the fetlock results from joint infection, improper shoeing, contraction of the flexor tendons, and subcarpal or suspensory ligament abnormality. Each of these produces its own characteristic appearances and stance. When the articular surfaces of the phalangeal bones are inflamed a variable degree of knuckling may reflect a voluntary effort to relieve pain.

In cases where radial paralysis has persisted for many months, the degree of tendon contraction resulting from flexion of the knee and fetlock may become so marked that there may be difficulty, after recovery from the paralysis, in getting the heel to the ground. Forced exercise then may produce flexor strain which adds to the general disability and may even terminate in permanent contraction. Rather than permit this to happen, one may weld a bar of iron, ½ inch thick, across the heels of the shoe, thinning and beveling it at the toe. After 2 to 3 weeks the bar is replaced by another, half its thickness, and after a similar interval the horse may return to a level shoe.

Fetlock lameness resulting from sesamoiditis, with distention of the superior sesamoid sheath, will produce knuckling directed toward the relief of pain. This knuckling may become chronic unless some measures can be taken to relieve the inflammation.

Clinical Signs: When the knuckling is due to shortening of the tendons or other structures situated behind the cannon, several degrees of the condition may be recognized:

1. The limb from the fetlock down is upright, with no flexion of the pastern.

2. The fetlock joint forms an open angle at its posterior border.

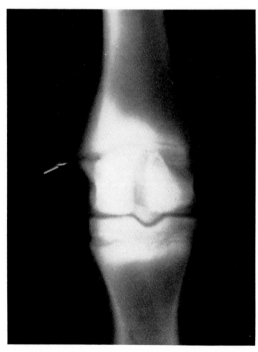

Fig. 24. Epiphysitis. Lesion simulates rickets. Radiograph by J. P. Manning, D.V.M.

3. The front of the fetlock projects in a forward direction so that a line dropped vertically from it would meet the ground in front of the toe of the foot.

Contraction of the deep digital flexor tendon will produce volar flexion of the limb from the fetlock down. The heel of the foot is lifted from the ground and weight is taken on the toe of the foot, or shoe, during walking.

Acute sprain of the subcarpal ligament may cause straightening of the phalangeal joints, but in most cases when shortening of this ligament occurs as the result of either acute or chronic inflammatory changes, the deep digital flexor tendon also becomes involved in the contraction. As a result, the type of knuckling corresponds with that just described.

When the superficial digital flexor tendon is contracted, either alone or in company with the suspensory ligament, the degree of knuckling may be slight or severe according to the amount of contraction, but the foot will remain flat on the ground without elevation of the heel. This applies mainly to cases in which the contraction is due to chronic changes resulting from tendonitis.

When any of the structures behind the knee, cannon, and pastern have been strained, there first will be knuckling with raising of the heel of the foot, sometimes entirely the result of the pain produced. Injury of the superficial digital flexor is in all probability the least painful of all these, and it is quite likely that in acute strain confined to this tendon, the heel may not be raised and the whole foot will rest on the ground. Usually, the trauma which produces sprain of the superficial tendon is so severe that it includes some of the other tendinous or ligamentous structures.

CONTRACTED TENDON

This term was once used chiefly to describe a condition of older draft horses which did heavy work on paved streets. From the constant pounding, one or both of the flexor tendons of one or more legs would shorten. Tenotomy of the affected structure offered a satisfactory solution. The term, "contracted ten-

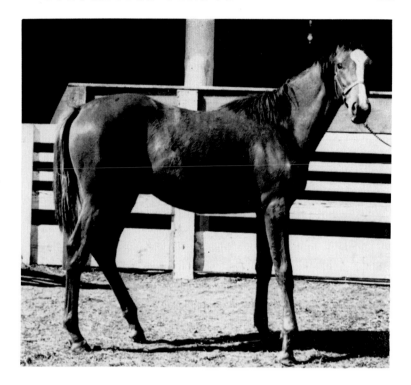

Fig. 25. Contracted tendon in yearling.

dons," today refers to a condition which has an enigmatic etiology and a miserable prognosis.

Among the light breeds which constitute most modern horse practices, it occurs almost entirely in horses less than 2 years of age, and in my experience (H.C.), most cases seem to appear in yearlings. This obviously removes the stress and strain of heavy work as an etiology. In these cases, the history usually will reveal that the affected animal has been standing with one or the other knee flexed more and more frequently. Inspection will show that the angle of the pastern is very steep, the ankle is twisted to the outside, and a corresponding deformity exists in the shape of the foot. Palpation almost always will reveal that the deep flexor tendon is under more tension than the superficial flexor tendon. The amount of pain, shown by the readiness of the horse to lie down, will depend on the amount of contraction, and arises chiefly from muscle spasm due to increased tension. When sectioned and examined, these tendons show a diffuse inflammation.

The contemporary theory regarding cause is that there is a disparity in growth rate between the metacarpal bone and the tendons. This is difficult to accept, since it would be a very narrowly selective disparity of growth that would involve one bone and predominantly one tendon in chiefly the front legs. The best evidence indicates that this is a hereditary condition.

Therapy, to date, has been useless. When the clinical signs and the history indicate this diagnosis, it is well to suggest the diagnosis and stall for time. The involved horses frequently are valuable animals and the owners will not be happy when euthanasia is advised. The condition is rare enough so that many people who have wide experience with horses have neither seen or even heard of it.

The best therapeutic approach is to immediately have plates put on the front feet. The blacksmith should trim the foot to correct the deviation, lower the heel as far as possible, and preserve the length of the toe as much as possible. The plates should be reset every 3 weeks and trimmed as previously described, because it is never possible to arrive at a decent foot on the first, second or even the third trimming. The object of this approach is to prevent further shortening of the tendon by increasing tension gradually. Further, by straightening the foot, joint damage is minimized. Pain may be relieved with the corticosteroids, or more often with phenylbutazone. At some point in this process the pain and discomfort to the horse will become so severe that humane considerations will dictate removal of the plates and trimming the toe down to a natural level. This will provide relief from pain and even what appears to be a remission for several months. However, the ankles will in all likelihood still be twisted and frequently osselets will form. When the process of contraction starts again, as it surely will, the practitioner is in a much stronger position to advise euthanasia.

Rupture of the Flexor Tendons

If complete rupture of any of the structures behind the cannon occurs when the horse is at full gallop, the animal usually falls and may turn a somersault. When the rupture is partial, the horse may pull up with difficulty on 3 legs while evincing considerable pain as shown by elevating the injured leg and shaking it. In complete rupture of the deep flexor, the fetlock descends and the toe of the foot turns upward, so that the back of the fetlock may rest on the ground. When complete rupture of the superficial flexor occurs, the fetlock sinks but the foot remains flat on the ground. When both flexor tendons rupture completely, the suspensory ligament ruptures also. The fetlock then sinks entirely to the ground and the toe of the foot turns upward.

In horses which have suffered previously from tendonitis, and in which there already is a marked thickening and increase in the amount of fibrous tissue normally present in the tendons, as well as in the metacarpophalangeal fibrous aponeurosis, the degree of breakdown occurring in the tendinous structures may be limited in spite of rupture of some of its component parts. Given complete rest, preferably in slings, such horses may make a useful recovery, but when conditions

compel the horse to make immediate use of its damaged limb, complete breakdown may ensue.

Treatment: All that usefully can be done therapeutically is to support injured tendons by elastic, adhesive bandages applied over a thick layer of cotton, or to encase the leg in a clay dressing made of finely powdered kaolin mixed into a stiff paste with vaseline and supported by layers of bandages. The heel can be built up when this is needed by surgical shoeing and thus the foot can be restored to a level position. More important, however, is that the owners of injured horses should be encouraged to await natural recovery with composure and without undue optimism.

Bowed Tendon

Bowed tendon is the horseman's term for severe strain of one or both flexor tendons. These ruptures do not produce a discontinuity of the structure. The severity of the lesion depends on the number of fiber bundles which are involved. There is a varying amount of subcutaneous extravasation of serum and blood. In appearance, the flexor tendons appear to arch backward from the knee to the ankle. The terms "high bow" and "low bow" refer to whether the lesion is mainly just below the knee or above the ankle. Actually, this is in no sense a pinpoint lesion and "high or low" makes little difference. The check ligaments are involved more often in high bows. There is a great deal of heat over the torn tendons and considerable soreness, accompanied by moderate to severe lameness.

Horses with excessively long and sloping pasterns are predisposed to strains of the flexor tendons. In race horses, early warning of injury usually is given by the evidence of heat over the tendons, pointing of the toe, soreness and slight thickening of the tendons on palpation, and by a degree of lameness. The tendons always should be palpated with the leg flexed, and the cannon bone parallel to the ground, so they can be felt in their entirety.

Early treatment involves liberal applications of cold water from a hose for at least an hour (preferably more) a day. The part should be bandaged and astringent lotion used overnight. Confinement to a stall is essential. When the inflammation has subsided (this usually takes several days of treatment) there are several lines of therapy which can be followed. Whatever approach is used, it cannot be emphasized too strongly that rest is an important adjunct of any treatment. Six months of complete rest is the minimum that can be considered sufficient. Violation of this maxim surely will reduce the effectiveness of any treatment used.

In the past few years a surgical treatment of bowed tendons has been used which consists of removal of the subcutaneous clots and fluid through a cutaneous incision. The advantage of this procedure is that it reduces the amount of adhesions formed along the tendons and, consequently, function is more likely preserved. Its disadvantage is that there is such a marked reduction in swelling and soreness that the owner or trainer will not carry out the confinement program faithfully.

The most common therapy is firing and/or blistering. I prefer to use a blister on show horses. Even if it is necessary to repeat the treatment, a clean leg can be produced with no external scarring to offend the eyes of the judges. Hunters, jumpers, and race horses must be fired to be reasonably sure that the tendons will withstand the strain of use. The area treated by firing or blistering should be from below the knee to above the ankle and from the lateral border of the metacarpal around to the medial border. Diathermy will be useful adjuvant therapy.

Wind Galls

Wind galls, or wind puffs, occur on both fore- and hindlegs. They are the result of strain and are inflammations of the great sesamoidean sheath. They appear as fluctuant swellings above the fetlock and occasionally under the pastern. Lameness will occur only when the acute stage of inflammation is present or when gross distention of the sheath is present. Therapy consists of cold water hosing and bandaging plus astringents at the onset. If, after 3 to 4 days of this treatment, swelling is still present, the excess fluid should be withdrawn and a corticosteroid injected be-

fore application of a bandage. This procedure can be repeated until the accumulation of fluid stops. Then the use of a liniment or, in the more chronic cases, an application of a paint will complete healing. Rest is important in the successful therapy of these lesions.

Inflammation of the bursae lying under the extensor tendons at the ankle will be seen rarely. These lesions may be distinguished readily from ankle joint synovitis or from osselets by palpation. Fluctuation cannot be felt behind the joint as in joint synovitis; alterations in the surface of the metacarpal bone are not present as in osselets. Therapy is the same as that outlined for wind puffs.

LAMENESSES OF THE METACARPUS AND METATARSUS

Splints

The articulations between the carpus (tarsus) and the second and fourth metacarpals (metatarsals) may be regarded as forming a part of the carpal (tarsal) joint, especially since they carry some part of the horse's weight. Owing to the fact that they are no longer complete, however, the weight placed upon them, especially in the forelimb, imposes a strain upon the interosseous ligaments which, in young horses, form the only connection between the bones. The pull upon these ligaments is conveyed to the periosteum of the large bones and results in inflammation and exostoses. The exostoses, called splints, occur most commonly on the second or medial metacarpal, or at the junction between the second and third metacarpals, and the deformity includes both bones.

Etiology: The etiology of splints is either trauma or concussion caused by working a horse on a hard surface which causes movement of the involved bones and periosteal tearing. It must be remembered, however, that splints in very young horses can be caused by mineral imbalances. Splints can be found on a majority of older horses although they will not, as a rule, cause trouble.

When unshod horses roamed soft, yielding plains, the small amount of movement occurring between the metacarpal (metatarsal) bones was of no great consequence. More time was available for natural fusion to take place, if this became necessary. Today, when horses race as 2-year-olds, or are engaged on regular roadwork, the pressure from the carpus above, combined with concussion from below, makes it necessary that fusion shall become complete much sooner than in the days before man and the horse entered into partnership.

Clinical Signs: Lameness first is manifested when young horses are taken from soft, yielding turf and are worked on hard roads. Although the bony lesions occur on either side of the limb, it usually is the medial side in which pain is more evident. Weight falls disproportionately on the medial plane of the hoof and concussion is directed upward largely from the inner wall of the foot, particularly in young horses. Splints on the medial aspect of the cannon are exposed to blows from the inner wall of the opposite foot; those on the outer side encounter less injury. The exostoses usually occur near the knee rather than at the lower end of the small metacarpal bone.

Arabians and Thoroughbreds suffer less severely from splints than do horses with heavier bodies. The most troublesome spints occur in heavy- and middleweight hunters and in polo ponies.

The age when splint lameness is most common is between 2 and 5 years, but if the union between the bones is not complete, this lameness may occur later in life. The more common form of splint lameness in older horses is due to repeated injury of an existing exostosis.

In young horses, limbs may be affected simultaneously or alternately, or only one limb may be affected and, in most cases, this will be associated with some pecularity of action which causes more weight to be thrown on one side of the foot than the other. Young horses may be intermittently or continuously lame for as long as a year due to splints. After recovery, unless the splints are damaged by the opposite foot, the lameness may never return.

Splints vary considerably in their location. The exostoses may appear at both the front and the back of the small metacarpal bone, producing what is termed a "peg splint," or they may extend across the back of the third metacarpal bone beneath the suspensory ligament. "Chain splints" comprise a series of small splints which develop at short intervals down the length of the small metacarpal bone. They do not always become active at the same time so that any one of them may cause pain at intervals.

The lameness caused by splints may persist for several days before localized tenderness can be detected, and this often seems to vary in its intensity from day to day. The lameness somewhat resembles foot lameness and it becomes more marked when the horse trots downhill and is more evident on hard roads than on turf. Although common in the forelimbs of young horses, splint lameness rarely is seen in the hindlimbs.

The smallest splints may be difficult to detect, but frequently they produce more pain than the larger ones. At first, splints will cause a lameness which is intermittent—absent when cold, present when the horse is worked. Occasionally, one will see a horse with a developing splint which appears to twist the lower leg to the outside when the leg is brought forward. When a splint has ankylosed and the inflammatory process has stopped, the location of the lesion will determine how much unsoundness is caused.

Diagnosis: The knee must be flexed with the cannon bone parallel to the ground to properly examine the leg for splints. In this position, the medial and lateral sides of both splint bones can be felt as well as the back. Pain on pressure can be produced with most early splints. Lesions at the backs and particularly on the inside of the splint bones will cause more obvious and persistent lameness because the flexor tendons and suspensory ligament will be damaged.

Treatment: There has been much debate about whether young horses recover from splints more rapidly when rested or given regular walking exercise. Freedom at pasture best answers the question, since the horse then can please itself, exercising enough to get food and resting when the splint is particularly painful. There is little doubt that light, regular exercise facilitates the fusion of the bones. In young horses, mineral intake should be checked and deficiencies corrected if they exist.

Firing is standard treatment for splint lameness in race horses. Counterirritation in the form of biniodide of mercury ointment, 1 to 16 or 1 to 20, applied over the painful area with the fingertips for 5 minutes once weekly, seems to produce a good effect, but the real remedy is time. Diathermy can be used advantageously in some cases.

Overworking a lame horse invites the formation of large exostoses. When these occur, they may be treated by subcutaneous division of their periosteal covering and incision into the comparatively soft new bone to encourage resorption. Alternatively, they may be punctured under local anesthesia by means of a pointed firing iron at a dull red heat, the puncture wound subsequently being filled with biniodide of mercury ointment. Some of the larger exostoses encountered in older horses may be removed by chisel under local or general anesthesia. Care must be taken not to injure the digital vessels or nerves.

After large splints have been removed, the horse should be shod with a shoe in which the iron of the inner branch is filed or beaten thin from above to below between the toe and the quarter. This shoe is nailed closely at the outer toe and calk. It carries only 2 nailholes in its inner branch, both near the heel of the shoe.

Bucked Shins

Bucked shins result from a tearing of the periosteum along the front of the metacarpal bone. The common digital extensor is very loosely tied down to the cannon bone in this region by fibrous bands. This condition is caused by excessive demands on the horse to exert itself physically. It is almost entirely an affliction of young running horses. There is a prevalent idea among Thoroughbred trainers that a horse must and will "buck his shins," so they set out to do it at the earliest date possible. Of all the ills the horse falls heir to because of our demands, bucked shins

are surely the most unnecessary and ridiculous. The idea that this is part of "toughening a horse up" to the strain of racing is exploded by the fact that this condition is almost unknown among Standardbred horses. The strain of racing is equally severe (if not more so) on harness horses, but because they are trained to fitness in a more reasonable period of time, this lesion does not appear. Anyone who deliberately sets out to produce pathology in a horse under his care with the idea that the result will improve the animal does not deserve the title of "horseman." But it is unfortunately true that many of our training methods serve more to break the horses down than build them up.

With bucked shins there will be heat, swelling, and tenderness along the front of the metacarpal. Lameness is present and the gait is short and choppy. Rest, application of cold water and astringent lotion until the heat and soreness are gone, then the use of a paint or a blister, constitute rational therapy.

LAMENESSES OF THE FORELIMB

Lamenesses Originating at the Knee

Anatomy: The knee joint is in reality 3 joints —radial-carpal, intercarpal and carpal-metacarpal. Flexion of the knee is accomplished by separation of radial-carpal and intercarpal joints in front while the bones remain in contact behind. Movement in the carpal-metacarpal joint is limited to sliding. The fibrous part of the joint capsule is common to all the joints, its limits being the articular margins of the radius above and the third metacarpal below. It is attached to all of the carpal bones. The synovial membrane forms 3 sacs, the radiocarpal sac, the intercarpal sac, and the carpometacarpal sac. The last 2 are connected.

Clinical Signs: When lameness of the knee occurs it is constant, and a spraddling gait is characteristic. Flexion of the knee is kept to a minimum and the foot is carried outward from the center line of the body so it can be brought forward without scuffing the ground. Varying degrees of heat and swelling will be present locally. The swelling will be either a diffuse edema or a discrete swelling caused

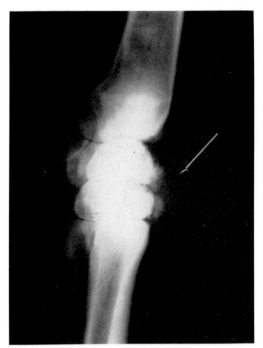

Fig. 26. Carpitis with rarefying osteoarthritis, exostosis, and narrowing of joint spaces. Radiograph by J. P. Manning, D.V.M.

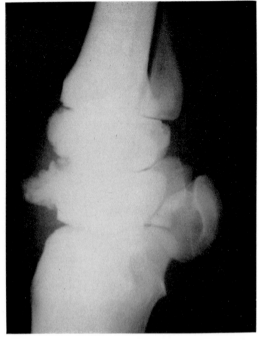

Fig. 27. Carpitis with abnormal new bone growth.

by increased synovia in one of the synovial sacs. The joint should be flexed and the joint margins explored by palpation. One should gain experience palpating the joint margins of the knee, because with practice a great deal can be learned by this procedure. When examining a horse for soundness, the fact that the horse has had carpitis will be evident even though the animal is not lame at the time. When flexing the knee for palpation, it is well to check how nearly the heel can be brought to the elbow. With a normal knee, the heel can be made to touch, or nearly touch, the elbow with little effort.

It always is wise to obtain radiographs of damaged knees. Fractures, particularly of the third carpal bone, may be present. Knowledge of the amount, position, and density of any proliferative calcium deposits and chips from them is important in planning treatment. The etiology in 80% of the cases of carpitis in race horses is overextension of the knee when the horse is worked beyond its capacity. Other causes include trauma from falls or concussion.

Treatment: Treatment of carpal injuries in-

cludes the application of cold water and astringent lotions until the heat is gone. If the excess synovial fluid has not begun to be absorbed within 48 hours, one can tap the sacs and inject a corticosteroid. Diathermy or the firing iron can be used to promote resorption of proliferative lesions and to speed healing. Surgical removal of calcium deposits is advisable in selected cases. Rest is imperative until reexamination shows that healing has been completed.

When a horse is observed with solid, proliferative calcium deposits which apparently are not causing trouble, one should let well enough alone. The calcium deposit if treated may become less solid and dense, but before resorption takes place a chip may break off. This obviously is a less satisfactory situation than having a sound horse with a lump on its knee.

TENDOVAGINITIS

Occasionally, a swollen knee will involve only the tendon sheath of the extensor carpi radialis muscle. This is readily diagnosed by palpation, particularly with the joint flexed. This lesion will not cause lameness. Immediate application of an astringent lotion under a fairly tight bandage often will be sufficient treatment. If, after several days, an edematous swelling remains in the area, the application of a liniment usually will remedy this. However, if the fluid is not resorbed, the tendon sheath should be aspirated, a corticosteroid injected, and further bandaging applied to the area.

Tendovaginitis involving the common digital extensor is rare. Diagnosis is obvious from the appearance and position of the lesion. Lameness is slight, if present at all. The treatment for this lesion is similar to that just outlined for inflammation of a tendon sheath.

Inflammations of the carpal sheath are fairly common in race horses. When this condition is encountered, care should be taken to ascertain that a synovitis is not present in the knee joint itself. This can be done by placing one hand on the front of the knee to detect fluctuation while palpating the swelling below the knee with the other. Since this is a sharply defined fluctuant swelling with little or no heat, and slight if any attendant lameness, it can be readily differentiated from a high bow of the tendons, which is characterized by a diffuse hot swelling. If possible, horses with carpal sheath inflammations should be rested for a time because this condition is the result of strain. If complete rest is not possible, a drastic reduction in work is indicated. Hosing the leg with cold water and bandaging it with astringents is adequate treatment for most cases. Unresponsive lesions should be aspirated and injected with corticosteroid. Chronic cases should be given complete rest and treated with diathermy or a paint.

Knee Spavin

High-stepping horses may injure the medial side of their carpi when turning at high speed. Ponies and race horses are most commonly affected. Chronic arthritis may result and greatly resemble spavin in the tarsal region. The prognosis in such cases is less favorable than in tarsal spavin since the normal movement between the carpal bones is considerably greater than between those of the hock, and ankylosis of the knee is therefore a crippling condition. When the disease is confined to the lower row of bones, joint movement may not be so greatly impaired.

The condition always produces marked swelling of the knee, and fibrosis. The knee usually is bent or slightly flexed and is incapable of full extension owing to adhesions between the articular cartilages and to the development of lateral exostoses. In addition to inability to fully extend the limb, the limb and foot make a circular sweep when moving forward, and the foot lands with the quarter coming to the ground first.

Elbow Lameness

Although not common, elbow lameness, especially the chronic arthritic type which occasionally occurs in aged horses, has on many occasions been mistaken for shoulder lameness. This happens because any inability to flex the elbow makes it very difficult to advance the limb, since knee and elbow work in unison.

Sometimes bruising of the cap of the elbow may give rise to inflammation of the bursa over the olecranon process which makes movement painful. Fracture of the olecranon has been recorded, but it is rare. Fracture through the elbow joint sometimes occurs during a race and usually involves the humerus which may be shattered without apparent trauma. This is due entirely to muscular incoordination. It is possible that rupture of the tendon of the triceps at its insertion on the olecranon can occur when a violent slip takes place. Diagnosis can be made in this case by noting the presence of heat, pain, and swelling. When the animal is moved, no weight is borne on the leg, and the elbow drops. Rest is the best treatment.

Capped Elbow

Capped elbows, or shoe boils, occur on the point of the elbow, and are inflammations of varying severity involving a bursa lying over the point of the olecranon. The cause is bruising of the elbow due to inadequate bedding, or much more commonly, to contact with a

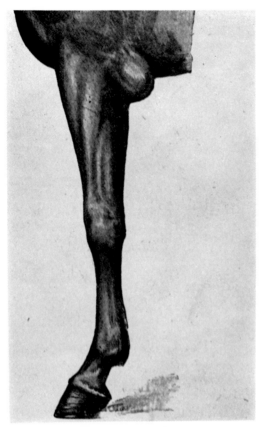

Fig. 28. Capped elbow.

shoe with heels or a foot which has been allowed to grow excessively. It will be seen most often in gaited show horses. The preventive measure for the first cause is obvious. For the second cause, a shoe boil roll should be used. This is merely a padded roll strapped around the pastern with sufficient diameter to prevent the heel's touching the elbow when the leg is flexed. Trotters with considerable action are protected with elbow boots when racing. Lameness occurs only during the stage of most acute inflammation, and is only transient. These lesions will vary in appearance from circumscribed, fluctuating swellings with little or no inflammation to a large inflamed area covering the entire elbow. Chronic cases show indurated swellings often with pouching of the skin at the elbow. All gradations between those described will occur depending on the amount of trauma and the chronicity of the lesion. Early cases will respond

well to icing and the use of astringent dressings for several days followed by the use of liniment. With the extensively inflamed lesions, care should be taken because they often will abscess. Parenteral antibiotics and enzyme preparations are indicated in addition to external treatment. Chronic lesions require surgical excision.

FRACTURE OF THE DELTOID TUBERCLE OF THE HUMERUS

Etiology: This is by no means an uncommon occurrence and the injury usually occurs when the horse passes through doorways or gateways. Occasionally it results from kicks, particularly in small ponies which are injured by larger horses. Muscular pull originating in the deltoid muscle may sometimes be responsible. When completely detached, the tubercle may be missing, but as a rule it is still held close to its usual position by fibrous tissue. It can often be taken between finger and thumb and moved backward and forward.

Clinical Signs: The signs of this fracture may at first be confused with those of radial paralysis. The knee and fetlock are flexed and the horse shows difficulty in advancing the limb. As in radial paralysis, the horse can place weight on the foot when it is brought forward and placed sole-downward upon the ground. After taking a step forward the horse is again unable to advance the limb. This condition can be distingushed from radial paralysis by the fact that in deltoid fracture the elbow does not drop. The deltoid process will make a fibrous union with the shaft of the humerus provided it is not completely displaced. In 10 cases observed by one of the authors (RHS), all recovered from lameness after periods of 6 to 10 weeks.

SHOULDER LAMENESS

Etiology: Shoulder lameness in horses is produced mainly by sprains and strains of the muscles which move the stabilizing ligaments, or of the bursae which lubricate the joint. The proliferative lesions of osteoarthritis are not common in this joint mainly because its angulation reduces the concussion of movement to a minimum.

Clinical Signs: The most striking of the muscle lesions is called "sweeny"; this lesion is an atrophy of both the supraspinatus and infraspinatus muscles following injury of the suprascapular nerve. There is little that can be done to remedy this appearance except to prevent obvious causes of trauma to the nerve. The affected animal should be allowed to rest for a period sufficient for regeneration of the nerve to take place.

Diagnosis: Muscular strains can be diagnosed by their contraction, tenseness, and soreness. Identification of the shoulder as the origin of lameness seems to present the greatest difficulty in these cases. Although shoulder lameness and foot lameness often are confused, differentiation is not difficult. The horse should be examined from the front with the animal standing squarely on both front feet to check its symmetry. Evidence of muscular atrophy should not lead promptly to a diagnosis of shoulder lameness since disuse and atrophy can occur with chronic defects of the leg. If the horse is moved in a straight line at a trot, the affected shoulder often will appear to be carried lower than the other. From the side, lack of motion in the joint can be seen. The leg is not brought forward as far as normal, although it is allowed to go back under the body in the usual way. When the horse is worked in a circle, the lameness will be most apparent when the affected limb is on the outside. As a routine procedure, the common digital arteries should be compared as to character of the pulse, and the foot of the affected limb should be examined.

Intertuberal (bicipital) bursitis sometimes can be diagnosed by pressing on the tendon of the biceps as it passes around the head of the humerus. When the horse is trotted up- and downhill, one with shoulder lameness is more lame going uphill. Shoulder lameness is constant or increases during use.

Treatment: The treatment for shoulder muscle pain involves the use of diathermy or moist heat. For joint pathology, the remedies include diathermy, the use of liniments, and internal blisters. Liniments applied with steam

have greater penetration. Internal blisters can be applied subcutaneously either in several sites over the joint, or by a single deep intramuscular injection behind the joint.

INFLAMMATION OF THE TENDINOUS BURSA OF THE BICEPS BRACHII

The biceps brachii arises from the coracoid process of the scapula. Its strong fibrous tendon passes over the bicipital groove of the humerus upon which its deep face is molded, and here a synovial bursa facilitates the movements of the tendon in the groove.

Lesions affecting this bursa may be slight but they often become chronic later. In the mildest type, there is inflammatory hyperemia of the bursal walls and an excessive secretion of flocculant synovia. In chronic cases, there is thickening of both the bursal walls and their synovial lining. Roughening occurs on the cartilagenous covering of the bicipital groove and also on the corresponding portion of the bicipital tendon. The biceps muscle may develop bony partitions throughout its length due to the deposition of lime salts. There is a record of one biceps muscle which became ossified throughout and fused with exostoses on the humeral shaft.

Etiology: The cause usually relates to trauma. The point of the shoulder, being the most advanced part of the trunk, is likely to come into contact with gateposts, or the rails of a jump, or to be injured in collisions. When trauma cannot be identified as the cause, one must bear in mind the possibility of bursal infection by Brucella, or other infectious organisms.

Clinical Signs: The type of lameness is typical of the condition. The horse is able to back, but is unable to advance the limb to its full extent, and in severe cases not at all. In an acute case, the affected shoulder is carried some distance behind the sound one and the knee is flexed with the foot carried well behind its normal position and rested on the toe.

When urged to move forward, the horse hops on the sound limb for a short stride, rests momentarily, usually grunts with pain, and carries the affected shoulder forward a short distance with the foot swinging behind the fetlock and without weight on it. During the next stage of movement the horse brings the hindfeet under the body to take some weight off the fore-end. It then rests for a moment on the toe of the lame foot, again advances the sound limb, and the process is repeated. The tempo is a little faster than the time it takes to read this account, but the movement forward is very slow and obviously causes a great deal of pain.

In mild cases of lameness, there still is some difficulty in advancing the limb which is carried a little behind its normal level so that the animal moves with a "3-cornered gait."

While the horse is standing, the foot of the affected limb may be rested on its toe with knee flexed, or occasionally it may be pointed a little forward with the foot flat on the ground. This is seen only in early cases and seldom when the lameness has become well-established. In these early stages, there may be some swelling visible at the point of the shoulder and pain is exhibited when digital pressure is applied to the area. One should always compare the effect of pressure on both shoulders in turn, since very few normal horses fail to resist any marked degree of digital pressure on the point of the shoulder.

In chronic cases, one may see a definite enlargement at the extreme point of the shoulder, made even more visible because of the increasing atrophy of all the muscles of the shoulder, particularly the supraspinatus and deltoid. In milder cases in horses which still are being worked, the lameness may be more pronounced when the horse is traveling uphill while it may be almost unnoticeable when the horse is returning downhill.

Pain will be shown when the foot is lifted, the knee flexed, and the foot drawn backward as far as possible. Once again, it is wise to compare the 2 forelimbs when exposed to the same procedure since many normal horses will attempt to rear when treated in this manner. In rare instances, the condition becomes bilateral and the gait then is similar to that observed in cases of laminitis when all 4 feet are affected. All 4 feet are drawn under the body and the horse refuses to advance either forelimb.

Farm horses suffering from a mild but chronic type of bursitis often continue to work for a considerable period before becoming markedly lame. Animals showing mild signs may be worked on ploughed land if they are shod with a ¾-inch bar, welded across both heels. This does not permit the foot to sink so easily into the soft earth as heels ordinarily do. Calkins are useless on soft earth so far as raising the heels is concerned.

Cases which are rested for 3 months either recover during that interval, or not at all.

Treatment: Apart from fitting a surgical shoe, the point of the shoulder may be blistered. Its inunction for 5 minutes with biniodide of mercury, 1 to 8 or 1 to 16 in lard, repeated every tenth day, appears to be beneficial. Corticosteroids may be helpful. In acute cases, older practitioners administered sodium salicylate and potassium iodide in an electuary. This treatment appeared to relieve pain although as in the case of the corticosteroids, the improvement continues only as long as the administration is continued.

INFLAMMATION OF THE TENDINOUS BURSA OF THE INFRASPINATUS MUSCLE

Etiology: The infraspinatus muscle occupies the fossa posterior to the scapular spine. It has 2 tendons of insertion. The outer passes over the external tuberosity of the humerus and may be subjected to strain during forced abduction of the limb. Such an accident may occur when a horse lands from a jump, or when a stallion has difficulty in descending from a mare. It can happen also as the result of a fall or sliding on slippery ground. Strain of this tendon causes injury to the wall of the bursa.

Clinical Signs: The clinical signs are rather striking and may be confused with those seen in "shoulder slip," in which the suprascapular nerve is involved. The horse shows pain when placing weight on the foot and when turning, but when walking straight there may be little or no indication of lameness.

In a week or fortnight following the injury or accident some degree of atrophy of the infraspinatus muscle is visible. This is manifested by flattening of the muscle as it lies in the intrascapular fossa. Most cases recover fully after 6 weeks' rest.

RADIAL PARALYSIS

The radial nerve is at its root one of the thickest nerves of the brachial plexus. It derives its fibers from the seventh and eighth cervical nerves and from portions of the first 2 thoracics. In common with other nerves of the brachial plexus, it emerges between the upper and lower divisions of the scalenus muscle, lying in fairly close proximity to the first rib. The dorsal roots of the plexus turn around the anterior border of the first rib, leaving on it a smooth impression close to its upper end.

The radial nerve passes in front of the long head of the triceps and enters the musculospiral groove of the humerus, lying on the brachialis muscle. Before emerging from behind the humerus it supplies the long and medial heads of the triceps and sends a long branch to the tensor fasciae antibrachii. It reaches the front of the elbow joint lying between the brachialis and the origin of the extensor carpi radialis. At this point it gives off branches to all the extensor muscles of the limb.

Injury to the radial nerve at the level of the first rib will therefore paralyze the extensors of the elbow, carpal, and digital joints.

Etiology: A great many causes for radial paralysis have been suggested. For a number of years the condition was considered related to a fractured first rib, and it is true that many cases of radial paralysis, which have been destroyed following a lengthy period of treatment, have been found at necropsy to have a fractured first rib. But more cases have not had evidence of fracture. It also must be borne in mind that a high percentage of cases ultimately recover, and many do not remain lame for longer than 6 to 8 weeks. It is unlikely that these would have shown evidence of a fractured rib had they been destroyed, so the percentage of the total cases associated with a fractured first rib probably is not so high as has been thought. Cases not associated with fracture, probably result from neural or muscle injury.

Neural injuries may include overstretching, tearing or bruising, any of which can occur when horses are cast. Many horses, when recovering from anesthesia, show difficulty in rising and once on their feet are unable to advance one of their forelimbs. In others, the signs of radial paralysis appear more slowly and first are observed a few days or a week after the operation.

In cases which make no progress after many months of treatment, hyperemia of the nerve often is observed at necropsy. There may be additional damage to the muscles of the forearm, which further complicates the clinical signs.

Clinical Signs: As might be expected, the horse is completely unable to advance the limb. The elbow hangs low as the triceps muscles are not functional and no longer are able to lift the point of the elbow toward the chest wall. If the forearm is lifted, so that the knee is advanced and raised, the cannon bone and foot still hang inert and pendulous. In a normal horse, the knee can be flexed only when the elbow is also flexed, but in cases of radial paralysis, lifting and flexing the elbow do not overcome the inability to advance the foot. Usually the foot is flexed from the fetlock with the result that not only the toe but some of the front wall of the foot also may rest upon the ground. If, however, the foot is carried forward by hand and placed on the ground flat upon its sole, and if pressure is now placed on the flexed forearm immediately above the knee, the horse will place weight on the foot and take one step forward. But, as soon as the body has moved forward over the forearm, the latter swings back to its original flexed position and can make no further move unaided.

In severe cases, the horse's back is arched and both hindfeet may be carried forward beneath the body in an effort to take some of the weight of the fore-end. Actually, this movement of the hindlimbs makes little difference in the rate of progress.

Prognosis: The dysfunction seldom is attended by pain and as a rule the horse continues to feed and maintain condition in other parts of the body. The muscles of the affected limb, particularly the extensors, atrophy.

Most cases of incomplete paralysis recover within a few months while others may require a year. Many of the long-standing cases are destroyed for economic reasons.

Treatment: The usual remedies for radial paralysis including massage, blistering, short wave therapy and electrical stimulation of muscles have been tried repeatedly without obvious results. There is no doubt that many affected horses would recover if they were given unlimited rest in a level field.

SUPRASCAPULAR PARALYSIS

The suprascapular nerve derives its fibers from the sixth, seventh and eighth cervical roots, passes into the space between the subscapularis and supraspinatus muscles, turns around the anterior edge of the scapula, gains its dorsal surface and is distributed to the supraspinatus and infraspinatus muscles. The infraspinatus is an abductor of the humerus and causes that bone to move away from the body and to rotate in doing so. The supraspinatus helps to extend the shoulder joint.

Etiology: Immediately below the lower end of the scapular spine and upon the anterior border of the scapula at this level, the suprascapular nerve is exposed to injury from blows, pressure or undue stretching.

Suprascapular paralysis commonly was encountered in country districts when horses were used for plowing, often with one foot in the furrow. The heavy collar bumped up and down on the edge of the scapula and the frequent change in its position and the placing of the forefeet tended to squeeze the nerve between the supraspinatus and the subscapularis muscles. The nerve also can be damaged when a heavy draft horse backs a heavy load for some distance. The condition has been encountered in polo ponies as the result of collision, and at one time this was common in cavalry horses. Tying a forelimb to a hindlimb prior to surgery also may cause stretching of the nerve.

When considering cases of peripheral paralysis, one must remember that practically all the motor nerves to the limbs issue from the spinal cord through a foramen. Spinal injuries may produce considerable effect upon a nerve such as the suprascapular.

Clinical Signs: The result of suprascapular paralysis is abduction of the limb. When weight is placed upon the foot, the shoulder revolves outward and the foot of the affected limb will approach nearer the midline of the body than will the foot of the sound limb. The loss of power in the supraspinatus muscle makes it more difficult to advance the limb. The toe of the foot which is moving forward may swing through the arc of a circle. It may require a few days or a few weeks before these signs disappear.

The lameness may diminish but the muscles overlying the scapula, especially the supraspinatus, atrophy rapidly. At first, the outer surface of the scapula looks flat. A little later, the muscles overlying the scapula will have atrophied to such an extent that the outlines of the scapula fossae and spine become visible.

The muscular atrophy may persist for 6 to 12 months, or longer. A small percentage of horses, especially those in which the nerve has been traumatized at the front edge of the scapula, never regain full use of the limb nor normal appearance of the involved muscles.

Treatment: To limit the onset of muscular atrophy as much as possible, the horse should receive daily walking exercise, or be turned out to graze in a level field. The front of the scapular region and its outer surface should be massaged daily, using a lubricating fluid such as camphorated oil to prevent undue friction. Blistering may be used but massage is better.

In early stages, warm counterirritants are indicated and short-wave therapy sometimes produces good results. An infra-red lamp, adjusted at a suitable distance from the skin, may be helpful but care must be taken as horses are far more susceptible to heat rays than are humans.

LAMENESSES OF THE HINDLIMB

The lamenesses encountered in the hindfeet and tendons resemble those of the forefeet, apart from the fact that hindfoot lameness is less common. Navicular disease rarely is encountered in a hindfoot and splint lameness is almost equally uncommon. Sesamoid lameness is fairly frequent in the hindlimbs but tendon injuries are less so.

The hock, which is probably the hardest worked joint in the horse's body, has its share of lameness.

STRINGHALT

In this condition, a hock is overflexed rapidly during progression. The point of the hock jerks upward and frequently the foot returns to the ground with undue force. One might suppose that the coordination between the gastrocnemius and the flexor metatarsi was faulty. It might be expected that such horses would develop a curb, but this is not often the case.

The condition may be uni- or bilateral; more often it is confined to one hindlimb. A somewhat similar condition has been observed in a forelimb but such cases must be very rare.

The etiology still is in doubt. It is believed that the seat of the disorder lies in the spinal cord. The condition often becomes worse with age. A few cases show improvement after division of the peroneus tendon, but others show none.

CURB

Curbs occur on the plantar surface of the hock a hand's breadth below the point of the hock. They appear to be a backward bulge of the tendons from what should be the normal straight line from hock to fetlock. Occasionally, one will see what is called a false curb. Although when viewed from the side there seems to be a swelling present, when viewed from above or closely inspected from the medial side, the normal straight line can be seen. Actually, this deceptive appearance is caused by an unusually large fourth tarsal bone. Horses with sickle hocks are predisposed to curbs. The condition results from a rupture of the plantar ligament of the hock at its insertion on the third and fourth tarsal bones, or a rupture of the calcaneo-cuboidal ligament. The etiology is strain from jumping, running, slipping, and other such stress.

Lameness due to a curb is constant and can be diagnosed in what might be called the sprain stage or as the horseman puts it, "before they have popped." In horses with hindleg lameness, particularly race horses, curb lameness should be suspected when the history reveals that the horse bears in or out when running at speed. Which way he bears depends on the leg affected (or most affected) because the horse tends to move the fall of this foot toward or across the center line of the body. This placement of a hindfoot between the forefeet also occurs in stifle lameness. A horse with a curb shows increased lameness after flexion of the hock, but not so dramatically as one with a jack spavin. The best way to determine whether the signs you see are truly a starting curb is to flex the hock and foot. This will slacken the flexor tendons sufficiently so that you can dig a finger down beneath them from either side. This will produce definite signs of pain if a curb is starting even though it is not visible. Very often when a horse has hock trouble, particularly curbs, the rear fetlocks will produce a cracking sound when walking.

Curbs should be fired. Any other approach only delays the eventual use of a firing iron, although inflammation should be reduced before firing. I use a diamond pattern with the short axis parallel to the ground. The long axis should extend well above and below the swelling. In the majority of cases, although the horse will become sound, the swelling never disappears completely. Four months' rest is a minimum requirement.

SPAVIN

It is not easy to find a definition of spavin which will include all the aspects of this condition. The horse owner ordinarily regards spavin as a bony enlargement on the inner side of the hock joint, often associated with lameness. If he were shown a sound hock and asked to place the tip of his finger on the site of a spavin he probably would be unable to do so.

The weak point in the definition accepted by the horse owner is that it often is very difficult to see or feel a bony enlargement in horses that are lame due to a spavin. Conversely, a horse with a large bony enlargement at the location of spavin may not be lame. Any stiffness related to such bony enlargements may be purely mechanical as a consequence of immobility due to the ankylosis between some of the small flat bones of the hock joint.

Bone Spavin

It is likely that reduction of hock flexion, which is so characteristic of bone spavin, is in reality an evidence of pain arising from movement of ulcerated joint surfaces present between these flattened bones. The exostoses which frequently develop on the joint margins tend to limit movement between these bones. Ankylosis can result in a serviceable hock which will operate without pain.

The horse with a well-developed spavin will often be free from painful lameness but one which is lame in the hock joint showing very little indication of spavin, undoubtedly will remain lame until an exostosis develops which is large enough to fuse the flat bones of the tarsus together and unite them to the metatarsals.

Bone spavins occur in 2 forms: true or "jack" spavin, and occult or "blind" spavin. True spavin is a periostitis which occurs at the medial joint margin of the head of the third metatarsal and on the medial surface of the fourth metatarsal. From there it may extend to the first, second and third tarsals, and the central tarsal. It seldom involves the fourth tarsal bone.

Occult spavin is a degenerative lesion of the articulations between any of the tarsal bones, or between the tarsals and metatarsals. Arthritis and ulceration of the articular surfaces are unaccompanied by exostosis of the joint margin. It can be diagnosed only from evidence of pain in the hock joint and limitation of hock flexion in the affected limb.

In both forms of spavin there is a tendency to place less weight on the heel of the foot. The toe of the shoe wears more rapidly, and this may be an indication of hock lameness, although this sign may accompany other causes of hindlimb lameness. In the forelimb, excessive toe wear often is seen in navicular disease and in tendonitis, but these conditions are encountered infrequently in the hindlimb, so the likelihood of excessive toe wear being due to spavin is increased. However, stifle and hip lamenesses may produce a somewhat similar appearance of the shoe on occasion, as will any condition which lessens hock flexion.

When the lesion is developing, this lameness will pass, frequently unmarked, unless the horse is worked excessively. As the lesion enlarges, the lameness observed when the horse is led from the stall will be more noticeable, and the animal will show more lameness when exercised.

In the case of jack spavin more often than blind spavin, the animal will have sound and lame days. There will be days when lameness is reduced or absent, depending on previous work, the weather, the state of the horse's digestion, etc.

Etiology: Spavin is regarded by some as a hereditary disease but statistical support for this contention is not convincing. Spavin is seen in all kinds of horses and especially in those used extensively on hard surfaces. When horses were the main means of transport, the majority of those suffering from spavin were heavy draft horses and horses used in harness and trotted on hard roads. Spavin is quite common in hunters, especially in the heavyweights, a point in favor of heredity as a cause.

The conformation of the hock itself appears to have little significance since many badly constructed hocks will remain free from spavin, though well-constructed hocks frequently become affected. The ease with which flexion is achieved between the tibia and the tarsus greatly reduces the amount of concussion transmitted from the ground to the hock. Although hock conformation may be thought to have little connection with spavin production, the degree of angulation of hock and stifle, and also straightness of the pasterns, may have a great deal to do with the amount of concussion to which the small bones of the hock are exposed. Concussion probably is one of the major factors in the etiology of spavin.

Clinical Signs: Lameness may exist for days or weeks before any exostosis is palpable. The horse comes out of the stable lame. The point of the lame hock is not lifted as high as a normal one. After a brief trot, the lameness usually becomes less marked, but in occult spavin, as well as in early cases of true spavin, there may be no improvement after exercise. When the horse is again trotted after a rest the lameness returns. If the lameness has been present for a week or 2, the toe of the shoe fitted to the lame foot will show a greater amount of wear (and brightness) than its opposite. This will depend upon the health of the opposite limb and whether both hind shoes were fitted at the same time.

When the spavined horse first leaves the stable it walks with most weight on the toe, and with the heel slightly raised, but after a trot the heel usually comes down to the ground. In lameness which has persisted for more than 2 weeks, the muscles of the lame quarter will be visibly flattened.

When the hindlimb is extended and the foot receives the weight of the body, a certain amount of rotation takes place between the small bones of the hock and the metatarsal bones. By flexing the hock and so lessening the weight upon the limb, and by bringing the toe to the ground first with the fetlock slightly flexed, this rotary movement, with its accompanying pain, is minimized.

Diagnosis: An excellent test for hock lamenesses is to flex it severely by holding the leg in such a way that the cannon bone is against the gaskin for 1 to 2 minutes, and then have the horse trotted as soon as the leg is released. The lameness is increased by this test if the hock is the origin of the lameness.

Jack spavin can be diagnosed by inspection of the lower anteromedial aspect of the joint. Stand in front of the horse and slightly to one side. An early jack spavin will appear as a rounding and thickening of the inner surface of the hock. Even before this is apparent to the eye, palpation, backed by experience and comparison with the other leg, will produce a definite impression of abnormal wideness at this point.

To determine the presence or absence of spavin exostosis it is necessary to be able to recognize the heads of the third and second metatarsal bones, and from this point trace with the tip of the finger, the outlines of the central and distal tarsals. There are prominences on the medial aspect of the hock which may act as landmarks. The largest of these, and the uppermost, is the medial malleolus of the tibia. Below this is the tuberosity on the medial aspect of the fibial tarsal and immediately below this are the fused first and second tarsal bones which are directly above the head of the second metatarsal. It is essential to be able to recognize these prominences, as well as the edges of the distal row of tarsal bones, before one begins to palpate for the presence of what may be quite small exostoses.

When palpating the lower and inner aspect of the hock, the prominent distal tuberosity on the inner aspect of the tibial tarsal can be located readily. The lower edge of this point marks the junction of tibial and central tarsals. The central tarsal has a very prominent rim, which can be followed by the fingertip. Slightly lower, one feels a groove which runs inward, backward, and upward. This represents the articulation between the central tarsal and the distal row of tarsal bones. A groove running vertically separates the fused first and second tarsals from the third tarsal which also carries prominent horizontal ridges. A horizontal groove separates the distal row of tarsals from the metatarsal heads.

In a thin-skinned horse, the cunean tendon (medial branch of the fibialis anterior tendon) can be felt running inward and downward from the front of the hock into the third tarsal in line with the chestnut.

It is important to recognize the ridges which run along the edges of the distal row and central tarsals. If these ridges are clear and well-defined, the grooves which lie between the ridges are distinct and free from calcareous deposit which blurs their margins, the examiner may feel sure that no exostosis is present. One may compare both hocks but should remember that the opposite hock may be more unsound than the one which is being examined.

Even if there are no exostoses, there is no guarantee, particularly if the horse is lame, that it is not affected with occult spavin. Confirmation of the diagnosis of occult spavin depends on radiographs. The diagnosis is made on the

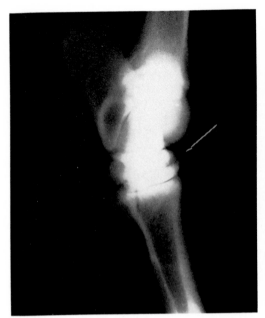

Fig. 29. Bone spavin. Lateral view. Radiograph by
J. P. Manning, D.V.M.

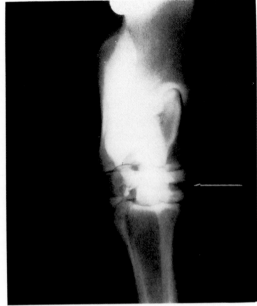

Fig. 30. Bone spavin. A.P. view. Radiograph by J. P.
Manning, D.V.M.

basis of reduction in joint space due to destruction of the articular cartilage unless ankylosis is present (Fig. 29, 30).

Treatment: When a spavin is just starting, the horse should be rested until the lameness ceases. The balance of the foot should be altered by cutting down the toe, leaving as much heel as possible, and putting heel calks on the shoe. A course of diathermy lasting at least a month should be given. If the involved animal is a race horse, following recovery from this initial attack of lameness it should be worked hard only when absolutely necessary to maintain fitness, but it should never be allowed to get out of condition because the strain of reconditioning the animal will surely bring a recurrence of lameness.

When the lesion is more advanced and spavin is visible to the naked eye, rest, altered shoeing, and diathermy is the regimen of choice. In the past, it was the practice to fire into the bone over a jack spavin to hasten ankylosis. This is considered by some to be a futile procedure. Since the cause of bone spavin is the strain caused by faulty conformation, ankylosis of one joint merely transfers the strain to the others. Perhaps surgical production of ankylosis of all the joints in the tarsus

except the tibiotarsal, would produce lasting relief. However, a jack spavin is a proliferative arthritic lesion and growth on the medial surface of the bones involved will continue even after ankylosis has occurred.

Running downward across the seat of spavin is a groove which accommodates the tendinous branch of the peroneus tertius which is provided with a synovial bursa. Many veterinarians believe that inflammation of this bursa is the primary cause of spavin formation and that section of the cunean tendon over the seat of spavin is excellent treatment.

There is no doubt that inclusion of the bursa in the inflammatory condition will accentuate the pain, but it is unlikely that it is the actual cause of spavin. Probably the irritation produced by tenotomy has a somewhat similar effect to that produced by firing and this may give temporary relief from pain. In selected cases, a cunean tenotomy will provide relief of varying duration and effectiveness. This leads to the fact that the horse with a bone spavin can never be considered absolutely sound, but that in most cases a varying period of useful work still can be obtained. These horses will have good and bad days, the bad ones slowly becoming more frequent. The condition is a day to day problem; therefore, preventive dosage of corticosteroid or phenylbutazone, starting 3 days before the date on which it is particularly desirous for the horse to be sound, usually will be helpful.

Bog Spavin

When movement of the leg is considered, the only effective joint in the tarsus is the tibiotarsal joint. All the other joints in the hock are restricted by ligaments to limited sliding movements. However, these movements play a part in the anticoncussion mechanism of the hindleg. The joint capsule, like that of the carpus, covers the entire complex of joints, but the synovial membrane is divided into 4 sacs. The 2 sacs of primary concern are the tibiotarsal and the proximal intertarsal sacs, which communicate with each other. Synovitis of either or both of these sacs causes distentions appearing on the upper lateral part of the joint and the lower anteromedial side of the joint. Accumulations of fluid in these membranes are termed bog spavins. Generally speaking, lameness related to these swellings is only slight and transient. On palpation, the fluid can be displaced from one sac to the other.

The importance of synovial distentions in the tarsal region depends upon 2 factors:

1. Whether there is any active inflammatory change in the tarsal articulation.
2. Whether the degree of distention interferes with flexion of the hock joint.

Unless they are very large and tense, these distentions seldom produce any marked degree of lameness.

Two other synovial distentions may be encountered in the hock region. One involves the tendon sheath of the lateral digital extensor on the lateral side of the proximal end of the cannon bone. The other affects the sheath of the long digital flexor on the inner side of the hock. Neither of these 2 conditions gives rise to lameness, and their presence should not cause the clinician to overlook some other source of lameness. As with bone spavins, insufficient angulation of the hindleg increases the amount of stress in the hock and predisposes to both bog and bone spavin. It might

be noted here that another lesion of the hock area is called a blood spavin. This is a varicosity of the saphenous vein.

Treatment: Unless the degree of distention in a chronic case is sufficient to produce clinical lameness it is not wise to attempt to reduce its size. Distention of the capsule which produces visible bulging may be regarded as a safety valve. If the bulging did not occur, the horse would be lame, and any attempt to reduce the swelling, especially if it were successful, might quite possibly provoke lameness. Bog spavins should be treated by immobilization and cold applications first. Bandaging the hock is difficult, but this should be learned. A cooling, astringent lotion should be used with the bandage. Several days of this treatment, followed by the use of a liniment, will produce the desired absorption of fluid. In cases that do not respond, the sacs can be aspirated and a corticosteroid injected. These animals will need prolonged rest, and diathermy will provide better supportive therapy than a liniment.

Some practitioners still advocate the injection of Lugol's solution. This is a painful treatment which at first increases lameness, and later causes a reduction in the amount of synovia secreted. Others advocate line-firing followed by blistering. None of these treatments is advisable in the absence of lameness.

Thoroughpin

Thoroughpins appear in what might be called the hollow area between the distal end of the tibia and tendon of the gastrocnemius muscle. They often appear to bulge on one side more than the other when viewed from behind. Thoroughpins result from strain on the flexor tendons as they pass around the hock. The consequence of the strain is an inflammation and filling of the tendon sheath. A horse with thoroughpins will be lame when the lesion first appears. After the lesion becomes chronic, the horse usually will be sound. Therapy is difficult because the location makes the application of pressure by bandaging difficult. Cold applications with or without the injection of corticosteroid are indicated at the out-

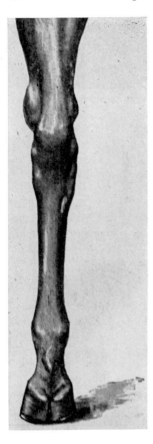

Fig. 31. Thoroughpin.

set of inflammation. My (H.C.) unhappy experience is that the use of paint or even a blister will almost always be necessary. Even this treatment will not be entirely successful.

CAPPED HOCK

A capped hock is an extremely unsightly blemish although it rarely causes lameness. It is the result of trauma, and generally occurs when a horse is thrown off balance in a van, or as a result of kicking in the stall when the animal hits the wall with the point of the hock. This vice is difficult to cure. Regular exercise can be of help; sometimes putting tail boards in the stall will keep the horse far enough from the wall so that the foot hits them rather than the hock. Good bandaging, or the use of hock boots together with careful driving, will reduce the danger of damage during transport. Also, the hay and feed tub should be so placed

in the stall that the horse cannot kick backward against a wall. Feed tubs should not be placed near those in the adjoining stall. Horses frequently will kick when eating grain, particularly when they are nose to nose with the horse in the next stall. When the injury has just occurred, cold water applications and astringent lotions frequently will be all that is necessary to reduce the swelling. When the injury is repeated a liniment may be needed after the cold application to completely reduce the swelling. In long-standing cases, or ones which frequently recur, repeated applications of a paint offer the best chance for a successful outcome. It often is impossible to effect complete reduction of the swelling in such cases. Surgery is not satisfactory therapy because the involved bursa is adherent to the underlying tendon.

RUPTURE OF THE PERONEUS TERTIUS

The peroneus tertius and tibialis anterior muscles assume an immense strain since they help maintain the rigidity of the hindlimb and act as antagonists to the gastrocnemius muscle. Despite use of the word, antagonist, the opposing muscles also act in perfect harmony to permit both flexion and extension of the hock joint. It appears that the gastrocneumius tendon is capable of taking more strain than the peroneus tertius, as rupture of the latter is a well-known form of equine lameness, but rupture of the gastrocnemius tendon, although comparatively common in cattle, is almost unknown in the horse. When it does occur, it usually is due to external trauma.

The peroneus tertius arises in common with the long digital extensor from the extensor fossa of the femur which is located between the trochlea and the lateral condyle. It travels through the notch between the anterior and external tuberosities at the upper end of the tibia where it is encased within the synovial membrane of the femorotibial articulation. The tendon passes down the front of the tibia superficial to the tibialis anterior and beneath the proximal annular ligament in company with the tendon of the long digital extensor muscle. The peroneus tertius bifurcates in front of the hock joint and the 2 portions run medially and laterally to the tendon of the tibialis anterior muscle. The medial portion is inserted into the third tarsal and third metatarsal bones immediately below the front of the hock joint, and the lateral part inserts upon the fourth tarsal and fibular tarsal bones. A portion is incorporated into the medial annular ligament which surrounds the tendon of the long digital extensor.

The tibialis anterior, which lies on the tibial surface, is continued by a single tendon which branches into anterior and medial portions. The anterior branch is attached to the third metatarsal and the medial branch to the first tarsal bone.

The small medial tendon of the tibialis anterior which passes obliquely backward over the inner surface of the hock in the shallow cunean groove, is considered a factor in the causation of spavin. It is provided with a small synovial bursa, which may become involved in the inflammatory changes connected with spavin. Dividing this ligament surgically is one of the treatments employed for the relief of spavin lameness.

The rupture which may occur is far more likely to involve the peroneus tertius than the deeper muscular tissue. The actual separation may occur close to the trochlea of the femur or near the middle of the tibial region.

Sometimes the rupture is complete, but more often the fibers are stretched and torn but still offer some resistance to the pull of the gastrocnemius.

Etiology: The commonest cause of rupture undoubtedly is slipping upon a slippery surface or on a soft surface when landing from a jump. When this happens the hock is fully extended with the foot carried behind its normal position. Any pull then contributed by the gastrocnemius will operate against recovery of the normal position of the limb. A similar injury may result when the horse lands on 3 legs after a jump with 1 hindlimb extended backward over the hurdle.

Rupture of the peroneus tertius also may be one of the hazards encountered when a horse is cast, and one hindfoot is drawn behind the body and held there, particularly if the rope holding it is firmly attached to a fixed object.

Any attempt to pull the limb free may then easily tear or rupture the muscle.

Clinical Signs: The signs exhibited when the rupture is partial differ somewhat from those shown in complete rupture. In partial rupture, the hock is straightened and the tip of the toe may be drawn back so that the horse tends to place weight on the lower part of the toe, immediately over the toe clip of the shoe.

There usually is some swelling in the midtibial region caused by extravasation of blood into the surrounding tissues. The condition is painful and the horse shows difficulty in bringing the toe forward sufficiently for weight to be placed on the sole of the foot. If it succeeds in accomplishing this, the horse then can take one pace forward, but encounters the same difficulty when it attempts to move the affected leg forward again.

In complete rupture, the picture is different. Being unopposed, the gastrocnemius muscle takes full charge and jerks the point of the hock upward and backward. The foot is lifted free of the ground and carried with the fetlock flexed but the hock extended. When the gastrocnemius relaxes, its tendon folds above the tuber calcis, giving an appearance of corrugation which is typical of the condition. Each time the gastrocnemius contracts the foot is kicked backward, and this occurs on every occasion the horse is moved forward.

Prognosis: The prognosis in cases of partial rupture is satisfactory and most cases recover completely in 2 to 3 months. In complete rupture the prognosis is doubtful and will depend upon the position of the rupture, the temperament of the patient, and the patience of the owner. Such a case will require a sling support for a considerable period.

Treatment: Even in partial rupture, a sling support is advisable, but if the horse can be kept in a level field in summer weather a light hobble applied around the heel below the fetlock and attached by a rope to a collar or neck rope, will enable the horse to place weight upon its foot and move slowly about the field. A mild biniodide of mercury ointment (1 to 15 or 1 to 20) may be gently rubbed into the anterior tibial region at intervals of 10 days.

TIBIAL LAMENESS

This type of lameness usually results from a kick on the inner side of the thigh, midway between hock and stifle. Sometimes it results from getting a hindlimb caught in a fence.

The tibia being almost subcutaneous, at this spot, is exposed to injury. It may suffer a star fracture or a depressed fracture, or the bone may be fractured without rupture of its periosteum. This may take the form of a fissure which subsequently may break down and form a complete fracture.

In other cases, infection may be introduced and an abscess of considerable size may form, or a sinus may develop leading to a splintered bone surface.

Injuries to this area generally are acutely painful and cause marked lameness, often attended by systemic disturbances. The degree of lameness often seems out of all proportion to the apparent severity of the injury.

PATELLAR LAMENESS

Apart from femoropatellar arthritis and superficial bursal enlargement, the commonest form of lameness associated with the patella is due to its luxation. When luxation of the patella occurs, it usually is displaced either upward or laterally. Medial luxation of the patella is rare in the horse.

UPWARD LUXATION OF THE PATELLA

The patella can be displaced only when the femorotibial joint is fully extended, not when it is partially or completely flexed, except in the few cases of congenital abnormality of the ridges and grooves of the femoral trochlea.

Since straight hocks and stifles became fashionable in race horses, luxation of the patella, particularly in growing stock whose bones have not fully developed, has become more frequent. The progeny of certain stallions are particularly predisposed, owing to the almost complete absence of stifle angulation.

Clinical Signs: The first sign of upward subluxation seen in the horse is a momentary locking of the hindleg when the animal is turned to be brought from the stall. This locking will become more frequent and pronounced until it occurs while the horse is being worked. The medial patellar ligament is stretched until it has lengthened sufficiently for frank dislocation to occur. Too straight a conformation of the hindlimb predisposes this disorder. A horse with moderately angulated stifle should be worked easily in as straight a line as possible, and never turned sharply.

In 2- and 3-year-olds, the patella may become partially luxated during a gallop and regain its position unaided. The only indication may be a sudden momentary fixing of a hindlimb in extension. This may persist during 1 or 2 strides (with corresponding loss of speed) followed by a return to normal, or the animal may be compelled to pull-up.

When the degree of luxation is more severe the horse is found with the hindlimb completely extended in the backward direction, the animal being completely unable to flex the limb at any joint.

When medial luxation occurs the limb is locked in flexion.

Treatment: To replace the patella a long rope is looped at one end and drawn over the head and neck until it rests in front of the shoulder. The free end of the rope is passed around the back of the pastern and then through the neck loop. While this is pulled upon by 1 or 2 men, the horse is persuaded to jump forward and the patella usually "clicks" back into place.

Subsequently, it is advisable to apply a suitable hobble and fix the rope to a collar or neck loop so that the limb cannot be extended in the backward direction. This rope should be kept in position for 24 to 48 hours, while the horse is confined. Diathermy or liniment can be used over the insertion of the medial patellar ligament.

The severely lame horse should be rested, a corrective shoe applied and the stifle treated by diathermy or subcutaneous blister, preferably the latter. Any horse disposed to patellar luxation should be regularly exercised to maintain tonus of the quadriceps femoris muscle which serves to maintain the position of the patella.

LATERAL LUXATION OF THE PATELLA

Lateral luxation occurs in foals which have congenitally absent or incomplete trochlear ridges. Sometimes the bony defect is less marked, and intermittent lateral luxation occurs in colts and fillies, as it does in cases of upward luxation. While the limb is extended in upper luxation, it is held in flexion in cases of lateral luxation.

The patella can be felt as a hard mass at the outer side of the joint. To replace it a rope is attached to the pastern and an attempt is made to pull the foot backward, while manual pressure is applied below the patella, pushing it upward and forward and inward.

STIFLE LAMENESS (GONITIS)

Etiology: Because of its extensive joint surface and marked angulation, the stifle joint is not a common site for proliferative arthritic lesions. Stifle lameness is produced by any mechanical factor which causes strains of the ligaments of the joints or damage to the joint surfaces. The commonest cause is overextension of the joint produced when the animal slips. The etiology for gonitis often is not known.

Clinical Signs: The horse with a painful stifle will carry the affected leg to or across the center line when moving so that its foot tends to fall behind the opposite front foot. Dropping of the quarter will not be as great as in hip lameness. Observation will show that the joint is not moved as much as normally. This lack of movement can cause the animal to scuff its toe because of the interaction of the joints of the hindleg. This is one of the most reliable signs of stifle lameness. Palpation along the medial edge of the joint margin of the tibia will reveal a thickening and rounding of the joint margin, and pain will be manifested in a large percentage of early cases.

In chronic gonitis, the horse attempts to avoid contact of the inflamed joint surfaces. To do this, it either flexes all the joints of the limb, or extends all of them. There is no alternative to these 2 positions since the stifle, hock and fetlock flex or extend in unison. Sometimes the foot is held off the ground with all joints flexed. Pain is experienced in advancing the limb and anything other than a slow walk becomes impossible. Any attempt to trot is made on 3 legs.

In chronic gonitis, the femorotibial articulation is usually the seat of lameness, and not only are the joint surfaces involved but also the interarticular disks of fibrocartilage and their ligamentous attachments. The head of the tibia shows ulceration, particularly in the neighborhood of the tibial spine, with corresponding ulceration of the femoral condyles. Osteophytes appear on the articular margins and the interarticular cartilages become degenerated and flake away so that the fluid contained in the cavities, in addition to being present in great excess, contains particles of the interarticular cartilages and bloodstained synovia.

In a small proportion of cases, ulceration may exist without increase in the secretion of synovia, especially in those cases which mainly involve the femoropatellar articulation.

When ulceration is present and the cartilages are involved, recovery is impossible. Many cases progress slowly, so that mild lameness may persist for some time and the horses often work for months until the diseased condition of the joint progresses to the stage when the animal is markedly lame and suffering pain.

Treatment: Intra-articular injection of corticosteroids and phenylbutazone to reduce pain and inflammation should be tried in conjunction with cold applications while the condition is acute. Diathermy is a logical supportive treatment.

For the common stifle lamenesses, rest is important. If the lesion occurs along the medial side of tibial joint margin, diathermy or a topically applied liniment will assist recovery. If evidence points to damage of the joint surface, injection of a corticosteroid followed by diathermy would be indicated.

Even the most modern treatments seldom delay the pathologic process for long. The older practitioners resorted to the administration of sodium salicylate and potassium iodide, and this treatment sometimes appeared to relieve pain, but then, as today, intractable lameness was the final result.

HIP LAMENESS

In horses, true hip joint lameness prob-ably is a rare condition since the region is well-covered by muscles and in a protected position. Damage to the external trochanter of the femur, however, is by no means rare and since this bony prominence overlies the hip joint it is probable that it is the origin for a great many lamenesses attributed as being in the joint itself. Bruising or fracture of the ex-ternal trochanter is followed by a shortening of the stride. The hindfoot of the affected side is often advanced with a circular swinging movement of the foot and lower part of the limb. The horse is said to "move away" from the affected side, a form of "3-cornered lame-ness." At rest, the horse is inclined to raise the heel and place weight on the toe.

Provided the skin is intact and no infection is introduced, fracture of the great trochanter usually heals by fibrous union. This may result in several months' lameness, but in the major-ity of cases recovery is complete.

In most lamenesses arising in the hip re-gion, the action is typical. The animal expe-riences pain, chiefly when it extends the joint, and the hip is held fixed at a slight degree of flexion, movement being confined as much as possible to the stifle and hock joints. This causes the horse to "hop" during each forward stride with the foot resting on the toe of the shoe.

TROCHANTERIC BURSITIS

The middle gluteal muscle arises from the outer surface of the ilium, from the iliosacral and sacrosciatic ligaments and from the gluteal fascia. It is inserted into the summit of the femur and the great trochanter. A synovial bursa facilitates the gliding of the tendon over the convexity of the great trochanter. Injury to this bursa and the cartilage of the great tro-chanter cause most of the so-called cases of hip lameness.

Clinical Signs: The clinical signs include pain and swelling with some distention of the bursa. Trochanteric bursitis often is called whirlbone disease. Its diagnosis depends on knowledge of the normal gait. The foot leaves the ground more slowly and the flight of the foot is slow. When the lameness is more severe, the foot is adducted during flight so that viewed from behind, it swings in toward the other hind foot, then out again, as it is put down. This gait is characteristic of hip lame-ness only. Occasionally, pressure applied over the bursa will produce pain. To differentiate from other causes of lameness, the foot should be examined carefully because hip lameness is not nearly as common as other hindleg disorders.

Treatment: Treatment consists essentially of enforced rest. Traditionally, an internal blister was used and this still is done successfully. A 2-inch needle is inserted at right angles to the skin above the greater trochanter. Corticoster-oids can be injected this way or directly into the bursa. Diathermy or ultrasonic rays can also be used in these cases.

PELVIC LAMENESS

Although injury to the floor of the pelvis, common in the cow, is seldom encountered in the mare or horse, there are 2 forms of pelvic lameness which are by no means rarities. Either may confuse the diagnosis of lameness if the possibility of pelvic injury is overlooked tem-porarily.

Etiology: The more common condition is in-jury to the tuber coxae, the external angle of the ilium. This bony prominence frequently suffers traumatic injury from falls or when the horse passes through doorways. The damage may be a mere bruising or it may involve frac-ture. When infection supervenes, portions of bone may become necrotic and require surgi-cal removal. In cases of simple contusion, the initial lameness may be slight or, occasionally, severe.

Clinical Signs: The signs greatly resemble those described for injury to the great tro-chanter of the femur; in addition, there is marked resistance to palpation of the tuber coxae. The horse shows difficulty in advancing the limb and places weight upon the toe of the shoe. Most cases in which there is no fracture, and in which necrosis does not super-vene, recover in a few days to a few weeks.

When fracture occurs the external angle of the ilium will be permanently lower than that of the sound side. The condition is referred to as "pin-down" or "knocked down hip."

The other injury, which may be very misleading unless a rectal examination is done, is fracture of the shaft of the ilium. The degree of lameness will depend on the type of the fracture. When complete, there will be overlapping of the 2 ends of the fractured shaft, great pain, and crepitation. When the shaft is fissured but not displaced, the horse dislikes placing weight on the foot, and it is quite easy to mistake the condition for foot lameness.

ILIAC THROMBOSIS

At one time, lameness arising from thrombosis of the iliac arteries at their point of origin from the posterior aorta was not uncommon. A similar condition has been encountered in the brachial artery, affecting the forelimbs. In either case, the occlusion is at first partial but later it may become complete. Bilateral iliac thrombosis has been reported.

Etiology: The etiology is uncertain. In some cases, strongyles are held responsible. The changes in the arterial endothelium also have been attributed to influenza and strangles but the evidence for this is inconclusive.

Clinical Signs: The first indication of iliac or brachial artery thrombosis is pain after or during a short trot. The horse sweats, appears distressed and usually is considered to have colic. Frequently, the animal attempts to lie down. Inability to move the affected limbs increases as the horse continues to move, but lessens rapidly if the animal is allowed to stand and rest for 10 to 30 minutes. The horse may then travel, perhaps a hundred yards, before the signs recur.

When the femoral artery is involved the pain may be present in the resting horse. When the external iliac artery is the site of thrombus, the blood supply to the gluteal and quadriceps muscles is impaired. The limb no longer can support weight, the stifle, hock and fetlock become flexed, and the signs exhibited when the animal is exercised resemble those seen in crural paralysis. In true iliac thrombosis, the horse may seem quite normal when in the stable.

Diagnosis: Diagnosis can be confirmed by rectal examination and a comparison of the arterial pulsation on either side. When the condition is bilateral, the comparison in pulsation can be made with a normal subject.

Although some horses have been said to have developed a collateral circulation and recovered, one might reasonably suspect the correctness of the diagnosis.

LUMBAR LAMENESS

Etiology: Although herniated intervertebral discs do not play an important role in equine lameness, a considerable amount of obscure lameness may be associated with changes occurring in the spinal column and/or in the muscles which lie over and below the lumbar region of the spine. In jumpers, steeplechasers, hunters, and even in horses which race on the flat, strain of the psoas and other sublumbar muscles is a fairly common occurrence.

Lumbar lameness may make its appearance in young horses used for racing, or in jumpers at any age, especially if they are overtrained or carry too much weight. Injury to the psoas muscles also may be caused by slipping. In horses more than 8 to 10 years of age, lumbar lameness may be complicated by spondylosis of the lumbar vertebrae. This may occur between any 2 of the bones or it may involve 3 articulations.

The bones of race horses preserved in natural history museums often show extensive ankylosis of lumbar vertebrae. This almost would appear to be the usual condition in aged horses and one which may cause no lameness whatever unless a bony union which had formed between 2 bones becomes separated. This results in pain and limits the ability to flex the spine.

Clinical Signs: In extreme cases, some pressure may be put on the spinal cord, with resulting lack of coordination of the 2 limbs, ataxia, and a disinclination to trot or canter. There may be partial or complete inability to lift the tail. This condition is sometimes referred to as "jink-back."

Such cases of partial paralysis commonly are encountered in jumpers. The earliest signs are a disinclination to jump. Horses which previously have jumped well, either refuse their jumps or take them in 3-cornered fashion, going obliquely across the jump rather than straight over it. At first, the disinclination may be more marked on some days than others. Weather sometimes may appear to play a part in increasing or lessening the discomfort, and a horse may jump on a warm day, yet completely refuse in wet, cold weather. The diagnosis may be assisted by palpation of the sublumbar region per rectum.

Prognosis: The prognosis depends on the cause, and on the condition of the lumbar articulations. Hunters and steeplechasers at 8 or 9 years of age suddenly may fade in their progress. If rested for 12 months, or even for 2 years, they may return to good form, but there always is a risk of a further separation of the ankylosed vertebrae.

EXTERNAL POPLITEAL PARALYSIS

This branch of the sciatic divides a little behind the lateral ligament of the stifle, into the musculocutaneous and anterior tibial nerves. The anterior tibial nerve supplies the extensor muscles in front of the tibia. Damage to it will produce paralysis of the extensor muscles of the hindlimb, and lack of opposition to the pull of the gastrocnemius. The limb therefore is carried backward, and the horse stands on the front wall of the foot with extreme fetlock flexion. When the musculocutaneous nerve also is involved the horse will be insensitive to a needle prick on the outer metatarsal region.

The limb cannot be brought forward voluntarily, but if the sole of the foot is applied to the ground by manual assistance, the horse will place weight upon it and take one step forward.

Recovery may occur but its course usually is protracted.

INTERNAL POPLITEAL PARALYSIS

The muscles at the back of the hindlimb, the gastrocnemius, soleus, deep and superficial digital flexors, and the popliteus are not functional during internal popliteal paralysis. The extensor muscles are unapposed and the foot is carried far forward at each step and returns to the ground with a jerk. Usually the neural defect is in the spinal cord and the prognosis is not good.

CRURAL PARALYSIS

The anterior crural nerve is derived from the lumbosacral plexus and supplies the quadriceps muscle which extends the femorotibial joint. During paralysis of this nerve, the stifle and hock are flexed, and there is absence of sensation on the inner aspect of the thigh. The affected quarter is carried lower than the other and this is seen readily during movement when the rear part of the body sinks at every step as the hock and stifle give way when weight is placed on the foot. The rectus and vastus muscles atrophy, and when the horse is moved they appear as thick cords.

The only prescription is exercise in a level, unobstructed field. If recovery occurs it will take several months.

H. CRESSWELL AND R. H. SMYTHE

REFERENCES

1. McCunn, J.: Vet. Rec. 63 (1951) 629-633.
2. Mitchell, W. M.: Vet. Rec. 61 (1949) 352.
3. Oxspring, G. E.: Vet. Rec. 15 (1935) N.S. 1433-47.
4. Pryer, A. A.: J. Army Vet. Cps. 2 (1931) 134.
5. Smythe, R. H.: Clinical Veterinary Surgery, Vol. 1.

CANKER

Canker basically is chronic hypertrophic inflammation of the horny frog. As the condition progresses, the deeper tissues become involved. The cause of the inflammation most often is irritation resulting from constant wetness of the foot. Urine-soaked bedding especially is apt to cause this condition. When the tissues become devitalized secondary infection occurs, though in some cases a direct injury to the frog permits entry of infective organisms into the deeper tissues.

Clinical Signs: The disease usually begins at the cleft of the frog; occasional cases begin at the junction of the periople of the heel and the corium of the frog. As the sensitive laminae become inflamed or infected, lameness is exhibited. The horny frog softens and enlarges, and a dark colored, odorous exudate often is noted in the crevices of the frog. As the process continues, the horny frog may be removed easily. The infection often spreads under the sole, and in advanced cases may penetrate under the bars and the wall of the hoof. Exuberant granulations often form under the loosened areas of the frog and sole.

Treatment: Treatment varies depending on the extent of the disease. In all cases, removal of the exciting causes is essential. In early cases, all loose frog and horn should be stripped down to healthy tissue and this may be all that is necessary for recovery.

More advanced cases require use of astringent preparations. Various astringent powders, such as tannic acid, boric acid, or commercially prepared astringents may be applied under a bandage after all loose frog and horn have been removed. Wet astringent packs may be used in place of powders. Formalin at ½% concentration, 1% copper sulfate solution, or 5% tannic acid solution often are employed. When the infection has been brought under control, as evidenced by hardening and drying of the frog and affected areas of the sole, shoeing with a leather pad over oakum and pine tar often is used. A moderate amount of exercise is beneficial.

Granulations, if present under the horny frog or the sole, must be removed or controlled. Excision by means of a scalpel or by actual cautery is the method of choice. Caustics such as calomel, butter of antimony, or a paste of sulfur and sulfuric acid may be used but their action is difficult to control. Astringents applied under pressure bandages are used as indicated, followed by shoeing to protect the area.

R. L. LUNDVALL

OSTEOCHONDROSIS DESSICANS FREE JOINT BODIES

Osteochondrosis dessicans is a term coined in 1905 to denote an osteochondritis which results in the splitting of pieces of articular cartilage and underlying bone into the joint cavity. Occasionally, the fragments are not detached completely. The condition occurs primarily in young animals before growth centers have closed. Most, but not all, cases appear to be post-traumatic in origin.

The term, osteochondrosis dessicans, is applied more loosely to free bodies (joint mice) located within joint cavities. Free joint bodies may result from a variety of other causes.

Etiology: Free bodies develop within joint cavities during the following conditions:

1. Osteochondrosis dessicans
2. Osteoarthritis
3. Synovial chondromatosis or osteochondromatosis

In osteochondrosis dessicans, the initial cause generally is trauma resulting in an ischemia and aseptic necrosis of bone. Excessive probing into joints with hypodermic needles is becoming an increasingly important cause of the condition. A needle may chip a small piece of the articular cartilage, causing a free body to form. It is interesting to note that almost every growth center may be involved in osteochronditis of growth centers. Varieties of this condition often are regarded as separate diseases, such as Osgood-Schlatter disease in which an epiphysial ischemia is an important factor.

In osteoarthritis, trauma again is a primary etiologic factor. The arthritic bony spurs may be fractured and isolated as free bodies in the joint.

In osteochondromatosis, a synovial membrane during a rather benign pathologic process may form osteocartilagenous bodies which extend into the joint cavity.

There also is some evidence that free bodies can form after the occurrence of hemorrhage into a joint cavity. In such cases, which often are associated with fracture of joint surfaces, blood is thought to clot, organize, and calcify to form the free body.

Clinical Signs: Since loose bodies may be cartilagenous or osteocartilagenous they may or may not be visible in radiographs. When lesions of osteochondrosis dessicans are visible, a sharply defined cavity can be observed in an adjoining bone from which the sequestrum arose (Fig. 32).

After the free body has become isolated in a joint it may continue to grow or it may be-

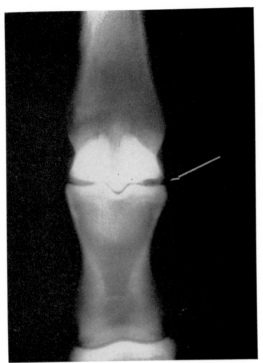

Fig. 32. Osteochondritis dessicans of the lateral distal condyle of the third metatarsus. Arrow points to darkened necrotic area. Radiograph by J. P. Manning, D.V.M.

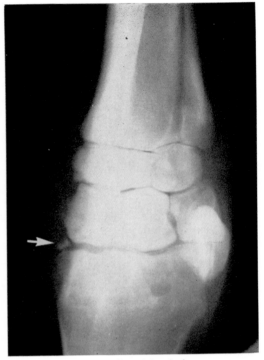

Fig. 33. Free joint body.

come fragmented. If the sequestrum becomes adherent to the synovial membrane, the animal may not show clinical signs of its presence. Generally, the larger the free body, the more likely it is to be confined to an area in which it will not cause signs. A partially attached body occasionally may cause signs, however (Fig. 33).

When the bony fragment floats freely in a joint it can restrict movement and cause intermittent locking and releasing of the joint. Pain, swelling and intermittent lameness accompany the presence of free joint bodies. Clinical signs generally are accompanied by serous effusion into the joint and hypertrophic synovitis.

Treatment: Rest and immobilization with a plaster cast are recommended in cases where the free body is not in a position to cause mechanical interference with the joint. The healing progress during conservative treatment can be followed radiographically.

Use of antiphlogistics and mild pressure dressings, applied immediately after an injury, will help control hemorrhage and inflammation, thus minimizing the development of deformities.

Arthrotomy for removal of the loose fragment is advisable in most cases. Surgery should not be undertaken, however, unless proper facilities for aseptic conditions are available. When surgery is undertaken for the removal of one loose body, more should always be suspected and looked for. Loose cartilagenous tabs and projecting marginal spurs should be removed to prevent the formation of additional free bodies. A bony fragment often may be difficult to locate since it moves quite freely within the joint.

The surgical incision should be made at right angles to the axis of the joint and as close as possible to the free body. Because access and visualization are limited in joint surgery it is desirable to enter directly over the area of pathology.

After removal of the free body and debridment of the area, hemorrhage should be controlled and the joint wiped clean before closure. At this point, antibiotics and anti-inflammatory drugs may be instilled into the joint. The joint capsule should be closely approximated. A tight suture line will prevent fistulas from forming.

After the operation, a mild pressure dressing is applied and the use of the joint is limited by confinement of the patient to a stall for 1 month, and then 3 months in a small paddock. After the suture lines have healed, radiotherapy is helpful in preventing recurrence of the condition.

OSTEOMALACIA (Adult Rickets) (Bran Disease)

Osteomalacia is one of a series of metabolic bone diseases which are characterized by a decrease in the mass of calcified bone, resulting from failure of calcium salts to be deposited in newly formed bone matrix. This is attributed to an inadequate concentration of phosphorus or calcium in the body fluids.

Osteomalacia presents the same histologic picture as rickets, except that it develops after epiphysial closure. The condition should be clearly distinguished from osteoporosis which is a failure of matrix production, and from osteitis fibrosa cystica which represents increased destruction of bone.

Etiology: The principal cause of osteomalacia is an inadequate concentration of available calcium or phosphorous in the body fluids. This can be caused by any or all of the following conditions:

1. A decrease in intestinal absorption due to dietary deficiencies, prolonged diarrhea, or lack of available vitamin D.

2. Increased urinary excretion of calcium and phosphorus due to renal tubular insufficiency.

3. Hyperphosphatemia—this is one of the major problems of race horses being fed a highly concentrated ration, heavy with bran and low quality roughage. The condition develops when the calcium-phosphorus ratio is reversed (some rations will provide an 8 to 1 ratio of phosphorus over calcium). The acid phosphate ions combine with calcium ions which are extracted from bone.[1] This creates a condition which can predispose the horse to a variety of other lamenesses.

Pregnancy or lactation will magnify the signs of osteomalacia by increasing the demand for calcium and phosphorus.

Clinical Signs: The early signs are skeletal pain and muscular weakness. As the condition progresses, gross skeletal deformities appear along with a loosening of teeth. The enlargement of the facial bones and contour has led to the descriptive term, "big head." In extreme cases, hypocalcemic tetany may occur.

Radiographic evidence of osteomalacia includes generalized radiolucency and pseudofractures which generally occur at the point where arteries impinge on the bony structure. These pseudofractures probably represent small fractures at stress points which fill in with an uncalcified matrix.

Blood serum may exhibit either a low or normal calcium level and/or a low phosphorous level with a high serum alkaline phosphatase, which is a reflection of the increased osteoblastic activity. In most cases, a negative balance of calcium and phosphorus can be demonstrated.

Pathology: The gross morbid anatomy of this condition includes softening and deforming of the bone, incomplete or pseudofractures, and pathologic fractures. Microscopically, there is an increased number of osteoblasts and a virtual absence of osteoclasts. There is an increase in width of the uncalcified osteoid seams.[2]

Treatment: Treatment requires vitamin D and calcium parenterally and in the diet, and a correction of the underlying causes.

R. H. BAKER

REFERENCES

1. Smith, Hilton, Atmore, and Jones, Thomas Carlyle: Veterinary Pathology. Lea & Febiger, Philadelphia, Pa. (1957) 628.
2. Cecil, Russell L., and Loeb, Robert F.: A Textbook of Medicine. 9th Ed. W. B. Saunders Co., Philadelphia, Pa., and London, England. (1955) 1450.

AZOTURIA

This condition, before the era of mechanized transport, was one of the most common and serious diseases of the working horse. It is known all over the world and still is seen frequently, though usually in a mild form.

Occurrence: Characteristically, there is an association with the occurrence of azoturia and a diet high in grain content, a period of rest for 1 or 2 days while on this ration, and then a return to work. Cases also develop as a sequel to casting for surgical procedures.

One common name for the disease arose because the period of rest for the working horse was usually the weekend, so that it almost invariably developed with the return to work on Monday. The Thoroughbred horse which is in the early stages of training also is subject to attacks of azoturia after a period of rest, but seldom are they as severe as those seen in draft horses. This probably is so because the rider notices the first sign of abnormality in the gait and immediately returns the horse to the stable before the condition becomes serious. Among the racing fraternity, the term "tied-up" often is used and usually refers to these milder cases of azoturia.

Clinical Signs: Mild attacks are manifested by signs of muscular weakness and pain, stiffness or incoordination, and tremor of the large muscle masses. These signs become more marked if exercise is continued and often are accompanied by profuse sweating which is interpreted as evidence of acute pain. Palpation of the affected muscles reveals their firmness, and pressure on them elicits evidence of pain. Should the condition develop further, the horse may go down and be unable to rise. The most severe form can develop quite rapidly if the animal is engaged in strenuous activity, such as pulling a heavy load. Associated with the damage to muscle fibers, there is liberation of myoglobin which later appears in the urine causing the latter to be discolored. Depending on the severity of the attack, the color may vary from a light brown to almost black.

Diagnosis: There usually is no difficulty in diagnosis because of the typical history and the clinical signs, particularly in the moderate to severe cases; mild cases, however, may not be so obvious. One may be assisted in making a diagnosis by determination of the urine creatine level, or the urine creatine-creatinine ratio, both of which are increased because of the

destruction of muscle cells and liberation of creatine into the blood plasma.

Prognosis: Recovery from azoturia depends mainly on the severity of the attack but generally animals which do not go down will recover with or without treatment, provided they are rested and given a light diet. The prognosis always is grave if the horse goes down.

Lesions: The precise cause of the muscle damage is obscure but is believed to be associated with large stores of muscle glycogen, and liberation on exercise of more lactic acid than can be rapidly converted in the carbohydrate cycle back to glycogen. The increased acidity in muscles, plus other unknown factors, probably results in coagulation of muscle protein, rupture and lysis of fibers, and the liberation of myoglobin.

As a sequel to the muscle damage, renal lesions develop and, in more severe cases, complete anuria may ensue. It is the renal damage, characterized by lower nephron degeneration, rather than the muscle lesions, per se, which causes death. Various theories for the cause of tubular necrosis have been proposed but, at present, the reasons are unknown. Our ignorance here is best covered by saying that the kidney damage may be the result of accumulation in them of unknown toxic products produced in the damaged muscles. A detailed discussion of the muscle and renal lesions is beyond the scope of this text.

Treatment: In horses which suffer mild to moderate attacks, recovery usually is uneventful. It is, of course, essential to give complete rest from work or training and to insure that the diet is reduced in carbohydrate content. In order to combat the accumulation of lactic acid and to minimize the formation of renal tubular casts, sodium bicarbonate should be given orally. The dosage will depend on the individual case but up to 6 ounces daily can be administered. Parenteral injections of 0.5 Gm. of thiamine hydrochloride daily appear to hasten recovery. When pain is severe, symptomatic treatment is indicated.

The prevention of attacks of azoturia involves a sensible relationship of muscular activity to the diet and rest periods. Any horse owner or trainer should be able to prevent further cases once he is aware of the cause of this disease.

D. C. DODD

THE "TYING UP" SYNDROME

This myopathy has been noted increasingly in recent years, particularly among race horses and light horses under heavy exercise or training. Its etiology is obscure and is thought by many to be a modification of classical azoturia or "Monday morning disease."

It appears to be more prevalent in mares than in geldings or stallions, and usually is associated with young animals in fat condition which are put on a rigorous training regimen. However, "tying up" can be seen in older animals, and in those which have been training vigorously. The condition also seems to occur frequently after the horse has been moved in a van or horse trailer. This may be so because transported animals become nervous and excited and burn up considerable quantities of muscle glycogen, or it may be due to a more direct nervous origin. This latter possibility cannot be discounted since nervous horses appear to be more prone to develop the condition.

"Tying up" also has been confused with physiologic muscle fatigue which can occur in horses that are trained excessively and do not possess adequate glycogen reserves. In muscular fatigue, however, there is not the characteristic hardness of muscle which is an outstanding sign of the "tying up" syndrome. There is considerable difference of opinion among practitioners and researchers as to the exact status of this condition. Some refer to it as a mild variation of azoturia and others as a specific entity. In any event, both conditions result from exertion and present similar clinical signs and lesions.

Etiology: In addition to the "nervous" theory mentioned previously, a number of other theories have been proposed regarding the etiology of this condition. The most probable one is that it is brought on by a spasm of the arterioles supplying the involved muscles, resulting in a decreased blood flow at a time when more is needed. This interferes with muscle function and secondarily results in an accumulation of lactic acid within the muscle cells. The disease apparently develops during the anaerobic phase of muscle metabolism. In the absence of oxygen, muscle glycogen is broken down to lactic acid to produce energy. As the acid environment in the working cell rises, there is a tendency for excess amounts to accumulate in the muscle cells and produce cellular damage which results in a release of myoglobin into the blood stream and from there through the urinary system. Since myoglobin is a much smaller molecule than hemoglobin, it is capable of passing readily through the glomerular filters. The pigment imparts a brownish color to the urine. Ordinarily, in "tying up" there is little damage to the kidneys, in contrast to azoturia which often produces severe renal damage. Actually, the exact nature of the syndrome is obscure and requires considerably more research before any definite statements can be made about its etiology.

Clinical Signs and Lesions: The signs consist of muscle rigidity and lameness affecting the muscles of the croup or loins, accompanied by pain, disinclination to move, a variable temperature, and myoglobinuria. The manifestations ordinarily appear toward the end of or after heavy exercise. Unlike azoturia, the condition seldom is characterized by renal damage, and the mortality is not high. Histologically, the affected muscle shows coagulation necrosis and hyalinization, with accompanying shredding and tearing of the muscle fibers. Grossly affected muscle is pale on cutting, but becomes pinkish-red upon exposure to air. The shredding of muscle fibers is not apparent in gross specimens.

Diagnosis: Diagnosis ordinarily is based upon clinical signs and history. A number of tests have been used or tried to determine the exact status of the syndrome. Serum glutamic oxaloacetic transaminase (SGOT) levels rise in both azoturia and "tying up." Lactic dehydrogenase levels also are above normal in both conditions. Serum potassium levels also rise (hyperkalemia) in both conditions. It is evident, at least from the chemical determinations, that azoturia and the "tying up" syndrome are essentially similar, although they might be of different causation. The essential difference appears to be the relative severity of azoturia.

Prognosis: The prognosis for most cases of "tying up" is good. Unless signs such as apparent myoglobinuria, colic, and severe lameness appear, the affected animal will recover in a relatively short time.

Treatment: Although an azoturia case should not be walked, a "tied up" horse can be moved for some distance providing care is taken not to move the animal too fast or for too long a period. A number of treatments have been suggested in conjunction with stall rest, reduction of the protein in the ration, catheterization of the bladder if necessary, and good nursing care.

Specific treatments include the following:

Calcium borogluconate (500 ml. of 20% solution administered intravenously), physostigmine, succinylcholine, physostigmine plus atropine, insulin, alkalization of the blood stream with sodium bicarbonate solution, thiamine, cortisone or corticosteroid derivatives, tranquilizers, and selenium. The plethora of treatments indicates a lack of basic knowledge of the disease.

Calcium borogluconate solution probably is worthwhile in those horses which show signs as a result of myasthenia or muscle fatigue rather than those with myoglobinuria.

Physostigmine and succinylcholine have been used for their respective potentiating and stimulating action on acetylcholine at the neuromuscular synapses. Atropine is used in conjunction with physostigmine to block the acetylcholine potentiation in the intestinal tract and prevent hypermotility and purging.

Insulin has been used with the object of restoring normal glycolysis.

Alkalization of the blood stream has been tried to neutralize the excess lactic acid in the affected muscle.

Thiamine aids the breakdown of lactic acid.

Corticosteroids have been employed for their anti-inflammatory and metabolic effects.

Tranquilizers have been used with some success in reducing the incidence in nervous animals being transported. This, however, is prophylaxis rather than therapy. Tranquilizers, however, may be used in severe cases which show excessive pain or colicky signs.

Selenium has been reported as an effective therapeutic and prophylactic agent in "tied-up" horses in New Zealand.

J. F. BONE

REFERENCES

1. Dodd, D. C., *et al.*, New Zealand Vet. J. **8** (1960) 45.
2. Hartley, W. J., and Dodd, D. C., New Zealand Vet. J. **5** (1957) 61.
3. Hartley, W. J., and Grant, A. B., Federation Proceedings **20** (July 1961) 2.
4. Brennan, B. F. *et al.*, Proc. 5th Ann. AAEP Conv., Dec., 1959.

CHAPTER 18

DIAGNOSIS AND SPECIAL TREATMENTS
OF LAMENESS

DIAGNOSIS OF LAMENESS

Introduction

It is not easy to define equine lameness. Everybody knows quite well what the term means, until asked to find words to describe it. Perhaps lameness is best defined as a condition in which there is a disturbance of the gait normally exhibited in any particular limb.

This may not altogether avoid some of the difficulties one may encounter. For example, after a day's hunting, or a grueling race over hurdles, a horse may exhibit general stiffness and soreness of muscles without the signs being confined to any particular limb. Toxic conditions or generalized illness may produce stiffness, while an allergic condition such as one that results in laminitis may cause the horse to be incapable of moving either forelimb. In other conditions a casual observer might assert that the horse seemed to be "lame all over," yet a horse in this condition does not conform precisely with our definition.

There are other difficulties to face. Is a horse which is stiff in a single limb truly lame? A horse stiff in a pair of forelimbs, or a pair of hindlimbs, may show less lameness than when one limb is affected. One may recollect the story of the horsedealer who, every time he sold, or resold, a certain spavined animal, prepared it for inspection by tapping the inner aspect of the sound hock with a mallet. The horse, lame on both hocks, showed less lameness than when only one was painful.

Age is associated with less action in the gait and it would sometimes be difficult to trace the stiffness to any particular limb. It even might have its origin in the spine. A horse may be lame in more than one limb at a time and the cause of the lameness may be similar in each limb, or it may be completely different. The lameness may exist in a pair of limbs, in 2 limbs of one side of the body, or it may affect 2 diagonal limbs.

Lameness may be a manifestation of pain, of mechanical inability to use the limb, or of both conditions combined. It may arise in a marked form from injury to a nerve, which also may remove all sensation from the seat of lameness. The pain may not be located in the limb at all. Horses show lameness when their ribs are injured, or when they suffer from pleurisy. An iliac thrombosis may be the cause, or an unsuspected growth on the end of the spermatic cord may produce lameness.

Many forms of lameness originate in the spinal column and may be associated with pressure on efferent nerves, or even upon afferent nerves in some instances, the cause being stenosis of one or more vertebral foramina. Such conditions may be hereditary, may arise from a vitamin deficiency in the dam or during the lifetime of the progeny. They also may result from repeated concussion, or from traumatic injury.

A fracture, a bone fissure, or an incomplete fracture in a foal (greenstick fracture), in which the periosteum remains intact, may produce marked lameness, and its site may be unsuspected until the fracture becomes complete. A lameness may appear quite suddenly and disappear nearly as quickly as it arose—or it may persist and result in subsequent malformation. Such may arise from a contusion and one of the most common causes is striking the inner surface of the fetlock with the opposite foot. In horses which step high the injury may be located on the inner aspect of the metacarpal bone just below the knee.

A suddenly occurring lameness often originates in the foot and may be produced by a penetrating foreign body which causes pain— or the immediate injury may cause only slight or temporary lameness, and the acute phase may not be manifested until several days later when suppuration within the foot produces severe pain.

Lameness may be intermittent, or it may vary in its severity at different times. A horse suffering from a developing spavin may leave the stable acutely lame. After 5 or 10 minutes of exercise, the pain may diminish and the lameness may almost disappear. Conversely, a horse affected with an articular lameness, such as true ringbone, may leave the stable very lame, improve a little as the stiffness wears off but become even more obviously lame after an hour's work.

Various conditions, as diverse as corns, curbs and arterial abnormalities, may produce intermittent lameness so that the horse may appear reasonably sound one day and visibly lame another.

Lameness due to chronic laminitis, edema of the limbs, and some joint conditions may be improved by turning the horse out to graze, or by providing daily exercise. Many horses which are persistently and slightly lame probably are more comfortable when given exercise than when rested.

Lameness in the horse may quickly give rise to muscular atrophy, contraction of the related foot, and general loss of condition. In many instances the lameness becomes aggravated markedly by the secondary condition, and on this account one always should consider whether absolute rest is indicated in the treatment of a specific lameness.

Extensive lameness of the hindlimb and occasionally of the forelimb may follow an attack of hemoglobinuria. This is due entirely to muscular atrophy which makes it difficult for the hindlimb to support the weight of the body, the damaged muscles being unable to hold the joint in extension.

DYNAMICS OF EQUINE LOCOMOTION

To understand the cause of lameness in the horse and its possible implications, one needs to know something of the dynamics of locomotion. Lameness in many cases is the result of repeated concussion, or due to failure of synchronization between a joint and the muscles which operate it. Such a failure not only is capable of producing injury within a joint but it may cause a large solid bone such as the femur or the humerus suddenly to shatter.

The forelimbs of the horse are more susceptible to concussion than the hind. The latter are protected by the constant flexion of the joints of the limb, the stifle and hock in particular, and by the fact that the stifle and hock joints work automatically in unison, so that by "squatting" a little the weight can be brought onto the hindfeet, the center of gravity carried back for some distance, and the weight of the body removed from the forelimbs.

A great many people fail to realize that the forelimb from the elbow down is completely locked into a solid rod when the horse is standing squarely on all 4 feet. The distal end of the humerus carries 2 cylindrical surfaces for articulation with the radius and ulna, and behind them lies a deep groove, the olecranon fossa. When weight is placed upon the foot, the free portion of the ulna (the olecranon) enters this groove, and through the arrangement of muscles and tendons in the forelimb this entry completely locks the joint. The only direction of movement possible in the elbow joint of the horse is one which is in a straight line with the rest of the limb. There are only 2 positions possible in this joint—it is either open or closed. When the forefoot is taking weight, the whole limb becomes a rigid structure. But when the horse flexes the joints of its hindlimbs so that its tail-end sinks nearer the ground, and especially when one hindfoot is carried forward a short distance, the weight is taken off the forefoot and transferred to the hindfoot. The elbow joint then again becomes capable of movement through an angle of 100°.

Due to this mechanical device, the elbow joint can move only when the carpus is flexed, so a horse is able to jump only when both forelegs are doubled under the body, and it is able to straighten the forelimbs to make a landing only after the feet are clear of the top rail. The old prints which showed horses clearing fences with their 2 forelegs stretched well out in front were fashionable, but highly unrealistic.

All of this has a marked bearing on concussion. The horse, carrying half a hundredweight of head and neck, is a front-heavy animal, and it almost is entirely dependent upon cooperation between the comparatively rigid fore-end and the highly flexible hind-end to preserve the forelimbs from damage due to concussion.

Commencing at the scapula, the suprascapular cartilage coupled with the flat undersurface of this bone and the loose areolar tissue between it and ribs cooperate to minimize some of the effects of the forefeet landing upon solid ground. The shoulder slides over the ribs, until it is pulled up by the muscles which attach it to the body. This action operates in the same way as the shock absorber of a car.

When weight falls upon the forefoot, the elbow automatically locks and the muscles and tendons, with the help of the suspensory ligament, brace the leg so that the knee and fetlock joints remain rigid and are unable to yield or double up, even when the whole weight of the body lands on one foot. In landing from a jump, one foot meets the ground first. The second foot, a fraction of a second later, lands a little in front of the first, not in an upright position but a little obliquely and at an acute angle with the ground, throwing a great strain upon the flexor tendons.

When the first foot lands the concussion is transmitted to it and is absorbed partly by the elasticity of the plantar cushion, especially when the method of shoeing permits the frog to make contact with the ground. The force of landing then travels through the various joints including the knee, which absorbs more concussion as the rows of small bones slide over one another. The elbow and shoulder joints, fortified by their muscles, each take up a little of the shock, and a great deal more is absorbed when the shoulder forms a more acute angle.

The second forelimb, which takes over after the first foot descends from the jump, does not receive as much concussion as did the first limb. Instead, the strain falls upon the tendons at the back of the cannon bone. The deep flexor tendon, being inserted into the under surface of the os pedis, prevents the toe of the foot from turning upward. This also is the moment when the crushing effect of the tendons falls upon the sesamoid bones behind the fetlock, and also upon the navicular bone.

The latter, wedged between the back of the os pedis and the ever-tightening tendon, must experience the sensations of a nut within the jaws of a nutcracker.

Not only do the forelimbs of the horse support a great deal of weight but they also play an important part in propelling, or perhaps it would be better to say pulling, the body in a forward direction. They have to travel in front of the body very rapidly and assume an acute angle with the ground, then, still rigid, revolve into the perpendicular and allow the weight of the body to swing above them, just as though they represented 2 spokes of a wheel. As soon as the hindfeet are planted firmly on the ground, the forelimbs have to be ready to shoot forward and repeat the whole process over again.

The forefeet also have to accept the responsibility of acting as the main brakes when the horse wants to check the momentum by preventing the rapidly moving body from overshooting the mark, getting off balance, and turning a somersault. This is of special importance when a horse lands from a jump at speed.

The one forefoot takes the weight and a great deal of the concussion, the second shoots forward to land a little in front of its fellow. This keeps the front end of the body from tumbling onto the ground, and at the same time permits the hindfeet to land well under the middle of the abdomen with both hocks flexed, and take all the weight for a moment off the forelimbs which have now locked at the elbow joints. The forelimbs then can advance into the next stride. This provides some idea of the amount of strain thrown upon the forelimbs, which are expected to act as rigid props during a great part of the horse's locomotor activities, while the hindlimbs are exposed much less to the effects of concussion since they are concerned mainly with joint flexion.

The forefeet are flatter in their soles, and the pasterns yield less than those of the hindlimbs. In most horses the frogs of the forefeet are much closer to the ground than are the frogs of the hindfeet, so that they more readily take the weight and cause expansion of the foot at the circumference, particularly at the heels, in a sequence of events which automatically produces constriction at the upper part of the hoof below the coronary band.

If a horse has upright pasterns together with an upright shoulder, there is little provision for the absorption of concussion, so it will be seen that conformation, both directly and indirectly, may play a considerable part in the production of wear and tear, with resulting lameness. A horse possessing this type of conformation not only will cause considerable discomfort to its rider but it also will bring about rapid deterioration of its own bones, joints, tendons and ligaments, with additional strain upon the sesamoids and especially upon the unhappily situated navicular bone.

In lighter horses, the strain and concussion travel up the limb to the shoulder. In the heavier, thickset draft horses which thump their feet upon the ground but are not exposed to the effects of galloping and jumping, the greatest damage resulting from concussion affects the feet, coronets and fetlocks.

When one appreciates the fact that the greater part of the lamenesses which the veterinarian encounters is the direct effect of concussion and strain, and that the underlying cause of these 2 injurious factors is related to faulty conformation which never can be overcome, one realizes the handicap under which he labors, and why treatment offers little hope of success in many cases.

It is only when he possesses at least an elementary knowledge of the dynamics associated with equine locomotion, that he can devise ways of lessening the effects of faulty conformation. He then endeavors by providing rest, suitable shoeing, changing the nature of the work and sometimes the weight of the load, and by giving relief by various means to the badly treated limbs to render the horse fit to carry on the work demanded of it. How successful the veterinarian will be depends to a very great extent upon the degree of cooperation that he receives from his client.

One of the greatest differences between human and veterinary medicine is that after a prolonged course of treatment the human patient is satisfied, even thankful, if he can walk about with the aid of a stick. The veterinarian's client is satisfied only if the patient makes a 100% recovery.

FACTORS IN THE ETIOLOGY OF LAMENESS

It would appear a little strange, perhaps, to associate the lameness within a horse's limb with some defect of the internal ear, but in some cases there may be a traceable connection. We have noted already that a defect within the spinal column may cause lameness, since it carries the spinal cord and provides access to all the nerves which regulate the movements of the limbs. Both these structures, the ear and the spine, are related closely to balance and the synchronization of body movements. Apart from concussion and direct traumatic injury from external sources, both direct causes of lameness, it is likely that incoordination or lack of harmony in the cooperation of muscles may be the factor responsible for the greatest proportion of the remaining cases of lameness.

The causes of lameness associated with direct trauma include blows, and bruising from any form of violence, often from kicks or collisions. To these we must add strains of tendons, ligaments or muscles (many of which may be caused indirectly by muscular incoordination) and the results of falls (which may cause lameness not only by contusion but also through unbalanced muscular contractions), wounds and punctures, burns and scalds, treads, fractures, and various other accidents. External violence is a common and very obvious cause but it probably is not the most frequent one. Stumbling, false steps, sharp turns, starting and pulling up, landing over jumps, stepping into holes, and slipping may account for many of the accidental causes of lameness. Sometimes these arise in an unexpected fashion. Two horses may collide without undue force during a race. One horse is pushed to one side, and to prevent falling on its hindquarters it quickly abducts the hindlimb on the side opposite to that on which it received the blow. The uncontrolled degree of abduction may fracture or dislocate the hip joint of the limb, or shatter the femur. This may occur despite the fact that no direct injury was received on this side of the body.

Sprains of ligaments, tendons and muscles are not so frequently the result of simple stretching as is imagined often. These tissues usually are capable of withstanding far greater strain than is encountered under normal working conditions. The majority of strains of tendons and ligaments, together with the tearing of muscles, can be attributed to faulty balance, false steps, bad timing, stumbling, or slipping. The resulting lameness is due to the effects arising from a lack of muscular coordination, which may exist only for a fraction of a second. During that brief period, weight may be thrown suddenly and unexpectedly upon a tendon or a ligament, or even upon the muscle operating the tendon. This may cause even greater damage when the ligament, stretched excessively, forms an intrinsic part of a joint.

The lameness produced will be the direct result of an unrestrained pull upon one group of muscles in the absence of a compensating contraction of the opposing group. This will expose various structures to severe stretching, or may create a sudden pull upon some portion of a bone. Since the muscular action is not restricted by normal coordination, the various structures involved may be overstretched, torn, or ruptured. A bone treated in this fashion may sustain a fracture.

Tendons are dependent for their soundness upon the elasticity of the muscles attached to them, and upon the normal restraints imposed upon the degree and rapidity of their contraction.

In the ordinary course of joint movement both the extensors and flexors of a joint contract at the same time, with emphasis on the force exerted by the group in control of the movement. If, however, one group undergoes contraction, only to find itself unopposed by the other group, the joint which the 2 groups flex or extend will fail to operate gently and slowly but will proceed to open or close with a snap. This may result in stretching or tearing of ligaments, or damage to the synovial membranes, while in some cases 1 of the bones forming the joint may break. In young horses, or in foals, the damage may occur at the epiphysis.

A horse prancing or running upon hard ground may shatter or split a pastern bone merely by bringing the sole of the foot into contact with the ground at a moment when the muscles of the limb temporarily fail to synchronize and permit the bones of the fetlock, pastern and foot to assume an abnormal relationship to one another. The resulting effect upon the structure injured is almost similar to that which would be produced by violence from outside the body. In a similar manner, a horse may attempt to jump a bank, and a portion of the earth of which the bank consists may crumble at the moment the hindfoot seeks support. By this means, the calcaneo-metatarsal ligament is unduly strained and the horse may then develop a curb.

In young horses in which the small metacarpal bones have not yet fully united with the main digit, concussion produced by road work, jumping, or exercise on solid turf may give rise to disturbances in the adjacent periosteum. This causes lameness which usually disappears after union between the large and small bones has become complete. The production of osteophytes may cause the development of a bony enlargement immediately below the knee, and although the original lameness may have disappeared, the horse still may be subject to intermittent disabling lameness every time the new growth of bone is bruised by contact with the inner surface of the opposite hoof, or its shoe.

Lameness also may result from excess weight, especially in heavy breeds of horses and ponies. Dartmoor, Welsh ponies, and the like remain perfectly sound when they have to work hard to obtain a small feed of grass, but are apt to become overweight and develop lameness due to chronic laminitis if they are housed and fed on grain and hay.

Lack of care and infrequent attention to the preparation of the foot and removal of shoes predispose to corns, though faulty foot conformation and the type of action also may play their respective parts. It is noteworthy that corns, laminitis, split pasterns, and strained flexor tendons rarely are encountered in the hindlimbs. This is true because the hindfoot does not strike the ground with the degree of force exerted by the forefoot. While the forelimb becomes locked and rigid when the foot descends and the weight falls upon it, the hindlimb regularly yields by increasing flexion of the hock and stifle joints as soon as the foot takes on the weight of the hind part of the body. In the forelimb, the only joint which yields is the shoulder joint, and this, unfortunately, is situated at the upper end of the limb. Whether or not the buffering effect exercised by this joint is exhibited, will depend entirely upon the acuteness of the angle which the scapula forms with the humerus.

There are a number of other factors which have a considerable bearing upon whether a horse will continue sound or develop lameness. Undoubtedly one of the main considerations is the amount of care and attention paid to the shoeing. Shoes provide an artificial bearing for the foot of the horse and while they may be highly beneficial, they often are a necessary evil. A considerate owner and a practical blacksmith can do a great deal to prevent the development of certain kinds of lameness. Many more horses would continue to work and stay sound if shoeing knives had never been invented, and the use of the rasp had been encouraged as a substitute. Bars and soles too frequently are stripped away, heels lowered, and feet trimmed to fit the shoe, instead of the shoe being forged to fit the foot.

Some owners avoid calling the blacksmith until shoes become loose and fall off, and horses have been injured because in casting a shoe they have stepped on their toe clips. Currently many horses are rested too long at one time, then grievously overworked over a relatively short period. After this they are again put into storage until required for use. Often, too little attention is paid to the nature of the surface upon which horses are expected to gallop, and also to the weight they are expected to carry. Mares which are too lame to work and are suffering from the effects of poor conformation seldom are wasted. Instead, their faults are perpetuated by breeding from them. There probably is no surer way of achieving bankruptcy.

R. H. SMYTHE

FUNCTIONAL ANATOMY OF THE LIMBS

The limbs of the horse serve 3 major functions in locomotion: weight-bearing, propulsion, and anticoncussion. Some idea of the amount of work performed may be had from the estimate that a 1,000-pound horse cantering at 11 miles per hour for one hour expends 3,000 foot tons of energy, requiring roughly the equivalent of 3 horsepower. To produce at the same rate, a 200-pound man would have to run up the Washington Monument in one minute (about 10 m.p.h.) which is possible, but not for long. But in terms of useful work (load moved), most horses can develop one horsepower for only 3 to 4 hours.

Locomotion, therefore, might be considered as an orderly progression of columns of articulated levers, each of which subserves the functions of weight-bearing, propulsion and anticoncussion in varying degrees depending on the conformation of the horse, the load carried or drawn, the gait, and the position of the limbs at any given instant. During locomotion these columns, either singly, or as lateral or anterior-posterior bipeds, are alternately lifted and advanced; they receive and distribute the body weight falling on them, and impart the needed propulsive force before being again lifted to repeat the cycle.

Normal functioning of the limbs is related closely to their structure, and disturbed function to deviation in form. Thus while the fore- and hindlimbs function in harmony with one another, it is necessary to consider them separately. And because of the similarities of the fore- and hindfeet, and the special functions they perform, the feet will be treated as a third entity.

THE FORELIMB

The center of gravity of a well-formed horse falls close to a vertical line through the xiphoid cartilage of the sternum, roughly about 6 inches behind the elbow. Projected to the ground this places the forefeet much closer to the center of gravity than the hindfeet—closer in fact than the 55% of weight borne by the forelimbs would suggest. This, of course, is due largely to the weight of the head and neck.

The fact that the forelimb from the shoulder down is relatively straighter than the hindlimb from the hip joint down may be related to the advantage of a more perpendicular column of bones in bearing weight—and to the greater incidence of affections of the forefeet. Moreover, the hindlimbs are alternately rested by shifting the weight in normal standing, but each of the forelimbs bears its full share of weight almost continuously.

In addition, the forelimb bears the full weight of the body for an instant in certain gaits, and for the heel to be planted on the ground the limb from elbow down must be practically straight. So, though weight bearing is favored by bone-to-bone transmission of force in a straight column, anticoncussion becomes a relatively more important factor. Some of the force is dispersed by the angulation of the elbow and shoulder joints, most of it by the anticoncussion mechanism (to be discussed with the foot).

The unique adaptations of the forelimb to its supporting function, and the assumption that a true joint was required for effective propulsive movements, have been stressed by many writers. Long ago, however, it was demonstrated that in the gallop one forelimb will propel the body as much as 10 feet and in so doing raise it 4 inches vertically as well. It seems unnecessary to belabor the point further; obviously, fore- and hindlimbs form a synchronous propulsive mechanism. Various components of this mechanism, however, can conveniently be considered along with the weight-bearing function.

THE SHOULDER

The broad and flattened upper third of the scapula provides ample attachment for the extrinsic muscles of the limb which secure the shoulder to the thorax. In particular, the serratus ventralis, with its extensive rib attachments, serves as a more or less sling-like arrangement to suspend the thorax between the scapulae and distribute weight over a broad area.

Although the serratus and pectoral muscles (with others) normally prevent much lateral

movement (abduction) of the shoulder, a fair degree of cranial-caudal movement is permitted—and indeed is favored by the mode of attachment of the shoulder to the thorax. This union, though mainly muscular, i.e., nonbony, can be regarded as functioning as if it were a true joint; the large amount of areolar tissue between the distal part of the scapula and the thorax permits gliding movements as freely as if this were a large, well-lubricated joint. The forward movement of the entire shoulder joint so permitted may not be of particular consequence in slower gaits, but with maximum effort an appreciable lengthening of stride might well be the difference between win, place, and also-ran. Even at a walk, the first phase of forward progression is advancement and elevation of the shoulder.

The length of the scapula, which is directly related to height of the withers, to a large degree determines the absolute extent of forward movement of the shoulder. A long shoulder also tends to be more oblique, thus favoring the muscles which produce its movement, and concussion is also thereby reduced. Obviously, a horse with a relatively vertical scapula would tire more easily and be more tiring to ride because of direct transmission of shock to the thorax. (The same would be true of other joints which are more vertical than optimal.) A long shoulder relative to length of the humerus favors maximum displacement (extension) of the latter with the least muscular effort.

It is perhaps significant that shoulder affections are often characterized by a swinging-leg lameness, i.e., they are likely to interfere with this essential first phase of progression although not of sufficient consequence to cause a supporting-leg lameness. The short steps and refusal to lift the foot far enough are suggestive of the importance of normal elevation and advancement of the shoulder in locomotion. Fracture of the neck of the scapula, although relatively infrequent, is probably the most severe interference with locomotion that can occur in the shoulder region. Earlier, when fistula of the withers was not uncommon, detachment of the scapular cartilage resulted in incoordination of movement by interfering with the normal rotatory action of the scapula in which the cartilage serves as a more or less fixed pivot. Injury to the suprascapular nerve, which is predisposed by its passing over the cranial border of the neck of the scapula, may result in atrophy of the supra-and infraspinatus muscles, or "sweeny."

The shoulder joint, while of the ball and socket type, admits little but flexion and extension because of limitation of other movements, principally by the pectoral muscles which keep the limb strongly adducted. Other than minor reinforcements of the joint capsule, ligaments are absent, and dislocation is prevented by muscle tonus, the large head of the humerus, and the cohesion of the synovial joint surfaces.

The usual scapulohumeral angle is about 120° (not 90° as is sometimes stated); in flexion it may be reduced to 80°, in extension enlarged to 145°. Though full extension is desirable in producing a long stride, overextension while standing is prevented by the weight of the body. Flexion is limited by the biceps brachii tendon which passes over the extensor surface of the joint and attaches to the distal end of the scapula.

The Arm

The relatively short humerus, especially by comparison with the shoulder, facilitates rapidity of movement and conservation of energy; it also permits the foot to describe an arc of a larger circle than would be the case otherwise. Although too complex to permit full consideration, in forward progression—either from a standing position, or at the end of a stride—when the foot leaves the ground both shoulder and elbow are flexed to elevate the foot, then extended to lengthen the stride.

The normal angle of the elbow joint is about 150° when standing; at this point it is very nearly maximally extended by the triceps muscles, which thus are an essential factor in weight-bearing. Further extension is limited by the insertion of the biceps tendon on the proximal end of the radius. The biceps is a key structure in the so-called stay apparatus in that its scapular tendon stabilizies the shoulder joint, and its long tendon (lacertus fibro-

sus) continues to the proximal cranial border of the large metarcarpal bone, thus helping to prevent flexion of the carpus while standing. Depending on the obliquity of the humerus in relation to the scapula (normally about 120°), the elbow can be flexed through about 55 to 60°.

Stability of the elbow is provided by the strong medial and lateral collateral ligaments and the long transverse axis of the humeral condyles. Both factors prevent movements other than flexion and extension. In flexion the lower limb is moved slightly outward, i.e., lateral to the vertical axis of the limb while standing, because of the slight obliquity of the articular surfaces of the elbow joint. The long axis of the humerus however, is parallel to the median plane of the body; if the elbow is displaced laterally, the foot will be turned inward (cross-footed) and may result in "speedy cutting"; with medial deviation of the elbow, the foot will turn outward (crooked-legged).

Concussion is transmitted from the radius (the ulna being incomplete is not involved) via the humeral condyles to the shaft. That the humerus is relatively short and heavy may be related to the fact that at rapid paces most of the body weight impinges on the elbow joint surfaces with less opportunity than at the shoulder for dissipation of force by spring-like flexion. With the elbow extended, angulation of the condyles places them in direct line with the radius.

The bicipital bursa (bursa intertubercularis), which facilitates play of the biceps tendon in the intertubercular groove at the proximal end of the humerus, may be the site of inflammation (bicipital bursitis). The bursa is vulnerable because of its exposed position and because of the great stress imposed upon it inasmuch as a major part of the body weight is supported by the biceps tendon, which prevents undue flexion of the shoulder joint.

The Forearm

In animals adapted for speed, the forearm, by comparison with the more distal part of the limb, should be long; though a long distal segment would further increase the stride, the advantage of having a relatively longer forearm to elevate the foot would be lessened. Moreover, as the foot hits the ground with the forelimb extended in full stride, part of the force resulting from the body weight is expended upon the ground and part upon the distal limb, which is roughly perpendicular to the weight vector. Inasmuch as some degree of flexion of the foot is essential in propulsion, the mechanical advantage of a short cannon relative to the forearm is a distinct aid in this phase of locomotion. Therefore, a long forearm is essential to a long stride, and the resulting greater length of the muscles acting on a relatively short cannon effects a more forceful traction and rapid recovery of the limb. The long axis of the radius should be perpendicular to the ground and parallel to the median plane of the body.

The Carpus

The anatomic foot (hand of man) begins at the carpus (knee), which is composed of the radiocarpometacarpal articulations. The radiocarpal and intercarpal joints essentially are pure hinge joints; the carpometacarpal joint is of the arthrodial (gliding) type. In aggregate, the carpal bones present numerous inclined planes which serve to disseminate concussion. In extreme flexion of the knee the dorsal articular surfaces of the radiocarpal and intercarpal joints are widely separated, thus facilitating injections into the voluminous radiocarpal synovial capsule and that of the intercarpal joint. The latter sac communicates with that of the carpometacarpal joint.

The carpal extensors and flexors and the digital extensors are provided with synovial sheaths which extend from 2 to 4 inches above the carpus to the proximal end of the metacarpus. The digital flexors are enclosed in a common carpal synovial sheath beginning 3 to 4 inches above the carpus, extending through the carpal canal, and terminating near the middle of the metacarpus. Bands of carpal fascia form annular ligaments which prevent displacement of the tendons.

The transverse diameter ("thickness") of the carpus is related to sureness of gait; narrowness is indicative of a tendency to stumbling. Width of the carpus (dorsal-volar diameter) provides greater articular surface and increased leverage for muscles acting on the joint. The long axis of the carpus is in direct line with the forearm and metacarpus; forward deviation ("kneesprung"), as in contracted flexor tendons, is a serious defect because of the instability of the joint. Scars on the dorsum of the knee are mute evidence of falls on this account. Deviations backward or to either side may interfere less with utility but frequently produce an ungainly gait and may lead to progressive breakdown of the limb.

Normally the larger medial condyle of the radius produces an obliquity of the radiocarpal articulation which displaces the foot laterally in extreme flexion, thus avoiding contact with the forearm or with the opposite extremity. Inadequate obliquity, or deviation of the carpus laterally, causes the toe to turn in and may result in interfering.

The Stay Apparatus

In man, most of the body weight in standing is borne by the column of bones of the relatively straight leg, muscular energy being used mainly to fix the ankle, knee, and hip joints rather than to support weight. In the horse, however, the flexed position of these joints and the corresponding ones of the forelimb would require considerable muscular energy to prevent collapse under the body weight. The ability of the horse to stand for days or weeks at a time thus makes it obvious that an additional mechanism is involved. This is the so-called stay apparatus, which is best developed in the forelimbs—undoubtedly as a concomitant of the fact that these limbs bear more weight than the hindlimbs. The alternate resting of the hindlimbs may also be an explanation (or a necessary result) of the lesser development of the stay apparatus hind than fore.

Much of the weight of the trunk is supported between the forelimbs by a sling-like arrangement of the 2 serratus ventralis mus-

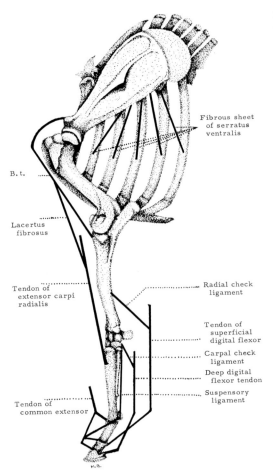

Fibrous sheet
of serratus
ventralis

B. t.

Lacertus
fibrosus

Tendon of
extensor carpi
radialis

Radial check
ligament

Tendon of
superficial
digital flexor

Carpal check
ligament

Deep digital
flexor tendon

Suspensory
ligament

Tendon of
common extensor

Fig. 1. The stay apparatus of the forelimb. Redrawn from Sisson and Grossman by M. Bharawaj.

cles, each composed of several fascicles attached to the more anterior ribs. When in effect, the horse "sinks" into this hammock, much of his weight is supported by strong bands of connective tissue investing each muscle fascicle. The weight is thus mechanically transferred to the scapula and thence to the other bones of the pectoral limb. At rest, the shoulder joint is fixed in a relatively flexed position, the elbow in an extended position, both joints being stabilized by the antagonistic actions of the triceps and biceps muscles. The tendon of the biceps runs from its scapular attachment through the belly of the muscle to its radial attachment. Thus when maximally extended (by shoulder flexion and elbow extension), the weight falls on the biceps tendon

rather than on its fleshy portion. In addition, the biceps has a long superficial tendon, the lacertus fibrosus, which attaches to the tendon of the extensor carpi radialis, thus taking weight off the fleshy part of this muscle and aiding in keeping the carpus extended.

The relatively abrupt change of direction of force at the fetlock because of the angle of the pastern places considerable stress on this joint, the tendency being to cause sinking of the fetlock. But rather than causing the entire body weight to fall on the digital flexor muscles, the latter are aided by 2 check ligaments. The radial, or superior, check ligament—morphologically the radial head of the superficial digital flexor—runs from the distal part of the radius to the tendon of the latter muscle. The subcarpal, or inferior, check ligament is a continuation of the strong volar carpal ligament to the deep flexor tendon. Without these, dorsal flexion of the fetlock could be counteracted only by contraction of the flexor muscles, but with the latter relaxed, weight is transferred directly from their tendons to bone.

The fetlock is further supported by the suspensory ligament, which is the (ligamentous) interosseus medius muscle. This is attached proximally to the distal row of carpals and proximal border of the large metacarpal. Above the fetlock it splits into 2 branches which pass forward and downward to join the common digital extensor tendon. Collateral ligaments detached to the proximal sesamoids prevent excessive dorsal flexion ("sinking") of the fetlock by transfer of force to the metacarpal and carpal bones. The fetlock itself is stabilized by these and other sesamoidean ligaments (Fig. 1).

THE HINDLIMB: RUMP AND THIGH

The practically immobile sacro-iliac joint may be considered an adaptation for propulsion and weight-bearing. The acute angle, some 35 to 40°, formed by the shaft of the ilium with the sacrum, together with the horizontal projection of the ischium, i.e., a wide ilio-ischial angle, makes for a long and gently sloping croup which is desirable for both beauty and speed. A horse with a croup more horizontal than desirable may be capable of great speed, but only for short distances when carrying minimum weight. Conversely, an oblique croup is advantageous for heavy work at a slow pace. Excessive width of the croup (transverse pelvic diameter) results in a swaying motion during locomotion, thus wasting energy better expended in forward progression. Excessive narrowness limits freedom of movement of the limbs, and the limited abduction may result in interfering.

The hip joint is of the ball and socket type, but movements other than flexion and extension are rather limited in normal locomotion. Abduction in particular is limited by the short powerful abductor muscles, the round ligament of the hip (ligamentum teres), and the accessory ligament (peculiar to equidae) from the prepubic tendon to the head of the femur. These factors, together with the heavy musculature, also account for the relative infrequency of hip dislocation. Kicking laterally also is restricted; few horses "cow-kick."

A relatively vertical femur in the normal standing position—inclined about 80° from a horizontal plane through the stifle—is conducive to speed by allowing for a relatively wide coxofemoral angle. Even at a gallop the stifle is not extended much beyond (behind) a vertical line through the hip joint; thus the limited excursion of the femur, only some 30°, is used to maximal advantage in advancing and elevating the limb. With a femur that is too oblique, i.e., with a smaller coxofemoral angle, flexion is limited—with consequent shortening of stride—and propulsive power in extension is reduced.

The Stifle and Leg

The stifle consists of the femoropatellar and femorotibial joints. The extensive joint capsule of the femoropatellar articulation is attached ½ to 1 inch above the articular cartilage of the femoral trochlea and pouches upward 2 to 3 inches under the quadriceps femoris. It usually has a small communication with the medial, and occasionally with the lateral, femorotibial synovial sac. The medial and lateral femoro-tibial joint capsules usually do not communicate with each other, and are partially separated into upper and lower compartments by attachment to the corresponding menisci. The medial sac pouches upward about a half-inch over the femoral condyle; the lateral sac pouches downward about 3 inches under the peroneus tertius and long extensor muscles.

Congruence of the femorotibial articulation is enhanced by the medial and lateral menisci, or fibro-cartilage discs, fragmentation of which may produce "joint mice," which may interfere with normal joint action. The large medial ridge of the trochlea, together with the greater strength of the lateral straight patellar ligament, predispose against medial luxation of the patella. Lateral luxation, following rupture of the medial ligament, is characterized by abnormal flexion of the stifle. Rupture of the middle patellar ligament results in locking of the patella above the trochlea.

Stability of the stifle is effected by the expanded joint surfaces and the strong collateral ligaments, together with the extensor action of the quadriceps femoris upon the tibia via the patellar ligaments. The latter provides for an important function of the stifle in rendering the limb firm and rigid when the foot is on the ground. Mechanical advantage is such that only moderate contraction of the quadriceps is necessary to maintain extension, and with the patella fixed on the upper part of the trochlea, flexing of the hock or stifle cannot occur unless the foot is first flexed—as is the case in normal locomotion.

Paralysis of the femoral nerve, which supplies the extensors of the stifle, if unilateral (as from local injury or tumor pressure) results in "dropped stifle"; if bilateral (as in azoturia), the animal usually is unable to stand. The stifles cannot be extended, and the horse sinks under its own weight.

In the normal standing position the angle of the stifle is about 150°. The joint cannot be completely extended, i.e., femur and tibia brought into a straight line, mainly because of limiting action of the cruciate and collateral ligaments.

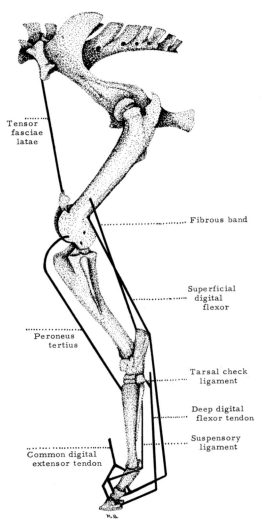

Tensor
fasciae
latae

Fibrous band

Superficial
digital
flexor

Peroneus
tertius

Tarsal check
ligament

Deep digital
flexor tendon

Suspensory
ligament

Common digital
extensor tendon

M. B.

Fig. 2. The stay apparatus of the hindlimb. Redrawn from Sisson and Grossman by M. Bharawaj.

THE HOCK

The hock forms the center of the major movements of the hindfoot, it being upon the point of the hock (tuber calcis) that the energy of the powerful extensor muscles of the hock which propel the body are attached. Although composed of 3 articulations: tibiotarsal, intertarsal and tarsometatarsal, the only appreciable movement—extension and flexion— occurs at the tibiotarsal joint. In the standing position the articular angle is about 150°. Full extension is limited by the collateral ligaments; flexion is checked by contact of the cannon

with the leg as the stifle is also flexed, and by "stops" on the anterior border of the tibial articulation which abut against "rests" on the tibiotarsal bone. In extreme flexion the tibial articular surface is raised from contact with the tarsal trochlea except along its anterior border; this apparently is related to the incidence of osseous pathology at or near this point.

The obliquity of the tibial tarsal trochlea ridges causes the stifle—and consequently the limb distal to it—to be carried laterally as the hock is flexed. This trochlear obliquity, which is found only in equidae, apparently is related to the caudal extent of the rib cage, i.e., this lateral movement of the limb prevents the stifle from hitting the ribs. Anatomic appearances to the contrary, during flexion of the hock the tibia and cannon remain in the same plane.

Another peculiarity is that the stifle and hock must function stimultaneously. When the stifle is extended the hock is automatically (mechanically) extended by the tendinous superficial digital flexor via its attachment to the tuber calcis. When the stifle is flexed the tendinous peroneus tertius (flexor metatarsi) mechanically flexes the hock. These 2 muscles, so-called "tendo-ligaments," are important parts of the stay apparatus of the hindlimb, i.e., they keep the limb extended with a minimum of muscular effort while standing at rest. However, unlike the situation with the forelimbs, the hindlimbs are rested alternately, one after the other being slightly flexed so only the toe touches the ground forward of the weight-bearing limb. This apparently explains the freedom from navicular disease in the hindfeet; the horse rests one forelimb (by "pointing") only when the foot is already affected.

The subtarsal check ligament, a continuation of the joint capsule to the deep flexor tendon, is less well-developed than its homologue in the forelimb; it may be absent—and usually is in the mule. The superior check ligament is absent, being rendered nonessential by the tendinous nature of the superficial flexor. Support of the fetlock is the same as for the forelimb (Fig. 2).

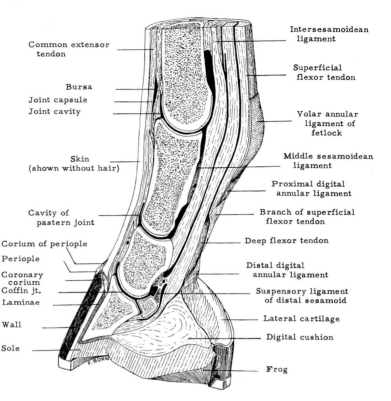

Common extensor tendon

Bursa

Joint capsule
Joint cavity

Skin
(shown without hair)

Cavity of
pastern joint

Corium of periople

Periople

Coronary
corium
Coffin jt.
Laminae

Wall

Sole

Intersesamoidean ligament

Superficial flexor tendon

Volar annular ligament of fetlock

Middle sesamoidean ligament

Proximal digital annular ligament

Branch of superficial flexor tendon

Deep flexor tendon

Distal digital annular ligament

Suspensory ligament of distal sesamoid

Lateral cartilage

Digital cushion

Frog

Fig. 3. Sagittal section of horse's foot. Original drawing by F. Born.

Concussion is concentrated wherever there is an abrupt change of direction of the limb at the time force is applied. The energy not absorbed by the anticoncussion mechanism of the forefoot is transmitted by a straight column of bones to the upper part of the forelimb; some is absorbed by the gliding action of the carpal bones, part by a spring-like action of the shoulder joint, and the remainder by the nonbony union of shoulder to thorax.

Conversely, energy in the hindlimb is transmitted to a flexed hock during impact and propulsion, and the greater the flexion the smaller is the articular surface (tibiotarsal) for receiving, dissipating and transmitting it. As in the carpus, some energy is absorbed by the small bones of the joint, but much of it would appear to be directed against the unyielding tarsometatarsal articulation. At any rate, it apparently is significant that spavins occur on the medial aspect of the distal row of tarsal bones and the large metatarsal; inasmuch as the medial "stop" on the anterior border of

the tibial articulation hits its "rest" on the tibial tarsal bone before the lateral, it is here that energy is concentrated and, apparently, directed downward.

Contrary to the rigidity characteristic of the hock, the stifle is provided with 2 resilient menisci which also confer some mobility upon the joint. Moreover, the angulation of the stifle and hip joints and the fact that they are stabilized to a greater extent by muscular action, facilitate distribution and dissipation of the shock transmitted above the hock.

THE FOOT

"No foot, no horse!" This aphorism, attributed to the ancients, has been repeated by writers on the horse since the age of printing. But with de-emphasis of the horse in recent years, physiology texts have omitted locomotion altogether, and anatomies devote less space to the foot than to, for example, the heart—which in large animals may have somewhat less clinical significance than the foot. Moreover, with the apparently increasing tendency to divorce structure from function, little can be found in print on the physiology of the foot of the horse.

The foot of the horse offers an unparalleled example of an intimate relation of structure to function. Five major functions, themselves interrelated, can be considered more or less separately: 1. Resistance to wear and tear. 2. Propulsion of the body. 3. Support of body weight. 4. Reduction of concussion. 5. Return of blood to the heart.

Resistance to Wear and Tear

The foot is encased distally by the hoof, which is composed of a highly organized and keratinized (cornified) epithelium constituting the epidermis. Keratin is the substance characteristic of horns, claws, nails and hair, as well as the hoof. The fundamental form of the hoof and arrangement of the epithelial cells are genetic characteristics, but at birth the hoof is relatively soft and little keratinized. The fact that the hoof becomes dry (after being immersed in fetal fluids) explains the initial keratinization—as well as the deterioration of the hoof if the horse stands in wet bedding for long periods. With use of the foot, friction becomes a stimulus to increased epithelial growth, and inasmuch as epithelium is avascular, as its thickness increases the outer layers (divorced from their blood supply) it becomes impregnated with keratin and dies. A similar process, but to a lesser extent, occurs with the body epidermis.

The horny substance of the hoof is not an amorphous mass of tissue; rather, it is composed of parallel horn tubes, each consisting of several concentric layers of keratinized epithelial cells. The outermost cells of the tubes are perpendicular to the rest and form intertubular horn which effects a strong union of the horn tubes. Increase in length of the wall is effected by addition of cells to the horn tubes at the coronary band; thus the horn at the toe is the oldest and most highly keratinized.

Although nonliving, the horn substance is normally elastic and tenacious even some distance from the coronary band, where it is soft and yielding. In humid climates, or in horses running on wet pastures, the horn remains relatively soft; under excessively dry conditions, or in interference with blood supply to the foot, the horn becomes exceedingly hard and brittle and may crack or chip off. Conversely, as noted before, standing in wet bedding or the like for long periods will result in deterioration of the horn by maceration of the epithelial cells.

Rate of horn growth is greater in warm climates, or in summer as compared with winter, and requires adequate nutrition and absence of foot pathology for optimal increase and keratinization. The hoof frequently bears evidence of systemic illnesses in the form of rings or ridges indicating unequal zones of growth. Under average conditions about 8 months are required for horn deposited at the coronet to reach the ground surface; i.e., the hoof is replaced this often. After loss of an entire hoof, as in ergot poisoning, a new hoof will be formed, but care is necessary to prevent injury and infection. In the unshod horse under optimal conditions—as in the wild state—growth is proportional to wear. But in the shod horse wear is prevented, and thus periodic trimming of the hoof is essential.

The outer surface of the hoof is covered for the most part with a thin layer of periople which consists of soft tubular horn. The periople is thickest at the coronet where it merges with the hairy skin; beyond this it becomes keratohyaline in nature—thus forming the so-called "hoof varnish." More distally it scales off, leaving a thin layer of cells, the stratum tectorium, which may be entirely lacking at the toe. The keratohyaline nature of the periople protects the newer horn of the wall from excessive drying; thus where this is removed by rasping, the wall tends to become brittle sooner than it should. Such a hoof is liable to cracking or chipping at the ground surface and complicates shoeing by limiting the placement of nails. Conversely, covering the hoof with an impervious dressing may result in a sodden hoof by preventing normal loss of water by evaporation.

PROPULSION OF THE BODY

The foot acts only mechanically in propulsion, the active agents (muscles) having their fleshy portions above the carpus or hock. Related to propulsion, however, is the form of the toe, its sharp wedge—somewhat more oblique fore than hind—being adapted to "digging in," especially in loose soil. The angle of the wall at the toe is about 50° for the forefoot and 55° for the hindfoot, and at the heel 100° and 95° respectively, but these measurements are subject to variation. The toe is the thickest part of the hoof, partly because of its inherent nature and partly because of increased stress imposed during locomotion. On hard or gravel-like surfaces the toe tends to wear in proportion to the rest of the ground surface of the wall (unshod foot). The wild horse of the plains manages quite well without having his feet trimmed. But on soft ground, or with considerable standing in the stable (shod or not), the toe tends to increase in length at a greater rate than the rest of the wall. This may be attributed to the horny substance being tougher at the toe and to the modeling of the hoof resulting from the body weight being borne more by the heels than the toe.

SUPPORT OF BODY WEIGHT

That the horse is adapted to traveling on at least moderately hard ground is evident from the heavy body mass which must be supported on the relatively small ground surface of the foot. The fact that the hoof is considerably larger in diameter than the pastern and cannon makes it evident that the horse is singularly ill-adapted for boggy conditions; e.g., a horse becomes mired easily by comparison with an elephant. The same is true in loose sand where the sharp hoof cuts deeply by comparison with the camel which has an expansible footpad.

In part because of the relatively small size of the hoof, and partly because of the stress of rapid travel over hard ground, a complicated mechanism for distribution of body weight and reduction of concussion is essential. Except for the specialized attachment of the distal end of the foot to the hoof wall, the entire weight of the horse would be transmitted to the few square inches of sole over the bottom of the third phalanx. In acute founder, with separation of this bone from the wall, it is not uncommon for the third phalanx to penetrate the sole.

The attachment of the third phalanx to the wall is by means of about 600 primary laminae, running parallel from the coronary border to the free edge of the third phalanx, which are intimately adhered to the periosteum. Each lamina bears 60 to 120 secondary laminae arranged in a feather-like pattern. These sensitive laminae (laminar corium) interdigitate so intimately with similarly arranged insensitive (epithelial) laminae of the wall that in a normal foot the laminar corium will be torn from the periosteum before a separation of the laminae is effected (as in mechanical removal of a section of wall).

These several thousand laminae provide a bearing surface of about 8 square feet for each extremity. The distribution of the weight of a 1,200-pound horse would, therefore, be on the order of about 4 ounces per square inch of attachment instead of the several hundred pounds per square inch (several times this momentarily during locomotion) if the union were a simple one. Further, the laminae on the dorsal aspect of the hoof are longer than those at the quarters or heel; thus support is greatest where the most stress occurs, i.e., during the final phase of propulsion the entire weight falls on the toes.

By means of the laminae the weight of the body is transferred to the wall of the hoof. The inflection of the bars posteriorly affords additional stability to the hoof wall without decreasing its essential expansibility, and increases contact with the ground surface, thereby increasing traction. The sole, being normally concave, bears very little weight except at its junction with the wall. However, the sole does descend slightly when weight is placed on the foot; this is an essential part of the anticoncussion mechanism.

THE ANTICONCUSSION MECHANISM

The structural adaptations of the foot to reduction of concussion offer perhaps the most striking example anywhere in the body of the relation of structure to function. Most of the force in impact of the foot comes at the heel, thereby putting pressure on the footpad (frog) in a normal foot. The frog itself being of a resilient, rubber-like consistency, absorbs some shock and transmits the rest to the digital cushion within the hoof. Distribution of energy to the deep part of the digital cushion is effected by the spine of the frog. The wedge-shaped mass of fibrous and elastic tissue composing the digital cushion absorbs shock and transmits it in all directions. Part is directed against the lateral cartilages which move laterally and, together with compression of the frog, spread the bulbs of the heel—thus accounting for expansion of the wall at the heel. In a healthy foot, this movement can be palpated just above the coronary border, over the lateral cartilages.

The inflection of the bars at the heel has been noted as providing stability of the wall without interfering with flexibility—as would be the case if the wall were complete. The lateral cartilages have sensitive laminae (laminar corium) on their outer surface, and so provide a flexible union of sensitive and insensitive laminae at the posterior (expansible) part of the foot. Ossification of the lateral cartilages (sidebone), probably resulting from uncompensated-for concussion, may produce a painful lameness, in part due to the lessened expansibility of the foot.

The digital cushion also transmits energy to the pedal joint, which is a complex formed by the second and third phalanges and the distal sesamoid, or navicular bone. The latter receives support from the deep flexor tendon passing below it, which better enables the joint to withstand the force applied to it. This 3-bone plus tendon complex results in greater reduction of concussion than if only a 2-bone joint were involved. Friction is reduced by the navicular (podotrochlear) bursa. Ringbone, which—like sidebone—apparently results from uncompensated concussion, interferes with normal function both mechanically and by the production of pain.

The incidence of navicular disease is indicative of compression of the navicular bone; that this occurs almost exclusively in the forefeet may be related to the lessening of concussion by the flexed hock (which thereby suffers) and the alternate resting of the hindlimbs. Navicular disease forces the horse to take weight off the affected foot. The compressive force of propulsion at the toe is distributed to the third phalanx by the extensive laminar attachments over the broadly convex and inclined dorsal surface of the third phalanx.

The angle of the pastern, about 140° for the forelimb and 145° for the hindlimb, together with the suspensory mechanism of the fetlock, provides for considerable diminution of concussion. A horse with relatively straight pasterns tires easily and is tiresome to ride. At maximum speed, dorsal flexion may be so great as to permit the fetlock to practically touch the ground, thus imparting a spring-like action to the joint as weight is lessened. Cutting of one or more of the supports to the fetlock results in sinking of the joint and greatly reduces this function. Most important in this respect is the suspensory ligament, which possesses considerable elasticity; the deep flexor tendon and, to a lesser extent, the superficial flexor also contribute. Together, the flexor tendons bear most of the weight at the fetlock; rupture of both results in extreme dorsal flexion, even with the suspensory ligament intact.

It usually is stated that the sole does not bear weight; this is essentially the case, but that it is not quite true is indicated by the fact that the sole normally descends slightly under impact of the body weight. Being concave on the ground surface, this force is transmitted peripherally to the wall, thus further expanding the wall at the heel. Normal thickness of the sole is maintained by a flaking off of the superficial layers and does not require contact with the ground.

The entire anticoncussion mechanism depends on the pliability of the horny substance of the wall, for without this the hoof would soon shatter and render this elaborate mechanism of little use. As indicated before, the stay apparatus also may be considered an integral part of the anticoncussion mechanism.

RETURN OF BLOOD TO THE HEART

Expansion of the foot when bearing weight has an important and necessary bearing on the circulatory mechanism of the foot and return of blood to the heart. For its size, the portion of the foot enclosed within the hoof has a richer blood supply than any other somatic structure. This has a direct bearing on the production of founder (laminitis), with separation of the sensitive and insensitive laminae resulting from inflammation, by the action of toxins produced elsewhere (as in overeating or metritis).

Though the force of the heart is adequate to bring arterial blood to the foot, the dependent position of the foot makes it physically impossible for venous return to be accomplished unaided. That the foot itself acts as a pumping mechanism can be observed if one of the plantar or volar veins is cut; blood spurts from the vein when weight is placed on the foot and stops when the foot is lifted.

It is evident, therefore, that as the internal structures are compressed by weight being placed on the foot, venous blood pressure in the vast plexus within the hoof is raised substantially above that in the more distant veins. The efficiency of this pumping mechanism is further demonstrated by the fact that there are no valves in the veins nearer than the middle of the pastern. It is, therefore, little exaggeration to say that the horse has, in effect, 4 auxiliary hearts.

The nerves to the foot are purely sensory (other than vasomotor), and, of course, are of considerable importance in the production and detection of lamenesses. Exteroceptive fibers transmit pain impulses, and proprioceptive impulses are responsible for an awareness of position of the feet—essential "knowledge" during locomotion over any but completely flat surfaces, and without abrupt turns. Although the nerve supply to the foot is not immediately essential to its normal function under optimal conditions—this being the result of coordinated muscle action above the level of the feet—

progressive deterioration is the usual consequence of complete neurectomy. This may be due in part to loss of the vasomotor mechanism, but mainly to damage to tissues incurred as a result of loss of sensitivity.

J. F. SMITHCORS

CONSIDERATION OF THE LAMENESS CASE

Before treatment is administered it is necessary to first discover the source or sources of the trouble. Hence, diagnostic ability is a prime requisite in the treatment of lameness. In establishing a diagnosis, the practitioner seldom has recourse to x-rays or laboratory assistance, and his work is done principally by physical examination. Therefore, a thorough knowledge of the physiology of locomotion is essential; memorizing facts without understanding principles is of no practical benefit.

In order to determine the reasons for certain signs shown by the subject, knowledge of physiology often gives important clues to the type and location of lameness. If one observes that an animal assumes a certain position while at rest, such knowledge enables the examiner to determine the specific ailment. For instance, in acute tendinitis, the resting patient maintains the affected member in volar flexion because this position permits relaxation of the inflamed tendon. Likewise, various abnormal positions such as adduction, abduction, undue flexion or pointing of a limb or its parts, have their special significance and must be taken into account during the course of an examination.

In the examination of lame horses, the cause often is not obvious and a systematic method of diagnosis must be pursued. In all obscure lamenesses a methodical and thorough examination of the horse according to an established procedure is necessary to determine the nature and source of the affliction.

HISTORY

The first thing to be given consideration in any history is the fact that the history itself is not always dependable, due either to lack of accurate observation or to willful deceit on the part of the owner or attendant. The experienced veterinarian has learned how to obtain information in a manner best adapted to the client—either by direct questioning or by subtle suggestion—and draws out evaded facts essential to make a diagnosis. He also has learned to make allowance for misstatements made to hide unpleasant facts of neglect or abuse. For instance, suppurating quittor, complicated by a large amount of granulation tissue, cannot be an acute or recently developed disorder. In complicated conditions, or chronic disturbances which cannot be deemed sufficient cause for marked lameness, accurate history may be a great aid to diagnosis. A case of an aged animal, recently lame, with a small exostosis on the first phalanx and a history that the bony deposit is of long-standing, should cause the veterinarian to seek the source of trouble elsewhere.

Visual Examination

A careful visual examination of the patient should be made before it is approached. The novice is prone to hasty examination by palpation, and does not realize how much may be revealed by careful scrutiny of the animal. In this way he is led to false conclusions which often are avoidable. Too much emphasis cannot be placed on the importance of a thoughtful visual examination before the horse is approached. In this examination, type, conformation and temperament of the animal are taken into account, for each of these qualities is in itself a determining factor in predisposing to certain ailments and in exerting a favorable or unfavorable influence upon existing conditions and recovery. Malformation of a part, or asymmetrical development of the body as a whole, may render an animal susceptible to certain affections which cause lameness. A sickle-shaped hock predisposes the subject to curb, and an animal having powerful and well-developed hips together with imperfectly formed hocks, will be predisposed to bone spavin.

The matter of temperament cannot be disregarded in diagnosis, for in some instances it is the chief determining factor in the outcome of the case. A nervous, excitable horse may, under some conditions, be expected to show disturbances which more lethargic fellows escape. Nervous horses, for instance, are more prone to azoturia and are more incapacitated by tendinitis. The placid horse often recovers from certain bone fractures which can be successfully treated only when the patient is sufficiently docile to remain confined to a sling for weeks.

Due allowance should be made for restiveness shown by nervous animals when their surroundings are strange or unusual. In such instances, even pathognomonic signs may be masked to such an extent that little sign of pain or discomfort is shown. In these cases, the horse should be given sufficient time to adjust to the environment, or it should be removed to a more suitable place for examination. Horses quickly detect notes of friendly reassurance in the human voice and often can be calmed by being spoken to quietly but firmly.

By visual examination, one may detect the presence of various swellings or enlargements, such as characterize bruises and strains of tendons, particularly when the inflammation is acute. Inflammation of the plantar ligament in curb is detected readily when the affected member is viewed in profile. Spavin, ringbone, quittor, and other conditions may all be observed from certain proper angles. The fact that the skins of most animals are pigmented and covered with hair, precludes the easy detection of erythema by visual examination, consequently this indicator of inflammation is not often used in examining horses.

The expression of the face often is indicative of the gravity of the condition. The facial expression of a horse suffering from tetanus, azoturia, or acute synovitis is readily recognized by the experienced eye, and upon this fact alone, a presumptive diagnosis and prognosis can be made.

Attitude

The position assumed by the horse at rest often is characteristic of certain affections and this, of course, should be noted at once. The manner in which the weight is borne by the resting animal should be given close attention, and if the attitude is abnormal or peculiar the reason should be found. If weight-bearing causes signs of pain, the affected limb will invariably be favored and held in one of a number of positions. The foot may contact the ground squarely and yet the leg may remain relaxed and free from pressure; volar flexion in such cases is indicative of inflammation of a part of the flexor apparatus. If the condition is painful, the position of the afflicted part is shifted frequently, but in all cases the injured portion is held in a state of relaxation. Here, knowledge of anatomy enables the observer to determine which structures are purposely eased. In all conditions where extreme pain results in the constant desire of the animal to keep its foot off the ground, examination should be made for local cause. Septic inflammation of the feet, such as nailprick and navicular disease, and newly made wounds where nerves have been severed and their ends exposed to pressure or irritation, will produce this sign. "Pointing" affords a comfortable position in some lamenesses. In navicular disease or unilateral foot lameness, one may observe the horse bearing weight on the sound foreleg, while the other is planted well-ahead. In bilateral foot lameness, weight may be shifted frequently from one foot to another.

In chronic cases, where there is no marked pain, the horse often stands squarely upon both front feet. In some cases of hip or shoulder involvement, complete relaxation of all parts of the affected limb may be noticed. In brachial paralysis, the pectoral portion is held limply. If the patient is made to move, it is apparent there is lack of innervation to the part. When contusion has caused acute inflammation, the horse tries to keep the part inactive. With active and painful inflammation of the prescapular lymph nodes and adjacent structures, the scapulohumeral joint is extended. This results in flexion of the elbow and carpal joints.

There are some bilateral conditions that are so painful during weight-bearing that the horse shifts weight from one affected leg to the other. An example of this may be observed in a case of acute bilateral gonitis. In acute laminitis of the forefeet a peculiar and characteristic position is assumed. The hindfeet are brought under the body sufficiently to relieve weight on the forefeet, and the horse assumes a squatting position with the forefeet extended.

In each abnormal position assumed by an animal, it may be deduced that the subject is attempting to obtain relief from pain, and further examination is made more effective because of this preliminary visual examination which has not annoyed the animal by manipulating unaffected structures.

It has been presupposed that the person making a visual examination for diagnostic purposes will remember that in the normal animal weight is borne equally well with both forelegs, and that this is done without shifting from one to the other; and that the pelvic limbs do not support the body in this manner. Normal horses shift their weight from one hindleg to the other and the relaxed leg rests in a state of flexion with the toe on the ground and the heel slightly raised.

EXAMINATION BY PALPATION

In nearly every case where lameness exists, examination of the affected parts by palpation or manipulation is necessary before an accurate conclusion may be drawn. In making this kind of examination one needs to exercise good judgment or he will fail to gain a correct impression of the actual conditions. Here, as well as in other conditions where physical examination is made, one should approach the horse in a manner that will not excite or disturb it enough to cause resistance or objection to the examiner, thereby masking the evidence sought. Nervous and unbroken horses may often be unsatisfactory subjects for palpation. The practitioner should acquire skill as a horseman (if he is not already possessed of such) and learn to handle each case in a manner best suited to the temperament of the animal.

By palpation, one can recognize hyperthermia and this, in lieu of dependable history, is at times sufficient to determine the duration of an inflammatory reaction. By comparison of parts of the affected limb with analogous parts of the other limbs, increase in surface temperature may be determined. In this manner, when examining a case of suspected laminitis or other inflammation of the feet, one may arrive at a fairly accurate conclusion without employing other means. Throbbing vessels are not always easily recognized, particularly if the horse has chronic lymphangitis. In some instances, where a moderate degree of lameness exists and the cause is obscure, the recognition of hyperthermia may be the deciding factor in establishing a diagnosis. In cases of sprained ligaments in the phalangeal region, because of the dense character of the structures involved, little if any evidence of the cause of lameness other than local heat, may be found 24 hours after the injury occurs.

In order to determine the degree of hyperthermia with fair accuracy, one must make due allowance for external conditions such as the amount of hair or dirt covering the area. All dirt should be removed, if practicable, so that the diagnostician's hand may contact the inflamed structures. If the operator's hands are chilled, tactile temperature determination is not dependable, and such an examination is of little value when the horse's feet are wet or when the examination is made hurriedly.

Often one is impressed by the fact that a horse shows hypersensitivity to palpation. Some animals, in anticipation of pain at the touch of an injured part, will withdraw or resist the approach of the practitioner. This sensitiveness is more apparent in horses which have been subjected to previous manipulation or treatment. No better example of this reaction can be seen than in cases of "shoe boil," or capped elbow. In animals treated with vesicants, hypersensitivity should be expected.

Unscrupulous dealers once made use of vesicants in various ways, often intentionally to cause lameness which would appear about 24 hours after sale. The new owner, dissatisfied, was willing to dispose of the animal at a sacrifice, thus enabling the original owner or his agent to regain possession at less than the animal's real value.

Some nervous horses, because of the way the practitioner approaches, are prone to flinch and show pseudohypersensitivity. Young ones not accustomed to being handled are likely to be skittish, and one must not hastily conclude

that a part is painful because the subject resents even gentle digital manipulation. In instances of this kind, one should compare sensitivity by manipulation of different parts of the horse's body. By exercising patience and good judgment, it is possible to distinguish between abnormal sensitivity. Here again, the examiner needs skill as a horseman and ability to evaluate individual temperament under conditions which exist at the time he makes his examination.

By palpation alone, one can recognize the presence of fluctuating enlargements. One may not only recognize such conditions, but distinguish between kinds of fluctuant masses. Through differences in density, the presence or absence of hyperthermia, and the quality of the mass one can determine, for instance, that an enlargement is an abscess rather than a tumor or a hematoma. Edematous swellings can be recognized by their characteristic indentation on pressure. With training, it is not hard to recognize postoperative or posttraumatic edemas that may or may not cause lameness, and to distinguish between an acute infection, a more or less benign edema, or an extremity swollen because of the existence of a chronic ailment. Since the outcome of these dissimilar ailments may be different, it is necessary to develop a trained, discriminating, tactile sense fortified by a knowledge of pathology in order to correctly interpret, evaluate, and prognose.

Fibrous tumors sometimes are located in the distal portion of the medial side of the tarsus —exactly over the site of bone spavin. When the affected member is supporting weight, such tumors cannot be distinguished from exostoses; but as soon as the affected leg ceases to bear weight, the nature of the enlargement can be recognized because it can be slightly displaced by digital manipulation. Displacement of an exostosis, of course, is not possible. A necessary qualification in evaluating exostoses is to be able to judge its nearness to articular structures, the extent or area of its base, and its exact position since these facts affect both treatment and prognosis.

Periarticular ringbone, because of the size and location of the lesion, may constitute a condition which cannot be relieved in one horse, but in another, because of the distribution of the osseous deposits, the condition may respond to treatment. In the examination of exostoses of the tarsus (bone spavin), it is particularly important to determine whether or not the spavin involves the tibial tarsal bone near the trochlea, for if this articular surface is involved, complete recovery cannot result despite the most skillful attention.

PASSIVE MOVEMENTS

Wherever it is possible to gain confidence of a horse to the extent that it will relax sufficiently to make possible passive movement of affected parts, much can be learned. By passive movement one may differentiate between fractures, luxations and inflammation of ligaments that have been injured, particularly in the phalangeal region.

In fractures, when pain does not prohibit relaxation, by gently moving an extremity in various directions one can produce the peculiar grating of newly broken bone (true crepitation). A horse with a phalangeal fracture, showing pain and tensing of the structures about the fractures, can be examined by anesthetizing the parts with a local anesthetic injected into the nerves proximal to the fracture. It is best to deposit the anesthetic at 2 closely situated sites along the course of each nerve. In some multiple fractures of the first or second phalanx this is absolutely necessary. Otherwise, pain produced by manipulation causes the horse to keep the tendons so tense that crepitation may not be detected.

False crepitation is a vibrating feeling caused by passive movement of articular portions of bones such as the metacarpo-phalangeal joint. This is observed when the horse permits the parts to remain in a state of complete relaxation.

Attempts to recognize the hypersensitivity of inflammation in the shoulder or hip by passive movement are not productive. Because of the bulk and weight of the parts, as well as the resistance the animal offers, no accurate conclusions can be drawn. Horses nearly always resist the placing of members in any position that is unusual or uncomfortable, therefore, such practice is useless because one can not distinguish between normal resistance and flinching.

OBSERVING THE CHARACTER OF THE GAIT

In order to determine degree of lameness as well as its character, it is necessary to observe the horse in motion. The degree of inconvenience or distress exhibited by a lame animal is manifested by the character of the lameness. When much pain is exhibited there is disturbance of respiration, sweating may be noticeable, and in some instances signs of nervous shock are evident, particularly in nervous animals that anticipate being punished when approached and, consequently, make every possible effort to move when urged to do so. A horse should be moved only enough to cause it to exhibit the degree of lameness present. If a marked impediment is manifested, it is not necessary to cause the horse to be exerted to the extent of inflicting unnecessary pain. Further conclusive examination is made by palpation.

To cause a horse to move, an assistant may simply lead it with a halter and compel it to walk a few steps. In this way, a swinging or supporting lameness or a combination of the 2 conditions can be determined. When the cause of lameness is not apparent, it is necessary to have the horse moved farther than a few steps and at different gaits. Depending on the character of lameness as well as its intensity, one needs to exercise the animal in various ways, but this should not be overdone.

The first thing to identify in the lame horse in action, is the lame leg. If this is not readily visible, the leg or legs which are at fault must be discovered by further examination, and to do this, word pictures convey little of value. Long practice is the only route by which one may become proficient, and this experience can be gained only after the fundamental principles of diagnosis have been mastered.

For a careful study of supporting lameness involving a forelimb, the horse is driven or led toward the examiner. If a hindleg is to be observed, the animal is moved away from the examiner. In swinging lameness, the horse should be moved past the examiner. In this lameness, making the horse step over a bale of hay or other obstruction can help a differential diagnosis. Horses with a swinging lameness ordinarily will balk but those with supporting lameness will not. In every case, examinations are best if the practitioner can view the patient from a little distance. Visual examination cannot be successfully executed in difficult cases if the practitioner is too close to the animal.

The average horse is best observed on a moderately loose lead, rather than being ridden. A close grasp on the lead may interfere with head movements. Nodding of the head with the placing of weight on a sound limb indicates supporting lameness of a foreleg and serves to indicate which leg is lame.

When supporting lameness involves a hindlimb the head is raised at the time weight is placed upon the sound leg. Here the long axis of the horse's body may be likened to a lever of the first class. The posterior part of the body, at the time weight is taken upon the sound leg, is the long arm: the forelimbs are the fulcrum, and the animal's head is the weight which is lifted. The head movements of a horse at a trot, in supporting lameness of a front leg, synchronize with the removal of weight from a lame leg to the opposite one, if it is sound; but in the pelvic limb lameness, the head is thrown or jerked upward as weight is placed on the sound member. This nodding movement is opposite in the 2 instances and often may be hard to evaluate.

In pacing horses, since front and hindlegs of the same side are advanced at the same time, nodding of the head occurs in supporting lameness with discharge of weight from the lame leg, and a dropping of the hip as weight is caught by the second pelvic limb. In observing animals that are limping (as in supporting lameness), one should particularly note the sacroiliac region in hindleg lameness, and the occipital region in lameness of the foreleg.

When a bilateral lameness exits (such as in some cases of navicular disease or mild laminitis) no nodding of the head occurs. The weight is supported for an equal length of time upon each 1 of the 2 legs, but the stride is shortened. The gait in such cases is peculiar, and the animal appears stiff and "choppy."

It is desirable in some cases to cause a horse to move from side to side. In other instances, it is made to walk or trot in a circle. If the circle is small it will employ the inner foreleg as a pivot. To augment the signs of certain lamenesses, it is necessary to have the patient walk backward. Each of these tests of locomotion points, in a more or less characteristic manner, to the site of a particular lameness.

Sprains, injuries of lateral ligaments of the extremities, ringbone, and certain foot disorders, are shown by a side to side movement or a pivotal movement. In fact, whenever it is possible to place undue tension upon a damaged structure, signs of pain are the response. In inflammation involving the lateral side of the phalanges, unequal weight-bearing resulting from standing on wedges or an inclined surface will cause undue strain upon the inflamed parts and result in a pain response.

When a horse with a supporting lameness is made to travel in a circle, and the affected leg is on the inner side, the lameness is accentuated because weight is borne by the injured leg for a greater length of time. The opposite, of course, is true if the lame leg is on the outside. In swinging lameness, because pain is increased at the time the affected leg is being advanced, signs are more apparent when the horse is made to travel in a circle with the lame leg on the outside.

Sometimes it is impossible to arrive at a definite conclusion as the result of a single examination. It then becomes necessary to see the horse at a later date. This is to be expected in rheumatic conditions and also in some foot diseases. In the examination of young animals, unused to harness and to other strange encumbrances, one must make allowance for impediments of gait, which are not disease conditions. Such conditions are termed "false lameness." Young mules that are not well-broken to harness, are difficult subjects for examination and in some cases it is necessary to have them led or driven a considerable distance before one can definitely interpret the nature of the impediment in their gait when lameness is not pronounced. Mules are especially difficult to examine satisfactorily since their normal rebellious temperaments result in resistance whenever a strange person approaches. In such cases—if an examination does not reveal the cause of trouble—rest must be recommended and further examination made at a later date.

SPECIAL METHODS OF EXAMINATION

After completing a general examination, it occasionally is necessary to employ additional diagnostic procedures. The use of nerve blocks may be indicated in phalangeal lameness, or progressive nerve blocks may be required in unusual lamenesses of the upper leg. Various shoes are employed in order to shift the weight from one part of the foot to another, thus changing the gait. The use of wedges, hoof testers or a hammer to determine the presence and degree of sensitivity occasionally is indicated. Such methods of examination are not dependable in themselves, but are valuable when used in conjunction with other technics. No examination for lameness is complete without removing the shoe and examining the sole of the foot.

Diagnosis by exclusion may be a final resort when recognition of the cause is particularly difficult. In this instance, the exclusion of possible conditions, one at a time, after an analysis of the signs generally enables the practitioner to eliminate all but the disturbing element.

J. V. LACROIX

This section was taken from a volume, *Lameness of the Horse*, by the same author.

OTHER MANIFESTATIONS OF LAMENESS

When lameness has been present for only a few days, there may be already some indication of atrophy developing in the muscles of the affected limb. This becomes increasingly evident as the period of lameness lengthens and it may be possible to estimate the time during which the affliction has existed.

The atrophy may not be generalized but may be confined to small groups of muscles. For example, any lameness which makes it painful for an animal to advance a forelimb will result in slight atrophy of the extensor muscles of the forearm as early as a week to 10 days after the onset of lameness. A little later, the suprascapular muscles will become somewhat flattened, and after a fortnight some difference may be observed between the outlines of the 2 forelimbs around the shoulder joint. The sound shoulder will look to be the fuller of the 2 and the lame one a little less rounded. The bones forming the joint in the affected limb may be better defined in outline. When this is pointed out, the inexperienced observer will at once presume that this difference in shape of the 2 shoulders must indicate that the affection lies in this region, and will forthwith diagnose shoulder lameness when the real site of the trouble may lie in the foot, or coronet, or may be associated with some injury to the nerve supply to the limb.

A careful scrutiny for bursal enlargements is always indicated, and when one clearly is evident it should be remembered that it may not be the actual cause of the lameness. A bursal enlargement where the neck joins the withers is sometimes the precursor of a fistula in that region.

Frequently, quite obscure lesions give rise to lameness. These include a growth developing on the severed end of a spermatic cord even years after castration, or a thorn embedded in a muscle or other part of a limb. In horses which are stabled, one of the most serious injuries occasionally overlooked, is a small puncture in the heel inflicted by a fork.

The signs of muscle atrophy, foot resting, drooping of the point of an elbow through loss of function of the triceps muscles, wasting of the suprascapular muscles, prominence of the point of the shoulder in suprascapular paralysis, inability to extend the limb in radial paralysis, and sinking of the point of the hock are all signs perfectly easy to observe, and each one of them tells its story to the trained observer even before the horse is moved from the stable. When the horse is taken out, a further assortment of clinical signs may be manifested. For instance, one must be constantly on the lookout for such abnormalities as abduction or adduction of the limb, or any part of it, for anything unusual in the placing of the feet as they come to ground, any inclination to "brush," or, conversely, to throw a foot outward, or any tendency to overreach.

In adduction, the limb is drawn toward the body in an unnatural manner. This may arise from a desire to relieve pain, or from some loss of function of the abductor muscles, which can no longer control the movements of the limb. In abduction, the limb is carried away from the body with the result that the foot travels through the arc of a circle outside its usual path of flight. Once again, this may be through a desire to relieve pain, or it may be due to lack of power in the adductor muscles. Sometimes abduction occurs when a painful abscess lies in the axillary or inguinal regions. Bruising of the sternum, lymphangitis, a contused hip, obturator paralysis, scirrhous cord, arthritis of the knee or hock, mastitis, pubic injury, or even a cracked heel, may at times produce abduction.

In the hindlimb, the hock and stifle joints operate in unison. Flexion of one necessitates flexion of the other, just as in the forelimb the knee and elbow joints work in harmony. An excessive degree of flexion of a hock must be accompanied by a similar degree of bending of the stifle joint. A straight stifle and a straight hock always go together. It may even be difficult at first to decide whether a horse is lame in the hock, stifle, or both. Similarly, a damaged knee limits elbow movements. When it causes pain to flex the elbow, as in arthritis, or when a capped elbow is present there will be corresponding difficulty in advancing the knee. Sound limbs travel in pairs, alike in every movement. If the point of 1 hock in lifted higher than the point of the other hock, the reason may be that 1 of the 2 is overflexing, as in stringhalt, or that 1 is underflexing, as in spavin. It is important to determine which of these is the case.

Some of the long-standing lamenesses associated with changes in the flexor tendons, produce such recognizable forms of knuckling of the fetlock that the site of the lameness within the tendinous structures can be recog-

nized at a glance. The early signs of tendon pathology may require prolonged and careful examination, however, before any definite diagnosis can be made.

One forefoot may, on occasion, appear at each step to travel a little further than its fellow. The toe is raised and the foot tends to descend upon its heel. At first glance the observer may be almost certain that the cause is a contusion or injury located at the region of the coronary band, immediately in front of the foot. One should not jump to conclusions and must take adequate steps to confirm suspicions before making a decision.

A fracture may be suspected, even in the absence of crepitus or deformity, owing to the degree of swelling and pain whenever movement is attempted, as well as by the fact that the horse attempts to fix the joint immediately above and below the injury. X-ray examination should be employed to confirm or refute the diagnosis when doubt exists.

When the horse is led, it is easy to observe whether it travels in a straight line, or if it adopts a "3-cornered gait." In certain neck injuries, in rheumatic myositis, and in cases of stiffness arising from various causes, the horse is unwilling, or unable, to follow a straight course. This same 3-cornered gait also is noticeable in true shoulder lameness, in which the horse advances the lame shoulder a little more (or less) slowly than the sound one.

One also should pay attention to the degree of flexion exhibited in various joints. The point of each tuber calcis normally attains the same level, and is raised at the same speed as the other. In cases of spavin in which lameness persists, lack of flexion may be observed in the box stall as well as out of it. After a little exercise, the signs of lameness may disappear, an indication that one must always begin to seek the cause of lameness in the "cold horse," not in one which has been exercised and "warmed-up" prior to the examination.

Old horses not infrequently develop a restrictive arthritis of the elbow joint. The foot is scarcely lifted from the ground and the horse crouches a little. The animal, so affected, seems to shuffle along rather than step out. This condition is seen less frequently now than years ago, but it is easily recognized and is one of the lamenesses accompanied by excessive head-nodding. When both elbows are affected at the same time, the condition may be confused with the signs shown in some cases of chronic laminitis.

Lymphangitis, in its early stages, may produce a puzzling type of lameness, until one introduces the hand into the inguinal or axillary regions and observes the marked limb abduction which is exhibited immediately. In these cases, the fetlock and cannons usually will exhibit edema before swelling becomes evident higher in the limb.

Lameness associated with damage to the flexor tendons often is accompanied by knuckling of the foot or at the fetlock, and sometimes with a lowering of the position of the fetlock joint. Frequently, there is a raising of the heel from the ground when standing. Many race horses and hunters exhibit quite obvious contractions of tendons, thickening and bowing, and yet when the true cause of their lameness is discovered, it often proves to have no connection with the chronic tendon deformities, but to be a foot injury or some form of lameness situated above knee level. It should be remembered that at least 75% of all causes of lameness are located below the knee and of these another 75% lie below the fetlock.

SUGGESTED PROCEDURE FOR ROUTINE EXAMINATION

It is well to ascertain first that the horse has not been exercised immediately prior to the examination, and it always is wise to make the preliminary observations unhurriedly, while the horse is at rest in its stall. Notice any tendency to point a foot, how the animal stands, and whether its weight appears to be evenly distributed.

Take heed of any tendency to change feet often, so that the weight falls upon opposite feet in turn. Notice, too, if one foot is partly raised at the heel or if the horse shows a tendency to rest upon the toe of one foot.

The animal should be moved slowly from one side of the stall to the other and any peculiarity of gait or tendency to lift one hock

higher than the other should be observed. Notice any tendency to knuckle at the knee or fetlock, any dropping of the elbow, whether each limb rests in its natural position and whether the animal appears to stand quite comfortably.

When making a detailed examination of the lame horse, the veterinarian should develop the habit of examining every case in a thoroughly systematic and routine manner, never jumping to rapid conclusions, and making a habit of examining every part of the affected limb before arriving at a decision. The horse should be brought out of the stable slowly and gently, without in any way exciting it. Once outside, permit it to stand quietly for a minute or 2, then let it start away at a slow walk. This is not a horse's best pace, and often will enable one to observe some peculiarity of gait which might be masked in an excited animal being hustled along at a fast trot. After it has walked 20 yards, have the horse turned and jogged back at the slowest trot possible, with the head rope as slack as is compatible with the safety of the attendant. On this trip, watch the head of the horse, not its limbs. Now have it turned again and trotted gently away from you and once more watch its quarters, and not its limbs. The head of the horse nods when the sound foot comes to the ground. The quarter of the horse drops when the sound foot comes to the ground. This is a general rule, and must be accepted as such. Cross lameness may confuse the pattern of action.

When the horse returns let it stand a minute, then have it trotted slowly away and back, and as it leaves watch the hindlimbs, and as it returns watch the forelimbs. Finally, have the horse backed and then turned each way in short circles. Next, stand away from the front of the horse a few yards and look at it but do not touch it. Notice the 2 shoulders and the 2 forelimbs and compare their outlines. Go a little closer and look at the feet, coronets and fetlocks very carefully to see if they are exactly alike. Note particularly if one forefoot appears larger, higher, narrower or flatter than the other. Observe whether both feet stand squarely upon the ground or whether one shows a tendency to lean to one side. Pass to the side of the horse and, from a distance of some yards, observe stance and general conformation while noting any obvious abnormalities, wounds, scars or harness marks.

Now go behind the horse, at least 12 feet. Observe the level of the quarters to see if the tuber ischii are level. Note the development of the muscles of the quarters and observe if one side is flatter than the other. Let your glance travel down the hindlimbs and observe any hock enlargements, swollen fetlocks, and any signs of grease or cracked heels. Take another look at all the feet and observe their type, whether they are flat feet, upright "pony" feet, and whether they have good heels, or if these are so flat that the bulbs of the heels come close to the ground. Remember always that feet, good or bad, should be in pairs which match. Two bad feet may travel better than a good and bad one. If you are now quite certain which is the lame leg, you may commence a closer detailed examination.

Always examine the foot first and take a little time in so doing. Using a light hammer, commence by very gently tapping the sound foot. In doing this do not alarm the horse. Pat his neck and talk to him from the side at which you propose to work. Then, stoop and place a hand lightly above his knee to steady the leg and prevent any nervous jerking of the limb when the foot is struck. Tap the front of the wall, very gently and once only, with the hammer. Do not endeavor to beat a rat-a-tat-tat, this will frighten the horse and tell you nothing. After a second or two, tap each quarter gently, then each heel. When you have gained the confidence of the animal, you may tap a little harder if it is likely to help your decision.

If the horse shows a greater degree of tenderness in the foot of the lame limb than in its fellow, clean out the foot, scrub the sole and frog with soap, water and a brush, and tap around the sole very lightly with the hammer. If one area shows more evidence of a painful reaction than the remainder, trim off the surface of the sole with a paring knife, particularly between the angles of the bars, to determine whether corns are present and then, using a large pair of blacksmith's pincers, gently squeeze the sole all round at intervals by grasping the wall and edge of the sole just inside the white line. If this leads you to suspect one definite area, have the shoe removed and trim out the nail-holes nearest to it in circular fashion with your searching knife. If you are certain the lameness is not centered in the foot, observe the coronets again at close range, note any disparity in size and shape by comparing the 2, then stand at one side of the horse (not in front) and palpate both coronets very gently with the tips of the fingers. Observe whether they are absolutely identical, take note of any bony enlargement, however small, and try to identify it with the particular bone involved, endeavoring so far as you are able, to determine whether it has an articular origin or if it appears to be unassociated with a joint. Examine the lateral cartilages and note the degree of their flexibility, first with the horse's foot firmly on the ground, then with the foot held backward with the knee fully flexed.

Place a finger in each heel and notice any enlargement, tenderness or the presence of cracks or fissures, or of a moist exudate. Examine each part of the limb slowly, carefully and minutely as your hands travel up it. Now, note the appearance of the flexor tendons and their outlines, whether they are flat and straight-edged or if they are thickened, hard or soft, and whether their posterior line is bowed from above to below. Let your second finger and thumb pass between them and the bone while you palpate the edges of the suspensory ligament, then at the higher part feel the check ligament. Run your hand down the tendons to the fetlock, observe its flatness or roundness and any evidence of bruising on its medial surface. Examine the sesamoid region, feel each bone independently and note any enlargement. Try to differentiate by touch the superficial and deep flexor tendons, and always compare those of either limb to note any disparity. Feel each splint bone carefully throughout its length, note any exostoses, and if any are palpable observe their shape and their disposition in connection with the tendons or carpal joint. Feel the front surface of each knee, notice any scars, skin adhesions or swelling, then palpate the carpal sheath and compare the 2 limbs if any synovial distention is suspected.

Next, note the extensor and flexor muscles of the forearm to observe any signs of atrophy. Feel the elbow joint and, by lifting the limb, flexing and extending it, observe the movement of both the elbow and shoulder joints. Observe the bodies of the triceps for fullness, firmness, atrophy and tone, and at the same time look closely at the muscles overlying the scapula to observe any evidence of hollowness on either side of the scapular spine suggestive of muscular atrophy. Also palpate the mastoido-humeralis muscle as it passes below the cervical bones. In lameness of any duration in which there is pain on advancing the limb, a marked atrophy of this muscle will become evident.

Now examine the area overlying the tendon of the biceps as it passes over the bicipital groove in the humerus. This area usually appears a little sensitive to pressure, but you may note undue heat or swelling and whether the one side appears more sensitive than the other. Lifting each foot in turn and drawing it backward toward the flank will accentuate any signs of such tenderness.

You may now have the horse walked or gently trotted again while you note its gait afresh in the light of whatever you may or may not have discovered during your examination. Observe whether the pain or discomfort shown appears more marked as weight falls upon the foot (supporting-leg lameness) or whether it is more obvious when the horse is lifting the leg, advancing the foot and extending the shoulder joint (swinging-leg lameness). This is equivalent to determining whether the lameness is associated with concussion or with muscular movements involving flexion or extension of a joint. Supporting-leg lameness is usually connected with abnormality below the knee or hock, swinging-leg lameness with that occurring above them.

You now may make your final examination of the limb, and if there still is doubt as to whether the lameness is in the foot you may consider performing a nerve block. This, however, is an operation which should never be done too readily if it can be avoided. If you decide to make use of it and find that the lameness definitely is located in the foot and

is of some duration, and if you are unable to detect any exostoses in the coronary region which might indicate the seat of lameness, you also may consider the advisability of making an x-ray examination of the foot, which will afford some indication as to the condition of the navicular bone.

In the case of the hindlimb a similar examination is conducted. You will note in the same way the condition of the feet, whether the toe of the shoe is unduly worn. Notice the heels, fetlocks, tendons, posterior edge of the hocks and the tuber calcis, and carefully palpate the hocks, particularly on the medial surfaces, for bony or bursal enlargements. Feel carefully along the inner edge of the tibia for signs of soreness, note the degree of development of the second thigh, and then, with due care for your own safety, pass the hand up into the flank and thigh and examine the scrotal or mammary regions and the inguinal glands.

Next examine the stifle. Observe any bursal enlargements, laterally or in front of the joint; grasp the patella in your hand, note its position and the degree of firmness of attachment. Now have the hindfoot lifted and the joint flexed and extended while you still keep a hand on the patellar region. Observe any discomfort caused during movement, and if such appears to exist, compare with the other stifle by handling it in the same manner. Note any sound or sensation of creaking, knocking or crepitating. Next run your fingers carefully over the femur and palpate the great trochanter. Press above it deeply to determine any painful condition of the hip joint and lay your ear against the hip while the leg is moved gently with the foot off the ground. Observe the development of the gluteal muscles and note any atrophy or swelling. Atrophy usually indicates either a faulty nerve supply or loss of muscle tissue arising from disuse.

If after examining the limb in detail you are still undecided as to the site and cause of lameness, make a rectal examination to determine the condition of the pelvis, the iliac shafts, sacrum and pubis, and observe the degree of pulsation on either side within the iliac arteries. Feel carefully within the abdomen for the presence of a large neoplasm and palpate the under surfaces of the lumbar bones so far as you are able to reach. Press gently upon the muscles on either side of them and observe any indications of pain. Notice also the presence of any glandular enlargements in the pelvic area.

If by now you have discovered the cause of the lameness this is a matter for congratulations. If you have not done so, do not be discouraged. You will not be establishing a precedent. Every experienced practitioner has been equally unfortunate many times.

R. H. SMYTHE

This section, "Clinical Examination of the Lame Horse," was extracted from the same author's *Clinical Veterinary Surgery* Volume I pp. 194-198, by permission of the publishers, Crosby Lockwood, London, and Charles C Thomas, Springfield, Illinois.

COUNTERIRRITATION

INTRODUCTION

One of the oldest remedies used in equine practice is counterirritation for the treatment of lameness. Despite modern innovations, technics, drugs, and equipment, this long-time approach to a perpetual problem is still the treatment of choice of many equine specialists. Justifiably regarded by some as a carry-over from the Dark Ages, this drastic treatment continues in wide use not only because of the legendary powers ascribed to it by horsemen, but also because of the actual over-all benefits it provides.

Counterirritation apparently achieves its success through the reactivation of circulation and, consequently, of the healing process of a chronic injury. It would be difficult to describe the exact extent to which this explanation is true, but it can safely be said that the increasing of circulation to an injured area will expedite the removal of products of inflammation—edema, exostosis, scar tissue, etc.

Most of the modern methods of treating muscle and joint injuries, such as irradiation, ultrasonics, radiotherapy, diathermy, hydrotherapy, etc., also achieve at least some degree of their effectiveness through stimulation of circulation. These methods, however, have one or more of the following drawbacks: they entail the use of expensive, elaborate equipment, re-

quire its use over a long period of time, and present the adaptation difficulties associated with use of equipment designed for human treatment.

Modern anti-inflammatory drugs, such as the corticosteroids, enzymes, and phenylbutazone, give promise of providing at least a partial solution to the problem of treating equine lamenesses. Improved surgical technics likewise have brightened the picture. However, these innovations are, for the present, tools to be used with, rather than as substitutes for, counterirritation. Until a more satisfactory method of treatment than any now available is devised, the economics of the horse-racing industry will continue to indicate the use of counterirritation as a standard treatment procedure.

Several forms of counterirritation are used commonly. Most artistic, and believed by a large number of practitioners to be the most effective, is the firing—the polka dot pattern puncturing of the epidermis with a cherry-red heated metallic point, or the quilted pattern of a heated bar drawn across the skin. Blistering, which can be the most drastic method, is the application of a vesicant—either as a paste or as a liquid—to produce skin lesions resembling those of second- or third-degree burns. Leg paints generally are irritant-containing liquids of varying strengths; they are applied when cutaneous exfoliation without vesiculation is desired. Counterirritants also may be administered hypodermically. In this method, an injectable irritant is diluted in a suitable vehicle.

The selection of method or methods of counterirritation will depend primarily upon the type and severity of the injury, the depth of penetration desired, and the time required for complete healing. A further consideration is the amount of time the owner or trainer is willing to allow for the animal's recovery. In this instance it might be noted that a distinctive firing pattern is a permanent signature of a veterinarian's work, and if an injury so treated recurs because insufficient recovery time was allowed, it is the veterinarian who gets the blame for the treatment's failure. The quality of the available nursing care, the temperament of the animal, and the climatic conditions also may influence the selection of method of application. The possible future use of the animal likewise may affect the choice. In certain horse show classes and in some jumping events there is discrimination against firing scars.

The degree of counterirritation desired may vary widely. It can be controlled by selection of method and by the amount of force with which it is applied. The degree of reaction can be predicted to some extent by a consideration of climate, and by the color and thickness of the patient's skin. Warm weather will increase the action of the counterirritating agent, and thin, light-colored skin generally is more sensitive to counterirritants.

Counterirritation should never be used to treat an acute injury in which vascular engorgement already exists. To do so would cause an excessive reaction in the affected area, and would result in further congestion of the capillary circulation. Edema, excessive tissue destruction, and possibly necrosis, sloughing, and permanent damage may ensue. The inflammation coincident with acute injuries must first be allowed to subside with complete rest, application of poultices, hydrotherapy, liniments, ultrasonics, and anti-inflammatory drugs. It has been noted, however, that joint injuries treated intra-articularly with corticosteroids do not respond favorably to subsequent treatment by counterirritation. The injured tissue must repair to as near a normal state as is practical, or until an apparent plateau of healing has been reached. Healing would, of course, continue beyond this point, but at a very slow rate. This cooling-out period may require from 2 weeks to 3 months, depending on the type and degree of injury.

Firing

Firing is one of the most controversial forms of veterinary surgery practiced today. Some veterinarians and horsemen consider it to be unnecessary geometric mutilation; others consider it the most reliable available treatment for many of the common ailments of the leg. It is the preferred method of counterirritation among practitioners specializing in race-track work. Of all the counterirritation methods, it probably is the easiest to control. Depth and severity of effect are readily adjustable within the same pattern in any area. Penetration may vary from a barely perceptible skin tattoo to a bone-searing pit, according to the will, and to some extent the skill, of the operator. Firing also has the advantage of leaving a permanent reminder to the animal's handlers that an unsoundness once existed and that any abuse of the animal while in training may lead to a recurrence of the injury. This indelible reminder of past troubles also may work to the owner's disadvantage should he wish to sell the animal at some future date. However, on the race tracks, firing scars generally have little influence on a prospective buyer's decision if the horse is training soundly and running well.

It behooves the veterinarian to use all his artistic skill in applying the firing pattern, for it is his permanent signature, often distinct from those of his colleagues, and constantly noted by owners and trainers for the duration of the animal's racing career.

Equipment: Heated nails, pitchfork tines, and converted soldering irons were used in the past as surgical instruments for the performance of the firing operation. Unfortunately, they still are used, often without the benefit of anesthetics, by horsemen in foreign lands and in remote sections of our own country. More professional, and far more convenient, are the commercially available firing irons equipped with a variety of interchangeable points and heated by fuel combustion or electricity. None, however, is without at least a few disadvantages.

The ether iron is the oldest type of fuel-combustion apparatus still in wide use today. Its proper application requires the skill of a master. It is tricky to start, even with the added convenience of a propane torch to provide the preheating necessary for proper fuel pressure. The ether supply of the tank located in the handle of the apparatus often is insufficient for completion of an extensive firing operation. Since the tank cannot be refilled until the iron has cooled, it is common practice for operators to carry in reserve 1 or 2 extra, filled irons. The agate containing the tiny orifice is the heart of the machine, and a fickle heart it can be. The open ether flame is a fire hazard in the stable area, just as are the occasional explosions which occur. The mild jet-like roar of the burning gas may or may not disturb the patient. But in spite of these difficulties, the uniform heat maintenance of the point and the ease of maneuverability of the unit make it the favorite of many veterinarians, who would not trade it for any other type of firing iron.

The simplest firing instrument available is the electric high-frequency cautery unit, which operates on standard 110-volt current. Heat to the needle tip is controlled by either a 3- or a 5-position rheostat within a large carrying case, and a spring-loaded ON-OFF squeeze switch in the handle. The newer models operate in complete silence. In spite of precautionary fusing and grounding, annoying electrical shocks occasionally surprise the operator. These may occur even in relatively new machines and on dry ground. After prolonged continuous use, the handle may become uncomfortably hot. The iron is connected to the carrying case by a large, somewhat awkward cable. Nevertheless, the relative safety, the speed of preparation, and the ease of operation make this the most popular type of firing instrument in use today.

Application: For the treatment of chronic injuries in which the reduction of an accessible exostosis is indicated, "point," or "pin," firing is the method of choice. In this procedure, the depth of penetration can be increased, where desired, by refiring the same holes. The outer edges of the holes should be at least ⅜" apart to preclude the sloughing of patches of skin, especially if circulation is increased further by the immediate application of a blistering agent to the area. Care should be exercised to avoid penetration of joint capsules, synovial sheaths, blood vessels, and nerves.

Bony enlargements, such as osselets, splints, ringbones, and bone spavins, are most amenable to firing. It should be emphasized, however, that x-ray examination is a valuable aid in diagnosing the exact nature and location of an ailment. The "obvious" splint may be a fracture callous of improper healing. The "obvious" ringbone may be an overriding of the first phalanx on the second because of a torn suspensory ligament. What appears to be a calcified carpus may be a slab fracture. Firing

has often received the blame for unexpected poor results when actually the diagnosis was at fault.

It is common practice on the race track to fire "bucked shins" (periostitis of the metacarpus). The results are somewhat inconsistent, as often is the rationale for performing this operation. Poorest results in treating this little understood but very common ailment occur after firing an injury which is still in the acute phase, or when the horse is returned to training without allowing sufficient time to heal, or from firing when the shins are only slightly affected. For some reason, shins which have "bucked out" completely, *i.e.*, those which have become much enlarged and very painful, often recover, after treatment, without further difficulties, but those which are treated during the first mild signs often recur. Firing does enforce needed rest, and in recurrent injuries may serve after other methods have failed.

The value of firing for the treatment of injuries to tendons and ligaments is open to considerable debate. In some cases, particularly those in which the damage is so slight as to be undetectable after the horse has been "cooled out," custom and the owner's insistence may play a large part in the decision to perform the operation. In such cases, firing should be done lightly to accomplish the necessary counterirritation with a minimum of tissue destruction. "Line," "cross," or "feather," firing— the drawing of a cherry-red heated bar across the skin to form patterns of parallel lines or quilted diamonds—is used most commonly for this. However, in chronic, enlarged, recurrent injuries of the suspensory ligaments or flexor tendons, in which excessive amounts of scar tissue are present and the chronic lameness demands drastic treatment, penetrating pin firing along with heavy line firing may be indicated. In old bowed tendons, obliteration of the tendon sheath actually may be desired. The percentage of these horses returned to racing is not high, and perhaps justification for such drastic measures lies in the fact that no other known treatment has proved superior.

Pin firing for the treatment of injuries to heavily muscled areas is practiced in some of the South American countries. The value of

Table 1.—Schedule For Firing

Ailment	Cooling Time	Type of Firing	Total Healing Time	Results
Ringbone	1 to 2 weeks	Pin	3 months	Good
Osselets	2 to 10 weeks	Pin	6 to 9 months	Good
Splints	4 to 10 days	Pin	3 weeks	Good
Bucked shins	1 to 2 weeks	Pin, light	3 to 4 weeks	Good
Carpitis	3 to 6 weeks	Pin	6 to 9 months	Fair
Spavin	2 to 3 weeks	Pin	6 months	Fair
Check ligaments	2 to 3 weeks	Pin	6 months	Fair
Flexor tendons, chronic	2 to 10 weeks	Pin and line	9 to 12 months	Fair to Poor
Flexor tendons, light	2 to 4 weeks	Line	9 to 12 months	Good to Fair
Tendon sheath above carpus	2 to 6 weeks	Pin	6 months	Fair
Plantar ligament	1 to 2 weeks	Pin	2 to 3 months	Good

this form of counterirritation is questionable, especially if the origin of the injury is deep below the skin surface. It is probable that the enforced rest required for the fired area to heal would benefit the original injury.

Procedure: The usual surgical procedures should be followed in the firing operation. The area is clipped, cleaned, and anesthetized. Tranquilizers are administered to the horse at the discretion of the veterinarian. Some practitioners apply a blistering agent to the fired area immediately after the operation. Several variables, among them the nature of the ailment, the degree of counterirritation desired, and climatic conditions, may influence the decision to do this. Many practitioners prefer instead to apply the more conservative and controllable leg paints. These usually are of the iodine-glycerine variety and are applied daily under bandages immediately after the firing and for from 2 to 3 weeks thereafter. The final exfoliation of the area may vary in thickness from that of onion skin to that of lemon peel.

During the first 10 to 14 days after firing, a cradle must be kept on the horse to prevent self-inflicted damage by biting or rubbing the affected area. After the painting is complete, the limbs are exposed to air for 4 or 5 days. The exfoliated tissue is then encouraged to drop off by the daily application of a "sweat," which is generally a mild, glycerine-containing compound applied under wax paper (or plastic sheets, oiled silk, etc.) and cotton to form an air-resistant bandage. The limb soon returns to a normal, though now patterned, appearance. The elapsed time is from 4 to 5 weeks from the firing date, and after

another week of rest the area will be ready for application of the first postfiring blister, if such is desired. Thereafter, blistering may be repeated at 6-week intervals until the horse is ready to return to training.

It would be well to note that except for very minor firing operations, such as the firing of a small splint on one limb, it usually is better to fire both limbs for the same ailment, even though only one has been injured. The reason for doing this is to balance the discomfort of the postfiring period so that the horse will not carry most of his weight on, and consequently perhaps breakdown in, the uninjured leg.

Barring the exceptions presented by individual cases, Table 1 represents some common ailments, their firing treatment, and general prognosis.

Blistering

In this method of inducing counterirritation, a caustic agent is applied directly to the skin. There is formation of vesicles, oozing of serum, drying and incrustation of the skin, and eventual sloughing of the exfoliation so formed. The usual blistering procedure involves clipping the area and, after protecting with a coating of petrolatum any adjacent areas which are contraindicated for blistering (behind the knees, above the bulbs of the heel, etc.), applying the blistering agent. The agent may be a paste, which usually is rubbed thoroughly into the skin, or it may be a liquid which is applied with a brush; the blister may be applied just once or on each of several consecutive days. The active ingredients may include 1 or more of such irritants as cantharides, red iodide of mercury, croton oil, strong iodine, muriatic acid, and coal oil in an appropriate vehicle. Some blistering agents should be left uncovered and others require daily bandaging.

When a severe blister is used, pain may be exhibited by the horse within minutes after it is applied. Tranquilizers and analgesics should be administered as needed. To preclude self-mutilation, the animal should be restrained by the use of a properly fitted cradle, a cross tie (halter-tied to 2 walls) or by haltering to a running wire above the animal's head and across the stall. Furthermore, he should be kept under close observation, for a clever horse in pain may find ways to elude restraint. Horses have been known to chew away skin, tendons, ligaments, and even pieces of bone, despite precautions. Permanent blindness from blistered corneas also has occurred. The acute pain may last from 6 to 24 hours. Twenty-four to 48 hours after application of the blister, vesicles form on the swollen limbs and beads of serum coalesce to form streams running down the legs. This wet phase will last for 3 to 4 days, and gradually will be replaced by drying of the serous exudate. As the drying continues, the edematous swelling subsides and the skin becomes incrusted with a layer of hard scurf. This exfoliation gradually separates from the new skin and hair below it. Four to 5 weeks after the blistering date the scurf is shed and the limbs resume their normal appearance. The application of a sweat will shorten this final stage. Seven to 10 days after the skin has returned to normal, the limbs are ready for repetition of the blistering process, should this be indicated.

The necessity for severe blistering is highly overrated by some horsemen and this practice is open to considerable question. There is no practical way to stop the action of a blister once it has been applied and the signs of its ultimate severity have appeared. Soap and water bathing, bandaging, and enzyme and corticosteroid injections may help. The successive administrations of moderately strong blisters will accomplish more in the long run than will the drastic action of severe blisters. It is wise to be conservative in the application of

the first blister to an animal, for only in this way can potential hypersensitive reactions be avoided.

Some favorable results recently have been achieved by the application of strong caustics or acids through a patterned stencil attached to an area. The healed pattern resembles that of the pin-firing operation. Simpler methods involve use of a mild application or a milder blister, perhaps even a so-called 3-day blister. All types of commercial products are available.

The daily use of leg paints similar to the after-firing paint is a conservative way to obtain varying degrees of exfoliation without vesication. In many cases, the animal is not withdrawn from training during the process, however, and the degree of counterirritation is considerably less than necessary for the proper treatment of a serious ailment.

Injectable Counterirritants

Injection of caustic agents to produce counterirritation is viewed by some as a clean and effective remedy in the treatment of certain injuries. It has the advantage of deep penetration and usually does not leave scars. The amount of nursing care required is less than for firing, blistering or painting. Moderate swelling generally is seen for a few days immediately following injection, but with mild daily exercise this subsides within 7 to 10 days. This method is best applied to injuries deep in heavily muscled areas of the hindquarters or back. Shoulder injuries respond fairly well to subcutaneous injections. In injuries to bony regions, as the knees, shins, and ankles, the results of this method of treatment are unpredictable. Excessive scar tissue swellings may occur and may be permanent. Abscess formation and sloughing occasionally may be seen in or about tendons and ligaments. Once the caustic agent has been injected, there is no means of controlling its action. Iodine in a vegetable-oil base is the most commonly used agent.

Counterirritant Formulas

Formulas for counterirritation compounds are regarded by some horsemen as priceless possessions. Broad and magnificent are the healing powers attributed to certain prescriptions. The main difference between these elaborate formulas appears to be the number and combination of volatile oils added. The basic ingredients are quite similar. A few simple, but effective, prescriptions are listed:

After-fire Paint or Leg Paint:
1. Phenol - - - - 2 oz.
   Glycerine - - - 2 oz.
   Iodine (7%) - 12 oz.

Paint daily for 21 days. Use bandages.
2. Kerosene and pine tar, equal parts.

Apply with brush for 21 to 30 days. No bandaging is required.

Blistering Agents:
1. Paste: 20% red iodide of mercury
           80% petrolatum

Apply once with rubbing. Change bandages daily.
2. Liquid: Turpentine - - - - - - 1 oz.
           10% tincture iodine - 4 oz.
           Croton oil - - - - - 15 drops

Apply with brush for 1 to 3 days as needed. Bandage.

Sweat:
   Glycerine and alcohol, equal parts. Apply daily. Bandage with wax paper, oiled silk, or plastic sheets under regular cotton bandages.

Injectable Counterirritant:
   Dissolve 2.5 drams iodine crystals in 1 pt. warm olive oil. Mix thoroughly. Inject 10 to 20 ml. throughout area.

J. L. Temple

BANDAGING

The application of bandages is a very important phase of equine therapy. Very often veterinarians do not become proficient in this skill due to the fact that around the race track grooms do most of it, and become exceedingly proficient in the technic. There are many types of bandages, and many types of materials are used in their manufacture. I will describe some

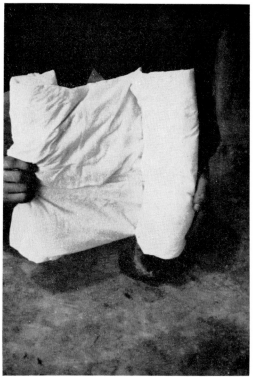

Fig. 4. Step 1 in the application of the standing bandage.

of the most common of these and the condition for which they are used.

The Standing Bandage

The standing bandage which usually is made of Canton flannel, is approximately 7 inches wide and 10 feet long. This type of bandage usually is used after firing, blistering, or when preparing a horse for shipping. It is applied over sheet cotton. Usually 5 sheets of cotton are folded to the desired length; a quilted pad is then rolled on, and the bandage applied over the pad as in the illustrations (Fig. 4-7).

Cold water bandages are used to reduce inflammation. They consist of a knitted type of bandage 4 inches wide, which usually is rolled over the affected area and to which cold water is applied with a hose.

The Running Bandage

The 4-inch Ace elastic bandage is applied and used as a running bandage. This gives support to the tendons and yet allows for maximum flexibility. In the case of a low bowed tendon, this bandage usually is applied from the hoof head up to a point just beneath the knee. It is most important that this bandage be applied by an expert as the tension and pressure must be even or the bandage itself may cause a bowed tendon if it should slip or roll. Clasps are supplied with this type of bandage; it is advisable, however, to use adhesive over the top of the clasp as there always is danger that it may slip (Fig. 8).

The Cast Bandage

The cast bandage is applied over sheet cotton when maximum support is required, as for a tendon bowed near its middle. A 4-inch gauze bandage is applied just above the fetlock to just below the knee. This bandage should be rolled to approximately ¼ inch thickness, and then painted with an adhesive solution, such as L-180 latex solution (Gutta Percha Rubber Co.). The bandage then is painted with vinegar. This will act nearly like a cast, give about as much support, and yet have some flexibility. It may be left in position for 7 to 10 days while the horse is training, and also while he is running. It is extremely important that the tension and pressure be even, and that the bandage causes the animal no discomfort.

Medicated Bandages

Several types of medicated bandages are in common use. They include Viscopaste, a zinc paste bandage in a moisture-proof wrapping. It does not require heating and is applied without mess or waste. It is used in many cases to control edema after the removal of a cast. After drying, the bandage supplies a fair amount of support to the area. This bandage is made by Smith and Nephew Ltd., Hull and Welwyn, Garden City, England.

The Rundown Bandage

The rundown bandage is used when track conditions cause severe irritation to the posterior portion of the fetlock joint when the horse runs. Thick, orthopedic moleskin usually is cut in a manner to fit over the back of the fetlock joint. This is held in position either with duo-adhesive or Elastoplast (an elastic adhesive bandage, Smith and Nephew, Ltd.).

When the knee of a horse has been subjected to surgery or firing, it often becomes necessary to apply a bandage. This is done by first folding 5 layers of sheet cotton and applying them from the hoof head to just below the knee. This is then bandaged in position by applying a quilted pad and a standing bandage. Another roll of sheet cotton similar to the first one is now applied on top of the first and extended

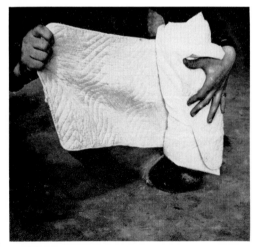

Fig. 5. Step 2 in the application of the standing bandage.

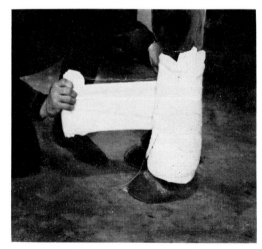

Fig. 6. Step 3 in the application of the standing bandage.

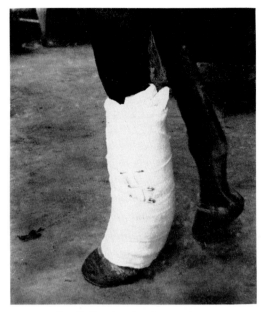

Fig. 7. Standing bandage applied.

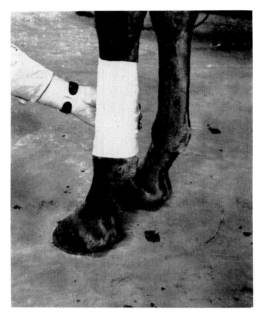

Fig. 8. Running bandage in position.

halfway or more up the forearm. This is then held in position by a "spider," which is made with a piece of strong duck material, the proper length to extend from below the knee to 7 or 8 inches above the knee. This material is torn in such a manner as to leave ties which may be secured behind the leg.

The Elastoplast bandage also is used on the front or rear leg. This is an adhesive bandage and is applied over a sheet of cotton; it is similar to the elastic running bandage but also has adhesive qualities.

PLASTER BANDAGES

Plaster bandages, 4 to 6″ wide, also are used over a newly bowed tendon and changed every 4 or 5 days for 2 weeks. These Cellona or Gypsona-Extra bandages harden extremely fast and are exceptionally strong and waterproof. They give excellent support for a bowed tendon, located either low, high, or near the middle.

ANTI-INFLAMMATORY AGENTS

The equine practitioner now has at his disposal a number of anti-inflammatory agents which, when used properly, greatly hasten the recovery of both chronic and acute inflammatory processes. Possibly the most widely known and the most extensively used of these is phenylbutazone (Butazolidin). This drug truly can be classed as a wonder drug. It has been observed that when it is used according to the manufacturer's directions there practically are no side effects. The product has been used successfully in the treatment of almost every type of inflammatory condition, as well as chronic rheumatoid conditions. Phenylbutazone is a most valuable aid in the treatment of obscure lamenesses when it is almost impossible to pinpoint the site of the injury. It has been used to good advantage in the treatment of both pleurisy and pneumonia in the early stages, as it reduces both the inflammation and the temperature. Many ocular conditions are improved with phenylbutazone due to its anti-inflammatory action. It is unfortunate that we cannot use this valuable agent at race tracks.

There are several other products similar to phenylbutazone which may be used in the treatment of both acute and chronic inflammatory processes. The commonest of these probably is Dipyrone (dipropal, 500 mg. per ml.) (Vitamix Corp., Philadelphia, Pa.). This product is extremely useful in controlling pain after bone and joint surgery. It has analgesic, antipyretic, and antirheumatic properties. It has been used quite successfully in controlling edema in the lower limbs when circulation has been impaired. It also is a valuable aid in the treatment of influenza. Dipyrone may be given either intramuscularly, intravenously, or subcutaneously.

Another product, Salzoline (Vitamix Corporation, Philadelphia, Pa.) contains Dipyrone-500 mg., physostigmine salicylate-0.6 mg., and atropine sulfate-0.6 mg. per ml. This product works well in acute inflammatory conditions accompanied by pain. The usual dose is 20 ml., given intramuscularly in 2 sites.

It would not be fair to overlook acetylsalicylic acid (aspirin) at this point. For many years, before phenylbutazone and the corticosteroids came into use, aspirin had a very important role in the treatment not only of inflammatory conditions affecting the joints, but also in the treatment of influenza, strangles, and pleurisy. It is administered in 60-grain tablets; usually 2 tablets 4 times a day are prescribed. Aspirin now is combined with dexamethasone and aluminum hydroxide gel and is used very widely in the treatment of rheumatic and arthritic conditions.

Possibly, the most commonly used and the most effective drugs in the control of inflammatory conditions are the corticosteroids. One of the most common of these is Azium (Schering Corp.), which is dexamethasone. This drug is distributed in injectable form (1 mg. per ml.). In acute conditions, such as tendonitis, periostitis, and laminitis, it may be used intramuscularly or given intravenously. It also is prepared in 5-mg. packets, which may be administered in the animal's food. This preparation is very effective when prolonged treatment is anticipated. Predef 2X (Upjohn Co.) is fluoroprednisolone acetate, and this product is used very extensively in the treatment of bursitis, tendonitis, and carpitis. It contains neomycin sulfate, approximately 5 mg. per ml. This is an exceptionally good product, and may be used in several ways, including the intra-articular route after synovial fluid is withdrawn and replaced with Predef.

Azium cannot be injected intra-articularly in cases of severe carpitis or "popped knee." Relief occurs, however, in a very short time after it is injected, and in many cases the effect will last for 7 to 10 days. It also is prepared in a bolus which may be crushed and given in the grain for prolonged periods. Azium also is a valuable aid in the treatment of pulmonary emphysema.

There are other forms of these steroids which are much longer-acting, such as Depro-Medrol (methylprednisolone, Upjohn Co.). This product may be used for intramuscular or intra-articular injections. When given via the latter route, it has been known to control inflammation and pain for as long as 4 weeks.

It must be pointed out that it is of the greatest importance that aseptic technic be used in the administration of these drugs, especially when intra-articular therapy is administered. All syringes and needles should be autoclaved. The area of injection should be thoroughly scrubbed, and then painted with either iodine or Merthiolate. Many of these drugs are prepared in ointments which are most effective when treating cutaneous conditions due to allergy. Prednisolone ointments when applied liberally to cracked heels effect a cure or great improvement in 48 to 72 hours.

DIATHERMY

Short wave diathermy has a beneficial effect when used to treat deep-seated injuries such as shoulder lamenesses, or lamenesses affecting the forearm, knee, or fetlock joints. It is exceptionally effective in treating affected areas over the neck. I do not use this mode of therapy extensively, however, due to the fact that the equipment is heavy and necessitates the presence of an operator with the animal while treatment is being given. The pads used in treatment are not adapted for use in horses, and it usually is necessary to improvise some method of immobilizing them, such as the use of adhesives. I usually expose the area to be treated for 20 minutes, 3 times a day, using heavy felt pads between the animal and the electrode. Most animals tolerate this treatment very well.

E. N. Anderson

RADIATION THERAPY

INTRODUCTION

Radiation therapy, whether produced by an x-ray machine or with the use of a radioactive material, as radium or cobalt-60, is useful in the treatment of many types of equine lamenesses. Most lameness is the result of tendinitis, bursitis, tenosynovitis, arthritis, periostitis, myositis, or any combination of these conditions. All of these conditions can be benefited by radiation therapy. For some, radiation is the treatment of choice, for others it is very useful, and there are conditions which are improved only in small measure by radiation.

Much of what happens in freshly injured tissues is not visible grossly and can be seen only in tissue sections examined microscopically. When trauma occurs in any part of the body certain tissue changes always occur. These represent the body's attempt to repair and are referred to as inflammation. The cardinal signs of inflammation (swelling, heat, pain, and some loss of function) are present in varying degrees. The blood vessels in the area become dilated and there is an increased flow of blood to the injured part. This is followed by a temporary slowing in the rate of blood flow. At this time, the white blood cells gradually accumulate along the walls of the blood vessels. Certain of these white blood cells pass through the blood vessel walls as the increased size of the vessels' intracellular spaces, due to their dilation, makes this migration possible.

Shortly after migration of leukocytes begins, the inflamed areas are densely packed with phagocytic cells. They ingest and remove cellular debris caused by the injury. Red blood cells in large numbers follow the leukocytes through the vessel walls and cause the surrounding tissues to become swollen and to contain more fluid than normal. It is after this acute response that tissue regeneration, pus formation if infection is present, and eventual resolution and repair take place. To some degree, all of these changes occur in any inflammatory response to trauma.

MECHANISM OF ACTION

Treatment of lameness is directed toward removal of as much swelling as possible, to provide relief from pain, to restore function of injured tissue, to limit the amount of connective tissue deposited, and to eliminate calcium deposits. The most sensitive cells in the body to x-radiation are lymphocytes. Radiation causes early nuclear disintegration of these cells and with their destruction and the resultant decrease in pressure, pain tends to lessen or disappear. Beyond this relief of pain, the disintegration of lymphocytes serves to liberate certain antibodies and enzymes contained within their cell bodies, thereby making these agents more available for body defense than they were while in the intact cell. Their presence speeds the phagocytosis of cellular debris and bacteria which may be present. There is microscopic evidence that the action of phagocytes is increased shortly after radiation treatment, and that this increased activity continues for several days.

Thus, it is readily apparent that radiation therapy can be useful in the treatment of most traumatic inflammations. The logical and ideal time—and in practice this opportunity is rarely presented—to use this type of therapy is at the peak of the leukocytic infiltration into the involved area. In other words, it should be administered as soon after the animal shows signs of lameness as possible.

In old, chronic injuries, however, radiation therapy may be of value because of other properties which the rays possess. It is well-known that radiation exposure is followed by a diminution of excessive connective tissue and calcium deposits which often are associated with chronic inflammation. Though normal tissue is not affected by proper doses of x-rays, abnormal tissue may be wholly, or in part, removed by the increased circulation induced in the damaged area by x-radiation.

METHODS OF ADMINISTRATION

There are 2 commonly used methods for administering radiation therapy to horses: 1. With the large, permanently installed x-ray machine, and 2, by using radioactive materials, such as radium or cobalt-60. Each method has certain advantages, as well as certain disadvantages. The x-ray equipment is costly, requires a large area for installation, and must be properly shielded to prevent injury to personnel working around or near it. Its use also requires that the animal must be transported to the machine. Its advantages include the shortness of treatment time required, its incorporation of necessary safety features, and its ability to deliver accurate dosage to any area regardless of the thickness of the part to be treated.

Radioactive materials can be taken to the animal and thus treatments can be given at the race track or farm. Danger is involved in the handling and transporting of radioactive materials, however. Should any be lost, a great deal of time and money may be spent in their recovery. Recent A.E.C. (Atomic Energy Commission) rulings and new public health laws in many states make it doubtful that it will be legal much longer to transport or use radioactive materials away from a fixed lead-lined or concrete stall. An x-ray treatment takes less than 10 minutes, but 12 or more hours are required for the average dose of radioactive material. Consequently, it seems likely that radioactive substances will have a restricted use in equine practice in the future.

I stopped using radium therapy in 1947 in favor of the x-ray machine. A General Electric Maximar 220 unit is used in my practice. This unit was designed for industrial use and is mounted as an industrial unit. This makes the machine much more flexible than the units with the usual mounting for medical use. The unit operates at 200 kvp. Our standard filter is 1 mm. of aluminum plus ½ mm. of copper. Treatment is given at a focal-skin distance of 50 cm. At 10 milliamperes, 33 roentgens are delivered per minute with a half-value layer of 1.1 mm. of copper. Thus, a dose of 200 roentgens as measured in air is given in 6 minutes. If doses are expressed in RADS (1 RAD represents tissue absorption of 100 ergs/Gm.), about 270 RADS may be given to the center of a knee in 6 minutes.

The focal-skin distance used permits us to keep the machine far enough away from the animal to prevent injury to it or the equipment. The industrial mounting makes it possible for the operator to follow the movements of the animal in any direction. Heavy leaded panels and hardwood planks restrict the animal's movement to a minimum. The horse is held by a halter shank passed over the leaded panel, and the holder, while on the other side of the panel, observes the horse through a heavy leaded glass. A lightweight curtain is drawn on the other side of the horse, away from the tube side, and a heavy oak plank interferes with his coming in contact with the x-ray unit. Noise and confusion are kept to a minimum when the machine is being used, and no one but the operator and the handler are allowed in the treatment room when therapy is being administered.

The x-ray machine is calibrated annually by a licensed radiation physicist and safety checks are made periodically. A film badge monitoring service for all personnel engaged in radiation work is a necessity, as are proper records of every case treated.

Use of Radiation Therapy for Lameness

Radiation therapy has been used with varying degrees of success in many types of lameness. In general, the acute phase of the disease is more amenable to this therapy than are chronic conditions. The veterinary radiologist rarely sees cases of acute lameness, however, as most horses which are presented have long-standing lamenesses which have been treated unsuccessfully with various drugs and methods. In locations where radiation therapy has been used for many years, more suitable cases are presented for treatment.

Conditions Treated

Shoulder Lameness (Bicipital Bursitis): Injuries to the point of the shoulder can result in acute bursitis. For such cases, 3 or 4 exposures to 100 roentgens are often all the treatment that is needed. In the chronic stage when the bursa is thickened or calcified, more exposures and larger doses are required (a total of 1200 to 1500 roentgens in a series), and the results are less satisfactory.

Carpitis: This term includes acute or chronic inflammation of the carpal joint, and may involve any or all of the anatomic structures of the joint. Cases of acute inflammation without bone damage or torn ligaments will respond well to small doses of radiation. Chronic cases with calcification or ossification involving one or more carpal bones can be aided by x-ray exposures of 1200 to 1500 roentgens. Many surgeons routinely use radiation therapy after surgical removal of bone fragments from a knee. This is done to discourage new calcification which so often follows orthopedic surgery in the horse. Other veterinarians prefer to irradiate an injured knee in order to hurry the reduction of inflammation prior to firing. For each condition 300 to 600 roentgens are sufficient.

Splints: The soreness of beginning splint formation is relieved by radiation therapy. If it is desired to fire the splint after radiation, no problem is presented, and time often is saved in this manner.

Tendon Injuries: Early cases of bowed tendon are definitely aided by radiation therapy. Much of the swelling associated with this injury is reduced and blood clots are partially or completely absorbed. Following irradiation, the tendon may be immobilized or fired as desired. Some, or most, of the fibrous thickening in an old bowed tendon and its sheath will be absorbed following radiation therapy, and this aids in restoring normal motion of the tendon. In the acute condition, doses of 150 roentgens to a total of 750 roentgens are given. In chronic cases, doses of 200 roentgens usually are given twice weekly for a total of 1600 roentgens. In all tendon injuries, radiographs should be made to rule out possible fractures of the splint bone.

Osselets: In the acute stage before new bone formation has appeared, radiation therapy may be used as the only treatment or as an aid in reducing inflammatory changes before firing. Chronic osselets can be reduced in size and some degree of motion restored to the area following irradiation.

Many animals are now treated by irradiation after firing is performed. This is done to reduce the acute swelling following the firing operation. Irradiation will greatly shorten the time that the horse must be kept from training.

Sesamoiditis and Injuries to the Suspensory Ligament: Good radiographs are most important in diagnosis of these conditions. Radiographs with great contrast, in order to show cracks or fractures in the sesamoid bones, often

will be inadequate for demonstration of soft tissue pathology in the area. Other radiographic technic is used to demonstrate soft tissue thickening and beginning calcification in the suspensory ligament that will not be seen when the sesamoid bones are overexposed. So 2 sets of radiographs are taken using different technics.

Treatment of these conditions requires doses of 600 to 900 roentgens in acute cases and doses of 1200 to 1500 roentgens in chronic cases with calcification or ossification.

Ringbone and Sidebone: When these conditions are in the early, formative stage, irradiation plus rest may be of considerable benefit. Small doses are indicated.

Navicular Disease: In the early phases of this disease, in the absence of a fracture, radiation therapy is the treatment of choice. If the bursa has become calcified, the bone eroded, or affected with periostitis, treatment is of little avail.

Hock and Stifle Inflammations: Injuries in this area, in the absence of fracture, may often be treated successfully by radiation. If noncastrates are presented for treatment, the owner should be advised about the possibilities of radiation damage and written permission obtained before treating the animal.

RADIATION HAZARDS

Health hazards related to radiation therapy are threefold. First, there is the possible overexposure of personnel engaged in giving the treatments and in handling the animal at the time of treatment. This danger can be avoided by proper shielding of the radiation equipment, through routine checks by a radiation physicist for leakage, by proper indoctrination of all people working with the radiation equipment, by the use of film badges, and by keeping unauthorized persons away from the area. A red light should be lit outside the building or shielded room when the machine is ON, and it should be impossible for anyone to get into the radiation area after the treatment has been started unless the machine is first turned OFF.

The second hazard involves the animal and is related to overexposure or improper treatment. If the machine is calibrated frequently, the operator knows the roentgen dose per minute at a given machine setting and a given distance. Thus, if the timer is working properly and is correctly set at the beginning of the exposure, no trouble should be expected provided the animal remains at the proper distance from the tube. If the animal moves, the machine must be turned off and the patient is repositioned. The timer then is reset allowing for the treatment already given.

Great care must be taken to insure that the proper filter is in place before each treatment. A treatment given unintentionally without a filter constitutes malpractice. The animal will feel nothing, but the number of roentgens given will be increased greatly. The rays will be absorbed largely in the skin and superficial tissues and cause a severe burn and slough that may never heal.

The third danger involves the detrimental alteration of genetic structure. It never is wise to expose the hindquarters of a mare or stud. No one knows the exact extent of this hazard because the horse is not suitable for research of radiation injury. It is almost impossible to produce sterility in the bitch and, in our experience, puppies born after heavy exposure have always appeared to be normal. Carlson has had the same experience. I have reported about the treatment of several hundred horses over a period of 10 years with no evidence of sterility or abnormality in the offspring. It must be repeated that every precaution always has been taken to avoid direct exposure of the gonads of intact animals.

M. Thom.

REFERENCES

1. Adams, O. R.: Lameness in Horses. Lea and Febiger, Philadelphia, Pa. 1962.
2. Carlson, W. D.: Veterinary Radiology. Lea and Febiger, Philadelphia, Pa. 1961.
3. Delario: Roentgen, Radium, and Radioisotope Therapy. Lea & Febiger, Philadelphia, Pa.
4. Murphy: Radiation Therapy. W. B. Saunders Co., Philadelphia, Pa.
5. Schnelle, G. B.: Radiology in Small Animal Practice. 2nd Ed. The North American Veterinarian, Inc. Evanston, Ill., 1950.
6. Tavernor and Vaughan: Radiology of horses and cattle. Brit. Vet. J. 118 (1960).
7. Thom, M.: Radiation therapy in equine lameness. Paper presented at the Sixteenth International Veterinary Congress. Madrid, Spain. 1959.

CHAPTER 19

DISEASES OF ALLERGY

NEONATAL ISOERYTHROLYSIS

Neonatal isoerythrolysis is a hemolytic anemia and icterus of newborn foals and mules resulting from isoimmunization of the mare against erythrocytes of the foal during pregnancy. The disease has been described as icterus gravis, jaundiced foals, hemolytic disease, isohemolytic disease, icteric foals, hemolytic icterus, and hemolytic anemia. The name, neonatal isoerythrolysis, was proposed by Hagan and Bruner.[1]

History: The concept that neonatal isoerythrolysis was caused by isoimmunization during pregnancy was developed and investigated independently in France, England, and the United States. Caroli and Bessis[2] ascertained that hemolytic anemia and icterus of newborn mules were caused by isoimmunization against erythrocytes of the donkey. Bruner *et al.*[3,4,5] found that an isoimmunization of pregnancy was responsible for hemolytic anemia and icterus of Thoroughbred foals. Similar findings were reported by Coombs *et al.*[6] and Parry *et al.*[7] in Thoroughbreds. Isoerythrolysis is somewhat analogous to the Rh disease of human infants, except that no definite blood type has been incriminated and development of the disease is entirely postnatal. Observations on serology, hematology, clinical features, lesions, and treatment were recorded by Doll *et al.*,[8,9,10,11] Brion,[12] Saint Martin,[13] and Cronin.[14,15]

Etiology and Pathogenesis: Isoimmunization may occur naturally,[2,3,7] be induced by blood transfusion, or by use of vaccine containing horse erythrocytes.[10] Natural isoimmunization results from passage of fetal erythrocytes or their components into the maternal tissues during pregnancy. The mechanism of transfer of fetal erythrocyte antigens has not been determined. Placental disease with possible adhesions and anastomosis of fetal and maternal circulation has been suspected. An abnormal placentation or other pathologic process appears to be necessary for natural isoimmunization. Most mares are not immunized after bearing many foals with blood incompatible with their type. Naturally immunized mares are not resensitized consistently during subsequent incompatible pregnancies. Although some show an increase of circulating antibody during the last 4 months of gestation, most mares do not have additional antigenic stimulation from subsequent incompatible pregnancies. Mares sensitized by equine tissue vaccines rarely develop additional antibody from bearing an incompatible foal.

Isoimmunization occurs when the fetal erythrocyte type is different from that of the mare. The fetal erythrocytes contain antigens corresponding to those of the stallion. Several erythrocyte antigens are involved but they have not been identified for lack of a standard system of typing equine blood. Antibody developed against the fetal erythrocytes is concentrated in the colostrum, usually at a titer 4- to 8-fold higher than in the mare's serum. The fetus is not affected *in utero,* as there is no transplacental transfer of antibody in horses.

Excluding other disease, foals are born healthy and are unaffected until they ingest colostrum. The colostral antibody is absorbed from the intestine, then attacks and destroys the foal's erythrocytes. Mares develop both agglutinating and hemolytic antibodies. Both types may be present, but frequently only agglutinating antibody is detectable. Hemolytic antibody with absence of agglutinating antibody has not been observed. Hemolytic antibody causes intravascular hemolysis and the agglutinating antibody causes clumping of erythrocytes, resulting in their removal from the circulating blood and their destruction in the liver and spleen. The severity of the disease is related to the type of antibody present, the antibody titer of the colostrum, the volume of colostrum secreted and ingested, and possibly to the antigenic mosaic of the foal's erythrocytes.

Hemolytic antibody is associated with more acute and severe anemia. Severe anemia, in turn, is associated with colostrum having high antibody titer, but also may result from a large volume of colostrum with a low titer. The antigenic mosaic of the foal's erythrocytes may have an important influence on the severity of the disease, especially when isoimmunization resulted from a preceding pregnancy by a different stallion.

Clinical Signs: Foals are healthy when born, nurse the mare and are active for a short period. In 12 to 36 hours after birth, they become dull, sluggish, weak, do not nurse, and may become prostrated. The heart and respiratory rates are increased, particularly after exercise. The mucous membranes are pale during the first 24 hours. Icterus appears in 24 to 48 hours and becomes progressively more intense within 4 to 6 days. The temperature is normal or subnormal. Citrated blood samples show marked reduction and agglutination of erythrocytes. Serum and urine are not discolored during the first 24 hours, but usually may be tinged with hemoglobin in very acute cases. Icteric discoloration of serum occurs after 24 to 48 hours and yellowish discoloration of urine is constant.

The course is variable. Foals may die from acute anemia in 12 to 36 hours. Most fatalities occur on the third or fourth day, but fatal issue may be delayed for 8 to 10 days.

Lesions: Anemia and icterus are constant. Foals dying in less than 24 hours are anemic only, though icterus is observed after 24 hours and becomes progressively more severe with increased age. The blood is pale. Erythrocytes are agglutinated, particularly in foals under 3 days old, but often are not in foals aged 5 days or more. The color of the urine varies from light yellow to a port wine color. Enlarged, turgid spleens are observed in foals dying under 72 hours. The spleens usually are not enlarged in foals surviving 5 days or longer, except in those that recently received transfusions of incompatible blood. Histologically, the internal organs show only simple degenerative changes in acute cases. Centrilobular necrosis occurs in the liver of protracted cases. Erythrophagia occurs in the spleen and liver.

Diagnosis: Clinical diagnosis may be presumed from an early afebrile weakness and prostration associated with anemia, increased pulse and respiratory rates, and agglutination of the foal's erythrocytes in their own plasma. Confirmation of diagnosis is made by agglutination tests using serum from the dam and erythrocytes from the stallion siring the foal or another suitable donor. Erythrocytes of the affected foal are not suitable for agglutination tests because of antibody adsorbed to them. They may be employed for diagnosis by testing in equine antiglobulin serum, in which agglutination establishes that the maternal antibody is adsorbed to the surface of the foal's erythrocytes.

Serum of the mare is diluted in 2-fold series. Erythrocytes from the stallion or donors are washed 3 times in 10 volumes of physiologic saline and used as a 50% suspension. Equal volumes of serum dilutions and cell suspensions are used for plate agglutination tests. Readings are made in 3 to 5 minutes. Tests should be controlled by use of erythrocytes from the mare for appraisal of rouleaux formation. Colostrum or milk is tested for agglutinin by the same procedure. Agglutination of the stallion's erythrocytes in serum of the dam at dilutions of 1:2 or greater indicates that isoimmunization has occurred. Further support of the diagnosis is obtainable by demonstrating unabsorbed circulating antibody in the foal's serum, and by use of the antiglobulin serum.

Prognosis: Severity and outcome of isoerythrolysis are related directly to the anemia and destruction of erythrocytes, which in turn are related to the volume, titer, and type of antibody in the colostrum. The most valuable index of the foal's condition is obtained by daily erythrocyte counts. The erythrocyte count may drop precipitously to 2,200,000 to 3,000,000/cmm. within 12 to 24 hours. It may recede gradually and reach lowest levels in 4 to 5 days. It may drop precipitously and start increasing after 36 to 72 hours, or remain at low levels for 4 to 6 days before recovery is initiated. Foals that maintain erythrocyte counts of 6,000,000/cmm. or higher do not need transfusion therapy. Those maintaining erythrocyte counts between 4,000,000 and 6,-

000,000/cmm. may be expected to survive, and transfusion is not desirable unless the anemia is protracted. Erythrocyte counts of 3,000,-000/cmm. or less are at the borderline of fatal issue, and transfusion is necessary to insure survival of the foal.

The presence of free, unabsorbed maternal antibody in the foal's serum at 24 to 48 hours after birth indicates that the anemia may become more severe, that recovery will be slower, and that there is greater urgency for exsanguination transfusion. Absence of free maternal antibody in the foal's serum usually indicates that destruction of blood will be less severe and recovery more rapid. Intravascular hemolysis and hemoglobinuria are associated with more severe disease and indicate urgency for large-volume exsanguination transfusion. Projecting severity of the disease from the titer of mare's serum is unreliable because of variation in the volume of colostrum secreted. In general, however, isoerythrolysis may be expected to be more severe when the titer of the mare's serum exceeds 1:8 to 1:16 than when it is at 1:4 to 1:8 or less. More severe disease may be expected when elimination of antibody in the milk persists for 24 to 48 hours or longer. Recovery of acutely affected foals is expedited by large-volume replacement transfusion within 24 to 48 hours after birth.

Treatment: Complete confinement until the erythrocyte counts approach normal range is essential in management of the affected foal. Many unobserved cases terminate fatally from exhaustion incident to the foal's running after its dam in paddock or pasture. Acutely affected foals, with erythrocyte counts falling below 3,000,000/cmm. within 18 to 48 hours, need large-volume exsanguination transfusions. This requires alternate infusion and withdrawal of 500 ml. volumes until 5 to 6 liters of the donor's blood is administered and an equal volume is removed from the foal. The entire 6-liter volume may be obtained safely from a single donor. This volume restores the erythrocyte count of the foal to 7,000,000 to 8,000,000/cmm. Replacement transfusion supplies erythrocytes not susceptible to the maternal antibody, and removes the foal's anti-body-laden erythrocytes and unabsorbed antibody in the foal's plasma. Response to a single large-volume exsanguination transfusion is more satisfactory than from repeated, small transfusions. Standard evacuated transfusion bottles are suitable.

Selection of donors involves finding a horse with erythrocytes that are not agglutinated by the maternal antibody. It requires matching of erythrocytes from prospective donors against serum from the dam of the affected foal. Technics are the same as employed for diagnosis. Rapid screening is possible by using equal volumes of citrated whole blood from prospective donors and serum from the dam of the foal. Bloods not showing strong agglutination are selected and the cells washed for final tests. By this procedure one usually can select a blood type similar to or identical with that of the dam of the foal, but incompatible for the foal. This system is employed because it is essential to transfuse cells that will not be affected by the maternal antibody absorbed by the foal from the colostrum. Its objective is overcoming the acute hemolytic crisis. In practical use, the transfusion alleviates the anemia for sufficient time for the foal to begin replacing its erythrocytes. Thoroughly washed erythrocytes from the dam may be used. Whole blood from the dam cannot be used because it contains the antibody responsible for the anemia. Transfusion of acute cases having free antibody in their plasma with cells incompatible with the maternal antibody may result in rapidly fatal issue.

The foal that is 4 to 7 days old and has no demonstrable free antibody in its plasma may be transfused with blood of its own type, or a type reacting with the maternal antibody. Use of equine antiglobulin serum after absorption of donor's cells in the foal's serum insures freedom from unabsorbed antibody and compatibility. Transfusion is desirable at this age when erythrocyte counts have not risen above 4,000,000. A single transfusion using 1 to 2 liters is adequate.

Colostrum or milk should be tested for antibody when the foal is under 36 to 48 hours old. If antibody is detected in the milk, the foal should be muzzled, fed from another source for 24 hours or longer, and the mare milked out hourly to remove additional antibody. Foals lose ability to absorb antibody from the intestine after 36 to 48 hours. If antibody is not detectable in the milk it is not necessary to interrupt nursing of the dam.

Prevention: Isoerythrolysis may be prevented by suitable testing of mare's serum before birth of the foal, or by correct management of known sensitized mares and their foals at foaling.

Serum from a mare with no history of isoimmunization may be tested against cells of the stallion 1 to 2 weeks before foaling. Agglutination of the stallion's erythrocytes indicates impending isoerythrolysis in a foal with the blood type of the stallion.

Mares with known isoimmunization continue to secrete antibody in the colostrum with successive pregnancies and isoerythrolysis may be expected in foals having a blood type against which the mare is immunized. Tests on serum of the mare do not enable precise prediction of a compatible or susceptible foal. A rise in antibody titer during the last 4 months of gestation indicates an incompatible foal and impending isoerythrolysis. Static antibody titers, however, do not insure compatibility.

Two alternatives may be used for the known sensitized mare. She may be bred to a stallion with a compatible blood type, and thereby produce a foal with cells not susceptible to her antibody. The second alternative is to breed indiscriminantly of blood type and manage foaling to prevent the disease. Foaling must be attended, the foal muzzled, and appropriate tests made before the foal is allowed to nurse. Erythrocytes of the foal are tested against serum and colostrum of the mare. If there is no agglutination the foal may be allowed to suckle colostrum. If the foal's erythrocytes are agglutinated it must be fed artificially and the mare milked out hourly until her milk is free of antibody before permitting the foal to nurse. Detectable antibody is eliminated from the milk of most mares after 8 to 16 hours of hourly milking. It may persist in the milk of some mares for longer periods. Foals may be returned to their dams after 48 to 72 hours, even though antibody is secreted in low titer. A nurse mare (foster mother) may be provided in lieu of milking by hand. Foals,

2 to 3 weeks old, may be employed for suckling colostrum from the sensitized mare while her foal is permitted to nurse another mare. Foals deprived of colostrum should be maintained on antibiotic therapy for 4 to 6 days to suppress bacterial infections. Colostrums may be collected from other mares, pooled, and preserved by freezing for feeding the foals of sensitized mares.

E. R. DOLL

REFERENCES

1. Hagan, W. A. and Bruner, D. W.: Infectious Diseases of Domestic Animals. 4th ed., Comstock Publishing Associates, Ithaca, N. Y., 1961.
2. Caroli, J., and Bessis, M.: Sur la Cause et le Traitment de L'ictere Grave des Muletons Nouveau-nes. Compt. rend Acad. Sci. 224 (1947) 969-971.
3. Bruner, D. W., Hull, F. E., Edwards, P. R., and Doll, E. R.: Icteric foals. J.A.V.M.A. 112 (1948) 440-441.
4. Bruner, D. W., Hull, F. E., and Doll, E. R.: The relation of blood factors to icterus in foals. Am. J. Vet. Research 9 (1948) 237-242.
5. Bruner, D. W., Doll, E. R., Hull, F. E., and Kinkaid, A.: Further studies on hemolytic icterus in foals. Am. J. Vet. Research 11 (1950) 22-25.
6. Coombs, R. R. A., Crowhurst, R. C., Day, F. T., Heard, D. H., Hinde, I. T., Hoogstraten, J., and Parry, H. B.: Hemolytic disease of newborn foals due to isoimmunization of pregnancy. J. Hyg. 46 (1948) 403-418.
7. Parry, H. B., Day, F. T., and Crowhurst, R. C.: Diseases of newborn foals, I. Hemolytic disease due to isoimmunization of pregnancy. Vet. Rec. 61 (1948) 435-441.
8. Doll, E. R., and Hull, F. E.: Observations on Hemolytic Icterus of Newborn Foals. Cornell Vet. 41 (1951) 14-35.
9. Doll, E. R.: Observations on the clinical features and pathology of hemolytic icterus of newborn foals. Am. J. Vet. Res. 12 (1952) 504-508.
10. Doll, E. R., Richards, M. G., Wallace, M. E., and Bryans, J. T.: The influence of an equine fetal tissue vaccine upon hemagglutination activity of mare serums: its relation to hemolytic icterus of newborn foals. Cornell Vet. 42 (1952) 495-505.
11. Doll, E. R.: Evidence of the production of an Antiisoantibody by foals affected with hemolytic icterus. Cornell Vet. 43 (1953) 44-51.
12. Brion, A.: Sur l'ictere hemolytique du poulain nouveau-ne. rev. de med. vet. 100 (1949) 229-235.
13. Saint Martin, A.: Prophylaxie et traitment de l'ictere du muleton. Rev. de Med. Vet. 103 (1952) 263-268.
14. Cronin, M. T. I.: Exchange transfusion in the foal. Vet. Rec. 65 (1953) 120-123.
15. Cronin, M. T. I.: Hemolytic disease of newborn foals. Vet. Rec. 67 (1955) 479-494.

QUEENSLAND ITCH

The disease known as Queensland Itch of horses has been recognized in Australia for many years, and now is considered to be an allergic skin reaction associated with attack by a species of Ceratopogonid fly. It is characterized by a chronic, recurring, intensely irritating, superficial dermatitis especially prominent about the ears, mane, withers and tail, and is most prevalent during the summer. Only certain individuals appear to be susceptible and many horses confined with affected animals on the same pasture never show signs of the disease. Affected animals rub against fences and gates to relieve the irritation, thus causing damage to property and injury to the skin. The disease is particularly serious among working animals as the desire to rub and bite the affected parts increases with rise in body temperature and with stimulation of the sweat glands.

Reports from overseas indicate that similar if not identical conditions occur in horses or mules in France (Henry and Bory, 1937; Vaills, 1946), in India (Datta, 1939), in Japan (Nakamura *et al.,* 1956; Ueno and Ishihara, 1957), in the Philippine Islands (Underwood, 1934), and in the United States of America (Alicata, 1936; Report of Georgia Costal Plains Experiment Station, 1947; Dikmans, 1948). As in Australia, only a portion of exposed horses is affected, and in these the disease is characterized by a dermatitis commencing in the early part of the hot season and continuing unchecked until the onset of cold weather.

Distribution and Incidence: The disease occurs in Queensland and northeastern New South Wales, and probably also in western Australia and Victoria. It seems to be confined largely to the summer rainfall areas of the continent and is most prevalent in Queensland where the highest incidence is seen in stock in the coastal and subcoastal regions. It appears to be absent in the arid central areas of northern Australia.

Signs of the disease usually become evident in the early part of the summer and continue progressively until the onset of cooler weather, when they gradually diminish. In chronic cases, however, lesions never completely disappear even during the winter months. The condition is most evident in the humid and hottest months of the year, namely January, February and March.

This allergic dermatitis is confined to horses, and animals of all ages are susceptible. Young animals, however, seldom show clinical signs although the condition has been observed in a 4-months-old Thoroughbred colt. Breed, sex, and color are of little significance in incidence. Some animals are never affected even though in continual contact with diseased animals,

and even when using the same harness. There does, however, appear to be a familial incidence which seems to be related more with the dam than the sire, as a higher incidence was found among the progeny of affected mares than among the progeny of apparently unaffected horses.

When affected animals are stabled at night or brought into stables for training, the lesions recede rapidly and, except in severely or chronically affected individuals, external manifestations disappear in 4 to 5 weeks. Complete recovery also may occur when animals which are showing signs are moved from one district to another.

Etiology: The disease is associated with the development of a cutaneous hypersensitivity to the bites of the sandfly, *Culicoides robertsi* (Fig. 1). Other species of sandflies (Ceratopogonidae) have been observed biting horses, but have not been implicated in this condition. Although microfilariae of *Onchocerca reticulata* have been implicated in the etiology of the disease overseas, there is no evidence to involve this parasite in Australia. Microfilariae have been recovered from the skin of both normal and affected animals.

Clinical Signs: The lesions of allergic dermatitis usually are confined to the dorsal regions including the butt of the tail, rump, along the back, withers, crest, poll, and ears (Fig. 2). In young animals the most frequent sites of lesions are the butt of the tail and the ears, and in many cases these are the only areas affected grossly. In older animals which have been exposed continually to the causal agent, additional lesions frequently are observed in the region of the withers and rump. Only in severe cases do the lesions involve the sides of the body, the neck, the face, and legs.

The most obvious sign is a continuous effort to relieve itching, particularly at night when animals will rub for hours against overhanging branches, leaning trees, fences or any suitable object.

During the initial stage of the condition there is formation of slight discrete papules on which the hair stands erect. These lesions are scattered over the dorsal surface of the body, but in severe cases also may be present on the sides of the body and on the neck. Lesions

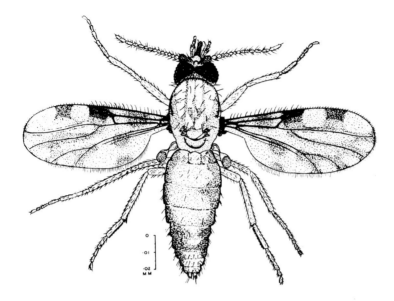

Fig. 1. Female *Culicoides robertsi.*

rarely are observed on the ventral surface of the body. Scaling, with loss of hair at the edges of the ears, is seen in almost every animal. The ragged appearance of the butt of the tail, so-called "rat-tail," and the loss of hair on the ears are the 2 most prominent lesions, and in some animals may be the only ones observed. Exfoliation of epidermal cells is pronounced, and conglomerate masses of cells appear in the exudate of serum and tissue fluids. The hair becomes brittle and crinkled, and in the vicinity of the papules it gradually is broken and shed. Loss of hair on the rump, withers, and mane is prominent.

Superficial abrasions, excoriations, and marked inflammatory reactions are produced by animals' rubbing, gnawing, and biting affected parts (Fig. 3). In chronic cases of some years' duration, the skin becomes thickened, dry, rough, and hairless in spots, and the formation of rugae, particularly in the region of the withers, is common.

The appetite is unimpaired and body temperature remains normal except when secondary bacterial infection of excoriations occurs. There may, however, be a loss of condition in aggravated cases through prolonged irritation, otherwise the general condition of the horse is unaffected.

Microscopic Lesions: The earliest change observed on microscopic examination is dilation and engorgement of the smaller blood vessels and capillaries of the corium. Varying degrees of serous effusion with some infiltration of leukocytes, particularly of eosinophils, result in the separation of collagen fibers. The cellular reaction, first evident as clumping of eosinophils around the smaller blood vessels and capillaries of the corium, gradually spreads through this tissue, but does not extend into the surrounding tissue to any extent.

Subsequent to the early papular stages, proliferation of the epidermal cells becomes pronounced, the horny layer being considerably thickened and consisting predominantly of parakeratotic cells.

There also may be some serous exudation with conglomeration of epithelial cells. Denudation of hair on these individual areas occurs through loss of these cell masses and by the rubbing associated with the intense irritation. As the lesions progress, a decrease in the cellular infiltration and in the edema usually is observed together with early evidence of mild fibrosis. The eosinophils tend to remain for longer periods. Some cellular infiltration, however, appears to be present at all times.

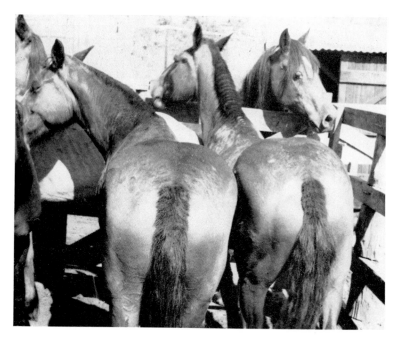

Fig. 2. Lesions at base of tail, croup, and withers.

In chronic cases of the disease extensive fibrosis, hypertrophy of epidermal tissue, and marked hyperkeratosis are evident, resulting in accentuation of skin folds on the crest, withers, and rump.

The histopathologic picture, however, frequently is complicated by trauma with formation of raw bleeding surfaces, and occasionally by secondary infection. In such instances, microscopic examination shows a typical inflammatory reaction and ulceration of the surface epithelium, which mask the earlier cellular reaction.

No pathologic changes have been observed on microscopic examination of the liver, spleen, kidney, and lungs of susceptible animals.

Diagnosis: Allergic dermatitis appears to be quite distinct as a disease entity among horses in Australia. Its restriction to certain animals, its seasonal prevalence, the predilection sites,

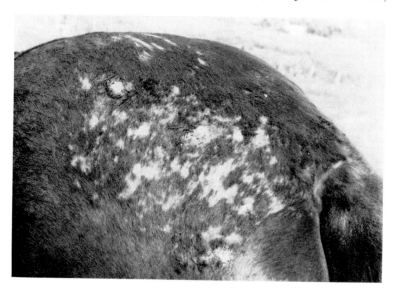

Fig. 3. Self-inflicted denudation.

and the characteristic early lesion are the main diagnostic features. The condition often has been referred to as psoroptic mange, a disease of horses unknown in this country, but which, in the initial stages, also affects the same dorsal areas. The "rat-tail" condition of allergic dermatitis could be confused with a dermatitis associated with infection by *Oxyuris equi*, particularly in young animals. Diagnosis of infection by the helminth is simple and is made by demonstration of creamy clusters of eggs on the perineum.

Treatment and Control: In the studies on etiology it was observed that the causative sandfly had a distinct seasonal prevalence. Adults occurred only during the warmer months. During the day they usually did not attack before about 4:30 p.m. and were most abundant during the early hours of the night. They disappeared shortly after daylight.

In a series of trials with susceptible horses, animals were housed in a screened shelter overnight from 4 p.m. to 7 a.m. and were permitted to graze during the remainder of the day. When confined in this manner from the early spring until the following winter, known susceptible horses remained free of the disease. It also was found that when horses showing lesions were confined in the screened shelter at night the disease disappeared within 3 weeks. The lesions reappeared, however, as soon as the animals were exposed again at night; the initial lesions appeared within 3 days after exposure.

A number of different materials including sump oil, lard, sulfur, and potassa sulfurata have been used by horse owners as external medicaments to relieve allergic dermatitis. Those with an oil base, when applied frequently, have produced improvement in the condition, probably because of their fly-repellent properties.

Observations on animals sprayed on their dorsal and lateral aspects with 1% DDT showed that complete protection from sandflies could be expected for 7 days. Weekly spraying with this concentration gave good protection in the majority of animals and, as a rule, lesions disappeared completely within 4 weeks after spraying was commenced.

During periods of heavy rain, it was necessary to use a 2% concentration to secure effective protection because of the rapid loss of DDT from the coat under such circumstances. The 2% concentration also gave better results on animals with short hair as DDT residues are lost more rapidly from animals with short hair than from those with long hair.

In man, desensitization is attempted by the frequent injection of the specific allergen in graded doses or the parenteral injections of histamine or histamine azoprotein. These treatments required a number of injections and thus would not be economical or practical except in exceptional circumstances.

The antihistamine preparations are reported to have effectively controlled hypersensitivity reactions in a large percentage of human patients. The antiallergic properties of these substances depend to a great extent upon the character, site, and state of the allergic manifestation for which they are employed. Antihistamines applied as creams or injected intramuscularly have relieved the irritation associated with this equine dermatitis, but were too costly for regular use.

R. F. RIEK

REFERENCES

1. Alicata, J. E.: No. Amer. Vet. 17 (1936) 39-40.
2. Datta, S.: Vet. J. 95 (1939) 213-222.
3. Dikmans, G.: Cornell Vet. 38 (1948) 3-23.
4. Georgia Coastal Plains Experiment Station, 27th Annual Report, pp. 37-41, 1947.
5. Henry, A. and Bory L.: Rec. Méd. Vét. 113 (1937) 65-78.
6. Nakamura, R., Matsuhashi, A., Yamashita, N., and Yamamoto, T.: Jap. J. Vet. Research 4 (1956) 81-88.
7. Ueno, H. and Ishihara, T.: National Institute Animal Health Japan Bull. No. 32, 1957.
8. Underwood, J. R.: Vet. Bull. U. S. Army 28 (1934) 227-236.
9. Vaills, J.: Rev. Méd. Vét. Lyon et Toulouse 97 (1946) 6-72.

ANAPHYLAXIS

Etiology: Anaphylaxis is a state of hypersensitivity which is induced by the parenteral injection of a foreign antigenic substance following which a suitable time interval is allowed to elapse. A subsequent injection of the same antigen may result in anaphylactic shock. Thus, most anaphylactic reactions do not occur naturally but are man-made. Substances other than complex proteins are capable of producing anaphylaxis. The reaction is produced by cell injury and release of histamine or a histamine-like substance. Severe reactions in animals frequently follow a single injection of foreign protein or drug to which the animal appears to be sensitized naturally or has become hypersensitized by unknown means. These cases usually are classified as serum sickness. The 2 conditions have similar clinical signs and are treated in the same way.

True anaphylaxis is a rare clinical occurrence in equines as most serums that might be repeated are of equine origin. It is possible that anaphylactic shock will follow repeated injections of leptospirosis or encephalomyelitis vaccines. In most cases, repeated vaccinations are spread far enough apart so that the animal becomes desensitized. Repeated injections of foreign protein for the treatment of ocular diseases may not only produce urticaria but anaphylaxis as well. Hypersensitivity to drugs may result in signs resembling anaphylactic shock. This usually occurs when drugs are given intravenously in concentrated solutions. Thus, the intravenous administration of 5 Gm. of aureomycin in 10 ml. of water produced severe anaphylactic shock in a 5-year-old mule. Concentrations of other antibiotics, neoarsphenamine, formalin, metaphen and several other drugs may induce an anaphylactic-like response. The same drugs when well-diluted and administered slowly are not apt to produce such reactions.

Serum sickness occurs following the injection of foreign proteins without previous sensitization. As biologics administered to horses usually are of equine origin, serum sickness is not apt to occur. This reaction may occur, however, after the injection of chorionic gonadotropic hormone made from the urine of pregnant women, or after the injection of sheep pituitary hormone.

Clinical Signs: The signs of mild cases of anaphylactic shock or serum sickness are dyspnea, incoordination, and edema. Edematous swellings occur around the head, the dependent portions of the body, and at the site of the injection. In serious cases, there is dyspnea, cyanosis, unsteadiness of gait, sometimes collapse and, occasionally, death. In severe cases, evidence of pulmonary edema and emphysema is present.

Treatment: Treatment consists of the administration of 10 to 15 ml. of adrenalin solution subcutaneously. Atropine sulfate, given subcutaneously in a 1/4-grain dose, is indicated. As it has been shown that histamine produces signs similar to anaphylaxis, antihistamine solution should be given.

PHOTOSENSITIZATION

Photosensitization, or light sensitization, is a condition in which an animal is rendered hypersensitive to sunlight by the presence in the blood stream and tissues of a photosensitizing agent. In animals, photosensitization may be: 1. Congenital, as in Southdown lambs or in congenital bovine porphyria, 2, primary or simple photosensitization due to the ingestion of sensitizing substances of plant or chemical origin, and 3, icterogenic photosensitization occurring when substances are ingested which damage the liver and prevent the elimination of phylloerythrin. Phylloerythrin then accumulates in the blood stream to sensitize the tender parts of the skin to sunlight. A review of the literature would indicate that equines suffer only from simple or primary photosensitization and not from the congenital or icterogenic types.

Etiology: Primary or simple photosensitization in horses occurs following the ingestion of certain legumes as pasture crops. The disease has been reported after ingestion of alsike or Swedish clover (*Trifolium hybridum*), alfalfa (*Medicago sativa*), red clover (*Trifolium pratense*) and burr clover (*Medicago denticulata*). The condition has also been reported in horses that were fed mainly with vetch (*Vitia sativa*). Several other plants, mainly the St. John's wort family, are capable of causing photosensitization but they usually are not ingested by horses.

Plants capable of producing light sensitization are classified as photodynamic plants. These plants under unknown circumstances contain fluorescent substances which resemble porphyrins and when absorbed they sensitize tissue cells to sunlight. The reason why or under what circumstances an occasional growth of forage will accumulate a sensitizing agent is not known. In one enzootic involving 28 young draft-type horses observed by me, the pasture was a new, lush growth of alsike clover. The incident occurred in the summer during brilliant sunshiny days and cool nights with heavy dew. Though the animals were no doubt sensitized by the ingestion of the clover, lesions appeared only on white, unpigmented areas in contact with the clover. Episodes of this nature have been termed "dew poisoning."

Clinical Signs: The signs of photosensitization in horses usually appear on the white or unpigmented parts of the skin. Lesions therefore often are confined to the extremities and face (Fig. 4). In piebald horses, lesions may appear on the white areas of the neck or body trunk. In the usual case, there is exudation of serum, matting of hair, and exfoliation of the superficial layers of the skin. Lesions produced by alsike clover frequently undergo necrosis, sloughing, and emit a foul odor. In the enzo-

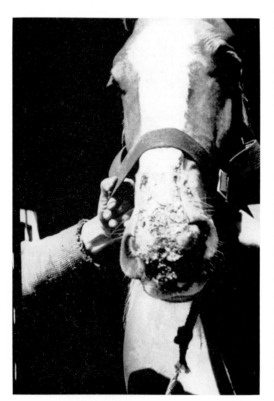

Fig. 4. Photosensitive reaction involving white area of muzzle.

otic previously mentioned where lesions appeared to be only on contact areas, the height of the clover could be measured by the extent of the lesions (Fig. 5). In clover disease affecting the white parts of the extremities, Fröhner[1] has reported stomatitis, icterus, and severe disturbances of consciousness with paresis. Painful lesions may develop about the mouth and cause inappetence.

Treatment: As soon as the condition is recognized, the animal should be removed from pasture or the diet changed to exclude the suspected feed. Affected horses should be placed in a darkened stable to protect them from light and insects. The stable quarters should be sprayed with insect repellents but such sprays should not be used on the affected animals. Topical treatment gradually will promote healing of lesions. When the affected areas are widespread, applications of carron oil or zinc oxide in oil are useful. For isolated necrotic lesions, cleansing them with 70% alcohol and following with the application of 5% sulfathiazole ointment is good therapy. A good medicament for topical application is an ointment containing a sulfonamide, an antibiotic, and a corticosteroid. The parenteral administration of corticosteroids also relieves pain and promotes healing.

Urticaria

Urticaria (nettlerash) is a skin eruption characterized by rounded elevations due to serous infiltration of the papillary and malpighian layers of the skin. The condition may be due to such systemic causes as the absorption of toxins from the digestive tract during gastroenteritis or constipation. Lesions of urticaria also may follow sudden changes in the diet or after the ingestion of certain feeds. This occurrence apparently reflects an idiosyncrasy of individual animals. Urticaria has occurred after grazing on clover or after ingestion of buckwheat. In one horse, a liberal feeding of carrots could induce profuse salivation and wheal-like skin elevations on the side of the neck and over the shoulders.

Urticarial eruptions may appear as a mild form of anaphylaxis due to parenteral injec-

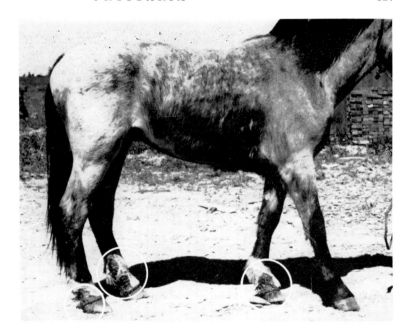

Fig. 5. Photosensitive reaction confined to exposed areas.

tions of foreign protein. Occasionally, eruptions follow the use of evaporated milk, condensed milk, hog cholera serum, or bovine serum as foreign protein therapy in the treatment of ocular diseases. Repeated injections of encephalomyelitis or leptospirosis vaccines also may cause urticaria. Nodular lesions occurring in strangles and dourine have been classified as infectious urticaria but these are primary or secondary infections of lymph nodes or ducts.

Local urticaria may appear after contact with certain plants which contain irritating chemical substances. The lesions produced by stinging nettles (*Urtica* spp.) account for the name of this condition. There are at least 108 types of vegetation capable of producing some form of dermatitis. Several of these species including nettles, poison wood, poison sumac, and poison oak produce urticarial-like lesions on the legs of fine-skinned horses. Apparently, only an occasional individual is susceptible.

In some horses, an allergic type of papillary swellings apparently is due to the secretion of insects. These lesions occur on the head, ears and side of the neck and are termed fly-bite dermatitis or allergy due to gnats.

Clinical Signs: Signs of urticaria appear very suddenly and disappear as rapidly. The swell-

ings of urticaria in the horse, however, tend to persist longer than in other species. There is a sudden appearance of wheal-like swellings from ¼ to 1½ inches in diameter over various parts of the body. The lesions occur principally over the neck and trunk of the body. In some cases, edema of the eyelids and lips is apparent, but generally edematous swellings are not as common in equines as they are in bovines and canines. Rarely, there may be edema of the mouth, perianal area, vulva or pharynx. Other clinical signs include evidence of discomfort and inappetence.

Treatment: In the treatment of urticaria the parenteral administration of adrenalin and antihistamines is indicated. Cases of urticaria tend to recover spontaneously. If the etiology appears to be dietary in origin or from contact with pasture plants or insects, proper control measures should be instituted. Cortisone has been found effective in the treatment of urticaria.

W. J. GIBBONS

REFERENCES

1. Fröhner, E.: Lehrbuch der Toxicologie, ed. 3 (1910) (quoted by Udall, 2).

2. Udall, D. H.: The Practice of Veterinary Medicine, Ithaca, N.Y. Published by the author. 1954.

3. Kral, F. and Novak, B. J.: Veterinary Dermatology, J. B. Lippincott Co., Philadelphia, Pa., 1953.

CHAPTER 20

DISEASES CAUSED BY PHYSICAL AND CHEMICAL AGENTS

PLANT POISONING

INTRODUCTION

When a horse dies suddenly and the true cause cannot be determined, a poisoning, either plant or chemical, frequently is suspected. This is a "catchall" diagnosis because most cases of poisoning cannot be determined accurately without laboratory analysis. People usually wish to avoid this expense and, therefore, willingly accept a diagnosis of poisoning.

If litigation is even a remote possibility, however, every effort should be made to obtain an accurate diagnosis. This is accomplished through a detailed history, a thorough examination of the living animal if possible, a careful postmortem examination, and a laboratory analysis if indicated.

It requires more than the presence of a poisonous plant in a given area to make a diagnosis of plant poisoning. There are hundreds of plants which have been incriminated as being poisonous to various species of livestock, including the horse. Most diagnoses of poisoning are not based on experimentation, but rather on field observation. In many cases, the observations are inaccurate or incomplete. Nevertheless, there are a number of plants which cause poisoning frequently enough to present good clinical evidence.

As with poisoning in general, there are very few clinical signs that are pathognomonic for a given plant poisoning. Therefore, it is essential that an accurate history be obtained. The plant in question must be available and there must be evidence that it has been consumed in sufficient quantity to cause toxicity. Many cases of poisoning will be seen only after death, thus a diagnosis must be made on the basis of postmortem findings. Here again, it is difficult to make an accurate diagnosis of plant poisoning because few plants cause distinctive pathologic lesions. In fact, many of them can kill an animal without producing gross changes.

It is not economically feasible, or in many cases possible, to isolate the poisonous principle or to run feeding experiments to determine the toxicity. A plant that is known to be toxic at one time may show little or no toxicity when dried or grown under different conditions. Therefore, the results of a plant feeding trial conducted under changed conditions may be misleading.

THE PREVENTION OF POISONOUS PLANT PROBLEMS

It is a general rule that poisonous plants are not palatable. Therefore, horses will eat them only if obliged to by such conditions as insufficient forage, mixing poisonous plants or seeds with hay or grain so that the animal is unable to separate the poisonous portions, or by putting poisonous plant clippings where a horse normally is used to eating.

If the horse-owner is on the alert for plants in his pasture which might cause trouble, these can be removed by digging them out, applying chemical weed killers, or if they are annuals, mowing before they go to seed. There is a special need to watch certain areas, as fence rows, ditches, and springs, because poisonous plants often are found in such areas. Certain plants are poisonous only during a particular season of the year. It may be necessary to remove horses from pasture during this time. In California, there is a particular problem with yellow star thistle (*Centaurea solstitialis*). In the late summer and fall when the native pastures are dry, care should be taken to provide animals with extra hay or supplemental forage, or they may eat the star thistle that grows during this time of the year. Occasionally it is necessary to remove animals from pasture because yellow star thistle is one plant for which horses will acquire a taste.

Sometimes animals are stimulated to eat certain plants because of mineral deficiencies. Plants high in nitrates have a salty taste, and thus may be palatable. If pasture is short, it is well to provide additional mineral supplementation.

Keeping poisonous plants out of hay is very difficult, because few people raise the hay they feed. It would be well, however, for the horse-owner to check the hay as he feeds it to make sure it is not too weedy. There are cases of livestock having been poisoned with oleander raked in the hay, baled, and fed. The difficulty in identifying this situation is that it is extremely difficult to get a good history. Usually not every bale is contaminated and all the contaminated bales may have been fed. Fortunately, most poisonous plants must be eaten in amounts of 1 to 3% of the body weight of the horse to cause toxicity. It is very unlikely that a horse will get this much in a bale of hay.

Hungry animals should not be turned into strange pastures, because they will be looking for anything to eat. If the first plants encountered are poisonous, they may be consumed. Lawn clippings or other plant cuttings should not be thrown into an area where horses are accustomed to eating hay. The lawn clippings themselves can cause colic and if they contain poisonous weed or plant leaves such as oleander, death can result. This particularly is true with young horses as they are more inquisitive than older ones and frequently will ingest potentially dangerous plants.

CLINICAL SIGNS OF PLANT POISONINGS

The observation of certain clinical signs in a sick horse suggests the possibility of a generalized toxemia. The central nervous system, the gastrointestinal tract, and the liver are frequent targets for the action of plant poisons. Most signs observed are produced by malfunction of these organs.

The signs of most plant poisonings include anorexia, dehydration, depression, emaciation, and dyspnea. Body temperature usually is normal or slightly below normal. In syndromes characterized by convulsions, the temperature may be elevated. Signs indicative of gastro-intestinal disease include: 1, diarrhea, 2, salivation, and 3, colic.

The character of the feces in diarrhea associated with poisoning varies markedly. They may be fluid, fetid, or hemorrhagic. Diarrhea certainly is not pathognomonic. Other conditions characterized by diarrhea include salmonellosis, chronic colitis, parasitisms, and heavy metal poisoning.

Salivation is not as common an observation in poisonings as is diarrhea, but it is produced by the physical stimulation of such plants as yellow bristle grass. Stomatitis of other etiology and choke are characterized by excessive salivation. These conditions must be considered in differential diagnosis.

Colic is a common ailment of the horse. Many predisposing factors and etiologic agents contribute to the production of this syndrome. An accurate history and a careful clinical examination to eliminate other causes are necessary when making a diagnosis of poisoning from the signs of colic alone. Considered with other evidence, however, the presence of colic may be significant.

Signs attributable to a deranged central nervous system include: 1, hyperexcitability, 2, muscular twitching, 3, incoordination, 4, paresis, 5, paralysis, 6, coma, 7, convulsions, 8, abnormal movements, and 9, peculiar positions assumed by the horse.

Hyperexcitability is seen in poisoning from *Datura* (Jimson weed) and *Nicotiana* (wild tobacco). However, it also may be noticed in horses with ticks in the ears, rabies, medicament reactions, meningitis, and liver malfunction.

Incoordinated animals may stagger and fall. They may assume peculiar positions such as pressing the head against objects or standing with the legs crossed. These same signs can be produced by injuries, lamenesses, septicemias, encephalitis, and toxemias associated with acute intestinal obstruction.

Partial or complete paralysis is seen in the terminal stages of many plant poisonings. Other conditions causing paralysis include injuries, abscesses, tumors, or hemorrhages of the spinal cord or brain.

Coma is another terminal sign of plant poisonings, but is seen as well in concussion or other injuries to the brain. Coma also results from overdosage of medicines such as tranquilizers and anesthetics.

Convulsions associated with diarrhea are the signs most indicative of poisoning. Convulsions or convulsive-like seizures are seen in many plant poisonings. But they also are seen in encephalitis, acute intestinal obstruction, and strychnine poisoning.

When the liver is affected, its normal function of detoxication is impaired. This allows the build-up of metabolic end products such as ammonia in the blood stream. The effect of liver malfunction on the central nervous system is characterized by a change in personality or temperament of the horse. It may become quite lethargic, and is said to have the "dummy" syndrome.

Occasionally an animal will die quickly with few signs noted. In such a case, caution is advisable in obtaining a history because observations by the owner may be inaccurate and the disease may have been of longer duration than reported. Sudden death also may be caused by circulatory collapse, anaphylaxis, electrocution, concussion, broken neck, and acute gaseous distention of the intestine or stomach.

These are just a few of the signs noted in plant poisonings. They are listed here, along with those of other conditions which must be considered in differential diagnosis, to show that a diagnosis of plant poisoning cannot be made without complete examination of the animal, coupled with a consideration of the history and all associated facts bearing on the case.

Treatment of Plant Poisoning

Since there are few specific treatments for plant poisonings, treatment in general will be discussed first, and specific treatments will be dealt with as related to the individual plant.

The first step in therapy is elimination of the source of the plant. To do this, the hay, grain, and pasture should be checked and changed if poisonous plants are present. There also is the possibility that well-meaning individuals have fed the animals at odd times, or have fed harmful substances such as oleander clippings. The water supply should be checked for sources of other toxic factors. Although plant poisonings are not associated with water consumption, some chemical poisonings may be.

Once the source of the toxic material has been removed from the feed, the next step is to remove the material in the intestinal tract of the affected animal. The general procedure is to give a laxative agent to hasten evacuation of the digestive tract. In general, a 1,000-pound animal should be given 1 to 1½ gallons of mineral oil, or a pound of magnesium sulfate, or 1 to 2 mg. of lentin to stimulate the intestinal tract to remove the material. If the animal has already eliminated excessively, the further administration of purgatives is not advisable.

In association with the attempt to remove ingesta from the intestine, efforts should be made to inactivate the remaining poison. Activated charcoal, Fuller's earth, bentonite, or tannic acid have all been used to adsorb various toxic agents, but these medicaments are not specific antidotes for any one poison. Their administration should be followed with another laxative to be certain that this material is eliminated from the intestine. If it remains, the poisonous substances may dissociate from the adsorbent and be taken into the general circulation of body fluids.

Assuming that the poison is inactivated, and an attempt has been made to remove it, the remaining treatment consists of the administration of detoxicants and symptomatic treatment. Nonspecific detoxicants that may be given intravenously include 100 to 500 ml. of 20% calcium gluconate, 500 to 1000 ml. of 10 to 50% dextrose, or 150 to 500 ml. of 25% sodium thiosulfate solution. These agents are considered to be universal antidotes and not specific for a particular poison. Calcium gluconate and dextrose supply energy and nourishment in addition to their action as detoxicants.

Symptomatic treatment must include sedation for hyperexcitable or convulsive animals. Barbiturates can be used. Tranquilizers, chloral hydrate, and magnesium sulfate combinations also are satisfactory sedatives. In severe diarrhea, it is necessary to maintain water and electrolyte balance. A 1,000-pound horse needs at least 20 liters (5 gallons) of fluid a day to maintain fluid equilibrium. This accounts for urine loss and insensible water loss only. The fluid requirements during heavy sweating or diarrhea may be doubled. Part of the fluid replacement may be given via stomach tube, though some may have to be given intravenously. Additional symptomatic remedies include intestinal emollients or protectants such as kaopectate or bentonite. If there is dyspnea, oxygen may be indicated.

PLANTS CAUSING HEPATIC CIRRHOSIS[5,6]

Three unrelated plants are included in this group because they each produce a similar clinical syndrome and postmortem picture. The poisonous principle is alkaloidal. Though the poisons differ in each species they do have a common pyrolizidine structure and they each produce cirrhosis of the liver.

Amsinckia intermedia (fiddleneck, tarweed, fireweed, buckthorn and yellow burr weed) (Fig. 1). These species and perhaps others of the genus are common in the western part of the United States. It is a common weed of wheat and other grain crops. The seeds are the most toxic part of the plant. Trouble develops when contaminated grain is threshed and screenings are fed to animals. The lesions produced by *Amsinckia* are similar to those produced by the other species and are included in this group, although the poisonous principle has not yet been isolated.

Various species of the genus, *Senecio*, are included as hepatotoxins. This is one of the largest genera known in the plant kingdom. Not all species of *Senecio* are poisonous or contain sufficient concentration of alkaloids to cause trouble. One which has been shown to be toxic is *Senecio jacobaea* (Fig. 2). There are many others that have been incriminated. These plants are known by the names of ragwort, groundsel, and "stinking willie." They are found over most of the west and midwest sections of the United States.

The Crotalaria species are found more commonly in the southeastern area of the United States. Two species known to be toxic are *Crotalaria spectabilis* and *Crotalaria sagittalis*. These plants also are called rattle box, rattle

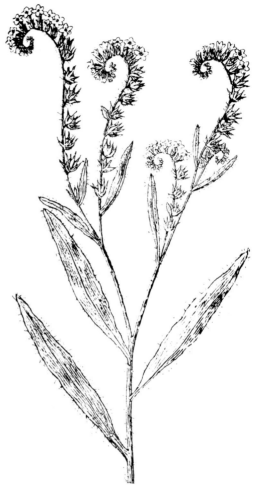

Fig. 1. Fiddleneck (*Amsinckia intermedia*). Photograph from "Weeds of California," W. W. Robbins, Margaret Bellue, and W. S. Ball. Calif. Dept. Agriculture, Sacramento, 1951.

weed, and wild pea. They belong to the pea family.

Poisoning by plants of the genus, *Heliotropium*, is not a problem in the United States; however, in Australia *Heliotropium* produces a clinical syndrome similar to *Senecio* poisoning in Australia.

Hepatic cirrhosis has been known for many years, and occurs world-wide. Only recently has the true poisonous principle been isolated and the plants in question definitely identified. *Senecio* spp. are the cause of Walking Disease described by Van Es in Nebraska. The same plant poisoning is called Winton disease in New Zealand, and it has been called Hard

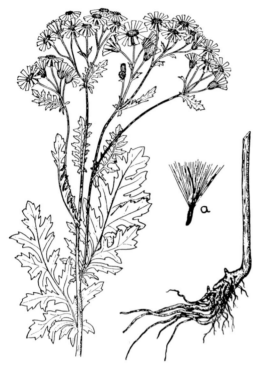

Fig. 2. Tansy ragwart *(Senecio jacobaea).* Photograph from "Livestock-Poisoning Weeds of Oregon," Helen M. Gilkey.

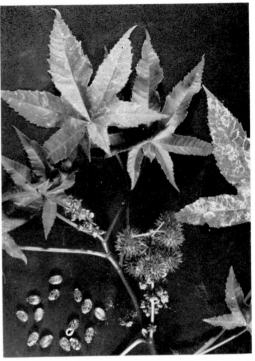

Fig. 3. Castor bean *(Ricinus communis).* Photograph from "Weeds of California," W. W. Robbins, Margaret Bellue, and W. S. Ball, Calif. Dept. Agriculture, Sacramento, 1951.

Liver disease and Walla Walla Walking Disease in the Pacific Northwest. The clinical signs of this condition are referable to the liver damage caused by the hepatotoxin.

The impaired liver function causes a typical disturbance of the central nervous system. Clinical signs include a staggering gait, aimless walking, pressing the head against solid objects such as fences or barns, mania, incoordination, or delirium. The animal may walk in circles, drag the rear legs, or hang the head and act sleepy. In some cases, there is severe intestinal irritation with tenesmus, diarrhea, occasionally a rectal prolapse, and colicky signs. The course of the disease usually is chronic. Once the liver has been sufficiently damaged, the animal loses condition rapidly and death ensues. The temperature usually remains normal.

Postmortem examination reveals a hard, fibrotic liver, usually smaller than normal. There may be generalized icterus, and ascitic fluid in the peritoneal cavity. There may be hemorrhages in the intestinal mucosa, or other evidences of enteritis.

Differential diagnosis must include consideration of all these plants discussed. In addition to plant poisoning other causes for such signs must be considered, such as rabies, meningitis, encephalitis, brain tumors, and abscesses.

Treatment is of little value because of the irreversible liver damage. The only solution to this problem is its prevention by eliminating access to *Amsinckia* screenings or to *Senecio* or *Crotolaria* plants in hay or pasture.

Castor Bean Poisoning[7,8]

The plant, *Ricinus communis* (Fig. 3), is the source of castor oil. It is called castor bean, castor oil plant, and palma christi. It is grown extensively in California and in the southwestern and southeastern states. The poisonous principle is a phytotoxin called ricin, a water soluble substance causing severe irritation to the intestinal tract. *In vitro,* ricin causes erythrocytes to agglutinate. Since this phytotoxin is a protein it is possible to develop a specific antiserum for this poisoning. Unfortunately, the antiserum usually is not available.

The poisonous part of this plant is the seed and the plant itself is relatively nontoxic. In addition to their commercial production, these plants are grown as ornamentals and may be found around corrals or barns where the animal has access to them. Poisoning usually is not a problem, except when new animals are brought into the area, or young inquisitive ones consume the beans inadvertently. All species of animals, including humans, are susceptible to poisoning by the castor bean. However, the horse seems to be the most susceptible. Various reports indicate that as little as 7 Gm. of the seeds have been sufficient to kill a horse. More commonly, it takes approximately 50 Gm. (150 beans) to kill a 1,000-pound horse. In comparison, the sheep is approximately 10 times and the ox about 20 times more resistant.

The syndrome produced by poisoning with castor bean seeds is characterized by signs of extreme irritation to the intestinal tract. There is a typical latent period following ingestion of the seeds, ranging from a few hours to 2 or 3 days. When the signs appear they are acute in onset, and quickly become worse. At first, the animal is rather dull, then becomes a little incoordinated, and finally sweats profusely. There may be tetanic spasms of neck and shoulder muscles. Upon auscultation of the heart, a strong beat is detected which may shake the entire body. A characteristic sign is the profuse, watery diarrhea, usually with no hemorrhage. Colicky pain accompanies the diarrhea and is shown by grinding of the teeth, humping of the back, and kicking at the belly. As the syndrome progresses, there may be convulsions and finally death.

Two of my experimental cases deviated from this classic syndrome. Both horses were given a lethal dose of castor beans, 0.05 Gm. per pound of body weight. Approximately 12 hours later there was a marked rise in body temperature to 107 F. Associated with the fever were general depression, sweating, and slight colic. The pulse rate increased to 140 and a very strong heartbeat could be observed at a distance of 10 feet from the animal. Death occurred within 36 hours. There was little evidence of diarrhea until immediately before death in one animal; the other produced normal feces throughout the course. The lack of intestinal signs is not entirely explainable, but perhaps the dose was so high it killed before they could develop.

OLEANDER POISONING[9]

Nerium oleander (Fig. 4) is grown as an ornamental shrub in the southern part of the United States and throughout California. It is very beautiful, with flowers blooming much of the year. It is popular as a roadside ornament for the freeways of California. Oleander is an extremely toxic plant and has produced poisoning in humans who have used oleander sticks for food skewers. The poisonous principle found in this plant is a glucoside very similar to digitalis, and its effects upon the body are similar.

Cases of oleander poisoning occur when cuttings are placed where horses are used to eating hay, when they are fed lawn clippings containing oleander leaves, or when leaves are baled in hay and fed. A horse rarely will eat the leaves from the shrub. A dosage of 40 to 50 Gm. of green or dried leaves is sufficient to kill a 1,000-pound horse. Green leaves will average slightly less than 1 Gm. each.

Clinical Signs: The following description of an experimental case will provide a good picture of oleander poisoning: A 600-pound gelding was given 25 Gm., or approximately 30 ground oleander leaves by a stomach tube at 7:30 a.m. By 11:00 a.m. there was profuse diarrhea, and abnormalities were noted in the heartbeat. Every fourth beat was skipped and the heart sounds were indistinct. At 12:30 p.m. a systolic heart murmur was audible. In oleander poisoning, there is alternate tachycardia and bradycardia, and beat-skipping which is at first regular, then irregular and imperceptible. Various murmurs occur over the heart area, which cannot be localized because they seem to change periodically and occur with different beats. Heart action is alternately strong and weak, and occasionally the strong beats can be felt over the entire body.

By 3:00 p.m. the diarrhea had stopped and the animal was in lateral recumbency and threshing about. The mucous membranes were slighly cyanotic and the extremities were very cold, which is another characteristic of oleander poisoning. These signs probably are associated with peripheral circulatory collapse.

At 5:00 p.m. the heartbeat was more irregular, peristalsis had stopped and the extremities still were cold. The pupils responded to light, the pulse was weak and thready, but the colt was able to get up unassisted. At 6:30 p.m. the pulse was imperceptible, respirations were very shallow, and the extremities and ears were cold. The animal died by 7:30 p.m.

Death thus occurred within 12 hours after ingestion of the toxic material. The really characteristic sign associated with this poisoning is the extreme variation in the heartbeat and sounds. There usually is diarrhea and some straining in the early stages. Respirations may be increased in rate and depth. Pathognomonic lesions are not observed at postmortem. There may be evidence of gastroenteritis and some ascitic fluid, but these findings are not diagnostic.

There is no specific therapy for oleander poisoning. Supportive treatment, removal of gastrointestinal contents, and good nursing are indicated.

BRACKEN POISONING[11]

Bracken fern, or brake fern, is a plant common to woodland areas over much of the United States. Various species of the genus, *Pteridium* (Fig. 5), are known to cause poisoning in horses and cattle. The syndrome in each species is quite different. In the cow, the syndrome is characterized by hemorrhagic diathesis, whereas in the horse there seems to be a thiamine deficiency and central nervous system disturbances are noted. This poisoning usually is seen in the fall, when animals have been obliged to eat the only material which is still green, because other forage is gone. Horses also may be poisoned by eating bracken which has been cured in hay. An animal must consume this material over an extended period of time, perhaps 30 or even 60 days, before showing signs of poisoning. Signs may develop 2 to 6 weeks after the animal is moved from the pasture containing bracken fern. A horse may acquire a taste for bracken after eating it for some time. The poisonous principle affecting the horse is not definitely known, but is thought to be a thiaminase.

Clinical Signs: The first sign noted is weight loss and then the horse becomes unsteady when walking. This will progress to swaying, incoordination, and staggering, and the animal

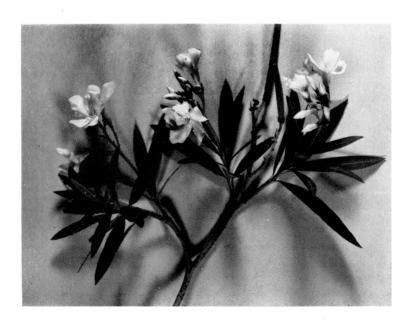

Fig. 4. Oleander *(Nerium oleander)*. Photograph from "Weeds of California," W. W. Robbins, Margaret Bellue, and W. S. Ball, Calif. Dept. Agriculture, Sacramento, 1951.

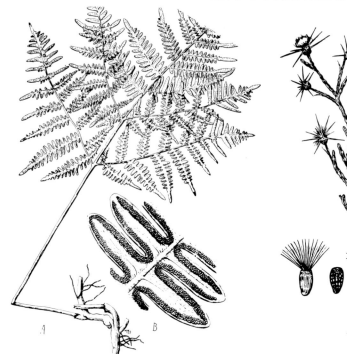

Fig. 5. Bracken fern *(Pteridium aquilinium)*. A—Frond and root. B—Underside of leaf showing spore cases.

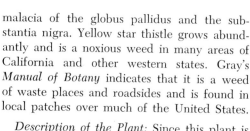

Fig. 6. Yellow star thistle *(Centaurea solstitialis)*.

may fall and be unable to get up. The temperature usually is normal or subnormal. Anemia may be present.

There are no significant postmortem lesions. Another plant, *Equisetum*, commonly called horse-tail or scouring-rush, produces a similar clinical picture which apparently is caused by a thiaminase. This plant may cause poisoning if meadow hay containing large amounts of the plant is harvested and fed to horses.

Treatment: Horses respond to intramuscular or intravenous injections of thiamine hydrochloride at doses of 200 to 1,000 mg.

Nigropallidal Encephalomalacia in Horses[12,13]

This disease commonly is called "chewing disease" or yellow star thistle poisoning. It was reported first in California in 1954 when a specific nervous disease of horses was associated with the ingestion of yellow star thistle, *Centaurea solstitialis* (Fig. 6). The toxic principle has not been isolated from this plant, but experimental feeding of it produces encephalo-

malacia of the globus pallidus and the substantia nigra. Yellow star thistle grows abundantly and is a noxious weed in many areas of California and other western states. Gray's *Manual of Botany* indicates that it is a weed of waste places and roadsides and is found in local patches over much of the United States.

Description of the Plant: Since this plant is not listed in reference texts of poisonous plants, a rather detailed description follows:* The plant is a member of the sunflower family *(Compositae)*. It is an annual. It usually grows to a height of 1 to 2½ feet and has rigid, spreading stems, which are branched from the base; the stems and leaves are more or less whitened with a loose, cottony wool. The basal leaves are 2 to 3 inches long and deeply lobed, appearing somewhat like dandelion leaves. The upper leaves are from ½ to 1 inch long, not lobed, narrow, sharply pointed, and extend down the stem at the base to form wings.

---

*Description by permission—Robbins, W. W., Bellue, Margaret T., and Ball, W. S.: *Weeds of California*. Calif. State Dept. of Agr., Sacramento, 1951, page 443.

The flowering heads are solitary at the end of branches and are about 1 inch long. The bracts of the head are armed with rigid spines from ¼ to 1 inch long. The flowers are bright yellow.

Clinical Signs: Horses must consume star thistle over an extended period of time, perhaps 30 to 60 days, in order for signs to appear. Once they do develop, the mortality is extremely high. A few animals which are affected only slightly will live if given satisfactory nursing care.

Onset is sudden. Frequently the owner will request veterinary assistance to remove a foreign body from the horse's mouth because of

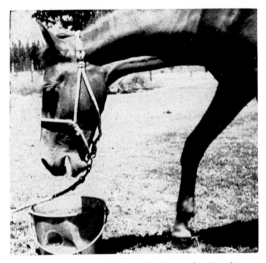

Fig. 7. Yellow star thistle poisoning—showing hypertonicity of facial and labial muscles.

its difficulty in swallowing, its chewing and spitting of food, or difficulty in prehension of food. The horse may push its head into water but be unable to drink. Even though there is paralysis of the muscles associated with prehension and swallowing, there is a hypertonicity of the facial muscles (Fig. 7), and affected animals will have a characteristic "wooden" expression. The muscles around the commissure of the mouth are also hypertonic. The tongue is not completely paralyzed and frequently is moved in and out of the mouth. The animal may go through characteristic chewing movements with no feed in the mouth or with feed in the lower part of the mouth,

but it is unable to push the food back into the molar area.

In the early stages, the horse may stand depressed, yawn frequently, and assume abnormal positions, but there is no apparent change in the gait. Usually the animal will remain at this stage and lose condition because it cannot eat or drink. It will die of starvation if no nursing care is given. Some cases will show an exaggerated central nervous system involvement characterized by pushing against objects, incoordination, falling down, and semiconvulsive seizures. This, however, is not the rule. Most cases exhibit pharyngeal and glossal paralysis and subsequent starvation. Experimental animals have been observed for varying periods of time to see if they might regain use of the swallowing mechanism, but this does not occur. Since the lesions of this disease include malacia of a vital area (Fig. 8), of the brain, the possibility of functional recovery is precluded.

In differential diagnosis, oral foreign bodies and other encephalitic conditions associated with pharyngeal paralysis must be considered.

MECHANICALLY INJURIOUS PLANTS

There are many plants which inflict cuts or puncture wounds when the horse comes in close contact with them. Thistles, cactus, and certain shrubs with thorns will cause mechanical injury. Usually this material is in the hay, when the animals consume it. These awns may work their way into various recesses (Fig. 9) in the commissures of the mouth, alongside the tongue, or between the teeth. They may also lodge in the nasolacrimal or the salivary ducts. If the animal is in an environment where awns are air-borne, they may become lodged in the conjunctival sac or ear, or even in the sheath. One severe case in my experience involved a mare which had foaled in a foxtail pasture and had not passed the placenta. She had some colic associated with after-pains and while rolling about in the pasture had filled the placenta with foxtails, which worked themselves into the vagina and uterus. Many hours were spent attempting to remove all of the awns from the uterus.

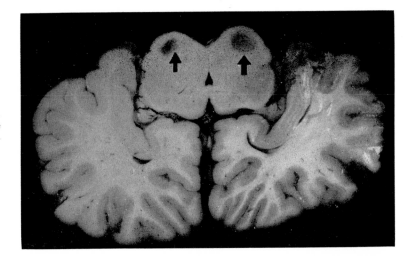

Fig. 8. Yellow star thistle poisoning. Area of encephalomalacia in the substantia nigra of brain.

Control consists of removing the source of the foxtails. If the hay is heavily contaminated with awns, it should be changed. If this is not possible, the owner of the horse must be cautioned to regularly remove the awns from alongside the tongue or wherever they may be lodged. After the awns are removed, the lacerated mucosa heals rapidly.

YELLOW BRISTLE GRASS

Yellow bristle grass (*Setaria glauca, S. lutescens*) (Fig. 10) causes an ulcerative stomatitis in the horse. The small, short, sharp, straight awns imbed themselves in the mucosa of the gums, the tongue, and the lips (Fig. 11), causing irritation and ulcer formation. The

ulcers may be 3 to 4 mm. up to 2 cm. in diameter. If the source of the material is removed they heal rapidly. Occasionally, debridement or cautery is indicated to initiate healing.

POISONING BY LUPINES

This is a large genus of plants. There are many lupines that are nontoxic. It is difficult for even a trained botanist to differentiate between the toxic and the nontoxic species. At certain times of the year, usually in the fall or winter when these plants are in the pod stage, poisonings can occur, particularly with sheep and horses. The poisonous principle is alkaloidal.

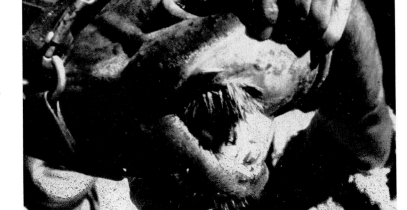

Fig. 9. "Foxtails" under upper lip.

These plants cause gastrointestinal irritation with accompanying diarrhea. The affected horse has a peculiar gait in which it lifts the feet higher than normal. In cases of acute poisoning there may be depression, weakness, prostration, and coma. Chronic lupine poisoning produces a toxic hepatitis syndrome.

There is no treatment that is of value in lupine poisoning.

LOCOWEED POISONING

In certain sections of the West, there are species of the genus, *Astragalus,* which are incriminated in a poisoning of horses called "loco-weed disease." Affected animals have abnormal gaits, wander in circles or in straight lines, act depressed, and may become convulsive and throw themselves to the ground. They may bump against objects or press the head against objects for varying periods of time. It is thought that alkaloids are the toxic

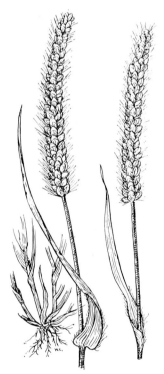

Fig. 10. Yellow bristle grass *(Setaria glauca).* Photograph from "Weeds of California," W. W. Robbins, Margaret Bellue, and W. S. Ball. Calif. Dept. Agriculture, Sacramento, 1951.

principles. Not all species of *Astragalus* are toxic, and it is difficult to distinguish the poisonous from the nonpoisonous.

SELENIUM POISONING

Various *Astragalus* species also are involved in another syndrome, that of selenium poisoning. For many centuries animals have been suspected of being poisoned by selenium-containing plants. The horse has been affected more than other species. Much confusion exists over selenium poisoning, and more study is required on the clinical aspect of this condition. There are certain plants which require selenium for their metabolism and they will cause selenium poisoning if consumed in large amounts. These plants include various species of *Astragalus, Stanleya* or "prince's plume," *Xylorrhiza* or "woody aster," and *Oonopsis* or the "golden weeds." If these plants are growing in a given area, it indicates that the soil is seleniferous. If consumed, they cause signs of acute poisoning. The central nervous system is affected, there are dark, fluid bowel eliminations, and there may be a temperature rise. The animals may die within a few hours to a few days.

Other plants are secondary selenium absorbers. They do not require selenium for their metabolism but if grown on selenium containing soil they will accumulate this material. They produce a chronic type of poisoning. In this category are plants such as common forage plants and common grains as oats, barley, and wheat. The chronic form in the horse sometimes is called alkali disease. It is characterized by the loss of hair and hoofs. These animals lack condition and become emaciated. There may be lameness, the haircoat is rough, and there may be a peculiarity of gait. The hoofs affected develop a crack at the top of the hoofwall resulting in a separation of the old hoof and new growth. Treatment involves removal of the animal from access to the selenium-bearing plants.

HYDROCYANIC ACID POISONING

Two types of plant poisoning which are very important in cattle and sheep are not a

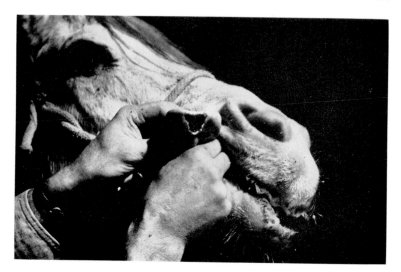

Fig. 11. Stomatitis and glossitis caused by yellow bristle grass.

problem in the horse. These are hydrocyanic acid poisoning and nitrate poisoning. It is possible for the horse to be poisoned with either of these but this occurs rarely.

NICOTINE POISONING

Many plants in the family, *Solanaceae* or potato family, are potentially poisonous. There are 3 alkaloid groups found in plants of this family which cause poisoning. Of these 3, the only one that poisons horses to any extent is the nicotine group. This alkaloid is found in various species of the genus, *Nicotiana*, called the wild tobaccos.

The syndrome seen in wild tobacco poisoning is similar to that due to the effects of nicotine. First, there is stimulation of the ganglia of the autonomic nervous system, followed by paralysis. Most clinical cases will be seen in the paralytic stage if they are seen at all before death. There is no treatment for this poisoning.

There are many plants which potentially are poisonous to the horse, but which give little trouble because horses usually are not placed in an area where these plants are found, or else the horse rarely eats them. These include *Datura*, Oak, Ergot, perhaps *Cicuta* or water hemlock, and *Conium* or poison hemlock, and perhaps many others.

M. E. FOWLER

GENERAL REFERENCES

1. Garner, R. J.: Veterinary Toxicology. Bailliere, Tindall and Cox, London, 1957.

2. Blood, D. C. and Henderson, J. A.: Veterinary Medicine, Williams & Wilkins Co., Baltimore, Md., 1960.

3. Smith, H. A., Jones, T. C.: Veterinary Pathology, Lea and Febiger, Philadelphia, Pa. 2nd ed., 1961.

4. Muenscher, Walter Conrad. Poisonous Plants of the United States, The Macmillan Co., New York, N.Y., 1951.

SPECIFIC REFERENCES

LIVER CIRRHOSIS

5. Van Es, L., Cantwell, L. R., Martin, H. M., and Kramer, J.: Nature and Course of the "Walking Disease" of Northwestern Nebraska. Exp. Sta. Bull. No. 43. University of Nebraska, Lincoln, 1929.

6. McCulloch, E. C.: Hepatic cirrhosis of horses, swine and cattle due to the ingestion of seeds of tarweed, *Amsinckia intermedia*. J.A.V.M.A. 96 (1940) 5-17.

CASTORBEANS

7. McCunn, J.: Castor-bean poisoning in horses. Brit. Vet. J. 103 (1947) 273-278.

8. Clarke, E. G. C.: Poisoning by castor seed. Brit. Vet. J. 103 (1947) 273-278.

OLEANDER

9. Wilson, F. W.: Oleander Poisoning of Livestock. Ariz. Agr. Exp. Sta. Bull., 59, 1909.

BRACKEN POISONING

10. Evans, E. T., Rees, *et al.*: Studies on bracken poisoning in the horse. Brit. Vet. J. 107 (1951) 399-411.

YELLOW STAR THISTLE

11. Cordy, D. R.: Nigropallidal encephalomalacia in horses, associated with ingestion of yellow star thistle. J. Neuropath. and Exper. Neurol. 13 (1956) 330-342.

12. Cordy, D. R.: Nigro-Pallidal Encephalomalacia (Chewing Disease) In Horses on Rations High in Yellow Star Thistle. A.V.M.A. Proceedings, 91 (1954) 149-154.

SETARIA

13. Bankowski, R. A., Wichmann, R. W. and Stuart, E. E.: Stomatitis of cattle and horses due to yellow bristle grass (*Setaria lutescens*). J.A.V.M.A. 129 (1956) 149-152.

SNAKEBITE POISONING

Occurrence: It is estimated that several hundred horses are bitten by poisonous snakes annually in the United States. Mortality estimates range from 10 to 30%. Morbidity is 100% and can be greatly reduced by proper treatment. These estimates are based on a recent Florida survey among practicing veterinarians,[1] the author's and his colleagues' personal experiences with rattlesnake bites, and a current, cross sectional poll of equine practitioners.

Poisonous snakes are found in 48 states. The most dangerous one, because of its size and aggressiveness, is the large rattlesnake of the genus, *Crotalus.* The pit vipers' (rattlesnakes, copperheads, and moccasins) toxin is mainly hemotoxic and proteolytic, causing rapid but weakening heartbeat and extreme local swelling.[2] The coral snake's venom is essentially a neurotoxin. This snake is not considered to be a major source of poisoning in the horse due to its less aggressive nature and limited geographic habitat.

Most bites occur during the first warm days of spring, and they may be expected throughout the summer. Occasionally, a horse is bitten during the winter months if the temperature rises enough to warm the snakes and to make them active. An Arizona practitioner can recall 3 such cases in a 20-year period.[3]

Clinical Signs: Horses are bitten most frequently on the nose and about the head, less frequently on the legs and chest. Nose and head bites are by far the most serious because of the tremendous swelling which rapidly follows a bite. Within a few minutes, the nose becomes edematous, the nasal mucosa swells, and later bloodstained, frothy exudate may hang from each nostril. The eyes are swollen shut and the ears are edematous and directed laterally. A severe dyspnea with stertorous breathing develops and is audible for a great distance. The extreme depression and helplessness make even unbroken horses very amenable to treatment.

Several factors influence the severity of snakebite in the horse. They are the size and particular kind of snake involved, the weight of the victim in relation to the amount of venom deposited, the area of the bite, and the condition of the horse. Face bites, as previously mentioned, are most dangerous. Most untreated horses will not die from snakebites, but the period of morbidity is a major consideration.

Diagnosis: Fractures about the head may be difficult to distinguish from snakebite, especially if occurring during warm weather in known snake-infested areas. Diagnosis of a fracture may not be confirmed for several days until swelling has receded and corroborative evidence such as a bone chip or a loose tooth is noted, or after one has resorted to obtaining radiographs.

Infectious diseases, particularly the strangles —influenza complex, may be confused with snakebite, but the presence of fever and purulent exudates helps in deciding that an infectious process is present.

Allergic or metabolic diseases characterized by edema of the head and legs such as purpura hemorrhagica may confuse diagnosis of snakebite. Diagnosis of purpura may be made on the basis of the edema's involving the legs and ventral abdomen as well as the head, and the presence of widespread mucosal hemorrhages. Bee stings, wasp stings, and bites of other poisonous insects may be difficult to distinguish from snakebite and may differ in degree of tissue reaction only.

Treatment: Treatment must include some of the following remedies depending on the time since the bite and the value of the horse:

Anti-inflammatory Hormones: The most useful drug to reduce morbidity and mortality in the horse is cortisone, its related analogs, and ACTH. This therapy was reported to be effective in cases of snakebite in 1956.[5] This report followed an earlier one concerning its use in humans by Hoback and Green in 1953.[6] With cortisone therapy the signs will subside and become milder; less tissue sloughing and necrosis will occur.

Antibiotics: Penicillin and streptomycin combination or broad spectrum antibiotics definitely are indicated as the bacterial flora in snakes' mouths have been shown to include coliform and enteric organisms.[7]

Antitoxin: Tetanus and gas gangrene organisms have been isolated from snakes' mouths, and therefore antitoxin is indicated.[1]

Antivenin: Specific antivenin therapy includes injections made into the site of the bite and systemically. This therapy is costly and its value greatly diminished in all but very early cases. The risk of an anaphylactic reaction must be recognized as the product is horse serum made by hyperimmunizing horses with a mixture of snake venoms.

Supportive Therapy: Saline and dextrose solutions, blood and blood substitutes, and vitamins to combat shock and dehydration and furnish nutrition are indicated. Epinephrine also is effective in combating shock and circulatory collapse. Calcium gluconate may be useful in reducing hemolysis caused by the action of the venom.

Enzyme Therapy: The parenteral administration of proteolytic enzymes to reduce swelling is indicated.

Surgical: A cruciate incision should be made ¼ inch deep over the fang marks and suction applied if the case is seen within a few minutes after the bite occurs. Tracheotomy may be a lifesaving procedure if severe dyspnea has developed. A local anesthetic will not be necessary to accomplish this.

Physical Measures: A tourniquet (usually rubber tube) is placed above the bite for 20-minute intervals, released for 2 to 3 minutes, and reapplied proximal to the swelling; the whole sequence should not exceed 2 to 3 hours. The indiscriminate use of tourniquets must be avoided. Ice packs and cold water applications will help prevent excessive swelling but their use should not exceed 2 to 3 hours as tissue destruction from freezing is a calculated risk in prolonged cryotherapy. Freezing with ethyl chloride or dry ice is contraindicated.

Antihistamines have been shown experimentally to have deleterious effects on mice[8] and dogs.[1] No work is reported in horses but it is a well-considered opinion that antihistamines should not be used in the horse.

Most veterinarians who have had considerable experience in treating snakebite consider the time involved between the time of the bite and the institution of treatment to be the most important factor in reducing mortality and morbidity. The breed of the horse has a bearing on the severity of the bite reaction. Thoroughbreds, Arabians, and other well-bred horses appear to be more susceptible to snake venom. If possible, the veterinarian should go to the bitten horse rather than having it ridden or brought in by trailer, as the movement and exertion involved lessen the chances for successful treatment.

Prevention: Rattlesnakes can be reduced in number through systematic, annual poisoning of squirrels and other rodents, and by grazing pigs on the pastures and fields where snakes are found.

C. H. Burger

REFERENCES

1. Parrish, Henry M., Scatterday, James E.: A survey of poisonous snakebites among domestic animals in Florida. Vet. Med. 52 (1957) 135.
2. Smith & Jones, Veterinary Pathology, Lee and Febiger, Philadelphia, Pa., 1957, p. 535.
3. Courtright, E. L., Cornville, Arizona: Personal communication.
4. Ahuja, M. L.: Snakebite. Current Therapy. W. B. Saunders Co., Philadelphia, Pa. and London, 1960, p. 719.
5. Burger, Charles H.: Special problems in pet horse practice. Presented to the California State Veterinary Medical Assn. Midwinter Conference (Jan.), 1956.
6. Hoback, W. W., and Green, T. W.: Treatment of snake venom poisoning with cortisone and corticotropin. J.A.M.A. 152 (1953) 236.
7. Parrish, H. M., McLaurin, A., and Tuttle, R. L.: North American Pit Vipers: Bacterial flora of the mouths, and venom glands. Virginia Med. Monthly 83 (1956) 383.
8. Schottler, W. H. A.: Antihistamine, ACTH, cortisone, hydrocortisone and anesthetics in snake bite. Am. J. Trop. Med. 3 (1954) 1083.

CHEMICAL POISONING

Introduction

Mention of the subject of poisoning immediately alerts one to the fact that the veterinarian must be able to recognize and comprehend the ramifications of a vast field of knowledge. An inclusive but simple definition of poisoning involves extension into such areas as animal husbandry, botany, biochemistry, pharmacology, physiology, and veterinary medicine and economics. Perhaps the most useful definition for our purpose is that of Guy (cited by Garner), modified to fit the circumstances.[14] A poison may be defined as any substance which, when applied to the animal body or introduced into it, can harm well-being or destroy life in a nonmechanical manner, irrespective of the temperature.

A poison may be classified according to source, kind of animal affected, the action on the animal, chemical and physical properties, and several other categories such as whether or not it is used as a commercial, industrial, or agricultural poison.[11,41]

As there are many complete and fine references available on the subject and many toxicologists spend most of their time in a small or restricted field of toxicology, no effort will be made here to discuss more than the chemical poisonings of special interest to practicing veterinarians who work mostly with horses. For a more complete treatment of the subject, Liegeois has written one of the better reviews of veterinary toxicology.[26] He has correlated the biochemic, pharamacologic and physiologic aspects of poisonings. Consequently an appreciation of the pathogenesis of toxic principles is obtained. Frear has provided an exceptionally well-written and complete account of the pesticides, including their specific actions, species tolerance, and most other facts concerning many of the newer industrial poisons.[11] Sax has written an exceptionally fine work—*Handbook of Dangerous Materials*—in which most of the important poisonous chemicals are given.[41]

ETIOLOGY OF CHEMICAL POISONINGS

Although malicious poisoning of horses has been reported in the literature and such instances still may occur from time to time, by far the greatest danger to horses arises from carelessness, human error in dosage of drugs, and plain ignorance of the hazards involved in the use of modern industrial and agricultural poisons.[35] Manufacturers are required to label their products and almost all of the presently available pesticides should pose no danger to animals if the labels are read and the directions followed.[50] Pertinent information also is readily accessible in the literature made available by the U. S. Department of Agriculture and state experiment stations.[46] Such publications as the *County Agent-VoAg Teacher* and many veterinary publications likewise contain helpful information.

Such old and well-known inorganic poisons as arsenite, the lead compounds, selenium, phosphorus, and such organic chemicals as phenol have been important animal poisons in the past, and will likely continue to be so. Newer compounds as the organic phosphates and chlorinated hydrocarbons have been developed and even such metals as mercury, lead, and arsenic now are contained in organic compounds of one kind or another.

Some toxic agents are very important in certain regions and are almost unheard of in other areas. Lead and selenium are examples. Arsenite and other forms of arsenic, once nearly discarded as insecticides, are now being used where the chlorinated hydrocarbons and organophosphates are failing because of the development of increased tolerance by insects or other pests. Important feed additives for certain species consist of modified forms of such elements as arsenic. Organic mercurial compounds have had wide use as seed disinfectants.[9] Potent medicinal compounds of antimony, bismuth, chromium, cadmium, silver, mercury, and copper are still in use.

Arsenic, because of its wide distribution and use, is perhaps the most common metallic poison to which horses may be accidentally or intentionally exposed. Other toxic metallic agents of this class are antimony, mercury, and bismuth, all of which have been used and are still used in paints, enamels, medicaments, and disinfectants. Poisoning by all of this group, except arsenic, is now rare in horses. Louw found that arsenic was detectable in the urine within 5 or 6 hours after a dose was given orally, and was eliminated for up to 8 days after a single dose.[27] Repeated doses show a definite cumulative action, and some forms of arsenic are more poisonous than others.[25] Arsenic is injurious to the capillaries, the gastrointestinal tract, the liver, kidneys, blood cells, and central nervous system.

The veterinarian must keep in mind the tendency for owners to feed an excessive amount of trace elements as the halogens, sulfur, and other agents which can act as antimetabolites to one or more other important elements of a balanced, adequate ration. Selenium, copper, iodine, zinc, manganese, fluorine, and perhaps other elements are required for proper nutrition but even a slightly larger amount than that required for good health may be deleterious. Selenium is perhaps the best example of this phenomenon.

Sulfur is required for good health of horses, yet, it is one of the elements that has been used excessively and often has been given in poisonous amounts.[14] It has been observed that horses could be killed by as little as 8 to 14 ounces of sulfur. Many horses have received much more than the lethal dose given here, but sulfur or its compounds such as hydrogen sulfide, sulfur dioxide, and carbon bisulfide are capable of causing dramatic clinical signs which can quickly cause the death of certain animals.

The chlorinated parasiticides such as DDT and BHC have had a wide range of usefulness. As horses are not considered to be food or dairy animals in this country, such compounds still may be used in parasite control programs. Though generally quite safe when used as recommended, all of the chlorinated hydrocarbon group except methoxychlor have a very wide range of toxicity for any given species.[11,14]

Relatively insoluble in water and readily soluble in fat solvents, chlorinated compounds have a moderately acute oral toxicity, and may be hazardous even in very low concentrations ingested over a period of time. All except methoxychlor are stored to some extent in the fat, and most of them are partially eliminated in the milk. Such compounds may constitute a dangerous hazard for the nursing foal. Horses vary considerably in individual sensitivity to DDT and BHC (and its isomers) so that no reliable minimum lethal dose can be set. Young animals are more likely to be hypersensitive to all of the chlorinated compounds than are mature horses in good health. The greatly increased sensitivity of emaciated, nursing ewes

that has been described probably applies also to mares, as well as to any other species.[38,44,50]

The tendency for parasites to develop resistance to DDT and BHC indicates a need for a different parasiticide rather than dangerously increasing the dosage of these agents above the usual recommendations.

The organophosphates are a relatively new group of pesticides. They range in toxicity from being so dangerous for mammals that they cannot be used at all, to such relatively safe varieties as malathion which virtually is nontoxic for horses as used under practical conditions. Jackson and others have shown that some of the organophosphates are more toxic than others.[20,44] Wills, Khan, and others have worked toward development of effective antidotes for such insecticides in horses, as well as for man and other animals.[14,48] Horses may show different clinical signs of organophosphate poisoning than those shown by cattle or other animals. Colic and general muscular weakness are the outstanding signs of this intoxication in the horse.[20]

Another hazard which is not generally appreciated, even by veterinarians, is the practice of using a nontoxic herbicide on poisonous plants and then allowing animals to have immediate access to the treated vegetation. In such cases, livestock owners are inclined to erroneously indict the herbicide. A veterinarian cannot afford to recommend leaving animals in a field or pasture where herbicides, insecticides, or fertilizers have been recently dispersed.

Pesticides which leave residues have strict recommendations as to where, when, and how they may be applied.[46] In some instances, such compounds may not be approved for use at all if meat-producing animals, dairy cows, or crops for human food are involved.[49,50] Horses might be victims of either careless disregard or of calculated risks with such potent agents.

CLINICAL SIGNS OF CHEMICAL POISONINGS

Although the chemical intoxications do not always cause a typical or characteristic syndrome in horses and ponies, nevertheless there generally are some definite signs which the experienced clinician will recognize. As the sick animals reflect one or more of the pharmacologic or pathologic actions of the poison, such can be recognized as being narcotic, corrosive, irritating, or hyperexciting.

If anoxia, for example, is the outstanding consequence of a poisoning syndrome, one must consider the possibility of nitrite, chlorate, prussic acid, carbon monoxide, or perhaps hydrogen sulfide poisoning, provided one can rule out severe anemia due to a hemolytic infection. Even though they will not be discussed here, one also must keep in mind such powerful depressants as chloral hydrate, magnesium, and alcohol, and such alkaloids as conine, because the anoxia might be caused by paralysis of the respiratory centers rather than being due to a direct effect on the oxygen-carrying ability of the blood.

A sharp division between the clinical signs caused by inorganic and organic chemicals is not easily made. Either group may cause an animal to exhibit signs referable to disturbance of the nervous system or show evidence of irritation of the gastrointestinal tract. Very often, a variety of signs is seen because the toxic agent has a general action which affects a number of systems at the same time.

Many poisons, both organic and inorganic, may severely damage the local tissues as well as cause a general effect. Strong alkalies and acids, some of the synthetic chemicals, and organic principles such as blister beetles (cantharidin), and snake or insect venoms are examples of powerful poisons which produce severe and often characteristic local lesions, as well as generalized effects.[5]

Many other harmful agents may damage important organs, such as the liver, and of importance here are such chemical principles as the chlorinated hydrocarbons, phosphorus, fluorides, and the heavy metals. One also may see either photosensitization or cachexia which may indicate that an intoxication is present as a consequence of liver damage.

An increasingly important phenomenon that is difficult for the veterinarian to handle under field conditions is known as the "interference" syndrome.[11] In this instance, no spectacular clinical signs are seen. Few, if any, horses die due to "interference" but the general health of an affected animal is not as good as it should be. Mares may not breed well, or they may lose their foals prematurely. Others deliver dead or weak foals. Young animals do not gain and grow normally, and there may be evidence of one or more nutritional deficiencies, especially in young horses just starting their training. Several of the infectious diseases must be considered or their presence ruled out before a diagnosis can be made.

During the "interference" syndrome, a horse suffering from what appears to be rickets, a vitamin A deficiency, or a hidden parasitism undoubtedly reflects the results of interference with enzyme activity which is vital to normal health and well-being. Such biochemic lesions, not revealed by the usual diagnostic procedures, must be interpreted in the light of the particular metabolic disturbance that is caused. Again, the finer points of the science of enzyme biochemistry are far beyond the scope of this discussion but some of the therapeutic measures for poisonings are very specific. Use is made of agents or principles which are efficacious because they are aimed directly at processes which would otherwise be irreversible. Some of the well-known and formerly difficult-to-treat poisonings, such as lead and arsenic, have yielded to such new biochemic methods of treatment.[5,19,20,26]

Some of the chronic, low grade toxicities still are poorly understood and are difficult to recognize and correct. For example, it may be difficult to determine when certain signs are due to malnutrition or intoxication. Anyone who has treated the chronic poisonings caused by certain plant principles, arsenic, lead, chlorinated hydrocarbons, or nitrites will readily appreciate the fact that these poisonous agents impair the function of the liver and other parenchymatous organs. Many of the signs of nutritional deficiency seen in affected animals are due to inability to properly utilize nutrients rather than to the lack of such in the ration, as often the owner practices what is considered to be excellent management.

If certain harmful agents are absorbed faster than the body can eliminate them, they are regarded as cumulative in nature. It often will require about as much time to correct such a poisoning as it took for the trouble to develop. This is very true of chronic nitrite syndromes.[6]

The veterinarian must realize that brood-mares and colts entering their first winter are likely to be more seriously affected by most chemical poisons than are fully mature horses in good health which are kept under usual maintenance programs. The one exception might be the aged animal, especially when the newer pesticide poisons are involved. Experience with other kinds of livestock supports this observation.[38]

Diagnosis of Chemical Poisonings

Diagnosis of chemical poisoning will depend upon the veterinarian's ability to evaluate the history, signs, and the environmental situation which exists. He should recognize or consider the things which tend to rule out infectious diseases. Certain poisonous plants, acute tympanites, rabies, electric shock from any source, massive prepatent parasitism, and other agents may cause a similar if not identical, syndrome to that caused by acute arsenic or acute insecticide poisonings.[5,6,7,11,15]

The history may be the most important thing to consider when one suspects chemical poisoning. There are no general signs which are characteristic of poisoning alone, but in most instances there is evidence which should serve as a guide for initial diagnostic procedures.[14] There may be 50 or more causes of gastroenteritis, however, which would be reflected as colic in the horse. There may be a score or more causes for convulsions or other signs of nervous system involvement. Often there is difficulty in distinguishing between muscular incoordination due to ingestion of a chemical poison and such conditions as rabies or nightshade poisoning. Anoxia may cause dyspnea as well as mental disturbances which vary from mania to coma. Anoxia, in turn, may be caused by such diverse agents as CO, SO_2, N_2S, NO_2, chlorate, both parasympathomimetic and sympathomimetic drugs, and many other materials.[8,41]

The diagnosis of poisoning often requires definite identification of one or more specific chemical compounds by analytical procedures. These can range from simple technics to very complex procedures.[47]

Treatment of Poisoning

Treatment includes both nonspecific and supportive measures as well as administration of the specific antidote, if such is available. Measures should be taken to remove or inactivate the poison and prevent additional absorption. If skin exposure due to spraying or dipping is a factor, the poison often can be removed by a thorough soap and water washing, though this is more practical with the smaller animals.

Severely and acutely poisoned animals generally do not recover regardless of the treatment used. Woodward, Law, Frear, and many others have given vivid descriptions of what happens when animals are either accidentally or intentionally poisoned.[11,25,49] Even though a specific and direct antidote is available and used, our experience indicates that animals which have received more than approximately 10 L.D.$_{50}$ amounts of a poisonous material do not recover, although there may be a temporary response to treatment. This has been observed by others.[14,25,38]

Chronically poisoned horses may respond to specific antidote therapy, especially when such poisons as arsenic and lead are the causative agents.[14,19] If vital organs, such as the liver, have been extensively damaged, however, the horse will not respond to treatment.

Sax and many others have shown that there is so much individual variation in tolerance within a species that any harmful agent may show a great range of toxicity between the minimum, maximum, and average lethal doses.[22,41] This is true of horses as well as of other species. Such variation makes it very difficult to offer specific guides pertaining to antidote dosages which will be effective for any given poisonous agent.

The "universal antidote" is useful as a first-aid measure for the poisons which act prin-

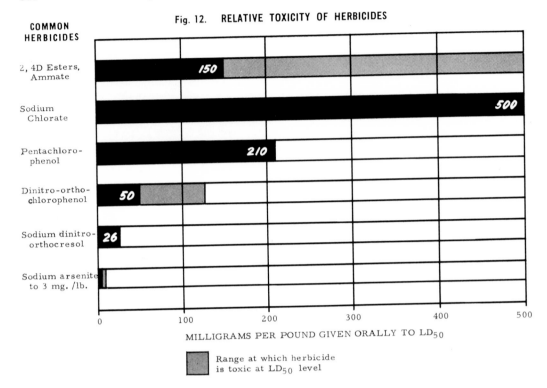

Fig. 12. RELATIVE TOXICITY OF HERBICIDES

cipally on the gastrointestinal tract. Its formula is: activated charcoal—50 parts

 light magnesium oxide—25 parts

 kaolin—25 parts

 tannic acid—25 parts

Usually, this antidote is given repeatedly (3 to 5 times) in enough tepid water to enable the use of a stomach tube. If gastric lavage is indicated, the "universal antidote" can be given and then promptly removed. The procedure can be repeated several times, if necessary.

 Supportive treatments include the use of fluids, electrolytes, calcium gluconate (almost always indicated in poisoning), the B-vitamins, stimulants or sedatives, and any agent that might help the animal survive until detoxication, elimination of the poison, and recovery can occur. Such treatment, including nursing care, may prove to be more important than antidote administration, but if a specific antidote is available its use is indicated.

 The antidotes for certain poisons, as arsenic, may not be as easy to use and as practical for horses as they are for man and smaller animals, but Bal has been used successfully in

horses.[3] In less acute arsenical poisoning, supportive treatment and good nursing care may be sufficient if the element is eliminated rapidly after the source is removed.[10,27]

 Arsenic preparations are indicated to counteract such intoxications as chronic selenium poisoning. According to Moxon, arsenic forms a nontoxic complex with selenium.[34] Other workers have successfully used sodium arsenite in drinking water at 5 parts per million.[17] Complex organic arsenicals and arsanilic acid have been used for the same purpose. Bal was discovered to be contraindicated because it increased the toxicity of the selenium for the kidney.[4] There are large areas in the U.S.A. where selenium toxicity is troublesome, but fortunately those areas are not now the same as those with large horse populations. The same can be said for fluorine and molybdenum.

 Most of the factual and specific data concerning chemical poisons, their action, and treatment are presented in the accompanying tables so that as much as possible can be covered in a brief, concise manner (Fig. 12, Tables 1-8).   A. A. CASE

Table 1.—Chlorinated Hydrocarbon Parasiticides

Name	Common Use	LD$_{50}$ Oral	Comments and First-Aid Measures
DDT and Chlordane	Sprays Dusts Dips	Acute—250 mg./kg.[38]	Poisoning in horses is rare if properly used. Dangerous in very low concentrations if a contaminant of feed or water. Most susceptible are very young, very old, and debilitated, gestating mares, and malnourished horses. Use calcium gluconate and supporting agents as necessary. DDT is secreted in the milk in large amounts.
BHC and Lindane	Dusts Dips Sprays	Acute—250 mg./kg. Chronic—low. Is cumulative. Very dangerous in milk.	BHC is unapproved for milking females and all meat animals, as it is eliminated in the milk and stored in the fat. Avoid use on the very young or very old animals, and avoid contamination of feed or water. Control convulsions with chloral-magnesium-barbiturate-type sedatives and use supportive treatment including calcium gluconate.
Heptachlor	Field spray and dust	Acute—90 mg./kg. Chronic—low. Is cumulative.	Most toxic of the BHC group of insecticides and too toxic for use on mammals. Use sedation as for BHC, and the same supportive treatment.
Methoxychlor	Dusts Sprays Dips	Acute—2800 mg./kg. or more. Virtually nontoxic if used as recommended.	Virtually nontoxic for horses under practical conditions. It is the least toxic of the chlorinated insecticides in common use. Approved for dairy establishments. Not eliminated in the milk and virtually noncumulative, yet is effective.
Aldrin Dieldrin Isodrin	Field or seed spray do. do.	Acute—50 to 55 mg./kg. Chronic—low. Acute—12 to 17 mg./kg. Chronic—low and cumulative.	Aldrin, Dieldrin, Isodrin, Endrin and others of this immediate group are too dangerous for use on mammals. Endrin is a dangerous contaminant, under certain circumstances, of other insecticides such as toxaphene if these are stored in "empty" Endrin containers. Used as either open field sprays on the nonfood crops (for man), on field crops, or as seed and seedbed insecticides, this group
Endrin	Field spray	Acute—10 mg./kg. Females Acute—35 mg./kg. Males	may be dangerous contaminants of feed or water supplies. In accidental poisoning, use sedation and liberal amounts of calcium gluconate and supportives as necessary.
Toxaphene (Camphene)	Dips or sprays (ticks)	Acute—60 mg./kg. Chronic—330 mg./kg. was LD$_{100}$ in 30 days for dogs. Horses probably the same.[38]	Toxaphene is one of the most effective agents against ticks and mites and is safe if properly used except for young colts, aged, or debilitated animals. Use with caution and treat symptomatically, with liberal use of calcium gluconate. This liver poison is a dangerous hazard if a contaminant of feed or water supply. Like any of the chlorinated poisons, certain animals of any species may show hypersensitivity to the usual dosage considered safe for mature animals, including horses.[44]

Table 2.—Poisonings Characterized by Gastrointestinal Disorder

Poison	Source	Toxic Level	Other Signs	Diagnosis and Treatment
Arsenic	Insecticides. Herbicides. Rodenticides. Wood preservatives.[3] Medicaments.[25]	Oral, acute—12 to 20 mg./lb.[25] Chronic—1 to 3 Gm. per day for 14 weeks to kill.[10,14]	Possibly, none in acute. Chronic—emaciation, in horses and mules. A marked resistance to post-mortem decomposition often is seen in arsenic poisoning.	Remove the source and give both symptomatic and supportive treatment. BAL has limited use in the horse. Reinsch test confirmed by Marsh test plus a high arsenic content of liver, blood, urine, and kidney tissue.
Lead (The most toxic are more soluble)	Paints. Insecticides. Medicaments.[14] Fallout from smelters.	Oral, acute—5 to 20 Gm./1000 lbs. Chronic—as low as 25 mg./lb., if repeated over a long period.[10]	Dyspnea with roaring. A central nervous disturbance similar to encephalomyelitis or rabies (paralysis of lips). Stiffness of joints. Lead sulfide line on gums. Weakness.[2,19]	Use 2% saline-sugar sol. of Ca-EDTA, intravenously at rate of 60 to 80 drops/minute q.s.1Gm./30 lbs. liveweight, once daily for 3 days, skip 4 days, repeat. Peracute and acute poisoning kill before one can diagnose or treat the condition.[14,19]
Selenium (Alkali disease)	Forage or grain grown on seleniferous soils.[40]	MLD is 1.5 mg./lb. as sodium selenite equivalent. Cumulative.	Loss of hair from mane and tail; softened and abnormal hoof; listlessness and emaciation; lesions in the kidney, liver, heart and spleen.	Remove from exposure; give supportive and symptomatic treatment and sharply improve the quality of the ration (increase the sulfur-bearing proteins). Many severely poisoned animals never recover.[32,35]
Organic Phosphates	Field and orchard insecticides. Miticides.	From less than 1 mg./lb. to 1000 mg./lb. From TEPP to Malathion.	Horses have colic, general muscular weakness, miosis, perspiration and, occasionally, profuse salivation.[20,45]	Atropine to effect and 2-PAM at the rate of 10 mg./lb., i.v., repeating as necessary each 2 hours until the intoxication is controlled.[48]
Phosphorus and Zinc Phosphide	Fireworks. Rodenticides.	1.5 mg./lb. for yellow phosphorus.[14] 10 to 20 mg./lb. for zinc phosphide.[37]	Violent colic, convulsions, garlic odor on breath. With zinc phosphide, the gas phosphine (PH_3) odor upon opening the stomach. Intensive petechial hemorrhages of serosa of bowel.[37]	Symptomatic and supportive; use of mucilaginous liquids; universal antidote. Treatment is not very effective.[37]
Phenol (Creosote)	Wood preservatives.	Acute—30 Gm. is lethal. Chronic—as little as 0.1 mg./lb. as a persistent contact irritant.[16,29,39]	Acute—depression, ataxia, convulsions, paralysis, and terminal muscular tremors. Chronic—contact burns, and slower changes with encephalitis.	Remove from exposure and give both symptomatic and supportive treatment. Treat the burns according to methods useful for any chemical burn.[16,39]

Table 3.—Poisonings Characterized by Nervous Manifestations

AGENT	SOURCE	TOXIC LEVEL	CHIEF SIGNS	DIAGNOSIS AND SPECIFIC TREATMENT
Chlorinated Hydrocarbons	Insecticides (dips, sprays) Field and tree pesticides	Variable and may be acute or chronic. From 10 mg./lb. to 2800 mg./lb.	Convulsions and colic, intermittent in type.	History of exposure. Sedate to effect. Symptomatic and supportive therapy. Chloral hydrate-magnesium sulfate or barbiturates to control the C.N.S. disturbance.[14,21,38]
Fluoroacetate[12] (1080)	Rodenticides	5 mg./lb. kills in a few hours.	Intermittent convulsions, colic, possibly diarrhea.	History of rodent eradication campaigns, plus a typical and rapid course. There is no effective antidote for horses.
Lead[2,14,25]	Paints	As low as 25 mg./lb. if constant intake of lead.	Convulsions. Recurrent laryngeal nerve paralysis (roaring).	Use Ca-EDTA and supportive treatment. Diagnosis by demonstration of lead in toxic amounts by analysis of blood, liver, kidney, urine; Hammond test.[49]
Organic Phosphates	Pesticides	From less than 1 mg./lb. to more than 1000 mg./lb.	Terminal-type convulsions.	Atropine and 2-PAM to effect. Diagnosis depends on history of exposure plus the severe colic and signs of parasympathetic stimulation.
Strychnine	Pesticides	1 to 2 mg./lb.	Typical convulsions.	History of exposure plus easily-induced convulsion. Control convulsions with chloral.[21]
Thallium	Rodenticides Insecticides	14 mg./lb.[14]	Tremors, dysphagia, depression, paralysis.	History of exposure. Intense hemorrhagic gastroenteritis, hepatitis, nephritis, and hyperemia of brain. Hammond test on urine. Only antidote of promise is diphenylthio-carbazone at 35 mg./lb. t.i.d. Not very practical for horses.
Antu[13]	Rodenticides	26 mg./kg. or 14 mg./lb. to kill in 8 hours at first dose.	Severe depression, death without convulsion.	No effective antidote, but sublethal and repeated exposure results in development of a tolerance which exceeds 4 times the initial lethal dose.

Table 4.—Poisoning Syndromes Associated with Sudden Collapse and Death

Toxic Agent	Source	Comments
Insect Venom	Wasps Bees Ants	Venom of bees contains complex neurotoxins and some contain formic acid. Generally, stings result in a local wound, cellulitis, and local reaction. If a swarm attacks a horse, then a rapid and fatal generalized reaction, collapse and death occur much as in man. Use adrenalin or equivalent agents as early as possible. Supportive and symptomatic treatment is indicated.[5,43]
Antibiotics and Other Injectable Medicaments	Commonly used therapeutic agents	Adrenalin hydrochloride or equivalent as early as possible after the emergency is recognized. Supportive and symptomatic treatment as indicated.[21]
Enzyme Inhibitors Anticholinesterases Antivitamins and Antihormones Producers of Carboxyhemoglobin and Methemoglobin	Drugs Bacterial toxins CO, CN (cyanogen), and many others	As with toxic gases, provide supportive therapy to keep animal alive until natural metabolism and elimination of poisonous principle occur. Nitrite, nitrobenzene, and chloroform poisoning may show mainly dyspnea, collapse, coma, and death unless immediate corrective action is taken. For curare and organophosphates keep the animal breathing, and use the specific antagonist. Cyanide poisoning, regardless of the source, requires immediate and specific treatment to effect. Almost all of this class of poisons are characterized by rapid detoxication and elimination, if the animal can be kept alive a few hours to a day. Antitoxins, if such are available, are specific and curative.

Table 5.—Classification of Poisons According to Toxicity
(likely single lethal dose when given orally)

Present Classification*	Milligrams Per Pound Basis	Common Equivalents for a 1,000-Pound Horse
6. Supertoxic	2.5 mg. or less	2500 mg. or about 1/14 ounce, or less
5. Extremely Toxic	2.5 mg. to 25 mg.	from 1/14 ounce to about 5/6 ounce
4. Very Toxic	25 mg. to 250 mg.	from 5/6 ounce to about 8 1/3 ounces
3. Moderately Toxic	250 mg. to 2500 mg.	from 8 ounces (½ pound) to about 5.5 pounds
2. Slightly Toxic	2.5 Gm. to 7.5 Gm.	from 5.5 pounds to 16.5 pounds
1. Practically Nontoxic	more than 7.5 Gm.	from 16½ pounds upward

The U.S.D.A. Classification for Pesticides and Other Agricultural Chemicals:
1. Highly toxic: To be labeled with a skull and crossbones, red lettering, and antidote given.
2. Toxic: Toxic, but not more than about one-tenth of the toxicity of 1; to carry warning, but not the skull and crossbones, nor the red lettered "POISON" of highly toxic.
3. Possibly hazardous: Labels must bear cautionary warnings only.
4. Substances considered free of dangerous properties. No special label information.

*Modified from data given by Gleason *et al.*, in *Clinical Toxicology of Commercial Compounds.*

There are various other classifications which are based on one kind of information or other but the veterinarian can fit most drugs and other compounds into this scheme. For instance, phenothiazine fits nearer to Class 4, than it does the moderately toxic group. Many veterinarians now know this fact, but when it first was sold commercially, phenothiazine was given a U.S.D.A. Class 3 instead of the more appropriate U.S.D.A. Class 2. To add to the confusion, Hodge and Sterner had used the opposite numerical system in 1943, by which they assigned Class 1 as supertoxic. When working with such potent drugs as anthelmintics, one would best use the mg./lb. or mg./kg. per liveweight basis.

Table 6.—Toxic Gases

Gas	Source	Toxic Concentration	Maximum Permissible Concentration	First-Aid Measures
CO	Motor fumes Fuel gas Manure pits	0.02 ppm. in 2 hours	100 ppm. a few minutes	Move to open air away from exposure. Sedate. Oxygen if indicated.
H_2S	Manure pits (liquid)	20 ppm. to start toxicity	20 ppm. is also MPC	Remove from exposure; fresh air, oxygen.
NO_2	Silo gas (upright)	10 ppm. if continuous 20 ppm. if 8 hours	10 ppm. is also MPC	Remove to open air, treat to avoid pulmonary edema. Oxygen.
NH_3	Fertilizer tanks Refrigerant	300 ppm. to poison	100 ppm. or less	Remove from exposure, provide symptomatic treatment. Ammonia can be a dangerous hazard in leakage from tanks near stables.
SO_2	Fumigant Refrigerant	3 to 20 ppm. affect eyes 20 to 50 ppm. will severely poison	10 ppm. MPC if a constant exposure 50 ppm. for 1 hour, 100 ppm. for 30 minutes	Remove from exposure; fresh air, protect the eyes. A dangerous respiratory irritant.
CS_2	Fumigant Solvent	70 ppm. to poison	15 to 20 ppm. MPC	Remove from exposure. Symptomatic and supportive treatment. Carbon disulphide is an extremely dangerous fire hazard.
HCN	Fumigant Accidents	20 ppm. a few hours	10 ppm. as CN. (very poisonous)	Remove to fresh air; can use specific antidotes as in cattle.
OZONE	High frequency generators	4 to 5 ppm. is toxic	0.1 to 1.0 ppm. is MPC	Remove from exposure, control pulmonary edema and bronchial obstruction.

Table 7.—Names, Sources, and Administration of Special Antidotes

POISONING	GENERIC NAME OF ANTIDOTE	COMMON NAME OF ANTIDOTE	DOSAGE AND ADMINISTRATION
Arsenic Antimony Mercury	2,3-Dimercapto-propanol	BAL or British anti-lewisite. (Nynson, Wescott, & Dunning Lab.)	1st day: 2.5 mg./kg., divide into 4 doses, im. 2nd day: 2.5 mg./kg., divide into 4 doses, im. 3rd day: 1.2 mg./kg., divide into 2 doses, im. 4th day: 1.2 mg./kg. im.
Lead	Disodium calcium ethylenediamine-tetraacetate	NaCa EDTA (Riker Labs.) CaNa EDTA (Jen-Sal) Havidote (Haver-Lockhart)	Dilute Riker's to 2% saline solution and give iv. at the rate of 60 to 80 drops/minute q.s. to dose of 1 Gm./30 pounds liveweight. Havidote is given iv., 50 ml./100 pounds liveweight, divided in 3 or 4 doses per day, for 2 or 3 days at a time.
Organo-Phosphate Insecticides	2-Pyridine-aldoxime methioide	2-PAM (Calif. Found. for Biochem. Res.)	2-PAM is given iv. at rate of 10 mg./lb., and repeated in 2 or 3 hours, if necessary. Also use atropine, iv. or subcut. at ¼ to ½ grain, to desired effect . . . may need more than usual dose.[38]
HCN or Prussic Acid	Trypan blue, dextrose, and sodium thiosulphate (As above)	Thiodex (Ft. Dodge) 2-PAM	100 to 200 ml., iv., or to effect; can be repeated if necessary. Can combine with 2-PAM.
Insect stings and Drug Shock Emergencies	Calcium gluconate or calcium lactate with dextrose and magnesium. Epinephrine HCl. Amphetamine sulfate, 5%.		Calcium gluconate with dextrose and magnesium 20% solutions given slowly, iv., to effect, usually 150 to 250 ml. Watch heart action. Can be given ip., sc., or im. Epinephrine injectable 1/1000, (Ft. Dodge) is given sc., 4 to 8 ml. Similar agents are given in a similar way.[5]

Table 8.—Toxicity of Rodenticides

Agent	Oral Dose Range for Acute Response	Action	Antidote
Antu[13]	12 to 36 mg./lb.	Pulmonary edema	None
Castrix[50]	12, or less, mg./lb.	Convulsant	Sedate to effect. Chloral-magnesium
1080[12]	0.22 to 0.75 mg./lb.	Convulsant and cardiac poison	None
Pival[50] and Warfarin	36 to 45 mg./lb., single 1 mg./lb., or less, repeated	Vascular shock and anticoagulant	Whole blood and vitamin K
Arsenic[14,25]	1 to 3 mg./lb.	Parenchymatous poison	BAL, plus symptomatic treatment
Barium Chloride[14,25]	50 to 100 mg./lb.	Parenchymatous poison	Symptomatic
Thallium[14]	27 mg./lb. to kill	Parenchymatous poison	None
Phosphorus[14]	0.5 to 2 mg./lb.	Parenchymatous poison	None
Zinc Phosphide[14]	9 to 18 mg./lb.	Pulmonary edema	None
Strychnine[21,25]	0.2 to 0.3 mg./lb.	Convulsant	Sedative to effect. Chloral-magnesium or barbiturate.

REFERENCES

1. Albert, Adrien: Selective Toxicity. 2nd ed. Broadwater Press, Ltd., Welwyn Garden City, England, 1960.
2. Allcroft, Ruth: Lethal doses of lead compared for horse, pig, and cattle. Vet. Rec. 63 (1951) 583.
3. Anon: Arsenical Poisoning. From Tifton Lab Notes, Ga. Vet. (Sept. 1953).
4. Belogorsky, J. B., and Slaughter, D.: Proc. Soc. Exper. Biol. of New York. 72 (1949) 196.
5. Buckley, Eleanor E., and Porges, Nandor.: Venoms. 467 pages. Publ. No. 44, A.A.A.S., Washington, D. C., 1956.
6. Case, A. A.: Poisons and antidotes. Ga. Vet. (Sept. 1960).
7. Case, A. A.: Toxicological Techniques for the Diagnostic Laboratory. The 63rd Ann. Proc. U. S. Livestock Sanitary Assn. (Dec. 1959). 389-393.
8. Daughtery, R. W., Wrong, R., and Christensen, B. E.: Studies in hydrogen sulphide poisoning. Am. J. Vet. Research 15 (1943) 254-256.
9. Edwards, C. M.: Mercury poisoning in a horse as result of eating treated oats. Vet. Rec. 54 (1) (1952) 5.
10. Fenestermacher, R., Pomeroy, B. S., Roepke, M. H., and Boyd: Lead poisoning, J.A.V.M.A. 108 (1946) 1.
11. Frear, D. E. H.: Chemistry of the Pesticides. 3rd ed. 469 pages. D. Van Nostrand Co., New York, N. Y. 1955.
12. Frick, E. J., and Boebel, F. W.: 1080 poisoning in horses. Vet. Med. 41 (6) (1946) 196.
13. Frick, E. J., and Fortenberry, J. D., Jr.: ANTU poisoning in horses. Vet. Med. 43 (3) (1948) 107-108.
14. Garner, R. J.: Veterinary Toxicology, Bailliere, Tindall & Cox, London. (Williams and Wilkins Co., Baltimore, Md. for U.S.) 1957.
15. Gleason, M. N., Gosselin, R. E., and Hodge, H. C.: Clinical Toxicology, Williams and Wilkins Co., Baltimore, Md., 1957.
16. Hammond, Paul B.: Creosote poisoning in the horse. Mod. Vet. Prac. Reference & Data Library, D-4-1.
17. Hendrick, C., Klug, H. L., and Olson, O. E.: Organic arsenicals in selenosis. J. Nutr. 51 (1953) 131.
18. Hodge, H. C., and Sterner, J. H.: Toxicity classes. Amer. Industrial Hygiene Assn. Quart. 10.4 (1943) 93.
19. Holm, L. W., Rhode, E. A., Wheat, J. D., and Firch, G.: The treatment of chronic lead poisoning in horses with calcium disodium ethylenediaminetetraacetate. J.A.V.M.A. 123 (1953) 383-388.
20. Jackson, J. B., Drummond, R. O., Buck, W. B., and Hunt, L. M.: Toxicity of organic phosphorous insecticides to horses. J. Eco. Entomol. 53 (4) (1960) 602-603.
21. Jones, L. Meyer.: Veterinary Pharmacology and Therapeutics, 2nd ed., The Iowa State College Press, Ames, Iowa, 944 pages, 1957.
22. Kerr, S. H., and Bragdon, J. E.: Relative toxicity to mammals of 40 pesticides. Agric. Chemicals. 135 (Sept. 1959) 44-45.
23. Kingry, S. H.: Coal-oil poisoning in the horse. Am. Vet. Ref.: (Apr. 1890) 14-16.

24. Knight, S. H., and Beath, O. A.: Selenium Poisoning. Bull. 221, Wyo. Exper. Sta. 1937.
25. Law, James: Textbook of Veterinary Medicine, Vol. II, 2nd ed., pp. 273-274. Published by the author at Ithaca, N. Y., 1905.
26. Liegeois, F.: Some modern aspects of veterinary toxicology. Rev. de Méd. Vét. 111 (1960) 594-620. English translation in Mod. Vet. Prac. Reference & Data Library, E5-85, 1961.
27. Louw, P. G. J.: The urinary excretion of arsenic in the horse. J. So. Afric. Vet. Med. Assn. 23 (1952) 107-109.
28. McNellis, Russel: Rattlesnake bite. J.A.V.M.A. 114 (864) (1949) 145-146.
29. Miller, Frank, and Beolin, V. S.: Creolin poisoning in horses. Am. Vet. Rev. 20 (1896) 218-220.
30. Miller, W. T., and Williams, K. T.: Minimum lethal dose of selenium as sodium selenite, for horses, mules, cattle, and swine. J. Agric. Research. 60 (1940 a) 163-173.
31. Miller, W. T.: Effects of feeding repeated small amounts of selenium as sodium selenite to equines. J. Agric. Research 61 (1940b) 353-368.
32. Moxon, A. L.: Alkali Disease or Selenium Poisoning. Bull. 311, So. Dak. 1937.
33. Moxon, A. L., Schuefer, A. E., Lardy, H. A., DuBois, H. A., and Olson, O. E.: Increasing the rate of excretion of selenium from selenized animals by the administration of p-Bromobenzene. J. Biol. Chem. 132 (1940) 785.
34. Moxon, A. L.: Selenium poisoning. So. Dak. Acad. Sci. Proc. 21 (1941) 34.
35. Nockolds, C.: Paris green poisoning in a horse. Am. Vet. Rev. 20 (1896) 343-345.
36. Parrish, H. M., Scatterday, J. E., and Pollard, C. B.: The clinical management of snake venom poisoning in domestic animals. J.A.V.M.A. 130 (1957) 548-551.
37. Petris, M. A.: Zinc phosphide poisoning in a mule. Vet. Rec. 68 (6) (1956) 414.
38. Radeleff, R. D.: Toxaphene poisoning: symptomology and pathology, Vet. Med. 44 (10) (1949) 436-442.
39. Reid, Charles H.: Sublethal phenol (coal tar creosote) poisoning in two horses. Calif. Vet. 13 (2) (1959) 28.
40. Rosenfeld, Irene, and Beath, O. A.: The influence of protein diets on selenium poisoning. J. Vet. Research 52 (Jan. 1946).
41. Sax, S. Irving, Schultz, W. W., and O'Herin, M. J.: A Handbook of Dangerous Materials. Book Division Reinhold Publishing Co., New York, N. Y. 848 pages. (1951).
42. Stiles, Walter: Trace Elements in Plants and Animals. 2nd ed., Cambridge University Press (New York Branch, for U.S.A), 189 pages. 1951.
43. Stitt, E. R., Clough, P. W., and Clough, M. C.: A Practical Bacteriology, Haemotology, and Animal Parasitology. 9th ed., The Blakiston Co., Philadelphia, Pa., 961 pages (1943).
44. Thorburn, J. A.: The control of ecto-parasites of domestic stock with toxaphene. J. So. Afr. V.M.A. 3:171-180.

45. Tracy, R. L., Woodcock, J. G., and Chodroff, S.: Toxicological aspects of 2, 2-dichlorovinyl dimethyl phosphate (DDVP) in cows, horses and white rats. J. Econ. Ent. **53** (4) (1960) 593-601.

46. U.S.D.A., Ento. Research Div., E. F. Knipling, Director. Insecticide Recommendations of the Entomology Research Div. Agric. Handbook No. 120, ARS-FES, 125-134 (Livestock), 138 pages. Washington, 25, D. C. (1961).

47. Von Oettingen, W. F.: Poisoning. Paul B. Hoeber, Inc. (Harper Bros.), New York, N. Y., 524 pages (1954).

48. Wills, J. H.: The use of 2-PAM in experimental parathion poisoning of horses. Federal Proc. **18** (1959) 1028-(25).

49. Woodward, George T.: The treatment of organic phosphate insecticide poisoning with atropine sulphate and 2-PAM. Vet. Med. **52** (12) (1957) 571-578.

50. World Health Organization: Monograph No. 16, J. M. Barnes, Toxic Hazards to Man, Toxicology of Pesticides to Man and Animals. WHO, Geneva, Switzerland.

SPECIAL REFERENCES ON PHENOTHIAZINE

1. Davey, D. G., and Innes, J. R. M.: The present position of phenothiazine as an anthelmintic. Vet. Bull **12** (1942) R 7-14.

2. Errington, B. J., and Westerfield, C.: Phenothiazine as an anthelmintic for horses and mules. Vet. Med. **35** (12) (1940) 688-693.

3. Errington, B. J.: Phenothiazine as an equine anthelmintic. Vet. Med. **36** (4) (1941) 188-193.

4. Fincher, M. C., and Gibbons, W. J.: Phenothiazine in emaciated horses. Cornell Vet. **31** (2) (June, 1941) 220-223.

5. Hatcher, W. L., Christian, T. T., and Smotherman, W. H.: Phenothiazine poisoning in horses. No. Am. Vet. **22** (3) (1941) 159-160.

6. Robinson, Virgil B., and Kays, John M.: Experiments with phenothiazine in treatment of horses for strongyles. Vet. Med. **36** (11) (1941) 557-559.

7. Schmidt, H., Christian, T. T., and Smotherman, W. M. A.: Is phenothiazine poisonous to horses? J.A.V.M.A. **99** (1941) 225-228.

8. Swales, W. E.: The use of phenothiazine in veterinary parasitology. Canad. J. Comp. Med. **4** (1940) 12.

9. Toynton, Clair: Effects of phenothiazine on equine blood picture. Vet. Med. **36** (9) (1941) 481.

10. Whitlock, J. H.: Toxicity of phenothiazine. No. Am. Vet. **22** (6) (1941) 351-352.

ADDITIONAL REFERENCES—TRACE ELEMENTS

SELENIUM

Beath, O. A.: Delayed action of selenium poisoning of livestock. Science 81/2112 (1935) 617.

Beath, O. A. *et al.*: Certain poisonous plants of Wyoming activated by selenium and their association with respect to soil types. J. Amer. Pharm. Assn., 23 (1934) 94-97.

Davidson, W. B.: Selenium poisoning. Canad. J. Comp. Med. 4 (Jan. 1940) 19-32.

Draize, J. H., and Beath, O. A.: Observations on the pathology of blind staggers and alkali disease. J.A.V.M.A. (June 1935) 753-763.

Dudley, H. C.: Toxicology of Selenium. U.S.P.H. Rep. 53 94-98.

Fairbanks, B. W.: Selenium poisoning. No. Am. Vet. 19/1 (1938) 22-25.

Moxon, A. L.: Alkali disease on selenium poisoning. Bull. 311, So. Dak. Sta. 91 pages (1937).

Moxon, A. L., and Rhian, M.: Selenium poisoning. Physiol. Rev. **234** (1943) 305-337.

Rosenfeld, Irene, and Beath, O. A.: The influence of protein diets on selenium poisoning. Am. J. Vet. Research **52** (1946).

Rosenfeld, I., and Beath, O. A.: The chemical changes in the tissues following selenium administration. Am. J. Vet. Research (Jan. 1946) 57.

Rosenfeld, I., and Beath, O. A.: The influence of various substances on chronic selenium poisoning. J. Pharm. & Exper. Ther. 91/3, 218-223.

Stenn, Fredrick: Alkali disease selenium poisoning. Arch. Path. 22 (1936) 398-412.

Moxon, A. L., and Rhian, Morris: Selenium poisoning. Physiol. Rev. 23 (1943) 305-337.

Durrell, L. W., and Cross, Floyd: Selenium Poisoning in Livestock. Bull. 382-A, Colorado Exper. Sta. June, 1944.

Stiles, Walter: Trace Elements. (189 pps), Cambridge University Press, Cambridge, England, 1951.

ADDITIONAL REFERENCES—ANIMAL VENOMS

Buckley, Eleanor E., and Porges, Nandor: Venoms, Publ. No. 44, A.A.A.S., Washington, D. C. 467 pages (1956).

Crimmins, M. C.: Facts about Texas snakes and their poisons. J.A.V.M.A. (Sept. 1927) 704-712.

Ditmars, R. L.: Snake bite among domestic animals. J.A.V.M.A. 47/4 (1939) 383-388.

Jackson, D., and Harrison, W. T.: Mechanical treatment of snake bite. No. Amer. Vet. 8 (8) (1927) 21-27.

Jackson, D., and Harrison, W. T.: Mechanical treatment of experimental rattlesnake venom poisoning. J.A.V.M.A. 90 (1928) 1928-1929.

MacNamme, J. K.: Physiological, pathological, and toxicological effects of snake bites on domestic animals. Vet. Med. 31/9 (1936) 376-381.

Merrill, E. D.: Snakes and poisonous plants in the tropical jungles. J.A.V.M.A. 102/792 (1943) 230.

McNellis, R.: Rattlesnake bite. J.A.V.M.A. 114/864 (1949) 145-146.

A reported case of death in a horse due to bee sting. Vet. Excerpts 3/5 (1943) 191.

Bee stings in horses. Vet. Bull. 14 (1944) 136.

ELECTRIC SHOCK

Electric shock is defined as the effects produced by the passage of an electric current through any part of the body.[1] Both lightning and man-made electricity are capable of producing electric shock. Although it does not cause a great economic loss to our horse industry, electric shock is a potential threat to the life of each individual animal. The destructive power of electricity usually is attributed to high amperage (rate of flow).[2] Animals can tolerate high voltage (pressure) if the amperage is low. Lightning is electricity with high voltage, estimated at 1,000,000 volts.[3] The electricity supplied to most stables has an amperage of 15 to 30 amperes and a voltage of 110 volts, but when an animal is well-grounded, it can and does kill horses.

Occurrence: In the United States, horses usually suffer lightning strokes during the summer months but they suffer from other forms of electric stroke throughout the year. Lightning travels from a cloud to the ground or from the ground to a cloud. It may strike a horse in an open field but is much more likely to strike him under a lone tree, near an ungrounded wire fence, or in a stable unprotected by lightning rods.

Accidental electrocution in the stable usually occurs as a result of animal contact with an uninsulated wire which is conducting electricity. The horse may rub or chew insulating material from an electric wire and expose the bare metal.

Low-hanging high tension wires and electric fences powered by improperly constructed fence chargers are hazards in pastures and exercise lots.

Pathogenesis: Although the animal's body as a whole is considered to be a poor conductor of electricity, nervous tissue is considered an excellent conductor.[3] This fact accounts for the commonly held opinion that death is caused by neuroparalysis resulting in respiratory and circulatory arrest.

Clinical Signs: Lightning stroke and other forms of electric shock usually are fatal. Affected animals often are found dead in an appropriate environment presenting the appearance of instantaneous death. The last mouthful of grass or hay may still be grasped between the incisor teeth. Most animals that survive electric shock make a complete recovery following a convalescence of several minutes to several months. The signs in these animals vary from a slight hyperexcitability to complete paralysis. Vertigo, nystagmus, impairment of vision, hyperesthesia, and general depression are the most constant manifestations.

Lesions: It may be impossible to find any postmortem changes attributable to electric shock in the cadaver. If the animal is necropsied in the field it will often be found in an attitude suggestive of sudden collapse. Rigor mortis develops rapidly but is of short duration. Burning or singeing of the hair, skin and underlying tissues occasionally is observed. The singeing may appear in an arboreal design or as a narrow line extending the entire length of one or more legs. These lines are indicative of the path of electricity from the animal's body to the ground. The viscera usually is congested and the veins are distended with uncoagulated blood. Extensive hemorrhages and bone fractures may be observed in violent lightning stroke, probably due to extremely high voltage. Negative, rather than positive, findings often are indicative of electric shock.

Diagnosis: A history of a sudden, unexplained death during a violent thunderstorm or access to an exposed wire conducting electricity suggests the possibility of electric shock. If a horse is found dead beneath a tree which shows evidence of lightning strike, or beside a fence which has wires welded to metal posts, such evidence, though circumstantial, is convincing. If several animals are found dead in close proximity to one another, the diagnosis is further justified. Singe marks, when present on the legs, generally are considered to be pathognomonic of lighting stroke.

As most animals are insured against lightning stroke and not against other causes of death, the veterinarian must be cautious in ascribing death to lightning. It is advisable, in most cases, to conduct a complete postmortem examination to rule out other diseases such as anthrax, blackleg, and peracute intoxications.

Treatment: Treatment of survivors consists of good nursing care and stimulants as indicated to maintain body functions.

Prevention: Wires carrying powerful electrical charges should be so located that they are not accessible to horses. Properly grounded lightning rods should be placed on all buildings in which horses are housed. Electric fence chargers should be properly constructed and installed. Home-made chargers are not acceptable.

Wire fences of any type attached to trees, buildings, and wood posts are hazards to livestock during thunderstorms and should be grounded. Metal fence posts may be interspersed between the wood posts at 150-foot intervals, or ¾ to 1 inch metal rods may be driven into the ground beside the wooden posts at similar intervals. These rods should be driven into the ground several feet and project several inches above the wooden post. Each line wire should be firmly attached to the metal rod with a pipe strap.

H. E. AMSTUTZ
R. C. HERSCHLER

REFERENCES

1. Dorland's Illustrated Medical Dictionary, 23rd ed., W. B. Saunders Company, Philadelphia, Pa., and London.
2. Garver, H. L., Lightning Protection for the Farm, Farmer's Bulletin, No. 2136, U. S. Department of Agriculture, 1959.
3. McConnell, W. C., Lightning Stroke, No. Am. Vet., 27 (1946), 220.

HEATSTROKE (HEAT EXHAUSTION)

Heatstroke or heat exhaustion was in previous years a common disease of equines during the summer months. Since mechanization has replaced most of the workhorses and mules, the incidence of heatstroke has decreased considerably.

Etiology: This condition in equines is caused more often by exposure to excessive heat, from overexertion in a hot, humid atmosphere, or from confinement in a hot, poorly ventilated place rather than from direct exposure to the sun. Inadequate water intake is a contributing factor. Horses overworked in hayfields on hot, humid days, when rain is threatening, may be subject to heatstroke. Saddle horses ridden for long distances on hot days may suffer clinical signs due to excessive exposure. Particularly susceptible are horses ill-conditioned to do the required work. Transportation in railway cars and trucks on hot, humid days when ventilation is poor may be a cause. Confinement in a hot, poorly ventilated stable after heavy work has been associated with heatstroke.

Mules seem less susceptible than horses but heatstroke has been fairly common and still occurs to a lesser extent in poorly conditioned mules used for work in tobacco and cotton fields. Occasional cases occur in horses confined in a small paddock without shade and exposed to the sun on days when the temperature approaches 100 F. The cause is due to overheating rather than to the direct effect of the sun's rays.

Clinical Signs: In horses that are ridden or otherwise worked, the initial signs are polypnea, weakness, stumbling, and sometimes refusal to continue working. The signs may not appear until the animal is stabled. Then depression, uneasiness, and refusal to eat are noticed. In all cases, sweating ceases and the skin becomes dry. This usually is an important sign of impending heatstroke. If the animal is forced to work after the initial signs develop, intense dyspnea, convulsions, collapse, and coma frequently occur. These signs may occur occasionally even when work is stopped if the animal is not cooled off. The diagnostic sign is hyperthermia, 106 to 110 F. or higher.

Other manifestations include congested mucosae, accelerated pulse rate, marked dilation of the peripheral vessels, and palpitation of the heart.

The course usually is short. Animals that are cooled and live for a few hours usually recover. Animals with convulsions and delirium die within ½ to 2 hours. During heat waves, the incidence and mortality may be high. Cases with a very high temperature, marked weakness, and delirium should be given an unfavorable prognosis.

In cross-country trials or steeplechase races, heatstroke should be differentiated from acute heart failure in poorly conditioned horses. In stabled horses, uneasiness and refusal to eat may lead the owner to suspect indigestion when the other signs are mild. The diagnostic features of heatstroke are high temperature and dry skin.

Lesions: When death occurs, rigor mortis and putrefraction develop early. The blood fails to clot and the superficial veins are greatly distended. Congestion of the lungs and brain is marked. The liver and kidneys are degenerated.

Treatment: Therapy for heatstroke of horses is aimed to reduce the high temperature by rapid cooling of the body, to adjust the circulatory disturbance, and to control convulsions and delirium. The animal should be placed in the shade and where there is a breeze when possible. If available, electric fans should be used to cool the animal. Its body should be sprayed with cold water. When a water hose is not available ice packs should be placed over the animal. When signs of disorientation are evident an ice pack should be applied to the head. The value of cold water enemas is debatable.

In heatstroke, blood is pooled in the peripheral circulation. The patient's visceral organs become deficient in body fluids (blood) and the intravenous administration of fluids is indicated. The Campbell formula of 10% saline solution has proved to be efficacious in the past. This solution consists of sodium chloride, 4%; sodium carbonate, 5%; potassium chloride, 0.05%; and magnesium chloride, 0.05%. The initial dose of 1,000 to 1,500 ml. is administered intravenously. Horses that will not eat are given a second intravenous injection after 1 hour, and a third injection 2 hours later. Within 15 minutes after treatment, most animals will drink large quantities of water. Their feet should be packed in ice to prevent laminitis.

When the Campbell formula is not available 3,000 to 4,000 ml. of physiologic saline solution containing 5% dextrose is useful. Another preparation which has proved beneficial is physiologic saline solution containing 10% calcium gluconate and 5% dextrose. This solution is administered in doses of 500 to 1,000 ml.

intravenously. Circulatory stimulants such as caffeine with sodium benzoate, 5 to 10 ml. (3.75 grains per ml.) depending on size, are administered subcutaneously or intravenously.

Horses that have recovered from heatstroke require gradual conditioning for work and frequently are unable to perform heavy work during the remainder of the hot weather season. Once affected, equines seem to be more susceptible to heat during the rest of the summer.

W. J. Gibbons

CHAPTER 21

NEOPLASTIC DISEASES

INTRODUCTION

A neoplasm is a growth of cells which serve no useful function, have no orderly structural arrangement and proliferate continuously without regard for the needs and demands of the body. Ordinarily, neoplastic cells bear some resemblance to the cells from which they arise.

CARCINOGENESIS

A number of theories about the origin of neoplasms have been advanced but none appear to be the complete answer. Heritable characteristics, viruses, chronic irritation, chemicals, bacteria, irradiation, hormones, and disorders of embryonal development have all been incriminated. It is a reasonable assumption that a majority of neoplasms arise in cells whose development is somehow distorted, and that all neoplasms depend upon some stimulus that produces a change from normal to uncontrolled cellular reproduction. A pre-existing susceptibility also is probably a prerequisite to the development of neoplasia. Since this susceptibility appears to be characteristic of species or of strains within a species, it can be presumed to have been passed in some fashion from parents to offspring. Heritability has been shown through laboratory animal experimentation; certain strains of animals and fowl have been bred for high susceptibility or resistance to neoplastic conditions. Although the neoplasms themselves are not inherited, the predilections appear to be.

Heredity, however, is not the entire answer since some tumors are obviously transmissible and have been shown to be of viral origin. The viral theory of carcinogenesis is not completely valid, although certain neoplasms are proved to be of virus origin and others show immunologic identity in that they are confined to certain species and cannot be transferred to another.

In recent experiments, a "tumor factor" which is apparently not viral has been isolated from neoplastic tissues. This factor, injected into susceptible laboratory animals, has resulted in the production of a wide spectrum of carcinomas, sarcomas, and benign tumors of skin, adnexa, and connective tissue structures of the body. Work with cellular constituents such as desoxyribonucleic acid (DNA) in the nuclei and ribonucleic acid (RNA) in the cytoplasm of cells has shown that there are virus types which selectively attack DNA or RNA and may result in the production of neoplastic cells. In the radiation spectrum, rays of the upper spectrum such as the actinic rays of sunlight, roentgen rays, alpha and beta particles, and gamma radiation have been shown to induce neoplasia. Whether or not these radiations act to weaken the cell and thus render it more subject to a carcinogenic agent or act directly is a point which has not yet been determined. Parasites, such as *Sarcocystis*, occasionally act as agents which set up conditions leading to neoplasia. In the horse, this has not been demonstrated, but studies of neoplasia in the horse are so few that such causation could easily have been missed.

Among the chemicals known to induce neoplasia, benzanthracene and methylcholanthrene have been outstanding. The application of these to skin of experimental animals has resulted in the production of tumors. The neoplasms produced are not all of similar type. For instance, application of these agents to the mammary glands of susceptible mice will regularly produce carcinomas though the application to the skin of fowl may produce cutaneous hemangiomas. The structural similarity of these chemical compounds to hormones and endocrine substances, particularly follicular estrogens, testosterone, lutean hormones, and the corticosterones has resulted in the belief that disorder in hormone metabolism may also act to produce neoplastic disease. Perhaps when more is known about the nature and function of cells we will be able to speak on carcinogenesis with more authority. It is a consummation devoutly to be wished.

CLASSIFICATION

Neoplasms are classified as benign or malignant depending primarily upon their invasiveness. A tumor which grows slowly and regularly and generally is separated from other body tissues by a capsule is classed as benign, but one which proliferates rapidly between or around normal cells or tissues and has the potential capacity for metastasis is malignant. Tumors which possess aberrant functional characteristics such as endocrine tumors, which secrete excess quantities of hormones, are usually benign.

It is the continued, uncontrolled cellular growth and reproduction which make neoplasms so dangerous to health and life; even the so-called benign tumors may mechanically impair the function of vital organs by pressure or displacement and damage bodily efficiency enough to result in impaired health and, occasionally, death. The metastatic tumors, however, are far more dangerous. Metastasis is the capability of some neoplastic cells to be transported from their original site via the blood stream or lymphatics to some other portion of the body where they form secondary tumors. Secondary tumors may be so numerous and extensive that virtually every organ in the body can be involved. Ordinarily, metastatic tumors will develop in organs which possess an extensive capillary bed such as the liver, lungs, kidneys, and spleen. Benign tumors, on the other hand, do not possess the ability to infiltrate tissues or to spread by metastasis. If, by some possibility, a segment of a benign tumor is carried by the blood stream or lymphatic circulation to another location, it does not survive. The exact reasons for these differences between malignant and benign growths are not known.

It should be emphasized that benign and malignant neoplasms are not divided by a rigid boundary. The terms are relative and there are all degrees of malignancy or benignity. Yet it is possible to predict, in most cases, the clinical behavior of a tumor from its gross and histologic features. The most effective aid in determining the course of a neoplasm is the characteristic life history of each tumor entity, insofar as such life histories are known. It is well-known that malignant melanoma of the horse is a metastasizing tumor that is invariably fatal within a short period of time. It is also known that an interstitial cell tumor of the testicles can readily be treated by castration and probably will not occur in another portion of the body. Such knowledge is valuable in making a prognosis and determining what therapy, if any, will be advisable or necessary.

NOMENCLATURE

The nomenclature of tumors is based upon the functional division of body tissues and the nomenclature of the cells and tissues of origin. A neoplasm is usually described by its tissue of origin followed by the suffix "oma." There is no set nomenclature that differentiates benignity from malignancy. One simply has to become familiar with the characteristics of tumors and their origin in order to recognize whether they are benign or malignant. For instance, a fibroma is a benign tumor of fibrous tissue, and an adenoma a benign tumor of glandular tissue, yet a hepatoma is a malignant tumor of liver tissue.

However, there are some general methods of describing certain malignancies. The body is divided into 2 major areas: one including the epithelial tissues, the other the remainder of the body tissues. Epithelium may be subdivided further into covering surface and glands. Malignant tumors of epithelial structures are known as carcinomas. The remainder of the body—the so-called "supporting tissues" which include connective, muscular, vascular, and lymphatic tissues—forms the origin of malignancies called sarcomas. These divisions form a broad primary base for differentiation. Finer classification depends upon subordinate functional and anatomic divisions of the body. For instance, a malignant tumor of glandular tissue will be called an adenocarcinoma, yet this term is not adequate to completely describe the lesion. A descriptive anatomic site must be added. Under this system, names can get quite complicated. For instance, a tumor of the supporting tissues involving smooth muscle is called a leiomyoma. If this tumor is malignant, it would be called a leiomyosarcoma and its specific nomenclature would depend upon the location of the smooth muscle fibers involved. Hence, we might have a "duodenal leiomyosarcoma."

It can be seen that the nomenclature of tumors can become somewhat ponderous. Yet this system is one which has been developed through years of trial and error and has been determined to best fit the needs of tumor description. However, this terminology alone is not sufficient to completely satisfy the requirements of the scientist and pathologist. Since tumors derive from individual cells or groups of cells, cellular classification also enters into the scheme. Tumors arising from special cells or cell groups may have their own specific names, such as mast cell tumor, Sertoli cell tumor, glioma, ependymoma, etc. This serves to further complicate the nomenclature as does the fact that tumors exist which are not traceable to any tissue found in the normal histology of an adult animal. Such tumors are referred to as embryonal types and possess the suffix "blastoma."

The resemblance which tumor cells bear to the normal cells from which they have arisen forms the basis for detailed classification and nomenclature in both veterinary and human pathology. Since there are as many different potential neoplasms as there are organs or specialized cells in the body, this classification is more of academic than practical importance. In neoplasia of horses, records indicate that almost every body tissue can be involved and a detailed classification thus would necessarily include the entire histologic spectrum of the body. And though it is nice to be able to accurately identify a tumor in its finest and most intimate detail, from a clinical and therapeutic viewpoint it is not necessary. It is sufficient to recognize a tumor as malignant or benign and to be able to give an adequate prognosis and therapeutic regimen for the patient.

GROSS CHARACTERISTICS

The gross appearance of neoplasms may not always be what is expected. The general conception that neoplasia is reflected by an enlargement or grossly apparent tumor-like growth is not always true. Some of the more malignant carcinomas and sarcomas may never reach great size before they kill the patient. In contrast, others may reach enormous size. These latter tumors are probably benign rather than malignant. In general, benign epithelial neoplasms tend to grow outward from the epithelial surface whereas malignancies often grow inward. Papillomas, or warts, are the most common and most obvious of the benign tumors and frequently reach enormous size with complicated branching and cauliflower-like projections upon their surface. If the tumor lies on a free surface and has a relatively thin neck in proportion to its size, it is in all probability benign. Tumors on a free surface which are flat and have a broad base, are more likely to be malignant. Ulceration suggests malignancy, but if a capsule is present the tumor is probably benign. Some benign tumors, particularly those near the surface of the body, may become ulcerated as a result of pressure necrosis or insufficient blood supply. Malignant neoplasms of the skin or mucous membrane often will ulcerate before they reach appreciable size.

Tumors encountered in visceral organs, such as the lungs, kidneys, spleen and liver, always propose the question of whether they are primary or metastatic, malignant or benign. The form of growth is usually significant. Primary neoplasms are seldom regular in shape or smooth in outline. Metastatic growths are almost always spherical. If more than one growth focus is present in a single organ, the condition has probably metastasized from some other site. Benign tumors usually will be encapsulated and circumscribed.

A cross-section of the cut surface of a tumor reveals it to be tissue of different color and consistency from the tissue surrounding it. The color usually is white or grayish-white. Melanomas ordinarily are black due to pigment-containing tissue although some may appear white or "amelanotic." Interstitial cell tumors of the testicles usually are yellow. Hemorrhage or numerous blood channels may impart a reddish color to a tumor and necrosis may cause blackish or brownish discoloration, and tumors of myeloid tissue may have a greenish color.

Tumor consistency may be harder or softer than the surrounding tissue. Lymphomas tend to be soft, homogenous and white. When cut, tumors may show hemorrhages, cysts, areas of necrotic tissue, or other structures which will aid in identification. Neoplastic tissue must be distinguished from inflammatory granulomatous lesions such as those produced by actinomycosis, tuberculosis, and exuberant granulation. This can be done occasionally through the clinical history or the location of the lesions, or by the presence of certain specialized structures within the lesion itself. However, most cases must await microscopic examination.

MICROSCOPIC CHARACTERISTICS

It is in tumor pathology and identification that the microscope and tissue sections have a peak value. Without these two tools, the identification and prognosis of many benign or malignant tumors would be difficult or impossible, and classification, characterization and knowledge of tumors would still be limited.

In general, neoplastic cells become more and more anaplastic or undifferentiated in direct proportion to their malignancy, that is, they return in an ever-increasing degree to a morphology simulating the embryonal state. Such undifferentiated cells appear to have a much greater ability to maintain themselves in unfavorable environments. However, the statement that anaplastic tumor cells are "embryonal" is only morphologically valid for they possess an uncontrolled power of multiplying and invading tissues that is not characteristic of embryonal cells or tissue.

There are accepted microscopic criteria which are used to estimate the degree of malignancy. The fundamental measure, of course, is the degree of anaplasia, or the extent to which the neoplastic tissue reverts to an embryonal form. The greater the anaplasia, the higher the malignancy. The manner of growth of a tumor is also of great importance. If metastases have occurred, or if the tumor shows an infiltrative pattern of growth, it is considered to be malignant. This is useful in diagnosing early stages of tumors, and gives some idea of the prognosis. The degree of cellularity is important. If the nuclei are closely spaced, indicating a large number of cells per unit area, this indicates malignancy. If the nuclei tend to be hyperchromatic, malignancy is probable. Numerous mitotic figures mean rapid growth and probable malignancy, although this is not an absolute criterion. Abnormal mitotic figures and division of a cell into 3 daughter nuclei instead of the normal 2 are indicative of malignancy.

A system of grading has come into common use to estimate the degree of malignancy of a given tumor, particularly of squamous cell carcinomas. Grade I is applied to a squamous cell tumor having epithelium well-differentiated into layers similar to normal. Grades II and III resemble the normal tissue less and less with Grade IV representing carcinoma in which scarcely any normal cells or structures exist. The malignancy increases directly with the size of the numbers, Grade I having the lowest malignancy and Grade IV the highest. Though grading may be useful, it has decided limitations since variations exist within different parts of the same tumor and patient response may be different. In dealing with malignancy, no hard and fast rules can be formulated for treatment or grade of malignancy. Each case must be handled as an individual problem.

INCIDENCE

The incidence of neoplasms is not high in any particular species and is relatively low in the horse, although tumors in the horse are not uncommon. A survey of about 1,500 equine pathology cases by the Armed Forces Institute of Pathology revealed a 9.5% incidence of neoplasia. This, undoubtedly, is much higher than would be encountered in practice since the tissues which are submitted to the AFIP are pathologic in the first place and, frequently, nothing but neoplasms are submitted. It is interesting, however, to review the neoplastic cases.

It is an accepted but erroneous belief that the malignant melanoma is the most common equine neoplasm. A survey of the literature indicates that squamous cell carcinoma outnumbers malignant melanoma at least 4 to

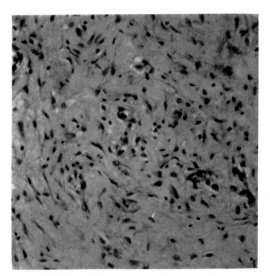

Fig. 1. Fibroma. Note loose, irregular arrangement of fibrocytes. x 150. AFIP #119670.

1, and that there are at least 4 other types of benign or malignant neoplasms which are more numerous.

It is interesting to note that of a total of 7,052 reported tumors in domestic animals, only 386 have been reported from horses as compared to 954 from cattle, and 5,315 from dogs. The study of equine neoplasia suffers from lack of clinical reports and pathologic material. This only can be obtained through the cooperation of practitioners. It is manifestly impossible with such limited data to produce anything but the barest outline of tumor types and incidence. Undoubtedly, in the future with greater use of diagnostic facilities at state and federal laboratories, a better accounting of equine neoplasia will be obtained.

CHARACTERISTICS OF EQUINE NEOPLASMS

The following descriptions of the known tumors of the horse list the outstanding diagnostic features from gross and microscopic points of view. This list is by no means complete and undoubtedly will be supplemented in future years as more cases are reported. Often, the pathologic report covers but a single case and, consequently, will not be as informative as those which include many cases.

BENIGN TUMORS OF SUPPORTING TISSUE

Equine Sarcoid

This peculiar growth is related to the fibroma, and possesses the histologic appearance of a neurofibroma or a moderately malignant fibrosarcoma with an ulcerated and bizarre epidermis that shows deep and irregular rete pegs. It occurs most commonly on the legs, head, and genitalia. The lesions are difficult to remove surgically since they have a tendency to recur. However, they do not metastasize. Evidence indicates that the lesion is capable of being transmitted from one animal to another. Similar lesions have been produced by exposing horses to bovine papilloma virus. See Chapter 4.

Fibroma

This tumor arises from fibrous connective tissue and may occur in a number of shapes and sizes. It can be found in almost any part of the body. Two subclassifications exist, the fibroma durum or hard fibroma in which collagenous tissue predominates, and the fibroma molle or soft fibroma which contains a higher percentage of cells and fewer collagenous fibrils. The collagenous fibrils and cells may show little or no orientation. A high degree of cellularity together with plump or stellate hyperchromic nuclei are indicative of malignancy (fibrosarcoma). Ordinarily, fibromas are benign and can be treated effectively by surgical excision (Fig. 1).

Leiomyoma

This is a benign tumor of smooth muscle cells. It has not been reported too frequently in the horse although it is not uncommon in other species. It is found principally in the digestive tract and organs whose tissues include smooth muscle. It is difficult to differentiate this tumor from a fibroma since the muscle cells usually are poorly defined. Distinguishing features include nuclei which have rounded ends and tend to lie parallel to one another. Special stains are useful in distinguishing this tumor.

HEMANGIO(ENDOTHELIO)MA

This tumor is usually benign and arises from the endothelial lining of blood vessels. It consists of mixed elements which include endothelial cells and endothelial-lined blood spaces filled with circulating blood. Subsidiary designations, depending upon the size and number of the blood spaces in ascending amount, are hemangioma simplex, hemangioma cavernosum, and hemangioma hypertrophicum. Deaths from this lesion are due to rupture of the blood spaces with resultant hemorrhage. A so-called malignant form is called hemangioendothelioma. It is probable that this designation is incorrect since anaplasia in sufficient amounts to produce malignancy probably would result in a structure indistinguishable from a sarcoma (Fig. 2).

LIPOMA

This benign tumor often is multiple and can conceivably occur in many places, although the recorded locations in the horse are in the mesenteries. The fat may be yellowish in color. The tumor mass is discrete and may be pedunculated. The size and shape of the fat cells show greater variation than normal. Ordinarily, visceral lipomas are diagnosed post mortem, and apparently they exert no detrimental effect upon the health of the animal.

OSTEOMA

This tumor shows a close relationship to the fibroma except that portions of its mass consist of bone. The bone appears as small islands or spicules surrounded by proliferating connective tissue. The degree of malignancy is determined by the anaplasia of the connective tissue. Malignant forms are called osteosarcoma. Osteomas must be differentiated from inflammatory exostoses. This is based upon the cellular architecture, the exostosis being more regular in its cellular arrangement. Leg lesions in the horse are almost invariably exostoses.

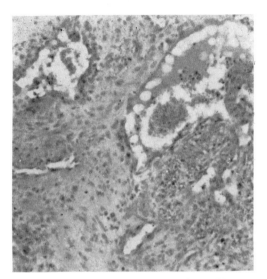

Fig. 2. Hemangioendothelioma. Note the proliferation of endothelial elements into the vessel lumen. x 120. AFIP #181273.

GIANT CELL TUMOR OF BONE

This tumor consists of large dark-staining fusiform nuclei associated with multinucleate giant cells. The cellular elements are imbedded in a fibrous stoma. The histologic appearance of the tumor suggests malignancy but clinical experience in other species indicates that it is usually benign.

CHONDROMA

This tumor differs from the osteoma in that cartilage is substituted for bone. The connective tissue cells, principally of fibrous connective tissue origin which surround the cartilage masses, differentiate into chondroblasts which, in turn, form more cartilage. The cartilage, however, is always surrounded by fibroblasts. Chondromas, like osteomas, may be malignant. The degree of malignancy is determined by the anaplasia of fibroblasts in the parts most divergent from normal.

MALIGNANT TUMORS OF SUPPORTING TISSUE

MALIGNANT LYMPHOMA

Among the neoplasms of the blood-forming tissues, those consisting of lymphoid cells are the most numerous. The malignant lymphoma is probably the most frequently encountered tumor in veterinary practice since it occurs in all the domestic species. In certain regions of the world, notably the United States, malignant lymphomas appear to be more prevalent. In South Africa, the condition apparently is rare.

The tumors usually are multiple and result in enlargement of lymph nodes in various portions of the body. In many cases, the spleen may be involved. The lymphoid organs are not invaded by metastases similar to those produced by other tumors, but instead are transformed virtually *in toto* into neoplastic tissue which possesses little or no normal histologic structure. Instead, the organ appears to be a monotony of lymphoid cells. Apparently, the malignant lymphoma is multicentric in origin and arises through a generalized transformation of normal lymphocytes into neoplastic cells. In addition to involving the lymphoid organs, the malignant lymphoma may invade practically any organ of the body. These invasions may take the form of discrete metastases or show, histologically, as infiltrations of neoplastic cells among normal histologic structures. Such infiltrations are common in the kidney where lymphoid cells may be interspersed throughout the stroma. In the intestine, malignant cells may be found infiltrated between the smooth muscle fibers (Fig. 3).

Two types of malignant lymphoma exist— the leukemic in which the total leukocyte count may rise to between 20,000 to 200,000 per cubic milliliter, and the aleukemic which does not show an appreciable rise in total leukocytes. It is not particularly difficult to differentiate the leukocytosis produced by malignant lymphoma from a leukocytosis associated with infection. This can be done by noting the morphologic differences between neoplastic and normal lymphocytes found in the circulating blood. In addition, the rise in the white cell count is due to an absolute increase in the number of lymphocytes.

A number of subclassifications of malignant lymphoma have been made. If the cells closely resemble normal lymphocytes, the tumor may be designated a lymphocytoma. If the cells are larger with a vesicular nucleus, considerable cytoplasm, and tend to resemble lymphoblasts, the tumor may be called a lymphoblastoma. A still more undifferentiated type is called the reticulum cell sarcoma. The term, lymphosarcoma, is used interchangeably with malignant lymphoma.

RHABDOMYSARCOMA

This term is applied to a malignant neoplasm arising from striated muscle cells, either skeletal or cardiac. These tumors are quite rare, although they have been found in all species of domestic animals including the horse. In some, the resemblance to striated muscles is obvious but the majority must be differentiated from fibrosarcomas or leiomyosarcomas by the recognition of an occasional fiber which contains cross-striations.

LEIOMYOSARCOMA

This is a malignant tumor of smooth muscle. It is not always easy to distinguish malignant smooth muscle from connective tissue since the muscle often is so poorly differentiated that it does not respond typically to special stains. One must rely largely on the fact that the muscle nuclei, though long and slender, have well-rounded ends and, together with their fibers, have a tendency to lie parallel to

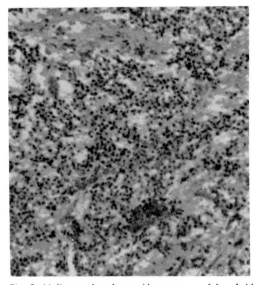

Fig. 3. Malignant lymphoma. Note masses of lymphoid cells. x 120. AFIP #134435.

each other although the composite band of cells and fibers may curve freely. Malignancy is evidenced by lack of differentiation, bizarre nuclei, hypochromatic nuclei, and numerous mitotic figures. Like other tumors, the degree of malignancy is dependent upon the degree of anaplasia of the muscle cells.

Liposarcoma

This is an exceedingly rare tumor which is characterized by areas of anaplastic fibrous connective tissue mixed with fatty tissue, and intermediate tissue in which only rudimentary fat cells with very small vacuoles are present (Fig. 4).

Malignant Myeloma

This is a tumor of bone marrow and is essentially similar to malignant lymphomas except that the cell of origin is the myelocyte of bone marrow and its earlier form, the myeloblast. A myeloma may be leukemic or aleukemic. The leukemia produced is called myelogenous or myeloid leukemia and shows a heavy concentration of cells of the myeloid series in the circulating blood. Though the myelomas are rare, they do occur in the horse and diagnosis depends principally on recognizing cells of the myeloid series in the circulating blood. Usually a majority of these are large, round cells with a moderate amount of cytoplasm and a fairly dark nucleus which is round or slightly indented. Certain myeloid tumors are composed of cells resembling plasma cells and are called plasmacytomas. Some myelomas have a greenish hue which, if faded, may be restored by oxidation with hydrogen peroxide. Because of their color, they have been called chloromas. Myelomas may appear in various organs, but particularly within the lymphatics. A careful search should always be made for a primary tumor site in the bone marrow. If such a site cannot be demonstrated, the correctness of a diagnosis of myeloma is questionable.

Fibrosarcoma

A fibrosarcoma and a fibroma are essentially similar in structure and differ only in the de-

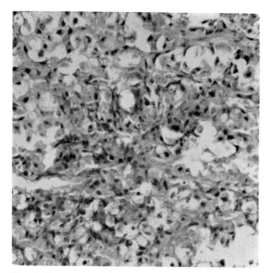

Fig. 4. Liposarcoma. Note the fat cells and the central focus of rapidly proliferating tissue. x 120. AFIP #119811.

gree of anaplasia of the fibrous connective tissue cells. The fibrosarcoma contains cells which are far more anaplastic than those found in the benign form of this tumor.

EPITHELIAL NEOPLASMS

As has been previously mentioned, a somewhat different nomenclature system exists for epithelial tissues. Since epithelium is subdivided into gland-forming and nongland-forming tissues, there are two cellular bases for nomenclature. Benign tumors of the nongland-forming tissues are called papillomas, and the malignant neoplasms are called carcinomas. For the glandular tissue, the term, adenoma, indicates a benign tumor and adenocarcinoma a malignant glandular tumor. The term, epithelioma, is occasionally used in older literature with an implication of malignancy. The basic simplicity of this characterization of epithelial tumors is quickly lost in a maze of subclassifications which exist in most textbooks.

BENIGN TUMORS OF EPITHELIAL ORIGIN

Papilloma

The term, papilloma, designates a tumorous projection from the skin. This is a benign neoplasm which has a core of fibrous connective tissue uniting it to a subepithelial base which provides nutrition (Fig. 5). Common sites of papillomas include the skin, particularly regions which are covered with stratified squamous epithelium without accessory skin structures and well-developed rete pegs. Papillomas may also be found in the intestinal tract or at the corneoscleral junction of the eye. The latter are often thought to be forerunners of squamous cell carcinomas. A subclassification of the papillomas is considered by some to include the polyp which is an inflammatory tumor-like growth which may be seen frequently in the nasal passages and in the lower bowel. Polyps may reach large size but essentially are not neoplastic. Histologically, a polyp consists of loosely arranged fibrous and mucoid tissue covered by epithelium and liberally infiltrated with leukocytes.

Adenoma

This is a benign, epithelial neoplasm derived from glandular tissue and is similar histologically to the parent organ. The glandular proliferation may be large or small, tubular or spherical. The epithelium extends to form

connection with the tissue from which it originated. However, this connection usually cannot be demonstrated. The epithelial lining is generally cuboidal or simple columnar. Any tendency for these epithelial cells to pile is an indication of malignancy. The lining is variable in contour and may form rounded bulges or may project into the lumen.

In some adenomas the acini become very large and, in addition, become filled with fluid. This variant is called a cystadenoma. In one form of this tumor, seen usually in the mammary gland, the epithelium and the fibrous stroma appear to share more or less equally in the neoplastic growth. Such a growth is termed a fibroadenoma or an adenofibroma depending on whether fibrous or glandular tissue is most apparent in the histologic section. Adenomas of the thyroid gland closely resemble normal tissue, but consist of round, lightly encapsulated nodules in which the neoplastic thyroid tissue can be seen to differ from normal in one way or another when the two are compared. Commonly, the acini of the adenomas are smaller and the lining cells are more highly chromatic than is the case with the nearby healthy thyroid. But the re-

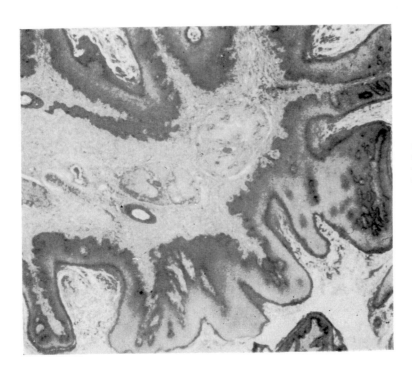

Fig. 5. Papilloma. Note the wrinkled proliferating thickened epithelium with essentially normal rete pegs and subepithelial connective tissue. x 30. AFIP #170184.

verse also may be true. The sharp difference in cell types betrays the adenomatous character of the area. Many thyroid adenomas are toxic, secrete thyroxin, and cause hyperthyroidism.

MALIGNANT TUMORS OF EPITHELIAL ORIGIN

ADENOCARCINOMA

This is the malignant form of the adenoma and shows much the same general structure except that the degree of anaplasia is much greater. An adenocarcinoma differs from an adenoma in that the epithelium is less normal and may show excessive proliferation into the acini either in several layers or in numerous papillary projections. The essential difference, however, is the power of the malignant cells to invade normal tissue. In more malignant forms, this basic characteristic is carried to a point where the cells fail to form glands at all and appear as solid masses of epithelium. Degree of malignancy can be determined by the degree of anaplasia, or lack of differentiation of individual cells. Anaplastic cells tend to be larger, rounder, and more hyperchro-

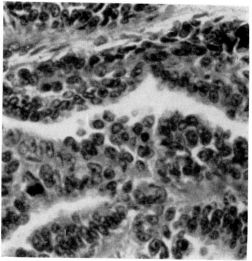

Fig. 6. Adenocarcinoma. Note the glandular appearance and cellular arrangement. x 300. AFIP #751113.

mactic than normal, and mitoses appear to be more numerous (Fig. 6).

CYSTADENOCARCINOMA

This is a malignancy in which certain of the acini of an adenocarcinoma form cyst-like spaces usually filled with a pink staining protein-like secretion (Fig. 7).

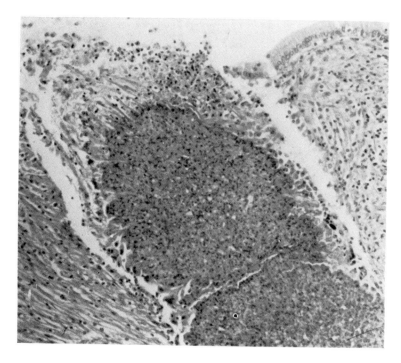

Fig. 7. Mucinous adenocarcinoma of rectum. The central section is neoplastic; note eroded epithelium and sloughing of neoplastic cells into rectal lumen. x 120. AFIP #838562.

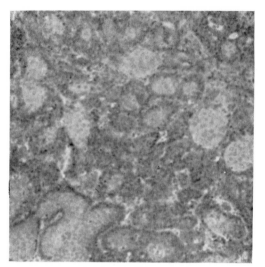

Fig. 8. Squamous cell carcinoma. Note islands and masses of irregularly growing epithelial tissue. x 75. AFIP #129905.

SQUAMOUS CELL CARCINOMA

This is the commonest form of carcinoma and is derived from the skin and from stratified squamous epithelium. It is particularly capable of metastasis and shows a close relationship to the epithelium from which it is derived, except that pigmentation and formation of rete pegs are not observed in the neoplastic cells.

The epithelium, however, is not restricted to the outer surface of the neoplasm. Epithelial masses and cords proliferate into and through the mass. Cross sections appear as islands of epithelium surrounded by stroma with the basal layer of the cells lying around the periphery. In the case of a cornifying tumor, the keratohyaline of the stratum corneum lies at the center of the epithelial mass, becomes quite dense, and forms a rounded, laminated structure known as an epithelial pearl which is diagnostic. In the more malignant forms, the epithelial masses consist of cells which are nearly uniform with dark, hyperplastic nuclei many of which are in the process of mitosis.

Occasionally, epithelial cells of a highly anaplastic carcinoma may assume a fusiform, or spindle, shape and it becomes very difficult to determine whether the tumor is a carcinoma or a sarcoma. Of some assistance is the fact that the cells of a sarcoma can, and usually do, form the walls of blood vessels within the tumor. Epithelial cells cannot do this and must be provided with enough interstitial tissue to form an endothelium for blood channels. The presence of this tissue is frequently an aid in identifying the more bizarre types of carcinomas. Also in sarcoma, are minute fibrils of

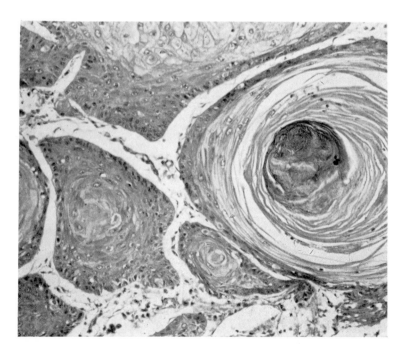

Fig. 9. Squamous cell carcinoma. Note reversed epithelial arrangement and enormous "epithelial pearl." x 150. AFIP #191666.

stroma which run between the cells, but in a carcinoma the cells merely rest beside each other (Fig. 8, 9).

BASAL CELL CARCINOMA

These are a group of epithelial neoplasms which are considered to arise from the basal cell layer, or stratum germinativum, of the epidermis. Clinically, basal cell carcinomas are locally invasive but rarely metastasize. They are also highly sensitive to radiation. The tumors tend to remain small but often ulcerate early. The arrangement of the cells varies but the cells themselves tend to be small to medium-sized, ovoid, and closely packed. The nuclei are small, round and darkly stained like those of the normal stratum germinativum. The cytoplasm is scanty and rather pale. Projecting spines or intercellular bridges are absent. Mitoses generally are rare.

In most basal cell carcinomas, the cells form solid masses which lie just beneath the epidermis, separated from it by a zone of connective tissue. The tumors are differentiated from squamous cell carcinomas by the lack of any gradation or transition from basal cells to the larger, paler, prickle cells, and by absence of any semblance of cornification. Basal cell carcinomas reportedly never contain melanin. Occasionally, cystic spaces which have the appearance of glands are found in basal cell carcinomas.

MISCELLANEOUS EPITHELIAL NEOPLASMS

At this point, the orderly classification of epithelial neoplasms becomes a confused aggregation of names, principally designed to identify the cells or tissue from which the neoplasm arises. It requires a considerable familiarity with nomenclature to recognize from name alone whether the tumor is benign or malignant.

HEPATOMA

In this neoplasm, the lobular architecture of the liver is disarranged. Normal, portal trinities do not occur and the cells show a staining

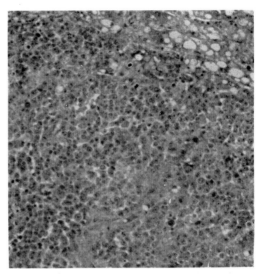

Fig. 10. Hepatoma. The small area of vaculated hepatic tissue in the upper right corner is being invaded by the mass of irregularly arranged rapidly proliferating cells of the tumor. Note the numerous mitotic figures. x 120. AFIP #611930.

reaction differing from that of the healthy tissue. Lipid infiltration may be pronounced. The tumorous tissue often is extensive, and is likely to show gross greenish or yellowish discoloration caused by bile which could not escape due to a lack of bile ducts. The cells are so highly anaplastic that they bear little or no resemblance to normal liver cells either in form or arrangement. Liver cell carcinoma is a synonym for this tumor (Fig. 10).

MELANOMA

Melanomas arise from melanin-forming cells. They may be classed as either benign or malignant, although the tendency is for any melanoma to become malignant. Melanin-forming cells occur chiefly in the skin but also are found in the pigmented layers of the choroid, retina, and ciliary body. Since the exact embryologic position of the cells is uncertain, and since some melanomas consist of cells arranged similarly to epithelium, they usually are included under the epithelial tumors. Melanomas are common in all species and though they frequently occur in the skin, they may be found in other portions of the body.

The histologic appearance of melanomas varies considerably. The cells may be filled

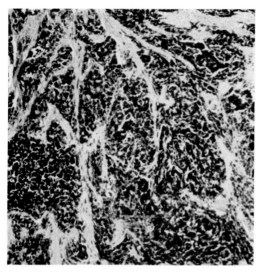

Fig. 11. Malignant melanoma. Note the characteristic "orange segment" arrangement. x 30. AFIP #482388.

with brown pigment to such an extent that little else can be seen, or at the other extreme, there may be no melanin at all, hence the name "amelanotic melanomas." The shape of the cells varies, sometimes within the same tumor, from round and polyhedral form resembling epithelium, to elongated fusiform cells similar to fibroblasts. In a typical melanoma, the fibroblastic-type cell predominates, and these fit neatly together to fill compartments shaped somewhat like the segments of an orange. The compartments are ordinarily enclosed by thin, fibrous trabeculae. The cytoplasm tends to be basophilic and when stained with mild hemotoxylin preparations, the nuclei appear a peculiar violet hue which reportedly is not seen in other than melanoma cells. When melanin is present, the diagnosis is relatively simple. In amelanotic melanoma, diagnosis must be based upon the morphologic and staining features (Fig. 11).

The modern view is to consider that all melanomas are either malignant, or potentially malignant. The grade of malignancy is represented by the degree of anaplasia, the number of hyperchromatic nuclei, bizarre forms, and mitotic figures. Lymphocytic infiltration is also considered to be a sign of malignancy.

Grossly, the melanoma is recognized by its deep black color and the inky pigment which diffuses from it into any watery medium with which the cut surface may come into contact. The amelanotic melanoma may be diagnosed only by microscopic examination.

In the horse, melanomas are particularly frequent in old, gray horses, although they do occur in horses of other colors. Their initial location tends to be confined to the perineal or perianal region from which they spread to the rectal and pelvic lymphatics and metastasize to the spleen, lungs, or other internal organs. Occasionally, melanomas may be found on the eyelids or other structures, such as the udder. Rarely, they may be allied with other tumors.

ADAMANTINOMA

This tumor arises from the enamel organ which is the embryologic forerunner of the tooth. The name indicates the hardness of the tumor which tends to form epithelial masses that have a peculiar horseshoe shape. Internally, the epithelial structures may vary from a single layer of small, dark cells like those of the deeper side of the enamel organ, to a many-layered epithelial island of larger cells in which pale, angular stellate cells or variable-sized cysts may be present. These represent the original central cavity of the developing enamel organ. The neoplastic mass grows from a dental primordium in either jaw to form a locally destructive tumor of considerable size. Though it is locally malignant, metastases seldom occur. Adamantinomas are among the rarer tumors of the horse (Fig. 12).

NEPHROBLASTOMA

This tumor arises near or in the kidney. It comes from the renal primordia from which the kidney is formed but which in early embryonal stages is not greatly different from primitive mesenchyme. An old name of little value histogenetically but suggestive of the microscopic picture is adenosarcoma of the kidney. The tumor consists typically of highly cellular fibroblastic tissue with scattered epithelial-lined glandular acini. In some specimens, the glands are scarce and difficult to find, but at the other extreme, they may be so numerous that the structure is suggestive of an adenocarcinoma. The tumor is not common in the horse.

HYPERNEPHROMA

This name has been used to define a neoplasm which arises typically near one end of the kidney and is characterized by columns of large cells with a clear, lipoid-containing cytoplasm. These cells were thought to be misplaced adreno-cortical cells, hence the name. The prevalent view today is that the tumor arises from the epithelium of the renal tubules. The tumor may be either benign or malignant but generally tends to be confined to the affected kidney.

PHEOCHROMOCYTOMA

The adrenal medulla is modified nervous tissue and is connected to the sympathetic nervous system. It gives rise to neoplasms of differentiated nerve cells, neuroblastomas, and ganglioneuromas, which will be discussed under the neoplasms of nervous tissue. Arising also from the cells of the medulla is the pheochromocytoma. This tumor commonly is brown on gross examination because of its pigment, hence the name. Synonyms include chromaffinoma and paraganglioma. If the tissue is fixed in chromium salts, the cells commonly develop a brown color which can be seen in microscopic sections, but there is no perfect consistency in this. The cells appear to be large epithelioid cells with central nuclei and abundant cytoplasm. Their outlines are indefinite as is true in the normal adrenal medulla. They are usually held in place by thin strands of fibrous connective tissue. Blood spaces usually are numerous. Pheochromocytomas are very infrequent in the horse.

GRANULOSA CELL TUMOR

The granulosa cell tumor arises from the stratum granulosum of the Graafian follicle of the ovary or from cells which are capable of forming that structure. The usual granulosa cell tumor consists of masses of epithelioid cells with round, central nuclei and considerable cytoplasm. In some, there are fluid-filled, open

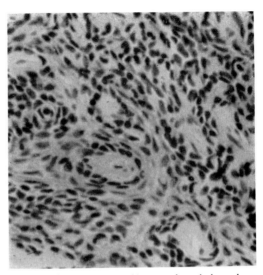

Fig. 12. Adamantinoma. Note oval and horseshoe-shaped cellular arrangement and small size and closeness of cells. x 300. AFIP #515211.

spaces which bear a resemblance to Graafian follicles. In others, a few cells cluster radially around a tiny space producing a rosette. In still others, the cells are distributed randomly and held in elongated or cylindrical lobules by thin fibrous trabeculae. Grossly, the granulosa cell tumor is usually rounded, smoothly encapsulated, and is attached to the ovary rather than included in it. The cut surface tends to be yellow in color (Fig. 13).

THECA CELL AND LUTEAL CELL TUMORS

Two other forms of ovarian tumor are the theca cell tumor and the luteal cell tumor. The theca cell tumor is composed of spindle-shaped cells which resemble the theca interna and externa of the Graafian follicle. The luteal cell tumor is similar to the granulosa cell tumor but is even more yellow. Its cells contain numerous lipoidal droplets and are microscopically suggestive of those of the corpus luteum. The tumors of the ovarian group secrete estrogen.

SEMINOMA

In the male, one of the three neoplasms peculiar to the testicle is the seminoma. This is believed to arise from the germinal epithelium of the seminiferous tubules. It is composed of large polyhedral cells with prominent round

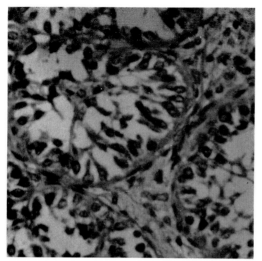

Fig. 13. Granulosa cell tumor. Note the preservation of follicular type architecture. x 300. AFIP #726507.

centrally located nuclei, not unlike spermatogonia. The nuclei of the seminoma have conspicuous chromatin bodies, a feature which aids in distinguishing this tumor from some types of malignant lymphomas. Mitotic figures are frequent. Fine trabeculae divide masses of cells into compartments. The seminoma is rare in the horse.

SERTOLI CELL TUMOR

The Sertoli or sustentacular cell tumor has not as yet been reported in the horse although there is no apparent reason why this tumor has not developed in this animal. As the name implies, the neoplasm arises from the Sertoli cells of the seminiferous tubules. Grossly, the Sertoli cell tumor consists of one or more nodules which may greatly distend the testicle and reach several times the size of the normal organ. The cut surface bulges and is gray to light yellow in color. This tumor is considered to be benign although rare anaplastic forms may spread into surrounding structures and may metastasize to the lymphatics. Reported Sertoli cell tumors occur almost exclusively in the dog.

INTERSTITIAL CELL TUMOR

The interstitial cell tumor, or Leydig cell tumor, arises from the interstitial androgen-

secreting cells of the testicles. The cells are larger and paler in cytoplasm and nuclei than the two preceding tumors. The cytoplasm contains large amounts of lipid which accounts for the pale and foamy character of the cytoplasm, and the distinctly yellow gross color. The cells form masses divided into compartments by fibrous trabeculae. Mitotic figures are seldom seen. This tumor would probably be seen more frequently if males were not castrated at a fairly early age. It has been reported to have occurred in a cryptorchid equine testicle.

THYROID CARCINOMA

Carcinomas of the thyroid are likely to be highly anaplastic and to bear no resemblance to their cells of origin. They may take the form of an adenocarcinoma with papillary projections extending into the glandular acini, or consist of solid masses of epithelial cells. The cells have central nuclei which are variable in size and color and are frequently bizarre, depending upon the degree of malignancy. These tumors invade nearby organs and tissues and metastasize to various organs, most frequently the lungs. The primary tumor is not likely to be large although some exert enough pressure on the trachea and larynx to interfere with breathing.

TUMORS OF INDETERMINATE CLASSIFICATION

TERATOMA

A teratoma is peculiar in that it contains tissue which is derived from more than one of the 3 primary germ layers. The great majority of teratomas occur in the reproductive organs, ovary or testicle, but a few are found in other regions of the body. They are usually found along the midline axis of the body while the patient is still young. Evidence indicates that teratomas develop early in fetal life. A teratoma may grow slowly or rapidly. In most cases, however, the growth is gradual. The different tissues within the teratomatous mass are arranged in no particular order. Most frequently encountered are connective tissue, cartilage and bone, epithelial structures, endoderm, skin, hair, and neuroglia. In one form, there is a cyst-like cavity lined with skin and filled with an increasing amount of hair. This is commonly called a dermoid or a dermoid cyst. Such cysts may contain teeth in which case they are called dentigerous cysts.

A true teratoma must show growth. Rarely one of its components may assume malignant qualities and show infiltration and metastasis, thus, in effect, constituting a carcinoma or a sarcoma. The fact that teratomas are usually located in tissues which in the embryo lie close to the median axis has been construed to mean that their origin is related to an abnormal development of the primitive streak. In general, the teratoma can be considered to be a slowly enlarging mass with benign characteristics.

MESOTHELIOMA

A mesothelioma arises from the mesothelial lining cells of serous membranes, particularly in the pleurae and peritoneum. These growths usually are in the form of diffusely disseminated nodules covering extensive areas of the membrane concerned. They may reach considerable size. In one case a horse had a mesothelioma weighing in excess of 200 pounds. Microscopically, the structures consist of rounded or papillary projections having a fibrous core covered by large mesothelial cells which bear a close resemblance to epithelium. It appears that either of these constituents can become dominant and develop into a neoplasm which may resemble a fibroma, or may consist of carcinoma-like masses of large epithelioid cells. Grossly, these neoplasms must be differentiated from actinobacillosis, tuberculosis and other granulomatous infections.

MYXOMA AND MYXOSARCOMA

The myxoma is composed of connective tissue which forms mucin. The nuclei tend to be round or stellate, the intercellular fibrils are bluish and show little organized arrangement. These tumors are always more or less malignant but the term, myxoma, generally is used despite that fact. The fact that myxomatosis in rabbits (a viral infection) closely simulates the development of the myxoma has given some supporting evidence to the viral theory of carcinogenesis.

TUMORS OF NERVOUS TISSUE

Neoplasms which arise from nervous tissue ordinarily occur in the brain and are derived chiefly from the neuroglia. Those having this source are known as gliomas. A glioma may be subdivided into a great number of groups or varieties. The classes commonly recognized are astrocytoma, glioblastoma multiforme, medulloblastoma, ependymoma, and oligodendroglioma. These represent the recognized types of glial tissue except for the microglia which does not form tumors. These classes are not sharply demarcated one from the other and some gliomas partake of the characteristics of more than one different class of cells.

Different rates of growth result in the terms, benign and malignant, although, technically speaking, all gliomas are benign since they do not metastasize to locations outside the central nervous system. However, infiltration to adjoining areas of the system is marked in some of the more malignant tumors, so that grossly and even microscopically, it may be difficult to discern their limits. In the horse, four neural tumors have been recognized—cholesteatoma, neurilemmoma, meningioma, and neurofibroma —and only these will be discussed.

CHOLESTEATOMA

This is a tumor-like formation consisting of layers of epithelial-like cells containing a great deal of cholesterol and other lipids. The tumor thus represents a cluster of pearls when examined microscopically. In the horse, these have been described in the choroid plexus and are considered to result from degenerative processes.

NEURILEMMOMA (SCHWANNOMA)

The neurilemmoma is considered to arise from the neurilemmal sheaths surrounding the axons of peripheral nerves. There is considerable variance of opinion as to whether this tumor should be distinguished from the neurofibroma which arises from the perineural con-

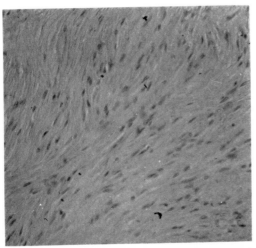

Fig. 14. Neurofibroma. Note regular arrangement and folded and whorled pattern. x 150. AFIP #235181.

nective tissue. The neurilemmona resembles the neurofibroma in general microscopic structure, but here and there areas are found in which elongated spindle-shaped nuclei are gathered together in rows. The nuclei lie practically parallel in a direction cross-wise to the row giving a palisade effect. This feature is the principal distinctive characteristic of this tumor. As would be expected, the growths are located along the course of the nerve or at a plexus or ganglion. In size, these seldom exceed a few centimeters in diameter, their growth is not rapid, and complete removal ordinarily is curative.

MENINGIOMA

The meningioma arises from the cranial or spinal meninges, presumably from the mesothelial cells which form their surfaces. In most meningiomas, the cells are plump and the nuclei are round, but there may be a tendency toward a whorled arrangement as in the neurofibroma. Occasionally, meningiomas form areas of bone. Rather commonly at the center of many of the whorls there is compressed hyalin or a calcified body grossly suggestive of a grain of sand. This form is sometimes called a psammoma, and the little granules are known as "brain sand." Grossly, the meningioma forms a more or less spherical, subdural mass which compresses but does not invade the underlying brain or cord tissue.

NEUROFIBROMA

This tumor arises from the fibrous connective tissue of nerve sheaths and usually is benign. It is recognizable, microscopically, by the scattered tight whorls of fibrous tissue which differentiate it from an ordinary fibroma. Grossly, the neurofibroma appears as a rounded subcutaneous mass, and may develop in any portion of the body although the cases in horses have been located in the head region. The malignant form, the neurogenic sarcoma, has not been reported in horses. Treatment is by surgical excision (Fig. 14).

QUESTIONABLE STRUCTURES

HAMARTOMA

A hamartoma may or may not be a neoplasm. The present consensus is that it probably represents a developmental anomaly rather than a true neoplasm. Hamartomas are seen in numerous organs such as the kidney, spleen, and lung as small, rounded, grayish nodules usually only a few millimeters in diameter. They are not encapsulated but may be separated from the adjacent parenchyma. Microscopically, they are composed of regular bundles of smooth muscles and connective tissue, and occasionally some fatty tissue. The tumors may reach the size of several centimeters.

KELOIDS

Keloids have often been confused with epithelial neoplasms although there is little if any similarity between the histologic aspect of this structure and that of a tumor. A keloid is a hypertrophic scar of the dermis which results from certain types of injury. It occurs with some frequency in horses and elevates the epidermis which frequently becomes ulcerated. The gross aspects of the keloid, therefore, could be confused with an epitheliocarcinoma. Histologically, however, a keloid shows a marked difference since it is made up of bands of eosinophilic collagen in which thinner collagen fibers and fibroblasts ramify. The skin adnexa are usually missing and the epidermis may be atrophied or ulcerated. Elastic fibers normally are very scarce.

J. F. BONE

REFERENCES

1. Abstract. Gastric cancer in a horse, J.A.V.M.A. **118** (1951) 51.

2. Abstract. Melanosarcomas in equine animals, J.A.V.M.A. **130** (1957) 48.

3. Abstract. A polyp on the vocal cord of a horse, J.A.V.M.A. **111** (1947) 315.

4. Anderson, W. A. D.: Pathology, 3rd Ed., Mosby, St. Louis, Mo. 1957.

5. Boyd, W.: A Textbook of Pathology, Lea & Febiger, Philadelphia, Pa. 1932.

6. Fisher, Alton K., A compact osteoma in the skull of a horse, J.A.V.M.A. **121** (1952) 42-44.

7. Howard, F. A., Granulosa cell tumor of the equine ovary, J.A.V.M.A. **114** (1949) 134-135.

8. Ogilvie, R. R., Pathological Histology, Williams & Wilkins Co. Baltimore, Md. 1957.

9. Reed, William O., Lymphosarcoma of the stomach of a horse, J.A.V.M.A. **114** (1949) 412-413.

10. Reid, Charles H., Mesothelioma, an unusual equine tumor, J.A.V.M.A. **124** (1954) 301.

11. Runnels, R. A., Animal Pathology, Iowa State College Press, Ames, Iowa. 1946.

12. Runnels, R. A., and Monlux, W. S. and Monlux, A. W., Principles of Veterinary Pathology, Iowa State University Press, Ames, Iowa. 1960.

13. Smith, Hilton A., Interstitial cell tumor of the equine testis, J.A.V.M.A.

14. Smith, H. A. and Jones, T. C., Veterinary Pathology, Lea and Febiger, Philadelphia, Pa. 1957.

CHAPTER 22

NUTRITIONAL REQUIREMENTS AND DEFICIENCIES

NUTRITIONAL REQUIREMENTS

GENERAL COMMENTS

The recorded information available concerning the feeding and nutrition of horses is very limited. Little research has been conducted in this field and many of the existing recommendations are based on empirical observations rather than controlled experimental studies. Current feeding practices for horses consequently are based, in part, on research done with other species. Thus, present standards and guides in horse feeding and nutrition are not adequate, and they are presented herein for use as a guide with the understanding that they are not exact and will need modification based on future experience and research.

Horse feeding and nutrition are complicated additionally because horses vary more in temperament and individual food requirements than any other class of livestock. The ration and feeding program which is satisfactory for one horse may not be adequate for another. Proper attention to each horse's particular nutritional needs may mean the difference between developing a winner or not. Individual needs, in addition, vary depending upon the animal's use and its owner's concern for optimum performance and appearance.

It must be emphasized also that feeding horses is as much an art as a science. The art consists in knowing the proper manner of feeding as well as how to ascertain each horse's individual requirements. The science, of course, is in knowing what to feed and how much to provide for the horse's basic nutritional needs. Thus, a good job of feeding horses will depend partly on the judgment of the feeder, his attention to details, and his desire to continually improve the job he is doing.

NUTRIENT ALLOWANCES

In the tables and discussion which follow, the currently recommended allowances are presented for the nutrients which are required in the equine ration. This information is intended to provide a basis upon which individual feeding programs can be developed. There is little reference to the physiologic effects of the various nutrients since such was not considered germane to the purpose of this book.

DRY MATTER

Table 1 gives the approximate pounds of dry matter which horses need daily. These requirements vary, depending on the energy needs and physical condition of the animal. The amounts should be altered if the animal either gains excessively or loses weight when fed the recommended amounts.

TOTAL DIGESTIBLE NUTRIENT (TDN)

The data in Table 2 give the TDN requirements for horses in pounds per day. The allowances should be regulated according to the physical condition of the horse. The TDN content in feeds will vary, and it is important to know its value to ascertain that the ration will supply the energy needs. Horses which are being used for hard work, racing, or nursing a foal have high energy requirements and will need rations high in TDN. The data in Table 2 can be used as a guide for determining these needs.

PROTEIN

To supply the protein needs of the horse, one must provide the essential amino acids. The value of a feed is determined largely by its amino acid composition, and how well it supplies the animal's needs for them. The horse is able to obtain some of its protein requirements from the action of microorganisms on cecal contents. Though the cecum is located at the end of the small intestines, which is the main area for the digestion and absorption of nutrients, there is considerable digestion and

Table 1.—Dry Matter (90% basis) Allowance for Horses in Pounds Per Day*

Weight of horses, lbs.	For growing horses with mature weights of							For mature horses at					
	600	800	1000	1200	1400	1600	1800	Mainte-nance	Light work	Medium work	Heavy work	For mares in last quarter of pregnancy	For lactating mares
	lbs.	lbs.	lbs.	lbs.	lbs.	lbs.	lbs.	lbs.	lbs.	lbs.	lbs.	lbs.	lbs.
200	6.7	7.2	7.5	7.7	8.2	8.5	9.0	—	—	—	—	—	—
400	9.1	9.9	10.2	10.4	11.0	11.8	12.3	6.2	8.2	9.4	11.0	8.6	12.3
600	10.2	11.7	12.3	13.3	13.4	13.9	14.4	8.5	11.0	12.8	14.8	11.7	16.7
800		12.6	13.8	14.7	15.8	16.6	17.0	10.6	13.8	15.9	18.4	14.4	20.6
1000			15.0	16.2	17.0	18.4	19.5	12.6	16.2	18.9	21.9	17.0	24.4
1200				17.1	18.4	19.5	20.8	14.4	18.6	21.6	25.1	19.5	28.0
1400					19.4	20.6	22.1	16.2	20.8	24.2	28.1	21.9	31.4
1600						21.1	22.7	17.8	23.0	26.7	31.0	24.3	34.9
1800							23.2	19.5	25.3	29.1	34.0	26.6	37.9

*The recommended allowances are taken from the National Research Council's Recommended Nutrient Allowances for Horses.[1]

Table 2.—Total Digestible Nutrient (TDN) Allowances for Horses in Pounds Per Day*

Weight of horses, lbs.	For growing horses with mature weights of							For mature horses at					
	600	800	1000	1200	1400	1600	1800	Mainte-nance	Light work	Medium work	Heavy work	For mares in last quarter of pregnancy	For lactating mares
	lbs.	lbs.	lbs.	lbs.	lbs.	lbs.	lbs.	lbs.	lbs.	lbs.	lbs.	lbs.	lbs.
200	4.2	4.5	4.7	4.8	5.1	5.3	5.6	—	—	—	—	—	—
400	5.7	6.2	6.4	6.5	6.9	7.4	7.7	3.9	5.1	5.9	7.3	5.4	8.8
600	6.4	7.3	7.7	8.3	8.4	8.7	9.0	5.3	6.9	8.0	9.9	7.3	11.9
800		7.9	8.6	9.2	9.9	10.4	10.6	6.6	8.6	10.0	12.3	9.0	14.7
1000			9.4	10.1	10.6	11.5	12.2	7.9	10.1	11.8	14.6	10.6	17.4
1200				10.7	11.5	12.2	13.0	9.0	11.6	13.5	16.7	12.2	20.0
1400					12.1	12.9	13.8	10.1	13.0	15.1	18.8	13.7	22.4
1600						13.2	14.2	11.1	14.4	16.7	20.7	15.2	24.9
1800							14.5	12.2	15.8	18.2	22.7	16.2	27.1

*These recommended allowances are taken from the National Research Council's Recommended Nutrient Allowances for Horses.[1]

Table 3.—Digestible Protein Allowances for Horses in Pounds Per Day*

Weight of horses, lbs.	For growing horses with mature weights of							For mature horses at				For mares in last quarter of pregnancy	For lactating mares
	600	800	1000	1200	1400	1600	1800	Mainte-nance	Light work	Medium work	Hard work		
	lbs.	lbs.	lbs.	lbs.	lbs.	lbs.	lbs.	lbs.	lbs.	lbs.	lbs.	lbs.	lbs.
200	0.77	0.93	1.04	1.06	1.22	1.28	1.39	—	—	—	—	—	—
400	0.57	0.80	0.94	1.03	1.16	1.43	1.50	0.31	0.38	0.46	0.52	0.46	1.01
600	0.45	0.65	0.77	0.93	1.13	1.33	1.49	0.42	0.52	0.62	0.72	0.62	1.37
800		0.54	0.74	0.87	1.05	1.23	1.44	0.53	0.65	0.77	0.87	0.77	1.70
1000			0.64	0.85	0.97	1.17	1.40	0.62	0.76	0.91	1.03	0.91	2.01
1200				0.72	0.95	1.11	1.34	0.71	0.88	1.04	1.18	1.04	2.30
1400					0.81	1.06	1.26	0.80	0.98	1.17	1.33	1.17	2.59
1600						0.86	1.18	0.88	1.09	1.29	1.47	1.29	2.87
1800							0.95	0.97	1.19	1.40	1.60	1.41	3.12

*These recommended allowances are taken from the National Research Council's Recommended Nutrient Allowances for Horses.[1]

Table 4.—Calcium and Phosphorus Allowances for Growing Horses in Grams Per Day***

Weight of horse	For horses with mature weights of													
	600 lbs.		800 lbs.		1000 lbs.		1200 lbs.		1400 lbs.		1600 lbs.		1800 lbs.	
	Ca*	P**	Ca	P	Ca	P	Ca	P	Ca	P	Ca	P	Ca	P
200	7.9	7.3	9.8	8.8	12.3	10.6	14.3	12.2	17.9	14.9	20.8	17.7	24.5	20.4
400	8.7	9.1	10.8	10.8	13.4	12.5	16.1	14.6	20.5	17.5	24.6	21.4	27.9	22.3
600	7.8	9.3	10.6	11.2	13.4	13.4	16.9	16.3	21.3	18.9	24.6	22.1	27.4	22.9
800			9.7	10.9	9.8	10.3	15.3	15.3	20.1	18.7	24.9	23.3	27.0	23.9
1000					11.6	12.9	14.7	15.4	17.8	17.8	22.6	22.6	26.5	23.9
1200							12.4	14.0	15.9	16.7	19.5	20.4	23.6	22.6
1400									14.1	15.8	16.8	19.6	21.1	22.0
1600											15.3	17.2	18.3	20.6
1800													16.8	18.9

*Calcium allowance per day in grams.
**Phosphorus allowance per day in grams.
***These recommended allowances are taken from the National Research Council's Recommended Nutrient Allowances for Horses.[1]

absorption from the large intestine of simple-stomached herbivores. Nevertheless, it is recommended that good quality protein rations, adequate in essential amino acids, be fed to horses. This should be done especially for young, growing colts, whose ceca may not have much bacterial enzymatic action during early life.

Table 3 presents information on the daily digestible protein needs of the horse. The data indicate that as the horse reaches mature size, its daily protein needs decrease. Growth elements of the body are high in protein, thus as physical maturity approaches the demands for protein decrease. Protein requirements at maturity are based on daily body needs.

The data in Table 3 also show that the harder the horse works, the greater will be his protein requirements. These needs will vary from those shown in Table 3, depending on the kind of work. The information indicates the unusual requirements for protein during the last quarter of pregnancy, and during lactation. It is very important that adequate protein be fed at that time in order to nourish the foal properly. Not only should the level of protein be adequate, but feeds containing high quality protein should be used in order to insure proper development of the foal.

If, for any reason, the foal does not get enough milk, then a good quality supplement should be added to the mare's milk. Dried skim milk of cows is an excellent feed for such a purpose since it closely resembles mare's milk. Some horsemen use calf starters or other high-nutrient supplements containing dried skim milk to fortify the ration of the foal.

The protein requirements shown in Table 3 are minimal needs. For valuable show and race horses, it would be well to exceed these suggested allowances in order to make sure that sufficient protein is available. If more protein is fed than is needed, the excess is converted to energy and consequently is not lost. Of course, this is an expensive way to supply energy since protein supplements are more costly than other energy-producing feeds. It is good insurance, however, against a possible lack of protein and will provide rapid and proper development of horses which are being prepared for show or racing purposes.

MINERALS

The necessity for feeding mineral supplements will depend upon the levels in the soil. It is as important to add minerals to the soil as well as to the ration in order to improve the quality of pastures and other crops grown thereon. Proper addition of minerals to the soil will increase the mineral content of the feeds as well as tonnage yield.

It should be emphasized that minerals are of the utmost importance in developing horses for show or racing purposes. These animals must have excellent bone development for good sound feet and legs. The old saying, "no foot, no horse," is still true today. Knowledgeable horsemen attribute good feet and legs to the provision of properly fertilized pastures as well as to the supplemental feeding of minerals which may be lacking in the feeds commonly used in the ration. Not only must all the essential minerals be provided, but they should be fed at the right level and in the proper proportion. Only then can horses develop good sound bone with minimal or no blemishes.

The minerals which are needed to perform important functions in the body are: calcium, phosphorus, sodium, chlorine, copper, iron, cobalt, manganese, iodine, zinc, potassium, magnesium, and sulfur.

Calcium and Phosphorus: Calcium and phosphorus are required for bone and teeth formation. They account for more than 70% of the mineral ash in the body. An inadequate supply of either will limit the utilization of the other. To obtain proper utilization of calcium and phosphorus, 3 requirements must be met: 1. Adequate quantities of calcium and phosphorus must be fed, 2, a certain ratio between them must be maintained, and 3, a sufficient amount of vitamin D must be supplied. The amounts and proper ratio of calcium to phosphorus for the horse are shown in Tables 4 and 5. The proper ratio is about one part of calcium to one part phosphorus, with some variation depending on the age of the horse. Vitamin D is needed for absorption and utilization of calcium and phosphorus.

A large excess of either calcium or phosphorus interferes with the absorption of the

Table 5.—Calcium and Phosphorus Allowances for Mares and Mature Horses in Grams Per Day**

Weight of horses, lbs.	Mature horses		Mares in last quarter of pregnancy		Mares during lactation	
	Calcium*	Phosphorus*	Calcium	Phosphorus	Calcium	Phosphorus
400	7.3	8.5	7.8	7.8	12.3	11.2
600	9.9	11.0	10.6	10.6	16.7	15.2
800	12.0	13.7	13.1	13.1	20.6	18.7
1000	13.7	15.4	15.4	15.4	24.4	22.2
1200	15.7	17.7	17.7	17.7	28.0	25.4
1400	17.6	19.8	19.9	19.9	31.4	28.5
1600	19.4	21.8	22.1	22.1	34.9	31.7
1800	21.1	23.8	24.2	24.2	37.9	34.4

*Calcium and phosphorus allowance per day in grams.
**These recommended allowances are taken from the National Research Council's Recommended Nutrient Allowances for Horses.[1]

other. With an excess of either mineral, the other tends to become bound as insoluble tricalcium phosphate which the horse cannot absorb. Similarly, excessive amounts of iron, magnesium, and aluminum in the ration should be avoided, since they interfere with the absorption of phosphorus by forming insoluble phosphates.

The information in Table 4 shows that calcium and phosphorus needs decrease as the horse reaches mature weight. Most bony deposition has occurred by then. Minerals are needed by adults mainly for maintenance of healthy bone and teeth, and for other essential metabolic functions.

The data in Table 5 demonstrate the importance of supplying higher levels of calcium and phosphorus during pregnancy, and especially during lactation. Adequate levels of calcium and phosphorus, as well as other essential minerals, are needed to insure proper growth and development of the foal.

Salt and Trace Minerals: Salt contains both sodium and chloride. It serves as a condiment and as a nutrient. When added to the ration, salt increases palatability. It also is essential to many body functions. Horses which are exercised severely need more salt since a considerable amount is excreted in sweat. It must be replaced or horses will shown signs of fatigue or heat exhaustion. If salt is not fed regularly, an abnormal appetite or craving for it often develops. This is followed by its ex-

cessive consumption which may result in digestive disorders, especially if adequate water is not available.

For best results, salt should be included in the grain ration at a level of 0.5 to 1.0%. Moreover, salt should be available free-choice in a mineral box in the pasture, in the paddock, stall, or wherever horses are kept. Horses will consume an average of 1 to 2 ounces of salt daily. They usually will ingest more salt if it is available in ground rather than in block form.

In certain areas of the United States (Great Lakes region, Pacific Northwest, and other areas), iodine deficiency has been reported in livestock. Unless iodine is supplied in the feed, foals are apt to develop goiter in these areas. Foals deficient in iodine usually are born weak, and are unable to stand and nurse (Fig. 1). Their breathing may be labored and the pulse rate high. There is some evidence that the incidence of "navel ill" in foals may be lessened by feeding iodine to the broodmare. However, more information is needed to confirm this possibility. Iodine is best supplied through the use of iodized salt.

Mineralized salt containing iodine, copper, cobalt, manganese, iron, and zinc is used by many horsemen since the trace mineral supplements add very little to the cost of the salt and provide insurance against possible deficiencies. The author is unaware of clinical manifestations due to a deficiency of many of

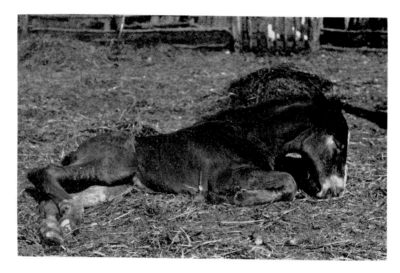

these trace minerals in horses. It is possible, however, that the rapid growth and early maturity demanded of race horses could increase the need for trace minerals. It is recommended that trace mineralized salt be furnished for horses, provided the supplemented minerals are not added excessively. Trace minerals might be helpful at low levels and will do no harm in case they are not needed. At high levels, however, they can be toxic or produce other harmful effects, and it is wise to remember that most mineral elements, if given in excess, will have harmful effects.

A lack of magnesium, potassium, and sulfur has not been shown to occur when well-balanced rations are fed to horses. Therefore, based on present knowledge, there does not seem to be a need to add these elements to equine rations.

This discussion concerning mineral needs indicates that one can supply the mineral requirements of the horse by using bone meal (or some other source of calcium and phosphorus) plus trace mineralized salt which contains iodine, copper, cobalt, iron, manganese, and zinc. The trace mineralized salt can be fed in one compartment and bone meal (mixed with about ⅓ salt to add palatability and to prevent moldiness) in the other compartment of a mineral box. The mineral box should be constructed to keep the supplement dry, and it should be placed low enough for the convenience of young colts. It always should be

kept full of clean, fresh mineral supplement so that horses can consume it at will. Many horsemen prefer to use a commercial mixture of minerals which has good palatability, is well-balanced, and contains the elements needed by the horse.

VITAMINS

Vitamins are important for growth and reproduction, and some are essential for maintaining horses in good health and condition. Unfortunately, very little information is available concerning which vitamins are needed, as well as what levels are required of those essential for the horse.

Vitamin A: Vitamin A is essential for the horse, and it is very important that an adequate level be provided. A lack of vitamin A may cause reproductive failure, nerve degeneration, night blindness, poor hoof development, a predisposition to respiratory infections, lacrimation, incoordination, keratinization of the cornea, progressive weakness, and possibly certain bone and joint disorders (Fig. 2).

Good quality, green pasture is an excellent source of carotene which the horse converts into vitamin A. Therefore, horses consuming enough good, green pasture should get an ample supply of vitamin A. Forages which are mature, or are exposed to rain during the drying process, lose considerable amounts of their carotene content. Much of this carotene ac-

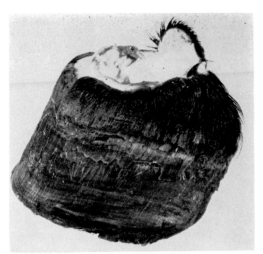

Fig. 2. Hoof of horse which died from vitamin A deficiency. Note scaling of periople. Courtesy of California Agricultural Experiment Station.

tivity also is lost during storage of the hay. The green color in hay or pasture is a good indication of its carotene level. Usually, the more green the color, the higher the carotene content.

The National Research Council[1] recommends 5.0 mg. of carotene per 100 pounds of body weight daily for both growing and mature horses. The recommendations indicate that this should be sufficient to build and maintain body reserves and to meet the demands of various physiologic functions, such as reproduction and lactation. Sager suggests that 4000 to 6000 I.U. of vitamin A per 100 pounds of body weight should be an adequate maintenance level.[8]

Vitamin D: This vitamin is needed by the horse for proper absorption and utilization of calcium and phosphorus. Foals occasionally will develop rickets due to lack of vitamin D, or of calcium and phosphorus. Most of the commonly used feeds, except sun-cured hay, contain little or no vitamin D. Fortunately, by exposing horses to sunlight, vitamin D is formed through the action of the sun's rays on certain oils in the skin. The skin contains the provitamin which is changed to vitamin D by the ultraviolet rays of the sun. Summer sunlight is more potent than winter sunlight in this respect. In areas where sunshine is lacking, it is advisable to add vitamin D to equine rations.

Experimental information is lacking on the exact vitamin D needs of the horse. The National Research Council[1] recommends that 300 I.U. of vitamin D per 100 pounds live weight daily should be adequate to meet the needs of the horse.

Vitamin E: The need for vitamin E supplementation has not been established. Well-balanced rations supposedly should have all the vitamin E needed. However, there may be conditions of stress or conditions in which the vitamin E is destroyed or used rapidly, and then supplementation is warranted. There are many breeders who feel that vitamin E supplementation will improve fertility of mares and stallions.

The requirements for vitamin E are not known. Ensminger has recommended the following daily doses of alpha tocopherol succinate in the feed: stallions and broodmares, 600 to 1000 I.U. beginning a few weeks before breeding; and 2,000 I.U. for race horses in training.[2] These levels can be used as a guide in case vitamin E supplementation seems warranted.

Vitamins C and K: There is no evidence to indicate a need for supplementing horse rations with vitamins C and K. As far as is known, the horse synthesizes all of its needs for these 2 vitamins.

B-Complex Vitamins: The requirements of the horse for the B vitamins have not been well-defined. It is known, however, that the horse needs many of the 11 B vitamins. The group includes: thiamine, riboflavin, niacin, pyridoxine, pantothenic acid, choline, inositol, para-aminobenzoic acid, folacin, biotin, and B_{12}. Thiamine is the only one of these vitamins for which the horse has shown a definite need of a dietary source. Supplementation needs for the others, therefore, are unknown. Under conditions of stress, as when horses are being prepared for racing purposes, it may be good insurance to enrich their rations with extra B vitamins. Hence, many horses are fed commercial protein supplements which are enriched with these vitamins.

There is some indication that periodic ophthalmia (moon blindness) may be due to riboflavin deficiency.[3] There is good evidence, however, that riboflavin is not the only factor concerned in the etiology of this condition. Nevertheless, there have been numerous reports of favorable responses following the administration of 40 mg. of riboflavin per day for prevention of periodic ophthalmia.

This discussion concerning vitamin requirements of horses indicates that little is known about the subject. Until more experimental information is obtained, each veterinarian will need to use his own judgment and relatively few scientific facts to determine whether or not existing conditions justify vitamin supplementation.

In lieu of specific information on the vitamin B requirements of horses the following levels which are recommended for the pig are listed. These can be used as a guide in case one wishes to advocate supplementation of equine rations.

Vitamins	Need per 100 pounds of body weight by the growing pig	
Thiamine	2.6	mg.
Riboflavin	5.3	mg.
Niacin	26.5	mg.
Pantothenic acid	23.8	mg.
Pyridoxine	2.0	mg.
Choline	2000.0	mg.
Vitamin B_{12}	.026	mg.

These levels which are adequate for the pig should also be appropriate for the horse. They probably are higher than his needs since the horse most likely will synthesize more of these vitamins than will the pig.

ANTIBIOTICS

There is some, if scant, information on the use of antibiotics for horses. Rosemere Farms at Ocala, Florida, have experimented with several antibiotics in their feeding program for young horses.[4] It was observed that the antibiotics used tended to promote growth. They also found, however, that it was necessary to increase the level of calcium, phosphorus, and other minerals in the ration to accommodate the extra growth, or skeletal troubles would result.

For cattle, swine, and poultry, antibiotics are most beneficial when the subclinical disease level is high. Similar experience might be anticipated on horse farms. The antibiotics may be beneficial, especially for young foals which do poorly because of malnutrition, infections, digestive troubles, or other stress factors. Caution is required in using antibiotics, and close observation of the horses also is necessary in order to properly evaluate their response.

PASTURE

An excellent pasture is one of the greatest assets a horse farm can have. Good horses and good pastures occur together. Pastures provide top-quality feed, exercise, and a natural environment for developing horses. Almost all of the leading horse farms have fine pastures which are well-fertilized, drained, and kept free of weeds. Pastures for horses should not be allowed to become too tall and mature. Neither should the pasture be allowed to be cropped too short if parasitic infection is to be controlled. Horses have both upper and lower incisor teeth, and if the pasture is short they will eat it to the roots. This is not only a good way to spread parasitic infection, but it also is harmful to the pasture. For good grassland development as well as parasite control, it would be ideal if the horses could be rotated to different pastures in order to rest each field regularly. In summary, the pasture should be kept lush and green—not too short nor too tall. It should provide shade, a source of clean, fresh water, and a mineral box.

Legume, grass, or legume-grass pastures are suitable for horses. Some grasses, during certain periods of the year, may be too laxative for horses which are exercised considerably. This can be controlled somewhat by the feeding of dry grass hay in addition to the pasture. Under certain conditions, it is best to keep broodmares and young colts on the forages which are laxative for horses being exercised or worked vigorously. If need be, pasture use may be restricted in order to give desired results for severely exercised horses.

Many horsemen agree that a lush, green pasture is one of the best guarantees for getting their animals bred. Hence, good grazing areas should be a must for breeding animals as well as for young stock. In addition to being an excellent source of protein, minerals, vitamins, and other nutrients, pasture greatly reduces the cost of raising horses. It must be emphasized that good pastures require an adequate management program to keep them highly nutritious, palatable, and productive. Horses crave green feed, and high quality pasture is one of the best sources. Temporary pastures of oats, rye, wheat, or barley, can be a welcome source of green feed when permanent ones are dormant. Cattle may be used to help fertilize pastures and to keep the grass cropped and short. This allows the horse to consume the young, tender grass which is preferred, and which is higher in nutrients. The cattle will graze the taller forage; beef cattle especially tend to graze well with horses when they become accustomed to one another.

Horses can be turned out on pasture at nights and on idle days. This decreases the amount of grain and hay which must be fed. It also gives the horses a chance to relax and exercise at will.

HAY

Hay is very necessary for a good feeding program. In many areas of the country, timothy is the standard or preferred hay for horses. There are some who will prefer to use only grass hays, whereas other horsemen will use legume or legume-grass hays also. The selection of hay to feed apparently depends on the preference of the feeder. Regardless of the kind, hay should be of top-quality and as free as possible from weeds, dust, and mold. The hay also should be leafy and green, indicating that it has a high nutritive value, and that it was cured properly. The final criterion of quality is the response obtained from the horses. If hay is too laxative or if the horses do not like it, another should be used. Soil, level of fertilization, and other factors will influence the effect that hay or pasture may have on horses.

Obtaining good quality hay is a serious problem on many farms, particularly when they are not equipped for making their own.

Moreover, the cost of shipping hay from any great distance is considerable; consequently, it is advisable to obtain high quality hay in a nearby locality if possible.

Horses can be fed too much hay. This will cause labored breathing and early tiring when they are worked heavily. Feeding of concentrates should be increased and hay feeding decreased as the amount of work and exercise increases. When roughage allowances necessarily are limited, it sometimes will be necessary to muzzle greedy horses to keep them from eating the bedding.

It is claimed that feeding alfalfa will increase urine output and also be laxative, consequently on some farms alfalfa is fed only at low levels, or only 2 or 3 times a week. In other areas, however, alfalfa is the only hay fed, and with good results. The difference in experiences with alfalfa may depend on the area where it was grown, its stage of maturity, and how it was cured. There are some who think that alfalfa is so palatable that horses will eat too much, and that impactions will result. Thus, they prefer to limit alfalfa to a reasonable amount, depending on the quality of the alfalfa and the horse. At any rate, alfalfa is a hay of excellent quality and its use must be gauged by the response obtained under existing conditions. Many horsemen prefer second or third cuttings of alfalfa since the first cutting sometimes is coarse and weedy.

Since a distended digestive tract is a hindrance to a horse's working or exercising hard, $\frac{1}{2}$ or more of the hay allowance can be fed at night. The remainder is divided between the other feedings during the day. If hay is fed only twice during the day, about $\frac{2}{3}$ of it is fed at night when the animal has enough time for its mastication and digestion. Lighter portions of hay are preferable when horses are shipped to the race track or when they are worked or exercised considerably.

The minimum roughage requirements of the horse are about 0.5% of its body weight. In other words, a 1,000-pound horse would require a minimum of 5 pounds of roughage. However, many horsemen prefer to feed at least a minimum of 1.0% of body weight or 10 pounds of roughage for a 1,000-pound horse. Since individual horses vary in stomach capacity, it is necessary to experiment to find the minimum roughage needs for each individual horse. It is important to determine the minimum roughage needs for horses being prepared for racing since as much TDN as possible should be fed. The least amount of roughage necessary is fed.

Methods of feeding hay vary. Many prefer to feed it in a low manger so that the horse will not inhale so much dust when eating. Others prefer to put hay on the ground, since they feel that racks or mangers can injure young animals.

GRAINS AND MOLASSES

The most used and popular grain for horses is oats. They are the standard with which all other grains are compared. Whole or rolled oats are used extensively. Oats are less concentrated than the other grains due to their bulky hulls. Thus, they tend to form a loose mass in the stomach, whereas some of the other grains tend to pack. For horses with poor teeth, or for young foals, it is best to use rolled or crushed oats. Bright, heavy oats, which contain a smaller percentage of hull, are preferred for adult, vigorous horses. Musty oats should not be used as they may cause colic.

Second to oats, corn is used most often for feeding horses in the United States. Most horsemen prefer to mix corn with oats in about equal parts. Corn should not be ground finely since it may form a mass in the stomach and thus cause colic. It can be cracked, ground coarsely, or rolled. Most horsemen feed corn only during the cool weather, and remove it when the weather gets warm.

Barley is used very extensively in many foreign countries. Many who use barley in this country prefer to mix it with oats in about equal parts. Because of its hardness it should be coarsely ground, or preferably rolled. There are some who prefer to soak the barley.

Wheat is not fed extensively to horses. When ground, wheat is rather doughy, and tends to pack with moisture. If used, it might best be rolled and mixed at a low level with a bulky feed such as oats or wheat bran. Wheat bran is used extensively for horses. It is valuable for its bulky nature and mild laxative effect. It usually is fed at levels of about 10 to 15% of the grain mixture.

Any of the grain feeds used should be of excellent quality and not moldy, dusty, or spoiled. Many horsemen prefer to have their grains steam-rolled in preference to grinding them. This gives a lighter ration which should result in less digestive disturbances.

Where mixing facilities are adequate or available, one can have 5 to 10% portions of molasses sprayed on the grain mixture during the mixing process. This sweetens the feed and makes it more palatable, thus encourages greater intake.

PROTEIN SUPPLEMENTS

Linseed meal is the most popular protein supplement for horses, probably because it is associated with the production of bloom and luster in the hair coat. Occasionally, however, one will hear complaints that the linseed meal available now is not as good in quality as it once was. Pelleted linseed meal and soybean oil meal also are used for horses. Other protein supplements have been used but there is little information about their nutrient value.

Commercial protein supplements which are well-fortified with minerals and vitamins often are fed by those who are developing horses for racing purposes. They feed their horses these supplements in excess in order to get as much weight for age as possible, and they are anxious that their ration be adequate in all essential nutrients. Linseed meal or other protein supplement, plus a commercial protein supplement in about equal proportions can be used for this purpose.

WATER

Horses always should have a good source of clean, fresh water. If they are deprived of water for any length of time, they should not be allowed to drink heavily at one time. This applies particularly to horses worked or exercised heavily. They should be allowed to cool off for a while before a considerable intake of water is allowed.

Table 6.—Approximate Percentage of T.D.N., Digestible Protein, Calcium and Phosphorus in Rations for Horses* (Based on air dry feed containing 90% dry matter)

Class of horses	Digestible protein	Total digestible nutrients	Calcium	Phosphorus
	%	%	%	%
Mature horses:				
Maintenance	4.9	62.5	0.17	0.19
Light work	4.8	62.5	0.17	0.19
Medium work	4.8	62.5	0.16	0.18
Hard work	4.7	66.7	0.16	0.18
Last quarter of pregnancy	5.3	62.1	0.20	0.20
Lactating mares	8.2	71.4	0.22	0.20
Growing horses:				
Up to 1 year	10.3	62.5	0.38	0.33
1 to 2 years	6.0	62.5	0.23	0.23
2 to 3 years	5.2	62.5	0.19	0.20

*These recommended allowances are taken from the National Research Council's Recommended Nutrient Allowances for Horses.[1]

There is a difference of opinion regarding when horses should be watered. Some think that they should be watered only before feeding whereas others think it should be done only after feeding. All agree, however, that horses should be watered frequently and regularly. When in doubt, it would be safest to provide water in small amounts rather than allow the animal to drink too heavily.

Water intake varies depending on the kind of work or exercise performed, the type of ration used, weather conditions, and other factors. It must be emphasized that proper water intake is as important as good feed.

PELLETING OF FEEDS

The pelleting of feeds for all classes of livestock is increasing. As equipment is improved and costs decrease, the use of pelleted feeds will increase even more. There are many advantages to be derived from using pelleted feeds. One is the elimination of dustiness. Those who have tried pelleted feeds for horses have been pleased with the results. It seems reasonable to predict that they will become more popular for equine feedings, and that their use will increase greatly in the future.

Pelleting the whole ration (grain and hay) has been tried, reportedly with good results.

Pelleting is an excellent way to feed dehydrated alfalfa meal. The use of 5 to 10% high quality, dehydrated alfalfa meal in equine rations should be beneficial. Alfalfa is an excellent source of vitamins, minerals, protein, and unidentified factors which can enrich many rations and increase their nutritional adequacy. If alfalfa meal is used, it should be of the highest quality. It should contain a minimum of 17% protein and 100,000 I.U. of vitamin A per pound. High quality alfalfa is comparable in food value to green pasture, and may be especially valuable during periods of the year when the pastures are dormant.

The data in Table 6 show the percentage of various nutrients needed in rations. This information is of considerable value in compounding rations.

SUCCESSFULLY USED RATIONS

Some rations which have been used successfully by various colleges and universities are presented as guides to use when comparing or computing rations. The following ration has been used with excellent results by the California Polytechnic College at San Luis Obispo.[5] It is fed to their young growing horses until they are sold as yearlings or 2-year-olds. It is combined with a mixture of 50% alfalfa and 50% oat hay, plus pasture.

Ingredient	Percent
Steam rolled oats	54.0
Steam rolled barley	20.0
Cracked yellow corn	10.0
Wheat bran	10.0
Linseed meal pellets	5.0
Steamed bone meal	0.5
Trace mineralized salt	0.5
	100.0

The following ration has been used with excellent results by Louisiana State University at Baton Rouge.[6] The ration is fed to all horses—pregnant and lactating mares, show horses, and developing foals. The only modification regularly made is that calf manna is added for the foals. The ration is fed with some permanent and some temporary pastures (red clover and rye grass). Bermuda grass hay is used whenever the pasture is short.

Ingredient	Percent
Oats, crimped	50.0
Corn, No. 2 yellow, cracked	14.0
Wheat bran	10.0
Alfalfa leaf meal	5.0
Linseed meal	7.5
Iodized salt	0.5
Steamed bone meal	0.5
Molasses	12.5
	100.0

The following rations have been used very successfully at Washington State University Hilltop Stables at Pullman.[7]

Stallions—900 to 1,200 lbs.

Ingredient	Ration 1 Percent	Ration 2 Percent
Steam rolled corn	10	—
Steam rolled oats	30	45
Steamed rolled barley	35	35
Linseed meal	10	11
Calf manna—Albers	6	—
Iodized salt	1	1
Steamed bone meal	1	1
Molasses	7	7
	100	100

Ration 1—is used during the breeding season and is fed at the rate of 1¼ pounds per 100 pounds body weight.

Ration 2—is used during the off-season and is fed at the rate of ¾ pounds per 100 pounds body weight.

Pregnant Mares—900 to 1,400 lbs.

	Ration 1 Percent	Ration 2 Percent	Ration 3 Percent
Steamed rolled barley	50	40	30
Steamed rolled oats	30	30	30
Soybean oil meal	11	11	11
Steamed bone meal	1	1	1
Iodized salt	1	1	1
Molasses	7	7	7
Wheat bran	—	10	10
Steamed rolled corn	—	—	10
	100	100	100

Ration 1—is used in early pregnancy and is fed at the rate of ½ to 1 pound per 100 pounds body weight.

Ration 2—is used in late pregnancy and is fed at the rate of 1 to 1½ pounds per 100 pounds body weight.

Ration 3—is fed during lactation. The amount fed will depend on the amount of milk produced and the amount the foal can consume without scouring.

Suckling Foals—100 to 450 lbs.

Steamed rolled oats	70
Linseed meal	11
Wheat bran	10
Molasses	7
Steamed bone meal	1
Iodized salt	1
	100

This ration is fed at the rate of ½ to ¾ pounds per 100 pounds body weight.

Weanling Foals—450 to 600 lbs.

	Percent
Steamed rolled oats	20
Steamed rolled barley	20
Steamed rolled corn	15
Soybean oil meal	11
Albers Sho Glo	25
Molasses	7
Steamed bone meal	1
Iodized salt	1
	100

This ration is fed at the rate of 1 to 1½ pounds per 100 pounds body weight.

Yearlings (Show and Sale)—600 to 1,000 lbs.

	Percent
Wheat bran	10
Steamed rolled oats	20
Steamed rolled barley	35
Albers Calf Manna	11
Soybean oil meal	15
Molasses	7
Steamed bone meal	1
Iodized salt	1
	100

This ration is fed at the rate of ½ to 1½ pounds per 100 pounds body weight for yearlings. The 2-year-olds are fed the same ration at the rate of ½ pound per 100 pounds body weight.

Hay Fed to Horses in Pounds per 100 lbs. Body Weight

	Alfalfa	Alfalfa Grass 40-60%
Stallions (a) breeding ..	1–1½	1–1½
(b) idle	¾–1½	¾–1½
Pregnant mares		¾–1½
Lactating mares	1–1¾	
Suckling foals	½– ¾	
Weanling foals		1½–2
Yearlings (show and sale)		½– ¾
2-year-olds	1–1½	1–1¾

The rations used by these 3 institutions are representative, and they can serve as a guide in developing rations for horses. Many modifications can be made depending on availability of feeds, the response obtained, as well as the likes or dislikes of the horseman.

Mashes of bran (sometimes of oats) are fed to mares shortly before and after they foal. The mare is then brought to full feed slowly after foaling. She should be fed enough grain mix to supply plenty of milk for the foal, and still keep her in a thrifty condition.

Some horsemen creep-feed their foals. Others prefer not to use a creep since this system makes it difficult to know whether or not a foal is eating. They prefer to feed the foals individually. Supplemental feeding usually is started when the foals are 6 to 8 weeks of age. The mare is confined while the foal is fed. On most farms the foals will be eating 6 to 8 pounds of feed by the time they are weaned.

QUANTITY OF FOOD (TABLE 7)

In addition to the levels of feeding advised by Washington State University the following levels are suggested as a guide in determining how much feed should be given to horses:

1. *For horses with light activity (1 to 3 hours per day of riding or driving).*
   (a) About ½ pound of grain mix and 1¼ to 1½ pounds of hay (or pasture equivalent) per 100 pounds of body weight.
2. *For horses with medium activity (3 to 5 hours per day of riding or driving).*

Table 7.—Daily Allowances for Mature Horses*

Body Wgt. lb.	Dry Matter—90% Basis		Total Digestible Nutrients		Digestible protein		Calcium	Phosphorus
	Maintenance	Work Light	Maintenance	Work Light	Maintenance	Work Light		
	lb.	lb.	lb.	lb.	lb.	lb.	Gm.	Gm.
400	6.2	8.2	3.9	5.1	0.31	0.38	7.3	8.5
600	8.5	11.0	5.3	6.9	0.42	0.52	9.9	11.0
800	10.6	13.8	6.6	8.6	0.53	0.65	12.2	13.7
1000	12.6	16.2	7.9	10.1	0.62	0.76	13.7	15.4
1200	14.4	18.6	9.0	11.6	0.71	0.88	15.7	17.7

Mares—Last Quarter of Gestation

Body Wgt. lb.		Dry Matter		Total Digestible Nutrients		Digestible protein	Calcium	Phosphorus
400		8.6		5.4		0.46	7.8	7.8
600		11.7		7.3		0.62	10.6	10.6
800		14.4		9.0		0.77	13.1	13.1
1000		17.0		10.6		0.91	15.4	15.4
1200		19.5		12.2		1.09	17.7	17.7

Mares—Lactating

Body Wgt. lb.		Dry Matter		Total Digestible Nutrients		Digestible protein	Calcium	Phosphorus
400		12.3		8.8		1.01	12.3	11.2
600		16.7		11.9		1.37	16.7	15.2
800		20.6		14.7		1.70	20.6	18.7
1000		24.4		17.4		2.01	24.4	22.2
1200		28.0		20.0		2.30	28.0	25.4

*Table, courtesy of Dr. H. H. Sutton.

(a) About 1 pound of grain mix and 1 to 1¼ pounds of hay (or some pasture equivalent) per 100 pounds of body weight.

3. *For horses with considerable activity (5 to 8 hours per day of riding or driving).*
(a) About 1¼ to 1½ pounds of grain mix and about 1 pound of hay (or some pasture equivalent) per 100 pounds of body weight.

In using this guide, the amounts are increased or decreased as the horse gains or loses weight excessively.

It should be stressed that overfeeding as well as underfeeding have been detrimental to many horses. The saying "The eye of the master fattens the beast" still is very true.

RECOMMENDED FEEDING PRACTICES

1. To develop top-quality horses, they should be fed as individuals after a careful study of each animal's peculiarities and needs. Some are slow and others are fast eaters. One animal may do well on only part of the feed required by another. Some will respond well to one caretaker and not to another.

2. The feces of horses should be observed frequently. They should be examined for consistency, unusual odors and abnormal color.

3. The feed boxes should be inspected frequently to determine the horse's eating habits. Feed boxes should be kept clean at all times. Moldy, old or spoiled feed should never be allowed to accumulate.

4. Animals always should be fed at the same time every day, including weekends.

5. Eating too rapidly can be controlled by using a large feed box and spreading the feed thinly. Another method is to place smooth rocks in the feed box, thus forcing the horse to eat slowly.

6. Rations should not be changed abruptly.

7. Caretakers should be instructed to work

quietly around horses and thus attempt to gain the animal's confidence.

8. Many prefer to feed horses twice daily and expect them to eat all of the grain ration in about 30 minutes. When an animal does not consume its grain ration rapidly it should be decreased gradually until the portion fed is eaten within 30 minutes or so. While at race meetings, horses usually are fed 3 or 4 times per day. A common practice is to feed an equal part of the concentrates at each of the feedings during the day.

9. It must be emphasized that quality of the feed is of utmost importance. Good commercial horse feeds are satisfactory for the person who has only 1 or 2 animals.

10. On days of idleness, the concentrate allowance for horses should be cut at least in half and the hay or pasture allowance increased.

11. In general, feeds that are too heavy will have a tendency to pack in the stomach. Feeds that are too high in fiber will tend to cause digestive disturbances, particularly in horses which are exercised vigorously.

12. The maintenance requirement of horses will represent about one-half of their daily needs. Consequently, the ration must be palatable in order to insure adequate consumption to meet maintenance requirements plus the other needs.

13. Horses develop a better appetite and their digestion and general well-being are improved when they get adequate exercise.

14. It must be noted that some horses work or run best when they are slightly underweight. Others need more size and conditioning to perform at their maximum. The level of feeding will vary with different horses, but the quality of the ration always must be high in order to supply the essential nutrients for sound bodies.

T. J. Cunha

REFERENCES

1. Pearson, P. B., Winchester, C. F., and Harvey, A. L.: Recommended Nutrient Allowances for Horses. National Research Council Publication. 1949.
2. Ensminger, M. E.: Light Horses. U.S.D.A. Farmers' Bulletin No. 2127. 1958.
3. Jones, T. C., Roby, T. O. and Maurer, F. D.: Am. J. Vet. Research 7 (1946) 403.
4. Heubeck, Elmer, Jr.: Feeding practices on Thoroughbred farms. The Blood-Horse Magazine. Page 16.
5. Bennion, L. L.: Personal communication. 1961.
6. Fowler, Stewart H.: Personal communication. 1961.
7. Ensminger, M. E.: Personal communication. 1961.
8. Sager, F. C. Feeding Horses. Stud Managers' Handbook, Lexington, Ky. 1958.

NUTRITIONAL DEFICIENCIES

Avitaminosis B

The vitamin B complex group is made up of 11 water soluble vitamins. They are heat-stable with the exception of pantothenic acid or its salt, calcium pantothenate. This group of vitamins is sensitive to light and many are oxidized easily. All are less stable in solution than in the dry state. The B-complex group is composed of vitamin B_1 or thiamine (aneurine), vitamin B_2 or riboflavin (lactoflavin), vitamin B_6 (pyridoxine), niacin (nicotinic acid), vitamin B_{12} (cyanocobalamine), biotin (also known as vitamin H, coezyme R, and Bios II), para-aminobenzoic acid (PABA), inositol (Bios I), folic acid, pantothenic acid, and choline. The ones of importance in equine nutrition will be discussed.

This group of vitamins is, in the main, synthesized in the alimentary tract of herbiverous animals. Recent experimental work, however, indicates that the availablity of the B-complex vitamins produced by synthesis in the large colon of the horse are not available to this animal. Colostrum is an excellent source of the B-complex vitamins for the newborn foal.[2] The vitamins in this group which are most important in equine nutrition are thiamine chloride, riboflavin, niacin, pantothenic acid, pyridoxine, biotin, and folic acid. It should be noted that a deficiency of any one B vitamin almost invariably is accompanied with a similar insufficiency of others.

Thiamine Deficiency

Deficiencies of thiamine occur in horses during heavy training, following high temperatures, during debilitating diseases and, of course, with insufficient intake. The classic example of primary thiamine deficiency in the horse is seen following ingestion of plants containing thiaminase, such as bracken fern and horsetail (*Equisetum* spp.).

Thiamine is active as a cocarboxylase in metabolism of fats, carbohydrates, and proteins and deficiency of this vitamin causes the accumulation of endogenous pyruvates. Although the brain is known to depend largely on carbohydrates as a source of energy, there is no obvious relationship between a lack of thiamine and the development of a nervous syndrome which characterizes this deficiency. Other signs of deficiency, such as inappetence and changes in the circulatory system, are hard to relate to the known functions of thiamine. The use of thiamine in the treatment of myoglobinuria may be open to criticism, but the accumulation of lactic acid in the affected muscles suggests that its use is justified.[2] Thiamine is readily absorbed from the intestines. Very little is stored, liver and heart muscles being the main depots. Excess is excreted in the urine. When absorbed, thiamine is converted, probably in the liver, into thiamine pyrophosphate (cocarboxylase). As such it acts as a coenzyme for several decarboxylating enzyme systems, the most important of which is probably decarboxylase. This enzyme is necessary for the decarboxylation of pyruvic acid, well-known as an intermediate stage in carbohydrate metabolism.[5]

Etiology: The classic cause of thiamine deficiency in the horse is produced by consumption of *Equisetum* spp. and bracken fern, which are known to contain large quantities of the antivitamin, thiaminase. Subclinical to clinical deficiencies may be caused by hard training or work. High temperatures and the debilitating diseases, such as infections and parasitism, also can contribute to avitaminosis B_1. Gross malnutrition invariably will produce a deficiency as vitamin B_1 is stored in the liver and myocardium for only short periods of time, probably not more than 2 weeks.

Clinical Signs: The signs of acute thiamine deficiency as seen in bracken fern and horsetail poisoning are incoordination, bradycardia, arching of the back, trismus, clonic convulsions, opisthotonus, and recumbency. The appetite usually is fair and the temperature normal. In the terminal stages, the temperature and pulse rate may rise above normal. In other cases, one may see muscular incoordination, inappetence, lethargy, and loss of stamina. These manifestations in the racing horse often are referred to as "tailing off." Abnormally fluid bowel eliminations also may be caused by thiamine deficiency. The hair coat usually becomes dull and the skin somewhat dry. Coprophagy in horses has been attributed to a deficiency of thiamine.

Diagnosis: In acute thiamine deficiency, the blood pyruvic acid levels are raised from the normal of 2 to 3 mcg. per 100 ml. to 6 to 8 mcg. per 100 ml. Myocardial deficiency often is seen. In the normal horse, the blood thiamine chloride levels are from 8 to 10 mcg. per 100 ml. but may be reduced to 2 to 3 mcg. per 100 ml. in a deficiency.[2] At necropsy, there is an interstitial edema of the myocardium, liver, and intestines.[2]

Sources: Vitamin B_1 is present in most all plants. Yeast and wheat germ are excellent sources. Milk, whole cereal grains, peanuts, molasses, and soybeans are good sources of vitamin B_1.

Treatment: The treatment dose rate for thiamine deficiency is 0.25 to 0.5 mg. per kg. of body weight administered daily until the clinical signs are no longer evident. In horses with myoglobinuria, 1.25 mg. per kg. of body weight are administered subcutaneously. Excessive doses can be toxic. The toxic signs are characterized by peripheral vasodilation, cardiac arrhythmia, depression of respirations with asphyxial convulsions, and death due to respiratory failure.

Control: The daily maintenance requirement of thiamine is from 30 to 60 mcg. per kg. of body weight. The addition of yeast, cereals, grains, and milk to the ration usually provides adequate supplies of this vitamin.

RIBOFLAVIN DEFICIENCY

Deficiency of riboflavin (vitamin B_2, vitamin G, lactoflavin) may occur under normal feeding conditions since most rations are low in this vitamin. Milk and actively growing green plants are fair sources, but the cereal hays and grains contain little or no riboflavin. Consequently, in most instances this vitamin must be supplied from a synthetic source. Little has been written regarding the synthesis of riboflavin in the intestinal tract of the horse.

Riboflavin is absorbed rapidly from the intestines or injection site and is distributed promptly throughout the body. Excretion is via the urinary system. The main organ of storage for riboflavin is the liver, however, small quantities exist in practically all organs. After absorption, it is phosphorylated into 2 coenzymes and these agents promote alternate oxidation and reduction reactions, often in conjunction with other enzymes containing nicotinic acid. Riboflavin has a direct effect on the metabolism of carbohydrates, amino acids, and aldehydes.[5]

Clinical Signs: Experimental diets deficient in riboflavin cause the following signs: anorexia, retarded growth, diarrhea, salivation, lacrimation, and alopecia. There may be areas of hyperemia around the oral commissures and navel. Riboflavin deficiency also has been indicted as a cause of periodic ophthalmia (moon blindness). Various types of ocular disorders have been attributed to a deficiency of riboflavin in other species. Microcytic anemia and certain nervous manifestations have been reported to occur in riboflavin deficiency.

Diagnosis: Diagnosis of riboflavin deficiency is extremely difficult. A history of questionable feeding practices for animals exhibiting characteristic clinical signs would indicate the potential value of a chemical analysis to determine the riboflavin blood level. It is most unlikely that deficiency of this or any water-soluble vitamin would occur exclusive of other concurrent deficiencies.

Sources: Of the natural sources of riboflavin, milk is the best one available. In order to supply adequate amounts of this vitamin, synthetic riboflavin ordinarily is used. Actively growing green plants are fair sources, so horses on excellent pasture usually are not deficient.

Treatment and Control: The daily maintenance requirement of riboflavin for the horse is from 2 to 4 mg. per 100 pounds of body weight, and in most instances this must be added as a synthetic supplement, or as dried whole milk.[5] Approximately 100 pounds of dried whole milk per ton of feed will supply the required amount of riboflavin. An intake of 40 mg. of riboflavin daily has been stated to prevent periodic ophthalmia. This intake

and even higher ones are of no value in treating the condition once it has become established. There is much controversy as to whether riboflavin has any effect in preventing periodic ophthalmia. Extensive field trials indicate, however, that it may be of value. Riboflavin is contained in sufficient quantities in parenteral and oral B-complex vitamin preparations.

NIACIN DEFICIENCY

Niacin (nicotinic acid, nicotinamide) also is known as the PP factor (pellagra preventing). Niacin deficiency is thought by some not to occur in the horse since it is believed that this vitamin is synthesized, absorbed, and utilized by this species.[1] However, horses in active training and on a protein-deficient diet, particularly a diet that is deficient in tryptophane, may develop evidence of niacin deficiency. Horses fed considerable corn, which is notoriously deficient in tryptophane, may show evidence of hyponiacinosis.

Niacin is absorbed rapidly after any route of administration. It is stored mainly in the liver, but only in small amounts. It undergoes methylation in the liver and is excreted in urine. After it has been assimilated, it is converted into nicotinamide. Nicotinamide is then combined in the tissues with adenosine, ribose, and phosphoric acid to form coenzyme I, diphosphoridine nucleotide (DPN), and coenzyme II, triphosphoridine nucleotide (TPN). These coenzymes act as hydrogen carriers for the oxidation-reduction processes in which they are essential. They act in conjunction with riboflavin coenzymes and are particularly important in carbohydrate metabolism. The essential amino acid, tryptophane, is a precursor of niacin, and dietary niacin is not required if sufficient tryptophane is present in the diet along with pyridoxine and vitamin E which are essential for this conversion.

Clinical Signs: The signs of hyponiacinosis are not well-defined in the horse, and probably occur only during a very low protein intake, or in horses fed a diet high in corn.

Diagnosis: If a hypoproteinemia and a negative nitrogen balance are demonstrated by blood chemistry, then hyponiacinosis probably is present.

Sources: The cereal grains are only a fair source of niacin. Yeast, legumes, and soybeans probably are the best sources. The optimum sources of synthetic origin are derived mainly from the alkaloid, nicotine.

Treatment and Control: The daily maintenance requirement is approximately 0.2 mg. per pound of body weight for parenteral or oral use. Nicotinamide should be used because it is utilizable immediately, and has few reactions. The parenteral administration of niacin produces a rapid, generalized vasodilation.[5] It should be administered at the rate of 100 to 200 mg. per day for the average horse. The ration should be adjusted to contain as much of the natural vitamin as possible.

PANTOTHENIC ACID DEFICIENCY

Pantothenic acid is a dietary essential for the horse since it is not synthesized *in vivo*. If there is a deficiency of riboflavin, there likely will be a pantothenic acid deficiency. It is found mainly in the form of calcium pantothenate which is very unstable in solutions having a high pH, and is readily destroyed by heat. It is the least stable of all of the B-complex vitamins and when cooked feeds are fed exclusively, a hypopantothenosis likely will occur. Deficiencies can occur in horses fed a ration primarily of whole cereal grains, or one consisting exclusively of oat hay or cooked feeds.

Pantothenic acid is absorbed readily from any route of administration. It is a component of coenzyme A, which is concerned with acetylation processes. This vitamin is essential for the conversion of acetates to sterols, and adrenal cortex necrosis is thought to be caused by a hypopantothenosis. Pantothenic acid is necessary for the acetylation of the sulfonamides and through its incorporation into coenzyme A it is involved with carbohydrate and fat metabolism. It also is necessary for the release of energy, for muscle contraction, and for other vital processes.[5]

Clinical Signs: Experimentally induced deficiencies of pantothenic acid are manifested by a rough hair coat, alopecia, retarded growth, usually a secondary pneumonia, and insufficiency of the adrenal cortex.[2]

Diagnosis: Diagnosis is based upon a history of a known lack of pantothenic acid intake, evidence of malnutrition, signs of adrenal cortex insufficiency, and asthenia. A diet consisting exclusively of oat hay or cooked feeds may be related to the characteristic clinical signs.

Sources: Sources of pantothenic acid include yeast, cane molasses, peanut meal, milk and milk by-products, and green grass. Pantothenic acid also is produced synthetically.

Treatment and Control: The daily maintenance requirements of pantothenic acid are between 100 and 200 mcg. per 100 pounds of body weight. About 200 mcg. per pound of body weight per day have proved effective in treatment and control. The addition of 10 to 12 Gm. per ton of feed is adequate.[2]

BIOTIN DEFICIENCY (HYPOBIOTINOSIS)

Biotin occurs naturally in most all plant and animal tissues. It is required in small amounts, and deficiencies are unlikely to occur, except during prolonged administration of sulfonamides or antibiotics. Avicidin, a biotin antivitamin, occurs in egg white. Experimentally produced deficiencies may result in posterior paralysis.[2]

VITAMIN B$_{12}$ DEFICIENCY

Vitamin B$_{12}$ also is known as cyanocobalamine. The occurrence of its deficiency has not been well-documented but it probably does not occur under natural conditions except during a primary deficiency of cobalt. Cobalt is necessary for the synthesis of cyanocobalamine. A deficiency is most likely to occur in racing animals, particularly those on a low protein intake.[2] Severe parasitic infections also may cause a vitamin B$_{12}$ deficiency.

Cyanocobalamine is absorbed readily following parenteral administration but it is doubtful that much absorption occurs from the gastrointestinal tract. After parenteral administration, some of this compound is bound to protein. Small quantities are stored in all tissues, but storage chiefly is in the liver. Cyano-cobalamine is an important factor in carbo-hydrate, protein, nucleoprotein, and fat metab-olism.

Vitamin B_{12} is essential for the synthesis of nucleoprotein. It also is necessary for mainte-nance of normal sulfhydryl levels in blood. Vitamin B_{12} is a methylating agent and affects fat metabolism in the liver. It is exceedingly important in maintaining normal hemopoiesis, in the maintenance of the neural myelin sheaths, and in protection of the liver from fatty degeneration caused by chlorinated hy-drocarbons and other toxins.

Vitamin B_{12} is important in the maintenance of ovum and sperm production. In general, it is involved in the maintenance of all tissues in which protein and nucleoprotein synthesis oc-curs, and where fat conversion proceeds.[5] Vit-amin B_{12} was referred to as the "animal protein factor" long before its chemical formula was revealed.

Clinical Signs: In a deficiency of vitamin B_{12} fertility may be impaired and, in studies of infertility, consideration should be given to the possibility of hypocyanocobalaminosis. Muscu-lar weakness, poor condition, and anemia are other clinical signs of a deficiency.

Diagnosis: A deficiency of B_{12} should be suspected when there is a history of cobalt deficiency and a lowering of the erythrocyte count. The presence of characteristic clinical signs in horses being fed subminimal protein rations likewise should prompt suspicion of a deficiency in vitamin B_{12}.

Sources: Liver is the best known natural source of B_{12}. However, milk and milk by-products contain adequate amounts. There is little or none present in green feeds. Vitamin B_{12} is a by-product of the antibiotic manufac-turing processes and practically all of the vita-min is obtained from this source.

Treatment and Control: The addition of co-balt to the ration usually will correct a sub-clinical deficiency. Vitamin B_{12} is administered routinely by the parenteral route to race horses and those being worked strenuously. It is used primarily to overcome anorexia, weakness, and anemia, and it has been used as an alleviating factor in some types of lameness. The dosage

ordinarily used is from 1000 to 2000 mcg. at biweekly to weekly intervals.[2]

Folic Acid Deficency

Folic acid also is known as pterylglutamic acid. Little is known concerning its deficiency and its action in the horse. A simple deficiency of folic acid in the horse has not been described as yet.

Deficiencies may occur when the diet con-sists solely of cooked feeds since heat will de-stroy folic acid. Prolonged administration of sulfonamides also may produce a deficiency.

Folic acid is absorbed readily from the in-testinal tract, and it probably is synthesized there. In combination with vitamin B_{12}, or cyanocobalamine, folic acid is involved in nu-cleic acid synthesis and in the production of nucleoproteins.[5] Folic acid is believed neces-sary for erythrocytic maturation.

Sources: The natural sources of folic acid are yeast, wheat, and green feeds. It also is avail-able as sodium foliate which can be given either orally or parenterally.

Treatment and Control: If a deficiency is suspected, the addition of natural feeds con-taining folic acid is indicated. Sodium foliate can be given either orally or parenterally at a rate of approximately 100 mg. per day for 4 to 7 days.

Choline Deficiency

Little is known regarding choline deficiency in the horse but it is likely that in liver dis-eases there may be less of this vitamin stored. Choline deficiency also may occur in cases of gross malnutrition, and in animals fed rations low in the essential amino acids, methionine and betaine.

Choline is absorbed readily from the intes-tinal tract or following its parenteral injection. This vitamin is distributed widely throughout the body but by far the largest amount is stored in the liver. Choline is involved in methylation processes, increases phospholipid metabolism in the liver, and is capable of pre-venting fatty changes in the liver. It is thought that choline will mobilize fat from an already fatty liver.[5]

Sources: Choline is a component of lecithin and is found in high concentration in most animal tissues, wheat, and soybeans.

Treatment and Control: Choline is employed in treatment as choline dehydrogencitrate or choline gluconate. The dosage for horses has not been well-established, however, this vitamin is relatively nontoxic and they probably will tolerate massive doses. Horses receiving a ration high in the essential amino acid, methionine, are not likely to have a choline deficiency as it is a precursor of choline. In the treatment of fatty degeneration or infiltration and other hepatic conditions, one of the salts of choline should be given orally along with a ration high in soybean oil meal. In cattle, a dose of 25 to 50 Gm. of choline salts is given either orally or subcutaneously. This dosage probably will be sufficient for the horse.[5]

VITAMIN K DEFICIENCY

Vitamin K is known as the antihemorrhagic vitamin. The classic deficiency of vitamin K is seen in sweet clover poisoning where toxic quantities of coumarin severely depress prothrombin levels and interfere with the blood clotting mechanism. Many industrial wastes also contain anticoagulants of the coumarin type. Subclinical deficiencies may occur in horses fed a ration of dried bleached hay or grasses for an extended period.

Vitamin K is synthesized in the intestinal tract from whence it probably is absorbed. It also may be supplied in the form of green forage or top-quality green hay. Absorption of vitamin K is dependent upon the presence of bile and fats in the intestines. Storage is mainly in the liver. Vitamin K is essential for the formation of prothrombin in the liver, and lack of it results in hypoprothrombinemia.

Sources: Green feeds are excellent natural sources. Menadione, the synthetic vitamin K, is used therapeutically.

Treatment and Control: In acute vitamin K deficiency, the administration of menadione is imperative; 100 to 400 mg. may be given in a 24-hour period, depending on the size of the animal and the severity of the condition. Menadione is used in conjunction with coagulants and vitamin C to control epistaxis in race horses. This same treatment also may be used postsurgically to control bleeding. Hemorrhage from trauma and rupture of the uterine arteries postpartum may be controlled by the use of menadione and the coagulant drugs. A supply of good green forage provides an adequate intake for the normal horse.

PYRIDOXINE DEFICIENCY

Pyridoxine, or vitamin B_6, deficiency seldom, if ever, occurs under natural conditions. After feeding experimental diets deficient in pyridoxine, one may see anorexia, retarded growth, apathy, dull hair coat, and alopecia. Some central nervous system disturbances also may be seen. Pyridoxine is the most stable of all the vitamin B complex group.

Under natural conditions, hypopyridoxinosis apparently occurs only when the ration is extremely deficient in pyridoxine and other B-complex vitamins.

Absorption, storage, and excretion of pyridoxine are very similar to niacin and riboflavin. After absorption, pyridoxine is utilized as an aldehyde in the formation of coenzymes, particularly codecarboxylase and transaminases which function in the metabolism of proteins and amino acids.[5]

Clinical Signs: Hypopyridoxinosis is accompanied by dermatitis, and there may be muscular weakness and nervous signs. Pyridoxine hydrochloride is a specific antidote for an overdose of cyanacethydrazide (Dictycide), a lungworm anthelmintic. This intoxication is characterized by inappetence and incoordination.

Sources: Sources of pyridoxine generally are the same as for other B vitamins. Though synthetic pyridoxine hydrochloride now is used in most instances, the cereal grains, milk, and molasses are fair sources.

Treatment and Control: If a deficiency is suspected, the addition of milk to the ration probably will remedy it. The daily requirement in the horse is not well-known. However, the injection of 50 mg. of pyridoxine hydrochloride 2 to 3 times a week will correct any deficiency that may occur.

Vitamin D Deficiency

A deficiency in vitamin D usually results from insufficient solar irradiation of animals or their feed. It is manifested by poor appetite and growth, and in advanced cases by osteodystrophies. A deficiency is most likely to occur in those areas in which there is a lack of ultraviolet irradiation. Cloudy overcast skies, smoke-laden atmospheres, and the constant stabling of horses prevent needed exposure to sunlight and are likely to promote the occurrence of avitaminosis D. Grazing animals, especially those feeding on lush, green cereal forage, often are affected with avitaminosis D because of an anti-D factor that is suspected to be present in this type of forage. Carotene has been shown to have an anti-D factor which virtually disappears from green cereal forage when flowering or blooming begins.[6]

Vitamin D is a complex of substance having antirachitic properties. Vitamin D_3 is produced from 7-dehydrocholesterol, which is contained in the mammalian skin when it is activated by natural solar irradiation or by ultraviolet light. Vitamin D_2 is present in sun-cured hay and is produced by ultraviolet irradiation of plant sterols.

Calciferol, or viosterol, is produced commercially by the irradiation of yeast. Vitamins D_4 and D_5 occur naturally in the oils of fish.[2] Vitamin D facilitates the deposition of calcium and phosphorus in bone and increases the absorption of these minerals from the alimentary canal. The effect of a deficiency of vitamin D is regulated by the calcium and phosphorus intake and ratio. Deficiencies of either or both minerals likewise influence the need for vitamin D. Minor functions of vitamin D include maintenance of efficient food utilization and calorigenic action. The metabolic rate is depressed when this vitamin is deficient. Disturbances of these functions probably are the basis for reduced growth rate and productivity in vitamin D deficiency.

Vitamin D also regulates the metabolism of calcium and phosphorous by reducing the rate of phosphorus excretion and increasing the rate of absorption and utilization of both elements. In vitamin D deficiency, the diaphysial side of cartilage develops osteoid tissue rather than bone.[3]

Clinical Signs: The signs of avitaminosis D closely resemble those of aphosphorosis. Since vitamin D regulates calcium and phosphorus metabolism, these deficiencies are interrelated. Animals suffering from avitaminosis D may show rickets, osteomalacia, retarded growth, nervous signs, lowered resistance to disease and parasitism, softening of the teeth, a general lack of stamina and well-being, and poor appetite.

Diagnosis: Diagnosis is based upon a history of insufficient exposure to solar irradiation, characteristic clinical signs, and lowered calcium and phosphorus blood levels. Avitaminosis D ordinarily produces a hypophosphatemia in its early stages and a hypocalcemia later. The plasma alkaline phosphatase level usually is elevated. The blood levels of these minerals will return to normal with treatment long before the animal shows any clinical improvement.[2] Radiographs which illustrate characteristic bony lesions will be of assistance in diagnosis.

Sources: Solar irradiation is a good source of vitamin D. However, when the sun is lower than 30° above the horizon, there is little effective irradiation. Feedstuffs exposed to solar irradiation are excellent sources of vitamin D. The longer that hay is sun-cured, the higher is the concentration. However, in our present methods of making hay, the speed with which it is cured, baled or pelleted makes this hay a rather poor source of vitamin D. Fish liver oils are high in vitamin D but are contraindicated in the horse. Irradiated dry yeast contains 9000 I.U. of viosterol per Gm., and is the simplest and cheapest method of supplying this vitamin. Milk is a fair source.

Treatment and Control: Horses require approximately 500 I.U. of viosterol per 100 pounds of body weight per day. Ordinarily the amount of vitamin D_2 in the ration is insufficient and the remainder must come from solar irradiation or by feed supplementation. Consequently, 1 Gm. of irradiated yeast should be added daily to a 1,000-pound horse's ration to supply enough viosterol, or vitamin D_2. Sunlight is necessary for treatment and control of

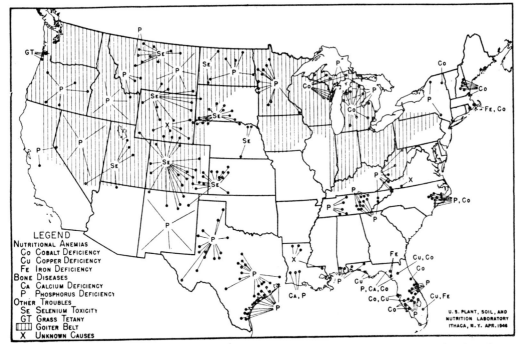

Fig. 3. Occurrence of mineral deficiencies in animals. The dots indicate the approximate location of the observed deficiencies. The lines not terminating in dots indicate a generalized area where specific locations have not been reported.

avitaminosis D. An injection of 1 to 2 ml. of viosterol in vegetable oil containing 500,000 USP units of vitamin D_2 will maintain a 1,000-pound horse for 30 to 60 days. Overdosing vitamin D_2 may cause calcification of the kidneys, blood vessels, bronchi, skeletal muscles, and heart. The signs of overdosing include drowsiness and muscular weakness. Extreme overdoses may prove fatal. Animals receiving vitamin D therapy should also receive adequate calcium and phosphorus intake.[2]

APHOSPHOROSIS

Aphosphorosis in horses as well as in other livestock is the most common nutritional deficiency in this country. All sections of the United States have phosphorus-deficient areas and these areas are pinpointed on the accompanying map (Fig. 3).

Drought, leaching rains, irrigation, and constant removal by cropping contribute to phosphorus deficit of the soil. Pastures lacking in phosphorus content usually are deficient in protein.[2] Horses are not highly susceptible to a primary aphosphorosis, but in phosphorus-deficient areas their growth is retarded, they are unthrifty, and subclinical osteodystrophies occur which tend to shorten their useful lives.

Etiology: Aphosphorosis occurs when the diet is totally lacking in minerals, and when an imbalance of the calcium-phosphorus ratio exists. This ratio is critical and must be maintained at 1:1 to 2:1 of calcium to phosphorus. An adequate supply of vitamin D is also essential for absorption of phosphorus. Occasionally, the horses may not utilize phosphorus properly. This may be a consequence of hypoparathyroidism or because phosphorus became insoluble in the intestinal tract through combination with oxalic, tartaric, or lactic acids.

Absorption of phosphorus may be decreased following the occurrence of diseases of the intestinal mucosa. An exceedingly high protein intake also may interfere with phosphorus absorption. An excess of calcium tends to chemically bind the available phosphorus and produce aphosphorosis.

Horses during active training, young growing stock, and pregnant and lactating mares require larger amounts of phosphorus in their diets than do other horses.

Phosphorus and calcium in combination with vitamin D and trace minerals are essential for the formation of bones and teeth. Phosphorus is present in the horse's body in the form of tricalcium phosphate (CA_3PO_4).[2] An excess of calcium intake combines with the available phosphate and removes this phosphorus from the body. An excess of calcium may even remove phosphorus that already has been deposited in bones and teeth.

Phosphorus is essential for the production of enzymes that are concerned with fat and carbohydrate metabolism, and the transformation of carbohydrates to energy. Phosphorus-deficient animals invariably are in poor condition and are unable to utilize fat and carbohydrates properly for growth and reproduction. A horse suffering from aphosphorosis will be deficient in energy, stamina, and speed.

The concentration of inorganic phosphorus in blood serum of horses ranges from 2 to 4 mg. per 100 ml. The intake of phosphorus must be in an available form to maintain this level, and the intestinal mucosa must be permeable to the phosphate ion, otherwise aphosphorosis can occur despite an adequate intake. The phosphates are of great importance in the blood buffer system. They also are necessary for the maintenance of proper electrolyte balance in blood and lymph.

Clinical Signs: Aphosphorosis is characterized by poor condition, lack of weight, weakness, rickets in young horses and osteomalacia in older horses, and anestrus in mares. Rickets may be recognized in the young foal or yearling by bony prominences at the costochondral junctions, crooked bones, enlarged joints, and supporting leg lamenesses. The cranium, pelvis, and mandible often are distorted. Osteomalacia in older horses is recognized by obscure lamenesses, enlarged and painful joints, varying degrees of posterior paresis, extreme fragility of the long bones, and the occurrence of exostoses in many places. A recurrent lameness of the forelimbs of the horse has been described as being caused by a primary calcium-phosphorus deficiency or an improper balance of these minerals.[4] Horses with sub-

clinical deficiencies will, after strenuous exercise, become lame on one or all legs. After rest, the lameness will disappear and no further trouble will be noticed until the animal is exercised again.[4]

A calcium deficiency, osteodystrophy fibrosa, can occur in horses fed a calcium-phosphorus ratio of 1:2.9 or greater. With a low calcium and high phosphorus intake the disease can occur within 5 months. Horses in strenuous training for racing are more likely to be affected because of the tendency to maintain these animals on unbalanced diets.

Diagnosis: Subclinical aphosphorosis is exceedingly difficult to diagnose but it occurs most often when the phosphorus level of forages is below 0.14% of the dry matter. When aphosphorosis is suspected, blood analyses should be made. A normal amount of serum phosphate does not preclude aphosphorosis, but if the phosphorus content of the ration is less than 3 mg. per 100 ml., aphosphorosis likely is present. Radiographs of the peripheral joints may show typical changes, such as rarefaction of bone and improper ossification.

Soil and feed analysis should always be made when aphosphorosis is suspected.

Sources: The accompanying table shows the calcium and phosphorus content of many commonly used mineral supplements.

Ca and P. Supplements	Ca%	P%
1. Raw bone meal (not recommended).	22.5	10.5
2. Steamed bone meal.	31.3	14.4
3. Dicalcium phosphate.	23.5	18.7
4. Spent bone black.	22.0	10.9
5. Ground limestone.	35.5	00.0
6. Oyster shell.	39.7	00.0

Other good sources of phosphorus for horses are wheat bran, cottonseed oil meal, and other oil meals. Cereal grains notoriously are deficient in this element. The calcium-phosphorus ratio can be maintained by adding a ration of high quality legume hay and supplementing this with a grain mixture containing 10% wheat bran, 10% cottonseed oil meal or other oil meals, and adding 1% bone meal.[3] Other good sources of phosphorus include: protein concentrates such as cottonseed meal, tankage, and wheat bran. Poor sources of phosphorus are roughage and hays, silage, fodder, and straw.

Treatment: If aphosphorosis warrants immediate alleviation, the intravenous administration of sodium acid phosphate, 1 ounce in 300 ml. of distilled water, is recommended.[2] Recurrent lameness may be treated with 1 or 2 intravenous injections of calcium, phosphorus, and glucose solution.[4] At the same time, these minerals are added to the ration. The use of calcium and phosphorus along with vitamin therapy has been recommended for the correction of a condition in race horses known as "tying up."

Control: The daily maintenance requirement of horses and cattle for phosphorus is 15 Gm. of phosphate equivalent. About 40 to 50 Gm. is considered optimal. Probably, the best source of phosphorus is steamed bone meal which may be given free choice, or by the addition of 20 pounds to a ton of feed. This supplies phosphorus and in the proper ratio, and in an available form. The calcium phosphates (monocalcium, dicalcium, and tricalcium) may be used either as a drench, by capsule, as a feed additive, or in the water. If monocalcium phosphate is used, 10 to 20 Gm. to 4 gallons of water is recommended or this amount is given in any other form. Dicalcium phosphate probably is best as it is the most palatable. A good ration includes 70% salt and 30% dicalcium phosphate. The use of bone black (purified animal charcoal N.F.) will supply a good source of phosphorus. The recommended dosage for tricalcium phosphate is 50 Gm. administered by any of the methods specified before. The use of raw or unsteamed bone meal should be avoided since there is the possibility of transmitting anthrax.

The ration should contain large quantities of wheat bran and oil meals as well as dried milk. Vitamin D should be supplied also and in adequate amounts.

The best method of preventing aphosphorosis is by the addition of available phosphorus to the soil on which forage is grown. All soils known to be deficient in phosphorus should be fertilized with a phosphorus-containing compound. The top dressing of pastures with superphosphates will correct most phosphorus deficiencies and it will also increase the protein yield of the forage.

LACTATION TETANY OF MARES

This syndrome also is known as eclampsia and transit tetany. It rarely is seen in the United States today but was prevalent during the heyday of the draft horse.

Etiology: Lactation tetany occurs when blood calcium levels drop below normal, sometimes as low as 4 mg.%. A hypomagnesemia also occurs, and the serum magnesium level may be as low as 0.9 mg.%. A predisposing factor is lactation. Mares on lush pasture producing large quantities of milk are most susceptible. During prolonged transit the mortality rate may reach 60% and in untreated animals a higher percentage may die. Mares observing foal heat or at weaning time usually are affected seriously, and the mortality rate is higher at these times.[2]

Clinical Signs: Profuse sweating, incoordination, stiffness of the extremities, rapid respiration, and dilation of the nostrils are common signs. A distinct thumping sound may be heard in the chest; this is thought to be due to a spasmodic contraction of the diaphragm. Trismus of the masseter and shoulder muscles may occur. The temperature is only slightly above normal. The pulse is normal in early stages, but later becomes rapid and irregular. The mare is unable to swallow and passage of a stomach tube is difficult or impossible. Urination and defecation are reduced. The mare usually becomes prostrate within 24 hours and experiences tetanic convulsions. Death commonly occurs within 48 hours following the onset of clinical signs.

Treatment: Rapid and complete recovery follows the intravenous injection of calcium solutions such as are used in parturient paresis. The voiding of a large quantity of urine is indicative of recovery. It must be remembered that the mare is more susceptible to calcium injections than the cow, and one should proceed with caution and with continuous cardiac auscultation. Too rapid administration of large quantities of calcium solutions will produce fatal heartblock.[2]

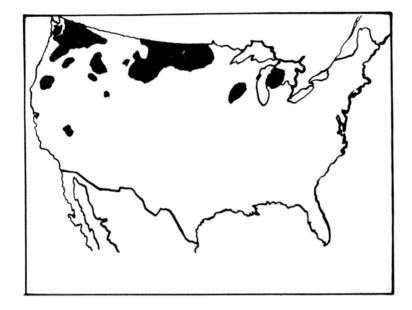

Fig. 4. Blackened areas show regions where iodine deficiency occurs in livestock in U.S.

IODINE DEFICIENCY

A deficiency of iodine occurs in most all continental land masses and is seen in sections of Great Britain, Europe, North and South America, and Australia. The deficient areas in the United States are shown in the accompanying map (Fig. 4).

Deficiencies in iodine most likely will occur where rainfall is heavy and iodine continuously is leached from the soil. Soils that are exceedingly rich in calcium or lacking in humus also are likely to be deficient in this element. The limestone soils notoriously are low in iodine. A heavy intake of calcium from any source will decrease intestinal absorption of iodine and thus contribute to an iodine deficiency. A ration containing 20% or more of linseed meal may produce an iodine deficiency.

Etiology: Iodine deficiency may be primary, due to deficiency of intake, or secondary due to a high intake of calcium, linseed meal, or thiocyanates which prevent the absorption and utilization of iodine. Thiocyanates are formed in the liver during the process of detoxication of the cyanogenetic glucosides found in some pasture and forage plants.

Clinical Signs: The cardinal sign of iodine deficiency is an enlarged thyroid gland which is produced as the result of a decreased production of thyroxine and stimulation of the secretion of thyrotropic hormone by the pituitary gland. The deficiency of thyroxine is responsible for the generalized weakness of the animal. In adult animals, there is a loss of condition, weakness, loss of libido, and long periods of anestrus may occur in the mare. Prolonged gestation periods have been reported in mares suffering from iodine deficiency. There is a high incidence of stillborn and weak foals. The foals have a normal hair coat and show little thyroid enlargement, but they are weak at birth and usually are unable to stand and nurse. There may be an excessive flexion of the forelegs and extension of the hindlegs. Adult horses living in affected areas have thyroid glands which almost invariably are enlarged. The glands often will pulsate with the normal arterial pulse. Obesity also is a common sign of iodine deficiency.

Diagnosis: The occurrence of enlarged thyroid glands and pulsation in the thyroid area is of clinical significance as is a history of animals having been in a known iodine-deficient area, or on a diet that would inactivate the available iodine intake. Normal blood levels for iodine range from 2.4 to 4 mcg. per 100 ml. of plasma. Horses that are on a continuous intake of commercial phenothiazine have an abnormally high blood level since commercially prepared phenothiazine contains large quantities of available iodine.

On postmortem examination, the abnormal thyroid gland will be grossly enlarged and myxedema usually is present. Histopathologic examination of such glands shows a definite hyperplasia. Stillbirths from iodine deficiency usually occur after a prolonged gestation period.

Treatment and Control: Treatment consists of administration of potassium iodide, the dosage being 2 Gm. for the average horse, or the addition of potassium iodate at the rate of 1 ounce per 300 lbs. of salt.[2] The addition of thyroprotein, an iodized protein and thyroxine, produces dramatic and quick relief of the clinical manifestations of iodine deficiency. This drug should be used only for immediate relief and not over prolonged intervals.[1] The organic iodides which contain available iodine also are effective as therapeutic agents.

Long-continued overdosing with iodides likely will produce iodism. The signs of iodism are especially noticeable in the mucous membranes of the eye, and the respiratory and gastrointestinal tracts. There is profuse lacrimation, serous nasal discharge, and scaly skin eruption with loss of hair. There may be palpitation of the heart, tremors, sweating, and loss of weight. The continued use of iodine after these signs are noticed may produce paralysis, blindness, and atrophy of the testicles and mammae.

R. S. JACKSON

REFERENCES

1. Dukes, H. H.: The Physiology of Domestic Animals. 7th ed. Comstock Publishing Associates, Ithaca, N. Y., 1955.
2. Blood and Henderson: Veterinary Medicine. Williams and Wilkins Co., Baltimore, Md., 1960.
3. Farquharson, J. F.: Clinical lecture.
4. Edmondson, A. H.: Mineral nutrition in the race horse. The J. of Applied Nutri. 10-3, 1957.
5. Daykin, P. W.: Veterinary Applied Pharmacology and Therapeutics. Williams & Wilkins Co., Baltimore, Md., 1960.
6. Pearson, Leonard; Michener, C. H. B.; Law, James; Harbaugh, W. H.; Trumbower, M. R.; Liautard, A.; Holcombe, A. A.; Huidekoper, Rush Shippen; Mohler, J. R.; Eichhorn, Adolph; Hall, M. C.; and Adams, John W.: Diseases of the Horse. U. S. Department of Agriculture, J. R. Mohler, Chief of Bureau, 1923.

WHITE MUSCLE DISEASE OF FOALS

The degenerative disease of muscle, known as white muscle disease or nutritional muscular dystrophy and by other designations, has been investigated most widely in sheep. It is known to occur also in calves, swine, rabbits, guinea pigs, chickens, and other animals. There is no doubt that the cause is related to a deficiency of vitamin E and/or selenium. Much active research is in progress at present to elucidate the mechanism of action of these two substances. Degeneration of muscle often is not the only manifestation of the disease and such changes as steatitis, hepatic necrosis, subcutaneous edema and hemorrhage, encephalomalacia, fetal resorption, infertility, abortion, and a decreased rate of growth have been described in various species.

With respect to the horse, white muscle disease has been described fully only in New Zealand.[1,2] There may have been one reported case in North America but, in this instance, there was not sufficient information on which to establish a definite diagnosis.[3] In Scandinavia, Alstrom has described a condition termed "Polymyositis."[4] The description of this disease is very similar to the reports of the New Zealand authors, and it appears that the 2 entities may have the same pathogenesis.

In New Zealand, white muscle disease has been recorded in foals varying in age from 2 days to 5 months, and usually has been fatal. Foals which have been submitted for necropsy invariably show a marked generalized steatitis. Most cases have been seen in Thoroughbred foals running with their dams on predominantly legume pastures. This is similar to the situation in lambs in which the disease occurs as affected lambs frequently are from ewes on a legume diet (clover and alfalfa).

Clinical Signs: Clinically, the onset of white muscle disease is rather sudden and, in some cases, foals which have not shown previous signs of illness have been found dead. As would be expected, muscular stiffness and difficulty in walking are manifested, and the foal may be unable to nurse. Palpation of the subcutaneous tissues reveals a diffuse layer of very firm subcutaneous fat. There also is a

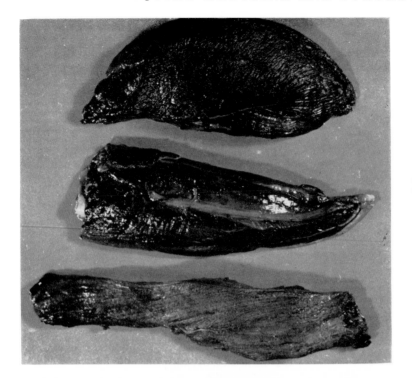

Fig. 5. Top, normal skeletal muscle; center, moderately affected muscle; bottom, severely affected muscle.

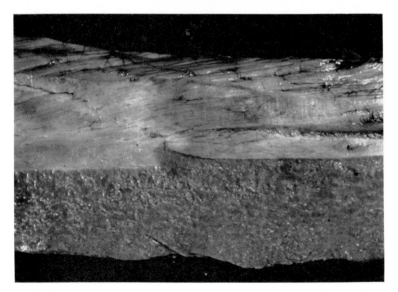

Fig. 6. Severely affected muscle.

pronounced firmness and thickening of the subcutaneous tissues beneath the mane. In acute cases, the foals have a dejected appearance, become prostrate, and usually die within 1 to 7 days. Some may excrete sufficient myoglobin in the urine to give it a brownish color. Inability to swallow is evidenced by the presence of saliva about the mouth, chin, and fore parts.

Lesions: At the necropsy of affected foals varying degrees of skeletal muscle lesions are seen. The damaged muscle may contain scattered whitish areas, or the entire muscle mass may be distinctly white. Muscles of the hindlimbs and shoulder usually show the most marked change. The lesions are bilaterally symmetrical and may be distributed throughout the body, including the tongue. All the body fat has a peculiar brownish color and is very firm; the subcutaneous fat may be 2 cm. thick. Muscles which grossly appear normal often show marked degenerative changes when sections are examined microscopically; in fact, the extent and severity of the lesions always are greater than appears to be the case from gross examination (Fig. 5, 6).

Treatment: Treatment of affected foals with as much as 1000 mg. of alpha tocopherol acetate per os daily generally has been unsuccessful, but a few cases treated with selenium have responded well. Because of the doubtful value of vitamin E and the good effect of selenium in lambs with white muscle disease, this substance should be given further trial. In New Zealand, injections of selenium have been given to pregnant mares on Thoroughbred breeding farms which have had a history of affected foals. The results apparently have been good inasmuch as no further cases have developed.

Particular care is indicated when a foal has to be hand-fed because of the danger of fluids entering the lungs and causing inhalation pneumonia.[3]

Where this condition is known to occur or once it has been diagnosed, prevention probably can be achieved by giving selenium either in the diet or by injection to pregnant mares.[2]

D. C. DODD

REFERENCES

1. Hartley, W. J., and Dodd, D. C.: N. Z. Vet. J. **5** (1957) 61-66.
2. Dodd, D. C., Blakely, A. A., Dewes, H. F., and Thornbury, R. S.: N. Z. Vet. J. **8** (1960) 45.
3. Jones, T. C., and Reed, W. O.: J.A.V.M.A. **113** (1948) 170-175.
4. Alstrom, I.: Skand. vet. Tidskr. **38** (1948) 593.

CHAPTER 23

REPRODUCTION

THE PHYSIOLOGY OF REPRODUCTION IN THE MARE

INTRODUCTION

The problems and difficulties that confront the horse breeder can be traced back to 3 primary reasons:

1. The mare was endowed by nature with a reproductive system that appears to be more complicated, but less stable, than that of other livestock species. For instance, her endocrine system concerned with production of gonadotropic hormones is of a high order, putting her, in this respect, close to the primates. At the same time, however, it also is unbalanced, working primarily on the FSH (follicle stimulating hormone)—estrogen side, while the LH (luteinizing hormone)—progestogen side is weak. For this reason, even under optimal conditions, the mare stays in heat for a long time which only the uninitiated would consider conducive to a good breeding performance. During pregnancy, her corpus luteum is so unstable that it is replaced by a complicated system of endocrine involvements. This situation is aggravated by a primitive type of placentation in an anatomically primitive uterus, taking place after an unusually long interval during which the embryo floats, more or less, in the lumen of the uterus.

2. Domestication has not completely liberated the mare from the effects of environmental and seasonal factors that regulated the breeding pattern of the wild and primitive horse. So, evolutionwise, the modern mare represents a transitional stage in regard to breeding habits. Modern breeding practices do not compensate for this property, but often work against the requirements imposed by nature such as the artificially restricted breeding season that falls partially into the natural nonbreeding season.

3. Selection for high reproductive performance has not been practiced in horse breeding to the same extent as in other kinds of livestock where a high innate fertility is a prerequisite for their economic utility. In horses, to the contrary, one frequently has to deal with individuals that, by their genetic make-up, are subfertile.

The following discussion is an attempt to integrate some of the phenomena of the physiologic functions in the mare with breeding practices.

THE BREEDING PATTERN OF THE MARE

THE BREEDING SEASON

Foals are born in every month of the year, which would imply that the mare is polyestrous and capable of reproducing the year-round. However, the difficulty of getting all mares to settle during the winter months, even under optimal nutritional and managerial regimens, supports the classic statement of Heape made as early as 1900, that the mare is a polyestrus animal with a tendency toward monestrum.[1] Others suggested that the modern mare represents a transitional stage of evolution from the monestrous to the polyestrus type.[2,7] A breed difference also is in existence. The more primitive breeds of northern origin in Great Britain, such as Shetland ponies, have a more restricted season than the more improved breeds such as the Clydesdales.[3] Certain individuals even of an improved breed still are monestrous, with a restricted breeding season, while others of the same breed are year-round breeders.

The environmental factors regulating the breeding season are only partially nutritional conditions. Neither are outside temperatures the sole influence, since also in the warmer regions of the northern hemisphere breeding seasons are in existence.[4] The most causal agent that instigates the onset of the breeding season in the spring, and causes its cessation in the fall, is the matter of available daylight. Experiments by Burkhardt in England have shown conclusively that in the anestrous mare, in the nonbreeding season, the initial stimulation of the pituitary and the ensuing activation of ovarian functions are brought on by the increase in daylight.[5] The ovarian changes that were observed under experimental conditions probably are typical for the changes occurring at the onset of the breeding season under natural conditions.

Mares of a seasonal breeding type were exposed to increasing periods of artificial illumination starting in January, the period of deep anestrus. After 2 weeks the effects of extra daylight were noted in ovarian stromal growth, and development of small follicles concomitant with increased vascularity of the cervix and vagina, and shedding of the winter coat. All treated mares came into estrus, on the average, 30 days before controls, and all mares settled to services given during the first estrual period. Control animals kept under normal farm conditions and one group that was irradiated with ultraviolet light did not come into full breeding condition until April, after a spell of warm weather. It was concluded that stimulation of the pituitary by increased daylight works through the eye.

The conclusion obtained from the experiment just described is supported by the investigations by Nishikawa et al., which gave essentially the same results concerning the initiation of breeding activity by increasing daylight.[6] In this experiment, to countercheck the affect of light, a group of mares was kept from November to February under conditions of decreasing light with the result that the onset of ovarian activity was delayed beyond the period of onset for the natural breeding season in most mares. A few mares did come into breeding condition at the normal time despite the decreased exposure to light. That decreasing daylight in the fall is a causative factor in terminating the breeding season was demonstrated by exposing mares to prolonged daylight from August into the fall. The mares not only maintained full ovarian activity, but also remained fertile.

In mares with a distinct nonbreeding season, the ovaries become hard and shrunken, with only small, nonfunctional follicles. Mares of the modern breeds generally do not go into deep anestrus. The ovaries do not regress into complete inactivity, but exhibit some degree of follicular growth. They go through a transitional stage in early spring when ovarian activity becomes intense on the estrogenic side, resulting in protracted heat periods. At this time their fertility is low. Thus, the appearance of the first heat period in the season does not coincide with, and is not an indicator of the onset of complete function of the reproductive system.

The fundamental reason for the sexual pattern of the mare, not only in regard to seasonal periodicity but also for the cyclic phenomena, is founded in the peculiar arrangement in the mare's pituitary, as suggested by Hammond.[8,9] The pituitary of the mare is particularly rich in FSH, but low in LH. As a result of this unbalanced production of gonadotropins, the mare is prone to have long heat periods because at times insufficient LH is produced to cause the mature follicle to ovulate. During the nonbreeding season, the activity of the pituitary as a whole is depressed, varying in degree from individual to individual and resulting in different degrees of ovarian activity from anestrus to subestrus. Later in the season when the activity of the pituitary rises, FSH still predominates over LH and only when sufficient LH is available does ovulation occur, and the heat periods become shorter.

The condition of the ovary in regard to receptivity to an impulse by gonadotropins also enters into the picture. In mares with irregular cycles, usually high amounts of gonadotropins are found circulating in the blood without provoking a proper response in the ovary.[10] The ovary of anestrous mares also does not respond to extraneous gonadotropins, but ovarian stimulation can be induced by first treating the ovary with small amounts of estrogen.[11] Under proper estrogen therapy, ovaries in shallow anestrus respond to estrogen alone, with complete follicular growth and ovulation, and the stimulated follicles contain fertile ova.[11,12]

THE ESTRUAL CYCLE

Seasonal factors in the form of daylight length, temperature, and nutrition continue their regulatory effects on the breeding mechanism into the breeding season by influencing the length of the estrual cycles and the fertility of mares. The length of the estrual cycle depends chiefly on, and varies with, the length of the estrual period. A comprehensive review of available data reveals that the average length of the estrual cycle is 19 to 24 days, but only 50 to 60% of the cases fall into this range, and shorter as well as longer ones are frequent.[7] A seasonal trend toward shorter cycles as the breeding season progresses is general, and is caused by a shortening of the estrual period. For instance, Trum in a study of more than 1,500 cycles in Thoroughbred mares found that 61% of the heat periods were 4 to 6 days long, but when arranged according to monthly occurrence, periods of less than 4 days' duration made up 44% of the periods in March, but 78% in July. Abnormally long heat periods of more than 10 days made up 18% in March, but dropped to 7% in April, to 2% in May, and did not occur at all in June or July.[13]

A correlation between the seasonal variation in duration of estrus and fertility seems to exist also. During early spring when estrual periods are long, fertility is low, but when estrual periods are of the normal 5 to 6 day duration in May and June, 50% of the services given during this period result in conception. The increase in fertility possibly is caused by two factors. In a short estrual period, the chances for serving the mare nearer to ovulation are better than in a long one. The other possibility is that the same extrinsic factors that regulate the physiologic mechanism leading to a normal cycle also directly stimulate factors favorable to conception. Since the short periods become established when the pituitary has regained its adequate production of LH, it is reasonable to speculate that this results in the establishment of more efficient corpora

lutea, and subsequently of a uterine environment more favorable for conception.

The stabilization of the LH-progesterone regulated phase of the cycle affects the duration of the entire cycle, and of the diestrual period. It has been stated that this latter phase regularly is 16 days because of the life span of the cyclic corpus luteum.[9]

However, a review of available data reveals that the diestrual period also is quite variable and may range from 5 to 22 days.[7,14] The long heat periods of the prebreeding season are followed by diestrus of a few days only because, due to lack of LH, follicles do not ovulate and are not converted into functioning corpora lutea. Even during the breeding season, the diestrual period is quite variable. Trum's data show that foaling mares have normal diestrual periods more regularly than barren, cycling mares, and that maiden mares have diestrual periods of less than 13 days. Trum has stated, "This variation in the interval between estrous periods makes the common practice of teasing mares only on specific days after the last service a precarious practice. It is possible to miss 50% of the mares by teasing on the fourteenth and twenty-first day after the last service. There is no correlation between the length of estrus and the length of subsequent interestrus." However, nursing mares occasionally go into prolonged diestrus. Britton and Howell noted that in such instances the length of diestrus was governed by the milk-producing capacity of the mare, heavy milkers staying in diestrus up to 6 months, and poor milkers for only 2.5 months.[15] Presumably in such cases, the pituitary principally is putting out lactogenic hormone at the expense of the gonadotropins. This is a regular phenomenon in the rat and sow, but it is rare in the mare, and as a rule the first diestrual period following foal heat is the same as in cycling, nonfoaling mares.[16]

Foal heat, or postparturient estrus, is a unique phenomenon of the mare and of such regular occurrence that it has to be considered a part of the breeding pattern. It does not occur in other domestic animals, but is said to occur in the camel.[17] The sow comes in heat within a few days after littering, but ovulation is absent.[17] In the mare, foal heat is complete with fertile ovulations, and as a rule, with the uterus in a progestational condition. This is possible because, as will be shown later, the ovary of the mare in the later stage of pregnancy does not contain a functional corpus luteum so that new follicles begin to develop as soon as the level of the estrogens and progesterone elaborated by the placenta drops low enough as not to exert an inhibiting effect on the pituitary-ovarian activity, and actually new follicles start to develop before parturition.[18] Furthermore, the postparturient uterus is capable of involution in a short time because of the primitive, loose, nondeciduate type of placentation in the mare which permits separation of the fetal placenta without major damage to the uterine endometrium. This, however, is not an infallible rule, as frequently restoration of the uterine epithelium is not completed at this time, and if breeding is practiced under such circumstances it may result in an increased occurrence of abortions.[13,20,21]

Onset of foal heat occurs at a rather regular interval after foaling even though it does not fall quite as constantly on the ninth day as believed generally by breeders. Trum had stated that between the seventh and tenth day after foaling 77% of the mares were in heat.[13] Seventy percent of the mares were in heat on the ninth day. He stated, "It is not possible to find so many mares willing to accept the stallion on any other specific day during the estrous cycle." On the other hand, intervals of greater length are not rare, and foal heat itself is of about the same duration as cyclic estrual periods.[7]

OVARIAN PHYSIOLOGY AND HISTOLOGY

During anestrus the ovaries are small and shrunken, and follicles are up to 1 cm. in diameter. At the start of the breeding season, follicles up to 2.5 cm. in diameter begin to appear. Burkhardt stated, "The chain of events in transition from anestrus to cyclic activity starts with an increase in stromal tissue due to an increased blood supply to the ovary and it can be recognized by palpation

before follicles become palpable.[5] The stromal growth coincides with increased vascularity of the cervix and vagina. It seems likely that estrogen secretion occurs as a result of stromal activity and that this is responsible for the changed appearance of the accessory genital organs before follicles can be palpated. Shedding of the coat seems to be closely related to the renewed ovarian activity." This observation could indicate that estrogen production starts outside of the follicles, and this is in conformity with other observations that it also takes place in the stroma, more particularly, in the interstitial cells.[22]

The origin of these interstitial cells and their relationship to other ovarian tissues such as the theca interna cells, as well as the role of these structures, still is a highly controversial issue.[23] Short offered evidence that the theca interna produces estrogen during the estrual cycle of the mare by converting progesterone into estradiol.[24] Burkhardt's observation would further imply that estrogen of extra-follicular origin stimulates follicular development, and this is supported by his own observations and those of others that administration of estrogen in proper form and dosage to mares in shallow anestrus will induce follicular maturation and ovulation, provided the follicles are at least 1.5 cm. in diameter when they are responsive to estrogen therapy.[5,8,9,11,12] During the transitional period from the nonbreeding to the breeding season, follicular maturation proceeds at a slower rate than during the breeding season resulting in the already described long heat periods due to insufficient LH. They rarely develop into large cysts, but in the absence of ovulation they regress without luteinization, as new estrual periods follow within a shorter time interval than would be possible in the presence of a functional corpus luteum. Large cyst-like follicles are found occasionally in the transitional stage from the breeding season to the nonbreeding season, but they too regress.[25] Such "autumn" follicles were described recently by Knudsen and Velle to contain a bloody liquid of gelatinous consistency, with an estrogen content (estradiol and estrone) lower than that of estrous follicles.[26]

The changes in the ovary during the estrual cycle have been described by several investigators.[18,27] The histologic changes during follicular growth and corpus luteum formation described by Harrison, and new information on the synthesis of hormones in the follicle by Short in regard to the endocrine functions of the granulosa and the theca interna cells, have contributed much to a better understanding of the physiology of the ovary.[24,28,29,30] According to Harrison, a number of follicles start to grow as early as 14 days before estrus begins, and 2 to 3 days prior to estrus a few of them enlarge more than the others.[28] During the early days of estrus, one of them enlarges rapidly to a diameter of 3 to 4 cm., but occasionally 2 very large follicles may be present in one ovary.

During this stage the most marked changes of histologic nature, and in regard to hormone production, occur in the theca interna layer. The theca interna cells now are well-vascularized, and by marked hypertrophy and hyperplasia they form a thecal gland. The granulosa cells, particularly those near the limiting membrane, are columnar with elongated nuclei, but play an inactive role. Harrison's postulation that it is the thecal cells that produce estrogen, and not the granulosa, was recently supported by Short, who also suggested that the estrogens in follicular fluid may have an intraovarian action in stimulating the growth of the granulosa cells, and that the follicular fluid is formed by filtration of plasma that contains the steroids secreted by the cells of the theca interna.[24,29]

The theca interna cells also have another function that was described by Strassmann.[31] He found that the theca interna cells proliferate eccentrically during the early growth of the follicle, forming a wedge-like "theca interna cone" that serves as "path breaker" for the growing follicle toward the ovarian surface. This wedge can be palpated in ovaries that are not too fibrous, and the presence of a well-defined cone has been suggested as an indication for approaching ovulation.[32]

The size of the mature and preovulating follicles is quite variable, and so is the size at which they ovulate.[13,14] Most often, they become softer just before ovulation. Ovulation is accompanied by a more or less sudden release of internal pressure, when not only the follicle, but the entire ovary becomes flaccid and soft.

Transformation of the follicle into a corpus luteum is rapid. According to Hamilton and Day, "Within 8 hours, the follicular cavity fills with a blood clot, and for 10 hours or so, it is soft and pliable to the touch until 24 to 30 hours after ovulation when it is plum-like in consistency. It becomes firmer and less conspicuous by palpation until, by about 4 or 5 days after ovulation, it is no longer palpable, but the ovary with the corpus luteum is normally about twice the size of the inactive ovary."[27] Harrison has described the histologic processes of corpus luteum formation in great detail.[28] The most significant features seem to be severe disintegration of the granulosa, invasion of the granulosa by theca interna cells, and beginning lutealization of the granulosa cells, all occurring in the first 18 to 24 hours. During the next 24 hours, the thecal gland has more or less disintegrated, and theca interna cells invade the folds of the collapsed follicle, which now have the appearance of trabeculae so that "the striking trabeculation of the mare's corpus luteum distinguishes it from the corresponding structure in other animals."[28] The trabeculae are next invaded by theca externa cells which make up their central core. The function of the trabeculae seems to be one of vascularization for the forming corpus luteum by the thecal capillaries.

By the fourth day the corpus luteum practically fills the follicle cavity, consisting principally of large, luteal cells with interspersed thecal cells. Theca externa cells of flat, spindle shape are also present.

The corpus luteum is fully developed and active by the tenth day, that is at a time when the fertilized ovum has already entered the uterus. It reaches its greatest size by the 14th day, continues to function actively to about day 17, then in the absence of fertilization ceases functioning but remains as an anatomic structure for 2 or 3 cycles. The detailed steps of its involution apparently were not investigated.

During its stage of activity, the corpus luteum produces principally progesterone, but no estrogens, according to Short.[24]

OVARIAN CHANGES DURING PREGNANCY

The mare is peculiar in that the corpus luteum initiated during a cycle in which conception took place, does not persist as a corpus luteum of pregnancy, but instead begins to regress at the end of the first month of pregnancy, and is replaced by a new crop of corpora lutea originating from a new wave of follicular development. These new follicles appear as soon as the 23rd day of pregnancy, that is at the interval of one estrual cycle. Follicle formation occurs at a rapid rate, with several follicles growing at the same time during the second and third month of pregnancy, when gonadotropic hormone in the blood becomes abundant. This hormone, as will be shown later, is derived from the endometrial cups in the pregnant uterus.

Ovulation in the additional follicles is a frequent occurrence. Amoroso and Rowlands observed it in 9 of 14 mares, 46 to 72 days pregnant, but corpora lutea also were formed in the absence of ovulation by luteinization of the theca cells, and they too are functional and their progesterone content was found to be high.[34,35]

From the fifth month on, new follicular formation no longer occurs and the existing corpora lutea begin regression into corpora lutea atretica, with the lutein cells decreasing in size and getting vacuolated. The ovaries now become atrophic and fibrotic, and eventually become smaller in size than the gonads of the fetus. They can be removed at 200 days of pregnancy without interrupting it.

Originally it was believed that the gestagenic system for pregnancy maintenance from here on was furnished by the fetal gonads because of their unusual size, not found in other species. In the light of newer investigations, principally by the California workers concerned with the gonadotropic hormones produced by the pregnant mare, it appears that the fetal gonads, in spite of their peculiar development, do not contribute to the mainte-nance of pregnancy but play a rather passive role.[37] Even though their biologic function is still obscure, their prenatal development is described here as an embryonic phenomenon specific for the equine.

THE DEVELOPMENT OF FETAL GONADS

At the period of gestation when the circulating gonadotropin in the mare is high and when the maternal ovaries undergo rapid follicular growth and corpus luteum formation, *i.e.*, between day 40 and day 100, the fetal gonads do not reveal a marked spurt of growth presumably because this hormone is not capable of crossing the placental membrane.[39]

The fetal ovary at the start of this stage contains small clusters of germ cells surrounded by epithelial cells arranged in a narrow cortical region, and the interstitial cells are confined to the medulla. In the fetal testes of this age, epithelial cords and interstitial tissue are distributed throughout the gonad.

Massive and conspicuous proliferation of the fetal gonads takes place in the following stage of gestation starting at about day 120 when the maternal ovaries begin to regress, the circulating gonadotropin is on the decline, and the estrogen in the urine and serum of the mare begins to increase. Their maximal development is reached in the eighth month, when estrogen output also reaches its highest level, but at this time gonadotropin has passed its peak for 2 to 3 months. For this reason, it is not clear which hormone stimulates the rapid, even though only temporary growth, of the fetal gonads. Clegg, Boda, and Cole suggested that some gonadotropin may still become available from the stores in the allanto-chorionic pouches from which it is released directly into fetal circulation, thus bypassing the placental barrier.[41] Others attributed the response by the fetal gonads to the action of estrogen affecting principally the interstitial cells in the gonads of both sexes.[39] This theory, however, would not quite explain why the gonads begin to decrease in size while the estrogen output by the mare is still high. One could speculate that by this time the gonads have become sufficiently organized and differentiated, and have become refractory to estrogen. They are now 5 to 7 cm. long, and are larger than the fetal kidneys. They weigh up to 150 Gm., twice as much as the maternal gonads which by now are devoid of lutein tissue and, apparently, are inactive as endocrine organs. The fetus itself now has achieved a crown-rump length of 45 to 65 cm.

Up to this time, from the third to the eighth month, growth changes in the fetal gonads concerned principally the interstitial tissue while the development of the germinal tissue was arrested.[39] In the ovary, the germinal epithelium lies over the cortex with short chains of germ cells growing into the cortex, and only a few oocytes located in the cortex are discernible. The testis now is covered by a well-formed tunica albuginea consisting of connective tissue, surrounding the interstitial tissue which contains very few solid germinal cords without cellular differentiation.[39]

After the eighth month comes the period of activation of the germinal tissue, concomitant with regression and breakdown of the interstitial cells and disintegration of the interstitial tissue. These processes result in reduction in size of the fetal gonads. In the ovary, small follicles now appear in the peripheral region of the medulla, and surviving interstitial cells enter into the composition of the theca interna of the newly forming follicles. At 9 months, the ovary is much smaller than it was at 6 months.[40]

The 9-month testis has developed a thick, well-vascularized tunica albuginea, and its interstitial tissue contains primordial, rudimentary seminiferous tubules.[40]

Near parturition, and in the newborn foal, the germinal epithelium extends only over a portion of the surface of the fetal ovary, the remainder being covered by peritoneum.[43] The germinal epithelium is distinguished by its dull gray appearance from the peritoneal surface which has a glistening character.[42] It forms a definite germ cell plaque that can be sliced off the surface of the ovary.[36] At birth the weight of the fetal ovary has decreased to about 20 Gm., principally due to the continued degeneration of the interstitial tissue,

and it now contains numerous follicles in the cortex.[36,43]

The testis at birth often has completed its descent into the scrotum, but it frequently happens that one testicle or both may be retained in the inguinal canal or in the abdomen for some months, and in other cases the testicle may return from a scrotal position at birth into the canal or abdomen.[42]

THE POSTNATAL OVARY

The organization within the fetal ovary is not finished with birth but continues into the postnatal life. With progressing, postnatal growth of the ovary, the germinal epithelium recedes further and is followed by the peritoneum with its underlying connective tissue and blood vessels. The original cortex now is covered and the follicles are mixed with the central stroma. Beneath the peritoneum is a thicker layer which is free of follicles, containing tortuous blood vessels and vestiges of the rete ovarii. Heavy tracts of connective tissue with large blood vessels reach into the interior where the follicles are distributed.[43]

In young mares, ovulation takes place anywhere on the surface covered by germinal epithelium. With advancing age of the mare, the ovary takes on a curved shape due to unequal growth at the poles that causes a progressively more pronounced bending of the ovary around the area covered by the germinal epithelium, and eventually this area forms a definite infolding designated as the ovulation fossa. Because of the thick peripheral layer of connective tissue everywhere else on the surface except under the germinal epithelium, in older animals the follicles can rupture only into the fossa.[43] The germinal epithelium eventually becomes a layer of short polygonal cells.[42]

The fully developed ovary of the mare is larger than that of any other domestic animal. It attains its greatest dimension during the third to fourth year, when in the resting stage it is 5 to 8 cm. long, and 2.5 to 4 cm. thick, with a weight of 40 to 70 Gm.[18] The size varies considerably during the estrual cycles, depending principally upon the dimensions of the cyclic follicle.

MIGRATION OF THE FERTILIZED OVUM

Information for the time required by the fertilized ovum to reach the uterus is scant. From available data it appears to be from 4 to 6 days. Hamilton and Day recovered a 15-cell morula in the uterine tubes 98 hours after ovulation, and one of similar dimensions in the uterus, 144 to 168 hours after ovulation.[27] Harrison also recovered one from the uterus at this stage and time.[28]

It is a peculiarity of the mare that ova preferentially migrate to, and implant, in the right horn. Thirteen of 15 pregnancies were found by Amoroso et al. to occur in the right horn, even though of 36 ovulations, 22 happened in the left ovary.[34] Even after twin ovulations which, incidentally, occur more frequently than is generally realized, both ova tend to transmigrate the uterine body and to implant in the right horn.[7,34,44] The cleavage stages of the fertilized ovum during its migration were described by Hamilton and Day.[17]

IMPLANTATION AND PLACENTATION

Even though the processes of implantation and placentation in the mare terminate in a placental system that is primitive, it still is a very complex process that cannot be fully described in the frame of this treatise. Also, Amoroso stated, "The structure and development of the fetal membranes and placenta of the horse at consecutive stages of pregnancy still await an exhaustive examination."[44] For the following discussion, the material was taken principally from Boyd and Hamilton, Amoroso, and Harvey for the purpose of bringing together those phases that are of more direct interest to the breeder.[44,45,46]

From this standpoint, it is important that a critical phase occurs in the very first few weeks of the initiated pregnancy. In contrast to many other species, in the mare the fertilized ovum after it has entered the uterus does not imbed into the endometrium by nidation, nor do the developing fetal membranes anchor the embryo to the uterus as they are formed. Instead the blastocyst remains free in the uterine cavity and eventually expands to fill the lumen.[45] The attachment of the membranes remains very frail, because they are held in position principally by pressure of the fetal fluids. At about the sixth week, the just-established chorio-vitelline placental circulation changes to the chorio-allantoic type, and this period is regarded as especially critical in development when the embryo is more likely to "slip" than at other times, as at this stage the attachment is weaker than heretofore.[44]

This precarious condition is aggravated by the fact that at this stage of pregnancy the ovaries undergo their new wave of activity and any derangement of the endocrine balance toward the estrogen side may contribute to the evacuation of the uterine contents. The attachment becomes firmer after the eighth week when the chorionic villi penetrate deeper into their mucosal folds, until at the 14th week complete attachment of the chorionic sac to the uterine mucosa is attained.[44] At this stage, the embryo has a crown-rump length of 15 cm., and the contact between the fetal membranes and the uterine mucosa now is so intimate that the uterine lumen practically is obliterated. Also at this time, the change-over occurs from the histotrophe-type of fetal nutrition to the hemotrophe-type, taking nutrient material circulating in the maternal blood by transmission through the now vascular villi.

Up to this stage, the embryo obtained its nutrient from the uterine milk, or histotrophe, derived from the breakdown of maternal tissue supplemented by secretions of the uterine glands and the intact portions of the uterine mucous membrane. This secretion accumulates in the space between the trophoblast and the endometrium. Starting with the seventh week it possesses, in addition, an unusually high concentration of the gonad stimulating hormone originally discovered in the pregnant mare's blood by Cole and Hart.[37] It is now considered to be the product of the so-called endometrial cups.[47] These structures originally were noted by Schauder, in 1912, as being present in the uteri of pregnant mares, and he associated them correctly with the formation of uterine milk, and as precursors of the pendulous hippomanes. Their gonadotropin production and other biologic performances were described by Clegg et al.[41] These cups are limited to the fertile horn and vary in size from a few millimeters to about 5 cm. in diameter. They form, invariably, in that portion of the endometrium in apposition to the chorion where the allantoic blood vessels fan out from the umbilical vessels over the allanto-chorion. The stroma cells in their vicinity undergo modification to form decidua-like cells. The cups develop their shape by the more rapid growth of the edges, resulting in a raised lip. They function in the first part of their existence as endocrine glands releasing the gonadotropic hormone into the maternal circulation, and in the later stages, as exocrine glands, releasing their product by desquamation into the space between chorion and endometrium. This sticky substance was noted by Aristotle floating in the amniotic or allantoic fluid and he called it, hippomanes. In many, but not all, endometrial cups, the accumulated secretion pushes out the allanto-chorion to form a sac-like structure hanging by a long neck into the allantoic cavity, the allanto-chorionic pouches. Clegg and co-workers believe that the content of these pouches, being rich in gonadotropin, is the source for the residual gonadotropin that stimulates fetal gonadal growth after the maternal circulating hormone has disappeared.[41] The endometrial cups appear approximately at day 40 of pregnancy and they are fully functioning to day 80, after which follows a period of desquamation that is completed by day 150. Thus their presence and activity closely follow the curve for circulating gonadotropin. The cups disappear by detachment into the space between the endometrium and the allanto-chorion, or they get into the allanto-chorionic pouch.

The fully formed placenta of the mare is of the diffuse, epitheliochorial type, and it is nondeciduate. The absence of an intimate fusion between the maternal and fetal placenta permits a flat and easy separation of the fetal placenta from the uterine endometrium at parturition so that delivery is effected usually in 5 to 15 minutes. For the same reason, any difficulty experienced in delivery is apt to cause death of the foal due to the disrupted connection between the maternal and fetal circulation.[48] Involution of the uterus in the mare generally is accomplished in a matter of days since the endometrium, on account of the nondeciduate placenta, is not greatly involved and does not require much repair. The effects of this on the onset of postparturient estrus, and the breeding at foal heat have already been discussed.

DURATION OF THE GESTATION PERIOD

The length of the gestation period of the mare generally is accepted in the horse breeding practice to be 336 days, and surprisingly little attention is paid to its well-documented variability that may range from 320 to 360 days.[2,7,17,19,50] Summer foals have a shorter gestation period, and vice versa, the longest gestation periods occur with winter foals. In one investigation, it was noted that parturitions in early spring terminating after a "normal" gestation period of only 330 to 340 days all produced stillborn and unviable foals, while during the same season, pregnancies resulting in healthy offspring had lasted 345 to 350 days.[7]

There could be several causative agents for this variation. The better nutritional condition of the mare bred in late spring may stimulate more rapid development of the fetus at the start, and again may hasten its final growth and development at the end of its uterine life. It also is possible that the same environmental factors which bring on the start of the breeding season, such as longer daylight, and the better balance of the endocrine system during the breeding season are responsible for a more favorable uterine environment, both at the start and at the end of gestation. Factors of a genetic nature also may be at play, and, all in all, very little is known about the mechanisms that terminate pregnancy.

HORMONES IN THE MARE

The role of hormones has been mentioned throughout the preceding discussion. In the following section a few more data are supplied in the form of a summary.

GONADOTROPINS (PMS)

PMS appears in the blood at about the 42nd day of pregnancy, frequently not until the 50th day, with a concentration of about 60 to 100 I.U. per liter. It rises rather abruptly to a level of 50,000 units from day 60, remains at this level for about 40 days, and then gradually drops off toward day 120, and practically disappears from circulation after day 150. There is a great variation from mare to mare, and pony breeds were reported to produce more potent serum, the level going up to 400,000 units per liter. With succeeding pregnancies, the titer of the serum gets progressively lower, but without affecting fertility.[51]

The biologic and chemical properties of PMS were studied by many investigators. Its value as a therapeutic agent for the treatment of infertility has not lived up to the original expectations.

ESTROGENS

The earlier investigations on the estrogens produced by the mare during the cycle and during pregnancy dealt principally with estrone, but the production of estrogens specific for the mare, such as equilin, equilenin, and hippulin, also was recognized.[14] More recent investigations have shown that besides these hormones, the urine contains also estradiol 17α and the "universal" estrogen estradiol 17β, estrone sulfate, and several derivatives.[29,30,38]

The urine of pregnant mares shows estrogenic activity by the 54th day, possibly of ovarian origin. The titer becomes high at the 100th day, up to 4000 R.U./liter, and markedly so from the 120th to about the 240th day (16,000 R.U./liter), after which it begins to decrease again. There is still some present until parturition. (For a review, see reference 38).

From day 80 on, estrogen also is detectable in the serum and it increases throughout pregnancy parallel with the concentration in the urine.[38]

The site of synthesis of estrogen during pregnancy presumably is the placenta. The fetal gonads originally implicated as the sole estrogen producers may contribute some during the peak of their growth period, but they are no longer considered the main source.

New information is available concerning estrogens produced in the cyclic follicle. Knudsen and Velle found that during the estrual phase, the estradiol level reaches a peak of 37.5 μg. per 100 ml. follicular fluid whereas in proestrus and diestrus the concentration is 6 to 7 μg., and in anestrus it drops to $\frac{1}{2}$ this level.[26] Estrone also is present, but at much lower levels. Another interesting observation made by these investigators was that in cases of cystic glandular endometritis, the ovary contained large follicles with an extremely high estradiol content of up to 190 μg. per 100 ml. "Autumn" follicles that persist at the end of the breeding season had a very low estrogen content, but during the nonbreeding season cyclic follicles that fail to ovulate on time are high in estrogen.

Short investigated the chemical nature of estrogens of follicles and corpora lutea.[29,30] In follicles, estradiol is the main component, in combination with 6α-hydroxy estradiol, and a small fraction of estrone. Androgenic steroids also are present. In luteal tissue, estrogen is absent, the main product being progesterone, with some 20α-hydroxy pregnenone and 17 α-hydroxyprogesterone. The enzymatic systems involved in the synthesis of these hormones were also investigated.

PROGESTERONE

Progesterone is produced not only by the cyclic corpora lutea, but also by the supplementary corpora lutea produced during pregnancy, even those that do not ovulate.[29] It still is an unsolved question where the progesterone originates in the later stages of pregnancy after the secondary corpora lutea become inactive following the 180th day of pregnancy. The urine after this time still contains several metabolites of progesterone, including pregnanediol. Since progesterone was found in the placenta in late pregnancy by Short, progesterone synthesis by the placenta is very likely.[38,52]

V. R. BERLINER

REFERENCES

1. Heape, W.: quoted by Eckstein, P. and Zuckerman, S.: The oestrous cycle in the mammalia. In: Parkes, A. S., Ed., Marshall's Physiology of Reproduction. vol. 1, pt. 1. Longmans, Green and Co., London, 1956. Chap. 4.

2. Berliner, V. R.: Seasonal influences on the reproduction performance of mares and jennets in Mississippi. J. Animal Sci. 1 (1942) 62, (Abst.).

3. Hammond, J.: Farm Animals. E. Arnold & Co., London, 1946.

4. Berliner, Victor: Horses and jackstock. In: Perry, E. J., Ed.: The Artificial Insemination of Farm Animals. 3d ed. New Brunswick. Rutgers University Press, New Brunswick, N. J. 1960. Chap. 10.

5. Burkhardt, John: Transition from anestrus in the mare and the effects of artificial lighting. J. Agric. Sci. 37 (1947) 64.

6. Nishikawa, Y.; Sugie, T. and Harada, N.: Studies on the effect of day length on the reproductive function in horses. 1. Effect of day length on the function of the ovary. Bull. Nat. Inst. Agric. Sci. (Japan) Sers. G. No. 5 (1952) 35, Animal Breeding Abst. 22 (1954) 103.

7. Berliner, V. R.: The estrous cycle of the mare. In: Cole, H. H. and Cupps, P. T., Eds.: Reproduction in Domestic Animals. vol. 1. Academic Press, New York, N. Y., 1959. Chap. 8.

8. Hammond, J.: The induction of ovulation in domestic animals. In: Engle, E. T., Ed.: The Problem of Fertility. Princeton University Press, Princeton, N. J., 1946. p. 60.

9. Hammond, John: Fertility. In: Parkes, A. S., Ed.: Marshall's Physiology of Reproduction. vol. 2. Longmans, Green & Co., London, 1952. Chap. 21.

10. Cole, H. H.: Hormonal control of ovulation. In: Engle, E. T., Ed.: The Problem of Fertility. Princeton University Press, Princeton, N. J., 1946. p. 74.

11. Burkhardt, John: Anoestrus in the mare and its treatment with oestrogen. Vet. Rec. 59 (1947) 341.

12. Berliner, V. R. and Scales, J. W.: Effects of stilbestrol on estrus of the mare. J. Animal Sci. 3 (1944) 431.

13. Trum, B. F.: The estrous cycle of the mare. Cornell Vet. 40 (1950) 17.

14. Andrews, F. N. and McKenzie, F. F.: Estrus, Ovulation and Related Phenomena in the Mare. Missouri Agric. Exper. Sta. Res. Bull. No. 329, 1941.

15. Britton, J. W. and Howell, C. E.: Observations on sterility. Vet. Med. 40 (1945) 264.

16. Cummings, John N.: A study of estrus and ovulation in the mare. J. Animal Sci. 1 (1942) 309.

17. Asdell, S. A.: Patterns of Mammalian Reproduction. Comstock Publishing Associates, Ithaca, N. Y., 1946.

18. Hammond, J. and Wodzicki, K.: Anatomical and histological changes during the oestrous cycle in the mare. Proc. Roy. Soc. B. 130 (1941) 1.

19. Britton, J. W. and Howell, C. E.: The physiological and pathological significance of the duration of gestation in the mare. J.A.V.M.A. 102 (1943) 427.

20. Williams, W. L.: The Diseases of the Genital Organs of Domestic Animals. 3d ed., W. L. Williams, New York, N. Y., 1943.

21. Jennings, W. E.: Twelve years of horse breeding in the army. J.A.V.M.A. 116 (1950) 11.

22. Diczfalusy, E. and Lauritzen, Ch.: Oestrogene beim Menschen. Berlin, Springer Verlag, 1961. p. 60.

23. Brambell, F. W. R.: Ovarian changes. In: Parkes, A. S., Ed.: Marshall's Physiology of Reproduction. vol. 1. pt. 1. Longmans, Green & Co., London, 1956. p. 481 ff.

24. Short, R. V.: Steroids in the follicular fluid and the corpus luteum of the mare. A 'two-cell type' theory of ovarian steroid synthesis. J. Endocrinol. 24 (1962) 59.

25. Burkhardt, John: Some clinical problems in horse breeding. Vet. Rec. 60 (1948) 243.

26. Knudsen, O. and Velle, W.: Ovarian estrogen levels in the non-pregnant mare. Relationship to histological appearance of the uterus and clinical status. J. Reprod. & Fertil. 2 (1961) 130.

27. Hamilton, W. J. and Day, F. T.: Cleavage stages of the ova of the horse, with notes on ovulation. J. Anat. 79 (1945) 127.

28. Harrison, R. J.: The early development of the corpus luteum in the mare. J. Anat. 80 (1946) 160.

29. Short, R. V.: Steroid concentrations in the follicular fluid of mares at various stages of the reproductive cycle. J. Endocrinol. 22 (1961) 153.

30. Short, R. V.: Steroids present in the follicular fluid of the mare. J. Endocrinol. 20 (1960) 147.

31. Strassmann, E. O.: The theca cone and its tropism toward the ovarian surface, a typical feature of growing human and mammalian follicles. Am. J. Obst. & Gynec. 41 (1941) 363.

32. Lensch, J.: Ovulation in mares. J.A.V.M.A. 132 (1958) 209.

33. Cole, H. H.; Howell, C. E. and Hart, G. H.: The changes occurring in the ovary of the mare during pregnancy. Anat. Rec. 49 (1931) 199.

34. Amoroso, E. C.; Hancock, J. L. and Rowlands, I. W.: Ovarian activity in the pregnant mare. Nature 161 (1948) 355.

35. Rowlands. I. W.: Anterior pituitary-like hormones. J. Endocrinol. (Proc.) 5 (1947) XX.

36. Cole, H. H.; Hart, G. H.; Lyons, W. R. and Catchpole, H. R.: The development and hormonal content of fetal horse gonads. Anat. Rec. 56 (1933) 275.

37. Cole, H. H. and Hart, J. H.: The potency of blood serum of mares in progressive stages of pregnancy in effecting the sexual maturity of the immature rat. Am. J. Physiol. 93 (1930) 57.

38. Catchpole, H. R.: Endocrine mechanisms during pregnancy. In: Cole, H. H. and Cupps, P. T., Eds: Reproduction in Domestic Animals. vol. 1, Academic Press, New York, N. Y., 1959. Chap. 14.

39. Amoroso, E. C. and Rowlands, I. W.: Hormonal effects in the pregnant mare and foetal foal. J. Endocrinol. (Proc.) 7 (1951) 1.

40. Davies, J.; Dempsey, E. W. and Wislocki, G. B.: Histochemical observations on the fetal ovary and testes of the horse. J. Biochem. Cytochem. 5 (1957) 584.

41. Clegg, M. T.; Boda, J. M. and Cole, H. H.: The endometrial cups and allantochorionic pouches in the mare with emphasis on the source of equine gonadotrophin. Endocrinology 54 (1954) 448.

42. Sisson, S. and Grossman, J. D.: The Anatomy of the Domestic Animals. 3d rev. ed. W. B. Saunders Co., Philadelphia, Pa., 1945.

43. Trautmann, A. and Fiebiger, J.: Fundamentals of the Histology of Domestic Animals. Comstock Publishing Associates, Ithaca, N. Y., 1952.

44. Amoroso, E. C.: Placentation. In: Parkes, A. S., Ed.: Marshall's Physiology of Reproduction. vol. II. Longmans, Green & Co., London, 1952. Chap. 15.

45. Boyd, J. D. and Hamilton, W. J.: Cleavage, early development and implantation of the egg. In: Parkes, A. S.: Marshall's Physiology of Reproduction. vol. II. Longmans, Green & Co., London, 1952. Chap. 14.

46. Harvey, E. B.: Implantation, development of the fetus, and fetal membranes. In: Cole, H. H. and Cupps, P. T.: Reproduction in Domestic Animals, vol. 1. Academic Press, New York, N. Y., 1959. Chap. 13.

47. Cole, H. H. and Goss, H.: The source of equine gonadotrophin. In: Essays in Biology. University California Press, Berkeley, 1943. p. 107.

48. Marshall, F. H. A. and Moir, J. C.: Parturition. In: Parkes, A. S., Ed.: Marshall's Physiology of Reproduction. vol. II. Longmans, Green & Co., London, 1952. Chap. 19.

49. Clegg, M. T.: Factors affecting gestation length and parturition. In: Cole, H. H. and Cupps. P. T., Eds.: Reproduction in Domestic Animals. v. 1. Academic Press, New York, N. Y., 1959. Chap. 15.

50. Dukes, H. H.: The Physiology of Domestic Animals. Comstock Publishing Associates, Ithaca, N. Y., 1943.

51. Day, F. T. and Rowlands, I. W.: Serum gonadotrophin in Welsh and Shetland ponies. J. Endocrinol. 5 (1947) 1.

52. Short, R. V.: Progesterone in the placentae of domestic animals. Nature 178 (1956) 743.

INFERTILITY IN THE MARE

THE ESTRUAL CYCLE

Most horse breeders are under the false impression that mares come in heat or accept the stallion all year long, at regular intervals, usually every 21 days. Some mares do follow this pattern, but they should be considered as the exception. During the year the great majority of mares seem to go through 3 different phases: a dormant phase, a period af adjustment, and a true breeding season. These 3 periods definitely are related to the season of the year, the environmental temperature, the amount of daylight, the type of feed or pasture, and probably some other conditions.

The dormant season lasts 2 to 3 months and usually occurs during the late summer, the fall, or the early winter. During this period, the ovaries do not seem to be very productive and the mare does not show signs of estrus, or if she does, the estrus (heat) is not proved clinically. Breeding at this time usually does not result in conception.

The period of adjustment may be very short and lasts through the months of January, February or March. This period is characterized by an irregular estrual cycle and unusually long heat periods.

The true breeding season, depending upon individuals and localities, may be considered in North America to begin in early March and extend to late July or August. During this period the heats are regular, with ovulation usually occurring every 21 days. The estrual periods normally last 7 to 8 days at the beginning of the season and become progressively shorter toward the end. During late June or July, some mares will exhibit heat for only 1 to 2 days.

ESTRUS

In the middle of the breeding season, a heat period usually will last from 5 to 7 days. It commonly is accepted that ovulation occurs during the second half of the period and toward its end. Andrews and McKenzie have recorded several cases when ovulation occurred after the end of the heat period.[1] This should be considered as the exception. From a clinical standpoint, the manifestations of the estrual period can be divided into 3 categories: changes in behavior, changes in the ovaries and the uterus, and changes in the cervix and vagina.

The only practical and efficient way to determine if a mare is in estrus or not is to observe her reactions when brought in contact with a stallion or teaser. If the mare is not in heat, she will violently resist the male; usually she whips her tail back and forth, kicks and even tries to bite. If in heat, she will stand straddle-legged, urinate, and assume the breeding position. The maximum evidence of receptiveness in the mare lasts 3 to 5 days. In the transitional periods before and after, the mare is said to be "coming in heat" or to be "going out of heat." To carry on a good breeding program and to reduce sterility cases to a minimum, checking the mare, or teasing, should be done every other day during the breeding season regardless of whether she has been bred or declared pregnant. A complete, detailed record of each mare's reaction should be kept for future reference. For Thoroughbred horses, because of the jockey club's regulations, and for most of the commercial breeds, the breeding season lasts from the middle of February until the middle of June.

CHANGES IN THE OVARIES AND UTERUS

Veterinarians concerned with horse breeding programs should routinely perform rectal examinations and be very familiar with the feel of the uterus, the ovaries, and the associated organs. The rectal examination should be performed in surroundings familiar to the mare so that she will be at ease. A chute or hobbles usually are not necessary, a nose twitch being the only means of restraint needed. The anus and the gloved arm should be thoroughly lubricated; a nondetergent soap, like Ivory, is a cheap and excellent lubricant. The arm is introduced gently into the rectum up to the shoulder and all fecal material is removed. Once in the rectum, one should identify the pelvic brim, the body of the uterus, the cervix, and then follow the body and the horns on either side to the ovaries.

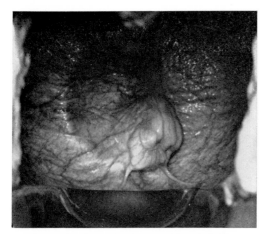

Fig. 1. Cervix during the interestrual period. The cervix is small, contracted, and erect. No secretions are apparent.

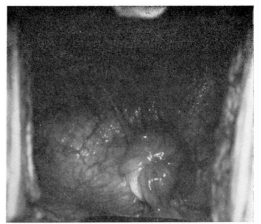

Fig. 2. Cervix at the beginning of the heat period. The cervix is still erect and begins to increase in size. The congestion is already apparent on several folds, the secretions are thinning and already visible.

The ovaries are located in the sublumbar region 5 to 10 cm. anterior to the upper portion of the iliac shaft. They are distinguished easily from fecal balls because of their definite consistency, and the limitation of their movement by the suspensory ligament and the uterus. Each ovary should be grasped gently between the thumb and the fingers and thoroughly palpated so that one becomes familiar with its size, shape, consistency, and surface irregularities.

When this examination is performed at the beginning of the heat period, a follicle is detected easily. It is the size of a hazelnut or a cherry, of tense consistency, and usually located on one of the apexes. Sometimes 2 or 3 follicles are present, but one usually is more advanced in development. If this operation is repeated every day, one will feel the follicle growing in size and losing its tenseness until the time of ovulation when it will be the size of a walnut or a small tangerine, and extremely fluctuating. It should be noted here that the essential sign of an imminent ovulation is not the size of the follicle but its degree of fluctuation. Some mares ovulate with a follicle the size of a cherry, though with others the follicle is the size of an orange, but all seem to have soft and fluctuating follicles immediately prior to ovulation.

After the follicle has ruptured one usually will feel a slight indentation in the ovary. Quite often the ruptured ovary is sensitive and the mare will show some response when it is palpated by lifting the corresponding limb. The day after ovulation the crater will start filling but the corpus luteum will not be palpable because this structure will not rise above the ovarian cortex.

CHANGES IN THE CERVIX, VAGINA, AND VULVA

When the mare comes in heat there is a slight relaxation of the pelvic ligaments. The vulva seems to be longer and less firm, and its mucosa is more congested, having a typical red appearance and increased secretions.

The most obvious changes observed in the mare during the heat cycle are the ones undergone by the cervix. The examination of the cervix is done under the same conditions of restraint used for the rectal examination. The external genitalia are cleaned thoroughly with a mild antiseptic solution and a clean and wet Caslick speculum is introduced. When the mare is not in heat, the cervix will be seen protruding into the vagina and standing erect above the lower spoon of the speculum. The cervical folds will be tight, the mucosa will be relatively pale, and the secretions will have a thick consistency which can be noticed as the

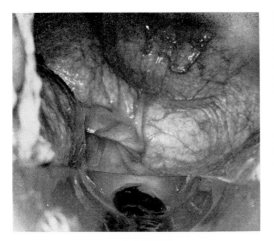

Fig. 3. Cervix toward the middle of the heat period. Notice its progressive enlargement.

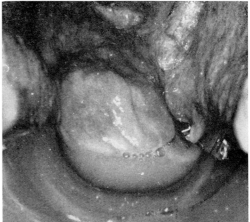

Fig. 4. Cervix immediately preceding ovulation. It has lost its tonus and lies flat on the lower spoon of the speculum. Notice the abundant fluid secretions.

speculum is removed. When the mare comes in heat one will notice that the cervical folds become slightly thicker and edematous, the colors changing from a pale pink to a darker shade. Quite often all the folds do not change color at the same time, some remaining pale, while others are pink or red, thus giving the cervix a striated appearance. The secretions become more abundant and more fluid during estrus (Fig. 1, 2, 3).

At the time of ovulation, the cervix has become 3 or 4 times its anestrual size. The congestion and the swelling of the folds are such that the cervix loses its tonus and lies flat on the bottom of the vagina, or on the lower spoon of the speculum. The over-all color is red and healthy. The secretions are abundant, clear, and fluid; however, they should not be so abundant as to form a small pool on the speculum. They are best checked after removing the speculum by touching the bottom of the lower spoon with a finger and slowly pulling it away. Quite often the thread so formed will not break before it reaches a length of 3 to 4 inches. At this time, the cervix is so relaxed that if one were to introduce the hand through the vagina, he very easily could penetrate the cervix with 2 or 3 fingers. If the same operation were to be performed during anestrus, one would have to exercise some pressure to

introduce a finger. It also should be noted that close to the time of ovulation the cervix is sensitive to excitation and often contracts when touched (Fig. 4).

After ovulation, the cervix returns slowly to its original size. The secretions become thicker and less abundant. The tonus returns relatively fast and the cervix, within 1 or 2 days, sticks out again like a finger. The congestion takes more time to disappear than it did to appear. If pregnancy has occurred, the cervix keeps getting tighter, the secretions thicker, and the vascularization less evident. Twenty or so days after the breeding, the secretions are thick, whitish, wax-like, and form a coating over a smooth and tight cervix closed by a cervical plug (Fig. 5, 6).

BREEDING

Very little needs to be said about the breeding itself except that when done at the opportune time, or time of ovulation, nature has provided the ideal physical conditions for copulation: abundant secretions which facilitate the penetration of the vagina and provide a proper medium for sperm, swelling and congestion of the mucosa for protection against trauma and bacterial infections, relaxation and opening of the cervix for direct projection of the sperm into the uterus.

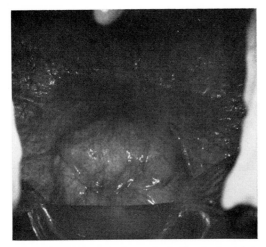

Fig. 5. Cervix toward the end of the heat period. Ovulation has occurred. The cervix is still much enlarged and is regaining its tonus.

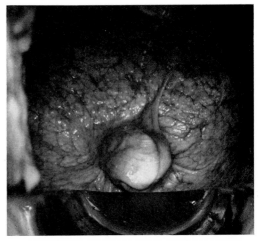

Fig. 6. Cervix of a pregnant mare, 45 days after service. The closed and erect cervix is covered by thick secretions which give it a smooth appearance.

PREGNANCY EXAMINATION

Different types of pregnancy tests are available to the practitioner but none is more rapid, accurate, and informative than rectal palpation. The rectal examination to determine pregnancy is performed in the same manner as the rectal examination of the uterus and ovaries. The operator introduces his hand into the rectum, locates the body of the uterus, and follows it upward on each side to the corresponding ovary to identify it definitely. He then takes the uterus in his hand with the thumb and the other fingers bent, and slides his hand underneath its anterior edge and palpates the whole uterus from one ovary to the other. While doing this, he carefully notes the consistency of the uterus and the presence or absence of the characteristic bulge indicative of pregnancy.

Listed in chronological order, the changes one would expect to find in a gravid uterus are presented:

1. At about 30 days, the uterus has great tonus, feels small, round, and hard. There is a noticeable bulge on one of the horns, usually on its lower third and about the size of a walnut.

2. At 35 days, the bulge still has a spherical shape and is approximately the size of a tangerine.

3. At 40 days, the bulge remains a spherical shape and is the size of an orange.

4. At 50 days, the enlargement is distinctly oval and is the size of a large grapefruit. It starts to enter the body of the uterus.

5. At 60 days, approximately ½ of the enlargement has entered the body of the uterus and is the size and shape of a football.

6. At 90 days, the whole uterus is enlarged considerably and the ventral part is now abdominal and cannot be reached.

7. At 5 months, the gravid uterus has grown in size and has fallen downward and forward to the extent that it is entirely abdominal, and usually cannot be reached. The characteristic findings at this time include the absence of a uterus in the place where one would usually expect to find it and an extreme tension of the broad ligaments which are being pulled downward and forward. The ovaries are displaced ventrally and sometimes are out of reach.

8. From 7 months to parturition, the characteristics of the broad ligaments and of the ovaries are the same but the fetus, now growing in size and moving when stimulated, can be detected more and more easily.

While performing a pregnancy examination, the practitioner should be careful not to mistake a distended bladder or the pelvic flexure of the left colon for a gravid uterus. A pyometra usually is distinguished from a pregnant uterus by its difference in consistency, the thickening of the walls of the uterus, and the lack of definite shape.

As described earlier, the vagina and cervix undergo some typical changes during pregnancy. However, these changes cannot be considered as having any diagnostic value and should not have any undue influence on the practitioner when he is doing a rectal examination to diagnose pregnancy. Some mares will be found to be in foal with a cervix typical of one during interestrus, but others will be found barren with a high and smooth cervix closed with a cervical plug.

LABORATORY TESTS FOR PREGNANCY

Among the numerous laboratory tests available to the practitioner, 2 have been selected for discussion because they are fairly simple, accurate, and useful during most of the pregnancy period.

The Friedman test is a biologic test to detect the gonadotropic hormone in the blood of pregnant mares. The test is considered to be 99% accurate between the 45th and 100th day of pregnancy. It is performed by injecting 10 ml. of the mare's serum into the marginal ear vein of a mature female rabbit which has been kept separated from all other rabbits for at least 21 days. The rabbit is destroyed after 45 hours and the ovaries are examined. In a positive reaction, one of the ovaries presents a typical graafian follicle of the shape and appearance of a small raspberry.

The Cuboni test is a chemical test designed to detect the presence of estrone in urine. It is considered to be 90% accurate from 120 days to parturition. It is performed as follows:

1. Place 5 ml. of urine in a test tube and acidulate by adding 1 ml. of concentrated hydrochloric acid.

2. Boil in a water bath for 10 minutes.

3. Cool under running tap water.

4. Add 6 ml. of benzene.

5. Mix by repeated inversion.

6. Evaporate to dryness in a 60- to 80-C. water bath.

7. Add 4 ml. of concentrated sulfuric acid and mix.

8. Replace in water bath for 10 minutes.

In a positive test, the solution shows a green fluorescence; in a negative test, it is a dull, reddish-brown to light green color.

CAUSES OF INFERTILITY

Infertility in the female, or failure to achieve pregnancy, is often related to one or several of the following etiologies: infectious, hormonal, anatomic, dietetic, or psychologic. In the equine species, psychologic factors have a minimal importance, and when apparent they usually resolve themselves with rest. The dietetic factors are extremely important, but apparently very little research has been done on this factor. The trace elements, minerals, and vitamins surely have their role and recently vitamin E has been strongly emphasized. However, no independent, controlled experimentation concerning the influence of this vitamin on reproduction has been published to my knowledge. Practice has shown that a well-balanced diet satisfying the basic needs of the body is essential to overcome a sterility problem of any origin. Consequently, dietetic and psychologic factors will not be discussed separately, but will be considered only when they have a specific influence on other factors.

INFECTIOUS PROCESSES

COITAL EXANTHEMA

Coital exanthema is an extremely contagious, viral disease which causes temporary sterility. The disease is said to be rather common in Germany but not so common in North America. It should, however, be considered as several isolated cases have been observed on this continent.

In the mare, the disease is characterized by the presence of numerous small vesicles, 1 to 3 mm. in diameter, on the vulvar and vaginal mucosas. The vesicles become pustules, then small ulcers. Because of these lesions, the vulva is congested, swollen, and extremely sensitive. A whitish discharge is observed to soil the buttocks and tail. The swollen vulva itches and causes the mare to stand with her back arched, to urinate frequently, and to switch her tail. After a few days, the clinical signs slowly subside and the lesions disappear, leaving nonpigmented spots which may last for several weeks.

The disease is very easily transmitted by contact, either directly during coitus or indirectly by the transfer of infected secretions or through the use of contaminated brushes, currycombs, or sponges.

As far as sterility is concerned, coital exanthema is only a temporary influence and does not leave any permanent aftereffect. A case of lasting complications or abortion has never been reported. It should be noted that the disease is different from the common, granular venereal disease of cattle, and transmission of the virus from horses to cattle, or vice versa, has not been observed except in one reported experimental case.

If needed, the treatment should be symptomatic as the disease is self-limiting. The affected animal should be quarantined for a period of 2 months. The disease does not confer any permanent immunity.

Dourine

Dourine is a trypanosomiasis of solipedes transmitted by coitus. The disease was introduced into North America in the late nineteenth century. At present, it has been almost entirely eradicated from the United States with the exception of isolated areas in Arizona and New Mexico. The infective agent is *Trypanosoma equiperdum*. This disease is discussed in detail in Chapter 7.

Bacterial Infections

Bacterial infection of mare's genitalia is fairly common and, in my opinion, responsible for 80 to 90% of the cases of persistent sterility. Special emphasis should be given to this cause for sterility in the mare. For clarity and practical value, the vagina and the vulva will be considered as a unit, then the cervix and uterus. Salpingitis in the mare apparently is very rare and has not been described as a clinical entity. The cases observed at postmortem examinations always have been as-

sociated with metritis and should be considered as a complication of this condition. Ovaritis also is very rare and has been diagnosed only at postmortem. The cases encountered seem to have resulted from tapping an ovarian cyst.

Vulvitis and Vaginitis: Acute vaginitis and vulvitis are relatively rare. They are caused by trauma or occur as postpartum complications, and they respond rapidly to topical treatment. They have no special bearing on sterility problems of the mare.

Chronic vaginitis is a very common condition, and is observed in so-called "wind-sucking mares." These mares, because of their anatomic predisposition and/or their general state of health, have vulvas which do not close properly. The labiae do not have normal tonus, and when the mare walks or trots air is alternately aspirated and expelled from the vagina. The condition usually becomes worse, the muscles lose tonus, and the vagina stays ballooned.

As described by Roberts, "Pneumovagina is predisposed by a conformation that includes a flat croup, elevated tail head, sunken anus, and small, underdeveloped vulvar lips that are pulled nearly horizontal by the sunken anus. It is also caused by lacerations, stretching or tearing of the vulvar muscles, or the vulvar or perineal body at the time of foaling."[21]

This condition usually is found in old, multiparous mares but it can occur in young mares, even in maidens. Poor physical condition is a predisposing factor as is relaxation of the vulva and of the pelvic ligaments during estrus. Some mares will show acute deformation of the vulva, and extreme "wind sucking" while in estrus, but will be perfectly normal if examined during the interestrual period. Others will exhibit the condition whether in or out of heat (Fig. 7).

In mild cases there are no apparent signs, with the exception of the obviously poor conformation of the vulva plus the fact that the mare is a poor breeder. If examined during estrus, the cervical secretions will have a frothy appearance which is very much increased after exercise.

In extreme cases, in addition to ballooning of the vagina, some fecal matter can be seen in the vulvar antrum and sometimes in the vagina. The cervical and vaginal mucosas will appear irritated. In some instances, the vaginitis is characterized by a thin discharge which is apparent at the ventral commissure of the vulva, and it usually soils the hindlimbs and tail.

Pneumovagina is conducive to sterility for 2 main reasons. The first is that subsequent to irritation of the vaginal mucosa and the presence of air-borne or fecal contaminants, a bacterial vaginitis, a cervicitis, and occasionally an endometritis develop. The second reason operates without the development of infection; the irritation of the vaginal mucosa causes a change in the pH of the genital secretions and, in so doing, inactivates sperm introduced during coitus. This opinion is at variance with several published statements in which the pH of the vaginal secretions is said to be unimportant in mares. Cases have been observed, however, in which mares, obvious windsuckers, were bred successfully after vaginal irrigation with sodium bicarbonate solution, or after introduction of sperm directly into the uterus following its collection from the dismounting stallion. Pneumovagina is corrected surgically by a well-known procedure identified as the Caslick operation. This procedure is described in Chapter 27.

Cervicitis and Metritis: Cervicitis and endometritis will be considered as one entity as their clinical signs, diagnosis, and treatment are similar.

In 1928, Dimock and Edwards published a study made in central Kentucky of 1,606 barren mares of which 587, or 36.55%, were found to have genital infections.[5] The causative agents of these infections were reported as:

Streptococcus genitalium (equi)	66.44%
Encapsulatus (Klebsiella) genitalium	10.22%
Miscellaneous infections	23.34%

Among the miscellaneous infections, Dimock and Bruner have isolated *Salmonella abortivo-equina, Corynebacterium equi, Shigella equirulis,* Micrococci, Streptococci, Staphlococci, *Escherichia coli,* and *Pseudomonas aeruginosa.* From my observations in recent years it seems that *Streptococcus genitalium,* or *S. equi,* still is responsible for more genital infections than any other organism, that *Encapsulatus genital-*

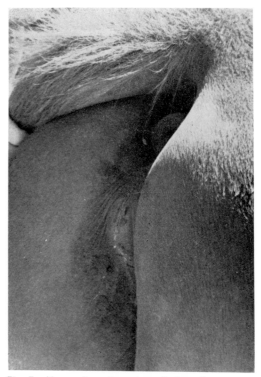

Fig. 7. Abnormal conformation of the vulva is conducive to pneumovagina.

ium is not as common as it was, but *Escherichia coli* and *Pseudomonas aeruginosa* are found much more frequently. *Proteus* spp., fungi, and yeasts also have been isolated from infected genitalia of mares.

Etiology: Most genital infections can be related to 1 of the 3 following causes: pneumovagina, foaling and postfoaling complications, and poor breeding practices. As already stated, pneumovagina usually is complicated by cervical and sometimes uterine infections because of the constant irritation of the mucosa and its exposure to airborne or fecal contaminants. Dystocias requiring lengthy manipulation or embryotomy usually are followed by uterine infection because of the tissue injury and contamination inevitably associated with such operations. The same is to be expected for abnormally long retention of placental membranes, 12 hours or more, and their extraction by careless operators. Abortions often are followed or accompanied by an endometritis; either the abortion was of infectious origin due to bacteria already present in the uterus or the uterus was exposed to the putrefying fetus for some time between the death of the fetus and its expulsion from the uterus.

Poor breeding practices seem to be increasingly responsible for the definite increase of genital infections. Most breeding farms follow some elementary hygienic practices, such as washing the mare's vulva and buttocks prior to breeding, but the stallion often is not washed thoroughly before and after services. Infection can be carried from one mare to another by the stallion, as Dimock observed.[5] Indiscriminant breeding of mares on the first estrus after foaling, 7 to 13 days postpartum, likely is responsible for a certain number of uterine infections. It is conceivable that tissues bruised during parturition and still in the process of involution would be very susceptible to infection introduced mechanically during service. It also has been observed that mares will conceive from a so-called "9-day breeding" even if the uterus has not returned to its normal interestrual state. The ultimate result of such breedings often will be early abortion, or the birth of a diseased or malformed foal plus the possible complication of a chronic uterine infection in the mare.

Indiscriminant use of the vaginal speculum by nonprofessionals who attempt to determine the time of ovulation is undoubtedly responsible for genital infections. Likewise, the practice of introducing the naked hand into the vagina to feel the cervix or to "open it up" by forcing 2 or 3 fingers through the cervical os must be indicted for cases of infectious cervicitis and metritis. The practice of depositing additional semen into the cervix after service or artificial insemination procedures, if not done with adequate precautions, can irritate and contaminate the cervical or uterine mucosas.

Clinical Signs: Whether acute or chronic, the cervicometritis usually is localized and without fever or other general signs of illness. Sometimes, infected mares will exhibit a discharge from the genital tract which soils the buttocks and tail but this sign is not constant. When cervicitis is present, the cervix is enlarged, slightly edematous, and a deep red color. The blood vessels of the vaginal wall are tortuous and enlarged. Quite often a discharge

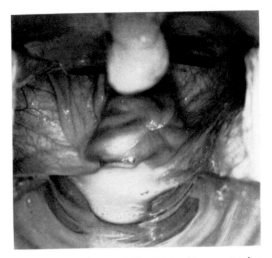

Fig. 8. Suppurative cervicitis. Thick white pus seeping from the cervix is visible on lower spoon of speculum.

is seen below the cervix, and sometimes this exudate is seeping from it. The exudate can be thin and clear, slightly cloudy, mucopurulent, or thick and yellow with whitish flakes of pus. In cases of *Encapsulatum genitalium* infections, according to Dimock, "certain changes are typical and characteristic of this infection. First and foremost is the character of the exudate. It always is thick, often containing many flocculi, exceedingly viscid and tenacious in consistency, and slimy to the touch. The color varies from a dull gray to a yellowish white. The visible portion of the vaginal, cervical membrane has a full reddish-brown color."[5]

In many cases of genital infections the signs are seen during the estrual period only; during the interestrual period the appearance of the genital tract may return to nearly normal. In view of this, mares should be examined during the estrual period only. Occasionally, mares will be found with a chronic uterine infection without exhibiting vaginal or cervical changes, even during the estrual period (Fig. 8).

Diagnosis: The diagnosis of genital infection is based on the clinical signs described previously plus a bacteriologic examination of the cervical secretions. Unless cervical exudate is obviously present during interestrus, the diagnostic examination should be done during the estrual period. The entire genital tract should be examined. The examination includes a thorough rectal examination of the uterus, fallopian

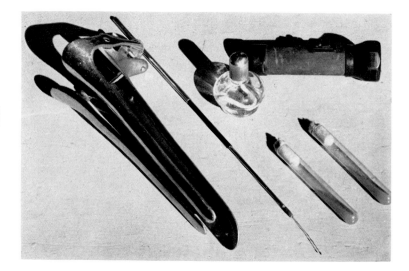

Fig. 9. Instruments used for culture of the cervical secretions in the mare.

tubes, and ovaries. A vaginal speculum then is inserted, and the vagina and cervix are inspected. Material for bacteriologic examination is obtained from the cervical os with a 5-inch platinum loop attached to a 20-inch holder. The loop is sterilized in a flame, introduced into the cervix, moved back and forth 2 or 3 times, and then withdrawn. If the loop has not touched anything after its removal it is used to inoculate 2 tubes of fresh culture media. If every aseptic precaution is applied and unfavorable surroundings are avoided, entirely reliable cultures can be obtained in this way (Fig. 9).

Solid agar medium should be used, as it is easier to handle and also easier to interpret when distinction must be made between contaminants and pathogenic bacterial growth. Some prefer to use a sterile, cotton-tipped applicator held in place with a Knowles forceps to obtain the sample, and to return to the laboratory for its inoculation into medium. This technic seems to be more complicated, and the samples are more apt to become contaminated. Dimock recommends the use of a horsemeat infusion agar slant as a culture medium.[8]

The inoculated culture medium should be placed in an incubator for 24 to 72 hours and read at 24-hour intervals. Streptococci grow readily but other organisms are slower.

Treatment: If the infected mare is found to be a wind-sucking mare, the treatment should include a Caslick operation, sexual rest for 1 or 2 heat periods, longer if possible, then bacteriologic examination of the cervical secretions. If infection still is present, antibacterial treatment should be instituted.

The mare should be treated only during estrus as at this time the cervix is open and the uterus is easily accessible. Extreme care should be exercised to avoid irritating the cervical and uterine mucosas with either the therapeutic agent or during its application. A low-grade cervicitis or endometritis easily can be transformed into a pyometra following irritation, scarring, and constriction of the cervix. Treatment should include adequate antibacterial medication as determined by a sensitivity test. It should be pointed out that the treatment of uterine infections is particularly unrewarding, and is a long, tedious process. Even when the drug of choice is found to be extremely effective *in vitro*, it usually is not so effective *in utero*.

The medicament should be administered both topically and parenterally to develop an adequate blood level. The addition of enzymes to the antibiotic is advantageous. Some advocate the use of steroids because of their antiinflammatory action. Estrogens have been recommended by others on the basis of their usefullness in similar conditions in the bovine. It has been demonstrated, however, that the cow's uterine environment is resistant to in-

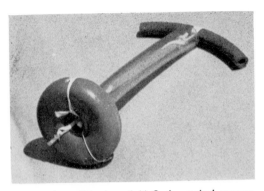

Fig. 10. A modification of McGee's cervical pessary. The part made with inflated human pessary stays in the vagina, the one inch plastic tube is in the cervix, and the transversal rubber tube lies in the uterus.

fection, even bacteriostatic, while in the follicular phase of the estrus cycle, but in the luteal phase, it promotes bacterial growth. Similar information should be sought in mares as this might provide clues concerning the reason many mares are hopelessly infected for years despite regular treatment.

At each successive estrus a bacteriologic examination of the cervical secretions should be performed unless the infection still is evident grossly. If the culture is positive, the treatment is reinstated. If negative, the mare is examined again on the following heat and bred only if the second culture is negative. Sexual rest is an essential part of the treatment and one should not breed an infected mare until it is certain that the condition has been cured. Coitus is irritating to the membranes and usually aggravates any pre-existing condition.

PYOMETRA

Pyometra is characterized by an accumulation of purulent exudate in the uterus, sometimes in excess of 2 or 3 gallons, and very often this is complicated by cervical atresia.

From the standpoint of future breeding success, a long-standing pyometra makes the prospect hopeless. The uterus is distended, the wall thin, flaccid, and atonic. The uterine epithelium is more or less destroyed and the mucosa is changed into a tough, thick membrane. Such mares are not treated successfully.

If the pyometra is a recent development, treatment may be attempted, but the outcome

should be considered with extreme reservation. Treatment for pyometra is similar to that described for endometritis, with special attention given to the cervix. Cervical adhesions should be ruptured and the cervix should be kept open to permit good drainage of uterine exudate.

McGee has described a very useful device to keep the cervix open.[17] It consists of a tube of vinyl plastic, 6 to 7″ long, containing a rubber band attached on each end to two ½″ plastic tubes, 4 to 5″ long, which are held at right angles to the longest tube. The device is introduced through the cervix with one of the ½″ plastic tubes held parallel with the main tube, then released when in the uterus. Once in place, the longest tube is in the cervical passage, with one end anchored in the uterus and the other end in the vagina. The device is left in place for 2 to 6 weeks before removal. The cervix then will be found to be smooth, and the adhesions healed. The pyometra in the meantime has improved considerably because of the constant drainage of uterine exudate. The condition then can be treated in the manner described for endometritis plus supportive estrogen therapy (Fig. 10).

HORMONAL DISTURBANCES

During the off-breeding season, which in North America extends from July or August till February or March, most mares present irregularities in their estrual cycles. Occasionally, as previously stated, there are very long periods of anestrus. Some authors have advanced the theory that mares were primarily monestrous animals and because of man's interference and other environmental factors they now can be classified as seasonally polyestrous. Some mares have regular estrual cycles throughout the year. These individuals should be considered as exceptional. It is good policy not to administer treatment to mares having irregularities in their estrual cycles during the off-season, as the nature and extent of their condition cannot be ascertained until the regular breeding season. It also should be considered that during the off-season their response to hormonal therapy is erratic.

During the breeding season, next to genital infections the most common cause of infertility in the mare can be attributed, in my opinion, to apparent or inapparent irregularities of the estrual cycle. These irregularities are thought to be of hormonal origin, and are treated accordingly. Very few controlled observations have been made of this phenomenon, and consequently its diagnosis and treatment are purely empiric. When considering irregularities of the estrual cycle, one should classify the mares into 3 groups, the first being foaling mares or mares which have foaled during or immediately before the breeding season. The great majority of these individuals establish a regular cycle immediately after foaling; their first ovulation is 9 to 13 days postpartum, then every 21 days thereafter. Any irregularity in these mares is highly significant, important to diagnose, and worth treating.

Barren mares, or mares which did not conceive during the preceding breeding season, usually take a longer time to establish a regular cycle, and before any therapeutic measures are initiated one should be sure that a regular estrual cycle is not established spontaneously. As a rule, it is best to wait until spring before undertaking any treatment. Sometimes, further delay is indicated if the winter and spring weather has been particularly inclement.

Maiden mares form the third group. They usually range in ages from 2 to 6 years. This group is very heterogeneous and extreme care and patience should be exercised with these animals. Some of these mares are too young or not sexually mature. Most of them have come from race tracks or show circuits, sometimes in poor physical condition, occasionally in a state of nervous frustration, and not infrequently suffering from excessive treatment with hormonal preparations or other medicaments. In any case, after the maiden mares' conditions have been evaluated, they should be given an opportunity to accustom themselves to their new surroundings and to establish a regular estrual cycle.

A diagnosis of hormonal disturbances of the estrual cycle should be based on the following: 1. Past behavior of the mare during the actual breeding season (this should be made available to the veterinarian by the farm manager as a detailed record of the mare's reaction while teased every other day during the breeding season), 2, a thorough rectal palpation of the uterus and ovaries, and a direct examination of the vagina and cervix, and 3, a detailed record of the findings.

The different types of hormonal disturbances can be classified according to their outward clinical manifestations into anestrus, abnormal estrus, abnormal interestrus, and apparently normal estrus.

ANESTRUS

Anestrus, or failure of the mare to come in heat, is one of the most common conditions encountered in practice. No attempt should be made to diagnose this condition unless the mare has been thoroughly examined and found to be barren. After it has been established that pregnancy is not responsible for anestrus, the mare should then be placed under observation for at least 3 weeks. She should be teased every other day and observed by a competent person. Examinations of the vagina and cervix, employing a speculum, should be made at frequent intervals to eliminate the possibility of silent heat. If the mare has not shown any sign of estrus during this length of time, it can then be assumed that she is in a state of anestrus.

Silent heat is a phenomenon exhibited by certain mares who fail to show outward signs of estrus while being teased, but nevertheless experience regular cycles and ovulations. In these mares, the cycle is determined by observation of changes in the appearance of the cervix and, if needed, by palpation of the ovaries. These mares are bred on the basis of such observations, and usually with success.

Anestrus can be related to infantilism. Infantile ovaries are small, sometimes the size of a pea or less, and hard to locate. Infantile ovaries often are accompanied with underdevelopment of all or part of the external or internal genitalia. The uterus may be found during palpation to have horns only 2 or 3 inches long. When a mare, 4 years old or more, is found with underdeveloped ovaries and uterus, the condition can be considered as hopeless. However, a younger mare with extremely small ovaries, but otherwise normal genitalia, should never be condemned as sterile as quite often such ovaries will respond to massage at regular intervals, or to hormonal injections of FSH (follicle stimulating hormone), 10 to 20 mg., or to pregnant mare serum, 2,000 I.U. every 2 or 3 weeks. Some authors have recommended biweekly doses of pregnant mare serum, 1,000 I.U. for 2 or 3 weeks. The results of either method have been erratic, but they should be evaluated on a long-range basis as sometimes favorable results are not evident until the following breeding season.

True anestrus, when occurring in a mare with a normally developed genital system, has been classified as deep anestrus and shallow anestrus. A deep anestrus often is characterized by the presence of small, hard, fibrous, and inactive ovaries. Such ovaries may have on their surfaces some nodules or even small, hard follicles up to 1 cm. in diameter. During the breeding season, deep anestrus is seen in maiden and barren mares, but more often in foaling mares. These mares usually exhibit "foal heat," but fail to establish the normal cycles subsequently. For still unknown reasons, foaling mare anestrus is more frequent in some years than in others, and it also occurs more often late in the breeding season. It is this irregularity which is responsible for the old and erroneous belief that breeding during "foal heat" was the only time to breed a foaling mare with any chance of success.

Britton *et al.* have advanced the opinion that anestrus is related to the activity of the mammary glands.[3] They report that anestrus can last up to 6 months in heavy milkers, and for an average of 2½ months in poor milking mares.

Treatment with hormones and by mechanical means usually is unrewarding as the condition corrects itself in a few months and the mare can be expected to have normal cycles the following season.

Shallow anestrus is more common and is found equally in maiden, barren, or foaling mares. The condition is characterized by healthy and apparently active, but temporarily arrested, ovaries. The ovaries are found to be normally developed, of a spongy or relatively spongy consistency, and with several follicles, occasionally as large as 2 inches wide. By re-

peated examination of the ovaries one will sometimes detect the appearance of new follicles or the regression of others, but neither maturation nor ovulation occurs. These ovarian changes may be reflected in the mare's behavior. When teased regularly the mare shows, at times, signs of impending heat which subside without developing further.

The prognosis of the condition usually is good, and affected mares respond relatively well to treatment. Mechanical stimulation should be used as much as possible, as this treatment seems to induce more natural heats and higher conception rates.

Mechanical stimulation is accomplished by transrectal massage of the uterus and ovaries, followed by introduction of 500 ml. of saline solution into the uterus. The uterine douche should be given as aseptically as possible. After thorough cleansing of the vulva, the gloved hand is introduced into the vagina, and the cervix is slowly and gently dilated with the index finger. Once the finger is introduced in the uterus as far as possible, a plastic insemination pipette connected to a 500 ml. saline vial is slid along the finger. When the tip of the pipette is in the uterus, the saline is allowed to flow, either under pressure or by gravity. Mares usually will come in estrus 3 to 4 days after the douche.

Another method of treatment is the tapping of ovarian cysts. This technic was very popular several years ago but is not practiced so widely now, probably because of the difficulty associated with doing it, the possibility of complications, and the inconsistency of the results. It is recommended that a minimum of 2 examinations be made over a weekly interval to determine which cyst should be tapped. The entrance is made through the cranial part of the vagina with one hand in the vagina guiding a long needle and the other in the rectum holding the ovary within reach. Some operators prefer working with one hand only and tap the cyst through the rectum.

Hormonal therapy also has been used with success to induce estrus. Diethylstilbestrol has been found to be very effective in 5 to 25 mg. doses though others recommend doses of 200 mg. The fear of inducing cystic development of the ovaries by using diethylstilbestrol has been overemphasized as there seems to be little danger of this if one limits the treatment to 1 or 2 injections. Pregnant mare serum in doses of 1,500 or 2,000 I.U., and successive doses of 15 mg. of FSH every few days also have been of value.

Pseudocyesis is another form of anestrus. It usually follows breeding, but can occur in mares who have not been bred. Affected mares behave like normally pregnant ones in their relations to the teaser, sometimes show a slight increase in weight and the healthy blossoming of the newly pregnant mare. On rectal examination, the uterus is found to have the consistency and tonus of a pregnant uterus. On direct examination, the vagina is found to have the typical appearance of pregnancy: pale mucous membranes, thick, whitish secretions, and a tightly closed cervix often covered by a cervical seal. If untreated, the condition can last 2 or 3 months, and sometimes up to 11 months or more. Some mares have been pseudopregnant for full term and have shown enlargement and waxing of the mammary glands. Evidence of pain, similar to foaling pain, has been observed at the time when the mare would have foaled if truly pregnant. The condition usually can be corrected with a saline douche.

Anestrus also occurs in thin, undernourished mares and is corrected once the animal is provided an adequate ration. Some overly fat mares often show manifestations of prolonged anestrus. Most of them have a hypofunctional thyroid gland as revealed by their blood P.B.I. (protein bound iodine), which usually is close to a value of one or below. If given thyroid extract or thyroprotein at regularly increased doses until the therapeutic level is established, these mares will lose weight and re-establish a regular cycle.

ABNORMAL INTERESTRUS

Some mares will be observed to "go out of heat" for 1 or 2 days in the middle of estrus and then show signs of estrus again. They are said to have a "split heat." In such cases, a follicle has matured rapidly, ruptured, formed a corpus luteum, and immediately afterward a new follicle has initiated another estrus. Split heats generally are 2 or 3 days longer than normal estrus and can be considered to be exceptional for an otherwise regular mare. Breeding is successful if performed during the second part of the split estrus. No treatment is required.

Some mares will have a short interestrual period, 5 to 10 days, probably because of a short-lived corpus luteum, which in the equine should last 21 days. This condition sometimes is associated with endometritis, but more often it is encountered in otherwise normal mares. In most cases, the condition will correct itself within a few estrual cycles. It usually does not cause sterility as affected mares have been known to conceive with or without progesterone injections at the time of breeding.

ABNORMAL ESTRUS

Early in the year, at the time of adjustment, one should expect to find barren mares having irregular cycles or very long estrual periods. As previously stated, the best course of action is to wait for these mares to establish a regular cycle spontaneously. Because of the relatively short breeding season of Quarter Horses or Thoroughbreds, it sometimes is difficult to wait for affected mares to adjust and to resist the request of the owner that something be done. Most Thoroughbred breeders are very eager to obtain foals early in the year, and want to breed their barren or maiden mares in February. It is best for the veterinarian to maintain that more harm than good can be done by early, or injudicious, treatment and that the administration of patience is the best therapy.

Most mares which have long estrual periods usually do not have a complete cycle. Upon examination of the ovaries, one invariably will find an enlarged follicle, the size varying from 1 to 4 inches wide, or occasionally larger. Other less mature follicles usually are present. Subsequent examinations often will detect further enlargement of the specified follicle. The cervix is found to be somewhat relaxed, sometimes it is atonic and open, pale in color, or it may be slightly inflamed. Cervical secretions are thin and not very abundant. Subsequent examinations usually do not reveal appreciable changes. Most of these estrual periods, in time, will terminate by ovulation which can be detected by rectal or vaginal examination. Massage of the cystic ovary and injection of a luteinizing hormone usually will bring the signs of estrus to an abrupt end within a week. The mare is to be expected to return to a normal cycle within 3 weeks. In very rare instances, cysts which do not respond to hormonal treatment have to be tapped.

Pseudonymphomania is relatively frequent. Some mares will be receptive to the male for long periods, usually during the first part of the breeding season but occasionally all year long, and still ovulate at regular intervals. No attempt need be made to correct the situation. These mares should be examined with a vaginal speculum regularly as the changes in the appearance of the cervix are quite evident. Once signs of an imminent ovulation are detected, they should be confirmed by rectal examination. Breeding at this time usually is successful. It is not uncommon to find a mare who will have conceived from such a breeding, and still be receptive to the teaser during most of her pregnancy.

True nymphomania occurs in various degrees, with or without cystic ovaries. Some mares will show signs of estrus constantly, and will accept the male if permitted, but breeding will be unsuccessful because of the mare's failure to ovulate. The ovaries will be found to be normal, or sometimes cystic. Often, a thorough examination will reveal an irritation of the clitoris caused by a foreign body such as grain, foxtails, or small balls of hair. Extraction of the offending material will result in reestablishment of a normal cycle. Clitoridectomy, as practiced in Europe, often is beneficial. Severe cases of nymphomania seem to be more often attributable to an established nervous pattern than to an endocrine disorder. An endocrine anomaly, however, can be the initial trigger. In nymphomanic mares, the ovaries are found to be small, hard, and shrunken. The mare constantly exhibits signs of estrus by switching the tail, squirting urine, and squealing. She usually refuses to receive the stallion, and if bred under restraint she does not conceive. Such mares are vicious, mean toward other horses, and sometimes toward humans.

Unfortunately, clitoridectomies, and even ovariectomies, often are not successful, as most of these cases do not respond to any treatment.

Apparently Normal Estrus

Some mares are presented to the veterinarian because despite having regular estrual cycles and adequate breeding, they fail to conceive though other mares bred to the same stallion conceive without difficulty. The first step should be elimination of the possibility of genital infection by making a bacteriologic culture of the cervical secretions during estrus. The second step involves examination of the mare rectally and vaginally every day or every other day during estrus to observe the changes taking place in the ovaries and cervix.

Some mares show signs of estrus and still do not ovulate. Rectal examinations of such animals will reveal follicles forming or regressing; sometimes no follicle can be felt. In these cases, the cervix undergoes a series of changes, but never shows the typical picture of ovulation: complete relaxation, congestion, and adequate secretions. Some mares occasionally will have such an estrus, usually in the early part of the season. When the condition is observed to recur, it usually can be corrected by injection of small quantities of FSH, 20 to 30 mg., immediately prior to the heat period. If the follicle is sufficiently developed, it may be successfully stimulated during estrus by injection of luteinizing hormone or of pregnant mare serum, 1,000 to 2,000 I.U. Ovulation usually follows within 24 to 48 hours.

In some cases, the follicle will be slow in maturing and ovulation will occur in 1, 2, or 3 days following estrus. Injection of luteinizing hormone during the heat period usually will be followed by a successful breeding.

Some mares will have a normal heat period with ovulation; they will have been bred at the optimum time by a fertile stallion and still will not conceive. One can then assume that implantation is not occurring. Successful treatment of this condition has been reported in cows injected with repositol progesterone immediately following breeding. To our knowledge, such observations have not been published about horses, and the practice in our experience has been unsuccessful. This difference might be due to the fact that placentation in the cow begins on the 11th day after ovulation, but in horses it occurs 8 weeks afterward.

ANATOMIC ANOMALIES

Malformation of the vulva as a condition predisposing to sterility already has been discussed in relation to the infected mare. As stated, the condition should be corrected surgically. Mares with a hypoplastic vulva usually have a poor breeding potential as the condition is evidence of undeveloped genitalia.

PERSISTENT HYMEN

Persistent hymen is a rare condition in mares. The hymen usually is formed of several vertical fleshy filaments at the junction of the vulva and vagina: these filaments are ruptured easily during coitus, but sometimes are still found in young mares. On some breeding farms, it is a common practice to rupture the hymen several days before breeding. Such is done not only to make the first service easier on the maiden, but also because of the fear that there is a greater change of genital infection when the hymen is torn during the breeding process.

A completely formed and thick hymen sometimes is encountered. Such a hymen is unusually thick, having the size, consistency, and appearance of the bladder wall. It may be perforated with a very small opening, but sometimes it is imperforate. When imperforate, it usually is very obvious when the filly lies down, as the hymen filled with uterine and cervical secretions, bulges through the vulva. The persistent hymen should be grasped with a pair of forceps and excised with scissors.

RECTOVAGINAL FISTULA (FIG. 11)

Rectovaginal fistula is a common complication of unattended foaling. It happens during delivery when the foal projects a hoof through the vaginal and rectal walls. The fistula may be a simple one varying in dimension from ⅛ inch or less to 2 or 3 inches. In some instances,

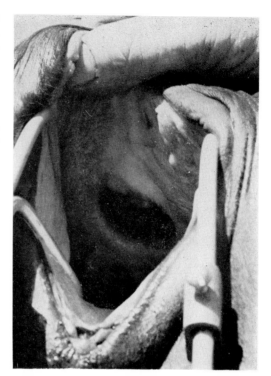

Fig. 11. Rectovaginal fistula. A common complication of foaling.

the tears extend to and involve the entire anus. The condition should be treated surgically as the mare is hopelessly sterile as long as the fistula is allowed to exist. Feces pass freely from the rectum to the vagina where they accumulate and seriously contaminate the vagina, the cervix, and often the uterus. A procedure for surgical repair of rectovaginal fistula is described in Chapter 27.

SINKING VAGINA (FIG. 12)

A sinking vagina sometimes is found in old multiparous mares which are in poor physical condition. Upon direct examination, one finds the vagina considerably below the pubic level, and usually filled with urine halfway to the cervix. Sometimes urine covers the entire cervix. The condition develops because of the poor muscle tone of the vagina and the elongated ovarian ligaments which allow the uterus to drop far below its normal level. Some mares will conceive despite the condition if the residual urine is removed from the vagina with

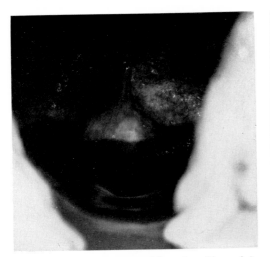

Fig. 12. Cervix nearly covered by urine. Observed in cases of sinking vagina.

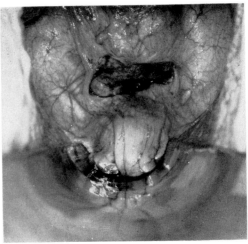

Fig. 13. Vaginal tear following coital injury.

aseptic cotton prior to breeding. In the majority of cases, the condition must be corrected before breeding. When observed in foaling mares the prognosis usually is excellent, as with sexual rest and an adequate feeding program the vagina and the uterus regain their original tonus. Old barren mares, who have this condition despite sexual rest and good physical constitution, should be treated surgically. The purpose of the operation is to narrow and elevate the vagina. This is best done with the mare on her back and under general anesthesia. A triangle of mucosa is detached from the roof of the vagina, the base at the level of the cervix and the summit at the vulva. The base should be from 1 to 3 inches wide, according to the extent of the necessary repair. Actual elevation of the vagina then is done by suturing the incised edges of the mucosa.

Injuries During Coition

Coital injuries are not uncommon in young mares. They result from breedings in which there is gross disparity in the size of the mare's and stallion's genitalia. The most common injury is perforation of the cranial part of the vagina. This type of injury is accompanied by abundant hemorrhage but it is not serious from the standpoint of future fertility. As a rule, suturing is not required. Sexual rest and main-

tenance of a high antibiotic blood level for a few days are sufficient. Such injuries can be prevented by interposing a breeding roll between the mare and stallion during service (Fig. 13).

Cervical Atresia

Cervical atresia is a common cause of infertility and it is difficult to correct. The healing of cervical tears which occur at foaling may completely or partially close the cervix. In isolated instances, the mare will be able to conceive if artificially inseminated. In most cases, however, the condition should be corrected prior to conception. Manual debridement and cauterization with silver nitrate have been tried but have not generally been successful. The best method of correction involves the use of the cervical pessary described for pyometra. When using the pessary, aseptic technic should be followed so as to avoid causing a cervicitis or endometritis.

Degeneration of the Uterus

Cystic degeneration of the uterine wall has been described by several authors. It is most likely to be a postmortem finding. The uterus will contain numerous, small submucosal cysts which are 1 to 5 centimeters in diameter.

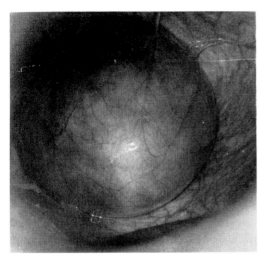

Fig. 14. Tumor of the cervix. This growth, probably a fibroma, was observed in a 12-year-old Thoroughbred mare with a 2-month-old foal.

The cysts are filled with a clear, amber fluid. The uterine wall will feel thick, soft, and spongy. A similar condition has been described in the dog and cow in which it had been associated with prolonged estrus and nymphomania. The condition apparently is of hormonal origin and is considered to render the animal hopelessly sterile.

IMPATENT FALLOPIAN TUBES

Occlusion of the fallopian tubes has not, to my knowledge, been described in the literature. The possibility of the condition should be considered, however, in those mares which fail to conceive and are otherwise normal. The patency of the tubes can be checked by inflating the uterus with gas during the anestrual phase while the cervix is closed and palpate rectally the distribution of the gas.

NEOPLASMS

Tumors of the genital tract in mares are rare and accordingly have very little bearing on sterility problems. They are described in Chapter 21 (Fig. 14).

INFERTILITY IN THE STALLION

INTRODUCTION

In 1950, Dimock reported the results of a 30-year study made in central Kentucky of 150 Thoroughbred stallions.[9] These 150 stallions were separated as follows into 5 groups according to their breeding records and semen quality:

47% were classified as having high fertility.

27% as having average fertility.

11% as having low or decreasing fertility; these were stallions 10 years old or more who had previously been classified as normal but were showing signs of declining fertility.

5% were showing increasing fertility. These were young stallions 4 to 7 years old whose fertility had been increasing considerably during the time they had been used for stud service.

10% were sterile from the beginning.

Fertility can be evaluated on the basis of the difficulty or ease with which pregnancy is induced in the female, *i.e.*, the number of services required to produce a live foal. A stallion should never be judged on the basis of his breeding a few mares. It should always be kept in mind that proportionately there are more sterile females than sterile males. A stallion which covers 40 to 45 mares a year will need an average of slightly more than 2 covers per mare to induce pregnancy in 70 to 75% of them.

The relatively low fertility ratio of the stallion is thought to be partly related to the fact that he is used to breed a mixed group of mares in a relatively short breeding season.

FUNCTION OF THE STALLION IN REPRODUCTION

THE GENITAL TRACT

The testicle is the essential gland of the genital tract. Its function is dual, being the site for both the formation of spermatozoa and the male hormones. The spermatozoa are formed in the seminiferous tubules and while slowly maturing pass through the collecting tubules, the rete testis, and the epididymis. The epididymis is divided into 2 parts: the head or receptacle for the tubules coming from the rete testis, and the tail which is a long, coiled, thick, single tubule of 50 meters or so continued by the vas deferens.

The epididymis secretes a nourishing fluid and acts as a reservoir for the spermatozoa. An average of 21 days is required for the spermatozoa to be formed and able to fertilize. Of these 21 days, 5 to 10 are spent in the epididymis. When ejaculation does not occur, the spermatozoa die and are absorbed.

Spermatogenesis is possible only when the testes are kept at a temperature below body temperature. This is made possible by the combined actions of the cremaster muscle and the scrotum.

Testicular function is under the direct control of the anterior part of the pituitary gland through the gonadotropic hormones. It is believed that the follicle stimulating hormone is directly responsible for spermatogenesis, and that the luteininizing hormone stimulates the growth of the interstitial cells and the production of testosterone. Testosterone regulates the development of the secondary sex characteristics and the growth of the penis and accessory glands. It probably is responsible for the appearance and maintenance of libido.

The accessory glands produce the fluid medium in which spermatozoa are carried into the female genital tract. Each gland apparently has a specific function but relatively little is known about their exact role. The glandular cells of the epididymis secrete a nourishing medium in which the spermatozoa can stay alive several days. The vas deferens and ampulla contain glands which add to the volume of the semen during ejaculation. The seminal vesicles of the stallion are large, 4 to 6 inches long and 1 to 2 inches wide; they are located at the base of the bladder on each side of the urethra and are thought to be the origin of the albuminous part of the ejaculate. The prostate gland lies on the neck of the bladder and surrounds the urethra. It secretes a thick, white liquid which gives the semen its characteristic odor and probably has an important part in buffering the total ejaculate, thus making it more suitable for spermatozoal viability. The bulbo-urethral glands lie on either side of the caudal part of the urethra and probably secrete the first part of the ejaculate which cleanses and neutralizes the urethra.

EJACULATION

Ejaculation is the act by which the semen is propelled into the female genital tract. Ejaculation can happen only after the penis is in a rigid state, or in erection. This is made possible by turgescence of the 3 essential elements of the penis: both corpora cavernosa, and the corpus cavernosus of the urethra. Turgescence results from the increased blood supply of the pudic and obturator arteries, and the slowing of blood outflow from the penis. Contraction of the smooth muscles of the corpora cavernosus, and the muscles of the penis are responsible for the constriction of the veins.

Erection and ejaculation are reflex acts whose neural centers are located in the lumbar portion of the spinal cord. They also are dependent upon psychic stimuli transmitted from the cerebral cortex.

The force for ejaculation probably starts in the epididymis and travels along the ductus deferens. At the same time, the accessory glands are contracting and forcing their secretions into the urethra. The semen is then transported along the urethra and expelled from the penis by rhythmic contractions of the urethral, ischiocavernosus, and bulbocavernosus muscles. In the horse, erection is relatively slow to appear, whereas ejaculation lasts only 10 to 15 seconds.

THE SEMEN

The complete ejaculate of the stallion measures between 60 and 300 ml. but lighter breeds often give a maximum of only 150 ml. According to Berliner, the ejaculate consists of 3 parts: 1. Close to 10 ml. of a thin, grayish fluid containing few or no spermatozoa, 2, the bulk of the semen, and 3, a portion, often missing or much reduced in lighter breeds, which is extremely white and of a gelatinous consistency.[2] It has been stated that this portion is extremely noxious for the spermatozoa, and probably is responsible for the short life of the equine spermatozoa *in vitro*.

The stallion ejaculates directly through the cervix and into the uterus. It has been theorized that the last part of the ejaculate is expelled while the penis becomes flaccid, and consequently is emitted into the vagina. This portion of semen could then function as a plug to close the cervix.

Opinions vary concerning the survival time of sperm in the genital tract of the mare. Neumann and Salzmann observed, during a series of postmortem examinations, that spermatozoa retain motility for only 28 to 36 hours.[19] Burkhardt, basing his observations on controlled ovulations and inseminations, concluded that the spermatozoa survive for 68 to 138 hours.[4]

Examination of Semen: The only absolute manner of determining a stallion's fertility is to demonstrate his ability to induce pregnancy. It is a common practice among breeders to try young and expensive stallions on a test mare before selling them. This practice is reliable, but it takes a long time, involves the fertility of the mare, and does not give an indication of the degree of the stallion's fertility. Examination of semen, however, can immediately provide some evidence of the degree of fertility, if any, and indicate the causes of infertility to some degree. When a young stallion is to be thoroughly evaluated, both methods should be used.

Collection of the Sample: There are at least 2 opinions concerning the best type of sample for semen examination. Some use the last part of the ejaculate, others the entire ejaculate. McLeod and McGee in their study of the semen of the Thoroughbred used whole ejaculate.[18] Dimock based his observations on examinations of semen collected from the flaccid penis at the time the stallion dismounted from the mare.[9] Haag after examining 175 dismount samples has concluded that the fertility of an ejaculation can be correlated to the quality of the dismount sample.[12] He also found that there does not seem to be any relationship between the spermatozoal concentration in the total ejaculate and in the last part of it.

Examination of semen remaining at dismount undoubtedly can provide an estimation of its quality and should be done routinely while examining stallions during the breeding season. It should be kept in mind that this method is totally inadequate to diagnose the causes of infertility as 2 essential determinations cannot be made: the quantity and quality of the accessory gland secretions and the total number of spermatozoa, which reflects testicular activity.

The total ejaculate must be collected during or after a normal service. The stallion may be fitted with a breeding bag or a rubber condom immediately prior to the breeding, and the sample collected from the bag when the stallion dismounts. Another technic involves the use of an artificial vagina into which the penis is diverted while the horse is mounting the mare. Either method provides a suitable sample, some horses responding better to one than the other.

The use of the artificial vagina requires experience in regulating the temperature and pressure of the device. It often is more suitable for young horses. The ejaculate should not be sampled after a long period of inactivity, or during the first time a young stallion is used as a stud, as such a specimen could not be considered representative of the horse's semen. The sample should be collected from the second or third ejaculate after several days of rest.

Characteristics of Semen: The collected specimen should be examined grossly and microscopically. Several chemical and bacteriologic tests also are indicated.

The total volume of the ejaculate should be carefully measured. As already stated, in lighter breeds a normal ejaculate should be between 50 and 150 ml. These limits can vary, however, for the same stallion depending on the frequency of use. In some horses which are breeding every day for a month or more, the total quantity of each ejaculate may diminish to 30 ml. or less. Other individuals kept under the same strenuous program will maintain their usual volume. A few days of rest for overbred stallions usually are sufficient to restore the total volume of the ejaculate to normal.

Special attention should be given to the viscosity of the semen. It normally has a consistency close to light mineral oil. If it regularly is found to be thin and watery, this is indicative of inadequate or hypofunctional accessory glands. The consistency often will improve after the horse is put on a better breeding schedule, and given more exercise and a better diet.

Sometimes the semen will be found to be extremely thick and gelatinous-like. This thick consistency of semen is attributed to oversecretion by the seminal vesicles and, as Berliner demonstrated, this secretion is relatively toxic to spermatozoa.[2] Many stallions with such semen, however, will be found to be fertile.

The turbidity of the sample will provide an estimate of the quantity of debris, cellular material, or mucus in suspension. It should not be excessive, as this would indicate the presence of some abnormality in the genital tract. In genital infections, pus cells in the semen plus occasional flakes of pus will cause the sample to appear cloudy.

A drop of semen should be examined microscopically at a temperature close to body temperature as soon as possible. An examination in the field is mandatory. The spermatozoa should be observed for motility. An estimate should be made of the number of motile spermatozoa and also of their type of motion. In a good sample, 90 to 95% of the spermatozoa will be alive at the time of collection, and their movement will be rapid and strong. Occasionally, some very fertile stallions are found to have sluggish and slow moving spermatozoa in their semen. Several standards have been suggested for grading the motility of a given sample. One of the most commonly used is the following:

Grade 0—No motility.

Grade 1—Spermatozoa exhibit weak, stationary or rotary motion.

Grade 2—Spermatozoa exhibit oscillatory and rotary motion. Less than 50% are active, no waves are formed.

Grade 3—Progressive and rapid motion of the spermatozoa, producing slowly moving waves. From 50 to 75% of the spermatozoa are active.

Grade 4—Vigorous and progressive movement with waves. From 75 to 90% of spermatozoa are active.

Grade 5—Vigorous and rapid forward motion; very rapid waves. Close to 100% of spermatozoa are motile.

Fertility and speed of movement are not necessarily closely related, but one can safely assume that semen with very active spermatozoa will likely be more fertile than semen not having this characteristic.

Studies of bovine semen have revealed that there is a constant relationship between longevity of the spermatozoa and fertility of the bull. The longevity of the spermatozoa is measured by the persistence of motility in a sample kept undiluted at 40 F. It is assumed that the same relationship exists with the stallion; equine spermatozoa are short-lived, however, and are very sensitive to changes in temperature. Consequently, equine semen should be examined at room temperature. A drop of the sample should be examined every 2 hours until motility is no longer observed. An average sample should show some evidence of motility after 8 to 10 hours. Some excellent samples will still exhibit weak motility after 24 hours.

The approximate total number of spermatozoa in the ejaculate should be recorded. This can be calculated by determining the concentration of spermatozoa, using a white blood cell counting chamber, in terms of concentration per ml. which can vary between 30,000 and 600,000. The total number of spermatozoa per ejaculate should be representative of testicular activity, and the concentration of a normal ejaculate can be considered to be inversely proportional to the activity of the accessory glands. Considering that the testicles produce spermatozoa at a constant rate, one can predict that a given horse will have the same total quantity of spermatozoa in each ejaculate. Experience has shown that such a prediction will not hold, and that the total number will vary, and often drop considerably when the horse is bred too frequently.

The semen also should be examined for abnormalities of the spermatozoa; this is best done with a stained sample. Several stains are available but one of the easiest to use is India ink. To prepare a slide, a drop of India ink is mixed with 5 drops of semen, and one drop of this mixture then is gently spread on a glass slide and allowed to dry. The slide is studied under oil immersion, and the abnormal spermatozoa are carefully examined and tabulated as a percentage of the total. Some spermatozoa will be tailless and some will have no head, some will have 2 heads, and others will have a twisted or bent tail. Dimock and McLeod estimate that a sample with 20% or less abnormal spermatozoa can be considered normal.[9,18]

The semen also should be examined for the presence of white blood cells. Too many of these cells are indicative of infection in the genital tract. From 1,000 to 2,000 white blood cells per ml. can be considered to be normal. A few red blood cells and epithelial cells are found relatively often but they usually are not significant, in reference to fertility.

When the concentration of the leukocytes is abnormally high, the semen should be examined for bacteria. In many cases, a Gram stain will reveal the presence of pathogenic bacteria. A bacteriologic culture should be done at the same time. It should be kept in mind that a semen specimen normally is not free of bacteria, and that the isolation of pathogenic organisms from contaminated samples often is difficult.

The pH of the semen sample should be determined, as any deviation from normal would reflect some change in the chemical composition of the semen and most certainly in the activity of the accessory glands. Dimock found that normal semen will have a pH between 7.3 and 7.8.[9] Presence of pus in the semen will alter the pH.

Haag has demonstrated that there is an inverse correlation "between the nonprotein sulfhydryl concentration of seminal fluid and the ability of that fluid to maintain motility of spermatozoa." He demonstrated also that there is a direct relationship between the quality of a given sample and the sulfhydryl level.[11] The titration of sulfhydryls is a relatively complicated process, but it is an additional way to ascertain the fertility of a stallion.

It should be stated in conclusion that several stallions have been observed to have apparently normal sperm but were absolutely unable to induce pregnancy.

CAUSES OF INFERTILITY IN THE STALLION

As in the mare, the problem of infertility in the stallion is extremely complex and is influenced by such factors as: infection, nutrition, psychologic attitude, genetic composition, and hormonal balance. These different factors are interrelated, possibly more so in the male than in the female. The testes, when under the continual stress of producing spermatozoa, are extremely sensitive to environmental influences, and the acts of erection and ejaculation are essentially dependent on proper balance of the endocrine and nervous systems. For the sake of clarity, each situation conducive to infertility in the male will be considered in relation to the factor which seems to have the strongest influence.

INFECTIOUS PROCESSES

Coital Exanthema: Coital exanthema follows a similar course in the stallion as in the mare. The lesions are limited to the genitalia and there is no systemic reaction. It is characterized by the appearance of small blisters, first on the glans and then on the body of the penis. These become pustules and ulcers in a few days. An infected stallion should not be used to breed as the condition is extremely contagious. The affected part should be treated topically by washing the affected areas with a mild antiseptic solution and cauterizing the lesions with silver nitrate.

Dourine: Dourine has been described in Chapter 7.

BACTERIAL INFECTIONS OF THE GENITAL ORGANS

In the stallion, inflammation and infection can be found at any level of the genital tract, from the testicles to the glans penis. Experience has shown that the 2 most common inflammations involve the testicle and the seminal vesicles with or without spreading to the adjacent structures.

Orchitis: Orchitis often is a complication of a systemic infection like strangles. Sometimes it is encountered as a primary condition, often due to trauma. In either case, the testes are swollen, warm to touch, and extremely sensitive. The condition often is associated with an epididymitis, and sometimes with an inflammation of the vas deferens and the ampulla. When these conditions are present they can be detected by manual examination; the affected portion of the genital tract is enlarged and sensitive. The condition can be so painful that the stallion will refuse to breed, but more often there is no interference with coitus. The semen may contain a great number of leukocytes, and in some cases clots of pus. The spermatozoa will be greatly reduced in number, have abnormal shapes, and their motility and viability will be sharply reduced.

The infective agent usually is a beta hemolytic Streptococcus. It can be cultured from the semen and often observed directly on a Gram stained smear of the semen.

The prognosis as to the future usefulness of an infected stallion should be guarded. The condition can become chronic, with the external signs slowly subsiding to the point where the testicle will return to normal size and lose its sensitivity. The gland will feel somewhat harder than normal, and adhesions sometimes will be present. The semen will have an abnormal quantity of pus cells, and the pathogenic organisms can be detected at times. The constant sign of persistent infection will be a rise in the number of abnormal spermatozoa which have poor motility and viability. As a result, the fertility of the stallion will be greatly decreased, and sometimes the animal becomes sterile. Even if the acute orchitis subsides completely with adequate treatment, one should expect some testicular degeneration to occur. The extent of the degeneration will be proportional to the severity and persistence of the orchitis.

Acute orchitis is best treated by generous use of cold water topically, and parenterally with a combination of enzymes and antibiotics based on sensitivity tests. Evaluation of therapy should be made more on the bacteriologic examination of the semen than on the clinical signs manifested by the horse.

Vesiculitis: Infections of the seminal vesicles are not uncommon in stallions. They sometimes are the result of systemic infections, as in the case of orchitis, but often their origin cannot be related to any apparent source.

In case of acute inflammation, one or both vesicles will be found on rectal examination to be greatly enlarged and sensitive. In many chronic cases, palpation of the sacs will not reveal any noticeable change; there will be some induration and a slight enlargement but no apparent sensitivity. In some cases, the stallion will be impotent and unable to ejaculate. More often, however, he will breed normally but the semen will be found to contain many leukocytes. Bacteriologic cultures will reveal the presence of pathogenic organisms. The bacterium most often isolated is a beta hemolytic Streptococcus; less often a Staphylococcus, Pseudomonas, or member of the coli group is cultured.

The fertility of the stallion is usually reduced during vesiculitis but he still will be able to induce some pregnancies, and surprisingly enough there will be few or no cases of vaginitis, cervicitis, or endometritis resulting from such breeding. However, a good number of the pregnant mares bred by infected stallions will abort at some time during their gestation or give birth to sickly, weak foals with very little chance of survival.

The prognosis should be very reserved when the condition is chronic. If an acute case is diagnosed early, however, there usually is good response to therapy. The treatment should include complete sexual rest and systemic antibacterial therapy, with the agent determined on the basis of a sensitivity test.

To my knowledge, infection of the prostate or of the bulbo-urethral glands has not been reported in horses. Occasionally, abscesses of the glans penis are encountered, most commonly in the fossa glandis. They usually respond to topical therapy. Sometimes, one will find a chronic corrosive induration of the processus urethrae which will not respond to repeated applications of various therapeutic agents and will require surgical excision.

NUTRITIONAL FACTORS

Testicular function appears to be extremely sensitive to changes in the animal's physiologic balance. A definite relationship exists between stallion fertility and the quality of the diet. Dimock stated that stallions suffering from nutritional deficiency usually are nervous, irritable, and difficult to manage.[9] He also referred to 2 stallions which improved considerably after having been fed a diet of a variety of "the best hays, mixed grains, and grasses without particular reference to the amount of any one element in the feed."

A subminimal nutrient ration results in testicular degeneration and atrophy. Sexual desire will diminish and eventually be nonexistent. The semen will show a decrease in the total number of spermatozoa and an increase of abnormal forms. If these changes are not checked they may become irreversible. Reid has observed that the same degenerative changes may appear in the accessory glands without being evident in the testes.[20]

Very little information is available concerning the relationship of nutrition and fertility in the stallion; most of our knowledge is based on extrapolation of observations in other species. It is safe to assume that a stallion should be given a well-balanced ration of mixed grain and hay and should have free access to succulent green grass. It has been suggested that stallions should not be kept too fat. It is difficult to find experimental evidence, however, that excessive nutrients would per se be detrimental to male fertility. In my opinion, most cases of low fertility in fat stallions are not attributable to excessive nutrients, but to lack of exercise. It should be emphasized that stallions need regular and rigorous exercise, especially during the breeding season. A stallion should be physically fit at the beginning and during the breeding season.

Data concerning specific avitaminoses are not available for the stallion. Vitamin A is considered essential for spermatogenesis. The B vitamins do not seem to have a specific role in fertility. Vitamin C is not emphasized as much now as it was several years ago as there is a lack of experimental evidence of its need and efficiency in sterility problems. The use of vitamin E for infertility has numerous supporters. Alpha tocopherol, which has the properties of vitamin E, has been given to stallions with some success, according to horse breeders. It is said to increase the libido and the quality of the semen. Results of controlled experiments concerning the efficacy of vitamin E for stallions have not been published, however. Reid

is quoted by Roberts as stating, "in few fields are there more opinions with less supporting evidence than in the field of sterility."[21]

The old practice of giving wheat germ oil to the stallion during the breeding season certainly is not detrimental and is useful as a general conditioner because of its high content of B vitamins. Fresh wheat germ oil also is rich in vitamin E. This vitamin is said to be destroyed relatively easily and there is no proof that the wheat germ oil has any vitamin E activity by the time it is administered.

PSYCHOLOGIC FACTORS

As previously stated, the male's participation in coitus is dependent, among other factors, upon stimuli from the voluntary and sympathetic nervous systems. Change of mood, habits, and the influence of former experiences often will be evident in the way a stallion performs. As most horses are hand-bred, the stallion's reactions will be complicated by the addition of this factor.

Training of a Young Stallion: The initial use of a young stallion as a stud is a very important step which can have a lasting influence on the subject's ability to breed. Though some young stallions know instinctively what to do when taken to a mare in heat, others will know that something should be done but that is all, and others are indifferent. The first rule which applies while breeding a young stallion for the first time is to use a patient and very receptive mare. If the female fights, squirms, or even kicks before, during, or after the act, some irreparable physical or psychologic trauma may be suffered by the male.

The second rule is to be extremely patient. A young stallion should be handled only by an experienced man. As McGee stated, there is no technic known for putting a stallion upon a mare unless he wants to mount.[16] It is the stud man's responsibility to encourage and coax the stallion at the proper time and discourage him in a proper way at the wrong time. No specific rule applies as this is determined by circumstances and personality.

A few suggestions concerning the procedure for initiating a young stallion follow: 1. The stallion should be allowed to become acquainted with the mare and tease her for a while at the teasing bar, 2, with the mare properly restrained, he should be brought to her rear and slightly on the left side, 3, he should not be allowed to bite and should be given ample time to get ready to mount the mare properly. The first service is usually done during the initial meeting and in 30 minutes or less.

A real problem is presented by young stallions who are mildly interested but do not attempt to mount the mare or have an erection. These horses should be tried repeatedly for a while; introduction to the mare should be repeated the following day or in the evening. In the meantime, the horse should be kept in a stall or paddock close to the mare. Some cases have been observed in which it took more than a week to initiate a young stallion.

In every instance the stallion should be given a well-balanced ration with a good supply of vitamin supplement to prevent possible nutritional deficiencies. Injections of B vitamins have proved to be helpful. Testosterone and luteinizing hormone, either of which theoretically should induce libido, produce disappointing results. Adrenal cortical extracts and steroids have been reported to be useful.

Breeding Habits: Many stallions have bad breeding habits which the stud man should know and take into consideration. Such habits often have been developed during their first use as a stud.

Some horses are extremely slow breeders; some have been known to require nearly 45 minutes to cover a mare. Various treatments and coaxing fail to accelerate the process. These stallions usually are very slow in mounting the mare and often have to cover her several times before ejaculation occurs.

A common cause of infertility in the stallion is inability to ejaculate. This often is not pathologic per se as the problem may simply be that the stallion has developed this breeding pattern and the stud man is unable to distinguish at what cover ejaculation occurs.

The person handling the stallion should be able to determine if ejaculation has occurred or not. It is the role of the veterinarian to explain to him how it happens and how it can be recognized. During ejaculation, the semen is propelled by rhythmic contractions of different muscles of the genital tract. This produces a pulse-like motion of the urethra. At the same time the tail moves up and down with each pulsation, probably when the contractions are transmitted to the tail muscles through the ischiocavernosus and the retractor penis muscles. This tail motion is called "flagging" by horse breeders and is considered evidence of ejaculation.

Some horses have been observed to refuse to breed mares of a certain color, and others have to be bred in special surroundings. Some bite the mare during the service, causing her to react defensively and to interrupt the cover; these horses have to be muzzled. The list of personal idiosyncrasies is practically limitless. It is the responsibility of the stud man, properly counseled by the veterinarian, to detect them and act accordingly.

Some stallions are nervous, mean, and hard to handle. These animals usually are bored and do not have proper alimentation. A good diet, plenty of exercise, and a regular routine are a must for stallions. They should always be handled by the same man, if possible. The handler should be observing, gentle, but firm. The great majority of mean stallions have developed their bad dispositions because of poor handling. They have never acquired a salutary respect for their handler. Some horses will perform better if kept isolated, and others will be more effective if they are put in a paddock where they can see mares and other stallions.

Masturbation: Nine of 10 cases of poor breeding performance and lowered fertility can be attributed to masturbation. Most horses do not masturbate in public; they do it at night or when alone. The stallion's owner or the stud man, if questioned, almost invariably will insist that his horse does not have this vice.

As a consequence of masturbation, the semen becomes thinner, the total sperm count drops considerably, and sometimes abnormal spermatozoa are increased in numbers. There is a noticeable decrease of libido and very often the stallion will have trouble ejaculating. Dimock stated that the habit, if prolonged, will have detrimental effects on fertility and that the associated lesions in some cases may be irreversible.[9] It has been my experience that masturbation by stallions can be stopped at any time, and that the animal will return to breeding condition in a relatively short time.

Masturbation can be prevented with the use of a stallion ring and cage or a masturbation harness. The rings are made of plastic and come in several sizes. The cages are made of light metal, resistant to corrosion. The ring is placed on the penis, one inch or so above the glans, and the cage is inserted around the glans. Both ring and cage should be the size of the relaxed penis. Their application prevents the stallion from achieving a full erection and ejaculation.

Some horses still manage to masturbate in spite of these devices; they should be attired with a restraining harness. The harness is complicated to install, but is very effective. It consists of a dented metal frame kept above the penis with teeth pointed downward. The teeth, by irritating the penis when the stallion tries to achieve erection, distract and hurt him, thus preventing ejaculation.

Ring, cage, and harness should, of course, be removed before breeding and washed carefully before being applied again immediately after breeding. If the horse is not bred regularly, they should be taken off at least once a week while the penis is examined for signs of irritation.

GENETIC FACTORS

The size of the genitalia is influenced by genetic factors. There are stallions whose penile size can create mechanical difficulties when they are bred to certain mares.

Testicular hypoplasia has not been reported in stallions; however, the condition probably is as common as it is in the bull. The testicles can be small and hard, or they may apparently be normal in size and consistency. The semen usually will have a low concentration of spermatozoa, a definite increase of abnormal forms (up to 50% or more), and a very poor viability. Horses observed with these characteristics have a poor fertility record. Their treatment with FSH, or gonadotropic hormone, does increase the sperm concentration and, in some cases, seems to increase fertility.

Some stallions have testicles which are held high and horizontal along the lower abdomen instead of hanging down in the scrotum in a slightly oblique position. The condition has been observed in bulls and has been associated with an important diminution of fertility. The stallions that I have observed with such anatomy had not bred any mares, consequently their fertility could not be evaluated.

Cryptorchidism, or failure of normal descent of the testicles, is a relatively common condition in horses. One testicle can be involved or both. The retained testicle may be in the inguinal canal or in the abdomen; in either case, it is not producing spermatozoa because of the temperature to which it is exposed. If the condition is unilateral, fertility is not reduced, but if the condition is bilateral, the stallion is sterile. Nervousness, irritability, and an increased libido are commonly observed in cryptorchid horses. These signs may be attributed to an increased secretion of male hormones by the nondescended testicle.

Monorchid horses should not be used for stud purposes as the condition is thought to be hereditary. In rare cases, continuous hormonal treatment with gonadotropic hormone, for a period of months, will influence the descent of retained testes. Testosterone has been used by some veterinarians for correction of retained testes. This hormone may be administered repeatedly, but with caution to avoid stimulation of undesirable libido. It is unlikely that hormone therapy for cryptorchidism will be successful when the retained testes are located intra-abdominally, or after puberty. One should not make a diagnosis of permanent cryptorchidism until the horse is at least 2 years old, as some testicles descend naturally up to that age.

Occasionally, sterile horses will be encountered which have normal libido, normal semen, and no history of past mismanagement or special illness. No explanation has been given for such an occurrence, but it may be related to some genetic factor.

Hernias, abdominal and inguinal, should be mentioned in a discussion of genetic influences on infertility. An abdominal hernia could mechanically hamper a proper breeding and an inguinal hernia might change the heat regulating function of the scrotum and thus diminish spermatogenesis. Both conditions are liabilities because of the constant possibility of strangulation. Stallions with inguinal hernias may be unwilling to breed due to the pain experienced as they attempt to mount.

HORMONAL FACTORS

The two essential signs which are evidence of a possible disturbance in hormonal regulation are a lack of sexual desire and a failure of spermatogenesis.

The lack of libido can be related to many different factors; masturbation and old age are the most common. Excessive sexual use also reduces the libido. I have observed this in 2 young Shetland stallions, who bred more than 30 mares when they were 2 years old. The following season both had a complete lack of libido, which resisted all treatments. They both resumed normal service 2 years later without further treatment. Some stallions which are used to breed every day and sometimes twice a day for a long period will show a lack of enthusiasm for the mare.

Whatever the cause, lack of libido should respond to hormonal treatment. Considering that injection of testosterone will produce libido in geldings, the same should hold true for stallions. Unfortunately, response to hormonal treatment is extremely erratic. Injection of testosterone sometimes does increase sexual desire. Injection of luteinizing hormone, or chorionic gonadotrophic hormone, seems to have a better long-range effect. Aphrodisiac preparations have been tried without any specific beneficial effect being observed.

Azoospermia is relatively uncommon and often is related to some pathologic factor. Both testes may be hypoplastic and not capable of producing spermatozoa. In this instance the condition may be irreversible. Azoospermia also could be attributed to some obstruction. Often the condition is evidenced by a marked decrease in spermatozoa, and sometimes by an increase of abnormal forms. Azoospermia seems to be related more often to old age. The logical therapy for azoospermia is repeated injections of FSH, or gonadotropic hormone, for an extended period. Testosterone is not recommended as a treatment for this condition.

OTHER PATHOLOGIC FACTORS

Neoplasms do not commonly invade the stallion's genitalia. However, their occurrence in cryptorchid testes is not unusual, and they occasionally occur on the penis and sheath where they mechanically interfere with the horse's ability to breed.

Bony or muscular lesions of the hindlimbs or back will have a definite effect on a stallion's ability to breed. Among the most common lesions of the hindlimbs are ringbones, occult or bone spavin, and fractures.

Occasionally a stallion will be kicked while mounting or dismounting a mare, and if the penis is kicked a hematoma might develop. The same condition may happen when the mare moves while being bred. A penile hematoma may be as large as a football. A stallion so injured should be given complete rest, and the affected parts should be treated with alternate cold and hot water applications several times a day. Systemic administration of enzymes often is beneficial and can shorten the period of convalescence considerably.

ABORTION

Abortion can be defined as the expulsion of the product of pregnancy before it is viable. About 30 days is the earliest date that pregnancy can be detected, and with very few exceptions, foals born one month before term cannot live. Consequently, abortion generally refers to loss of a fetus dead or alive between the first and the tenth months of pregnancy.

VIRAL ABORTIONS

Abortions due to virus are far more common than any other type of abortion. They have been described in Chapter 4.

BACTERIAL ABORTIONS (also see Chapter 5)

Salmonella: Salmonella abortus-equina was identified as being responsible for abortion in mares as early as 1893.[15] Abortions caused by this organism were relatively common in the last part of the nineteenth century and the first quarter of the twentieth. The disease was called contagious equine abortion. Because of the development and successful use of a bacterin, this type of abortion now seems to have been eradicated from the United States.

The equine practitioner should be aware of this disease because of the current failure to routinely use the vaccine. Several generations of horses exist today which have not had a chance to develop resistance to this infection. There is constant danger that the condition will reappear in an epizootic form because of the extreme contagiousness of the disease and the rapid movement of horses within and between countries.

The incubation period for this infection is from 10 to 28 days, after which the mare shows signs of a systemic reaction with fever, usually unnoticed, then she aborts. Abortion usually occurs between the sixth and ninth months of pregnancy, sometimes later. The mare often gives birth to a weak, infected foal which succumbs in spite of treatment. The abortion usually is sudden and without pelvic, cervical, and vaginal relaxation. As a result, the mare's genitalia is badly bruised and often the placenta is retained. The placenta is edematous, hemorrhagic, and contains areas of necrosis.

Secondary infections of the genitalia are common complications and often endanger the mare's breeding future. If metritis does not develop after a few days of vaginal discharge, the mare soon will be in breeding condition and able to have a normal pregnancy the following year. Other mares of the same band often will become infected by eating material contaminated by the discharges of the first mare. They will then abort. As many as 90% of them may lose their foals.

Diagnosis is made by isolating the specific organism from the exudates, the fetal membranes, or the fetus, or by detection of a serum agglutination titer that can vary between 1:500 and 1:5000.

A salmonella bacterin has been used with great success in the control of equine contagious abortion. Vaccination should be repeated every year. It always is recommended in case of an outbreak, but the immunity is slow to develop and many mares abort despite this treatment.

Streptococcus genitalium (equi): The same organism responsible for many cases of metritis and cervicitis in mares also is responsible for a large number of abortions. In one study, *S. equi* was isolated in 196 fetuses of 1,150 examined.[6] The infection usually is limited to the genital tract and is not transmitted by ingestion.

This organism does not cause epizootics of abortion. In a band of mares, abortion will be limited to 1 or 2 individuals. Often the infected mares will conceive with difficulty in the succeeding years, abort repeatedly, or produce weak foals.

The Streptococcus originally is present in the endometrium and then in the fetal membranes. After a short period the fetus and membranes are expelled. As the abortion often occurs before the fourth or fifth month of pregnancy, it often is unnoticed.

There is no available preventive for this infection. The only means of control involve good sanitary practices during breeding and foaling, routine examinations, and treatment of chronically infected mares and stallions.

Streptococcus equi can be isolated at the time of abortion from the mare, the fetal membranes, the fetus, and often from the umbilical cord.

Other Bacteria: Abortion in horses also has been related to infections with *Escherichia coli,* Staphylococci, *Shigella equirulis,* and *Corynebacterium equi.*[6] These abortions appear without pattern at any time during the pregnancy. Diagnosis of the cause for these abortions is made by isolating the pathogen from the fetus or fetal membranes.

Fungal Abortion: Three cases of Aspergillus abortion have been reported in mares.[13] In all 3 cases, the mares aborted their fetuses in the pasture, between the seventh and tenth months of gestation. In each case, the Aspergillus was isolated from the fetus.

Protozoal Abortions: Trypanosoma equiperdum has been indicted as the cause for abortion during the course of dourine.

Rickettsial Abortion: Leptospira pomona has been known to provoke abortions in horses.

Three cases, confirmed by laboratory procedures, occurred in late pregnancy and in places where infected cattle had been introduced.[14] The disease probably is transmitted through ingestion of material contaminated by urine or genital secretions from infected animals. The aborting mares usually do not have a febrile reaction. The fetuses are icteric and contain large quantities of dark red, thin fluid in the abdominal and chest cavities. The pericardial sacs of the fetuses contain a straw-colored fluid. Their livers and spleens are swollen and congested, and the kidneys are dark red, soft, congested, pulpy, and usually quite enlarged.

The Leptospira occasionally can be observed under darkfield examination of fresh abdominal fluids. They ordinarily cannot be demonstrated in other tissues.

The diagnosis of leptospiral abortion is confirmed by demonstration of a positive serum agglutination titer. As a rule, 2 titers should be compared. One sample is obtained at the time of abortion and another is collected 2 or 3 weeks later. Infected mares have had a rise of titer from 1:1000 to 1:10,000 within 14 days.

Infected mares usually recover from leptospiral abortion and can be bred successfully within a month or so and have a normal pregnancy. Leptospiral vaccine seems to provide good prevention but it must be given annually to animals living on infected premises.

ABORTIONS DUE TO NUTRITIONAL FACTORS

Very little is known about the influence of nutritional factors on abortion in horses. It is known that mares need a balanced diet to have a healthy pregnancy. Roberts stated, "Animals on a very low plane of nutrition abort as a protective mechanism to conserve their own body reserve."[21] It is likely that under normal conditions, horses never reach this low a nutritional plane, and mares generally will carry their fetuses to full term despite their being fed a very poor diet. In such cases, the foals reflect the deficiencies to which the mares have been exposed.

Vitamin A is known to have a specific function in pregnancy (probably in the develop-

ment of the placenta). Vitamin D, calcium, and phosphorus likewise fulfill specific needs during fetal development.

ABORTIONS DUE TO HORMONAL OR GENETIC FACTORS

Twins: The incidence of twins in horses is thought to occur at a rate of 1 to 2 per 1,000 births. It has been our experience, however, that during the past 10 to 15 years twinning has increased in Thoroughbred horses. It is now encountered in more than 5% of pregnancies. No explanation can be given for this fact, as the great majority of the mares in our practice which have had twins had not been given hormones at any time within 6 months of conception. The increased incidence of twins probably is of genetic origin, and may be connected with inbreeding practices.

Most twin pregnancies do not reach full term. One twin develops more rapidly, and progressively assumes the major portion of the endometrium available for placental implantation. When the other twin does not have a sufficient blood supply it dies, and this ultimately results in the expulsion of both feti. A twin abortion can occur at any time during pregnancy and seems to be strictly dependent upon the relative sizes of the fetuses.

Sometimes one of the fetuses dies very early, 1 or 2 months after conception, and for some reason is not aborted. In such a case, the mare has a normal pregnancy and at parturition an undeveloped and calcified fetus, 3 to 6 inches in diameter, is discovered in the placenta.

Most twinning can be detected when mares are examined for pregnancy before 55 to 60 days. It has been observed when a mare aborts twin fetuses in late pregnancy that the abortion often is preceded by an increase of mammary development. This may be related to the death of one of the twins.

Habitual Abortion: Some mares have been known to lose their foals during or before the fourth or fifth months of pregnancy when the abortion could not be related to an infectious cause. As most of these mares respond to progesterone therapy, it has been assumed that the cause of this condition is of endocrine origin. It is similar to the habitual abortion described in human medicine which is attributed to progesterone–estrogen imbalance.

The progesterone necessary for the maintenance of pregnancy in mares is secreted by the ovary for the first 5 months of pregnancy, then by the placenta.[10] It has been observed in human medicine that this transition in progesterone production is not always synchronized perfectly, and abortions occur at this time because of a decrease in the total progesterone secretion. For different reasons, the balance of progesterone and estrone also can be upset during pregnancy. In human medicine, this usually can be detected by titration of blood or urine hormones, and treated accordingly.

To our knowledge, no systematic study has been done in horses to determine the physiologic balance of progesterone, estrogen, and other related steroids at different stages of pregnancy. At present, the equine practitioner is unable to diagnose an impending abortion which reflects a hormonal imbalance. Considering that the imbalance usually is due to lack of progesterone, mares which abort regularly and are not infected should be treated with progesterone injections. A repositol-type of progesterone should be used; 200 to 500 mg. may be given every 3 weeks from the time that pregnancy is diagnosed until the last month. This procedure usually gives good results.

OTHER TYPES OF ABORTION

Without establishing a regular pattern, some mares lose their foals between the 40th and 60th day of pregnancy. This probably is caused by a lack of proper implantation, and possibly for other reasons.

Other mares will show signs of impending abortion in late pregnancy. There is excessive activity of the mammae often accompanied by some degree of pelvic relaxation. These mares often can be treated successfully with progesterone. It has been our experience that foals born of mares given progesterone, because of signs of impending abortion in late pregnancy, were not healthy and did not develop at the same rate as other foals of the same age. Consequently, from an economic standpoint, it seems more advisable not to treat a mare show-

ing signs of imminent abortion. Horses which are not healthy have little economic value, and mares usually can become pregnant without complication shortly following an abortion.

In a study of aborted fetuses it was concluded that the cause of death or abnormality could not be detected for 440 specimens of the 1,150 examined.[6] Some evidence of abnormality was found in 15 of the aborted fetuses and this could have been the cause of the abortion. If allowance is made for the abortions induced by some accident, it still must be concluded that many of these unexplained abortions might be due to genetic influences.

ABORTIONS DUE TO ACCIDENTAL FACTORS

Twisted Cords: A 1.04% incidence of twisted umbilical cords has been recorded in a series of fetuses.[6] The umbilical cord of the equine fetus makes 1 or 2 twists. In some, it has been found to be very edematous and have up to 20 twists. It has been theorized that twisting is caused by fetal turning in the uterus. This might cause a reduction of the blood supply and death of the fetus (Fig. 15).

Miscellaneous Causes: Trauma, such as kicks or falls, sustained during late pregnancy, often can result in abortions. The fetus often will have a lesion at the point of impact in cases of kicks.

The breeding of mares in advanced pregnancy often will cause abortion. This accident fortunately is not very common, but has occurred with uninformed breeders. Some pregnant mares show signs of estrus, but they usually refuse the male. These mares can be forced to breed and will abort within a few days, probably because the cervical seal has been ruptured.

Provoked Abortions: Abortion can be induced in mares by injection of large and repeated doses of estrogen. Unfortunately, such dosages of estrogen also will cause the development of cystic ovaries.

Abortion also can be induced mechanically by breaking the cervical seal and opening the cervix. Injection of 500 ml. of saline containing an antibiotic will at the same time minimize the danger of infection. It has been our

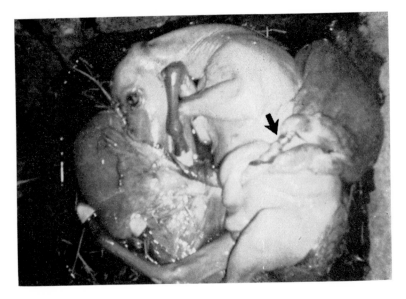

Fig. 15. Nine-month-old fetus with twisted cord.

experience that pregnancy is relatively difficult to induce within the 6 to 8 months following a provoked abortion.

P. LIEUX

REFERENCES

1. Andrews, F. N. and McKenzie, F. F.: Estrus, Ovulation, and Related Phenomena in the Mare. Bull. 329, Univ. of Missouri Agr. Exper. Sta.
2. Berliner, V. R.: The Biology of Equine Spermatozoa. The Problem of Fertility. Earl T. Engle, ed. Princeton University Press, Princeton, N. J., 1949.
3. Britton, J. W. and Howell, C. E.: Observations in sterility. Vet. Med. 40:8 (1945) 264.
4. Burkhart, J. H.: Sperm survival in the genital tract of the mare. J. of Agr. Sci. 39 (1949) 2.
5. Dimock, W. W. and Edwards, P. R.: Pathology and Bacteriology of the Reproductive Organs of Mares in Relation to Sterility. Bull. 286, Kentucky Agr. Exper. Sta. 1928.
6. Dimock, W. W., Edwards, P. R., and Bruner, D. W.: Infections observed in equine fetuses and foals. The Cornell Vet. 37 (1947) 2.
7. Dimock, W. W. and Bruner, D. W.: Barren Broodmares. Bull. 63, Kentucky Agr. Exper. Sta. 1949.
8. Dimock, W. W. and Bruner, D. W.: Notes on the procedure for handling the barren mares. No. Am. Vet. 30 (1949) 433.
9. Dimock, W. W.: Fertility and infertility of stallions. Circ. 68, Kentucky Agr. Exper. Sta., 1950.
10. Cole, Harold H., Howell, C. E. and Hart, G. H.: The changes occurring in the ovaries of the mare during pregnancy. Anat. Rec. 49 (1931) 3.
11. Haag, F. M. and Werthessen: Relationship between fertility and nonprotein sulfhydryl concentration of seminal fluid in the thoroughbred stallion. Fertility and Sterility. 7 (1956) 6.
12. Haag, F. M.: Evaluation of dismount semen in thoroughbred horse breeding. J.A.V.M.A. 134 (1959) 7.
13. Hensel, L., Bisping, W., and Schimmelpfennig: Aspergillus abortion in mares. Berl. u. Munch. Tierärzt. Wschr. 74 (1961) 15.
14. Jackson, R. S., Jones, E. E., and Clark, D. S.: Abortion in mares associated with leptospirosis. J.A.V.M.A. 131 (1957) 12.
15. Kilborne: U.S. Dept. Agr., Bull. 3, Bur. An. Ind., 1893.
16. McGee, Wm. R.: Veterinary Notebook. The Blood Horse, Lexington, Kentucky, 1958.
17. McGee, Wm. R.: Some diseases and related conditions affecting fertility in broodmares; Thoroughbred of California. 34 (1962) 5.
18. Mc Leod, J. W. and McGee, Wm. R.: The semen of the thoroughbreed. The Cornell Vet. 40 (1950) 3.
19. Neumann, O. F. and Salzmann, A. A.: The survival and rapidity of penetration of the spermatozoa in the sexual organ of the mare. trud. Labo iskusat Osemen Zivot (Mosk) 1 (1940) 317.
20. Reid, J. J.: Relationship of nutrition to fertility in animals. J.A.V.M.A. 114 (1949) 864.
21. Roberts, S. J.: Veterinary Obstetrics and Genital Diseases. Published by the author, Ithaca, New York, 1956.

BREEDING FARM PRACTICES

The equine breeding farm, particularly the Thoroughbred breeding farm, constitutes a field in which veterinary service of a high degree of excellence is in strong demand. The value of the animals justifies the use of many modern devices and drugs considered economically out of line in other fields. Consequently it is a common practice for competent veterinarians to be engaged as residents or at least on a contract basis on most of these farms. Many of the factors concerned in this work have been discussed previously, hence this article will briefly outline the routine of breeding farm practices with comments on some of the problems involved.

The ultimate goal of the breeding farm is to reach the utopia wherein a 100% normal, healthy foal crop is weaned each year. The first problem encountered in this process is, of course, getting the mares in foal. Mares are conveniently divided into 3 groups—maidens, barren mares, and foaling mares. In order to establish the heat periods of the first 2 groups it is common practice to commence a teasing routine about 30 days prior to the start of actual breeding. The breeding season starts in most instances in the first week of February in order that the first foals will be born as soon as possible after the universal birth date of January 1, which applies to all Thoroughbred horses. Teasing is conducted as a rule with the mare in a teasing chute (Fig. 16) or across a teasing gate. The teaser should be a tractable stallion who will not be excessively savage or irritate the mares during the teasing act. The mares are led into the chute or against the gate and the stallion is allowed to conduct the teasing process. The reactions of the mare are noted on the daily record form by the veterinarian in attendance. This procedure is continued every other day throughout the breeding season—usually from February 1 to July 1. The purpose of the preseason teasing of maiden and barren mares is to establish the heat cycles, detect abnormalities, note typical reactions, and afford time to correct any cyclical irregularities prior to breeding. It should be remembered that time is a limiting and important factor.

Maiden mares commonly fall into 2 groups—normal and anestrual. Normal maidens require very little attention and are among the best breeding mares of any group. The big problem among the maidens is anestrus or failure to exhibit heat periods to the teaser. Among Thoroughbred maidens much of this anestrual behavior is of a psychologic nature. Many of the fillies come to the breeding farm directly from training and are nervous and completely unaccustomed to the placid routine of the nursery. It is prudent to tease these mares gradually at first to acquaint them with the process and to rely on biweekly vaginal inspection to detect true estrus. The vast majority will show the cervical changes characteristic of estrus at least once a month and when this date is established, careful teasing under tranquilization usually will prepare them adequately for breeding.

Barren mares fall into 3 categories, namely: those that are normal, those with long estrual

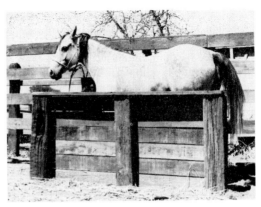

Fig. 16. Mare in chute ready for teasing.

periods, and those with signs of anestrus. It is this group of mares which are particularly benefited by preseason teasing to establish the group into which they fall. These groups are based on their psychologic reactions to the teaser. One may encounter a wide variety of individual differences. Close observation by the attending veterinarian, however, and the use of descriptive records on each animal, will enable him to separate the false estrual and diestrual periods from the true ones. His judgment in these matters should of course be verified by vaginal inspection. It will be found that many mares during the winter months are either in a state of anestrus or subject to very irregular periods, with the estrual periods predominating. As the season progresses, the overwhelming majority of these mares return to relatively normal cycles. Since it is the desire of the breeder to have his foals born as close to January as possible, it is imperative to settle as many mares as possible at an early date.

Anestrual mares are handled the same as anestrual maidens. Mares showing irregular periods or long estrual periods are the most difficult group to settle early. Vaginal inspection will reveal the true heat period in many of them and breedings at this time often will result in a good conception rate. Another group will show estrual periods without actually ovulating and will require either hormone (pregnant mare serum) therapy or more time to establish normal cycles. At any rate, the injudicious, haphazard breeding of these mares does more harm than good. In every case the estrual stage should be confirmed by vaginal inspection prior to breeding.

In some areas, the practice of manual dilation of the cervix in anestrual mares, so called "opening up," is popular. The veterinarian should not attempt this operation unless all other procedures have been tried. Cervical stimulation does have estrogenic effects but the danger of introducing infection in delicate tissues is constant. Infection of the cervical and uterine mucosae obviously is an important hazard that must constantly be avoided.

It is axiomatic that only healthy mares and stallions should be bred. The majority of the infections in mares are introduced at the time of foaling when the genital tract is partially bruised and most susceptible to the establishment of infection with the normal bacterial flora of the external genitalia. No less important in this regard is the habit of windsucking, predisposed by abnormally shaped vulvae and by tissue stretching with concurrent temporary paralysis following foaling. Should examination reveal this defect, surgical correction is indicated at once and breeding suspended until infection has been controlled. Many barren mares showing long estrual periods will develop infection if repeatedly bred during the long heats.

The estrual cycles of foaling mares are among the most regular of any class of mares. An occasional foaling mare will resist the teaser's attentions following the early ninth-day heat period; however these can usually be detected in estrus by vaginal inspection from the 25th to 35th days. The principal problem for the veterinarian concerns the owner's pressure for ninth-day breedings. Authorities in the field of equine reproduction have for many years almost universally been opposed to ninth-day breedings under any circumstances. This heat period, however, is almost as universally proclaimed by the breeders as the best time to breed foaling mares. In every instance, when adequate records have been maintained, the evidence is overwhelmingly against the practice. As a matter of fact, the so-called "foal heat" is considered by many authorities to be a cleansing function which removes the postparturient debris left in the uterus rather than a normal estrus period. The laxative effect of this ninth-day estrus on the nursing foal is a well-established phenomenon among horsemen which further indicates abnormality.

Conceptions following breedings during the foal heat are notoriously unstable, with an excessively high percentage of abortions, dead and diseased foals resulting. Incidentally, many records indicate a conception rate of from 30 to 40% in this period compared with 65 to 80% during following periods. Actually the objection to ninth-day breedings is that they aggravate existing infections which would ordinarily be removed by this estrus, and establish them in the uterus. The full effect may not be observed for the next several parturitions but eventually the practice will condemn the mare to the ranks of poor breeders. The easy settling mare thus is penalized by foal heat breeding, and one or more viable foals become lost to her reproductive record.

The veterinarian certainly must withhold from foal heat breeding any mares showing certain danger signs. These include difficulty in foaling, placental retention for longer than 1 hour, placentae weighing more than 14 pounds, dead or diseased foals, or any abnormal discharge following foaling. Any of these conditions definitely must eliminate the mare from foal heat breeding. If vaginal inspection on the seventh or eighth day shows a completely normal recovery from parturition and it is late in the breeding season, one may consider ninth-day breeding rather than let the mare skip a year. Under no circumstances, however, should it become a routine practice even in apparently normal mares.

Condition of the mare has a very definite bearing on the estrual cycles. There is an old saying among horsemen to the effect that mares will not breed until they shed their winter coats. It is true that these long-coated, thin mares show quite abnormal periods, usually long heats, and every effort should be directed toward increasing the nutritive level and all means should be used to get them in condition to breed.

The other extreme, the so-called fat mare, likewise is a poor breeder but tends toward the anestrual state. One often hears it stated that these mares are too fat to breed. Actually many, if not all of them, are suffering from a hypothyroidism, and are both fat and sterile for this reason. Characteristically, they show abnormal, hard fat deposits on the neck, withers, hips, and back. They tend toward exaggerated masculinity in their behavior and may even ride other mares. The external genitalia are juvenile. These mares are aided greatly by a 2-week course of thyroprotein, or iodinated casein added daily to their rations.

Breeding should be done in a quiet area with a minimum of external interference. It has been suggested that too much nervousness or excitement increases the adrenalin output and decreases the percentage of conceptions. Tranquilization often is utilized when the mare is not manifesting good psychologic heat or is unruly for some reason. The mare usually is restrained with some sort of breeding hobbles (Fig. 17, 18), or a twitch, or both. Her tail is wrapped and the external genitalia are thoroughly washed with soap and water and a mild disinfectant. The penis and sheath of the stallion are likewise washed immediately after service.

A variety of rituals often are performed on the mare immediately after copulation. Usually cold water is thrown on her rump and she is walked for several minutes. It is not known if these acts do any good but certainly they are harmless and need not be discouraged. The natural service may be reinforced by filling a 1/2-ounce breeder's capsule with semen from the vaginal floor and inserting the loaded capsule through the cervix. This practice must be done with sanitary precautions, and it certainly has value in mares with a chronic cervicitis where dilation is inadequate because of existing fibrosis. It also may be useful in aged mares with a tipped cervix.

One of the constant decisions a veterinarian must make on a breeding farm is when to breed a mare. It rather generally is believed that the sperm must be in the genital tract prior to ovulation, that the sperm remains viable in the tract for not much longer than 24 hours, and that ovulation generally occurs 1 to 2 days before the end of heat. When only 1 or at most 2 covers are permitted during a period, it has been determined that breedings on the second or third day of a normal estrus, or the second and fourth days, is most favorable.

In abnormal periods, vaginal inspection often is helpful in determining the ovulation time, as the characteristic changes become more pronounced as ovulation approaches. Many wasted covers and overworked stallions can be saved by attention to these details without sacrificing breeding efficiency or resorting to blind every day services. Individual records are helpful sometimes, as mares tend to maintain their breeding pattern over the years.

In general, no definite pattern can be established which will apply to all mares at all times. The veterinarian must study each ani-

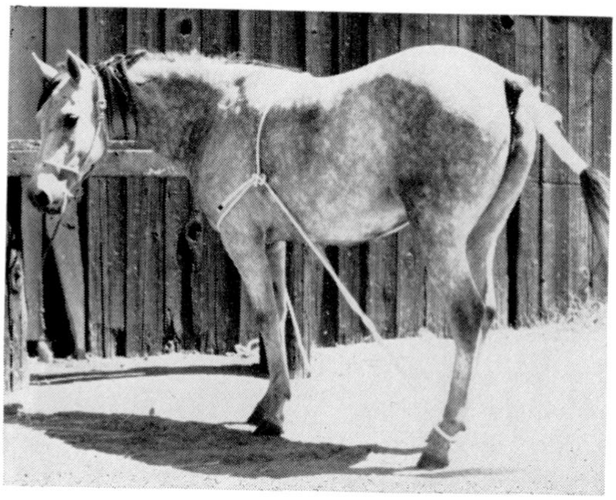

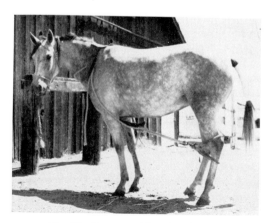

Fig. 17. Mare ready to breed. Restraint with a simple side line.

Fig. 18. One type of breeding hobbles.

mal's psychologic as well as physiologic characteristics in order to accomplish his purpose. Careful attention must be paid each mare during the teasing period. In anestrus mares, even minor variations in behavior often are justification for vaginal inspection. In many instances, these will be determined to be evidence of true estrus. Likewise, many mares will show false estrual periods in which all the behavioral evidence of estrus is demonstrated to the teaser despite an existing pregnancy of 30 to 90 days.

It has been stated that the majority of barren mares fail to breed simply because they have not had an opportunity to conceive. By this is meant that the mares have either been bred at an inopportune time in relation to ovulation during the cycle, or that teasing has been inadequate. For example, in the early portion of the breeding season many irregular mares may be in heat 5 to 7 days, then show a short diestrus of 8 to 10 days followed by another 5-day estrual period. When the older methods of teasing are followed, in which a mare is turned out for 15 days after the last breeding before teasing is commenced again, it can be seen that such mares would have passed through a second heat before being reteased. There is no substitute for every other day teasing until 90 days after the last breeding.

Teasing on every other day also catches so-called "split heats" wherein a mare shows signs of estrus for 3 days, then apparently goes out of heat for a day or 2, and back in for a final few days during which ovulation occurs and breeding is optimal. Finally, every other day teasing detects those mares which suffer early abortion or fetal absorption. This is a relatively common experience between the 45th and 90th days of pregnancy and easily is missed unless careful teasing is conducted. These early abortions occur during the time of implantation when hormonal control of pregnancy gradually shifts from the ovaries to the uterus. Any hormonal imbalance, or weakness in the developing embryo, may result in fetal death and abortion or resorption. Clinically, the mare simply comes in heat.

The moment of truth at the breeding farm is the act of parturition. This represents the culmination of the year's planning, breeding, care, and management of the pregnant mare. All the hopes and aspirations of the breeder and the justification of his selection of sire are wrapped up in the delivery of the new foal. Characteristically, parturition in the mare is violent and stormy, consequently veterinary service is urgently required for the 10% of foalings classed as abnormal. It behooves the veterinarian to become thoroughly familiar with every detail of the foaling act and, in particular, the signs of imminent labor, because of the necessity for early intervention in equine dystocia.

Much has been written of infallible signs indicating the early onset of labor; however, in practice one often finds that very few mares fit the classic descriptions. The accumulation of colostral secretions, the so-called "wax" on the ends of the teats, is said to indicate parturition within 48 hours. In a long series of records, only 50% of mares showed any wax whatsoever. There may be waxing, milk secretion or simply mammary development for a variable period of time. There usually is some vulvar enlargement and a relaxation of the pelvic ligaments prior to parturition. The mare may wander off by herself or be irritable with other pasture-mates.

Labor pains are initiated by restlessness, getting up and down, making a bed, sweating, and contractions of the abdominal muscles. Normally, these signs indicate impending parturition, usually within an hour. However, aged multiparous mares or mares with uterine atony may show such signs intermittently for several days or for as long as 2 weeks. It has been jokingly stated, but with more than a grain of truth, that when the amnion ruptures and the head and feet are presented at the vulvar orifice, foaling time has arrived.

Because of the difficulty in predicting the exact time of foaling and because of the violent nature of parturition in the mare, most breeders prefer to bring mares into the barn overnight for several weeks prior to their delivery date. They are watched during the night and the veterinarian is called at the earliest signs of labor. These precautions are necessary to detect early dystocia before delivery becomes virtually impossible or at least highly dangerous.

A rather commonly observed deviation from normal foaling is so-called delayed parturition due to uterine atony. It is not unusual to have 30% or more of mares in a band to be so affected. They will show mild or even severe labor pains lasting for several hours, then get up and stand quietly. There may be sweating over the shoulders, flanks or back, and an actual flow of milk. These signs may continue for several nights and be accompanied by an edema of the limbs and lower abdomen. Extreme discomfort and anorexia are concomitant. If allowed to progress untreated the foaling is delayed and in many cases accompanied by dystocia. Almost without fail the amnion is edematous and grossly overweight. Because the fetal circulation is thus impaired and the antibody-rich colostral milk is lost in the preparturient lactation, the foals frequently are born weak or are subject to early navel ill.

During the past 10 years, I have handled this problem by inducing labor in selected cases. The vast majority of these mares were past due 10 days or more, hence there was little danger of causing premature birth. These mares were examined vaginally at regular intervals and when there was evidence of cervical dilation and loosening of the cervical seal, treatment was instituted. When the cervix was dilated sufficiently to admit 2 fingers, 5 ml. of posterior pituitary extract was administered subcutaneously. Usually, labor commenced within 30 minutes and was completed within 1 hour. Occasionally a second injection was given when results were not apparent after 30 minutes. After delivery, it is a wise practice to administer 10 ml. of a penicillin-streptomycin mixture and at least 100 ml. of the dam's blood subcutaneously to the foal, to prevent septicemia.

The advantages of inducing labor are numerous but obviously timing is the crucial factor in this procedure. It enables the attending veterinarian to be able to be present and prepared to correct malpresentations and diseased foals. It provides the opportunity to examine the presentation at the time of the amnion's appearance when corrections are easy.

There is very little danger to mare or foal in this method of treating uterine atony as long as cervical dilation is present. With a completely sealed cervix there always is the possibility of uterine rupture following severe uterine contractions.

Upon the completion of delivery the attendant should soak the navel stump of the foal in a good, drying disinfectant, such as tincture of iodine, to prevent postparturient navel ill and hasten dessication of the cord. A few older horsemen prefer to tie the cord before it ruptures and then cut it below the ligature. It is the modern practice to allow the normal process of rupture to occur during the struggles of the newborn to rise. Many veterinarians routinely administer 10 ml. of a penicillin-streptomycin mixture to newborn foals. Certainly, it is an additional safeguard.

The mare and foal are left alone after parturition and the foal is allowed to rise to his feet and nurse unassisted. Note is made of the time of placental retention and once it is passed, the attendant should weigh and examine it carefully for evidence of pathologic changes indicative of infection. The late Dr. W. C. Williams often stated that inflammatory changes in the uterus are accurately mirrored in the equine placenta. Thus the veterinarian is able to obtain a picture of the health status of the uterus by this procedure and institute therapy at this early stage if indicated. Overweight placentae or the presence of gross abnormalities should definitely exclude the mare from ninth-day breeding.

Placentae are considered to be retained if not passed within 1 hour. Efforts at removal should not be attempted for at least 6 hours but should not be delayed longer than 8 hours. If the placenta does not come away rather easily, antibiotics should be administered intramuscularly and removal attempted in another 4 hours. The majority of retained placentae are quite light and friable, consequently any rough attempts at manual removal likely will tear the necrotic membrane, leaving small bits retained. These become important foci of infection which can lead to septicemia. For this reason, each placenta should be carefully examined to determine whether or not the entire membrane has been removed.

Finally, the mare should be examined carefully to determine whether any vulvar lacerations exist. If present, these should be sutured or clamped immediately and antibiotics administered parenterally. Postpartum is an extremely critical period in the reproductive life of the broodmare. Many apparently minor lesions, if left untreated, can develop into chronic disorders with important effects on the mare's future breeding ability. With exclusion of ninth-day breeding and antibiotic treatment of existing infections at this early time, excellent results are to be expected.

The first 30 days of the foal's life are critical ones, not only from the point of view of survival, but also because serious joint lesions may develop which tend to become chronic permanently crippling defects. The veterinarian's responsibility lies in exercising constant vigilance over growing foals and in the early detection and treatment of disorders. Diarrheas accompanying the ninth-day heat periods are to be expected and usually are mild. Occasionally, severe diarrhea is encountered due to bacterial infection and it requires prompt, vigorous treatment. Foals not infrequently are born with a wide variety of leg deformities, often of a serious nature. Although many of these are corrected spontaneously in time, the veterinarian should use any remedial devices necessary to hasten this process. Despite all efforts, some of these crippled foals remain deformed and valueless for life.

The care and management of stallions present many individual problems; however, ample exercise and a high nutritive level always are demanded. Monthly examinations of semen are advisable to determine the ability of the sire to maintain his breeding schedule. In general, it can be safely stated that overbreeding does more to shorten a stallion's reproductive life than any other single factor. For this reason, it becomes highly important to avoid nonindicated breedings and to be certain that each mare is in true estrus and free from infection prior to service. Double covers in a single day are permissible for vigorous stallions during the height of the season but this should not be overdone. An infinite variety of individual idiosyncrasies are presented by different stallions and the veterinarian should be alert to detect these if he is to insure a high conception rate. The knowledge of experienced studmasters can be invaluable in this regard.

J. W. Britton

ARTIFICIAL INSEMINATION

At present artificial insemination in the breeding of horses has only limited use. This is largely due to the fact that offspring resulting from artificial insemination cannot be registered in many horse breed associations. Its restricted use also is related to the limited viability of undiluted or diluted equine semen when it is stored. Shipping of equine semen for breeding purposes has not proved practical, but artificial insemination is used on some farms when 2 or more mares are to be bred to a stallion on the same day.

Collection of semen from a stallion may be accomplished by recovery of the ejaculate in a breeding bag applied to the erect penis before teasing. A more satisfactory method is to use an equine artificial vagina (distributed by Haver-Lockhart). A mare in estrus and the stallion are prepared as for natural service, with sanitary procedures being used to prevent contamination. As the stallion mounts, the erect penis is directed into the artificial vagina which is held firmly against the lateral pelvic area of the mare.

Equine semen must be handled carefully if sperm viability is to be maintained. At the time of collection, the semen should be kept as near to body temperature as possible.

The volume of semen ejaculated can vary from 20 to 500 ml; investigators have reported the average to be 130 ml. Stallion semen has been successfully diluted to 5 times, and it has been recommended that 20 to 30 ml. of diluted semen be used for each insemination. A conception rate of 85% has been obtained with semen stored in 5% glucose, 0.8% egg yolk diluter for 12 to 24 hours, and a 72% conception rate was obtained after storage for 48 hours.

In experiments with various diluters for stallion semen stored 4 days at 4 C., 5% reconstituted buttermilk in 5% glucose was found superior to higher concentrations of buttermilk in glucose, plain mare's milk or cow's milk, or egg yolk-glucose in the maintenance of sperm motility. A dilution of 1:4 gave slightly better results than dilutions from 1:1 to 1:7. The addition of 400 I.U. of penicillin and 1 mg. of streptomycin/ml. of diluted semen effectively controlled bacterial growth without adversely affecting the viability of sperm.

Fertility of stored semen has not been determined, but it has been estimated that fertility can be maintained in buttermilk-glucose diluter for 2 days. Because spermatozoa will survive 5 days in the reproductive tract of the mare, however, immediate insemination after collection is advisable. If more than 30 minutes may elapse between collection and insemination the semen should be diluted, and if it is stored longer than 2 hours it should be cooled gradually to 4 C.

The optimum time for insemination is based upon the imminence of ovulation as determined by rectal palpation of the ovary. Because the ovum is viable for only 5 to 8 hours after ovulation the optimum time to inseminate is shortly prior to ovulation. Breeders who practice artificial insemination attempt to inseminate between 6 to 12 hours prior to ovulation. One insemination per estrual period is the usual practice.

Mares may be inseminated by pushing a capsule of semen through the cervix. A better method is to use a plastic insemination catheter and syringe as is used in bovine artificial insemination. A speculum is used and the catheter is passed through the cervix.

Until better ways of storing equine semen are perfected, artificial insemination in equines will continue to have a limited use. The development of improved freezing methods for preservation of equine semen is currently under study. Preliminary reports indicate that with improved procedures stallion semen has been kept viable for 18 days.

W. J. GIBBONS

REFERENCES

1. Berry, R. O. and Gasder, P. J.: Viability of stallion spermatozoa influenced by storage media and antibiotics. Southwestern Vet. 13 (1960) 217-220.

CHAPTER 24

OBSTETRICS

DYSTOCIA IN THE MARE

Although contemporary veterinarians are far less often than formerly called upon to attend a case of difficult parturition in a mare, it has become even more important than ever before that every practitioner should be capable of delivering a foal. A lack of practice should never go hand in hand with a lack of knowledge, due to want of opportunity. The incidence of dystocia in any 100 foaling mares, under any conditions, will be considerably less than in an equal number of cows. But when difficulty in parturition occurs in the mare, it is a more urgent matter than it is in the cow. The mare normally foals quickly and silently, as far away from sightseers as possible. Her pains are strong and violent and she is susceptible to shock and to infection. Any hindrance to a rapid delivery adds to the risk that she will develop an acute laminitis, or a metritis, or that her afterbirth will fail to be expelled promptly.

The foal possesses a long neck and limbs relatively much longer than those of the calf. It is possible, therefore, for the head of the foal to be retained so that its muzzle rests on its stifle, far out of reach of the human hand. Nor is it at all rare for both hindfeet of the foal to protrude through the vulva of the mare, with the head and 2 forefeet following a little way behind. The mare, too, is a lengthy and deep-bodied animal, and the operator will be at an advantage if he is of medium height and has a small hand at the end of a long and slender arm. However, many good obstetricians are not blessed in this way but still contrive to obtain excellent results. Veterinary obstetricians often find that in foaling a mare, the enemy most likely to defeat their good intentions is sheer physical exhaustion. In the cow, the fetus usually is more active and more cooperative than the foal, which dies sooner than the calf if parturition is delayed. Not uncommonly, however, the foal is quite active while life remains in it.

Many mares behave as though suffering from colic and will sometimes throw themselves onto the ground quite violently, which may entail some risk if the arm of the operator is fully extended into the uterus at the time. Epidural anesthesia, and sometimes the administration of a tranquilizer, will make the proceeding easier, but when the foal is alive one must be careful in the choice of sedatives as they may endanger its life. There is a far greater risk of rupture of the uterus or vagina in the mare than in the more placid cow.

Obstetrical Instruments and Appliances

Speaking generally, it may be stated that the fewer instruments introduced into the uterus of the mare, the greater are her chances of survival. When metal appliances are employed, they should be used very carefully and by experienced operators. It may also be added that this sort of operator seldom has need of them.

Practices vary greatly in different localities. The type of stabling, the amount and quality of assistance available, facilities for provision of water of any kind, hot water, soap, and towels range from good to none. It is advisable to carry one's own soap and towels, clean pails, antiseptics and lubricants, and hope that hot water will be available on the premises. Concerning the all-important matter of lubricants, their use in sufficient quantity to smear inside the vagina, on the foal inside the uterus, and on the operator's hands and arms, will lessen his work and the risk for the patient. Lard may be inserted into the maternal passages, and many experienced practitioners relied largely on linseed gruel. A more modern lubricant and a very efficient one is a solution of gum acacia in water. Also available is a variety of antiseptic creams usually provided in tubes.

Rope or Chains for Traction: For the purpose of traction one may decide among cotton rope, nylon rope, and stainless steel chains,

Nylon ropes of small caliber and a high tensile strength now can be obtained. It is essential that they should be able to stand repeated and prolonged boiling and on this account cotton ropes may be superior. Moreover, cotton is soft and flexible. Ropes should be of assorted lengths, from 3 to 6 feet—a 4-foot length being suitable for general utility. At one end of each length of rope, an eye is spliced—a metal ring large enough to slip easily over the first finger may be even better. The other end is slipped through the eye to make a noose.

In addition, or in place of ropes, one may employ flat, metal obstetrical chains. Chains have many advantages: they never break, are easy to handle, and being flat do not cause unnecessary friction. In addition, hand grips are provided to hook on the chain so that one or more helpers can apply traction at the same time. Their only disadvantage is that being unyielding, they are more likely to cause fracture of the foal's limbs if traction is excessive, or if it is applied at an angle to the limb. Chains damage the vagina less than ropes and they have the supreme advantages of not absorbing fluids and being resistant to boiling as often as needed. Both ropes and chains should be carried in a container in which they are sterile, and should be dropped frequently into an antiseptic during use to remove discharges.

Hooks—Blunt or Pointed: Some of the most important instruments in the hands of a veterinary obstetrician are metal hooks. They may be either sharply pointed or blunt. Blunt hooks generally cause less damage to the foal but are inclined to slip, and if pulled upon by enthusiastic but inexpert helpers, may do a lot of damage. In fact, sharp hooks are safer in this respect. They rarely slip out of an orbit during traction, but if they do they may inflict serious damage to the arm of the operator if it is in the vagina at the time. A sharp hook inserted into the orbit at the nasal canthus may withstand a good deal of traction without injuring the foal in any way—in fact it usually is impossible after delivery for an onlooker to decide which orbit has carried the hook.

For the operator's own safety it is advisable that he, alone, apply traction to the rope attached to a sharp hook so long as his arm is within the vagina. He should grasp with his free hand the lower jaw of the foal as soon as it comes into reach. Any disadvantage pertaining to the use of sharp hooks is slight in actual practice, particularly as in the greater number of cases requiring their use, the foal will be dead. Foals do not withstand delay in parturition in the same way that calves do nor do they survive as much forced traction and pressure upon the thorax and abdomen during the process of withdrawal.

The Porte-Cord: An appliance, often very useful in a foaling operation, is a porte-cord. By means of this device a rope may occasionally be introduced to a position out of reach of the operator's hand. The best type is made of a flat steel spring, curved into a circle and provided with a finger ring at either end to which a cord may be attached. The steel spring need be only from 1 to 1.5 cm. in width. The longer the spring is, the better for use in a mare in which the foal's head or limb may be out of reach. When a head cannot be reached by the hand, a spring porte-cord can sometimes be inserted below or above some portion of the neck, and between it and the uterine wall.

A thin cord attached to the opposite ring may then be drawn through by hooking the finger into the first ring, when it reappears at the opposite edge of the neck. The cord can then be attached to the end of a rope or chain, and this too can be drawn through, and subsequently used to change the position of the neck and head. The cord attached to the ring of the porte-cord should be strong but thin, and approximately 6 feet long, so that some of it will still lie outside the vulva after the remainder has been passed around the foal's neck or body by means of the porte-cord. The rope or chain attached to the cord and drawn through in its turn, also should be 6 feet long. This will enable both its ends to be brought outside the vulva and held together while traction is applied upon the neck, head, the flexure of a knee or hock, in an attempt to bring the part itself—as well as adjacent portions of the body—into reach of the operator's hand.

Other Useful Appliances: Another instrument of value, when the foal already is dead, is the wire embryotome, which will effectively dismember a foal. The introduction of rigid steel instruments into the vagina and uterus of a mare, however, should be avoided if possible. One has to consider whether the risk will be greater if the foal is disarticulated, or if attempts are made to correct the position of the foal by manual manipulation. Some foals can be moved about with ease, if they are small and comparatively limp. Necks which have lain in the uterus, bent upon themselves for days or weeks, may become rigidly curved, while limbs may be tightly flexed at the joints and may resist all efforts to straighten them. These are cases in which the advantages of the wire embryotome are evident.

For purposes of more forceful traction that can be applied by hand, one should carry a set of small pulley blocks. One end of these should carry a blunt hook, to which a rope or chain can be attached, while to the other end a long chain is fastened by which the pulley may be anchored to some convenient fixed object. In addition, a clean steel crowbar about 4 to 5 feet long is an admirable instrument with which to apply moderate traction in difficult situations. It often is preferable to blocks.

Anesthesia

In obstetrical operations on large animals one cannot speak too highly of the advantages of epidural anesthesia. In the mare it controls the strong uterine and abdominal contractions which otherwise render the operation so difficult and exhausting to both patient and obstetrician. Relaxation of the uterine wall also makes it more easy to insert the lubricated hand and arm much further. In regard to general anesthesia a great deal depends upon the demeanor of the mare and whether the foal is alive or dead. If the foal is alive, a combination of epidural anesthesia with a moderately deep general anesthesia gives the best results in a mare which has to be cast.

Quiet mares usually are handled much more easily in the standing position; reliance is placed on epidural anesthesia and care should be taken to regulate the dose so that sufficient anesthetic is employed to control straining, but insufficient to cause the mare to lose the use of her hindlimbs and become recumbent.

When the foal is dead, one may use intravenous chloral hydrate, or a tranquilizer combined with epidural anesthesia. Chlorpromazine does not pass the placental barrier and can do no harm even when the foal is living. It produces medium to deep sedation in the mare in a dosage of 2 mg./kg. administered intramuscularly, but mares do not respond alike, and in some this dosage produces little effect. When successful, sedation occurs in 40 minutes and lasts from 5 to 8 hours. Pentobarbital sodium is able to pass the placental barrier and do harm to the foal. In any case, it is an uncertain anesthetic in the adult horse and recovery from its effects may be accompanied by hyperesthesia and excitement.

To keep a mare on her feet, yet reduce straining to a minimum, from 10 to 20 ml. of a 2.5% solution of procaine is injected into the epidural space, commencing with the minimum amount and adding a little every 15 minutes. One attempts to arrest the labor pains without causing the mare to stagger unduly on her hindfeet. The anesthetic fluid is injected into the first coccygeal space. This can be felt with the tip of the finger about an inch in front of the most anterior tail hairs.

In those cases in which the mare is recumbent or has been cast, it is advantagous to elevate the hindquarters. This practice enables the foal to drop or be propelled forward, makes more room for the operator's arm, and enables parts of the foal, formerly out of reach, to be handled.

Examination of the Mare

Before making the preliminary examination, the anus, perineum and vulva should be washed with warm water and soap containing a nonirritant antiseptic. The hands and arms must be repeatedly cleansed too, especially after handling materials outside the mare.

Before introducing the hand and arm for the first time, it is advisable to have the foreleg of the mare lifted from the ground and held there by an assistant who keeps the toe of the foot cupped between the fingers and palm of the hand, with the fetlock and knee completely flexed. If the operator inserts his right hand, the left foreleg of the mare is raised, and vice versa.

The first objective of the examination is to determine the exact position the foal is occupying within the vagina and uterus. This part of the examination should never be hurried. Having in readiness a good supply of sterilized cotton or nylon ropes or chains, one should first attach these to all available parts of the foal's body: to each fetlock presented, to the lower jaw, or to the head by means of a loop passed over the poll of the foal and drawn taut within the opened mouth. If the fetlocks cannot be reached, a rope may be passed around the flexures of the hocks, or below the knees, if this is possible.

The advantage of roping available parts is that in an animal as large and roomy as the mare, parts of the body at first within reach may easily be "lost" during attempts to move the foal into a more normal position. If parts carrying ropes "disappear" they can be recovered, if necessary, by gentle traction on the rope. It facilitates identification if each rope is tagged with a number, or if the free ends are marked with colored tape. By using one identification habitually for lower jaw, one for forelimbs, and a third for hindlimbs, much time and unnecessary exploration can be avoided.

Identification of Body Parts

Identification of various parts of the foal's body may be accomplished as follows: If the foal lies in normal anterior presentation one may feel the muzzle and mouth, the eyes, and the poll lying uppermost. The 2 forefeet will be presented with soles turned downward. If on the other hand, the soft soles are turned upward, one may presume that the foal is lying on its back. This will be confirmed if its lower jaw is found to be uppermost.

When identifying knees and hocks remember that knees and front fetlocks flex in the same direction, but hocks and hind fetlocks flex in opposite directions. Take care also never to mistake an elbow, reached by the fingertips, for the point of a hock—a mistake not so difficult to make as one might imagine.

More difficulty may be experienced in transverse presentations, when no limbs, or head or tail can be felt—only a solid body surface. In this case, one should try first to locate ribs or the solid spine. If the spine can be located, follow it with fingertips to determine where the base of the neck or the foot of the tail may lie. Having discovered this, one makes an attempt to propel the fetus lengthways in one or another direction so as to bring one end, preferably the posterior in most cases, within reach. Always count the number of feet or limbs presented so that twin pregnancies can be recognized promptly.

In a simple case in which no epidural anesthesia is being employed, introduce the hand between pains, and not when the mare is straining. Similarly, when exerting traction, pull with the pains, and relax between them, exerting only enough tension to keep any advantage gained from again being lost. Let the mare rest between her pains as she would do normally, and do not make straining on her part a continuous performance, which will exhaust the mare as well as the obstetrician. When the parturition is in danger of being delayed, and when the only hope of delivery depends upon manual extraction, proceed at once to administer epidural anesthesia.

Anterior Presentation: Dorsosacral Position

Many types of presentation are encountered in the parturient mare. Before considering the more common types of fetal dystocia, we must know the pattern of normal presentation in the dorsosacral position: the 2 forefeet of the foal lie on the floor of the vagina, or may protrude through the opening of the vulva. The foal's muzzle rests above the fore fetlocks. Both hindfeet will be out of reach.

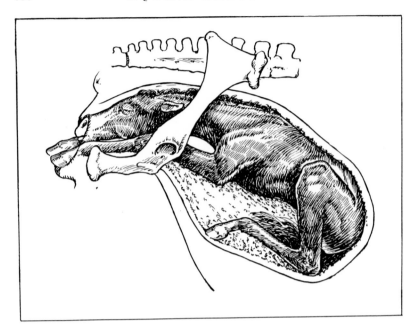

Fig. 1. Anterior presentation, dorsosacral position. Drawing by A. C. Shuttleworth, M.R.C.V.S.

The soles of the forefeet point downward; the poll of the foal is uppermost (Fig. 1).

Delivery may commence naturally, but the foal may be held in the pelvis by jamming of the hips or stifles, or both. Repel the foal a little, if possible, and cross the front limbs. Exert traction on these in a manner which will twist the body of the foal in spiral fashion.

If this fails, repel the body once more, endeavor to introduce a quantity of lubricant between the body of the foal and the vagina and, if this enables the hand to be introduced sufficiently far, carry some more lubricant into the pelvis, or smear it upon the stifles or hips if it is at all possible to reach them. Then apply traction to each forelimb in turn.

If this again fails, raise the hind parts of the mare either after casting, or by standing her at a lower level in front (even if it means digging a trench in a field, as has been done on many occasions). This enables the foal to be repelled further. More lubricant is inserted and rotation applied by tying a length of wood between the 2 forelimbs of the foal, and applying torsion by rotating the ends of the wood, before re-establishing traction.

When the foal is oversized and difficulty in delivery occurs, apply a quantity of lubricant around its head. Pass a length of rope over the poll and behind both ears, pass the free end through the eye of the rope, and tighten the loop by drawing on the free end so that the eye of the rope passes into the foal's mouth between its open jaws. Rope both forelimbs at the pasterns. Use plenty of lubricant to keep the parts free from friction.

Attempt to deliver the muzzle, then the poll, with the 2 forefeet either following, or lying on the vaginal floor near the vulva—and not slowly retreating into the uterus. After the poll is delivered, apply traction to each front foot in turn, introducing the hand as far as possible to guide the feet and prevent their tearing the vagina or vulva.

When the head and both elbows have emerged, keep steady traction upon both forelimbs and head so that delivery will not be checked with the hindquarters of the foal jammed within the mare's pelvis. If this should occur, treat as advised previously.

ANTERIOR PRESENTATION:
DORSOPUBIC POSITION

The presentation resembles the previous one with the exception that the foal is lying on its back, instead of upon its sternum, with the lower jaw and the soles of the forefeet uppermost. After applying plenty of lubricant, rope the head and both forelegs as before. If the foal is small and the mare roomy, repel the head and body slightly. Carry one forelimb across the head and neck until both forelimbs lie on one side of the thorax. Introduce the second finger and thumb into the orbits of the foal and rotate the head toward the side of the body on which the forelimbs now lie, attempting to get the poll uppermost. Introduce a hook into the lower orbit (the one furthest from the limbs as they now lie). Apply traction to the limb which was carried across the head and neck, and simultaneously upon the rope attached to the eye hook. This tends to set the front half of the body in its normal upright position. As the head emerges, try to keep it upright and apply traction now to both forelimbs. If the front portion of the body emerges in its correct position, the rear half should follow it. If it does not do so, apply lubricant to the hand and arm and endeavor to introduce it to make certain that one or both hindfeet are not extended forward.

If the foal is large and the mare is not, one should draw the 2 forelimbs outside the vulva and place between the cannon bones a short length of 4-inch board. Lash the cannon bones to this with rope. Draw upon head and feet simultaneously, at the same time applying torsion to the piece of plank in the hope of "spiraling" the foal through the vagina. The crowbar method of leverage gives good results in this case, and it may be advisable to attach the ropes high up on the bar so that the pull follows the line in which the foal is lying.

When the foal is in the dorsosacral position better results are obtained by pulling downward upon the forelegs. When in the dorsopubic position, uplift is required, otherwise the stiff spine is forced against the pubis of the mare. If no headway can be made, and if the foal is dead, it will become necessary to perform embryotomy and remove one forelimb and shoulder of the foal (the one which lies uppermost, or can be made to do so by gentle traction upon the leg rope and manipulation).

EMBRYOTOMY

Introduce the embryotomy knife (into the end of which a cord has been threaded) into the vagina or uterus with the first finger inserted through its ring. Carry the knife up to the withers and, with pressure and the aid of the cord, drive its point through the skin. By drawing gently upon the cord, incise the skin down the outer side of the limb to the fetlock. By traction upon the rope attached to the pastern, draw the fetlock outside the vulva, and with a scalpel incise the skin around the fetlock to meet the longitudinal incision. After a little dissection to make a start in the skinning process, grasp the skin between the fingers and palm of the hand and force the detached skin upward until the whole limb is skinned to above the elbow. Introduce the fingers, and eventually the whole hand, into the axilla of the foal and break down the areolar tissue. Now attach a chain around the limb above the knee, and fasten it to the steel bar, or have 2 or 3 men exert steady traction. With the hand in the vagina, assist the breaking-down process until the limb comes away completely, with scapula attached. Apply traction to the remaining limb and head, endeavoring also to induce some degree of torsion in the more favorable direction.

LATERAL DEVIATION OF THE HEAD

In this position, both forelimbs are in the vagina but the head is lying back in the uterus, possibly resting on the stifle or flank of the foal (Fig. 2). The more one pulls upon the forelimbs, the more tightly the head will become wedged. In this case, rope both front pasterns, and push the foal back into the uterus as far as possible, remembering that the further one repels the body, the nearer the head travels in the direction of the vagina.

Having done this, lubricate the hand and arm well, and feel for the mane of the foal. Follow this until you come to an ear. Grasp this and pull upon it in the hope that you will next feel an eye, or the orbit. If you do so, try to introduce a sharp hook into it, and draw gently upon this with one hand while you try to grasp the lower jaw of the foal so that you may turn the muzzle to face the vaginal passage. If you can do this, ask an assistant to repel the forelimbs while you draw upon the eye hook and the jaw. This should succeed in bringing the head into the pelvis. If this fails, amputate one forelimb and try again. In rare cases, it may be necessary to amputate both forelimbs.

In some cases when only the mane can be reached, a sharp hook can be driven into the skin of the neck or mane as far forward as can be reached. If traction is exerted on the rope attached to this hook, it may bring the head a little closer, so that a second hook can be inserted a little nearer the head—and so on, until an ear or orbit can be reached.

Anterior Presentation with Retention of One or Both Forelimbs

The head of the foal may be: 1. Free in the uterus, 2, firmly wedged in the vagina, or 3, hanging outside the vulva. The forelimb or limbs may be flexed at the knee or knees, or carried straight backward in full extension. In 1 and 2 the first essential is repulsion of the head, after which an attempt is made to find a knee. If grasping this and exerting pull upon it are insufficient, the end of a rope should be carried through the flexure of the knee and both ends of the rope pulled at the same time. The hand will feel for the foot; grasp it in the palm and steer it into the vagina. One then seeks the other foot in the same way.

When the head lies outside the vulva it will be swollen and edematous, and the foal will be dead. As the head cannot be replaced through the vulva and vagina, it must be amputated. An incision is made through the skin transversely across the forehead of the foal, and the skin is then dissected back over the neck region, leaving both ears in position. A rope is applied to this skin, using the ears to prevent its slipping off. A knife is now employed to amputate the head. The skin and ears are arranged around the stump of the neck, and tied there before applying repulsion, to avoid injury to the mare by sharp bones when the neck is again withdrawn. The procedure will now be as previously detailed.

When the head is firmly wedged in the vagina with no feet in sight, an attempt must be made, with the help of much lubrication, to pass the wire of the embryotome between the

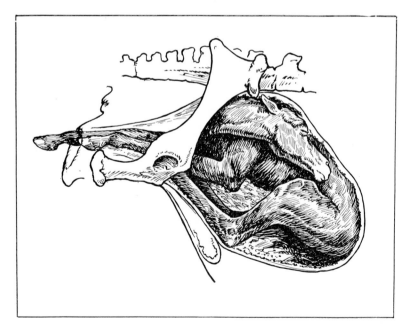

Fig. 2. Lateral deviation of the head. Drawing by A. C. Shuttleworth, M.R.C. V.S.

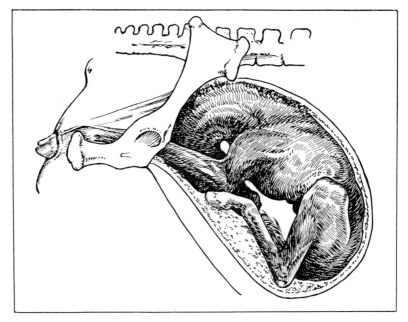

Fig. 3. Head deviated downward. Drawing by A. C. Shuttleworth, M.R.C. V.S.

poll and the vagina, until it lies behind the ears. The end of the embryotome is kept beneath the neck of the foal on the floor of the vagina and, with it in this position, the head is amputated. The stump is pushed back into the uterus and the limbs searched for and retrieved. Great care must be taken to protect the vagina from injury by the severed neck bones by covering them with the palm of the hand during their withdrawal.

Head Deviated Downward

When the poll of the foal lies below the pubic brim (Fig. 3), both forelimbs must be repelled, in a rigidly extended condition, into the uterus, after applying a rope around each fetlock. When using the forelimbs to effect repulsion, it is advisable always to extend them fully and, as though endeavoring to over-extend the foot, to push hard upon its sole with the palm of the hand.

To recover the head, a succession of sharp hooks may be inserted in the skin of the foal, or a spring porte-cord may be successfully employed to pass a rope beneath the neck. Usually, however, repulsion will bring some part of the head into reach of the hand.

Anterior Presentation: Dog-Sitting Position

The foal is doubled upon itself at the loins so that the head, the 2 forefeet, and the 2 hindfeet are all presented together. This is one of the most serious presentations encountered in the foaling mare. One must first determine which of the feet are fore- and which are hindfeet. In this presentation, if the 4 feet all belong to the same foal it will be necessary to run the hand along each cannon bone to determine whether a knee or a hock is encountered.

One should rope all 4 feet, apply a rope over the poll, and loop it through the open mouth. Having discovered the 2 feet which are provided with hocks, it is essential that these should be directed backward, so that the hindfeet will not become wedged during traction and tear the uterus or vagina.

If there is sufficient room within the uterus, push the foal back into it as far as it will go with safety. Try to flex the trespassing hindfeet at the fetlocks and apply pressure on the front of each fetlock joint in the hope that the feet will return to the uterus when traction again is exerted on the head and forelimbs of the foal.

If it is apparent that the hindfeet are still approaching the vagina, such efforts must cease. An attempt should now be made to repel the hindfeet, one at a time, by the use of a straight porte-cord. This instrument usually is made of steel, being a straight rod 1 to 1.5 cm. thick fitted with a "T" handle at one end and a large metal loop at the other. To be really effective the rods should be a little more than 3 feet long. The purpose of the metal eye is to enable the porte-cord to slide along the rope attached to the hind pastern of the foal after the rope has been threaded through the metal eye. Pressure can then be applied to the pastern, which will then fall back into its proper place in the uterus. By drawing the porte-cord gently back along the rope it can be removed from the uterus and vagina. The alternative, if all other measures fail, is to amputate both forelimbs (possibly the head also), repel the thorax and abdomen of the foal, and effect delivery by traction on the ropes attached to the hindfeet. In the case of a dead foal, this may prove in the long run to be the quickest method.

Figure 4 illustrates the dog-sitting position with the back presented.

POSTERIOR PRESENTATION: LUMBOPUBIC POSITION

When the 2 hindfeet are presented, with soles of the feet uppermost and no other feet within reach, the presentation may be regarded as being normal (Fig. 5). Unless delivery can be carried out fairly rapidly, there is considerable risk of the foal's dying during the process, or subsequently, owing to fluids being forced down the trachea and inhaled when inspiration commences.

In the lumbopubic position the foal lies on its back with the 2 hindfeet directed upward toward the roof of the vagina. If the foal is not abnormally large, traction is effected by block and pulley, first attaching the block high so that it lifts the feet upward. When both hocks have been delivered, lower the block and pull first on the level, then downward as the delivery proceeds.

The feet, in the early stage of delivery, must be held in the hands to avoid injury to the vagina or vulva. The points of the hocks also must be watched. Sometimes it becomes necessary to cross the hindlimbs as soon as they emerge through the vulva and, by pressing one limb downward and the other upward, de-

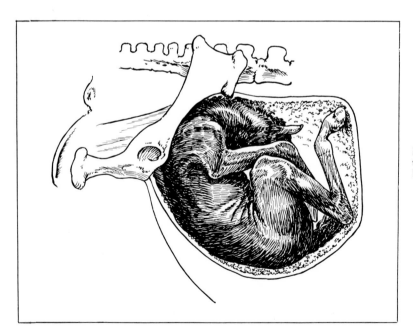

Fig. 4. Dog-sitting position with back presented. Drawing by A. C. Shuttleworth, M.R.C.V.S.

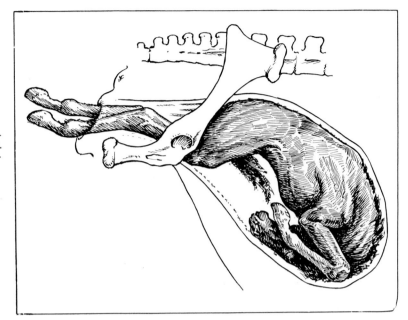

Fig. 5. Posterior presentation, lumbosacral position. Drawing by A. C. Shuttleworth, M.R.C.V.S.

velop a spiral movement of the body of the foal. This makes delivery much easier.

POSTERIOR, HOCK PRESENTATION

The buttocks and tail of the foal, and the points of both hocks, are presented. The hindfeet lie well-forward within the uterus. To raise each hindfoot in turn, first repel the foal's body by placing the palm of the hand beneath its tail and pressing firmly upon its hindquarters. Slide the hand quickly down a hindlimb into the flexure of the hock and draw the limb toward you. Then push the point of the hock upward, in the arc of a circle, so that the tuber calcis slides along the roof of the uterus, well-protected by being covered with your hand. Allow your hand to slide rapidly down the front of the cannon bone, grasp the fetlock, flex it, and draw the hindfoot toward you. Be very careful as you do this so that the point of the hock is not thrust through the uterine roof. Repeat in the case of the second hindlimb.

If the foal is large and cannot easily be repelled, try to pass a rope through the flexure of the hock. Lift the hock upward by traction on the rope with one hand, while the other hand enters the vagina and again attempts to force the foal deeper into the uterus.

Sometimes raising the hindquarters of the mare to a standing position is a great help. The danger to the mare in delivery of a foal from this presentation is twofold. One must prevent the point of each hock from tearing the roof of the uterus, and at the same time be equally careful to see that neither hindfoot becomes trapped beneath the pubic brim and punctures the uterus at this point when traction is applied.

POSTERIOR BREECH PRESENTATION

This presentation resembles the previous type but, instead of the points of the hocks being presented, each hindlimb is extended in the forward direction, so that nothing can be felt apart from the buttocks and tail of the foal (Fig. 6). Repulsion of the buttocks of the foal may sometimes convert this into a posterior hock presentation, but in a great many instances the hindlimbs appear to possess a marked rigidity and in such cases repulsion becomes impossible. It then becomes necessary to remove a hindlimb at the hip joint.

As an embryotome will be of little use in this case, the limb is amputated by means of the embryotomy knife, an operation requiring a good deal of skill. Briefly, the procedure is as follows: A lengthy incision is made in the skin overlying the hip joint. By using the knife, the fingers, and sometimes a chisel, the hip joint is exposed by a process of blunt dissection. The older practitioners used to cut through the ligamentum teres and extract the head of the femur from the acetabulum. Time can be saved and less energy expended by introducing a length of embryotomy wire around the neck of the femur and sawing through it.

From this stage, efforts are made to secure the upper end of the femur by a rope or chain and draw it (femoral head first) out of the vulva. Before doing this it is advisable to incise the skin of the hindlimb as far down as the stifle, if this can be reached. As the upper head of the femur is drawn by traction through the vulva, careful use of the embryotomy knife or a scalpel severs the soft tissues until eventually the whole limb is withdrawn, hip and stifle first, and hock and foot last. If the mare is roomy, it now may be possible to pass a rope around the front of the remaining stifle and withdraw the foal with the remaining hindlimb extended. If this proves too great a

risk, one must amputate the second hindlimb in the same way as the first.

Usually, this type of embryotomy is carried out under general anesthesia. The recumbent mare will need to be turned from one side to the other in order that the limb being operated upon is uppermost. It is very helpful in such cases if the hind parts of the mare can be elevated upon sacks packed tightly with straw.

TRANSVERSE PRESENTATIONS

In sterno-abdominal transverse presentations, the muzzle of the foal and all 4 feet are presented at or in the vagina (Fig. 7). The umbilicus and the umbilical cord are turned toward the operator. The presentation resembles the dog-sitting position but the foal lies transversely in the uterus instead of being upright. In most instances, it will be dead.

First, one should make sure that all the limbs belong to the same foal. Then decide whether it will be easier to repel the rear end of the foal, or to repel the head and forelimbs and effect delivery by traction upon the hindlimbs. Usually the latter method is the easier. The head and all 4 feet should be roped before commencing to repel one end of the body.

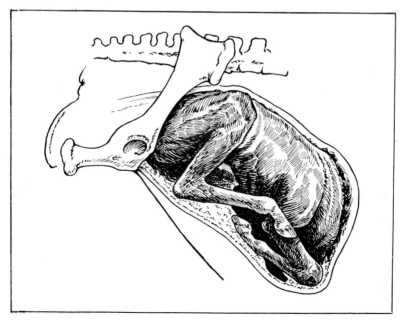

Fig. 6. Posterior breech presentation. Drawing by A. C. Shuttleworth, M.R.C. V.S.

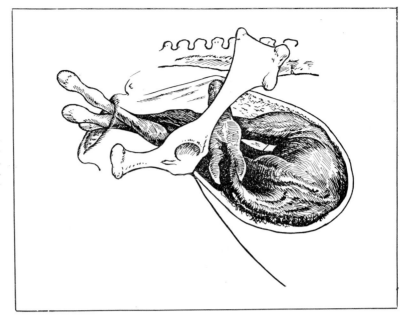

Fig. 7. Transverse presentation with all 4 feet presented. Drawing by A. C. Shuttleworth, M.R.C.V.S.

Here is a case in which the straight rod porte-cord may be of assistance. Fortunately, this type of presentation occurs more often when the foal is small than when it is particularly large. If the latter is the case, the remedy usually is amputation of one or both forelimbs, including the scapula, propelling the head and thorax in circular fashion, securing first one hock and then the other, and treating the case from this point as though it were the posterior hock presentation, previously described.

In cephalo-iliac transverse presentations, the belly of the foal faces forward, the reverse of that described in the sterno-abdominal type of presentation (Fig. 8). All that can be palpated is the ridge of the spine, or the ribs, or some other part of the body wall. This is a very difficult presentation to deal with, and the mare should be cast, the hindquarters raised, and a general anesthetic administered.

One should attempt first to discover which end of the foal's body is on either side, or, in other words, try to locate the mane or tail. When this has been accomplished, attempt to propel the front end of the body further in the direction in which it is facing, so as to bring the hindquarters into reach of the hand.

If these can be felt, but the hindlimbs cannot be manipulated, one may attempt amputation of the uppermost hindlimb at the hip joint in the manner already described.

If all attempts in this direction fail, try to make an opening between the ribs, remove one or more ribs, and then withdraw the viscera. If this does not enable the body to be propelled headfirst sufficiently to bring the hindlimbs into reach of the hand, one should make another incision through the opposite side of the body. Pass the end of the spring porte-cord through this hole, and try to direct it so that the eye at its extremity emerges above or below the foal's body, after passing between it and the inner surface of the uterus. If it does so it can carry the wire saw of the embryotome around one-half of the body, and this can then be severed. The same procedure is carried out on the remaining portions, until eventually the body of the foal is divided into an anterior portion carrying the head and forelimbs, and a posterior portion carrying the hindlimbs and the tail. The 2 halves are then removed separately, after determining which is the easier to withdraw first.

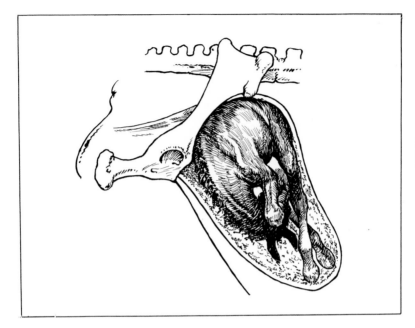

Fig. 8. Transverse presentation, back presented. Drawing by A. C. Shuttleworth, M.R.C.V.S.

TWIN PRESENTATIONS

When one foal is presented anteriorly and the other posteriorly, try, as a general rule, to first remove the foal presenting its hindlimbs. Repel the other foal as far as possible until the one being extracted fills the vagina. Be careful always to trace all the limbs, rope them, and make sure that the 2 limbs—whether fore or hind—selected for traction, actually belong to the same individual. If one foal happens to be considerably larger than the other (something which often happens), attempt to remove the smaller foal first.

COMPLICATIONS
ARISING DURING PARTURITION

Parturition may be accompanied by such developments as prolapse of the bladder, prolapse of the vagina, and rectovaginal fistula. Rupture of the uterus is an ever-present risk, and in an excitable mare it may occur before the arrival of the veterinarian. Uterine rupture usually results from the foal's feet being forced through some part of the uterus during straining, or when the mare throws herself to the ground. Rupture from muscular contraction also is a possibility.

When rupture of the uterus does occur, it is often (but not always) attended by some degree of hemorrhage through the vulva. Uterine contractions cease, the mare appears dejected, and often is covered with cold sweat. She may or may not show signs of acute colic associated with the onset of peritonitis. Her pulse will be weak and usually slowed, and her temperature, after an initial fall, will rise considerably if the mare does not succumb to shock immediately.

RUPTURE OF THE PREPUBIC TENDON

A complication which may have occurred during the last weeks or 2 months of pregnancy is rupture of the prepubic tendon of the rectus abdominus muscle. In this condition, the abdominal wall drops considerably, and some difficulty may be experienced in delivering the foal. If the obstetrician finds it difficult to reach the head or limbs in such a case, the mare should be cast and anesthetized, then rolled on her back to effect delivery, her limbs being supported on either side by bags packed with straw.

Prolapse of the Vagina and Bladder

Prolapse of the vagina is not a common occurrence as the weight of the foal tends to draw the vagina forward. When it does occur, the mare must be given an epidural anesthetic and elevated behind. Lubrication is needed especially in such deliveries. Prolapse of the bladder is a complication seldom encountered since epidural anesthesia has been practiced widely.

When the bladder becomes everted after passing through the urethra, its surface will be pink, the color of the exposed mucous lining. Urine will squirt out through the 2 ureters when the mare strains. This accident usually happens during delivery and the prolapse must be corrected before further traction is applied to the foal. If epidural anesthesia has not already been given, it should be administered immediately, as it prevents straining and a repetition of the prolapse after the bladder has been returned into its normal position. The bladder must be propelled back through the urethra and to do this without causing its rupture, one may first use the fingers to push the fundus of the bladder through the urethra, then follow this by pushing a wax candle, the end of which has been trimmed to roundness (or test tube, pessary, etc.), very gently through the urethra until the whole of the bladder returns to place.

Whenever parturition is attended by a good deal of manual assistance, it is advisable to administer antibiotics and, in cases in which a tendency to develop laminitis appears, to inject a full dose of an antihistamine.

Rupture of the Vagina

Rupture of the vagina may occur when a foot is pushed upward and through the vaginal roof as the mare strains. The foot may penetrate the rectum also, and appear outside the anus. Repeated straining causes a detachment of the structures between the rectum and vagina and the production of a rectovaginal fistula. When this occurs, feces enter the vagina and may collect there or be passed through the vulva. Curiously, although mares succumb from quite minor obstetrical injuries, a number of those developing this type of fistula survive. In some instances, the injury is not detected by the owner or attendant until feces and urine are discharged simultaneously through the vulva. The condition must be corrected surgically and this is not always successful.

Rupture of the Perineum

Tearing of the upper commissure of the vulva, and its extension in the direction of the anus, enable "windsucking" to occur—air being aspirated into the vagina and expelled. The vagina itself usually becomes dilated, and the mare fails to conceive to later services. Caslick's operation for the relief of this condition usually is successful.

Prolapse of the Uterus

Fortunately, this is a rare condition in the mare, but when it occurs it is serious. The mare exhibits signs of colic, lies down, and may roll and damage the uterus. Epidural anesthesia, combined with a sedative, is the first essential in treatment. The hindquarters must be raised to facilitate manipulation, and the mare should be restrained by service hobbles. After replacing the prolapsed tissue, the lips of the vulva are approximated with mattress sutures, but sufficient room is left at the lowest suture to permit the passage of urine. Antibiotics and an antihistamine should be administered.

Retention of the Fetal Membranes

In the mare, the fetal membranes should be expelled within a short period following birth of the foal. The time allowed differs with various practitioners, but it is agreed that at 6 hours they may be removed manually, and that 18 hours is the extreme limit of safety for the mare. If retained longer, metritis may occur and there is a considerable risk of the mare's developing acute laminitis. The administration of an antibiotic and an antihistamine is advisable in any case in which placental removal has been delayed.

Method of Removal: The fetal membranes may be hanging down to hock level, or merely showing at the vulva. It will be noticed that they consist of 2 main portions. The bulk of the membranes (allantois) is gray and comparatively thin. The lesser portion (chorion) is thicker, more resistant to traction, and of a light chocolate or reddish color.

The usual procedure is to introduce the palm of the hand between the chorionic portion of the membranes and the uterine wall to effect separation and withdrawal. As infection can be carried in by the hand, I adopt the following method which enables the membranes to be removed intact without inserting the hand into the vagina: Collect within the hand as much of the chorionic portion as possible. Wrap this around the gray membranes so that the free portion of chorion, now outermost, represents the layer previously adherent to the uterine wall. Now commence to twist the afterbirth, in a clockwise direction, keeping the chorion outermost, and at the same time exerting gentle traction to keep the membranes moving steadily out of the vulva. This torsion is continued until the whole of the afterbirth has been delivered.

As soon as this has been accomplished, the placenta should be examined to determine its completeness by opening the sac at the end which first protruded, and pouring a gallon of water into it. The membranes are lifted sufficiently high to let the fluid reach into the apices of the 2 uterine cornua. These should be intact so that the afterbirth holds water and appears something like a pair of trousers, the legs of which have been tied separately at the feet. If any portion is missing, the hand, well-disinfected, will have to be introduced into the appropriate cornu and the retained portion removed. It is rare, however, that any part remains when removed by torsion and gentle traction in the manner described.

R. H. Smythe

CHAPTER 25

PEDIATRICS

IMMEDIATE POSTNATAL CARE OF THE FOAL

Immediate care of the newborn foal, even one that is free of infection or disease, is essential for maintenance of the good health of this susceptible individual. Treatment of the umbilical stump with tincture of iodine or another good disinfecting agent should be done as soon as the cord is severed from the umbilicus. The umbilical cord should never be severed surgically except in extreme cases. It should be left intact, and in most instances it will sever itself when the major portion of placental blood has drained into the living foal. The placenta contains a high percentage of the foal's blood supply and if it is severed too soon, the fragile foal will begin life with a decreased amount of blood, making it more susceptible to infection.

If it becomes necessary to surgically disengage the umbilical cord, an indented area approximately 1 to 2 inches from the umbilicus, or the area where it would normally break, should be found. Sterile ligatures should be placed around the cord at this point and it is severed aseptically between the ligatures. Emasculators also may be used for severance of the cord.

It is the opinion of many equine practitioners, that antibiotics should be given to all foals immediately postnatal for their prophylactic effect. This has been done routinely for a number of years by the author and it appears to be a sound procedure. The antibiotic, dose, and number of treatments may be varied with the individual animal. Foals which are delivered in a weakened condition, of course, should receive more treatment than normal foals.

Neonatal isoerythrolysis is a rather common condition. It is discussed in greater detail in Chapter 19. The early detection of the agglutinating or hemolytic factors in colostrum is essential to prevent isoerythrolysis from occurring. It is a simple procedure to collect a few drops of blood from either the umbilical stump, or by venipuncture of the jugular vein. Normal saline is added to prevent coagulation and to suspend the erythrocytes. For every 1 ml. of blood, approximately 5 ml. of normal saline are added to make a good suspension of cells. The mare is milked and some of the colostrum is obtained, one drop of which is mixed on a slide with one drop of cell suspension. A cover glass is placed over the mixture and this is examined under low power at 5, 10, and 15 minute intervals. If there is no agglutination nor hemolysis present at the end of 15 minutes, the colostrum is safe for the foal. This may seem to be a rather inexact type of laboratory procedure but it has been used routinely for more than 500 foalings with excellent results.

Weak and diseased foals are always a disheartening sight. Most of them die in a short period of time. Occasionally, one can be saved if emergency measures are instituted at the time of birth or very soon thereafter. These foals should routinely receive oxygen therapy via either a resuscitator or an oxygen nasal tube, combined with artificial respiration if needed. This simple procedure sometimes will provide dramatic results. A transfusion of 50 to 100 ml. of the mare's blood may be given to the foal if there is no isohemolytic factor present. Antibiotics and/or chemotherapeutics are administered in large and frequent doses along with corticosteroids.

NURSING

A majority of normal foals will nurse within 3 hours after foaling. The more vigorous ones will nurse within 30 to 45 minutes. Foals which have not nursed at the end of 3 hours should be examined thoroughly to determine if a defect exists that prevents their doing so. The mare also should be examined at this time for evidence of mammary abnormalities which would make nursing difficult. If there are no pathologic conditions found in the foal or mare, it usually is wise to allow the foal another 2 to 3 hours before resorting to handfeeding.

Handfeeding usually is accomplished by milking the colostrum into a suitable bottle. Then, by using the index finger as a guide, teach the foal to suck on the attached nipple. Most strong and healthy foals present no problems in this respect. After they have learned to drink from the bottle, they should be taken at the next feeding time to the mare and introduced to the nursing procedure. Primiparous mares ordinarily have very small teats and this sometimes makes prehension difficult and the foal becomes discouraged. These mares also may be flighty and not stand still for nursing, and may even kick, thus discouraging the foal. Most flighty or kicking mares can be restrained by the use of ataractics or, if necessary, by the use of the twitch.

Patience with the mare and foal is essential. Some mares, particularly good milkers, may have a "caked udder" which is very sensitive. Such udders should be milked manually and the colostrum given to the foal in a bottle. Light massage is then applied to the tender udder.

Occasionally, primiparous or old mares may have little or no milk, but they usually will produce some after being stimulated by the foal's nursing. Complete agalactia causes a definite problem. It usually is met by allowing the foal to suck in the hope that the manipulation will stimulate milk production. Estrogenic hormones have been tried as lactogenic agents and varying results are reported. The use of a nurse mare, if one is available, is a satisfactory solution. However, the use of simulated formulas is equally as effective but one must remember that for the first week, the foal should be fed every hour, night and day. At the end of the first week the feedings can be given every 2 hours and then gradually lengthened as the foal becomes older until there are 4 feedings a day at one month of age.

The following formula is used by many nurseries:

    4 ounces of evaporated milk in 4 ounces of warm water.
    1 teaspoonful of Karo syrup.

A vigorous foal will consume with relish 8 ounces of formula every hour. If the Karo syrup has an undesirable laxative effect, one tea-spoonful of limewater should be substituted for the syrup for several days. At some equine nurseries a nanny goat in full production is satisfactorily used as a substitute for a nurse mare. It must be remembered that orphaned foals have not received colostrum and they should be maintained on high antibiotic levels for at least 7 days. Vitamin supplementation also may be indicated during this period. Orphaned foals need company. Some nurseries have satisfactorily used goats or small burros as company for orphaned foals.

Colostrum or the "first milk" is essential for any newborn animal. It contains antibodies in high concentration, and for the first 36 hours of the foal's life the intestinal tract is permeable to these antibodies. Acquired immunity is obtained from the colostrum during this period. Colostrum also has a high vitamin content and high food value plus a laxative substance that promotes intestinal elimination. Without colostrum, a foal begins life under a disadvantage. He is more susceptible to constipation and infections in his early days. Some nurseries remove colostrum from mares which have had dead foals and store it at deep-freeze temperatures for future use in foals who have not received colostrum. This is an excellent practice.

PREMATURE FOALS

Premature foals, as is the case of any premature animal, are not fully developed under the protection of intrauterine environment. The rate of growth of a fetus *in utero* is exceedingly rapid during the last 4 months of pregnancy. If the foal loses as much as a month of this rapid growth within the uterus, it usually is poorly prepared for exposure to the external environment. These foals will need special attention. Most of them are not breathing when they are delivered and often require oxygen therapy. Stimulants are advised, and certainly some type of incubation is essential because the temperature of premature foals may be as much as 2 to 3 degrees below normal. If any more body heat is lost by radiation, the foal surely will succumb. Feeding can be accomplished by the insertion of a stomach tube left in place so that 2 to 4 ounces of mare's milk or formula, or any medication that may be desired, can be administered at will. Intravenous feeding may be indicated. The majority of foals delivered 2 to 3 weeks prematurely are in good condition and are able to stand and nurse without help. If a foal is delivered more than 5 weeks prematurely this definitely is an abortion, and the foal almost invariably is dead. If alive, it will live only a few hours even with the best of care.

Premature foals should routinely receive antibiotics and vitamin supplements. Blood transfusions are indicated and the blood of the dam can be used if isohemolysis is not demonstrable.

SIGNS OF ILLNESS IN THE NEWBORN

Diarrhea

Etiology: The more common causes for diarrhea in newborn foals include dietary incompatibilities, foal heat, coprophagy, and infections.

Clinical Signs: Diarrhea in foals due to a dietary intolerance is commonly seen when the mare is an exceedingly good milker and the foal is a greedy type. Diarrhea usually is preceded by slight signs of colic. On auscultation, the intestinal tract will be found hypermotile with evidence of considerable fermentation. The fecal material will vary in consistency from a yellow, tenacious material to an almost fluid substance, and will have the characteristic odor of fermented milk. Usually there is no temperature rise and the foal will continue to overfill his digestive tract. If corrective measures are not followed, serious consequences may follow.

Diarrhea is common in foals for 3 to 5 days during the mare's "foal heat" period. These diarrheas seldom, if ever, are associated with a temperature rise or any serious gastrointestinal disturbance other than the diarrhea. The diarrhea begins and ends ordinarily with the signs of foal heat. Little damage is done, and the foal may even benefit from the laxative effect at this time.

Most foals are prone to be coprophagic. Their ingestion of large quantities of fecal material often produces diarrhea. Fecal material is foreign to the intestinal tract which is not ready to handle solid food, and this is the initiating cause of the abnormal eliminations.

Any foal with diarrhea should be examined and watched carefully as this is a common sign of septicemia and infectious gastroenteritis. A rise in temperature invariably accompanies infectious causes for diarrhea. Inappetence, colicky signs, lethargy, injected mucous membranes, rapid dehydration, and a rise in the leukocyte count also are seen commonly. The fecal material may be pasty but is most often quite fluid and has a putrid odor.

Many organisms have been incriminated as causes for diarrhea. The most common ones are *Actinobacillosis (Shigella) equili, Salmonella* spp., *Streptococcus* spp., *Escherichia coli, Corynebacteria* spp., and occasionally *Micrococcus aureus.* There probably are diarrheas of viral origin but these have not been clearly identified at the present time. Exposure to adverse weather conditions and other stresses may produce a transient diarrhea which, if untreated, may be fatal.

Treatment and Control: Control measures for diarrhea due to food intolerance are obvious but sometimes they are difficult to carry out. The heavy milking mare should be milked frequently and the foal may be muzzled. Control of coprophagy can be accomplished by muzzling or by the immediate removal of the mare's eliminations from the paddock. The parenteral administration of vitamin B-complex in foals has not seemed to alter their tendency to be coprophagic.

Good husbandry is essential for the control of all causes of diarrheas in the newborn foal. Treatments are many and varied. The use of large doses of intestinal protectives and antiferments plus anticholinergic agents is common. If there is temperature elevation or any signs of septicemia or infection, broad spectrum antibiotics and/or chemotherapeutic agents should be administered in high doses in addition to the symptomatic agents. As soon as possible the causative organism should be identified and its sensitivity to antibiotics determined. The choice of drugs should be guided by this finding. Large quantities of normal electrolyte solutions should be administered intravenously even before acute signs of dehydration appear. As much as 1000 ml. can be administered every 12 hours in a very young foal.

Constipation

Etiology: Constipation in newborn foals usually is present at birth or develops in a very short time thereafter. It is caused by a collection and hardening of meconium in the large intestines. The meconial mass may occur in a very small area or as much as 2 or 3 feet of colon may become impacted. The underlying and initiating causes of constipation and impaction are not well-understood.

Clinical Signs: A constipated or impacted foal almost invariably is normal at birth and will stand and nurse within a reasonable period of time. Evidence of straining and tail switching may occur, however, as soon as 3 hours postpartum. Many of these foals will have had normal appearing bowel movements soon after birth. The condition may not manifest itself in extreme cases until 2 to 5 days postpartum. Foals which do not receive colostrum in adequate amounts are more prone to become constipated than those which do. Digital examination of the rectum often will reveal the presence of a hard fecal mass.

Treatment and Control: Many practitioners routinely administer warm, soapy enemas to the newborn foal. This appears to be a good practice as it does aid in emptying the posterior part of the bowel, allows the free movement of meconium in the anterior colon, and initiates the habit of defecation. Administration of an enema and the passage of fecal material do not preclude subsequent constipation. Often sizable quantities of hard fecal material can be removed from the rectum with one finger. In simple constipation, repeated warm soapy enemas are indicated. The instillation of approximately 2 ounces of hydrogen peroxide glycerite rectally seems to have considerable value.[2] One to 2 ounces of equal parts of castor oil and mineral oil may be given via the stomach tube. The use of smooth muscle stimulants and derivatives of cascara sagrada may be indicated. Close supervision of the foal is absolutely necessary. There are many routine treatments which are as effective as those mentioned, but it must be stressed that constipation can develop into a serious condition if not corrected in a very short time.

For foals in which there is a true impaction, surgery is indicated and should be performed before the animal becomes semicomatose. Many foals can be saved by early surgical intervention which otherwise would be lost.

CLINICAL ENTITIES OF THE NEWBORN FOAL

Atresia Coli

Atresia coli is an anatomic deformity of the large intestine in which the large intestine consists of 2 sections without a connection between them. Extending forward from the rectum there are 1 to 3 feet of colon which end in a blind pouch, and from the large colon there are 2 to 4 feet of the small colon ending in another blind pouch. Several feet or even whole sections may be missing from the digestive tract.[1] Most of these foals are born normally, stand and nurse, and are apparently in good health for 8 to 24 hours. At this time, they develop severe colic and the severity increases despite any form of treatment. A pathognomonic sign of this condition is the failure of liquid or feces to be expelled following the administration of an enema.

McGee states that he knows of no successful treatment. He has attempted anastomosis on numerous occasions and even though the technical procedure was successful, so much of the intestinal tract was missing that a cure was not affected.[1]

REFERENCES

1. McGee, William R.: Veterinary Notebook. The Blood Horse, Lexington, Ky., 1958.
2. Brennan, H. H. and Laskey, F. M.: Personal communication.

Pervious Urachus

Pervious urachus is a rather common condition. The urachus is a small ureter-like structure within the umbilical cord that connects the bladder of the fetus with the allantois and through which fetal urine is excreted. This outlet usually is closed at the time the umbilical cord is severed, but in some individuals it may remain patent and urine will continue to drip from this opening. This is observed especially when the foal is micturating. This is not a serious condition but it does keep the umbilical stump wet and soiled. The majority of cases will correct themselves within a few days but some urachi must be cauterized daily with silver nitrate to effect a cure. The navel cord should not be ligated to correct this condition. It should be cleaned and cauterized daily.

Scrotal Hernia

Scrotal hernia is caused by a relaxed or enlarged inguinal ring which allows a loop of small intestine to herniate through it into the scrotum and inside the tunica vaginalis. It usually is noticed at the time of parturition or within a day or two later. Most scrotal hernias in foals will correct themselves in time. Rarely is surgery indicated except in cases of strangulation. When examining a male foal which is showing signs of colic, the scrotum always should be examined for the presence of a strangulated, scrotal hernia. If the strangulation has been of short duration, many of the hernias can be reduced manually. Surgical intervention is necessary if manual reduction is impossible.

Umbilical Hernia

A hernia at the umbilical opening may be present at birth or develop within 3 to 7 days. This defect is caused by an abnormally large opening in the abdominal wall or by the failure of the opening to close. The hernia may be from 3 to 12 cm. in diameter. An umbilical hernia seldom becomes strangulated and the majority will undergo spontaneous reduction by the time the animal reaches 12 to 14 months of age. The majority of these hernias can be completely reduced by hand but will not remain in the abdominal cavity. The application of mild blisters over the hernial site will facilitate their reduction. Clamps are used by many practitioners with excellent results. Some prefer surgical reduction and closure by using an overlapping type of suture through the linea alba.

Ruptured Bladder

Rupture of the bladder is not an uncommon condition in foals. The exact causes are unknown. Rupture probably occurs as a result of compression at the time of parturition or by extreme tension on the umbilical cord. One case has been seen that was attributed to anaphylactic shock caused by a bee sting. The powerful muscular contractions during the state of anaphylaxis were believed to have caused the bladder's rupture.

Clinical Signs: The foal appears normal from 12 to 24 hours following the rupture. There is little or no elevation of temperature at this time. There are repeated attempts to defecate and urinate with very little or no urine being voided. In 48 to 72 hours abdominal distention is noticed, and at this time the temperature may be elevated 1 to 2 degrees. Hyperpnea is evident at this time. The mucous membranes become pale, and the foal is unwilling to nurse. Toxic signs develop rapidly. Some foals may show blindness and many of them suffer severe convulsions. Paracentesis will reveal the presence of a large quantity of urine in the abdominal cavity. While the needle is in the abdominal cavity as much urine as possible should be removed. This immediately alleviates most of the signs, and undoubtedly makes the patient a better surgical risk.

Treatment: After the diagnosis is made, surgical correction of the defect should be done immediately. If surgery is postponed until toxic signs develop, the chances of recovery are greatly reduced. Most foals will recover completely, however, if surgery is performed before the animal has become moribund.

R. S. Jackson

CHAPTER 26

TRAUMATIC INJURIES AND THEIR TREATMENT

FRACTURES

INTRODUCTION

Most fractures encountered in the horse involve the bones of the limbs. Other fractures which are not infrequent in occurrence involve the mandible, premaxilla, ribs, cervical vertebrae, and certain of the pelvic bones.

Numerous factors influence the prognosis for fracture healing and the decision concerning whether treatment is justified or not. Immature animals will more likely recover from fractures than will adults. Aged animals usually respond poorly to treatment and often have delayed callus formation. Ponies have a better prospect for fracture healing than do the larger breeds, partially because of their lesser body weight, and partially because of their more docile disposition. Fractures of bones which bear weight directly warrant a poorer prognosis than fractures of those which do not. Fractures of the lower leg usually have a better prospect for healing than do those above the carpus and tarsus. Compound and comminuted fractures have reduced chances of successful repair.

The type of animal, the use to which it is to be put, the nature of the fracture, and economic considerations influence the decision as to whether or not fracture therapy is justified. Most horses have sentimental value or are valuable for breeding purposes and treatment of their fractures may be warranted even though permanent lameness should result. Lameness which is accompanied by constant pain may preclude the use of the animal for breeding purposes, however. With the expenditure of enough time and effort, healing of some sort may be expected for most fractures.

GENERAL CONSIDERATIONS IN FRACTURE REDUCTION

Fracture reduction consists of applying sufficient traction in the proper direction to effect proper alignment of the fractured ends of the bone. Early reduction of the fracture and its immobilization are important for prevention of further damage to the part. Delay in reduction and immobilization often results in a simple fracture's becoming compound or comminuted, thus decreasing the prospect of good healing. Considerable swelling from extravasation of blood and serum develops within a short time following occurrence of a fracture, especially one above the carpus and tarsus. This may make it necessary to temporarily immobilize the injured part and to postpone reduction until the swelling subsides. If reduction is performed when the fracture site is swollen, the orthopedic device may have to be modified several times to conform to the reduced size of the part.

The application of considerable traction usually is necessary to accomplish reduction of fractured, weight-bearing bones above the carpus and tarsus. The degree of muscular spasm at the site of the fracture dictates the amount of traction necessary. General anesthesia, and possibly the concurrent use of muscle relaxants, are necessary to accomplish good reduction of fractures.

Fractures of the forelimb usually are easier to reduce than those of the hindlimb because the former is much straighter. The heavier musculature of the hindlimb is not only stronger mechanically, but also presents greater opportunity for damage to soft tissue and consequent muscular spasm. Sufficient traction must be applied in the proper direction to secure alignment and correct overriding of the fractured ends. In the forelimb, traction is exerted in a straight line with the possible exception of the phalanges and the humerus where normal angulation should be maintained. In the hindlimb, traction is applied in the same manner for fractures below the tarsus. To reduce fractures above the tarsus, traction should be exerted parallel to the long axis of the affected bone with the limb partially flexed as in the usual standing position. In some instances reduction may be accomplished only with the limb fully flexed.

CLOSED REDUCTION

Closed reduction ordinarily is the method of choice for simple fractures. Comminuted fractures are not infrequent and, depending upon the location and the bone involved, usually may be reduced without penetrating the skin. Compound fractures must be considered infected. Careful cleansing and debridement of soft tissue, removal of loose bone fragments, and local application of antibiotics or sulfonamides must be performed prior to their reduction. This should be followed by the parenteral administration of antibiotics and/or sulfonamides.

The periosteum often reflects back from the ends of fracture fragments for a considerable distance. This especially is true of metacarpal and metatarsal fractures. Bone necrosis may result as a consequence of periosteal reflexion. Sequestra formation is common in such instances, particularly if the fracture is comminuted.

Radiographs should be taken of the fracture prior to and after reduction to insure proper alignment. Care must be taken to avoid having soft tissue interposed between the fragments, and their ends must be held in contact before firm callus formation will occur. Disruption of nerve and blood supplies distal to the site of the fracture may occur at the time of injury, or may result from movement of the sharp ends of the fragments. In most cases, loss of blood or nerve supplies cannot be determined for several days.

With the animal under general anesthesia it is possible to exert sufficient force by manual traction to reduce most fractures of the forelimb. Occasionally, reduction of fractures above the carpus is possible only with the aid of such devices as a block and tackle or a fetal extractor. Fractures of the humerus, however, tend to be forced out of alignment by traction applied in a straight line from the hoof to the body. Care must be taken to insure that rotation of the part distal to the fracture does not occur during the administration of traction. Fractures of the radius and humerus ordinarily cannot be fully reduced by the closed method, and some overriding is to be expected.

Difficulties often are encountered in the application of traction to the hindlimb. The normal angulation of the leg prevents application of traction on the leg as a whole. For fractures of the tarsus and below, traction may be applied at the hoof and at the tibia. If it is applied to the whole limb, angulation of the fractured ends will occur. It is not always possible to correct overriding of the fragments in fractures of the tibia and femur by closed reduction. If closed reduction is employed for these fractures, flexion of the limb is necessary to manipulate the fragments into alignment. Many fractures of the tibia and femur will heal with some shortening of the limb, even though there is considerable overriding, provided there is sufficient contact between the fragments.

OPEN REDUCTION

Open reduction is employed for certain fractures of the long bones of the limb. Exposing the fracture site also may be necessary to remove small fragments which may form sequestra. Open reduction is employed for fractures in which such technics as pinning, plating, or the use of screws are indicated. The fractures which commonly are reduced openly involve the proximal and distal portions of the femur and tibia, the olecranon process, and the radius and humerus. Fractures of the metacarpi and metatarsi occasionally may be reduced by this method to facilitate immobilization by plates, intramedullary pins, screws, or wire. Open reduction also is done in cases of nonunion when the fracture is complete and transverse, and in some compound fractures.

Strict aseptic technic must be followed when open reduction is done. Plates, intramedullary pins, or other internal fixation devices in themselves act as foreign bodies and tend to produce considerable tissue reaction. If infection is superimposed, osteomyelitis, bone necrosis, or loosening of the device may occur with resulting nonunion. The prognosis following open reduction ordinarily is not as good as when closed reduction is possible.

Surgical removal of the fragments is the treatment of choice for certain fractures. Examples are those of the second and fourth metacarpi and metatarsi, certain fractures of the proximal sesamoids, and small chip fractures, especially of the tuber coxae, the interdental spaces, and the carpus.

IMMOBILIZATION TECHNICS

General Considerations: Immobilization of fractures in the horse is complicated by the necessity of using devices sufficiently strong to withstand the mechanical force exerted by the muscles and the weight of the animal, and at the same time permitting ambulation. Many animals will not tolerate the severe limitation of movement imposed by a cast on the hindlimb or by a modified Thomas splint, and some especially resent being placed in a sling or a padded crate for an extended period of time. Decubital ulcers develop within a relatively short period if the animal is recumbent 50% or more of the time.

Immobilization of a fracture ideally should be complete. It may be necessary to permit some slight motion or some weight to be placed on the fractured ends to stimulate callus formation. Absolute rest of the part can result in poor callus formation or failure of the soft callus to calcify properly. Excessive irritation from too much motion also will result in poor callus formation or poor calcification. As a general rule it is essential that the first joint on either side of the fracture be immobilized. It is best, however, to immobilize all joints below the fracture and as many as possible above it. This requires the application of a full limb cast.

The period of time that the part must be immobilized will vary with the animal's age, state of general health and nutrition, the site and the type of fracture, the reduction and immobilization technics employed, and whether or not infection of the soft tissues or of the bones occurs. Incomplete fractures in very young animals may require only 1 or 2 weeks' immobilization. Simple fractures of the meta-

tarsus in aged animals may require 10 to 20 weeks' immobilization. Compound and comminuted fractures in adult animals may require 4 months' immobilization. Fractures repaired by open reduction usually require a more extended period of immobilization.

Splints: Splints are most useful for temporary immobilization of fractures of the lower limb to prevent additional damage to the part prior to final reduction. Splints also are used as supporting devices for varying periods of time following callus formation and cast removal.

Simple splints may be made of wooden strips of varying thickness depending upon the strength desired. Half-round aluminum plates shaped to fit the part, aluminum bar stock, or other materials rigid enough for the particular purpose also are used. The limb should be padded sufficiently so that the splint or the bandaging material does not interfere with circulation and cause pressure necrosis of the skin and deeper tissues. It is difficult to adapt a rigid bar to the limb and keep it in proper position. An excess of padding or an improperly fitted or contoured splint will allow the fracture to angulate or to override further.

If a splint is to be left in place for any length of time, the limb should be checked daily for evidence of interference with circulation and to insure that the splint has not slipped from its proper position. Interference with circulation is evidenced by coolness of the part distal to the fracture site and swelling above it. Pressure necrosis of the skin ordinarily occurs within a short time. This usually produces a rise in the local temperature of the part and of body temperature as infection and inflammation of the deeper tissues develop. As the necrosis progresses, odor is noted. If interference with circulation is not remedied, necrosis and sloughing of the distal parts may result.

Modified Thomas Splints: Modified Thomas splints are employed for certain fractures of the long bones. They are used alone or in conjunction with other immobilizing devices. These splints commonly are used to add support and help immobilize a fracture reduced with bone plates or intramedullary pins. A modified Thomas splint also may be used in conjunction with a plaster of paris cast.

Thomas splints are relatively easy to fashion and apply to the leg. The upper ring must be well-padded and fitted rather closely to the upper leg to lessen the possibility of skin ulceration caused by pressure or motion. Aluminum rod (⅜ or ½ inch in diameter) may be used for foals and small Shetland ponies. This material is relatively easy to shape. For larger animals, ¾- to 1-inch iron pipe may be used, since the splint must be strong enough to support a portion of the animal's weight. Much lighter and more malleable aluminum alloys also are available for the adult horse. The distal end of the splint can be fixed to the hoof wall by means of wires placed through it to a shoe.

There are several disadvantages to the use of a modified Thomas splint in the horse. The total length of the leg is increased considerably if the splint alone is used to maintain alignment, and to a slightly less degree if it is used in conjunction with a plaster cast. This causes difficulty in walking, and in rising when the animal lies down. The splint tends to displace the leg from its normal position in relation to the body when used for fractures above the carpus or tarsus. It also causes some distortion at the fracture site. In the hindlimb, it is difficult to maintain enough traction with a Thomas splint to keep the fracture immobilized after its reduction because of the normal angulation of this limb. When applied to the hindlimb of a mare the ring of a Thomas splint may interfere with urination and cause excoriation of the thigh. The pressure of the ring also may cause venous and lymphatic stasis, and edema of the prepuce and scrotum in males.

Casts: See p. 690 for discussion of the walking cast.

Slings: Slings are useful to aid an animal to regain its feet after reduction and immobilization of a fracture of the weight-bearing bones. They also may be used in conjunction with other immobilization devices to keep the horse in a standing position and still allow it to rest.

The successful use of a sling will depend upon the temperament of the individual animal. Not all horses will tolerate being confined in one position for long periods of time. Furthermore, if the animal must depend upon the sling to support its entire weight, interference with cutaneous circulation often results and digestive difficulties may develop. If a sling is to be used, it should be equipped with straps to prevent the animal from sliding forward or backward. If possible, the sling should be adjusted so that the abdominal band just contacts the body. Then, when the horse must rest a limb other than the fractured one, the weight is supported by the abdominal band. In the case of males, care should be taken not to restrict the preputial orifice because urine which accumulates beneath the abdominal band will cause cutaneous excoriation.

Padded Stocks and Crates: Padded stocks or crates may be used instead of slings to help support an animal with a fracture of one of the weight-bearing bones. They are used most often for fractures of the tibia, femur, radius, and humerus. Most animals will tolerate confinement in these devices much better than in a sling, and rarely will attempt to walk as they do in a sling. The width of the stocks should be adjusted so that they are in fairly close contact with the animal. One or more bars should be placed at the front to prevent the horse's moving forward. A padded bar also should be placed behind the animal and just in contact with it. The height of the rear bar should be such that the animal may sit on it, or lean back into it and thus rest the rear limbs. A canvas sling ordinarily is placed under the abdomen and not quite contacting it. This will prevent the horse from lying down or losing its footing, and will support it if necessary.

Stader and Kirschner-Ehmer Splints: External fixation by means of through and through pins and bars without the additional support of a plaster cast, Thomas splint, or other external device ordinarily is not successful in the horse. Even foals will manage to bend, break, or loosen the pins and dislodge the device. Through and through fixation by means of pins inserted transversely through the fragments, the pins then being locked in place by external bars, has been useful in certain types of fractures, especially those of the radius and the tibia (Fig. 1).

Reduction of the fractures is performed with the animal in lateral recumbency and with the affected leg uppermost. Either open or closed reduction technic may be used; the latter is preferable. After reduction, the alignment is maintained and overriding is prevented by tension applied with a block and tackle or other fixed apparatus. Four pins (2 through each fragment) are necessary to prevent rotation and angulation at the fracture site. The pins are inserted from the lateral side, care being taken to avoid the larger blood vessels and nerves. The external bars are used as guides when inserting the pins, so that the pins may subsequently be locked to the bars. The pins are allowed to protrude several inches on either side. A form-fitting plaster of paris cast is then applied over the limb. After this cast has hardened sufficiently, the bars are fitted to the protruding pins, the pins locked to the bar, and the whole incorporated in additional plaster. Pin cutters are used to cut pins which protrude excessively (Fig. 2).

Care must be used in applying this technic. The pins should be placed carefully so that they will meet the holes in the pin bars. This is the case particularly with the Stader splint. The Kirschner-Ehmer splint affords more latitude in this regard and almost eliminates the

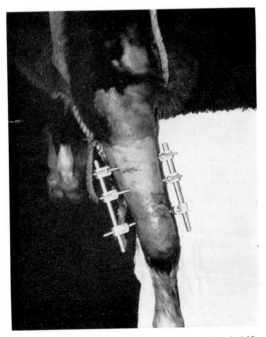

Fig. 1. Through and through fixation. After Reichel.[15]

problem. Fractures through the epiphyses cannot be reduced and immobilized by this technic without bridging the involved joint.

Intramedullary Pins: Intramedullary pins have been used with some success in the immobilization of certain fractures of the interdental spaces, of the metacarpi and metatarsi, radius, humerus, tibia, and the femur. Several difficulties attend their use. Most intramedullary pins are not sufficiently strong to withstand the muscular force applied, or to bear the animal's weight without some additional support. It is difficult to insert intramedullary pins into long bones without penetrating a joint cavity, and this may result in impaired function of the joint. Septic or aseptic bone necrosis and osteomyelitis may occur following insertion of intramedullary pins.

Solid, round intramedullary pins are used most frequently. When applied in the femur and in the interdental space the pin may be left protruding so that it can be removed in 6 to 8 weeks. If it is allowed to protrude through the skin some danger of infecting the medullary cavity exists, as infection can be disseminated through the tissues along the pin. If the pin is cut short and the soft tissues are closed over it, they may break down and expose the end, or the pin may drift slightly and be difficult to locate and remove later.

If the pin is to be left in place permanently, its length must be carefully measured. The pin is then inserted to within approximately one inch of the total length, cut off to the desired length, driven within the bone and countersunk. If driven in too far, pins have a tendency to drift through the distal condyle and interfere with joint motion. Permanent pins may bend prior to the fracture's healing. If this occurs a permanent soft callus, rotation, and permanent deformity of the bones result. Aseptic bone necrosis sometimes occurs.

Some intramedullary pins which have curved or otherwise machined surfaces are somewhat more difficult to insert. The advantages are that they do not drift as readily as the smooth round pins, and they minimize rotation of the fragments.

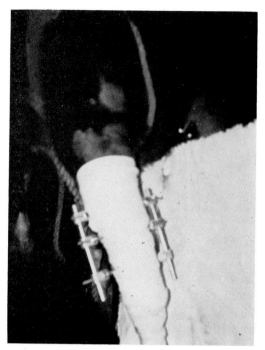

Fig. 2. Through and through fixation, first layer of plaster of paris applied.

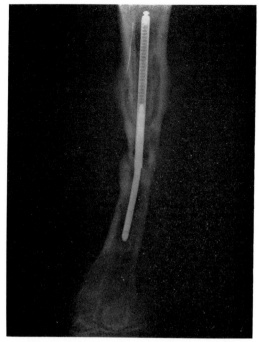

Fig. 3. Intramedullary fixation with Jonas pin. Immobilization with plaster of paris cast. Shetland colt.

Jonas pins and solid shuttle pins may be used to prevent angulation of fractures through the midshaft of certain long bones. The advantage of this device is that it may be inserted into the medullary cavity at the site of the fracture without interfering with either end of the bone or with the articular surfaces. A plaster cast or other external immobilization device is necessary for additional support when intramedullary pins are employed (Fig. 3).

Bone Plates: Bone plates of stainless steel or other electro-passive metals may be employed for immobilization of certain fractures. If used on the long bones of the leg, they are most applicable to fractures through the shaft. Each fragment should be long enough to allow 2 or more screws to be placed when fixing the plate. When bone plates are used, the fracture is reduced openly and then the plate is fitted to the contour of the bone. The periosteum may or may not be stripped from the surface prior to fixing the plate.

Several sizes of screws are necessary, since each one should penetrate almost completely through the bone, the point not quite penetrat-

ing the opposite cortex. Use of a depth gauge insures the proper selection of screws. If the screw is too short, some movement will result and bone necrosis may occur around the screw. The plate and screws should be of identical metal or electrolysis is likely to occur.

Plaster of paris casts or other external immobilization methods must be used in conjunction with internal forms of fixation. The plates and screws usually are removed after the fifth or sixth week, since the screws ordinarily begin to loosen after this length of time. A further period of enforced rest and immobilization is necessary after their removal.

Bone Screws: Screws alone are used for immobilization of certain fractures. Common examples are fractures of the olecranon process, "slab fractures" of the third carpal bone, and in sufficiently oblique fractures of long bones. Open reduction usually must be performed prior to placing the screws. On occasion, it is possible to accomplish reduction without penetrating the skin and then to insert the screw through a stab incision.

FRACTURES OF BONES OF THE FORELIMB

Third Phalanx: Fractures of the third phalanx occur relatively infrequently. The most common fracture of the third phalanx occurs perpendicularly through a wing. The articular surface of the coffin joint may or may not be involved. Acute supporting lameness is noted immediately after the fracture occurs and there is heat and sensitivity to pressure over the hoof. Radiographs are necessary to confirm the diagnosis. Displacement of the fragments ordinarily is not severe, since they are enclosed in the hoof. Treatment is limited to stall rest for several months, or a plaster cast may be applied from the foot to just below the knee to immobilize the phalanges. Healing often is incomplete and if this happens, chronic lameness may result from articular damage due to exostoses extending into the coffin joint or due to interference with the flexor and extensor tendons. Volar digital neurectomy may relieve the pain provided it rises from the posterior aspect of the bone. Fractures involving the wings and not the articular surfaces usually heal (Fig. 4).

Navicular Bone: Fractures of the distal sesamoid are not infrequent, especially in racing or in aged animals. The fracture may or may not be preceded by the classic signs of navicular disease resulting from degenerative disease of the bone. The signs of navicular fracture reflect an acute, supporting lameness immediately after the fracture. After confinement in a stall for several days the lameness usually is alleviated. Sensitivity to pressure over the middle third of the frog is noted. Radiographs are needed to confirm the diagnosis (Fig. 5).

Navicular fractures almost never heal. Relief of the resulting lameness is accomplished by posterior digital neurectomy. The success of this procedure depends upon the extent of damage to other structures, and whether or not the coffin joint is seriously involved.

Second Phalanx: Fractures of the second phalanx usually are comminuted and involve the articular surfaces. The prognosis is favorable, though much depends upon the type and location of the fracture. Comminuted fractures usually heal with a great deal of new bone formation and ankylosis of the coffin and pastern joints (Fig. 6).

Often severe damage to soft tissues occurs at the time the second phalanx is fractured or when the animal attempts to use the injured

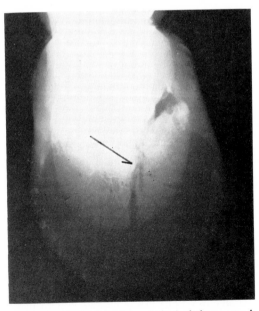

Fig. 4. Longitudinal fracture of third phalanx extending into the coffin joint. Radiograph by J. P. Manning, D.V.M.

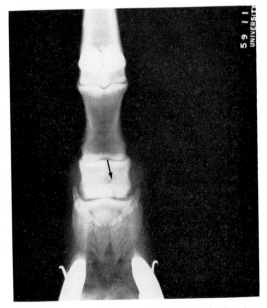

Fig. 5. Fracture of the navicular bone. A. P. view. Radiograph by J. P. Manning, D.V.M.

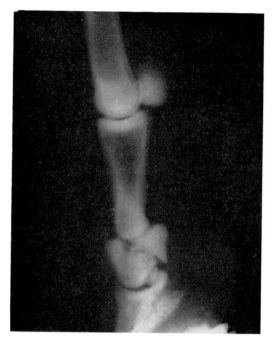

Fig. 6. Comminuted fracture of second phalanx.

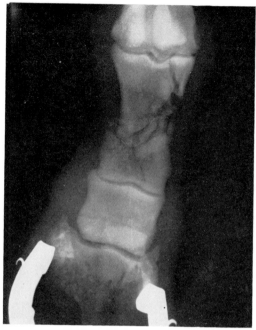

Fig. 7. Comminuted fracture of first phalanx.

limb before an immobilizing device can be applied.

Fractures of the second phalanx usually are reduced without opening the skin. The foot should be placed in as normal a standing position as possible, and traction is applied to the hoof wall until the fracture is reduced. The foot should be immobilized in this position. A full-limb plaster of paris walking cast is the usual method of immobilization. The cast should extend from the ground surface to immediately below the elbow.

The cast usually is left in place for an average of 4 to 6 weeks in immature animals, and from 6 to 10 weeks in mature ones. Radiographic evidence of a substantial callus and healing should be obtained before removing the cast.

Compound fractures of the second phalanx may be reduced after careful debridement. The skin wound may be packed with nonirritating bactericidal agents. Plaster casts often are used for immobilization. A window may be cut in the cast to permit access to the wound, but a pressure dressing must be used over the window to prevent edema and subsequent skin necrosis.

Therapeutic cautery (firing) has been used to increase the rate of partial resorption of large exostoses following healing, and to complete ankylosis of the pastern or coffin joints following fractures of the second phalanx.

First Phalanx: Fractures of the first phalanx are often comminuted, and commonly the articular surfaces of the proximal and distal ends are damaged. Longitudinal fractures and Y-shaped fractures of the proximal end occur, as do fractures of the proximal articular tuberosities. Compound fractures may be suffered if the animal is traveling at high speed when the fracture occurs (Fig. 7).

Reduction and immobilization of fractures of the first phalanx involve the same principles and basic procedures employed for similar injuries to the second phalanx. Screws have been used with some success to immobilize longitudinal and Y-shaped fractures. A splint or plaster cast should be used in conjunction with the screws to reinforce immobilization of the limb and to add support to it (Fig. 8).

Proximal Sesamoids: Fractures of the proximal sesamoid bones occur frequently in racing animals. The prognosis concerning future racing ability depends upon the location of the fracture, whether it is comminuted, and the size of the fragment(s). Conservative treatment rarely is successful in the case of race horses. Fractures that are badly comminuted, those that result in chips more than ⅓ of the sesamoid bone in size, fractures of the distal third, and those that are not surgically treated for some time after the fracture occurred have a poor prognosis.

Fractures of the ventral portion of the sesamoids often result in one or more slab-like fragments. These commonly interfere with the motion of the fetlock joint and if not removed within a relatively short time will cause arthritic lesions. In some cases excessive bone is produced in fractures of the dorsal part of a sesamoid. Small chip fractures of the dorsal portion occasionally resorb in several months. Their resorption may be accomplished by therapeutic cautery (Fig. 9, 10).

Surgical removal of fragments of the dorsal portion is not difficult. The incision is made between the suspensory ligament and the third

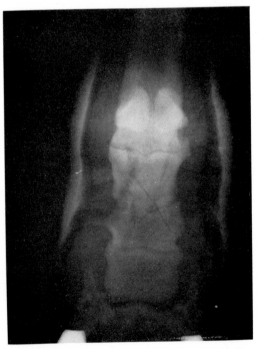

Fig. 8. Comminuted fracture of first phalanx 10 days after immobilization in plaster of paris cast. Ankylosis of fetlock joint resulted as fracture extended into the joint.

metatarsal bone beginning just above the tip of the sesamoid and extending down to the level of the fetlock joint, or slightly below. After the joint capsule is opened, slight flexion of the fetlock joint aids detection of the fragment or fragments. The fragment is removed with as little damage as possible to the suspensory ligament and other soft tissues. Either stainless steel suture or fine chromic catgut is used to close the joint capsule. The subcutaneous tissues are closed separately with the same materials, and the skin is then united. The animal is given penicillin for several days prior to surgery, and this is maintained for 8 to 10 days following surgery. Most surgeons believe that some exercise is advisable beginning the day after surgery to prevent adhesions. Phenylbutazone has been used postoperatively to prevent swelling and to relieve pain.

Fragments of the distal portion may be removed through an incision extended below the joint and at the same site as that used for removal of dorsal fragments, or the approach may be from the posterior aspect. The latter seems more difficult since more soft tissue damage may result and difficulty may be experienced in locating the fragment. The same pre- and postoperative care is applied as for removal of dorsal fragments (also see p. 694).

Third Metacarpal: Fractures of the third metacarpal are quite common. The site and the type of fracture influence the method of treatment and the prognosis to a great extent. The fact that the bone is not covered with a mass of muscle and is relatively accessible permits various reduction and immobilization technics.

Simple transverse fractures through the midshaft, or comminuted fractures in the same location having only 1 or 2 fragments, should be given a good prognosis. Closed reduction and immobilization with a plaster of paris cast usually are employed for these fractures. Traction is applied to the foot for reduction and the cast is then applied. It should be inspected daily for swelling, odor, and breaks in the plaster. If necrosis occurs the cast should be removed and reapplied, or some other method of reduction and immobilization should be used.

Simple transverse fractures occasionally re-

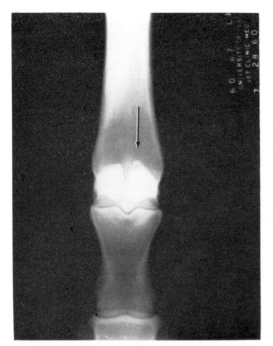

Fig. 9. Fetlock joint, fracture of lateral proximal sesamoid bone. A. P. view. Radiograph by J. P. Manning, D.V.M.

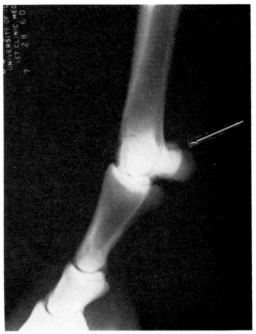

Fig. 10. Lateral view of fracture in Fig. 9. Radiograph by J. P. Manning, D.V.M.

sult in nonunion. This occurs when soft tissues become interposed between the fragments, when immobilization is not achieved, or when there is insufficient contact of the fragments. If this occurs, open reduction and other stabilization technics may be indicated. Jonas pins, shuttle pins, and bone plates often are used in such cases. Removal of the soft callus and the grafting of autogenous bone have been done with good results.

Comminuted fractures of the shaft with multiple fragmentation have a poor prospect for repair with the exception of those cases occurring in immature animals.

Simple fractures through the distal epiphysis are common in young animals. Closed reduction is relatively simple in these cases. This fracture may be confused with luxation of the fetlock joint unless a careful examination is made. These fractures commonly are immobilized with a plaster cast applied from the ground surface to a point close to the elbow. Assessment of healing and indication for cast removal are based upon radiographic evidence. These fractures generally require from 4 to 6

weeks before healing sufficiently to permit removal of the cast.

Fractures of the proximal epiphyseal junction occur less often than those of the distal. Treatment is the same. Fractures through the proximal portion of the shaft often are comminuted and may extend into the proximal articular surface. A form-fitting plaster of paris cast, applied after closed reduction, is the usual method of treatment.

Compound and compound, comminuted fractures of the metacarpus should be given a poor prognosis. Since the soft tissue essentially is limited to the suspensory ligament and the flexor and extensor tendons, interruption of the blood or nerve supply at the site of the fracture is common. Because of the arrangement of the tendons, the leg distal to the fracture tends to displace laterally, with the fractured end(s) penetrating the medial surface. If the wound is not badly contaminated and extensive soft tissue damage has not occurred, careful cleansing of the area and topical application of an antibacterial powder or paste may be followed by reduction and immobilization in a plaster cast. If it is necessary to leave a window over the site of the fracture to permit dressing of the wound, pressure packs must be used to prevent edema and skin necrosis from occurring. Systemic antibiotic therapy for an extended period usually is indicated to prevent or control osteomyelitis.

Second and Fourth Metacarpals: Fractures of the second and fourth metacarpals occur infrequently, except in racing animals. Since these bones are not primarily weight-bearing, the consequences are not immediately serious but chronic lameness may result. Fractures usually occur in the distal third of the bone and the associated signs vary widely depending upon the nature of the fracture and the amount of soft tissue damage. Lameness usually is exhibited several days following the fracture and is related with swelling at the site. The lameness and swelling recede with rest, but recur with exercise (Fig. 11).

Considerable exostosis may develop at the fracture site. Diagnosis of the fracture may be made by observation of the typical doughy swelling and by palpation, and it should be confirmed with radiographs. The fragment distal to the fracture should be removed surgically. This should be done prior to the formation of the exostosis.

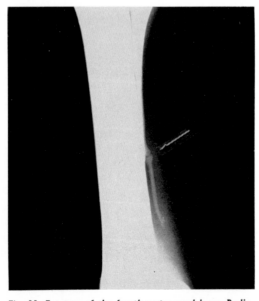

Fig. 11. Fracture of the fourth metacarpal bone. Radiograph by J. P. Manning, D.V.M.

The surgical procedure may be performed in a standing or recumbent position. It involves exposure of the bone and removal of the periosteum with the fragment. The subcutaneous tissues should be approximated with stainless steel or fine chromic catgut sutures. The skin is sutured with nylon or stainless steel. Pressure bandages are used for 10 to 14 days following surgery. Primary union should be achieved although some filling of the leg over the surgical site may be expected.

Carpal Bones: Fractures of the carpal bones are infrequent, except as a complication of fractures of the third metacarpal or the radius, or fractures of the third carpal bone in race horses. Treatment of those occurring as a complication of fractures of the radius or third metacarpal bone is difficult and often unsuccessful.

Fractures of the third carpal bone usually are of the "slab" variety and fractures of the other carpal bones are of the "chip" type. Open reduction and fixation by means of screw(s) or surgical removal of slab fractures of the third carpal are the preferred methods of repair. The treatment of chip fractures also involves surgical removal of the fragments.

Radius: Fractures of the radius are not infrequent. The bone is fairly well-protected by the musculature of the arm, and except in animals with osseous fragility severe force must be applied to produce a fracture. Many fractures of the radius are comminuted, but relatively few are compound (Fig. 12).

Reduction of radial fractures is difficult because of the overriding of the fragments and the swelling that ordinarily occur. Considerable traction is necessary to effect reduction. A combination of immobilization methods is used most successfully. Internal fixation plus external devices such as plaster casts or the modified Thomas splint are commonly utilized.

Ulna: Fractures of the shaft of the ulna usually occur in conjunction with fractures of the radius. Treatment of ulnar fractures is essentially the same as for fractures of the radius. If the shaft of the ulna alone is fractured, no treatment other than several months of confinement in a stall may be necessary.

Fracture of the olecranon process occurs fre-

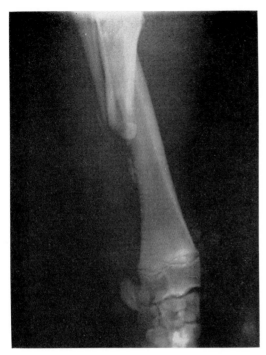

Fig. 12. Fracture through midshaft of radius. Typical
overriding of fragments.

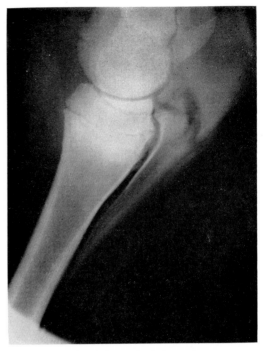

Fig. 13. Fracture of olecranon process.

quently. Extreme swelling and acute lameness occur within a short time after the fracture is sustained. Palpation is difficult, and crepitation may not be noticed because of the swelling. Diagnosis may be difficult until the swelling subsides or until radiographs are taken (Fig. 13).

The prognosis for ulnar fractures depends upon whether or not articular surfaces are involved. Those not involving the articular surfaces and not resulting in sequestra formation may be given a good prognosis. If articular surfaces are involved, permanent lameness usually results.

Treatment of an olecranon fracture depends upon the type and its location. If the displacement is not extreme, confinement to a stall for several months may be all that is indicated. Reduction and immobilization are difficult unless the fracture site is exposed surgically. If the fracture results in a large fragment that is displaced considerably, open reduction and fixation by means of one or more stainless steel screws are indicated. This should be followed by several months of enforced rest.

Sequestra formation and bone necrosis are common sequelae of olecranon fractures. The extreme force which produces the fracture plus the displacement due to pull of the triceps muscles often disrupt the blood supply. If the fragments are not fixed, or if multiple fragmentation occurs, bone necrosis and multiple fistulous tracts may develop. Surgical removal of the necrotic fragments may be successful. If the main portion of the olecranon is involved, the prognosis for a reasonably sound animal is not good, as the attachments of the triceps muscles are involved.

Humerus: Fractures of the humerus are relatively infrequent. The bone is heavy and well-protected, and severe force is necessary to produce a fracture in a normal animal. Spiral or oblique fractures of the shaft are the most common type, and simple fractures of the shaft or at the junction of the proximal condyles and the shaft occur occasionally. Considerable overriding may be present with the distal fragment pulled posterior to the proximal one. Flexion of the leg is necessary to reduce the fracture. Securing proper alignment of the fragments and correction of overriding are extremely difficult.

In colts and smaller breeds reduction may be accomplished after exposure of the fracture site, and immobilization can be obtained with intramedullary pins. The pin usually is inserted through the lateral surface, just above the deltoid tuberosity. When it is necessary to insert the pin through the proximal articular surface, permanent lameness often results. Additional support from a sling or a padded crate is necessary following open reduction and immobilization.

Scapula: Fractures of the scapula are not common, though they do occur more often than fractures of the humerus. Most are simple fractures which involve the neck of the scapula and they result from trauma to the lateral side or to the point of the shoulder. Occasionally, fractures of the spine of the scapula are seen.

The prognosis with regard to future soundness is poor as it is almost impossible to accomplish reduction and immobilization, and in most cases there is concurrent damage to the shoulder joint. If the spine has been separated from the main portion of the bone, nerve damage and atrophy of either or both the infraspinatus or the supraspinatous muscles often result. Sequestra also are frequent sequelae.

Fractures through the neck of the scapula commonly cause the proximal fragment to override forward. Diagnosis is difficult unless the animal is examined before swelling occurs, or when it subsides. Diagnostic radiographs of this area are difficult to obtain because the limb must be extended a considerable distance to provide a view of the neck and a portion of the body.

Scapular fractures may heal in docile animals which will tolerate a padded crate or sling, or will protect the leg for an extended period of confinement.

FRACTURES OF THE BONES OF THE REAR LEG

Fractures of the phalanges, distal and proximal sesamoids, and the second and fourth metatarsals are treated in the same manner as the corresponding fractures of the forelimb.

Third Metatarsal: Fracture of the third metatarsal is the most common fracture of the hindlimb. The technics of reduction and immobilization are almost identical with those employed for corresponding fractures of the third metacarpus. One factor that influences reduction and immobilization is that the limb should not be completely extended during reduction because this tends to cause angulation at the fracture site. The limb should be placed in as nearly a normal standing position as possible. Traction is then applied at or just above the hock and at the hoof. The limb then is immobilized so that the normal angulation in a standing position is preserved. If it is immobilized in an overextended position the animal will have difficulty standing or regaining its feet after lying down.

Separation of the proximal epiphysis from the shaft is not infrequent in young colts. The prognosis is good unless the fracture is compound or the hock joint is involved. Swelling of the hock is apt to be extreme, and a temporary cast frequently must be applied until the swelling subsides before reduction and immobilization can be accomplished.

Fractures of the third metatarsal bone which extend into the hock joint warrant a poor prognosis for recovery with a functional joint. Swelling and pain are extreme. Some animals die from shock within a few days after the fracture. Others lie down and refuse to rise, or will not tolerate a cast or other immobilization device. They develop decubital ulcers, and die of subsequent infection within a few days. A temporary cast often must be applied to immobilize fractures extending into the hock joint until the swelling subsides and reduction can be accomplished. Most animals are ambulatory following reduction and immobilization of fractures of the metatarsal bones. A few may require additional support from a sling or padded crate.

Tarsus: Fractures of the tarsal bones occur infrequently, with the exception of fracture of the fibular tarsal bone (tuber calcis). If fractures of the tarsal bones occur, they usually are the result of a severe blow such as a kick, or of a twisting strain. Considerable soft tissue damage and swelling occur. The prognosis is poor with regard to future function of the joint; ankylosis usually results. Pain is severe and many animals refuse or are unable to regain their feet, or to stand after being aided to their feet. Plaster of paris casts are employed for immobilization and additional support is provided by a padded crate or a sling. The cast should extend from the ground surface to as high above the hock as is possible. It ordinarily is not possible to immobilize the stifle joint. Consequently, some motion occurs at the fracture site and there is a corresponding delay in healing.

Fractures of the fibular tarsal bone have a fair prognosis when they occur at the upper epiphyseal junction or through the shaft alone, without injury to the articular surfaces. If the fracture is simple and without much displacement it will heal after extended rest with or without the support of a sling or padded crate. Plaster casts, if applied, should extend from the ground surface to well above the hock. Modified Thomas splints may be used alone or in conjunction with the plaster cast. Open reduction and fixation of the fragment to the main portion of the shaft with one or more stainless steel screws are employed infrequently. Some interference with normal motion usually results from these fractures.

Compound fractures of the fibular tarsal bone have a poorer prognosis. Sequestra formation often occurs and extended treatment is necessary before healing takes place. The insertion of the gastrocnemius tendon complicates the healing of any fracture of this bone.

Tibia: Considerable difficulty is encountered in reduction and immobilization of tibial fractures. Because of the angulation of the leg and the swelling that results shortly after the fracture occurs, good apposition and proper alignment of the fragments are difficult. It may be necessary to apply a temporary splint until the swelling subsides before closed reduction and immobilization are possible.

Fractures through the shaft are the most common type in adult animals, and those through the proximal or distal epiphyseal junctions are most frequent in immature animals. If the site of the fracture is the lower one-third of the shaft or the distal epiphyseal junction,

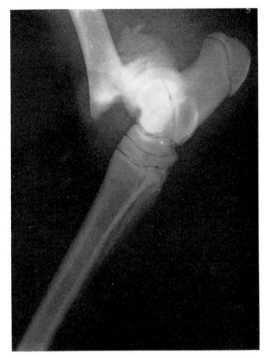

Fig. 14. Fracture at distal epiphysis of tibia in colt.

overriding may produce injury to the hock joint. A fracture through the proximal epiphyseal junction commonly results in overriding of the distal fragment (shaft) posteriorly, with the proximal condyles continuing to articulate with the femur (Fig. 14).

Fractures through the shaft, though not compound originally, often become so in several days after the animal attempts to bear weight upon the limb. The proximal fragment usually penetrates the skin of the medial surface, since the heavy musculature of the gaskin and the accompanying swelling tend to bow the fractured leg inward.

Closed reduction and immobilization of tibial fractures with a plaster cast frequently are attempted. A Thomas splint can be used in conjunction with this. Reduction must be accomplished with the leg partially flexed, and usually it is not complete. Combinations of internal and external fixation also may be used.

Fractures of the epiphyses or of the proximal or distal portions of the shaft with overriding into the hock or stifle joint usually result in permanent lameness.

Menisci: Fractures of the menisci of the stifle joint usually result from a crushing type of injury imposed by external violence to the area or by a twisting strain causing total or partial luxation of the joint. Diagnosis is difficult because of the soft tissue swelling that often occurs and because of the difficulty in palpating the area. Prior to the swelling or after it subsides, it may be possible to hear grating sounds as the joint is flexed and extended. Lameness is prompt and severe and the animal will flex the joint with difficulty. If only one meniscus is crushed, medial or lateral angulation of the joint may be noted.

Diagnosis is confirmed by radiographs. Both latero-medial and antero-posterior views should be taken. The normal separation of the distal end of the femur and the proximal end of the tibia will be absent or decreased.

The prognosis for recovery of function is poor. Ankylosis often results and is accompanied by atrophy of the thigh muscles, especially of the quadriceps group.

Patella: Fractures of the patella alone occur rarely. They usually are found in conjunction with a fracture of the distal end of the femur. The patella normally is fairly mobile, and considerable force is necessary to fracture it. Crepitation may be detected in patellar fractures but soft tissue swelling of the area usually is extreme and palpation is difficult. Diagnosis is made or confirmed with radiographs.

The prognosis with regard to recovery with normal joint movement is poor. Interference with stifle joint movement and atrophy of the quadriceps group of muscles are usual sequelae.

Treatment of patellar fractures usually is limited to enforced rest. The use of supporting and immobilizing devices such as a Thomas splint or plaster casts is of doubtful value. Attempts made to immobilize these fractures by means of stainless steel screws have had limited success.

Femur: Fractures of the femur are relatively common. Considerable force must be exerted in the case of normal animals to produce a fracture. Osseous fragility is suspected in fractures in which the bone literally "explodes" into multiple fragments. Fractures at the distal epiphyseal junction are most common in immature animals and these are followed in frequency by fractures of the proximal epiphyseal junction and neck, then by fractures through the shaft. In adult animals, comminuted fractures of the shaft are observed most commonly.

The diagnosis of femoral fractures may be difficult because of the muscle mass and the soft tissue swelling which occur within a relatively short time. Diagnostic radiographs are difficult to obtain in larger animals. This especially is so for fractures of the proximal third of the femur.

Fractures at the distal epiphysis may simulate displacement of the patella since the distal end of the shaft tends to override anteriorly, fixing the patella and the stifle joint. The distal condyles continue to articulate with the tibia in the stifle joint. The animal may be able to partially support its weight on the affected limb (Fig. 15).

Fractures through the femoral shaft may be simple or comminuted with few or many fragments. There is extreme swelling, and inability to support weight on the affected limb is noticed immediately. Crepitation may be masked by the soft tissue swelling.

Fractures through the proximal epiphysis or the neck of the femoral shaft occur most often in young animals. Radiographs of the area often are worthless, making diagnosis difficult. The animal may be able to partially support the weight on the affected limb. These fractures must be differentiated from luxation or subluxation of the coxofemoral joint, but crepitation may be detected by rectal palpation.

Healing of fractures through either the proximal or distal epiphysis may occur in young animals without any treatment except confinement to a box stall. Permanent lameness results, however, as the shaft overrides anteriorly in case of a distal epiphyseal fracture and posteriorly in most cases of fracture through the proximal epiphysis. Union without alignment occurs and there is excessive callus formation or a false joint. Atrophy of the large muscles of the area is a common sequel.

Reduction of femoral fractures is difficult. In most cases, reduction and alignment are possible only with the leg flexed, since extension tends to cause angulation of the fragments. Closed reduction with partial approximation and alignment of the fragments may be accomplished for fractures through the shaft. It is almost impossible to keep the fragments in proper alignment if this technic is used. Simple fractures through the shaft may heal with a certain amount of angulation and shortening of the leg if the animal is supported in a sling or a padded crate for several months. This is especially true for young animals.

Open reduction offers a reasonable chance for good approximation of certain fractures of the femur. Simple fractures through the distal third of the shaft are most amenable to this approach. The fracture site is exposed through the lateral or anterior surface. Reduction is accomplished with the limb in flexion.

Large, Jonas-type intramedullary pins have been used in small colts to maintain reduction and alignment of femoral fractures. Additional support by means of slings, padded crates, or a modified Thomas splint is necessary. The Thomas splint, however, tends to cause angulation at the site of the fracture.

Open reduction and introduction of a permanent intramedullary pin which is inserted through the distal end of the femur have been done for distal epiphyseal fractures and those of the shaft. After open reduction with the leg in a flexed position, the pin is inserted through a slit in the skin over the distal condyles or by an extension of the original incision. The pin should be measured for length so it may be countersunk and left in place permanently. It is inserted through the trochlear groove. Antibiotics and corticosteroids ordinarily are administered both systemically and intra-articularly following this procedure. Enforced rest for several months is necessary. Smaller animals and foals of the larger breeds are best suited for this type of reduction and immobilization because it is difficult to introduce a pin sufficiently strong to bear the weight of a large animal.

Bone plates have been used in a number of femoral fractures but the results were poor. The plates and screws alone are not sufficiently strong to bear the animal's weight. Additional restraining and immobilization de-

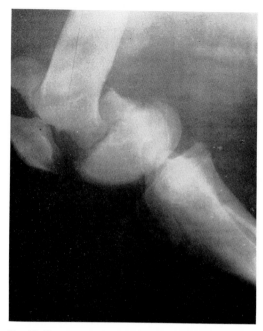

Fig. 15. Fracture at distal epiphysis of femur. Note that stifle joint articulates but that proximal fragment impinges upon patella, locking stifle joint.

vices are difficult to apply. Wiring of fragments with stainless steel wire in conjunction with the use of plates likewise has not been markedly successful.

Miscellaneous Fractures

Coccygeal Vertebrae: Fractures of the coccygeal vertebrae occur infrequently. If not reduced and immobilized by bandaging or splinting, a crooked tail often results. Corrective surgery consists of severing the appropriate muscles if it is necessary to straighten a crooked tail. In some instances, surgical removal of a vertebra or fragment is necessary.

Compound fractures of the coccygeal vertebrae are rare, but if they do occur, necrosis of the tail distal to the site may result. Amputation or sloughing is the usual outcome.

Sacrum: Fractures of the sacrum usually are the result of the animal's rearing and falling over backward, or the result of a blow to the sacral area. Diagnosis is difficult although rectal palpation may reveal the extent of the injury. Partial or complete paralysis of the rear quarters may result from damage to the nerve supply at the time of the fracture, or from subsequent swelling. The prognosis depends upon the extent of the damage to the bony tissues, and to a great deal upon damage to nerves.

Treatment frequently is limited to enforced rest, supportive measures, and nursing. In some cases, it is possible to force the displaced fragments back into proper position by manipulation through the rectum. Compression of nerves by the adjacent soft tissues may be relieved by intravenous administration of hypertonic glucose solution. Diuretics also may be of some value in reducing the swelling.

Pelvic Bones: Fracture of the tuber coxae is common. Considerable lameness and swelling of the soft tissues occur in most cases. Depending upon the size of the fragment, the lameness may be temporary or permanent. Treatment depends upon the extent of the injury and the type of fracture. Simple fractures with only a small fragment require no treatment. Simple fractures with a large fragment may be reduced, then immobilized by fixing the fragment to the main portion with a screw. There always is danger of introducing infection when this is done. Many cases are best treated by aseptic drainage of any hematomas 5 to 10 days after the injury and allowing the fragment to unite the ileum without surgical intervention.

Bone necrosis and sequestrum formation are not uncommon, even with a simple fracture, because the fragment loses its blood supply. The prognosis for fractures of the tuber coxae will be poor if bone necrosis results, as not only the fragment but the body of the ileum may be involved. Draining fistulous tracts often result. An extended period of treatment may be necessary, and curettage and removal of sequestra plus large doses of a broad spectrum antibiotic may be needed before healing occurs. Fistulous tracts and necrosis of the ventral surface of the ileum occasionally result from migration of necrotic and infectious material downward under the pelvis or between the muscle layers. Drainage of this area is difficult.

Fractures of the shaft of the ileum are seen on occasion. The diagnosis may be difficult, even with rectal palpation. Treatment ordinarily is limited to confinement in a stall.

Multiple fractures of the bones of the pelvis are not infrequent. Crepitation may be noticed before soft tissue swelling occurs, and rectal palpation often will reveal the extent of the damage. If the pelvis is not so badly comminuted that support of the rear quarters is impossible, or if the fractures do not extend through one or both acetabuli, most will heal after enforced rest. Interference with normal gait or distortion of the pelvis may result depending upon the degree of bone displacement.

Fractures of the tuber ischii alone are rare, due to their relatively protected position. Treatment of these fractures is limited to stall rest and removal of sequestra.

Lumbar Vertebrae: Fractures of the lumbar vertebrae usually result from accidental falls, accidents in transport, or as a consequence of casting. The last 2 lumbar vertebrae are involved most often. Paraplegia is immediate if the spinal cord is severed or badly damaged. The paralysis may progress gradually if there is extravasation of blood into the spinal canal or if edema of the cord results. Diagnosis is difficult unless considerable displacement of the spinal column has occurred.

The prognosis is poor if the paralysis persists. Under the best of circumstances some permanent nerve damage may result and cause an impairment of gait.

Treatment is limited to stall rest and supportive treatment. Hypertonic solutions, given intravenously, and diuretics may be indicated to relieve fluid compression of the spinal cord.

Thoracic Vertebrae: Fractures of the thoracic vertebrae rarely occur except in cases of extreme violence. Complete posterior paralysis or immediate death may result depending upon the site of the injury.

Rib Fractures: Fractures of the ribs are not uncommon. Their diagnosis usually is not difficult unless considerable soft tissue swelling has occurred. The clinical signs vary widely depending upon the site, type of fracture, and whether or not the pleura has been penetrated. Most simple fractures are not treated. If the pleura is penetrated and the lung is damaged by the rib fragment, coughing will occur and frothy blood may appear at the nostrils. The peritoneum may be penetrated if the last 4 or 5 ribs are fractured.

Compound fractures which also penetrate the pleura are not infrequent. Such wounds must be closed promptly before collapse of the lungs occurs. Systemic administration of antibiotics may be necessary to control a subsequent pleuritis and/or pneumonia.

Compound or comminuted rib fractures often result in necrosis and sequestra formation, and osteomyelitis of the main portion of the rib. Chronic costal fistulae frequently occur. Removal of necrotic bone fragments and the affected portion of the rib dorsal to the fracture site usually is necessary. Removal of the rib distal to the fracture down to the costochondral junction also is indicated. The periosteum of the medial face of the rib should be carefully preserved to prevent opening the pleural or peritoneal cavities.

Cervical Vertebrae: Fractures of the cervical vertebrae usually involve one of the first 3 vertebrae. The signs vary considerably depending upon whether or not the spinal cord has been injured, or if only the lateral processes are involved. Crepitation may or may not be observed. Torticollis often results from soft tissue or nerve damage. A peculiar, stiff gait is noted occasionally, and a superficial examination of the animal may lead one to make a diagnosis of laminitis.

The prognosis for cervical fractures depends primarily upon the extent of damage to the spinal cord and the persistence of torticollis. If the spinal cord is severed, death is immediate. Incomplete severing of the cord and fractures extending into the spinal canal without causing immediate damage to the cord may produce paralysis and death later due to its compression by extravasation of blood. Radiographs usually are necessary to differentiate fractures of vertebral processes from luxations, subluxations, and torticollis due to muscle spasm.

Treatment usually is limited to fracture reduction by manual manipulation and immobilization by means of a cradle or neck stick. Swelling of the soft tissues and torticollis often prevents straightening of the neck. Confinement to a stall and provision of food and water at a height at which neck motion is limited are often the only treatment needed. Torticollis may be relieved in some instances by hot packs and injections of a local anesthetic into the affected muscles.

Fractures of the dens of the axis occasionally occur. If not immediately fatal due to damage to the spinal cord, recovery from such fractures may occur but continued sensitivity over the poll and inability to move the head properly are common sequelae.

Nasal Bones: Fractures of the nasal bones are infrequent. When they do occur, hemorrhage from the nasal passages usually is profuse. Their treatment is limited to reduction by digital manipulation and control of the hemorrhage. Packing one nostril with gauze occasionally will provide sufficient immobilization until swelling of soft tissues occurs and holds the fragments in position.

Premaxilla: Fractures of the premaxillae are not infrequent. Separation at the symphysis may occur, but usually this is seen in conjunction with a fracture at the interdental space of the corresponding side. The prognosis of such fractures usually is good, except that the incisors may be lost if the injury is severe. Closed reduction by digital manipulation and immobilization by wiring the incisors together are usually sufficient to obtain satisfactory healing. Removal of sequestra and loose incisor teeth may be necessary.

Unilateral fractures through the interdental space usually require no treatment other than provision of soft feed and removal of sequestra that may form. Bilateral fractures through the interdental spaces result in lowering of the upper incisors. Occasionally, these fractures may be reduced without exposing the fracture sites. Soft feed should be provided for several weeks. Wiring the corner incisors to the first cheek teeth may immobilize the fractures sufficiently. Stainless steel pins can be inserted just lateral to the corner incisors to immobilize the fractures. Sequestra formation is common since small fragments often occur at the fracture site.

Facial Bones: Fractures of the facial bones are comparatively rare. Sequestra formation and infection of the various sinuses often result from such fractures. Curettage and removal of sequestra and draining the sinuses may be necessary.

Mandible: Fractures of the mandible through the symphysis and through the interdental spaces are treated in the same manner as those of the upper jaw. Chip fractures with subsequent sequestra formation are common following improper use of a bit.

Fractures through the body of the mandible usually are caused by severe external violence, or are a consequence of bone necrosis due to alveolar periostitis. The diagnosis may be difficult unless radiographs are taken because the masseter muscles prevent palpation and detection of crepitation. Examination of the mouth may reveal that the upper and lower incisors are not in alignment, or a break in the continuity of the table surface or in the alignment of the cheek teeth may be noticed.

Provided there is little displacement, treatment can be limited to feeding and watering through a stomach tube for 7 to 10 days and following this by feeding foods which require little mastication for several weeks. Wiring the cheek teeth together across the site of the fracture may immobilize it and permit healing with little permanent distortion. Removal of any sequestra that form is necessary. If the fracture is the result of alveolar periostitis or if this develops at the site, removal of the affected tooth is necessary.

Fractures through the ramus of the mandible result in severe swelling and considerable pain. Radiographs often are required to establish the diagnosis. Treatment usually is limited to feeding and watering through a stomach tube until the animal can swallow soft feeds.

Fractures of the coronoid process of the mandible are difficult to diagnose without radiographs. Tetanus may be suspected because the animal is reluctant to open the mouth. It is necessary to use a stomach tube to provide feed and water for some time. Permanent interference with normal masticatory motions usually results from injury to the temperomandibular articulation. The teeth subsequently must be dressed at frequent intervals. Intraarticular injections of cortisone preparations may be of some value in limiting the arthritic changes in the joint.

R. L. Lundvall

REFERENCES

1. Beckenhauser, W. H.: Fractures of the mandibular symphysis in a cow. J.A.V.M.A. **129** (1956) 103.
2. Beckenhauser, W. H.: A practical large animal splint. J.A.V.M.A. **132** (1958) 284-288.
3. Carney, J. P.: Rush intramedullary fixation of long bones as applied to veterinary surgery. Vet. Med. **47** (1952) 43.
4. Churchill, E. A.: Surgical removal of fractured fragments of the proximal sesamoid bone. J.A.V.M.A. **128** (1956) 581.
5. Dollar, Jno. A. W.: Regional Veterinary Surgery and Operative Technique. J. F. Hartz Co., Toronto, Canada, 1912.
6. Franks, E. R.: Veterinary Surgery. Burgess Publishing Company, Minneapolis, Minn., 1959.
7. Hendricks, John W.: Treatment of tibial and radial fractures in large animals. Cornell Vet. **41** (1951) 219.
8. Henig, H. F. and Walker, J. D.: External fixation of fracture in a colt. J.A.V.M.A. **124** (1954) 113.
9. Jenny, J.: The management of bone and joint injuries in large animals. Vet. Scope VI (1961) 9.
10. Kirk and Hamilton.: Fractured legs in horses. Vet. Rec. **19** (1949) 244.
11. Lundvall, R. L.: Observations on the treatment of fractures of the long bones in large animals. J.A.V.M.A. **137** (1960) 308.
12. O'Connor, J. J.: Dollar's Veterinary Surgery; General, Operative, & Regional. Alexander Egar, Chicago, Ill., 1931.
13. Pallister, E. F.: Surgical treatment of the fractured splint bone. Proc. Book A.V.M.A. (1953) 390.
14. Pettit, G. D., and Wheat, J. D.: Distal epiphyseal fracture of the femur in a Shetland pony. J.A.V.M.A. **138** (1961) 13.
15. Reichel, Ernest C.: Treatment of fractures of the long bones in large animals. J.A.V.M.A. **129** (1956) 8.
16. Riley, W. F. and Brinker, Wade O.: Intermedullary fixation in fractures of the equine metacarpal. J.A.V.M.A. **137** (1960) 597.
17. Wheat, J. D. and Mullenax, P. B.: Surgical treatment of fractures of the proximal sesamoid bones in the horse. J.A.V.M.A. **132** (1958) 378.
18. Whitford, Eugene L.: Fracture of the metatarsus in a Pinto stallion. J.A.V.M.A. **137** (1960) 58.

THE WALKING CAST

A walking cast provides a maximum amount of fixation for fractures below the knee and hock and permits the animal to be ambulatory and weight-bearing on the affected limb more than 75% of the convalescent period. This prevents unfortunate sequelae and complications, such as injury of the opposite or sound limb, decubital ulcers, muscular atrophy, and osteoporosis. Because the horse is comparatively comfortable he is more willing and able to exercise in the stall, thus stimulating circulation and appetite.

A well-nourished and comfortable patient is essential during the long convalescent period. Psychosomatic factors should not be overlooked. If a horse finds his cast uncomfortable because it is ill-fitting or cumbersome he may become discouraged and "give-up." Those who know horses are aware of the fact that constant or repeated unpleasant stimuli worry some animals so much that there is rapid mental deterioration which is reflected almost immediately by degenerative somatic signs.

Approximately 80% of fractures which occur in the horse are located in the extremities below the knee and hock. It is important, then, that the surgeon be familiar with the materials and methods which are most suited to treat this large category of fractures.

Veterinarians are accustomed to using a variety of equipment, materials, and methods for correction of orthopedic disorders. Chief among the available materials is plaster of paris. When the physical and chemical properties of such a material are well-understood, it is much easier to expertly and skillfully execute its application. Although it is not necessary, an inherent artistic sense is helpful when applying a cast.

Plaster of paris is anhydrous calcium sulfate which is impregnated into crinoline bandages. When water is added to it, heat is generated as the anhydrous calcium sulfate crystallizes to form gypsum. It is best to buy bandages of good quality, sealed in moistureproof containers with a manufacturing date not exceeding one year. Once a satisfactory brand of plaster has been found it is wise to continue its use. Certain differences exist between brands because of manufacturers' latitude in prescribing the composition of the product. A difference can be noticed in the setting time, the number of bandages needed for a given situation, the durability, and the degree of interference with radiography.

Presently, plaster with several different setting times is available. For our purposes, the medium-setting plaster serves best. If fast-setting plaster is used for a full leg cast there is too much opportunity for premature setting of the cast, resulting in poor adhesion of the successive rolls of plaster and, consequently, in a weak cast.

Although the product's composition has largely established the maturation process of freshly applied plaster, the following factors are influential in modifying the setting time:

Delays Setting Time

Cold water°
Soft water
Addition of borax or sugar to water
Bandage too wet

Hastens Setting Time

Hot water
Hard water
Table salt added to water
Rubbing the cast

The purposes in casting include: 1. To prevent pain by reducing muscle spasm, inhibiting movements of the fragments, and enforcing rest of the affected parts, 2, to facilitate healing, 3, to maintain proper position and alignment of the fragments, 4, to prevent deformity not only of the injured part but also of the opposite limb, (if during convalescence, sufficient weight is not borne by the injured limb, harmful changes can occur in the sound one) and, 5, to obtain functional restoration of the injured limb.

Surgical Preparation: The hair is thoroughly cleaned and dried. Boric acid powder then is dusted over the entire limb including the sole of the foot, and the hair is carefully smoothed in the direction of its growth. Boric acid powder has some bacteriostatic properties, and it also provides a slick surface over which the cast is applied. When this procedure is followed there is less opportunity for the hair to be turned back on itself, thus serving as a source of irritation and folliculitis.

To achieve stabilization, traction, and correction of fragment angulation while the cast is being applied, wires are attached to the heel of the foot. When the animal is in an atonic state, as in recumbency or under general anesthesia, the pastern and coffin joints are flexed. This must be overcome during casting for 2 reasons. First, the horse will be more comfortable while wearing the cast if the foot is in approximately the normal standing position. Second, flexion of these joints usually tends to prevent good alignment of fragments in fractures occurring below the knee or hock.

°Optimum temperature is 95 is 105 F.

The aforementioned wires are placed in the following manner: a ⅛-inch drill is placed 1 inch anterior to the point of the heel, ½ inch above the sole surface, and directed at a 45° angle toward the white line of the sole. A similar hole then is drilled 1 inch anterior to the first one. This is done on both the medial and lateral sides of the foot. Baling wire is threaded through the 2 holes (on the same side of the foot) to form a block "U". This procedure is repeated on the other side of the foot. The 4 ends of the wires may be twisted together in order that a rod may be inserted between the strands. An assistant, by pulling on this rod, creates enough tension at this point to lower the heel and extend the toe to a nearly normal position. By correcting the flexion in this manner the fragments are brought to closer apposition.

The specifications given here as to size and quantity of casting materials are for full-limb casts. It is felt that such a cast is best, even for a fracture of the second phalanx. Immobilization and stability of the limb are much improved in this way. The cast should never

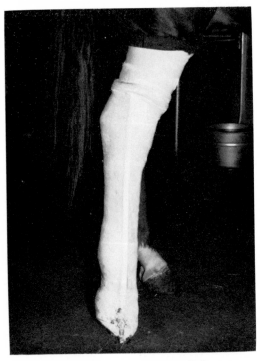

Fig. 16. Walking cast on rear limb.

end at or near the middle of a long bone because enough leverage may be brought to bear at the top of the cast to cause tissue necrosis or even a new fracture at this point. On the forelimbs, the cast should invest the foot and be carried upward to a point just below the elbow. On the rear limb, the cast should be carried upward to a point just below the stifle (Fig. 16).

An appropriate-sized stockinette, already rolled and sterilized, is started over the wire and foot and rolled (not pulled) to a point several inches above the intended high point of the cast. Then a single piece of ⅛-inch felt, cut to follow the contour of the limb, is placed on its anterior aspect. A similar strip is prepared and placed on the posterior side of the limb. At no point should the 2 strips meet. There should be at least a 1-inch separation between the strips at the point of their closest approximation. This point usually is in the metacarpal or metatarsal areas. Over the joints or bony prominences, such as the angles, knees, and hocks, the 2 strips will be separated by 2 or more inches. In these areas, diamond-shaped pieces of felt are cut and fitted over the lateral and medial sides of the joints. It is very important that overlapping of padding does not occur. When applied in this way there is room for some swelling under the cast, immobilization is better, and the lack of bulges or irregularities in the padding reduces points of possible irritation. The 2 strips plus the pieces over the prominences are secured with just enough 3-inch gauze bandage to hold them in place.

At the intended upper limit of the cast a 4-inch wide piece of felt should completely invest the circumference of the limb. This prevents skin irritation by the rough, sharp edges of the cast.

The fracture site then is manipulated to insure proper positioning of the fragments. The limb and the correctly positioned fragments are held in place by an assistant who applies traction on the previously installed wires.

For full-limb casts in adults, 6-inch plaster rolls should be used. The rolls are handled in the recommended manner. The first roll should be squeezed thoroughly to remove the excess water. If too wet, the roll will soak the felt and thus predispose the growth of mold. Too much water also may cause delayed setting of the inner layers of the cast and thus reduce its strength. The first roll of plaster is particularly important because it must provide enough tension to eliminate all dead space, thus insuring the closest fit possible. Subsequent rolls are merely rolled over the first layer smoothly and evenly.

It is best to start the first roll in the middle of the metacarpus or metatarus and proceed to apply the roll spirally to the upper limit of the cast. This will use all or nearly all of the roll. The second roll is started 3 to 4 inches above the beginning of the first one and is rolled spirally to the foot where it completely invests the foot and sole. The remaining rolls begin where the preceding one ended. Each roll must be started with a 4-inch overlap. Each spiral of the bandage should overlap the preceding spiral by 2 inches. Repeated figure of 8's are made over each important joint (ankles, knees, and hocks) to increase the strength of the cast at these points. To further increase the cast's strength, one roll of plaster may be layered up and down from the top of the cast to the toe. This should be applied to the anterior surface. Succeeding rolls are placed in the usual spiral fashion.

Twelve rolls of 6-inch plaster should be sufficient for a full-leg cast. After the application of 8 rolls, a previously prepared walking bar is put into place. The bar should be long enough to reach within 6 inches of the top of the cast. Its width should barely accommodate the foot and leg plus the plaster applied. It should conform roughly to the shape of the limb and foot (Fig. 17). The walking portion of the bar is placed ¼ inch below the sole of the foot and as near the center of the foot as possible. The top of the bar is secured in place with 2 or 3 turns of plaster bandages. The roll then is turned on its edge so that the bandage is laid just above the top edges of the bar in a rope-like fashion around the cast. The ends of the bar then ride against this ridge of plaster

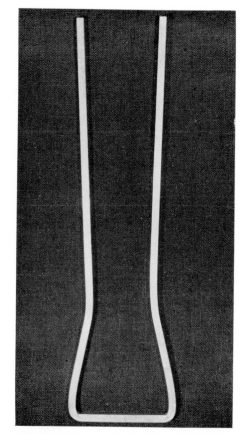

Fig. 17. Walking bar made of light, durable aluminum alloy. Malleable, but strong, and bent to conform to shape of limb.

and become the place which receives most of the weight transference. Two or 3 additional rolls of plaster are applied over the remaining portion of the bar to hold it firmly in place. Approximately 30 minutes are needed before the cast has sufficient rigidity to support an animal's weight. The wires used for traction are cut as close as possible to the plaster at the foot.

In addition to the foregoing the following procedures are advised:

1. Each layer of plaster should be gently rubbed to insure good contact and adhesion of layers, 2, assistants should prevent, during the construction of the cast, a downward bowing of the limb or rotation of the foot when traction is exerted, 3, should it become neces-

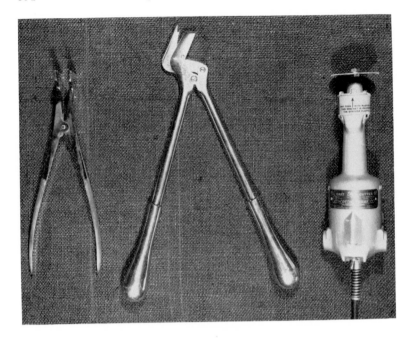

Fig. 18. Instruments used in removal of plaster of paris casts: cast spreaders, cutters, and oscillating saw.

sary to handle, lift, or move the limb before the cast has set, the palms of the hands should be used, as indentations made by fingers are reflected to the inner surface of the cast and may create a source of irritation, 4, chewing or gnawing of a chest almost always indicates that severe irritation exists beneath the cast. Such a situation demands removal of the cast and application of a new one before tissue necrosis develops, 5, the walking cast may be used in combination with other types of splintage, such as plates, screws, pins, etc., 6, the removal of a walking cast is facilitated by the use of cast spreaders, cutters, and an oscillating saw (Fig. 18).

L. E. Johnson

REFERENCES

1. Cozen, Lewis: Office Orthopedics. Lea and Febiger, Philadelphia, Pa., 1950.

2. Howorth, M. B.: A Textbook of Orthopedics. W. B. Saunders Co., Philadelphia, Pa. and London, 1952.

3. Speed, J. S. and Smith, Hugh: Campbell's Operative Orthopedics. 2nd ed. C. V. Mosby Co., St. Louis, Mo., 1949.

SURGICAL REMOVAL OF SESAMOID FRAGMENTS

In 1956, Dr. E. A. Churchill first reported about a series of cases involving surgical removal of sesamoid fracture segments.[1] This type of fracture is very common in both Thoroughbreds and Standardbreds, both trotters and pacers. The lateral and medial sesamoids of both front and hindlimbs apparently are equally susceptible to fracture. In a series of 38 sesamoid fractures presented for surgery, 20 were basal fractures and 18 were apical.

Etiology: Trauma undoubtedly is a factor in the etiology. There are many severe fractures of sesamoids, however, in which there is no external evidence of trauma. Churchill suggested that "fatigue which causes the horse to rely on basic skeletal structures rather than muscular activity," is an etiologic factor. Wheat has stated that a consideration in sesamoid fractures is "the unequal tension applied to the sesamoid bones when the foot strikes the ground in an unbalanced position."[2] Jockeys and trainers have reported that their horses showed the initial signs of lameness when bumped in a race or when changing leads. The fact that many hindlimb sesamoid fractures occur when the animal is not close to other participants in a race supports the theory of unequal tension caused by fatigue or an unbalanced position.

Anatomy: The proximal sesamoids ossify from a single center. They are situated close behind the distal end of the third metacarpal or metatarsal and are attached at the base to the first phalanx by the distal sesamoidean ligaments. Their flexor surfaces are covered by cartilage which fills the space between the two bones and forms a smooth groove for the deep flexor tendon. The abaxial surface is concave and provides attachment to part of the suspensory ligaments.

The distal sesamoidean ligaments may be regarded as digital continuations of the suspensory ligament. The sesamoids are incorporated into this superior stay apparatus by which the fetlock is supported and concussion is absorbed. A knowledge of the regional anatomy of the distal sesamoidean ligaments is essential for successful surgery in this area.

The distal sesamoidean ligaments are 3 in number:[3]

1. The superficial sesamoidean ligament is attached above to the base of the sesamoids and the intersesamoid ligament; below it attaches to the proximal end of the second phalanx.

2. The middle sesamoidean ligament is triangular. Above, it is attached to the base of sesamoids and the intersesamoid ligament; below, its deep face attaches to the triangular rough area of the volar surface of the first phalanx.

3. The deep or cruciate sesamoidean ligaments arise from the base of the sesamoids, cross one another, and attach to the proximal end of the first phalanx. The superficial and middle sesamoidean ligaments are of great importance in the surgical repair of basal sesamoid fractures.

Clinical Signs: When improper or faulty healing of basal sesamoid fractures occurs, the first clinical sign observed is an upward or dorsal displacement of the distal end of the first phalanx. This ringbone-like effect or up-ward displacement indicates that the basal attachment of the superficial and middle sesamoidean ligaments has been impaired. This sign is the basic reason for a poor postoperative prognosis. As a rule, the smaller the fractured segment of the sesamoid and the less displacement, the better the prognosis.

Many cases have been reported in which rather large segments have been fractured, but with little or no displacement. Some of these animals have raced successfully after only a few days of rest.

Many times the horse may show very little lameness during a race. He may stop shortly or show some lameness when "cooling-out," but the owner generally will not be concerned until the next day. At the end of 24 hours, depending on the severity of the fracture, the animal may be standing on 3 legs, or pointing the injured one. The ankle usually is swollen and hot. The acute inflammation and lameness may subside only to recur with exercise. At times, the joint is warm and swollen, and may show evidence of chronic inflammation. The volar or plantar surface of the fetlock may have a triangular appearance suggesting that spreading of the intersesamoidean ligaments has occurred.

Pain may be elicited on palpation or when pressure is applied by flexion. In cases of apical or abaxial surface fracture, pain is shown when pressure is applied over the branch of the suspensory ligament. In cases of distal or flexor surface fracture, pain is most intense when the pressure is applied at the base of the sesamoid.

Diagnosis: Diagnosis may be made by palpation and detection of crepitation at the fracture site. Positive diagnosis is dependent, however, on radiography. Anterior-posterior, lateral-medial, medial-lateral, medial-oblique, and lateral-oblique views are obtained. These 5 views are absolutely necessary; more may be useful to fully estimate the size and exact position of the sequestrum. Remember that the nearer the sesamoid is to the cassette the smaller will be its shadow. Extreme care should be taken to assure that the positions of the cassettes are clearly marked. When contemplating surgery it is imperative that the operator know not only which sesamoid is fractured but also the position and size of the chip. This information allows one to make an intelligent selection of the most practical site for removal of the sequestrum.

Prognosis: It is agreed that the optimum time for surgery is 10 to 20 days after the initial injury. However, cases have been operated as long as 18 months following injury and have recovered to race successfully.

Fractures of the apical and abaxial portion of the sesamoids are most accessible, most easily removed, and have the best prognosis, which is about a 65% chance for success. Basal fractures and fractures involving the flexor surfaces are less accessible; more ligament damage is done at the time of fracture and during removal of the sequestrum. The chances for successful recovery and return to racing form are about 30 to 35%.

The sesamoid has only a small amount of periosteum and a limited blood supply. Normal healing is slow and sometimes only a fibrous union occurs. Bone fragments originally showing very little displacement may separate and migrate. These migrating fragments will never heal. If nature achieves a fibrous "false joint," the resulting fibrosis and calcification interfere with the normal range of joint movement.

Surgical Technic: Removal of sesamoid sequestra, as in all orthopedic procedures involving a joint, must be done under strict asepsis. The leg should be washed, clipped, and soaked in an antiseptic solution. It is preferable to do this 24 hours prior to surgery. During the 24-hour period preceding surgery, antibiotics are administered and the patient is given a laxative diet. Tetanus antitoxin also is administered during this period.

The patient is tranquilized, and the volar nerves are blocked proximal to the surgical site. The operative area is again scrubbed and the site is draped. The incision for the apical, abaxial, and those basal fractures involving any part, except the inner or flexor border, is made between the suspensory ligament and the volar border of the third metatarsal or metacarpal. The distal end of the second or fourth metatarsal (metacarpal) is a good landmark. The proximal end of the skin incision should extend to within an inch of the distal end of the splint bone. A straight vertical incision will cause a minimum amount of injury to nerves and vessels. Continue the skin incision downward to the level of the articulation of the third metatarsal (metacarpal) bone and the first phalanx. Reflect the skin freely in order to obtain plenty of working space.

The subcutaneous tissues should be incised down to the annular ligament of the fetlock and reflected in the same manner as the skin. The annular ligament is incised in an arc which roughly coincides with the shape of the condyle at the distal end of the third metatarsus (metacarpus). This elliptical incision allows maximum access to the sesamoid's articular surfaces. Rongeurs, dental elevators, right angle periosteal elevators with a cutting edge, and ¼-inch straight chisels have proved invaluable in removing the sequestra. Even though displaced, the sequestra invariably are tightly adhered to the intersesamoidean and distal sesamoidean ligaments. Care and restraint are advised when removing the segments so that there is a minimum of intra-articular damage.

Fragments of the distal outer border of the sesamoid often may be removed through a liberal incision, such as described, without cutting the distal sesamoidean ligament connecting the abaxial surface of the sesamoid and the proximal end of the first phalanx. Basal sesamoid fractures are usually T-shaped and have 2 or 3 segments. It is imperative that all of them be located and removed. The remaining fracture line should be curetted or smoothed with a bone file.

A surgical technic has been described in which the operator cuts through the intersesamoidean ligament and removes the fractured segment through the dense fibrous tissue. This approach necessitates flexing the joint and abducting the flexor tendons. In my opinion, this procedure is necessary only when the fracture involves the basal or the inner (flexor) border of the sesamoids.

The joint capsule and pericapsular tissue are closed with stainless steel, interrupted sutures. Care is taken to cut the suture material as close as possible to the tie, so as to prevent any loose ends from causing tissue reaction. The annular ligament is closed with double 0 chromic catgut. The subcutaneous tissues are approximated with a continuous suture, using the same material. The skin is closed with double 0 silk, using a continuous stitch.

Postoperative Care: No skin or intra-articular medication is used postoperatively. Aseptic technic and the preoperative preparation are relied upon to achieve first intention healing. Phenylbutazone is used routinely to allay postoperative pain and to encourage weight-bearing on the operated leg. The fetlock joint is wrapped in an Ace elastic bandage which is reset every 12 hours. The aseptic pack is left in place, however, for 72 hours after surgery.

Complete stall rest is advised for 7 days. The stitches are removed on the eighth day. When healing is complete, mild glycerine and alcohol sweats are applied. Regulated exercise is recommended for 60 days. A period of 6 months' abstinence from hard work has proved to be the usual convalescent period required.

D. L. PROCTOR

REFERENCES

1. Churchill, E. A.: Surgical removal of fracture fragments of the proximal sesamoid bone. J.A.V.M.A. **128** (1956) 581-582.

2. Wheat, J. D., and Rhode, E. A.: Surgical treatment of the fractures of the proximal sesamoid bones in the horse. J.A.V.M.A. **132** (1958) 378-381.

3. Sisson, S., and Grossman, J. D. The Anatomy of the Domestic Animals. 4th ed. W. B. Saunders Co., Philadelphia, Pa. 1953.

WOUNDS AND THEIR THERAPY

INTRODUCTION

Probably no other species of domestic animals is subject to such an awesome variety of wounds as the horse. A large proportion of any equine practice, exclusive of race track work, involves treatment of traumatic wounds. Because of his evolutionary background during which the horse survived principally by running from danger, the modern horse instinctively will panic under pressure and often run blindly. Consequently, thunderstorms, loud unusual noises, etc. often will be followed by a rash of calls to treat wounded horses.

The most common instrument responsible for wounds in horses is barbed wire but an infinite variety of wood, glass, metal, and other objects frequently is incriminated. Bearing these facts in mind and remembering that the horse is remarkably helpless and unable to take care of himself, the practitioner often is able to offer suggestions which will eliminate many hazards and materially decrease the incidence of wounds. For example, horses often will fight across a fence but will graze amiably together in the same field.

CLASSIFICATION OF WOUNDS

In general, wounds are classified as follows:

1. Abrasions are wounds in which only the surface layers of the skin are destroyed by friction, leaving a sensitive area exposed. Falls on gravel or rough soil, rope burns, and scraping the shins on the tail gate of trailers during loading or unloading are the chief causes of abrasions. These wounds are very sensitive, hemorrhage little if at all, and heal more slowly than would be anticipated. They may lead to such complications as granulomas or excessive fibrosis (Fig. 19).

2. Incised wounds are produced by sharp instruments, such as a scalpel during surgery or accidentally by glass, tin, and similar sharp objects. The edges are cleanly cut and there is a minimum of tissue trauma. Incised wounds, particularly those that are inflicted accidentally, may seriously damage the deeper tissues, sever blood vessels, nerves, muscle, tendon, and abdominal or thoracic viscera. They cause a variety of signs. Hemorrhage is apt to be more persistent and serious in incised wounds than in other types.

3. Contusions occur most commonly from falls, kicks, and similar trauma. They are characterized by loss of continuity without actual separation of tissue. Thus, bruising and hematoma formation within the underlying soft tissue and only minor abrasions of the skin constitute the usual contusion. The importance of contusions depends upon the degree of damage to underlying tissue. A small surface wound, for example, on the medial aspect of

the radius with minor underlying bruising may actually mask a linear radial fracture which often will not become a complete fracture for several days (so-called deferred fracture). The vast majority of contusions heal by resolution and absorption of the extravasated blood and lymph.

4. Puncture wounds produce many serious complications in horses. They commonly are caused by a nail or splinter penetration of superficial tissues. Dirt, manure, and other foreign material are carried into the depths of the wound. Obviously, the seriousness of these wounds is related to the favorable environment created for multiplication of anaerobic organisms. Penetrating foreign bodies may invade such vital tissues as tendon sheaths, bursae, joint cavities, or even the chest and abdominal areas and cause serious complications.

5. Lacerations probably comprise more

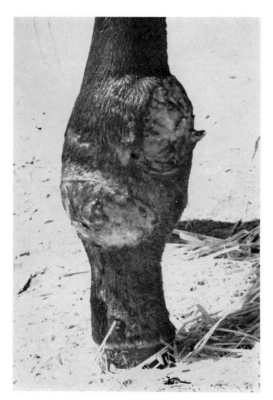

Fig. 19. The result of an untreated abrasion of the ankle. The surrounding tissues have sloughed leading to open joint, suppuration, and tendon sheath infection.

wounds than any other type. They differ from incised wounds in that the edges are torn and irregular, hemorrhage is not so profuse, and they are slower to heal. Barbed wire is the most frequent cause of lacerations in horses although many other objects may cause them. When there is tearing away of tissue, the laceration is termed an avulsion. There may be extensive tissues loss, particularly in barbed wire wounds of the anterior aspect of the forearm, with surprisingly little pain (Fig. 20).

SPONTANEOUS WOUND HEALING

In order to fully appreciate the body's proficiency in wound healing, some knowledge of the process of tissue repair is important. It also is important that the veterinary clinician be able to distinguish between normal and complicated wound healing. This especially is true for extensive lacerations in which natural debridement proceeds slowly for the first week and leads the uninformed to ill-advised interference.

Wounds of the horse generally heal by first intention or by granulation. First intention healing is the ultimate, and the aim of the surgeon should be to have all of his incisions heal by this method. Such healing repairs a simple incised wound relatively free from infection, its edges maintained in apposition with a minimum of movement, and absence of a local circulatory disturbance. Early in the healing process there is union of the wound edges by coagulum and leukocytic invasion of the blood clot. Shortly thereafter, connective tissue cells multiply, and fibroblasts and small capillary buds grow into the coagulum and replace it. At the same time, epithelial cell proliferation has bridged the incision.

There should be no discharge from such a wound unless irritant antiseptics have been utilized, in which case the work of regeneration will be increased and will result in more extensive fibroblast proliferation, a wider fibrous band between the wound edges, and a more lengthy healing period. When antiseptics are applied as frequently as recommended, inevitably gaping of the wound occurs. Similarly, should pyrogens be introduced at the time of incision or at a later date, an inflammatory reaction ensues and is accompanied by discharges and a suppurative softening of the coagulum, and gaping will occur.

If the wound is sutured, swelling will be more severe because of inadequate drainage. Wounds, which fail to heal by first intention because of infection or due to irritant antiseptics, must heal by granulation.

Healing by granulation is the most common method of wound repair in horses. Granulation tissue is a simply constructed new tissue composed chiefly of capillary vessels and fibroblasts. This reddish, granular, insensitive tissue which bleeds quite easily grows inward and upward from the depth of the wound. Leukocytes are liberated from the new capillaries and they phagocytize contaminants on the surface of the wound. Once the granulation tissue has filled the gap in the wounded area, the surface becomes impervious to bacterial invasion and infection is prevented. Gradually, epithelial cells multiply and bridge the gap filled by granulation tissue, which eventually becomes less vascular and more fibrous until the healing process is completed (Fig. 21).

Healing of wounds in the horse may be delayed by a number of factors. The presence of foreign bodies is a common cause for delayed healing. These contaminants may be bits of wood, metal, dirt, wire, or fragments of fractured bone or cartilage. Healing seldom is completed until such material is removed.

Another common cause of delayed healing is excessive movement of the wounded area. For this reason, many wounds below the knee and hock fail to heal properly and quickly. Wound irritation by insects likewise interrupts the normal healing process.

Probably the most important deterrent to adequate healing is the use of harsh and irritating disinfectants on wounds. This is an old custom and it is one of the most serious problems the veterinarian encounters, particularly during the first week of healing when the surface cells which have been destroyed are being sloughed. Well-meaning advisers usually will suggest or actually use a variety of drugs to overcome the "infection." About all

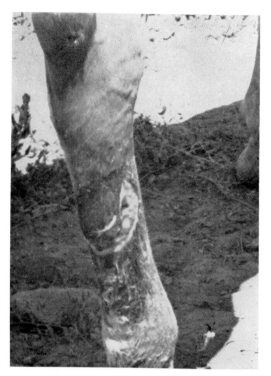

Fig. 20. Typical laceration of the metatarsal region caused by a kick. The superficial tendon is involved.

that most of these agents accomplish is to dessicate and cause further necrosis of the delicate granulating tissue and thus retard healing. Topical therapy should be limited to the use of a saline solution which may be gently flushed over the wound twice daily to placate the owner and wash away the wound secretions.

Biting, rubbing, or licking of the wound obviously may lead to serious delay in healing. When this occurs some restraining device should be applied. The horse sometimes can be controlled by the use of a cradle, a bib, a side stick (a pole from the halter ring to a surcingle), or by cross-tying the head in a tie stall. When the horse bites or chews at a bandage or cast, the application of some deterrent such as oil and cayenne pepper on the bandage may be preventive.

WOUND COMPLICATIONS

The overwhelming majority of wounds heal in routine fashion by the granulation process.

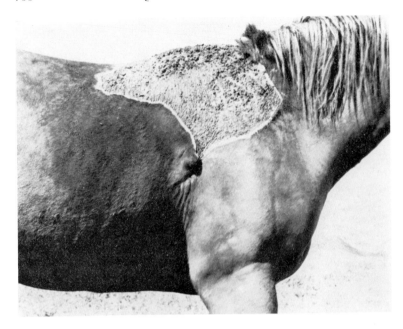

Fig. 21. An example of an evenly granulating wound, 6 weeks after avulsion of the skin. Treated by antibiotic injection alone.

The veterinarian must remain constantly alert, however, for early signs of an infinite variety of complications. One of the most important points in the management of horse wounds is the ability to distinguish between normal and abnormal healing. Initially, a wound may be complicated by hemorrhage, shock, or both. Neither is as important in the horse as in the human patient where shock is a particularly serious complication. With the exception of wounds involving the larger vessels such as the carotid artery or jugular vein, fatal hemorrhage seldom occurs in horses. Even profound bleeding from extensive wounds usually ceases as the blood pressure drops, and before death ensues. Hemorrhage from wounds should be checked, of course, as soon as possible by compression with forceps, ligature, or packing the wound with gauze. Arterial bleeding is characterized by spurting of bright red blood and is more serious than venous or capillary hemorrhage. Arteries always should be ligated to prevent recurrence of bleeding. Secondary hemorrhage may occur up to 48 hours after the initial bleeding has been controlled. It is seen most commonly following routine castrations. Wounds should be checked frequently for the first 48 hours when hemostasis in any form has been required in the initial treatment.

Shock occasionally is a complication of severe and extensive wounds, particularly when there has been loss of tissue. Typically, there is profound depression of all body functions. Abdominal wounds, either surgical or accidental, almost always are complicated by shock and the surgeon should be continually aware of this danger. Whole blood, plasma, and blood extenders are useful in the treatment of horses showing signs of shock, those with a history of serious blood loss, and those suffering from extensive trauma. (See Chapter 3.)

Imperfect drainage frequently is a serious complication of many wounds. Virtually all wounds of the head, neck, withers, and back drain poorly by reason of their location, and often become necrotic. Antibiotics and gauze drains are essential in the treatment of any dorsal wound. A rather large percentage of puncture wounds are complicated by imperfect drainage. Infection becomes entrapped in the depths of the wound, leading to abscess formation or cellulitis. Many skin wounds develop undermining infection because skin flaps are so located that they interfere with drainage. For such wounds, the surgeon should establish as complete drainage as possible on the initial visit. It is well to remember that large draining wounds heal more rapidly and completely than smaller, poorly drained ones.

One of the most commonly encountered complications of horse wounds is the presence of foreign bodies. It is extremely embarrassing to the clinician to treat an open wound and offer a good prognosis, only to have the client call back several weeks later to say that the wound has failed to heal. Re-examination almost always will reveal an offending foreign body. The most frequently encountered foreign bodies are pieces of wood and bone sequestra; however, bits of glass, metal, wire, and other objects may be present. An important part of the initial examination is a thorough exploration of the depths of any wound to ascertain the presence of a foreign body. Favored locations for foreign bodies are chest, axillary, groin, and mouth wounds.

In one case, a 6-inch piece of wood nearly an inch thick that had penetrated the tongue was removed from the space between the mandibular rami. This horse had been wounded 6 weeks prior to admission to the hospital. His wound had been treated topically by the owner but it had failed to heal. On examination, there was a small fistulous opening between the mandibular rami, some thickening of both rami, tremendous enlargement of the tongue, inability to swallow, persistent choke, emaciation, and diarrhea. Under general anesthesia, the tongue was incised and the wooden stick removed. The foreign body was surrounded by a thick fibrous capsule. Recovery was uneventful and complete.

Trauma inflicted over bony protuberances, such as the cannon bone, hip, face, etc., may result in small chip fractures which act as foreign body sequestra. These often cause draining fistulae which resist healing until the offending bits are removed surgically. Chronic, draining wounds should immediately arouse suspicion of foreign body involvement.

Infection is, of course, a major complication of all wounds. The environment under which horses are maintained, particularly when kept in stables or corrals, is especially conducive to the establishment of infection in wounds. Puncture wounds are particularly susceptible to the entrapment of infectious organisms at the bottom of the wound. Such wounds furnish an ideal environment for the bacteria which cause tetanus, gas gangrene, and cellulitis. Tetanus follows puncture wounds in the horse so frequently that it is considered gross negligence for the veterinarian not to routinely administer tetanus antitoxin when they occur.

Cellulitis is a very serious complication of wounds. It results from the spread of a virulent infection throughout the surrounding subcutaneous tissues. There is a hot, painful swelling of the area accompanied by fever, depression, and anorexia. The wound discharge becomes more serous in nature and septicemia may ensue. Prompt treatment with broad spectrum antibiotics, hot topical applications, and supportive agents is indicated. When the invading organism is less virulent or when there is more adequate drainage and more resistant subcutaneous tissue, suppuration usually occurs. This process is more easily controlled than cellulitis, and frequently responds to systemic antibiotic therapy alone.

Infection at the base of a wound may remain localized and form an abscess as the external wound heals. This is likely to happen following deep puncture wounds or when foreign bodies are present. The character of the exudate in an abscess depends a great deal on the invading organism as well as its location. All abscesses characteristically reach a stage, however, when they soften the tissues to such an extent that they "come to a head." Some deeply situated abscesses may not be capable of complete drainage because the point of exit is too small or the channel through which the pus must travel is too narrow. Abscesses in the shoulder region are often of this nature and a persistent draining sinus may develop.

By definition, a sinus communicates with an abscess in any part of the body, whereas a fistula communicates with an endothelial lined body cavity. In practice, these definitions are of little significance because common usage has established such terminology as fistulous withers which, in fact, is a complex sinus in many cases.

The most common sites for abscess formation in the horse are the submaxillary and parotid regions and the feet. Abscesses should not be confused with hematomas. Abscesses develop slowly and are characterized by evidence of heat, tenderness, reddening of the skin, and are rather firm to the touch. Hematomas develop rapidly and are cold, painless, and fluctuating during the first week of their development. Hematomas are most commonly found on the chest, hips, and flanks.

Abscesses should not be incised before walling off has occurred, otherwise the infection may be distributed to the surrounding tissues and/or systemically. Liberal incisions are indicated for drainage of abscesses while the cavity is healing from its depths. Caution also should be exercised in opening a hematoma too early. At least 7 days should be allowed before incising one in order to give the ruptured blood vessel an opportunity to clot firmly and thus eliminate the danger of recurrent hemorrhage.

An important and almost universal complication of wounds below the knee and hock in the horse is the formation of exuberant granulation tissue. Granulation tissue, which is indispensable in the repair of most wounds in horses, has some of the characteristics of neoplastic tissue. Its basic cell is embryonic and, given the right environment, it overgrows in rough, grape-like masses known as granulomas. These clinically resemble a benign neoplasm.

The basic requirement for the development of exuberant granulation tissue is a wound in an area where the skin is closely applied over bone or tendon and in a part which is difficult to immobilize. Therefore, wounds below the hock and knee (particularly below the front of the hock and back of the knee), the front of the rear fetlocks, and the feet are particularly susceptible. Infection may sometimes be a contributing factor, although in my opinion this is not as important as the mechanical factors involved.

The mechanical factors include inelasticity of the skin, because there is little subcutaneous tissue, and continual movement. They stimulate granulation tissue to develop beyond the limits of the original wound defect until it overgrows the epithelial borders and continues as an uncontrolled neoplastic-like growth known as "proud flesh." The fact that application of pressure bandages to such wounds successfully prevents granuloma formation lends support to this theory.

Foreign bodies also may stimulate development of granulomas. Once a granuloma has developed, it tends to recur unless completely excised. The wound then is handled as a fresh lesion.

TREATMENT OF WOUNDS

Until recent years, an infinite variety of pharmaceutic agents has been vigorously championed for the treatment of wounds in horses. These drugs have varied from cod-liver oil to every new antiseptic produced in the laboratory. A great deal of reliance has accompanied the spraying, dusting, flushing, sprinkling, or soaking of these chemicals on any wound. More recent evidence quite clearly demonstrates that these preparations not only fail to destroy the invading organisms in many instances but that they actually retard the activity of leukocytes, phagocytes, and other cells active in the regeneration of wounded tissue. In short, they do more harm than good in many cases.

Tradition has dictated the application of some form of antiseptic or "healing" preparation to all open wounds and its violation amounts to malpractice in the opinion of many laymen. Nearly every horseman has some noxious mixture which has been used for generations and has become a fixture in his medicine chest. Actually, the fact that horses' wounds heal so well despite the use of these drugs demonstrates the considerable reserve of healing power inherent in the beasts.

Modern medical practice encourages the treatment of wounds by systemic administration of antibiotics and sera. A minimum of therapy is given to the wound itself except for cleansing it with warm saline solution, applying necessary bandages to immobilize the injured area, and eventually exposing the area to heat to increase local blood circulation. Good nursing care often is the determining factor in cases of severe and painful wounds.

The treatment of wounds involves certain principles which apply generally. Infection should be controlled on the first visit by the intramuscular administration of tetanus antitoxin and an antibiotic. A favored antibiotic for equine wounds is the combination of penicillin and streptomycin. This should be given daily for 4 to 5 days.

After antibiotic therapy has been initiated, the surgeon should examine the wound thoroughly. It should be determined which tissues are injured, and a careful search for foreign bodies should be made. To do this, it may be necessary to gently cleanse the wound with cotton swabs soaked in warm saline solution. After the examination is completed, all foreign material should be removed mechanically or rinsed from the wound. It often is better not to clip the hair around the wound if it is short because of the danger of contaminating the wound and establishing centers of infection and irritation. Long hair may be grasped with forceps or the fingers and removed with scissors. The presence of hair on the skin surface is not nearly the deterrent to epithelization that might be suspected. Areas of skin which are badly lacerated and lacking circulation should be removed.

Most incised wounds should be sutured and many lacerated wounds likewise benefit from suturing. As many sutures should be used as are required for good apposition and drainage should be provided. Suturing should include as much skin as possible in order to establish firm skin contact. Good approximation of skin can be aided by the application of retention sutures. Either interrupted or mattress sutures may be used.

Puncture wounds should never be sutured; instead the external opening should be enlarged to provide adequate drainage.

Wounds of the lower extremities seldom benefit by suturing and generally are better treated with either pressure bandages or encasement in plaster of paris casts. Healing proceeds quite well under the cast or bandage, the pressure of which adequately prevents granuloma formation. The advantages of the plaster cast include restriction of the development of exuberant granulations and reduction of the handling and rewrapping of the wound. It prevents the use of irritant disinfectants, and allows uninterrupted use of the horse in most cases. Antibiotics routinely are given intramuscularly during the first 4 or 5 days following initial therapy. The casts need not be heavy; two or three 5-yard by 4-inch bandages usually suffice, and they can be left in place for 2 to 4 weeks, depending on the severity of the wound. A light sheet of cotton is applied under the cast. This method is especially useful for wounds of the foot, particularly wire cuts across the heels. This is an area difficult to bandage except with plaster, and without pressure bandaging deformed feet with large scars are likely to develop.

Caution must be exercised when the possibility of an open joint exists. It is more prudent to treat these topically and immobilize the area with a bandage until the joint closes, and then apply a cast. Owners must be cautioned not to be alarmed by the fetid slough and discharge from the top and bottom of the cast. So long as the patient shows no increased lameness or systemic reaction, the cast should be left undisturbed. Most of the fetid discharge is simply the slough of the necrotic surface cells, and on examination one will find a healthy, firm, granulating surface under the cast.

Exposed joints, characterized by the discharge of straw-colored joint or bursal fluid, require prompt treatment. Antibiotics and, when economically feasible, cortisone preparations are given systemically. When allowed to remain untreated, marked systemic signs and evidence of extreme pain develop. Infection increases the severity of the signs and renders the prognosis less hopeful. Ulceration of the joint surfaces and ankylosis are common sequelae.

Rest, under tranquilization if necessary, is indicated for cases with exposed joints. Antibiotics are used to flush the joint cavity and these are combined with intramuscular administration of antibiotics. The affected joint should be bandaged to minimize movement.

Occasionally, the healing process of a large granulating wound in which there has been extensive loss of tissue will appear to stop. This is called regeneration fatigue. The use of an irritant such as scarlet red, tincture of iodine, or even a light mercury blister often will stimulate the epithelial edges to regain their regenerative powers and complete the closure.

Most wounds of horses heal more firmly and thoroughly when light exercise is prescribed. Wounds treated with absolute rest often heal more rapidly than when exercise is allowed but the resulting scar is prone to break down or develop serious underlying adhesions.

Wounds of Special Regions

Head: Wounds of the head are not infrequent in the horse and usually are inflicted by barbed wire, by rearing while being loaded in trailers, or by poorly constructed mangers or hayracks. The skin over the poll and face is rather closely attached to the bone and has a poor blood supply. For this reason suturing should be done early before excessive gaping and dessication occur. When the suturing is accomplished promptly these wounds usually heal quite well, leaving a minimal scar. Even though large flaps of skin are removed surgically or avulsed during the accident, healing by granulation usually will remedy the defect without excessive scarring. When the facial bones are exposed, a bland ointment or moist packs should be employed to prevent excessive dessication. Horses' ears occasionally are split by barbed wire and, if untreated, will heal with an appreciable slit. As the cartilage heals very slowly and imperfectly, many surgeons prefer to allow the ear to heal naturally rather than to suture the laceration. For severely lacerated or split ears one may suture the edges of the skin and not include the cartilage. Such attempts to repair should include the use of protective bandages and other immobilizing devices.

Wounds of the eyelids occur rather commonly in the horse. The torn portion usually hangs freely from the lid and it soon becomes dry and wrinkled. Early suturing is essential for successful repair and should be attempted even though a portion of the lid is badly torn. No portion should be trimmed away until the wound has been allowed to heal as far as possible. Re-examination at this time will indicate whether further surgery, such as plastic repair, is desirable. Even badly torn lids often repair remarkably well when sutured promptly, and antibiotics are given intramuscularly. Occasionally the wound is so extensive as to cause dessication of the cornea, and keratitis. When early suturing is impossible, one should freshen the edges of the fragments and suture them in as normal position as possible (see Chapter 15).

Wounds of the nostrils occasionally are inflicted by nails or other protruding objects in the stable. When the cartilage is involved, as it frequently is, it should not be included in the sutures. These wounds heal quite rapidly because the area involved is highly vascular.

Wounds of the tongue are frequent in horses and most often these are caused by unskilled or rough use of a spade bit. Rarely, the tongue is cut by pieces of glass, tin, or other sharp objects accidentally included in the feed. These wounds usually are undetected at the time of their occurrence and are not discovered until the tongue is examined during such procedures as floating teeth or performing physical examinations. If detected early, suturing with strong nonabsorbable material results in good recovery. If these wounds are untreated, the tongue may heal in a twisted or constricted shape. Plastic repair is possible even for old, severe tongue wounds, although it seldom is requested.

Neck: The seriousness of neck wounds is not related to superficial wounds, which heal readily, but to the involvement of deeper structures such as the vagus nerve, carotid artery, jugular vein, esophagus, and trachea. Wounds involving the vagus may cause immediate death, but if less severe, laryngeal paralysis and roaring may ensue. Wounds of the jugular furrow may expose the jugular vein without actually involving it. These wounds should be sutured, and if the wound is large it may be necessary to ligate the vein above and below the wound to prevent its spontaneous rupture during the healing process.

When the carotid artery is perforated, it obviously is necessary to provide immediate surgical aid to prevent fatal hemorrhage. The artery should be compressed with a forceps and double-ligated above and below the wound after first separating the vagus trunk, which should not be included in the ligatures.

When the trachea is torn it may be necessary to perform a tracheotomy below the wound in order to achieve adequate healing.

Esophageal wounds are quite serious and have a host of possible complications. There may be constriction at the point of healing with accompanying dilation above it. More frequently, an esophageal fistula develops and there is a continuous discharge of saliva and feed through the external opening. These can be corrected surgically. Many esophageal wounds heal quite readily even when the wound in the esophagus is an inch long. Suturing should be conducted carefully and completely, and in many cases it becomes necessary to enlarge the skin wound to prevent imprisonment of feed particles in the wound.

Axilla: Wounds in this region are fairly common and often result when a horse tries to jump a barbed wire fence and lands astride it. Branches or sticks of wood cause wounds of the axilla in many instances. Characteristically, these wounds result in the development of extensive subcutaneous emphysema because of the suction-like movement of the parts. It is common for these wounds to enlarge but this simply insures better drainage. Only occasionally are the large axillary vessels torn. If this should occur, it becomes necessary to pack the area with gauze until hemorrhage is controlled. Whenever wooden objects cause the wound, one should make a detailed examination to be certain that no foreign body remains lodged in it. When no complications exist, axillary wounds heal quite rapidly. The subcutaneous emphysema generally is disregarded, as the entrapped air is absorbed in due time. Recovery is remarkably complete, even for extreme lacerations, except in the presence of the easily overlooked foreign bodies.

Thorax and Abdomen: Wounds of these 2 body cavities are classified as penetrating or nonpenetrating. The latter are of no special significance and are treated by application of the general principles already outlined. Penetrating wounds of the thorax are caused by horns, collisions with wooden fences, stakes, etc., or by hard falls which result in a compound rib fracture. Penetrating thoracic wounds of the horse are quite serious because the resulting aspiration of air into the chest cavity (pneumothorax) may cause complete lung collapse. The mediastinum of the horse is fenestrated behind the heart so that air entrapped on one side will pass to the other. Thus, complete pneumothorax and pulmonary collapse, as well as extensive bilateral pleural infection, are more frequent than not following perforation of the thoracic wall. Hence, penetrating wounds of the thorax demand immediate institution of intramuscular antibiotic therapy and complete closure of the wound in the hope of controlling infection and obtaining resorption of the air and correction of the pneumothorax.

Penetrating abdominal wounds, of course, permit a wide variety of possible complications depending upon the organ or organs involved. Most commonly, the intestines are involved with peritonitis or ventral hernia being primary complications. Often there will be a minor external wound or a hematoma with bruising of the skin surface, yet a rent of considerable extent can develop in the musculature and result in ventral hernia. In any event, abdominal wounds should be sutured carefully, uniting the torn musculature with sutures inserted through the fascial covering and closing the skin firmly with stout mattress sutures.

When the abdominal cavity has actually been perforated, the horse should be anesthetized and placed on the sound side. The protruding organs should be cleansed thoroughly, rinsed with warm saline, and then carefully returned to the abdominal cavity. One should not hesitate to enlarge the skin opening with a scalpel and to tear the musculature with the fingers in order to facilitate replacement of prolapsed tissue. After replacement of the viscera, every effort should be made to suture the peritoneal surfaces, using absorbable catgut.

When an extensive laceration has occurred or the wound has existed for some time, the peritoneal lining may be difficult to locate, in which case the sutures should penetrate the deep muscle layer. When the peritoneal surfaces are held in apposition, they unite strongly in a very short time and effectively seal the abdominal cavity from further external insult. Finally, the superficial muscles and then the skin may be united. Systemic antibiotic therapy should be instituted immediately and it is wise in most cases to administer blood plasma or extenders intravenously to prevent shock. The bulky portions of the diet should be greatly restricted for several days in order to reduce the weight and pressure on the weakened tissues.

Dorsum: Wounds of the back, withers, croup, and tail are of significance because it is difficult to establish adequate drainage for them, and because they may be accompanied by vertebral fracture. When the heavy dorsal fascia is exposed it becomes an ideal site for bacterial invasion and cellulitis. The anaerobic organisms, such as the tetanus and gas gangrene species, are especially likely to become established here. These infections, therefore, should be guarded against by the administration of antitoxin and antibiotics.

Forelegs: Barbed wire lacerations of the forearm are encountered commonly. These may be quite extensive and contain avulsions of the extensor muscles. In other cases, a large portion of the muscle may be hanging down over the carpus. Healing occurs quite readily, even when avulsion is a complication, although there often is a noticeable dragging of the limb or evidence of difficulty in advancing it for some time after the wound surface has healed. It often is worthwhile to attempt suturing the torn muscle fibers, and in severe cases when the value of the horse justifies the procedure, good results have been obtained by encasing the entire limb in a plaster cast and confining the horse to a tie stall for several weeks.

Wounds of the front of the knee are not infrequent. They occur as a consequence of falls, stumbling, etc., and may present several important complications. Tendon sheaths, the joint structures, or both may be involved, granulomas may develop here or cicatricial adhesions may occur and cause some loss of movement. The use of systemic antibiotics should be continued until synovial discharge has ceased. Bandaging or plaster casts will inhibit exuberant granulation tissue formation. The adhesions that tend to form between the skin and bone can be materially reduced by digital massage, using stimulating liniments, and by exercises to stretch the contracted skin.

Wounds of the metacarpal region may include the arteries, veins, tendons, and ligaments of this region. When the superficial flexor is involved, the foot is placed flat on the ground but there is extreme knuckling of the fetlock, whereas severing of the deep flexor tendon causes the toe to point upward when weight is placed on the foot. Should either tendon be involved special treatment is required. Division of the deep flexor tendon is most serious, and requires a special shoe with a posterior extension to accept the weight. In either case, the leg should be wrapped in plaster to hold the severed ends of tendon in as close an apposition as possible. When the synovial sheaths are involved, antibiotic therapy should be instituted. Serviceable recovery is possible in most cases.

Wounds of the fetlock and pastern present no particular problem except that joint movement presents a complication. Flexion of the fetlock renders healing in a normal manner virtually impossible unless pressure bandages or casts are used. Occasionally, one will find a wire cut in the region of the pastern joint which causes a degenerative arthritis of the joint clinically indistinguishable from ringbone. This development should be handled in the same manner as a ringbone.

Feet: Wounds of the feet are among the most commonly encountered traumatic injuries of the horse. Nail penetrations of the sole and frog produce marked lameness and are among the most frequent causes of tetanus. The nail may be accidentally inserted during shoeing or it may be picked up from the ground. In many of the latter instances the nail simply penetrates the sole and then is withdrawn, leaving only a small hole as the wound. These wounds usually cause severe and sudden lameness with typical signs of inflammation.

The wound may be located easily by cleaning the surface of the sole and applying hoof testers to detect the sensitive area. This area is then thoroughly pared with a hoof knife until the hole is located. Usually thick black pus will exude from the opening. The opening should be enlarged and all undermined sole removed. It may be necessary to remove the shoe in order to locate the wound if it has been caused by a shoe nail. Tetanus antitoxin and antibiotic therapy should be instituted and the hoof should be kept in an antiphlogistic dressing for several days.

Nail puncture wounds respond well to treatment unless the wound involves deeper structures. Wounds at the toe may fracture the os pedis and cause a bone sequestrum to act as a foreign body. Radiography is helpful in the diagnosis of this condition.

Wounds around the point of the frog or anywhere in the middle third of the sole may puncture the navicular bursa or fracture the navicular bone. This is the most serious wound of the foot and it may become necessary to resort to surgery to achieve correction. Antibiotic and cortisone therapy has materially reduced the gravity of this condition. Treatment is based on the general principles outlined for opened joints.

Wounds of the posterior third of the foot are never so serious. Because of the spongy nature of this portion of the foot (frog and digital cushion), drainage often is difficult to establish and wounds in this region frequently establish a sinus opening at the coronary band above the initial wound opening. Intramammary ointment tubes of penicillin-streptomycin are convenient for treating these conditions. Not infrequently, toe or quarter cracks become infected and present similar signs with the sinus eventually draining from the coronary band. In these cases, lameness is never so acute and the course may be prolonged for months before the sinus finally becomes established.

Serious wounds of the heels and coronet are not uncommon when horses attempt to paw through barbed wire fences. These may be extremely serious when the wire slips medial to the lateral cartilage and extends to the center of the frog, thereby exposing such vital tissues as the joint capsule, digital tendon sheath, and lateral cartilage. Even in relatively simple lacerations of the foot, its constant movement results in unsightly deforming scar formation if left untreated. When the wound extends through the coronary band, deformities of the hoof or quarter cracks may occur. Such areas become a constant source of irritation and are susceptible to infection. These wounds require thorough debridement including the ragged areas of torn coronary band. The hoof wall under the wounded coronet should be thinned with a rasp to relieve the pressure during healing. Antibiotic therapy and tetanus antitoxin are administered and the entire foot is firmly encased in a plaster cast to hold the edges of the wound in apposition. If the wound is several days old and gaping when first observed, it may be necessary to excise the granulating flaps. This procedure greatly reduces the size of the resulting scar.

Hock: Severe lacerations of the flexor surface of the hock caused by barbed wire are common in the horse. Again serious complications from open joint and granuloma formation are not infrequent. The excessive movement of the joint predisposes to the development of exuberant granulations. Although these joints are difficult to bandage, attempts should be made to do so. When the joint has been penetrated or exposed, antibiotic therapy must be commenced as early as possible and if inadequate drainage is a factor, this should be corrected. Antiphlogistic treatment also is of value. Small granulations frequently can be controlled with copper sulfate which is applied as a paste under a pressure bandage for 48 hours.

J. W. BRITTON

CHAPTER 27

SURGICAL PROCEDURES

INTRODUCTION

Cosmopolitan surgery is an appropriate and descriptive name for the material presented in this chapter. Obviously the authors have drawn on many varied experiences and references (local and foreign) and with typical Yankee ingenuity have added elaborations of their own. A diversity of methods, opinions, and conclusions is bound to exist in any book with multiple authorship.

The editor of the surgery section believes that there often is a fine line between fact and opinion, and though not always in complete agreement the experiences and accomplishments of the authors have demonstrated evidence of success with the reported procedures.

Some [authors] have emphasized fundamentals and detailed descriptions, but others have excluded them in the belief that the reader has already reached some degree of surgical competency.

There are obvious omissions but these concern matters considered to be of a routine nature, and they already have been documented in existing texts. Future editions of this volume will include these descriptions, together with such refinements as time and progress permit.

As a result of these pages it is hoped that the reader will be able to face difficult surgical situations with a feeling of facility and confidence.

L. E. JOHNSON

CASTRATION

Castration is one of the most common surgical procedures that the veterinarian is requested to perform. The reasons for castrating a horse are many and varied. One reason is to increase the animal's tractability, particularly that of a mean or studdish horse. A gelding performs much better than a stallion, whether used for racing or as a draft horse. This particularly is true when the animal is used with or near mares. Following castration many dangerous stallions have a changed disposition and become quite tractable around humans. Elimination of certain secondary sexual characteristics such as an overdeveloped crest may be desirable in many animals. The poorly bred or inferior animal should be castrated to avoid transmission of undesirable characteristics. Finally, organic disease of the testicle such as a Sertoli-cell tumor is definite indication for castration.

It is advisable to make a complete examination of the scrotal area to ascertain that the testicles are present and that there is no evidence of hydrocele or hernia. Special precautions must be taken if hernia is suspected, or a prolapse of omentum or bowel may follow castration. Presence of cryptorchidism eliminates the prospect of using the standing castration technic.

Castration in the standing position has the advantage of avoiding injuries which may occur in casting a horse. It also is possible to operate in this manner with only one assistant who holds the horse by the head, whereas usually 2 or more assistants are required when the animal is cast. The time needed for the standing castration is less than that required for castration after casting.

If the animal is difficult to handle, an intravenous injection of a tranquilizer, such as Promazine at a dose of ¼ to ½ mg. per lb. of body weight, may be helpful in quieting the horse. Preparatory to surgery, the scrotum is thoroughly cleansed with a surgical soap. The sheath is washed and if a cage or ring is on the penis it is removed. The scrotal skin is painted with an antiseptic, as tincture of Zephiran. Local anesthesia of the skin is obtained with a 0.5 to 1.0% procaine solution, using a 22-gauge needle and a 10 ml., 3-ring tonsil syringe. An attendant restrains the horse with a twitch applied on the upper lip during the initial injections, which are the most sensitive. The skin injections are made midline over each testicle in a linear fashion. Usually

10 ml. of local anesthetic is sufficient for each testicle.

The 3-ring syringe (which provides complete control at all times during injection) then is used, with a 5-inch sharply beveled 18- or 19-gauge needle attached, to puncture the anesthetized area over the testicle. The needle is directed upward through the testicle, and after reaching its dorsal aspect 2 or 3 ml. of procaine are deposited. The needle then is advanced further into the posterior part of the spermatic cord and the remaining 7 or 8 ml. of procaine are deposited there. As the anesthetic is injected, the subsequent swelling can be felt between the forefinger and thumb. It must be remembered that the anterior portion of the spermatic cord contains the spermatic artery enclosed in the pampiniform plexus of veins. To inject the local anesthetic in this area is useless from the standpoint of obtaining anesthesia.

Both testicles are injected in this manner and the animal is turned loose in the stall for 15 minutes while anesthesia develops. Immediately preparatory to surgery the twitch is applied again to prevent the animal from moving and complicating the surgery. The skin is painted with Zephiran and the testicles are checked to determine if anesthesia is adequate.

The surgeon usually stands on the left side of the horse in the flank region and grasps both testicles in the left gloved hand. An incision is made through the anesthetized skin, dartos, tunica vaginalis, and into the testicle. The incision is made with a #12 Bard-Parker blade on a #3 handle. The 2 incisions are made in rapid succession and the scalpel is laid aside. The left testicle is released and the right one is retained in the left hand. A right angle kidney pedicle clamp is applied with the right hand to the pampiniform plexus directly above the testicle. The other testicle then is grasped and similarly clamped. This is done to avoid and control hemorrhage. The tunica vaginalis then is grasped with an Iowa membrane forceps (a long curved Allis forceps used in gynecological surgery). With light tension, using the left hand, an 8- or 10″-curved scissors is used to separate the tunic from the main portion of the cord, particularly in the posterior

portion where it forms the scrotal ligament. This permits removal of a greater length of cord. With this accomplished, the spermatic cord is completely exposed and the emasculator is applied above the pedicle clamps. A satisfactory emasculator is the Hauptner. This is a German-made emasculator which completely crushes before it cuts and separates the testicle from the cord.

The emasculator is left on the left testicle while the opposite one is prepared. Just prior to removal of the emasculator a large Ochsner forceps is applied to the anterior portion of the cord, or pampiniform plexus, and allowed to remain in place until the following day. This procedure will help avoid the occurrence of postoperative hemorrhage. Both cords are handled in the same manner.

Tetanus antitoxin is administered either before or after surgery. I prefer to tie the horse for 30 minutes immediately after surgery to prevent his running around the stall.

Adequate exercise must be provided postoperatively. It is preferable to accomplish this by jogging or trotting to obtain a massaging action on the operated area and sheath. It is better to exercise twice daily rather than once over an extended period. Thorough cleansing of the operated area daily to remove exudate, and application of a suitable antiseptic will materially assist in avoiding postoperative complications, such as infection and swelling of the sheath and scrotal area.

The described technic represents a combination of various technics which have been used in the past.

W. O. REED

CASTRATION IN RECUMBENCY

Because most surgeons are right-handed the horse should be cast on his left side. After the skin over the scrotal area is prepared for surgery, the bottom or left testicle is grasped and drawn to the bottom and posterior part of the scrotum where it is immobilized with the left hand. A 4-inch-long incision is made 1 inch lateral to the median raphe through the skin, intervening tissues, and the tunica vaginalis.

As the testicle emerges through the incision, it is grasped with the right hand while the middle finger of the left hand is thrust through the mesorchium. Care should be taken not to twist the testicle at this time, as this may cause loss of orientation in reference to the location of the large blood vessels supplying the testicle. These vessels are always in the anterior part of the cord. A pair of Oschner forceps is inserted along the cord to a point where the tunica vaginalis may be grasped. After it has been set on the tunic, traction is exerted and the tunica vaginalis is withdrawn through the incision. Another Oschner forceps then is used to grasp the opposite side of the tunic. With the middle finger of the left hand penetrating the mesorchium and the 2 Oschner forceps held between the thumb and index finger of the left hand, traction is exerted on the forceps to expose the maximum amount of tunica vaginalis. With the right hand, the subcutaneous tissue around the tunic is separated. This is done so that a minimum of 4 inches of tunica vaginalis is freed of extraneous tissue. The emasculator then is placed around the tunic and its contents and closed, thus removing the testicle. The emasculator should be left in place for a minimum of 1 minute to provide maximum hemostasis. The emasculator may be left in place while the right or upper testicle is prepared for removal.

On occasion the surgeon may wish to exercise his prerogative of establishing positive hemostasis by ligating the spermatic artery and vein. This deviation in method is used when it is felt that the crushing action of the emasculator will not be sufficient to prevent excessive postoperative hemorrhage. Likely candidates for ligation are animals in whom there is an enlargement of the blood vessels supplying the testicles, e.g. the aged stallion, one who has been used for breeding purposes, stallions with testicular tumors, etc.

Ligation is easily accomplished by slightly modifying the previously described technic. At the point when the operator holds the testicle and both Oschner forceps in the left hand, a pair of blunt scissors is placed over the edge of the tunica vaginalis between the two forceps and pushed well up into the inguinal canal. By splitting the tunic in this way, the blood vessels are laid bare on the anterior side of the cord and are easily accessible for ligation. The ligature should be placed high enough on the cord so that it is not disturbed when the emasculator is used.

One of the most important features of this operation is the provision of drainage. It is said that horses never die from overdrainage of a castration wound, but only from underdrainage. With this in mind, the skin incision on the left side is enlarged in the direction of the inguinal canal until it is approximately 8 inches long. The incision on the right side is enlarged in the same manner.

Postoperative care includes the administration of 1500 units of tetanus antitoxin and recommendations to the owner as to exercise. Exercise should be provided twice daily for a period of 1 week. At each exercise period the horse should be trotted for 20 minutes or a mile, whichever comes first. In this way, drainage is encouraged, thus reducing the possibility of ascending infections, swelling or edema, and pain.

CRYPTORCHIDISM

A cryptorchid is a horse whose testicles have not decended. Synonyms are ridgling, original, and high-flanker. The diagnosis of cryptorchidism can be difficult, particularly if the horse has had several owners. The problem arises when the horse has been purchased as a gelding and then is found to be "studdish." Examination of his scrotum may reveal scars on both sides causing the veterinarian to wonder whether only one testicle was removed, whether both are retained, or if one testicle was removed, which one is retained. Rectal palpation can be helpful in such instances. Location of a testicle in this way eliminates the need for surgical exploration of both inguinal canals. If a canal is explored without doing a rectal examination and a cord stump is found within the canal it may be assumed that the retained testicle is located on the opposite side. Since more than 50% of retained testicles are found to involve the left side, this should help in deciding which inguinal canal to explore first.

Technic: Cryptorchidism may be unilateral or bilateral, but most cases are unilateral. Two operative sites are available for surgical intervention. A grid incision may be made in the flank (see page 725). Alternatively, the incision may be made through the scrotum. When the left testicle is retained, skin and fascia of the left scrotum are incised. The incision should be ample to readily permit passage of the operator's hand. There is no further need for a knife after the original incision is made because the tissues of the canal are easily separated with the fingers as the canal is explored. Failure to find the testicle within the canal necessitates breaking the peritoneum and entering the abdominal cavity. The testicle commonly is found to have an elongated attachment on the medial-posterior quarter of the internal inguinal ring. Should it not be located here, the surrounding area must be examined. Rolling the animal to the side being explored may force the testicle toward the ring. After it is located, the testicle is withdrawn through the canal to the exterior for emasculation.

In true cryptorchidism, there is no tunic on the testicle (but those of high-flankers do), nor is the epididymis attached closely to the testicle. Therefore, extreme care should be taken to make certain that all of the epididymis is delivered through the incision before emasculating the testicle.

Entrance into the abdominal cavity necessitates packing the canal with gauze. This is best done by using a gauze pack 1 yard wide and 3 yards long. The gauze is folded so as to be 6 inches wide and 3 yards long. Care should be taken to avoid placing any part of the pack in the abdominal cavity because it may adhere to the intestines. It is inserted only to the edge of the internal ring. The gauze is placed in the canal in an orderly accordion-like fashion so that it may be removed with ease. One suture placed through the skin of the scrotum and the end of the gauze pack is sufficient. Twenty-four hours later, the skin

suture is removed and 1 yard of the gauze is pulled from the canal and cut off. One yard is removed on each of the 2 succeeding days.

Pre- and Postoperative Care: It is best to withhold bulk-producing feed for at least 36 hours prior to surgery. The patient may have grain and water, however. By reducing the bulk, it is easier to locate the testicle. It also reduces the chances of postoperative hernia. Postoperatively, the animal is kept standing and partially fasted for 72 hours to reduce the chances of hernia. On the fourth day, the horse may be released in the stall and fed small amounts of hay again. The usual postoperative medication includes tetanus antitoxin, three million units of long-lasting penicillin every 72 hours for 2 doses, plus 1¼ Gm. of dihydrostreptomycin every 6 hours until a total of 15 Gm. have been given.

High-flankers present no special problems and they are castrated in the usual manner. On occasion, it is difficult to palpate a testicle high in the inguinal canal when the horse is standing. While in the recumbent position and under general anesthesia, there is enough relaxation, however, so that the testicle may be palpated. Rarely is it necessary to pack the canal or take the postoperative precautions recommended for cryptorchidism.

L. E. JOHNSON

CASTRATION OF FOALS

Detailed references in past literature concerning early castration are difficult to find. Vague mention of castration at an early age was made by O'Connor in 1938 and the technic was described in detail by Formston in 1951. It was also described by me in 1960. This present report refers to experiences over the past 10 years in which more than 400 colts, all aged between 15 and 24 weeks, were castrated. The majority of these animals were offspring of a breeding herd of Thoroughbreds crossed with Welsh or New Forest ponies. They roam, virtually wild, on marshland in Great Britain.

Though castration of the horse generally is advocated at the age of 1 or 2 years, there are certain advantages in castrating at an early age in special circumstances. Anesthesia may be given safely with little help, and risks to man and patient are minimal. The procedure has been found to be ideal when large numbers are to be castrated at one time.

Technic: A mask similar to the Cox-type inhaler is used. It is made of canvas and therefore is lighter, easier to handle, and more easily tightened to fit the different head sizes of young colts. The subject's nostrils are lubricated with vaseline. A lead rope is attached to both sides of the halter usually, but not necessarily, with an assistant on each lead. The mask is then slid under the face bands of the halter enclosing the upper and lower jaws, and fastened over the poll. A swab soaked with 4 to 8 drams of chloroform is inserted into the mask, and the end is laced tight. (The efficacy of chloroform as a general anesthetic is appraised in Chapter 2.)

Anesthesia is started in the standing position. There normally is some struggling but this can be controlled easily, especially if the halter ropes are relatively long and the animal is allowed to remain reasonably free to move. The ropes should be kept taut and the assistants should stay about 5 feet from the head, on each side and slightly forward. This permits good control of the colt with little risk to either the assistants or the animal. Usually within 3 to 6 minutes, the horse sinks to the ground. One assistant controls the head with the animal in lateral recumbency. As soon as the patient is reasonably relaxed, *i.e.*, with the tail limp and the corneal reflex barely present, a looped rope is attached to the uppermost hindlimb. The limb is then pulled forward. If the halter leads are long, one of them can be passed under the neck and over the front of the withers and used to tie the upper limb.

The surgical site is prepared in the normal manner and the testicle, within the scrotum, is held between the index finger and thumb. An incision is made through skin, dartos, and fascia thus exposing the testicle. The tunica vaginalis is incised, the body of the testicle gripped, and the scrotal ligament severed. The vascular portion of the cord is ligated as high in the inguinal canal as possible, using No. 2 chromic catgut, and the cord is severed below the ligature with an emasculator.

The manner of ligation is a matter of choice; it may be a transfixing ligature or a modification which "beds" the ligature by clamping forceps on the area intended for ligation, releasing them and then tying the ligature over the pressed tissues. This modification tends to prevent slipped ligatures and enables the operator to obtain maximum tightness of suture tie.

The stump is returned to the inguinal canal and the other testicle is removed similarly. The scrotal wound is not sutured. The operative site is cleansed and the hindlimb released. Tetanus antitoxin can be injected at this time. The mask is then removed and the foal should be on its feet unassisted within 4 to 10 minutes. It is feasible to castrate as many as 6 colts an hour with this procedure. After the operation and recovery from anesthesia, the foal is returned to the mare. As a general rule the scrotal swelling is negligible. Small hematomas occasionally occur but are best left alone.

D. G. LEWIS

REFERENCES

Dollar's Veterinary Surgery, 3rd ed., 331.
Formston: Vet. Rec. **63**:2 (1951) 18.
Lewis, D. G.: Vet. Rec. **72**:11 (1960) 212.

LARYNGEAL VENTRICULECTOMY

This operation is performed for the relief of clinical signs arising from paralysis of the muscles controlling the arytenoid cartilages (particularly the left one) of the larynx of the horse. In this condition the left recurrent nerve undergoes degeneration which results in paralysis of the vocal cord (see Chapter 14). The relaxed cord and arytenoid cartilage obstruct inspiration and produce a noise when the horse is exercised beyond a walk. This noise may be slight and high-pitched (identifies a whistler), or it may be a deeper tone (identifies a roarer).

The operation is intended to cause a firm and complete adhesion of the arytenoid cartilage and vocal cord to the medial face of the thyroid cartilage. This is the normal position during forced inspiration when air passes unrestricted.

Diagnosis of the condition is best accomplished by laryngoscopic examination. A right angle scope 1 mm. by 17 inches in length (American Cystoscope Company) is used. With the larynx adequately illuminated, examination of the typical roarer will reveal paralysis of the left arytenoid cartilage and the left vocal cord. With the aid of a twitch, sufficient time can be taken to observe the movement and position of the arytenoid cartilages during each inspiration. If a laryngoscope is not available, exercise may produce characteristic signs of laryngeal hemiplegia, but these signs may have other causes. The diagnostic signs in the exercised horse are dyspnea and a roaring sound made during inspiration.

Although surgical correction for laryngeal hemiplegia can be done with the horse standing, many surgeons prefer to administer a general anesthetic and to position the animal on his back. Inhalation anesthesia may be used satisfactorily. It is administered through a 28-mm. endotracheal catheter. It might seem that the presence of a catheter would hamper the surgeon but this is not the case. The head should be extended but not unduly so.

After the area has been cleansed and prepared for surgery, a longitudinal incision is made through the skin and fascia over the larynx as nearly as possible on the median raphe commencing at the anterior extremity of the thyroid cartilage and extending downward and backward to the region of the first tracheal ring. The incision is made with a #10 Bard-Parker blade on a #3 Bard-Parker handle. The sterno-hyoideus muscle then is separated on the median line with the scalpel and by blunt dissection down to the crico-thyroid membrane. This structure is triangular in form and is bordered anteriorly and laterally by the thyroid cartilage and posteriorly by the cricoid ring. It is possible to mistake the space between the cricoid and first tracheal ring for

the crico-thyroid membrane. This is avoided by careful palpation of the triangular crico-thyroid membrane whose apex is directed forward and whose lateral borders are sharply defined by the hard borders of the alae of the thyroid cartilage. The base of the triangle rests upon the more elastic borders of the cricoid cartilage.

After having identified the crico-thyroid membrane it is incised on the median line through its length. A Rigby retractor is used to expose the larynx. Preference for this instrument is based upon the fact that its blades are longer and wider, thus providing better exposure. A glove stretcher forceps then is used to grasp and tense the mucous membrane of the ventricle. With the glove stretcher forceps inserted into the saccule and with mild tension being applied, an incision is made on the median margin of the saccule with a #15 Bard-Parker Blade on a #7 handle. The incision is made as far as possible both anteriorly and posteriorly. The Rigby retractor then is removed and the index finger of the left hand is inserted into the saccule and with mild pressure being exerted between the incised saccule and the rim of the ventricle, the mucous membrane is separated and everted.

The Rigby retractor is inserted again into the wound and an 8-inch Carmalt forceps is used to grasp the incised margin of the mucous membrane. With a gentle twisting action of the Carmalt forceps in the left hand the mucous membrane is exposed, cut, and removed with a 7"-sharply curved scissors. The excised mucous membrane should be stretched over a gloved finger or thumb immediately and carefully examined to determine if the entire saccule has been removed. If it has not been entirely removed, the remaining mucosa should be grasped with either a Carmalt or Allis forceps and removed.

The next step is very important. It involves the use of electric cautery coupled with a Bucy-Frazier aspirator. The purpose of this procedure is to completely remove blood by suction and, at the same time, to control continuing hemorrhage with electric cautery. This is done with the aid of a metal tongue depressor and with the Rigby retractor in position to expose all of the surgical area. Cauterization enhances complete adhesion of the operated site. Some surgeons also remove the prolapsed vocal cords at this time. This is done by grasping one end of the affected cord with a Carmalt forceps and removing its entire length with a curved scissors.

If a cordectomy is performed, cautery with the Bucy-Frazier apparatus is done again. It is preferable not to operate the right side of the larynx if it is normal. The operative site is left open for drainage.

An immediate postoperative danger is acute laryngeal edema, which causes respiratory distress. Careful observation is made to detect this complication. If dyspnea does occur, a laryngeal tube may be inserted temporarily. The operative wound is dilated by using a clean tongue depressor and spreading the lips of the operative area, to improve the air flow, thus relieving the patient. In persistent cases, a tracheotomy may be performed and a tracheotomy tube inserted.

Aftercare consists of thoroughly cleansing the operative site twice daily and the application of a suitable mild antiseptic. It is preferable to confine the horse as long as 30 days for adequate healing. At the end of this time, the animal can be exercised lightly.

W. O. Reed

HERNIAS

Introduction

In the broad sense a hernia is the protrusion of a loop or portion of an organ or tissue through an abnormal opening. Nearly all hernias in the horse are located in the region of the abdomen. They are either internal or external and the latter occur much more frequently in the horse. An external abdominal hernia is a protrusion of a portion of the abdominal contents through accidental or enlarged natural openings in the abdominal wall into the subcutis. The skin and usually the peritoneum remain intact and cover the protruded contents.

All hernias have a ring or opening, contents, and sac. The ring consists of the tissues at the opening in the abdominal wall. The contents usually are the small intestines although other tissues such as the omentum may be included. The sac is composed of the skin and the thickened parietal peritoneum. One often refers to the neck as that part of the sac which is continuous with the ring.

Abdominal hernias are commonly classified according to location, contents, condition, and cause:

1. Location – umbilical, inguinal, scrotal, and ventral. A ventral hernia occurs in the linea alba or at points of the abdominal wall other than the inguinal or umbilical openings.

2. Contents—intestinal (enterocele), urinary bladder (cystocele), omental (omentocele), etc.

3. Condition—reducible, irreducible, strangulated, gangrenous, etc.

4. Cause—congenital, acquired, traumatic, incisional, etc. A hernia thus may be identified as a congenital, reducible, umbilical enterocele.

Umbilical and scrotal hernias which appear at birth or shortly thereafter usually are congenital, and some are considered to be inherited—especially scrotal hernias. Any defect in the abdominal wall predisposes acquired abdominal hernias. Such defects are caused mainly by trauma and abscesses. Straining may be a precipitating cause of herniation as may any external force or trauma.

Clinical Signs of Abdominal Hernias

Umbilical and ventral hernias commonly appear as spherical enlargements and have a definite ring or opening which is palpable. A similar but somewhat elongated swelling in the inguinal region which may be extended to involve the scrotum also is readily recognized. The scrotum will be markedly enlarged either unilaterally or bilaterally.

Hernias may become irreducible due to adhesions or when the contents are too large to return to the abdominal cavity. If strangulation occurs there is evidence of acute inflammation. The enlargement becomes edematous, firm, and painful. The strangulated tissue becomes darkened and necrotic. When signs of digestive disorder and intestinal obstruction occur, death follows rapidly.

DIAGNOSIS OF ABDOMINAL HERNIAS

Palpation will distinguish a reducible from an irreducible hernia. The important thing to identify is the condition which causes the latter to be irreducible. This often is determined during surgery. One can easily detect adhesions if they are present. Darkened and hemorrhagic intestines are evidence that strangulation has occurred.

An enlargement at the umbilicus may be an abscess, cyst, tumor, or hematoma. Aspiration of their contents will aid in differentiating these conditions from hernias.

Rectal palpation always should be made, especially on young stallions showing colicky signs. By so doing, one may detect a portion of the small intestines entering the internal inguinal ring. Through careful manipulation this often may be replaced into the abdominal cavity.

PROGNOSIS FOR ABDOMINAL HERNIAS

The size and location of the hernia and the age of the animal must be considered when making the prognosis. It seems a logical assumption that large hernias would have large rings but this is not always true. In many umbilical or ventral hernias, constant abdominal pressure forces the contents to undermine the skin. This results in a large hernial mass with a relatively small ring.

It is well-known that umbilical, inguinal, and scrotal hernias, when present at birth or shortly thereafter, may disappear spontaneously by the time foals become yearlings. This may occur provided that the hernial ring is not excessively enlarged or that its contents are irreducible. An acquired umbilical hernia with a 3- to 4-inch ring in an older animal warrants a more guarded prognosis than one with a smaller ring in a yearling. It should be pointed out that hernial contents may be strangulated at any time. This is particularly true

of scrotal hernias. For this reason many surgeons advise early correction of all hernias.

Inguinal and scrotal hernias, because of their location, are subjected to trauma which causes inflammation and pain. This may result in adhesions and an irreducible hernia.

Recently acquired hernias are more dangerous than those of longer standing; this is due to the lack of a well-formed ring in the former. Accidental hernias are more serious than those occurring through natural openings. In hernias through other than natural openings the rings usually are more narrow and slit-like, thus strangulation and adhesions are more likely to occur.

CORRECTION OF ABDOMINAL HERNIAS

The objective in the treatment of hernias is to replace the protruded contents to their normal position, and to prevent recurrence.

The most rigid aseptic precautions must be followed if herniorrhaphy is to be successful. It will be assumed, therefore, in the description which follows that presurgical preparation, sterilization of instruments, drapes, and gloves, as well as restraint and anesthesia have been done carefully.

Many methods have been described for the surgical correction of hernias. The size of the hernial ring, type of hernia, age of animal, and condition of the abdominal wall all have a direct influence on the choice of the method selected.

UMBILICAL HERNIA

In years past, the application of blisters and the injection of irritants were used extensively to correct umbilical hernias. Success with these methods depended upon their ability to stimulate scar tissue formation which filled the ring. These methods were used on small hernial rings approximately an inch in length. Success was not only lacking in many instances but it was much more difficult to reduce the hernias subsequently due to the excessive induration following such treatment.

Metal skewers were employed in another method which falls into the same category.

After reducing the hernial contents, 2 skewers were inserted at right angles to each other. They passed through the skin and peritoneal sac, then through the sac and skin on the opposite side. They were positioned as close to the ring as possible. A heavy cord or suture was then wrapped several times around the neck and between the skewers and abdominal wall. At each wrap moderate tension was placed on the suture and the final wrap was tied securely. The long ends of the skewers were cut and the remaining ends bent into small loops to prevent injury to the surrounding skin. The objective of this technic was to stimulate scar tissue formation in the ring. The necrotic sac would eventually slough.

A satisfactory method for hernias with small rings is to place a few horizontal mattress sutures through the neck of the sac. They should be so spaced that approximately a quarter of an inch remains intact between them. This allows sufficient blood supply for the sac and at the same time the pressure of the sutures will stimulate sufficient scarring to close the ring. The sutures should be removed in about 20 days.

Metal clamps have been used successfully on hernial rings that are as large as 3 or 4 inches in diameter. The clamp is placed over the sac which is pulled between the 2 adjacent bars after it is ascertained that the parietal peritoneum is included. The clamp is manipulated to insure that no intestines are retained within the sac. It is forced as close to the ring as possible, then tightened by the bolts and wing nuts which are on each end. The clamp should not be set too tightly as it is likely to cut the skin and this should not occur before scar tissue has had time to develop. The bars should only exert enough pressure to arrest circulation. The clamp may be held in position by a wide bandage circumscribing the abdomen, and it usually is left in position until sloughing occurs. Daily examination of the animal should be made postoperatively.

A more acceptable variation in the use of the clamp from that described involves the addition of sutures in the neck of the sac. These are placed immediately under the clamp or through the long slit-like opening in each bar. A baseball or cobbler's stitch is made by using a long straight cutting needle on each end of the suture. Umbilical tape is very satisfactory although other types of suture may be used. Starting at one end a needle is inserted approximately a quarter of an inch in from the edge of the sac. The suture is pulled halfway through, then the other needle is placed in the skin opening where the first one emerged. This half is pulled through its entire length, thus

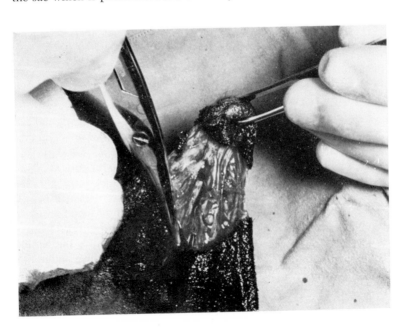

Fig. 1. Tension placed on isolated skin reduces danger of lacerating peritoneal portion of sac during blunt dissection.

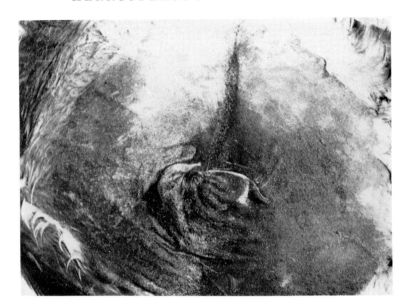

Fig. 2. Presurgical appearance shows amount of redundant skin comprising hernial sac.

forming a snug loop around the skin at the end of the sac. This procedure is continued across the entire neck. Sufficient tension is applied during the suturing to arrest circulation. The suture is then securely tied. The clamp may be left in position but it usually is removed.

Still another satisfactory method of hernial reduction is to make two elliptical incisions, starting and ending together over the convex surface of the sac. This produces an elliptical island of skin (Fig. 1). The amount of the skin removed should be slightly longer than the size of the ring. This particular step is taken to eliminate the considerable amount of redundant skin remaining at the end of the operation when the skin sutures are placed (Fig. 2).

The skin is separated by dissection from the underlying thickened peritoneal portion of the sac which should be completely exposed. Still further dissection should be done to expose the fascia for an area of approximately an inch beyond the entire circumference of the ring. From this point one of several technics can be used to close the ring. A method sometimes used in reduction of umbilical hernias is to place a purse string suture in the neck of the sac, then completely invert the sac and tie.

Open reduction of umbilical hernias is done frequently. Any of several methods is satisfactory. The sac is exposed in its entirety as described before. It is completely excised with the exception of a small portion which is left as a flap on one side of the ring (Fig. 3A). The flap should be trimmed so that it is 1 or 2 inches wide at the center and tapers at each commissure. The amount of flap depends on the size of the hernial opening. The hernial ring is closed by placing a series of mattress sutures through its edges. The illustration makes it appear as if the sutures were farther from the edge of the ring in the center than at the commissures. Actually the shape of the flap accounts for the appearance. The needle is passed inside through the entire wall. It is carried outside within the ring and entered into the opposite wall from the outside. It then is carried a quarter of an inch parallel to the ring edge and inside the wall. The needle then is passed through the wall to emerge outside. Next it is crossed to the original side and introduced inside the wall. It is directed outside opposite the point of original penetration (Fig. 3B). When these sutures are properly tightened and tied, the edge of the ring and flap overlap the opposite side. Interrupted sutures

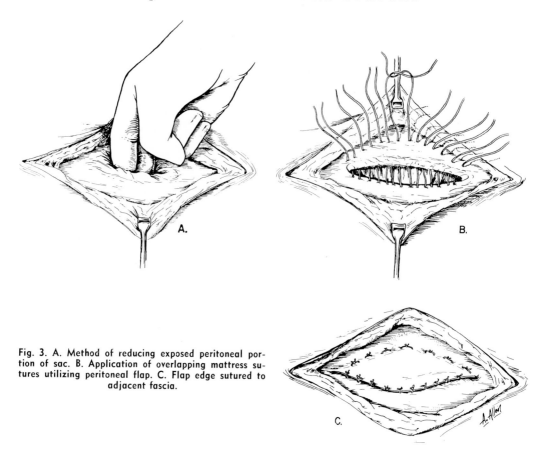

Fig. 3. A. Method of reducing exposed peritoneal portion of sac. B. Application of overlapping mattress sutures utilizing peritoneal flap. C. Flap edge sutured to adjacent fascia.

placed along the edge of the flap secure it to the abdominal fascia (Fig. 3C). This reinforces the area considerably.

Another procedure used when the ring is large makes use of stainless steel gauze. Exposure and extirpation of the hernial sac including a narrow (¼-inch) strip of the edge of the hernia ring are done. The wire gauze is cut to proper size, threaded with several stainless steel sutures placed about ¼ inch in from its edge, and then inserted into the abdomen and positioned immediately under the ring. The wire gauze should extend from ½ and ¾ inch beyond the circumference of the ring (Fig. 4). The free ends of the wire sutures are secured with forceps and brought through the fascia about ¼ inch from the edge of the hernial ring. Right- and left-handed Deschamps forceps are very useful for this purpose (Fig. 5). The end of the suture is threaded through the eye of the instrument and by rotating the wrist the instrument is pushed through the fascia, carrying the strand of the suture with it. This process is repeated with the other end of the suture. Forceps are again placed on the 2 ends. This entire process is repeated for each suture. After all are placed, they are tied individually. This technic holds the screen firmly against the peritoneum and internal surface of the fascia and ring. Connective tissue eventually will cover it. Some operators prefer to close the ring first, then place the mesh over the area and attach it to the fascia with a continuous suture around its circumference.

Ventral Hernia

The procedures used for repair of umbilical hernias apply generally for ventral hernias.

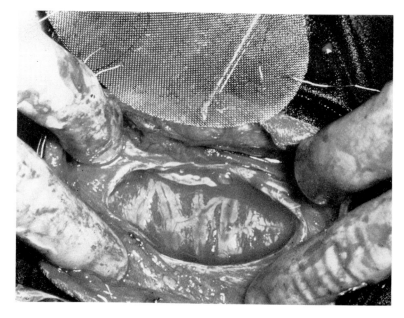

Fig. 4. Exposed ring with wire mesh screen containing cable wire sutures, prior to insertion into peritoneal cavity.

The latter, if long-standing, also have a definite ring developed. They usually are no more serious than reducible hernias in other locations.

If of recent origin, the ring usually is not well-developed and early repair is essential. The main difference is in closure; usually, ventral hernias require separate suturing of the tissue layers.

INGUINAL AND SCROTAL HERNIA

Inguinal and scrotal hernias have so much in common that they might well be discussed together. A 3- to 4-inch incision is made over the scrotum and parallel with the midline. It also may be made directly over the inguinal ring. The tissues are separated by dissection to isolate and free the testis within its parietal peritoneal covering. This should not be incised. The dissection is continued to expose the cord

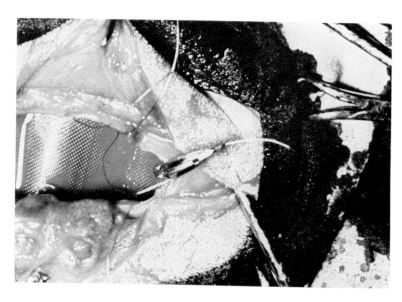

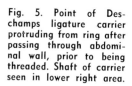

Fig. 5. Point of Deschamps ligature carrier protruding from ring after passing through abdominal wall, prior to being threaded. Shaft of carrier seen in lower right area.

to the external inguinal ring. By twisting the testis and cord, any contained intestines are forced into the abdominal cavity, providing the hernia is reducible.

Any one of several methods may be used to apply a transfixation ligature to the cord as close to the ring as possible. The testicle and cord then are removed with an emasculator. The cord stump should be included in these sutures as it helps close the ring. A sterile gauze pack may be placed in the canal for 24 hours. If a pack is used, a single skin suture is sufficient to hold the skin in place. Granulations usually develop and recovery is uneventful.

It is preferable to use subcutaneous sutures to obliterate any cavitation rather than to employ packing. The operation is completed with the application of skin sutures. They ordinarily must be removed unless subcuticular sutures are applied.

Aftercare should consist of moderate exercise and a daily check on temperature and general attitude. Tetanus antitoxin should always be given following surgery.

Incarcerated and Strangulated Hernias

Incarcerated hernias are corrected by any of the previously described methods of open reduction. In addition, one must remove the cause of incarceration. If adhesions are present, they must be carefully dissected to free the incarcerated tissues. If the ring is too small, it must be enlarged.

When strangulation develops, an immediate operation is necessary. If operated early, the strangulated intestines may only be congested. If it appears safe to replace them, this should be done after correcting the cause of the developing strangulation. In instances when strangulation has caused thrombosis of mesenteric blood vessels, intestinal resection is necessary.

The congested or anastomosed intestines should be manipulated as little as possible when they are replaced. They should never be pressed through the ring. This can be avoided by exposing a sufficient amount of healthy gut, then manipulating it in such a manner that the injured portion will pass through the ring in nearly a straight line.

Anesthesia for Hernia Operations (also see Chapter 2)

General anesthesia is required for any procedure involving open reduction and repair. Any one of several anesthetic agents or combination of agents may be used depending upon the preference of the surgeon and the requirements of the particular case.

J. F. Bullard

FURTHER DISCUSSION OF HERNIOPLASTY

Hernioplasty has few, if any, antecedents in the field of surgery. Historically, references to hernias may be found to occupy a prominent place in the earliest medical writings. The primitives of long ago, realizing the disabling properties of hernias, devised a crude truss. By using over the defect packets of leaves which were secured by thongs of hides or vines, they were able to afford themselves some degree of relief.

As time and knowledge increased, so the methods of hernial repair improved. Man eventually discovered metals and almost immediately applied them to the old problem of hernia repair. Petronius, in 1565, attempted the implantation of gold plating as a substitute for tissue in the repair of abdominal defects. Other investigators tried silver, platinum, aluminum, brass, nickel, and many other metals and alloys. Only in the past few years have surgeons used metals, which are sufficiently physiologically inert for implantation into living tissues. These metals are vitallium, tantalum, and a special kind of stainless steel. Still more recently, the surgeon's armamentarium of tissue substitutes has been enhanced by various types of plastics.

In the horse, the majority of hernias occur at the umbilicus. These usually are present at birth and if still present after the first 3 or 4 months, they generally require some sort of surgical treatment.

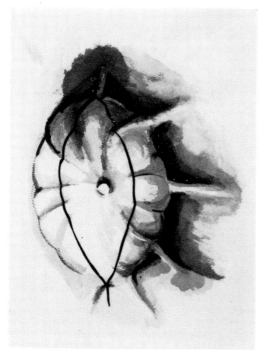

Fig. 6. Skin excised over hernial sac.

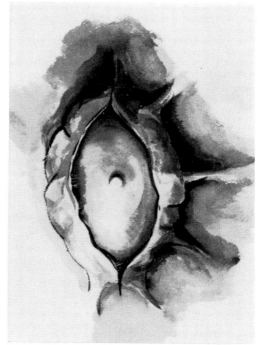

Fig. 7. Exposure of hernial sac.

The etiology, classification, and some treatments for hernias have been presented in the preceding discussion. The following is intended as an addition to the surgical procedures for repair. It deals with 2 different methods of repair.

The first method is referred to as the overlapping technic and enjoys wide usage and success. The second method is a new procedure designed to fit special situations. It involves the use of sliding fascial flaps.

For proper repair of a hernia 2 requirements must be satisfied. They are: 1. Obliteration of the hernial sac, and 2, repair of the defect. The methods to be described satisfy these 2 requirements.

OVERLAPPING METHOD

After proper preparation of the surgical site, draping of the field, and administration of a general anesthetic, an elliptical piece of skin is dissected from the hernial sac (Fig.

6, 7). The hernia should not be reduced during this procedure since distention of the sac facilitates dissection. After the entire sac has been completely dissected free of the skin and abdominal wall (Fig. 8, 9), the intact sac and its contents are pushed into the abdominal cavity (Fig. 10). An Eisele needle #428-2, a noncutting, half-circle needle, is threaded with a 15-inch double strand of #2 extra chromic catgut in preparation for placement of the overlapping mattress sutures (Fig. 11).

The suture should be started ½ to 1 inch from the edge of the ring and is carried through the entire thickness of the abdominal wall on both sides of the ring. A finger is placed in the inverted sac to determine the depth of the needle in the wall of the abdomen; this also prevents the inadvertent inclusion of intestines with the suture. The width of one suture should be approximately 1 inch with ½ inch between individual sutures. After the sutures are placed, all the ends are pulled simultaneously to effect the overlap (Fig. 12).

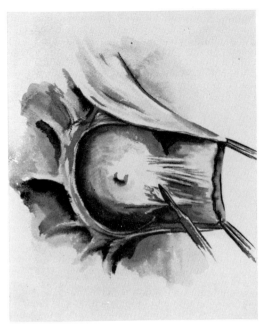

Fig. 8. Sac is dissected from skin and abdominal wall.

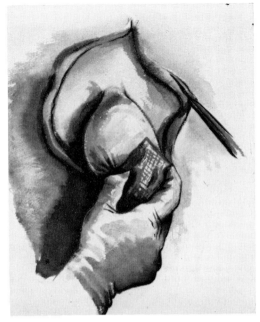

Fig. 9. Sac freed of attachments.

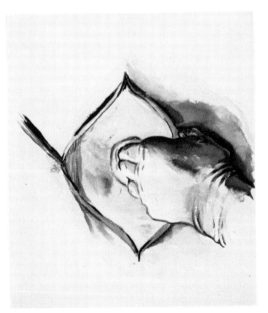

Fig. 10. Hernial sac is replaced into abdominal cavity.

While an assistant maintains tension the sutures are tied individually. Since there is tension on the sutures when they are being tied, care must be taken to maintain firm contact between the overlapped portions of the ring. Interrupted sutures, using the same needle but a single strand of the same catgut, are placed between each overlapping suture. This not only insures good apposition of the overlapped tissues but prevents the escape of any portion of the hernial sac.

The advantages of this method are as follows: 1. Should wound disruption occur for any reason during convalescence the abdominal contents are protected by the intact sac, 2, the invaginated portion of the sac heals together, thus adding some strength to the repair, 3, there is minimal contact with the peritoneal cavity (it is possible to put all sutures extraperitoneally by pushing the peritoneum away from the ring edge), 4, it satisfies the 2 criteria for satisfactory hernia repair, and 5, it requires less time than some modifications of this method.

REPAIR WITH SLIDING FASCIAL FLAPS

Most umbilical hernia rings in the horse are oval with only slightly thickened, pliable edges, thus lending themselves well to the overlapping technic. There are situations, however, when almost the reverse is true. The

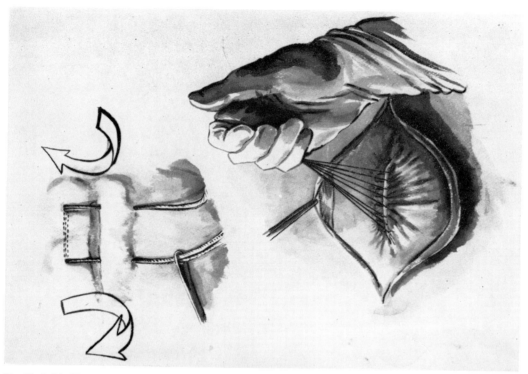

Fig. 11 (left). Placement of overlying mattress sutures.

Fig. 12 (right). Sutures tensed to effect overlap.

rings may be found to be round, thickened to such a degree as to be osseo-ligamentous in character, and so rigid as to make the overlapping technic virtually impossible.

It is for this latter group of conditions that the fascial flap method was designed. In this procedure the fascia of the abdominal tunic is used to repair the defect and to maintain obliteration of the sac. The ring itself plays only a passive role in the repair.

Technic: Dissection of the hernial sac is carried out as described for the overlapping method. After the sac has been completely freed from the abdomen and surrounding tissues, dissection of the skin and subcutaneous tissues is carried laterally (on both sides of the ring) for a distance slightly in excess of half the diameter of the ring. The fact that the abdominal tunic and the ventral sheath of the rectus muscle blend at this point is of only academic interest since they are clinically indivisible. If one is repairing a hernia with a ring 4 inches in diameter, dissection should be carried laterally a distance of 2½ inches on

either side of the ring in order to provide an equal amount of fascia from both sides to cover the defect. At this predetermined point an incision is made through the abdominal tunic starting 2 inches anterior to the ring and extending to a point 2 inches posterior to the ring. A similar incision then is made on the other side of the ring (Fig. 13). Through these incisions one may see fibers of the rectus muscle. Since the rectus muscle has not been disturbed and because it also has a dorsal sheath, no weakening of this area may be expected. Also, the incisions fill in with fibrous tissue which aids in repairing the damage.

By using a noncutting needle as previously described and #2 extra chromic catgut, interrupted sutures are used to draw the fascia together over the ring and invaginated sac (Fig. 14). The sutures are placed through the fascia only and at a point adjacent to the ring. All muscle tissue and the ring are excluded in the suture pattern. Between the elasticity of the fascia and the gaping of the incisions adequate tissue is obtained to cover the defect.

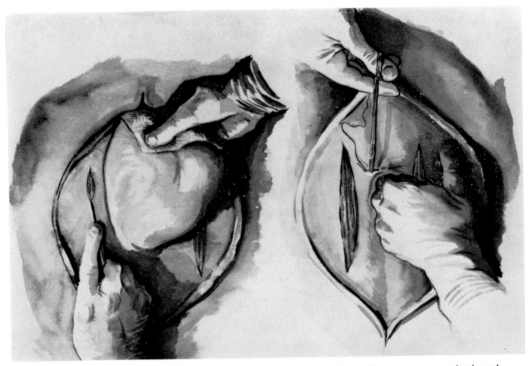

Fig. 13. Exposure and replacement of hernial sac. Two incisions on either side of ring are made through the abdominal tunic prior to suturing.

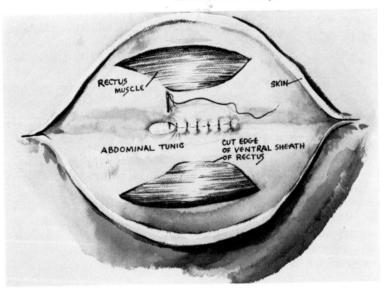

Fig. 14. Closure of abdominal tunic over hernial ring.

If the defect is unusually large and it is felt that additional strength is needed, metallic or plastic gauze may be sutured over the repair. Eventually, such appliances become ensheathed in dense fibrous tissue which acts as an added buttress against the abdominal contents.

A routine closure of the skin is used.

L. E. Johnson

LAPAROTOMY BY THE GRID INCISION

A grid incision provides easy access to the abdominal cavity with the least tissue disturbance and a minimum of suturing. The incision is placed to take advantage of the anatomic arrangement of the muscles which comprise the flank.

The purpose of using the flank as an operative site ordinarily is to circumvent some undesirable characteristic involving the usual or orthodox site. Familiarity with this approach, however, often induces one to use the procedure more and more frequently, even for the uncomplicated situation. Ideally, this approach is used for such surgical procedures as removal of testicles retained in the abdominal cavity, ovariectomies, palpation of abdominal contents, and possibly for the reduction and repair of scrotal hernias.

The advantages of the grid incision are as follows:

1. A minimum of surgical technic is needed.

2. After the initial incision is made through the skin and subcutaneous fascia, the knife may be discarded. Passage through the various layers of muscles is by blunt dissection.

3. Because the muscles are not divided surgically but only separated in the direction of the fibers, there is no temporary nor permanent loss of strength in the area.

4. The possibility of a postoperative hernia is greatly reduced, even in the event of wound dehiscence.

5. Wound closure requires skin sutures only.

6. The saving in time is increased because there is little need for attention to hemostasis.

Technic: It is best to use general anesthesia. The flank of choice is prepared for surgery. An 8"-incision is started midway between the tuber coxae and the last rib. The upper limit of the incision is at a level with the tuber coxae and it is carried distally for the prescribed distance. This is the only time when hemostasis is required. After the hemorrhage in the skin is controlled, an incision is made through the subcutaneous fascia in the same direction and for the same length as the skin incision. The fibers of the external oblique muscle are thus exposed as they pass downward and backward. The fibers are separated easily with the fingers for a distance of 6" to 8". This places the opening through the externus at an angle of 45° to the skin incision. Directly beneath the external oblique muscle the fibers of the internal oblique muscle may be seen running downward and forward at a 90° angle to the former muscle. The internal oblique also is divided easily with the fingers, thus revealing the transversus. The fibers of this muscle extend approximately dorsoventrally. They also are separated, together with the peritoneum, by the fingers. This places the opening through the transversus parallel, or nearly in line, with the skin incision.

From the foregoing it is apparent that no two adjacent incisions are parallel. In order for a hernia to develop, viscera would have to follow a circuitous course. Moreover, the musculature of the flank is tightened (in support of the abdomen and its contents) when the horse assumes a standing position. This action results in obliteration of the slit-like openings in the muscles. Therefore, closure of the wound is accomplished by suturing the skin only.

Aftercare consists of the usual restriction of physical activity, and the selection and administration of antibiotics which may be indicated. Four weeks is the usual convalescent period.

L. E. JOHNSON

SURGERY OF THE CARPUS

Carpal surgery in the horse first was done as a routine procedure in 1957.[1] This type of surgery, to be acceptable and successful, must be done aseptically as contamination of the carpal articulation jeopardizes the future usefulness of the racing animal. Unruly patients, however, can disrupt all efforts to maintain asepsis. Therefore, carpal surgery should be done with operating table restraint, or with the horse under general anesthesia and in an environment devoid of dust and insects. Strict adherence to these basic needs soon made a routine procedure out of the once forbidden surgical invasion of an equine joint cavity.

X-ray examination of cases which are presented for firing of the carpal area generally is necessary in order to give an intelligent prognosis. Fractures, sequestra, osteophytes, or osteochondrosis dissecans are considered to be poor prospects for successful firing. "Calcification" is a broad term that has been used to describe all of the mentioned lesions and their sequelae. The inadequacy of firing in cases of calcification led to an enthusiastic reception of the first reports concerning the use of gamma radiation for relief of clinical signs related to articular calcification and inflammation.[2] The sources of gamma radiation include the relatively soft gamma rays in x-rays and radium. Because of the danger of contamination, radium was superceded by the hard and relatively safe gamma radiation provided by the radioisotope, cobalt-60.[3]

Gamma radiation is relatively efficient in the treatment of carpal injuries. It prevents excessive calcium formation around fractures and actually causes some resorption of calcified tissue.[4]

INCIDENCE OF CARPAL LESIONS

In a series of 111 surgical cases there were 33 which involved the carpus. Almost ⅓ of the total cases presented for surgery in one equine practice involved removal of sequestra in the carpus, or of calcifications in the carpal or radiocarpal articulations.

In another series of 102 cases for which carpal surgery was done, the right leg was affected in 63 cases, the left leg in 34 cases. This difference was influenced by the practice of counting the removal of extensive calcifications which required 2 incisions as 2 separate cases. The locations of the fractures or calcifications were as follows:

Radial carpal bone, right	42	
Distal end of radius, right	8	
Third carpal bone, right	13	
	63	Total
Radial carpal bone, left	17	
Distal end of radius, left	11	
Third carpal bone, left	6	
	34	Total

Other carpal areas of both limbs	5	

CARPAL INJURIES

Etiology: Kicks, accidents in starting gates, accidents in stalls, and racing contribute to the etiology of carpal fractures. I am dubious about the importance of nutrition, heredity, or other diseases in the etiology of carpal fractures. Their incidence indicates that they are caused by trauma and the stress of racing. Whether it is induced by rapid starting, as when the Thoroughbred breaks out of the starting gate, by changing leads, by overextension of the carpus due to cupping of the racing surface, or to the stress created by "toe grabs" on racehorse plates is a matter for conjecture. One may wonder whether the percentage of right and left leg involvements would be reversed if racing were done in a clockwise direction.

Clinical Signs: The usual carpal fracture or calcification is characterized by pain on flexion or during palpation over the joint. The knee is warm to touch, particularly on the morning after a hard workout. Swelling may or may not be present; usually there is some increase in synovia.

The animal may be lame and refuse to change leads. He may bear out or lug in, particularly on the turns. Some horses take a few bad strides or become lame when "cooling-out," but are sound again until subjected to hard workouts. Many animals race successfully on such a fracture for the greater part of a season. As a result, this chronically inflamed area becomes infiltrated with a tremendous amount of calcium. Blood-tinged synovia is almost pathognomonic of a fracture or severe articular damage.

Diagnosis: The diagnosis is based on the clinical signs, the results of arthrocentesis, and radiographs. Routine radiography of suspicious carpal abnormalities will reveal osseous pathology that the owner, trainer, or attending veterinarian may not have suspected.

The x-ray examination should include a minimum of 5 views: anterior-posterior, 45° medial oblique, 45° lateral oblique, latero-medial, and a latero-medial with the carpus flexed.

Medicinal Therapy: Phenylbutazone, systemic corticosteroids, and salicylates allay the clinical signs. Aspiration of the increased synovia and injection of steroids intra-articularly are effective but they are only palliative measures.

SURGICAL TREATMENT OF CARPAL LESIONS

The prognosis for surgical repair is related to the size of the sequestra, the amount of joint surface involved, and the amount and location of calcification. A very good prognosis may be given for joints with little change in the character of synovial fluid and in the joint capsule linings, and when there is little or no calcification. Very large sequestra and calcium proliferations have been removed successfully, and the animal has regained its former racing ability.

Sequestra involving joint surfaces and articular cartilages, and the presence of grossly abnormal synovia and synovial membranes, indicate a poor prognosis. Treatment of diffuse osteophytic formations, osteochondrosis dissecans, and calcifications underneath the extensor tendons has a poor prognosis.

Preoperative Preparation: The patient is treated for parasites, if indicated. Normal temperature, a good appetite, and normal hematocrit values should be present at the time of surgery. The lungs are auscultated carefully prior to surgery. If the animal is insured, permission to operate must be obtained or the insurance is automatically void.

The patient receives no food for 12 hours prior to the operation. Two-and-a-half grams of Aureomycin are given intravenously, and 1500 units of tetanus antitoxin are injected intramuscularly. The operative area is clipped and covered with a wet 1:500 bichloride of mercury pack.

If halothane is used for anesthesia, 30 ml. of Relaxans are given for sedation ½ hour prior to removing the horse from the stall. If local anesthesia is to be used, a combination of 250 mg. of promazine hydrochloride and 25 ml. of Relaxans is administered intravenously before taking the patient from its stall.

In the area used for surgical preparation, the sterile dressing is removed and 2% procaine is infiltrated in a semicircle above the operative site. A tourniquet is applied and the animal is placed on the operating table. The operative area is shaved, scrubbed, rinsed with alcohol, and draped. The radiographs are studied and the extent and site of the incision are determined. A reference specimen for consultation is helpful.

Additional radiographs should be obtained just prior to surgery. To precisely locate a small sequestrum it is imperative to know the exact angle from which the x-rays were taken. The radiograph reflects the view from the cassette—not from the x-ray tube. If the radiographs indicate extensive involvement, the condition invariably is found to be even more extensive when the joint is opened.

Surgical Technic: A liberal incision is made over the affected area and the skin is reflected on each side of the incision. The fascial layer then is incised and reflected in the same way. Sufficient access to the joint capsule should be provided in order to avoid unnecessary trauma to the edges of the incision while removing sequestra or calcium fragments. The large cutaneous and subcutaneous blood vessels are avoided. They should be ligated, when necessary, to maintain a dry operative field. Tendons and their sheaths should not be disturbed.

The joint capsule is opened and the synovia is allowed to drain. The joint capsule is grasped with a rat-tooth forceps and the edges of the incision are abducted to provide a good view of the carpal articular surfaces. A periosteal elevator is used as a probe to explore for possible hairline fractures. It also will serve as an elevator to remove the smaller sequestra.

A thorough examination is made of the structures adjacent to the fractured segment. Hairline fractures with no displacement often can be found. All sequestra must be removed, as well as osteophytes and calcium deposits. Periosteal elevators, gouges, curettes, rongeurs, chisels, mallets, and bone files are surgical instruments which are used to advantage.

The joint capsule and overlying fibrous tissue are sutured with stainless steel sutures. Double O chromic catgut is substituted for wire sutures if the opening is adjacent to a tendon. The fascial layer is closed with double O catgut and the skin with double O silk. A pressure bandage and sterile compresses are used to cover and support the wound in uncomplicated cases. If the incision has been extensive and much trauma to the joint surfaces has occurred, a plaster cast is applied over the carpal area. Such a cast prevents the animal from chewing at the operative area or otherwise traumatizing the wound. The plaster cast is left in place for 8 days.

Postoperative care involves confining the horse to a stall. Ten million units of Combiotic (a penicillin-dihydrostreptomycin preparation) are given every 24 hours. Phenylbutazone is administered at the rate of 2 Gm. daily for its analgesic effect. If a plaster cast is applied, dry sterile packs are placed beneath it. If a cast is not used, the sterile packs are replaced every 48 hours and the elastic pressure bandage is reset every 12 hours to prevent its slipping or tightening.

Without exception, first intention healing has resulted by following the described procedures. Pressure sores frequently are caused by the cast, but they heal when Furacin dressings are applied.

Gamma radiation has been useful in preventing recurrence of calcium deposits. Its anti-inflammatory action has helped to restore the mobility of the carpus by reducing soft tissue reaction. The total radiation dose is 1000 roentgens, given over a 6-week period.

One should not advise that the patient be turned out in pasture. Controlled exercise is recommended. The horse is "hand-walked" for the first 60 days. During this period a mild glycerine and alcohol, or iodine and glycerine, sweat is applied before and after the gamma radiation treatments.

During the period from 60 to 120 days after surgery, the patient is walked under saddle for a maximum of 3 miles daily. The sweat

may be applied repeatedly. Hydrotherapy is helpful during this period.

During the third 60-day period the animal is walked, jogged, and then galloped up to a maximum rate of 1 mile in 2 minutes. The knee is bandaged in an Absorbine brace. After 6 months the patient is ready to breeze and should be able to race 6 furlongs within the next 45 days.

D. L. Proctor

REFERENCES

1. Jenny, Jacques and Reed, W. O.: Personal communication.
2. Thom, M. G.: X-ray Therapy in the Horse. Proceedings of A.V.M.A. Convention. 1959.
3. Johnson, L. E.: Fifth Annual Proceedings A.A.E.P. 1960. Radiation Panel.
4. Proctor, D. L.: Fifth Annual Proceedings A.A.E.P. 1960. Radiation Panel.

TENDINITIS

Pathology of Bowed Tendons

Over the years bowed tendons have caused the retirement of more horses from racing than any other pathologic condition. Because acute tendinitis does not cause mortality, there have been few opportunities for postmortem examination of the involved tissues. It was theorized by orthopedic surgeons, however, that tendinitis in the horse was pathologically the same as tendinitis in man. The "Snap Thumb" operation, in which the annular ligament and tendon ring of the superficial flexor are opened to allow free movement of the inflamed deep flexor tendon, is dramatically successful in humans. Consequently, this surgical procedure was adapted to the horse and was performed on a series of cases since 1956.

As surgical intervention for bowed tendons became more common, it was apparent that tendinitis was a misnomer. The terms, "peritendinitis" or "fibrinous synovitis," are more nearly descriptive of the condition referred to clinically as bowed tendon. In only 7 of 89 cases was there a separation or lack of continuity of the tendon fibers. In 5 of these cases, the insertion of the carpal check ligament was torn from the deep flexor tendon.

It was reported at the 1962 meeting of the American Association of Equine Practitioners that histologic sections from clinically bowed flexor tendons revealed that the pathology actually involves the tendon fibers. It is agreed that in a certain percentage of so-called bowed tendons there is pathology of tendon fibers. Both their disruption and necrosis have been observed. In the series of 89 cases, careful preoperative examinations and observation of the gross appearance of the tendons during surgery have convinced me, however, that tendon pathology is present in only a relatively small percentage of clinically bowed tendons. In my opinion, the basic lesion in the bowed tendon case exists in the peritendinous structures, not in the tendinous fibers proper.

A close scrutiny of the available histories of the operated cases reveals that 35% of the animals that went back into training suffered bowed tendons in the nonoperated leg. This raises a question about whether the stress factors or faults in conformation that caused the first tendon to bow, also caused similar lesions in the second leg. It is possible that the tendency to suffer a bowed tendon in the previously sound leg is due to the animal's inclination to protect the operated leg, thus putting unusual stress on the sound one.

The enlarged peritendinous fibrotic tissue seen in the "ham bone" bowed tendon represents tissue reaction to torn synovial structures and leakage of synovia into the tissues adjacent to the flexor tendons. Tearing of the resulting fibrotic adhesions during the stress of hard work aggravates the peritendinous inflammation, and may cause additional formation of large amounts of fibrotic tissue. This tissue encompasses the flexor tendons, forms adhesions, and limits motion. The theory that bowed tendons are caused by leakage from torn synovial structures gives rise to a regimen of treatment that has stood the test of time and has enabled many such injured horses to race again after only 6 weeks of rest.

TREATMENT OF TENDON INJURIES

Immediately after it is recognized that an animal has suffered a tendon injury it is stood in ice boots continually for 7 days. The anti-inflammatory action of the cold hydrotherapy is supplemented by the administration of corticosteroids locally and systemically. Enzymes also have been used. This phase of treatment is followed by supportive bandaging over a mild leg paint or sweat, and controlled exercise. If this treatment is to be at all successful, it should be started as soon as the bowed tendon is discovered.

Once the inflammatory products become organized a certain amount of adhesions always develop. Consequently, the condition tends to recur when the animal is subjected to stress. Sweating, blistering, firing, and resting for as long as a year are treatments that have been repeated over the years and with little or no success. The percentage of recoveries has been estimated to be as low as 5 to 10%. When the fibrosis is not too extensive or has not been present more than 90 to 120 days, the surgical removal of adhesions, in contrast, offers a 20 to 25% chance of returning the animal to racing form successfully. The surgery must be done aseptically and the healing must be by first intention. I have never seen a horse recover racing form after surgery unless the healing was by first intention. Delayed union results in formation of new adhesions.

Surgical Technic: Under strict asepsis, a liberal incision is made on the lateral posterior aspect of the metacarpus, over the area of fibrotic enlargement. The skin and then a layer of subcutaneous tissue are reflected carefully. The annular ligament is incised and dissected from the underlying structure. It is at this point that a line of cleavage can be found in the majority of cases. By following this line by careful blunt dissection the operator usually can locate and remove the mass of fibrosis and adhesions that prevent free movement of the flexor tendons. At this time an elevator or the operator's gloved finger may be used to insure that all adhesions between the superficial and deep flexor tendons are removed or broken down. Adhesions between the tendons and the

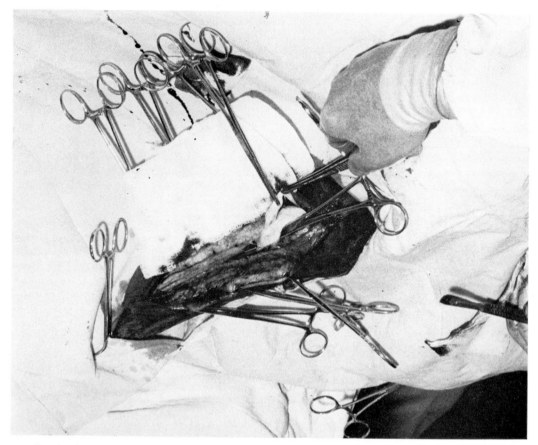

Fig. 15. Surgical repair of bowed tendon. Thumb forceps hold the cut edge of the annular ligament. The hemostats are thrust through the ring of the superficial tendon.

annular ligament are treated similarly. If free movement of the deep tendon through the ring of the superficial tendon is prevented by adhesions or fibrosis, the offending tissue must be removed. It may be necessary to incise and open the ring of the superficial digital flexor tendon to allow free movement of the deep flexor tendon at that point (Fig. 15).

A 2-layer closure is made by using double 0 catgut in a continuous suture in the subcutaneous tissue. The skin is closed with double 0 silk by a continuous suture. Tension sutures are placed as needed, using a vertical mattress stitch and #2 silk. The entire metacarpal area is placed under an Ace elastic compression bandage.

Postoperative Care: The animal is walked on the third postoperative day. Regulated exercise is maintained for 30 days postoperatively. A minimum of 6 months of rest is recommended before the operated leg can be subjected to the stress of hard work. The application of repeated sweats in many cases will cause the leg to return to normal size and appearance.

D. L. PROCTOR

REPAIR OF RECTOVAGINAL DEFECTS

A mare is quite subject to lacerations of the vagina and rectum because of the speed with which parturition takes place. Her expulsive efforts are so great that it is not uncommon for a foot of the foal to be forced through the roof of the vagina and into the rectum.

Two major conditions in this area require surgical correction. First, a rectovaginal fistula which is formed when a rent exists between the rectum and vagina, but the anal and vulvar sphincters are still intact. Second, a 3rd-degree perineal laceration in which the sphincters have been torn and a common opening exists for both the rectum and vagina. The surgical approach is different for each type. First and 2nd degree perineal lacerations only penetrate the vaginal or vulvar mucosa and submucosa. They rarely require surgical correction. If the dorsal commissure of the vulva is torn a Caslick operation will correct this.

RECTOVAGINAL FISTULA

The classic operation as described by Forssell is satisfactory.[6] The mare is prepared for surgery by withholding all hay for 4 to 6 days but grain may be given. Minimizing the amount of feces passing through the rectum is paramount to success in this operation. A saline cathartic will aid in removing material from the intestinal tract.

Surgical Technic: From 15 to 20 ml. of 2% procaine is given epidurally. The rectum is

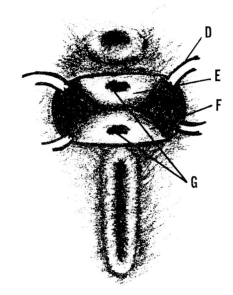

Fig. 17. D, retractor; E, rectal floor; F, vaginal roof; G, lacerations in rectum and vagina.

emptied and the perineal area is cleansed thoroughly. A 4- to 6-inch incision is made horizontally between the rectum and vulva (Fig. 16). This incision is continued forward

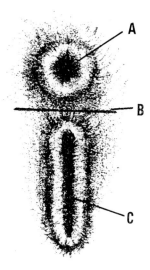

Fig. 16. A, anus; B, line of incision; C, vulva.

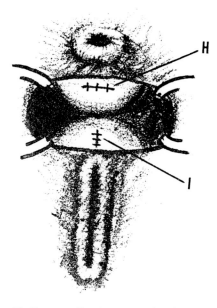

Fig. 18. H, suture line in rectum placed perpendicular to long axis; I, suture line in vagina placed parallel to long axis.

1 to 2 inches beyond the anterior border of the fistula (Fig. 17). As much tissue as possible should be left on the rectal surface.

The rent in the rectum is closed first and in such a way that the incision line is at right angles to the long axis of the rectum. In this manner less stress will be placed on the suture line (Fig. 18). A Lembert-type suture is used so that the rectal mucosa is inverted into the lumen of the rectum. Care should be taken that the suture does not penetrate the mucosa. Heavy, nonabsorbable suture material such as silk, stainless steel, or one of the synthetic materials should be used and removed at a later time. The vaginal tear is closed with a suture line that is parallel to the long axis of the vagina (Fig. 18). The initial skin incision is closed with simple interrupted or vertical mattress sutures.

A sterile gauze pack is placed between the 2 layers. This is replaced every other day after the wound is cleansed gently with sponges.

Bulk-producing feed must be withheld for 1 to 2 weeks. Bran mashes can be given and are desirable. In 10 to 14 days the sutures can be removed and the wound allowed to fill with granulation tissue. Parenteral feeding may be necessary.

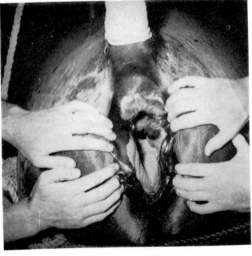

Fig. 19. Mare prepared for surgery.

REPAIR OF PERINEAL LACERATIONS

The preoperative preparation is the same as for rectovaginal fistula (Fig. 19). Many surgical approaches are used but a modification of Gotze's technic as reported by Straub and Fowler gives satisfactory results. Long-handled instruments are necessary to work at the depth of some lacerations (Fig. 20).

Surgical Technic: An incision, parallel to and ¼ inch anterior to the mucocutaneous junction of the vulva, is started at the dorsal border of the vulvar mucosa and extended ventrally as far as is necessary (Fig. 21). Generally, the incision is made about ⅓ of the height of the vulva in small lacerations, and almost ½ in severe lacerations. The mucosa, along with some submucosal tissue, is separated from the perivaginal tissue to make a flap extending from the vulva diagonally to the area where the rectum and vagina are clearly separated (Fig. 22). The same procedure is followed for both sides. The flaps on both sides should be as symmetrical as possible. Any scar tissue resulting from unsuccessful attempts at repair or from healing processes should be removed, for it hampers healing. The ventral borders of the rectal mucosa then are freshened.

A long needle holder and a No. 00 half-circle needle are used to place the individual sutures which, first, go deeply through the vaginal mucosa to include perivaginal tissue and then emerge through this tissue in the region of musculofascial defect (Fig. 23). Next, the suture is placed deeply in the submucosal layer of the rectum on one side without penetrating the lumen. The suture then is advanced to the other side where the submucosal layer of the rectum is penetrated. The suture then is placed in the perivaginal tissue and through the vaginal mucosa to the vaginal lumen. The suturing technic is completed by passing the suture through both flaps of vaginal mucosa and back to the starting point where it is tied.

It is of utmost importance that the ties are pulled tight so that no slack remains. The rectal mucosa from both sides thereby is pulled together as well as the vaginal mucosa. To facilitate easy removal, knots are tied into the ends of the individual sutures, starting with

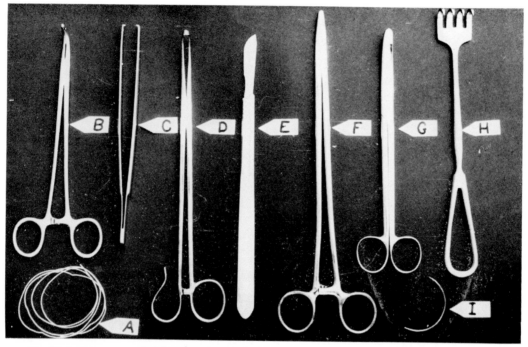

Fig. 20. Instruments needed for operation: A, 0.40-mm. nylon suture; B, 9-inch full-curved hemostat; C, 7-inch thumb forceps; D, White tonsil-seizing forceps; E, scalpel; F, 10½-inch needle holder; G, 8-inch curved scissors; H, rake retractor; I, No. .00 half-curved surgeon's needle.

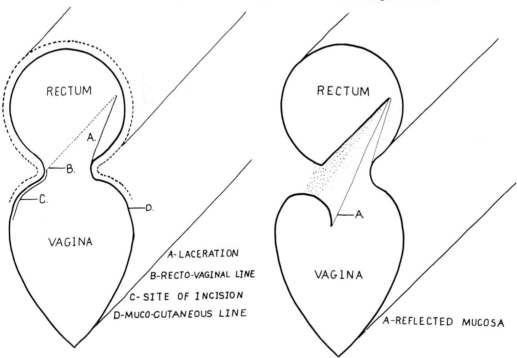

RECTUM

A.

B.

C.

D.

VAGINA

A-LACERATION
B-RECTO-VAGINAL LINE
C-SITE OF INCISION
D-MUCO-CUTANEOUS LINE

Fig. 21. Diagram of operative site.

RECTUM

A

VAGINA

A-REFLECTED MUCOSA

Fig. 22. Mucosal flap reflected.

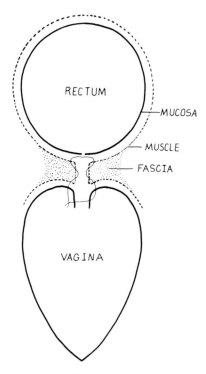

Fig. 23. Suture pattern.

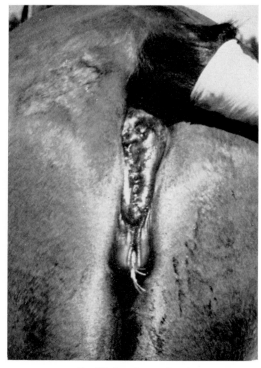

Fig. 24. Repair completed.

one, etc. These sutures should be cut 4 to 6 inches long so that they can be grasped from outside the vulva for removal; however, they should not be so long that they accumulate filth or tail hairs. Sutures should be placed about ¾ of an inch apart. When all have been placed, the rectal mucosa should be examined carefully for sutures that can be palpated. Any palpable ones should be removed and need not be replaced if the other sutures are placed properly.

With the new shelf completed, care should be taken to furnish a good connection between it and the sphincter ani. This is accomplished with single mattress sutures placed into the sphincter muscle and deeply in the upper portion of the vulva, thereby avoiding a possible pocket directly in front of the sphincter. The ends of the sphincter muscle must be freshened before suturing. The upper part of the vulva then is closed, either by simple interrupted sutures or by vertical mattress sutures (Fig. 24).

Aftercare is similar to that given following

repair of rectovaginal fistula. The sutures are removed in 8 to 10 days. Occasionally, the vulva is too small for natural breeding following surgery but the mare can be bred artificially, or the vulva can be enlarged by episiotomy. Episiotomy may be necessary prior to a future parturition and preparations must be made for this eventuality.

This suture pattern is adaptable to any perineal laceration and provides a thick, strong shelf between the rectum and vagina with a minimum of suturing. The suturing method also can be adapted to the repair of rectovaginal fistulas.

M. E. Fowler

REFERENCES

1. Bemis, H. E.: A new operation for rectovaginal fistula. No. Am. Vet., 11 (1930) 37-40.
2. Dollar, J. A. W.: Regional Veterinary Surgery and Operative Technique, William R. Jenkins Co., New York, N. Y., 1912.
3. Farquharson, James: Surgical treatment of third degree perineal lacerations. No. Am. Vet., 24 (1943) 220-225.
4. Faustka, K.: Beitrag zur Kenntnis und Operationstechnik der Dammrisse bei Stuten (Contributions to the knowledge and operational technique for third degree perineal lacerations of mares). Ztschr. Tiermed., 16 (1912) 515.

5. Flemming, George: A Text-Book of Operative Veterinary Surgery. Vol. II, William R. Jenkins Co., New York, N. Y., 1908.

6. Forssell, Gerhard: Eine neue Operationsmethode der Fistula Rectovaginalis bei der Stute (A New Operational Technique for Rectovaginal Fistula in the Mare). Collected Papers from the Veterinary Institute, Stockholm, Sweden, 1927-1928.

7. Frank, E. R.: Veterinary Surgery. Rev. ed. Burgess Publishing Co., Minneapolis, Minn., 1953.

8. Goetze, R.: Dammrissnaht, vulva und scheidenvorhofplastik bei stuten und kuhen (A plastic operation for rupture of the perineal seam, the vulva and the vaginal vestibule in mares and cows).

9. Goetze, R.: Die operation des kompletten dammrisses beim rind (The operation for the perineal laceration in the cow.) Deutsche tierärztl. Wchnschr., 37 (1929) 181-183.

10. Goetze, R.: Die Operation des vernarbten Dammrisses beim Rind und beim Pferd (The operation for chronic perineal lacerations in the cow and in the horse.) Deutsche tierärztl. Wchnschr., 49 (1941) 339-341.

11. Goetze, R.: Dammrissnaht, Plastik der vulva und des Scheidenvorhofes bei Stuten und Kühen. 4th ed. M. & H. Schaper, Hannover, Germany, 1952.

12. Greenway, L.: Surgical correction of a rectovaginal fistula in a mare. Canad. Vet. J., 1 (Feb., 1960) 69-70.

13. Habel, Robert E.: The perineum of the mare. Cornell Vet., 43 (1953) 249-278.

14. Liess, J.: Dammriss bei Kuh und stute (Perineal tear in the cow and mare). Berl. u. Munch. tierärztl. Wchnschr. (1936) 611.

15. Merillat, Louis A.: Veterinary Surgical Operation. 2nd ed. Alexander Eger, Chicago, Ill., 1917.

16. Pires, Antonio: Contribucion al estudio, en las yeguas, del habito de tragar aire, de la fistual recto vaginal y de la cloaca recto vaginal (Contribution to the study in mares of the habit of "windsucking" of the recto-vaginal fistula and third-degree perineal laceration). Rev. Fac. agron. y vet. (Nov., 1947) 248-298.

17. Straub, Otto C., Fowler, Murray E.: Repair of perineal lacerations in the mare and cow. J.A.V.M.A. 138 (June 15, 1961) 659-664.

CASLICK'S OPERATION FOR "VAGINAL WINDSUCKING" (PNEUMOVAGINIA)

It is estimated that the greatest single cause for sterility in the mare is a low-grade vaginitis induced by poor conformation of the vulva. Such a statement presumes, of course, that operators of breeding establishments practice acceptable preventive therapy and hygiene.

The chief factors influencing vulvar malfunction are:

1. Age. As the mare grows older there is loss of tone in the musculature of the area and tissues of the vulva, resulting in gaping or opening of the lips. Such a condition permits entrance of air and bacteria into the vagina, thus predisposing it to infection.

2. Distortion of the vulva. This may be due to tumors and old lacerations or injuries acquired at previous foalings.

3. Displacement of the vulva. This condition usually is found in the aged mare. In such a mare it is not uncommon to find the upper ⅓ or even ½ of the vulva to be pulled forward over the edge of the ischium. In such an instance the vulva rather than being vertical is now partly horizontal and consequently receives added infective material during defecation.

The diagnosis of possible vaginitis is based upon:

1. Visual examination of the vulva.

2. Examination of the vagina with a speculum.

3. Most important of all is a bacteriologic culture of vaginal mucus or exudate.

The treatment most often is surgical and medicinal.

Preoperative Preparation: Feces should be removed from the terminal rectum and the tail is bandaged. The vulva, perineum, and surrounding area should be thoroughly cleansed. Vigorous scrubbing is not recommended since the exterior of the vulva is thin-skinned and sensitive. Neither should strong antiseptics be used as they may irritate the skin and cause eventual exfoliation of tissue. A 3-minute scrub with Phisohex-soaked gauze sponges is sufficient. The area then should be thoroughly rinsed.

Anesthesia: An epidural anesthetic may be given or the intended line of incision may be infiltrated with 2% procaine using a fine-gauged needle (23-gauge).

Restraint: Considering the individual temperament of the mare to be operated, appropriate measures for restraint should be taken. To support the anesthetic, one may use breeding hobbles, a twitch, tranquilizers, 300 ml. of a 7% solution of chloral hydrate i.v., or 15 ml. of Nembutal i.v.

Technic: The objective here is to remove a thin strip of tissue (⅛ to ¼ inch in width) from the edge of the vulva extending from the dorsal commissure to a point 1½ to 2 inches from the ventral commissure. This should leave ample opening at the ventral commissure for urination. Throughout the length of the incision this strip of tissue is removed from the vulva at the junction of the skin and mucous membrane. Though either a knife or scissors may be used to remove the tissue, the latter usually is preferred. When using a scissors it is most convenient to start at the estimated distal limit of the incision and cut upward. The reverse is done when using a knife. A similar strip of tissue then is removed from the other lip of the vulva.

The 2 fresh wound surfaces are brought together with metal skin clips or some nonabsorbable suture such as medium-sized Vetafil. A suitable needle for this purpose is the relatively small ½ circle, cutting needle (Anchor #1834-4). Tetanus antitoxin and such antibiotics as may be indicated by the bacteriologic cultures are administered. Healing should be complete in 10 days at which time the sutures or clips may be removed.

At breeding time it usually is necessary to incise the surgical adhesions between the lips of the vulva to permit entry by the stallion. After breeding, the wound edges are brought together again and allowed to heal.

The owner must be warned to have the adhesions cut again just before foaling in order to prevent serious complications.

L. E. JOHNSON

DENTIGEROUS CYST

A dentigerous cyst, or cystic temporal odontoma, is characterized by a slowly enlarging mass measuring 2 to 6 centimeters in diameter and usually located on the mastoid process of the petrous portion of the temporal bone. However, the growth may also occur on the forehead or in the paranasal sinuses. A true dentigerous cyst is unique in the horse and seems to enlarge with the rest of the dental tissues. The lesion is observed most commonly during the period of dentition in the first 2 years of life; however, horses of all ages may develop a cyst.

Etiology: Some confusion exists as to whether the dentigerous cyst should be classified as a congenital malformation or a true neoplasm. Moulton considers the lesion to be a congenital malformation representing an errant dental follicle which has its origin in the bronchial cleft.[1] In support of this theory, the cyst does not appear to metastasize or undergo malignant changes.

On the other hand, Smith and Jones classify the structure as a teratoma.[2] Since a true teratoma must demonstrate active growth, however, it would be more accurate to consider the dentigerous cyst to be a congenital malformation.

Clinical Signs: The first observable sign of a dentigerous cyst is an enlargement near the base of the ear. As the mass increases in size a fistula is formed to the skin surface and a thick, clear fluid is discharged. The fistulous opening is usually located on the anterior border of the external ear. The cyst frequently becomes infected through the fistula and the exudate may become suppurative. The fistula may be located directly over the tooth or several centimeters away from the actual cyst. Upon palpation, the mass is found to be a soft, fluctuating structure of variable size. When the cystic fluid has escaped via a draining fistula, however, a depression can be palpated and in some instances a tooth can be felt in the cavity beneath the skin.

Systemic signs are rare unless a tooth grows into the cranial cavity and causes an increase of intracranial pressure.

Diagnosis: The diagnosis of a dentigerous cyst usually is made on the basis of physical findings and the location of the enlargement. When a fistulous tract is absent, it may be necessary to differentiate the cyst from an abscess, hematoma or supra-atlantal bursitis. When the diagnosis is uncertain one should first attempt to aspirate the thick, clear fluid characteristic of a dentigerous cyst. During the aspiration procedure, the cavity should be probed in an attempt to locate the errant tooth. Differentiation usually can be made between a dentigerous cyst and supra-atlantal bursitis on the basis of clinical findings and the location of the lesion. In questionable cases, the aspirated fluid should be cultured for *Brucella abortus*, and the brucella agglutination test should be performed.

Lesions: The mass usually contains the crown or root of a tooth enclosed within a cystic cavity. In most cases, there is a single, irregularly shaped tooth resembling a molar. Some dentigerous cysts, however, may contain multiple teeth. In some instances, the teeth are secured in alveoli, but most of them are loose within the cavity. Histologically, the cells lining the cyst are composed of stratified squamous epithelium. The errant tooth appears to be normal in that it contains enamel, cementum, and dentine. Dentine usually is present in the greatest amount. The fluid within the cyst will vary in character, depending upon whether or not infection is present. In the case of an infected dentigerous cyst, purulent exudate is present.

Treatment: The only satisfactory method of treating a dentigerous cyst is by surgical excision. In some cases, the surgery may be accomplished with the animal in a standing position while under sedation or tranquilization. Promazine hydrochloride administered intravenously provides satisfactory control of well-mannered subjects. The surgical site, in addition, should be thoroughly infiltrated with a local anesthetic. It may be necessary to use a general anesthetic in some horses.

The surgical site is prepared. In the absence of a fistulous tract, an elliptical incision is made directly over the enlargement and the cyst is removed by blunt dissection. Care must be taken not to puncture the cyst since its dissection is more difficult when the structure is collapsed. In the event that the resulting cavity cannot be obliterated by suturing, an absorbable gelatin sponge may be inserted. Chromic catgut is then used to approximate the subcutaneous tissue, and the skin is sutured separately with interrupted, horizontal, mattress stitches.

If a fistulous tract is present, the incision is started at the fistulous opening and is continued toward the main portion of the cyst. After removal of both the cyst and fistulous tract, the wound is closed as previously described. By removal of both the tract and the cyst it is possible to obtain healing by first intention. If the cyst is located beneath the auricularis muscles, care must be taken to avoid severing them or their nerve supply, or the carriage of the external ear will be affected.

In the event that the lining of the cyst cannot be removed, it is advisable to destroy the remaining cystic epithelium by electrocautery, silver nitrate, or by packing the area with 7% tincture of iodine. The pack may be removed after 48 hours, and the ventral 1 inch of the incision is left open to enhance drainage.

Prognosis: In uncomplicated cases in which excision of the cyst is complete, the prognosis usually is good. Possible complications include excessive swelling due to accumulation of fluid, and infection. In these events, proper drainage and supportive therapy must be instituted.

R. C. HERSCHLER
H. E. AMSTUTZ

REFERENCES

1. Moulton, J. E.: Tumors in Domestic Animals, 2nd ed., University of California Press, Berkeley 4, 1961.
2. Smith, H. A. and Jones, T. C.: Veterinary Pathology, Lea and Febiger, Philadelphia, Pa., 1961.

SURGICAL REPAIR OF ENTROPION AND ECTROPION

ENTROPION

Inversion of the lids, particularly the lower lid of foals, usually occurs bilaterally but there may be a marked difference in severity between the 2 eyes. Entropion frequently is associated with blepharospasm. Relief of this condition occasionally is obtained by the instillation of a few drops of topical anesthetic if during its anesthesia the lid is massaged, drawn down, and stretched a little with the fingertips. When this does not succeed, one may evert the lid by means of skin sutures without incising the skin below the palpebral margin.

In adult horses, entropion may follow shrinking of the eyeball, such as may happen after an attack of periodic ophthalmia or during a debilitating condition in which the postorbital fat disappears.

Treatment: In the first method of treatment in the foal, without preliminary clipping the skin below the affected eyelid is washed with soap and water, dried, and carefully wiped with alcohol. A 2% procaine solution is injected subcutaneously at the involved site. A straight triangular needle is threaded with nylon suture and introduced through the skin, ¼ of an inch below the lower edge of the eyelid, and carried upward and subcutaneously, avoiding the orbicularis muscle, to emerge through the skin of the eyelid slightly below its lower margin. From 2 to 3 sutures are inserted, a quarter of an inch apart, and these are tied just tightly enough to free the eyeball of contact with the edge of the eyelid.

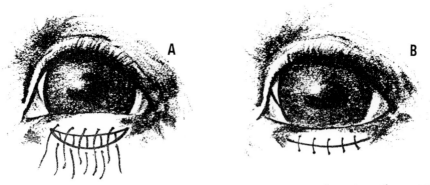

Fig. 25. A technic for correction of entropion. A—preoperative appearance, B—postoperative appearance.

For the next few days, a topical anesthetic is applied to the eyeball 3 times daily and penicillin ophthalmic ointment is squeezed into the conjunctival sac between these applications. If the foal is not unduly disturbed by the sutures, the antiseptic may be omitted provided the blepharospasm is remedied.

When corrective surgery is employed for entropion in the foal after more simple measures have failed, the skin below the lid is clipped, washed, and swabbed with alcohol. Injection of a 2% procaine solution provides suitable local anesthesia.

The skin segment to be removed should be long enough to correct the deformity, but should not be carried beyond the terminal parts of the lid when it is positioned normally over the eyeball. The skin may be removed with a sharp scalpel, or picked up in a tissue forceps and removed with a curved scissors. The former method usually is preferred as the quantity of skin to be removed may be judged more easily. Usually a strip 2 to 5 mm. wide (according to the severity of the condition)

and 2 cm. long is ample. The extremities of the excised area should be tapered to avoid puckering. Some operators undermine the skin between the incision and the edge of the eyelid with the scalpel, before suturing. The incisions should be sutured when blepharospasm exists, otherwise they may be permitted to heal unsutured. Suturing, however, provides immediate relief.

Suitable suture material is blue nylon, and the sutures should penetrate all the skin layers, and be drawn just tightly enough to approximate the edges of the incision (Fig. 25).

ECTROPION

Ectropion is rare in the horse, and when present it usually has followed laceration of the lid, or of the skin below it, with resulting cicatricial contraction. To remedy this defect, a satisfactory surgical technic is illustrated in Figure 26. A triangular wedge of skin is removed, as shown, from the lower lid at the lateral canthus.

R. H. SMYTHE

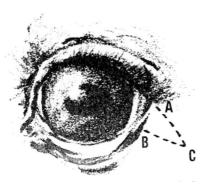

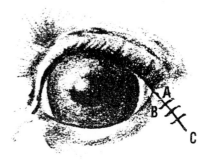

Fig. 26. A technic for correction of ectropion. A, B, C indicate outline of triangular area to be excised.

EQUINE DENTISTRY

Introduction

Dentistry in horses ordinarily is performed with two ends in view: to improve physical condition and to relieve pain. Cosmetic dental surgery in horses has not achieved any popularity and probably never will, owing to the peculiar manner in which the equine teeth compensate for wear. Although drilling cavities in equine teeth has been popular in certain circles (cf. bishoping), the filling of cavities has not. Equine dentistry has thus been confined to correcting irregularities in the dental arcade, to the extraction of teeth, and to certain surgical procedures aimed to reduce infection and restore oral health. Orthodonty, except in its most basic form, has not been and probably will not be practiced upon the equine patient.

Dental examination and correction of defects are important factors in the early training of all breeds of horses. In older animals, dentistry is less important as a training aid and more important in maintaining the physical condition of the animal. It should neither be slighted nor downgraded by the equine practitioner.

The equine dental arcade is wonderfully adapted for the mastication of herbage and the preparation of plant material for digestion. Like most mammals, the horse has 2 sets of teeth during its lifetime. One is deciduous: "milk teeth" which ordinarily begin to erupt through the gums about a week after birth, some of which are functional over a period of approximately 4½ years. These teeth consist only of incisors and premolars. The other set, or "permanent teeth," begin to appear at about 10 to 12 months of age with the first molar teeth, and at about 2½ years of age begin to progressively displace the temporary teeth commencing with the central incisors and the first premolars (Fig. 27). By 5 years of age all of the deciduous teeth have been shed and the horse is in possession of a complete permanent dental arcade (Table 1).

Table 1.—Eruption of the Teeth

Teeth		Eruption
A. Deciduous:		
1st incisor	(Di 1)	Birth or first week
2nd incisor	(Di 2)	4 to 6 weeks
3rd incisor	(Di 3)	6 to 9 months
Canine	(Dc)	
1st premolar	(Dp 2)	Birth or first
2nd premolar	(Dp 3)	2 weeks.
3rd premolar	(Dp 4)	
B. Permanent:		
1st incisor	(I1)	2½ years
2nd incisor	(I2)	3½ years
3rd incisor	(I3)	4½ years
Canine	(C)	4 to 5 years
1st premolar (wolf tooth)	(P1)	5 to 6 months
2nd premolar	(P2)	2½ years
3rd premolar	(P3)	3 years
4th premolar	(P4)	4 years
1st molar	(M1)	9 to 12 months
2nd molar	(M2)	2 years
3rd molar	(M3)	3½ to 4 years

The periods given for P 3 and 4 refer to the upper teeth; the lower ones may erupt about 6 months earlier.
From Sisson & Grossman, *Anatomy of the Domestic Animals.*

The nomenclature of the equine teeth has always been subject to some confusion, and rather than compound it I shall adhere to the classification proposed by Sisson and Grossman with one explanatory note. The premolar teeth are numbered from 1 to 3 in the deciduous arcade and from 1 to 4 in the permanent arcade. Positionally, however, the second permanent premolar is the homologue of the first temporary and replaces it in the arcade. Similarly the third permanent replaces the second temporary and the fourth permanent replaces the third temporary premolar. The first permanent premolar is the so-called "wolf tooth" and is inconstant. It appears (usually in the upper arcade only) at about 5 to 6 months of age, and may be shed together with the first temporary premolar. If it remains it usually is extracted because it serves no useful purpose and may predispose to irritation and infection of the buccal mucosa through irritation by the bit.

All permanent equine teeth, with the possible exception of the canines, are continuously erupting teeth, *i.e.* they are constantly being pushed out of the alveoli by slow proliferation of cancellous bone beneath their roots. This is a continuous process throughout the life of the animal and is a natural adaptation to compensate for wear. The process continues in the absence of wear, and teeth which have none opposing them may grow considerably longer than adjacent teeth in the arcade.

The surfaces of the teeth have various names which are descriptive enough once the anatomy of the mouth is understood. The terms "buccal surface," "lingual surface," "labial surface," "table surface," and "interdental surface" are sufficiently obvious not to require definition. Of all these, the table or wearing surface of the teeth is the one of primary interest in equine dentistry.

Dental Equipment

Practitioners fortunate enough to obtain a surplus U.S. Army Veterinary Corps Equine Dental Set, together with its canvas roll, need not worry about equine dental instruments for the remainder of their professional careers except for compound molar cutters. And if one has enough muscle to compensate for the lack of a compound fulcrum even this last item is not necessary. There are a variety of dental instruments produced by various manufacturers that will, more expensively and occasionally more efficiently, compensate for the lack of war surplus equipment.

The choice of instruments depends a great deal upon the personal likes, dislikes, and practice of the practitioner. It would serve no useful purpose to list all possible equine dental instruments which have been manufactured. The ones shown in the accompanying illustration (Fig. 28) indicate most of the items included in a complete set.

For routine dentistry, a good set of floats, a pair of offset bone cutters, a screw driver, a set of medium-sized extraction forceps, a core-hardened steel root elevator, a twitch, a length of ⅜"-woven cotton rope, dental wax, and a good mouth speculum will suffice.

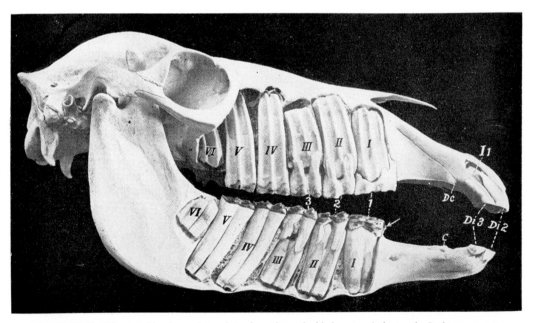

Fig. 27. Skull of 2-year-old colt, sculptured to show the embedded parts of the teeth. Both permanent and temporary cheek teeth are shown. The upper first premolar ("wolf-tooth") is present, but not visible; the lower one is indicated by the arrow. Temporary chief premolars are numbered 1,2,3; permanent premolars and molars are designated by Roman numerals; Dc., upper temporary canine; C, lower permanent canine, which was not ready to erupt; Di 2, Di 3, second and third temporary incisors; I 1, first permanent incisor, not quite ready to erupt. From Sisson and Grossman's *Anatomy of the Domestic Animals.*

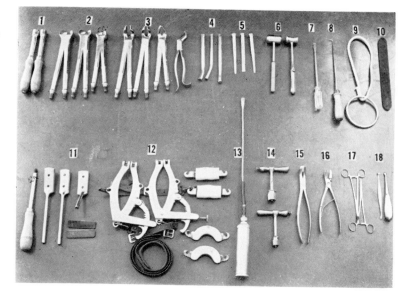

Fig. 28. Set of equine dental instruments:

1. Handles
2. Molar cutters
3. Extraction forceps
4. Repellers
5. Bone chisels
6. Mallets
7. Screw driver
8. Dental pick
9. Twitch
10. Farrier's rasp
11. Floats
12. Speculum
13. Flashlight
14. Trephines
15. Rongeurs
16. Bone cutters
17. Splinter forceps
18. Curettes

RESTRAINT

The principles of good restraint outlined in Chapter 2 apply particularly to dentistry since the operator is in a disadvantageous position most of the time. Physical restraints such as a twitch or a war bridle may be used, but occasionally their employment is a detriment since they can block the working area. A speculum is necessary at times but this instrument, too, can be awkward and its use requires an extremely well-mannered horse in full possession of his faculties. Whether or not a speculum should be used upon an alert and untranquilized horse is a moot question. Many veterinarians believe that horses object to a speculum more than they do to minor dental surgery. Palpation of cheek teeth by inexperienced persons, however, can result in lacerated knuckles and crushed fingers if it is done without mechanical aids, and major dental surgery, such as extraction or repulsion of teeth, requires a speculum.

Chemical restraint provides a better way to control horses for minor dentistry, although even with tranquilizers or sedatives there will be an occasional excitable animal upon which the drugs have no apparent effect. Such horses may have to be confined in stocks and given sedatives for satisfactory restraint.

Major dental procedures such as cutting molars, removing supernumerary teeth or repelling infected molars should be done with the horse under general anesthesia. Major dental surgery cannot be casually approached and performed in the field as fairly extensive preparation is needed.

EXAMINATION OF THE TEETH

Certain principles should always be kept in mind and an orderly sequence followed when making a dental examination. These can be summarized under five main headings:

1. Don't hurry.
2. Examine the animal and its actions from a distance.
3. Take the history.
4. Examine the external lesions (if any).
5. Examine the mouth and teeth.

It is impossible to make a satisfactory examination of a nervous, frightened, or stubborn horse. Therefore, one must take every precaution not to increase the animal's natural suspicion and distrust of strangers. It is rare when a horse will permit a dental examination without suitable preliminaries to convince him that the examiner intends no harm. For painful dental disorders this may be impossible without the aid of ataractics or anesthetics.

The incisor teeth should be examined first by rolling back the lips and examining the exposed incisors visually. Note the angle of the bite, and any external abnormalities. Check deciduous incisors for looseness if evidence indicates they are about to be shed. Open the mouth by reaching into the interdental space and withdrawing the tongue, or by applying opposing pressure on the upper and lower lips. Check the animal's age as it can be an important clue to disorders which may be encountered in further examination of the mouth and dental arcades.

Examination of cheek teeth without a speculum is not difficult once one has mastered the technics, and the examination is simpler, neater, less objectionable to the patient, and more impressive to the owner. Two methods may be employed. In one, both hands are required; in the other only one hand is used. Each method has its advantages and disadvantages and should be carefully evaluated by the individual practitioner before it is employed.

In the 2-handed method, to palpate the right side of the dental arcade approach the horse from the left, and with the right hand part the left labial commissure, reach through the left interdental space, grasp the tongue, and withdraw it through the left side of the mouth. A light cotton glove on the right hand will facilitate this manipulation and keep the tongue from slipping. The horse will open his mouth and tend to pull back which gives one a good chance to observe the table surfaces of the upper incisor teeth and the right upper cheek teeth. A flashlight held by yourself or an assistant will facilitate this examination. Still holding the tongue in the left labial commissure, pass the left hand between the right half of the dental arcade and the cheek, knuckles toward the cheeks and palm toward the teeth. Palpate the upper and lower cheek teeth with the fingertips. As long as the tongue is held in the commissure of the lips, the horse (ordinarily) will not close his mouth and one's fingers will be left intact. But do not be laggardly in the examination. It annoys the horse to have

his tongue clutched for long periods in an examiner's hand while each tiny ridge and cavity of his premolars and molars are examined. When finished on the right side repeat the process for the left using opposite hands and labial commissure. Persons with large hands and knobby fingers may find this technic unsatisfactory.

For experienced operators, the one-handed technic is more suitable. It also is applicable to otherwise manageable horses who dislike speculi or tongue-holding. The horse is approached from the front, and the right side of the mouth is palpated by inserting the right hand into the right interdental space with the palm facing laterally (Fig. 29). The back of the hand should be slightly flexed and should lie between the lingual surface of the cheek teeth and the tongue. This will force the tongue between the left rows of cheek teeth and keep the horse from completely closing its mouth. The hand is advanced into the oral cavity, the thumb and forefinger are used to palpate the buccal, lingual, and table surfaces of the teeth (Fig. 30). During this examination one should also palpate the buccal mucosa, the gums, and the right lateral side of the tongue. The left side of the mouth is examined in the same manner, using the left hand. There is danger of being bitten when using this technic, particularly if one is careless. The operator's hands may be scratched by sharp edges of the upper cheek teeth; this ordinarily results from failure to palpate the outside of the cheeks prior to inserting one's hand into the horse's mouth.

The cheek region around the labial commissures can be readily palpated by placing the thumb in the commissure with the ball toward the buccal mucosa. Wolf teeth can be felt by inserting the thumb or forefinger into the interdental space and palpating the first upper and lower cheek teeth on the close side. Do not attempt to palpate the premolars on the opposite side of the jaw to the one in which your finger is inserted. Wolf teeth will be felt as much smaller ones anterior to the definitive anterior premolar. Since wolf teeth may occur

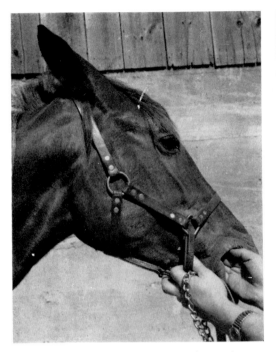

Fig. 29. Position of hand entering the mouth.

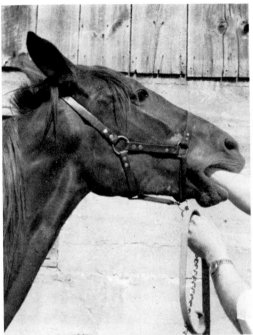

Fig. 30. Hand in mouth examining area of 4th upper cheek tooth.

in either the upper or lower jaw, both upper and lower arcades should be examined. At the same time the jaws are examined for wolf teeth the first definitive premolars should be palpated for protuberances and sharp edges. It is in this area that the bit draws the cheeks or tongue against the teeth, and sharp edges of the first premolars can cause painful lacerations.

No examination is complete without a history. This may be taken before, during, or after the examination according to the examiner's discretion. Preferably, it should be done prior to examination. All pertinent information should be gathered. Though some of this will have to be discounted, information regarding eating habits, "quidding," refusal to eat, unusual carriage of the head, excessive tossing or shaking of the head, refusal to drink cold water, and pulling ("lugging") against the bit will give clues about where to look for damage or disease. By correlating the history with the age of the horse, a presumptive diagnosis often can be made prior to examination.

DENTAL ANOMALIES

By far the most common dental problems of horses are those which are produced by anomalies in structure and number of adult teeth, bone structure of the jaws, and by abnormal shedding of deciduous teeth. Infective processes involving the teeth are relatively rare, and tumors or cysts are even less frequently encountered. The following anomalies are ones which may be encountered in practice, although a person would have to examine many thousands of horses before he would ever see them all, and the chances are slim that any practitioner will encounter more than a few of them in a lifetime of practice.

Abnormal Shedding

Abnormal shedding of the deciduous teeth is probably the most common dental defect in horses. The resulting anomalies are usually observed in animals less than 5 years of age, although an older animal will occasionally be affected. Specifically they involve dental "caps," retained temporary incisors, and retained temporary premolars.

Dental Caps: Dental caps are deciduous cheek teeth which remain attached to the permanent teeth after the permanent ones have erupted. The deciduous teeth are ready to be removed when the separation between them and the permanent teeth can be palpated. This separation can be felt on the medial surface of the lower arcade and the lateral surface of the upper arcade. Retention of caps, however, may be so persistent and complete that the line of separation cannot be felt. Deciduous teeth will sometimes be movable on palpation but even if they are not loose, once it has been definitely determined that the permanent tooth has grown beyond the gum line, the cap should be removed. It is best not to attempt to remove caps if it requires a great deal of effort to loosen them. Age and signs of pain generally dictate removal of offending caps.

In the lower arcade, medium-sized forceps should be applied and the cap rocked loose and removed. Caps on the upper arcade can best be removed by inserting a common screw driver blade into the junction between the cap and the permanent tooth, and prying the cap loose. The extracted tooth should be examined to make sure a portion of it has not broken off and remained in the jaw, since it may not only hinder eating but cause the permanent tooth to grow unevenly, cause inflammation around the gum area, and predispose to infection.

The removal of dental caps should be accomplished before the mouth is dressed, or floated, as sharp edges or points are sometimes present on the underlying permanent teeth. By removing deciduous teeth at the proper time, the permanent teeth can grow normally, and there is less probability that training will be interrupted due to mastication difficulties or interference with the bit. This is particularly true between the second and third year of life when the first deciduous premolar becomes loose.

Retained Temporary Incisors: Retained temporary incisors are similar to dental caps except that they may remain embedded more or less firmly in the gums and the permanent incisors erupt behind them rather than push them out of the jaw. Ordinarily these teeth are loose and can easily be removed with a pair of dental forceps, but occasionally the tooth will have to be loosened with a bone gouge or dental elevator. The cavity should be searched with a probe or splinter forceps to make sure all fragments of tooth are removed, otherwise inflammation and infection may ensue from the irritation produced by the fragments. Occasionally the gum may have to be incised under local anesthesia and dental fragments removed. The surgical lesion will ordinarily heal without suturing although 1 or 2 interrupted sutures of nonabsorbable material may be placed in the gum to appose the divided tissues. Sutures should be removed before 10 days. Most horses do not object too severely to this procedure, and removal can be accomplished with minimal restraint.

Retained Temporary Premolars: Retained temporary premolars are deciduous teeth which inhibit the eruption of the underlying permanent teeth. Any cheek tooth may be involved but the first premolar of the lower arcade is most commonly affected. The condition is ordinarily seen in animals 2½ to 3 years old, but may also be found in older horses. It can usually be diagnosed by the presence of a bony enlargement on the ventral portion of the horizontal ramus of the mandible directly beneath the permanent premolar. In the absence of alveolar periostitis or dental caries, this diagnosis can be confirmed by radiographs.

Treatment involves the removal of the deciduous premolar. This can usually be done with the patient standing and restrained with a twitch. It occasionally is necessary to use local anesthesia or to place the patient in lateral recumbency either on a table or on the ground. A heavy dental forceps is used after having incised the gum from around the deciduous tooth and loosened it with a root elevator.

SUPERNUMERARY TEETH

This category includes wolf teeth and excess numbers of incisors or molars.

Wolf Teeth: Of these anomalies, wolf teeth, or first permanent premolars, are by far the most common. These may be shed at the same time as the second deciduous premolars, and whenever they are present they should be removed as they are often a source of irritation and can make training difficult. There is a common superstition among horsemen that these teeth are capable of affecting the horse's vision. There is no evidence to support this contention, but since wolf teeth are a source of irritation and since many horsemen place a great deal of importance on their removal, they should be extracted whenever encountered. It is advisable to remove them intact, but if they are broken in the process the portion left in the jaw seldom causes difficulty.

There is no single satisfactory method for removal of wolf teeth, and the method used often will be dictated by the size of the tooth, the angle of growth, and the position of the tooth in relation to the second premolar.

Deciduous teeth often are held with such tenacity that the corresponding permanent tooth becomes impacted. When this occurs in the upper arcade and involves a permanent premolar whose root is immediately beneath the floor of the maxillary sinus, alarming signs may appear. There is swelling over the sinus wall and evidence of pain is exhibited when the area is percussed. This apparently reflects an exaggerated physiologic reaction which accompanies the teething process.

Removal of the cap provides almost immediate relief to the patient. When the impediment to normal eruption has been removed there is a gradual reduction of pain and swelling over the sinus. Rarely does a sinusitis develop which requires surgical drainage or medicinal therapy.

Retained caps commonly occur in pairs. Therefore after removing one, the corresponding tooth on the opposite arcade should be examined carefully. If a cap is found it should be removed.

One method involves use of a rongeur or bone cutter, particularly one that is double-faced and off-set; however, an ordinary bone cutter is satisfactory. The tooth is palpated with the thumb or forefinger and the bone cutter is applied posterior to the finger between

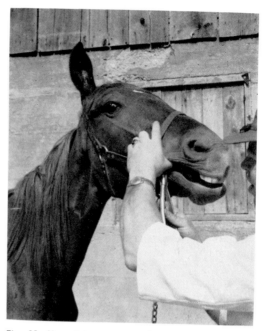

Fig. 31. Use of bone cutters in removal of premolar tooth.

the first and second premolar with the flat face toward the second premolar (Fig. 31). As it is applied, it is guided into place with the thumb or forefinger palpating the tooth. The instrument is placed high enough so the points will close ¼ to ½" above the gum. As the forceps are closed, they are given either a rotating twist or a prying motion by moving the handles posteriorly. If properly done, this will loosen the tooth with a minimum of pain to the horse and a minimum of effort by the operator. The tooth can then be removed with the fingers or forceps.

A canine root elevator works well for this operation and is used in the same manner as the bone cutters. A root elevator must be quite strong, however, and it is difficult to obtain one that can withstand the pressure. An ordinary screw driver also may be used in the same manner as the root elevator, but it does not fit the tooth as well and must be employed more carefully to prevent injury to the roof of the mouth. In horses that resist any manipulation of the mouth, the area around the first premolar may be anesthetized with a local anesthetic. This may be accomplished by injecting a 2% procaine solution into the gingival area through a fine-gauge needle. If one is working on a group of horses, an anesthetic dental ointment containing butyn sulfate or some other topical anesthetic may be massaged into the gum around the tooth every 10 minutes or so until the area is sufficiently anesthetized to remove the tooth without causing any sensation to the horse.

Supernumerary Incisors: Supernumerary incisors are not uncommon and are apparently the result of division of the permanent tooth buds. In some cases there may be a complete double row of incisors, but more often there will be only 1 or 2 extra teeth (Fig. 32). Treatment depends upon how the teeth develop. If they tend to wear more or less evenly and cause no apparent trouble, they should be left alone. If, however, the extra teeth become elongated, they should be cut off or extracted to prevent damage to the mouth. The type of operation depends upon the location of the teeth and the judgment of the veterinarian. Frequently, the owner will wish to have supernumerary incisors removed for cosmetic reasons, and it may be necessary to accede to his request even when there are no other reasons for extraction. The technic of extraction is the same as for normal incisor teeth except that extra care should be taken to prevent infection of the cavity and involvement of the remaining teeth.

Supernumerary Molars: Supernumerary molar teeth occasionally occur. Their position in the dental arcade is inconstant but ordinarily they are found posterior to the third molar tooth in prolongation of the normal dental arch in either the upper or the lower jaw. Less frequently they may appear buccal or lingual to a normal molar. Usually, the supernumerary molars are paired. If possible, they should be extracted. If this is not possible, they should be cut at regular (usually annual) intervals to prevent injury to the soft tissues and bone of the opposite jaw.

ABNORMALITIES OF TOOTH STRUCTURE

There are a number of abnormalities of tooth structure which can be found in horses. Most of these become apparent either at postmortem examination or after skulls have been prepared for anatomic specimens. Abnormalities which do not apparently interfere with function or mastication should, if detected, be watched but left alone.

Abnormalities of structure which result in excessive wear, cavities, or erosions may lead to decay or peridontal infections. In general, it can be said that serious abnormalities usually involve the cheek teeth and more frequently involve the first molars more than any other. This may be due to the fact that the first molar is the first fully-formed permanent cheek tooth

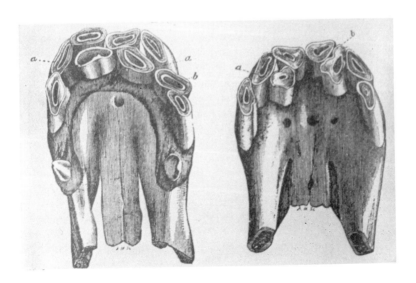

Fig. 32. Supernumerary incisor teeth. From Huidekoper's *Age of the Domestic Animals.*

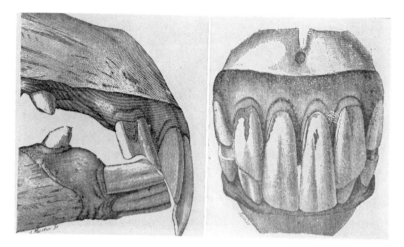

and has not had as much time for its development prior to its eruption. But whatever the cause, the first molars are likely to be softer, more prone to decay, and less well-formed structurally than the other cheek teeth. Treatment depends upon the degree of damage. In severe cases with associated infection, extraction is frequently the only recourse.

Sharp Enamel Points: Sharp enamel points, particularly on the lingual borders of the table surface of the lower cheek teeth and on the buccal borders of the upper cheek teeth, are structural abnormalities that ordinarily occur from defective or unequal wear. This is a common dental defect, and ordinarily easy to correct. The points tend to interfere with mastication by lacerating the tongue or buccal mucosa, and are ordinarily revealed by refusal to eat, restricted eating, "quidding," excessive salivation which may be so severe that the animal drools, and holding the head to one side while chewing. External palpation of the cheeks over the lacerated area will elicit pain. In longstanding cases there may be mild to severe ulceration of the torn mucous membranes of the mouth and tongue. Enamel points are removed by floating. The projecting points are rasped down with a few strokes of the float. In affected animals, floating should be repeated at regular intervals.

Projecting Teeth: Projecting teeth may or may not be a defect of structure. Ordinarily they are not, but are merely the result of growth uncompensated by wear. They usually occur as the result of excessive wear of the opposing tooth, extraction, or improper apposition of teeth in the upper and lower jaws. The teeth most often affected are the second upper premolar and the third lower molar, and often are associated with brachygnathia, or parrot mouth. In these cases the projection, formed by unequal wear, takes the form of a sharp point that can be seen readily or palpated. Projecting molar teeth also occur where the opposing molar has been extracted or is so soft that it wears excessively. Elongated lower molars, if untended, can cause considerable damage to the hard palate.

Projecting teeth can result in difficult mastication, loss of condition, and impactions of the gut due to improperly chewed food. The presence of grain and coarse material in the feces is indicative of this anomaly. Palpation will readily reveal the affected tooth or teeth. Treatment involves cutting off the projecting portion of the tooth, and rasping the surface level with the other teeth in the arcade. Treatment must be repeated from time to time or the condition will recur.

ABNORMALITIES ARISING FROM BONE DEFECTS

The spectacular conditions of parrot mouth (brachygnathia) (Fig. 33), undershot jaw (prognathia) (Fig. 34), and shear mouth arise from defects in bony growth of the jaws.

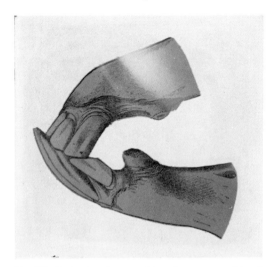

Fig. 34. Undershot jaw resulting from prognathia of lower jaw. From Huidekoper's *Age of the Domestic Animals.*

Parrot Mouth: In parrot mouth the upper jaw is relatively longer than the lower. Whether this is caused by excessive growth of the upper jaw or defective development of the lower (as the Greek name indicates) is immaterial. The deformity is congenital and may be heritable, and the horse is considered to be unsound. The defect principally involves the incisor teeth although there may be a concomitant involvement of the cheek teeth with projection of the first upper premolars and last lower molars. Less often, there may be an associated shear mouth. Since the incisor teeth are in abnormal apposition, abnormal growth of the teeth ensues. The lingual edges of the lower incisors may become elongated and sharp, and lacerate the gums and hard palate, but more commonly the lower incisors tend to prolong the line of the lower jaw and the labial edge of the upper incisors becomes long and sharp and lacerates the lower lip. From the front the horse appears "rabbit toothed," with the upper central incisors showing the greatest elongation. From the side, the position of the incisors gives the appearance of a parrot's beak. Secondary infections, digestive disorders, and impactions frequently occur as sequelae to this condition. Parrot mouth can be alleviated to some degree by regularly dressing the teeth with a float and farrier's rasp, but eventually the horse will

actively resent such treatment and the improvement effected ultimately will not be worth the fee. Ordinarily, for the sake of both the owner and the horse, euthanasia should be advised at that time.

Undershot Jaw: Undershot jaw (prognathia) is the opposite of parrot mouth. This condition primarily involves the incisors also. Associated with it are projections of the first lower premolars and last upper molars resulting from imperfect apposition of the cheek teeth. Shear mouth is not a sequel. Instead, the table surfaces of the cheek teeth tend to lose angulation. A horse with an undershot jaw is unsound, and treatment is the same as for parrot mouth, and the same ultimate results ensue.

Shear Mouth: Shear mouth arises when the difference in width between the upper and lower jaw is excessive. In a normal horse the upper arcade is always wider than the lower, and a slight excess of this inequality results in excessive angulation of the table surfaces of the cheek teeth and the development of long, extremely sharp edges. This condition may be seen in horses of any age, but is more common in old animals where irregularities in wear and age changes involving the shape of the lower jaw combine to produce this defect. Only 1 or 2 cheek teeth or all of the premolar and molar teeth may be involved. It may be unilateral or bilateral. The signs and lesions are similar to those associated with sharp enamel points, but are more severe. Treatment is usually unsatisfactory. It involves cutting and rasping to secure as normal an alignment as possible. Postoperative treatment involves placing the horse on hard feed in the hope that this will postpone recurrence of the condition. It seldom does.

ABNORMALITIES RESULTING FROM
IRREGULAR WEAR

The 3 major conditions resulting from irregular wear are wave mouth (undulating table surfaces), step mouth (step-formed table surfaces), and smooth mouth (smooth table surfaces). These conditions all involve the cheek teeth and are characteristically found in aged horses. Irregular wear may also involve the incisors with the production of an irregular or V-shaped bite in the incisor group, but this seldom is more than esthetically unpleasant, and if there is no functional or associated derangement of the cheek teeth, the incisors should be left alone.

Wave Mouth: In wave mouth, the cheek teeth show an undulating or uneven arcade. The greatest deviation usually occurs at the level of the first molar. In severe cases the teeth in one arcade may be worn level to the gums, which permits the opposing molar to lacerate the gingiva and predispose to alveolar periostitis or gingivitis. If the history indicates that mastication is normal and the arcades meet complementary to each other, nothing need be done except floating. If mastication is abnormal, however, or if there is much salivation or "quidding" of hay or grass and dropping it from the mouth, an attempt should be made to even out the arcades by use of the dental rasp and compound molar cutters. In most cases this is best accomplished under general anesthesia with the horse in lateral recumbency and with a speculum applied. In mild cases, however, the procedure can be accomplished with the horse standing and confined in stocks or a stall. Treatment of severe cases is seldom satisfactory despite adequate removal of the projecting portions of the wave.

Step Mouth: In step mouth there is a sudden variation in the height of individual premolar and molar teeth. This may be due to unequal wear of opposing teeth in the dental arcade, or it may be a sequel of extractions. The signs of this condition are similar to those of other dental disorders, but malnutrition and emaciation are usually more evident since a step-mouthed animal cannot chew food properly. Treatment involves leveling the projecting teeth and must be repeated at regular (usually annual) intervals.

Smooth Mouth: Smooth mouth is normally found in old horses, although it rarely may be encountered in young animals. The table surfaces of the teeth have become smooth through either complete erosion of the crowns, or through defects in the lamellar arrangement of enamel, cement, and dentine. Individual teeth or the entire arcade may be affected, although an animal is not ordinarily called smooth-mouthed until at least a majority of the teeth are involved. The smooth table surfaces of the teeth prohibit proper grinding of plant material. The signs associated with this condition include colic and poor condition. Smooth table surfaces can be discovered readily by palpation. In young animals, smooth mouth may occasionally be caused by improper floating. It reflects lack of knowledge of equine dental anatomy and physiology. There should be no need to belabor the point that table surfaces of cheek teeth should not be filed smooth when an animal is floated. However, the warning should be mentioned much in the spirit of adding "Danger" to a sign reading "Explosives."

Treatment of smooth mouth in old animals and in young animals with defective teeth is useless. Feeding soft mashes and chopped feed to young animals that have been mishandled will give the teeth an opportunity to re-establish their normal rough table surfaces (Table 2).

ABNORMALITIES FROM MISCELLANEOUS CAUSES

Fractures or Fissures: Fractures or fissures are fairly common. These may be the result of trauma or congenital defects. Trauma is the principal cause. In the incisors this is usually the result of accidents. In the molars, traumatic fracture is ordinarily caused by biting on some hard material such as a stone. Fractures which extend as far as the root usually will predispose to alveolar periostitis. Such teeth should be extracted once a diagnosis is made. Fractures which do not involve the base of the tooth can be treated by removing the broken part and dressing the rough edge with a file or float.

Injuries to the Mouth: Occasionally, severe injuries involve the mouth. The most common are injuries to the incisor areas caused by kicks or other severe blows. These are best handled by using common sense and cleaning the wound thoroughly. The teeth that can be saved should be given every opportunity to reseat

Table 2.—Dentistry for Horses

Age	Examine for:	Necessary dentistry:
2 to 3 years	1. 1st premolar vestige (wolf teeth)	1. Remove wolf teeth if present
	2. 1st deciduous premolar (upper and lower)	2. Remove deciduous teeth if ready. If not, file off corners and points of premolars
	3. Hard swelling on ventral surface of mandible beneath 1st premolar	3. Examine with x-ray. Extract retained temporary premolar if present
	4. Cuts or abrasions on inside of cheek in region of the 2nd premolars and molars	4. Lightly float or dress all molars and premolars if necessary
	5. Sharp protuberances on all premolars and molars	5. Rasp protuberances down to level of other teeth in the arcade
3 to 4 years	1. 1, 2, 4 and 5 above	1. 1, 2, 4 and 5 above
	2. 2nd deciduous premolar (upper and lower)	2. Remove if present and ready
4 to 5 years	1. 1, 4, and 5 above.	1. 1, 4 and 5 above
	2. 3rd deciduous premolar	2. Remove if present and ready
5 yrs. and up	1. 1, 4 and 5 above.	1. 1, 4 and 5 above.
	2. Uneven growth and "wavy" arcade	2. Straighten if interfering with mastication
	3. Unusually long molars and premolars	3. Unusually long molars and premolars may have to be cut off if they cannot be filed down

themselves and become useful again. Teeth that are broken completely away from the alveolus or are split to the roots should be removed.

As much of the torn gingiva as can be apposed should be sutured in place and if the mandible or maxilla is fractured, fragments of bone must be removed and fixation of the fracture should be accomplished by any method which will allow the process of prehension and mastication of food to be as near normal as possible. It always is good procedure to obtain both a lateral and dorso-ventral radiograph of the area to ascertain the extent of damage to the osseous structure, to aid in determining the prognosis, and to help determine fixation procedures.

TUMORS

Tumors involving the teeth and oral cavity are exceedingly rare. In the horse, the tumors involving the oral cavity and teeth include the pseudo-odontoma which is, in reality, a bony exostosis that can better be characterized as chronic ossifying alveolar periostitis. True neoplasms include odontoma, adamantinoma, osteosarcoma, and squamous cell carcinoma. For descriptions of the last 3 neoplasms see Chapter 21.

Odontoma: An odontoma is a benign tumor of dental tissue usually involving the base of a tooth. The condition may be present and cause no trouble except for swelling around the base of the tooth. It can be misdiagnosed as chronic ossifying alveolar periostitis and its true nature discovered only when an attempt is made to extract it. Extreme resistance to removal is encountered and the jaw can be fractured if forcible efforts are made to remove the tooth. In cases where the tumor is causing no inconvenience to the horse, it is advisable to leave the tooth alone. Since the bulk of an odontoma lies beneath the gum line, surgical removal is quite difficult and may involve splitting the tooth and removing the fragments, or removing the external alveolar plate to gain access to the tumorous mass.

INFECTIONS

Dental Caries: Dental caries specifically refers to a localized, progressive molecular disintegration of the enamel of a tooth followed by a more widespread bacterial invasion and decay of the underlying dentine. The process essentially involves removal of inorganic material which leaves the exposed organic material of the dentine open to bacterial invasion. There is considerable doubt that this condition exists in equines. If it does occur, it probably is secondary to alveolar periostitis.

Dentinal infections do occur, but their pathogenesis is not the same as true caries. More properly, such conditions should be referred to as "decayed teeth." Because the dentine of worn, complexly folded teeth of horses is already exposed, the initial infection results in a small pit or cavity on the table surface which expands toward the pulp cavity until the pulp is affected and alveolar periostitis ensues.

Early cases of decay seldom are seen in practice. Those which are presented for treatment are usually so advanced that nothing can be done to save the tooth. It is advisable to wait until an active case of alveolar periostitis develops before attempting to remove the infected tooth, since the decay is usually so extensive that the visible portion of the tooth has been virtually reduced to a shell of enamel and cement that is hard but brittle. Attempted extraction of the decayed tooth at this time probably will result in its fragmentation, leaving the root embedded in the alveolus. Removal is much more readily accomplished if as a result of alveolar periostitis the deeper structures are loosened.

Decay is readily recognizable if it is present, since it has a very distinctive odor that is not easily forgotten. When palpating the teeth on initial examination, the affected tooth can sometimes be identified by an inflamed gum around it, or by discovering that it has not erupted normally to meet its opposing tooth. If the decay is long-standing and the tooth is impacted, there is usually an enlargement of an overlying sinus.

A unilateral malodorous discharge appears at the nostril of the affected side when an upper cheek tooth is involved, or there is enlargement of the ramus of the mandible in the region of the affected lower cheek tooth. One must be careful to differentiate between decay and impaction of a lower tooth or failure to shed a lower deciduous tooth. Occasionally a polyp may be found medial to an affected upper cheek tooth. If this is found, it is well to withhold a prognosis until a biopsy is taken and a pathologist's report obtained, as these growths can be extensions of neoplasia of the sinuses or turbinates, and dental surgery under these circumstances could well be disastrous. A radiograph of the affected area is always valuable in assisting diagnosis and prognosis.

Once a definite diagnosis of caries is established, and the tooth is determined to be removable, it can be extracted.

Alveolar Periostitis: Alveolar periostitis is probably the commonest dental infection of equines. The disease is essentially an inflammation of the alveolar periosteum and may be produced by a number of pus-forming pathogenic organisms. All teeth in the dental arcade are susceptible, but infection of the cheek teeth is more frequent. The teeth most often involved are the fourth premolar and the first molar. Involvement of the incisors usually is secondary to traumatic injury.

The etiology is varied. Anything which exposes the alveoli to bacterial invasion may give rise to the disease. Gingival injuries, separation of gums and teeth, material between the teeth, cracks or fissures, imperfectly formed infundibuli, and extensive decay processes may form routes of infection. The condition of the horse appears to have some connection with alveolar periostitis since it seems to be more prevalent in young horses in poor condition. Age and associated tooth wear can also be predisposing factors.

The symptomatology is variable. Often the animal will show only obscure signs, such as poor condition, lethargy, reluctance to eat, avoidance of cold water, or abnormal carriage of the head. When the molars of the upper arcade are involved, the first sign may be a unilateral, purulent, flaky nasal discharge that has the fetid odor of necrotic bone. Occasionally a fistulous tract will develop between the maxillary sinus and the outside. Here again, the purulent discharge will be fetid and contain flakes of necrotic material. Involvement of the lower teeth may result in sufficient swelling around the roots that the enlargement is visible on the outside. A suppurating dental fistula may form along the sides or ventral border of the mandible. It should be noted that all external fistulas are not products of dental involvement but periostitis should always be suspected in their presence. Other signs include peridontal gingivitis, recession of the gum from around the infected tooth, and the presence of pus. In severe cases, the tooth will be loose in its socket and held in position only by the pressure of adjacent and opposing teeth. If displacement occurs, it will be buccal or labial in the upper teeth and lingual in the lower.

The diagnosis of alveolar periostitis should be followed by thorough and careful examination of the adjacent teeth and the entire gum line of the oral cavity. Treatment is removal of the affected tooth, ordinarily by extraction.

Chronic Ossifying Alveolar Periostitis: Chronic ossifying alveolar periostitis (pseudo-odontoma) is a condition more commonly encountered in horses less than 5 years of age. It is characterized by an exostosis involving the alveolus around the root of the affected tooth. The fourth upper premolar most frequently is involved. The exostosis is slow to develop, but ultimately may attain considerable size. The condition results from a low-grade alveolar periostitis. The affected tooth fails to develop normally and the exuberant bone formation may greatly hinder its removal. When ossifying periostitis involves a permanent tooth prior to or shortly after eruption, the tooth may fail to develop. Ordinarily such teeth must be removed by repulsion following their surgical exposure.

Dental Fistula: A dental fistula arises from alveolar periostitis or from secondary infection following traumatic injury to the teeth. Fistulas involving the maxillary sinus with subsequent nasal discharge are much more common than those which empty through tracts extending to the face. The affected tooth or teeth should be removed and the fistulous tract dissected out if it is external.

SURGICAL PREPARATION

In performing dental surgery care should be taken to insure adequate restraint, anesthesia, and preparation. Restraint has already been discussed elsewhere in this book, as have general and local infiltration anesthesia and surgical preparation. The technic of administering local nerve blocks for dental surgery, however, is quite important and should be described in some detail.

Nerve Block of the Upper Arcade: To eliminate sensation in the upper teeth, the infraorbital nerve must be blocked. The right and left infraorbital nerves supply the entire upper dental arcade. The nerve's function is blocked by depositing local anesthetic around the nerve at the maxillary foramen, which is located on the anteroventral aspect of the orbit about one inch medial to the edge of the orbital ring (Fig. 35).

A 4½-inch, 16-gauge hypodermic needle is inserted below the zygomatic arch at a point approximately 1 inch below the lateral canthus of the eye. The line of the facial crest should be palpated to determine the location of the bony arch before the needle is inserted. The needle is inserted anteromedially until the point strikes the orbital portion of the palatine bone. With experience, it is not difficult to hit the maxillary foramen on the first trial, but ordinarily the point of the needle must be moved around until it strikes the nerve as it enters the maxillary foramen. The horse will jerk its head when the nerve is struck.

If blood flows from the needle, it is an indication that the maxillary artery or vein has been penetrated. The character of the blood

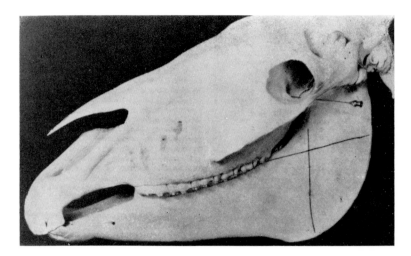

Fig. 35. Needle is shown in proper position to block the infraorbital nerve. Lines on mandible intersect at approximate position of mandibular foramen.

will indicate which vessel is involved. Since these vessels lie below the nerve, the needle should be slightly withdrawn and the point directed upward.

When the nerve has been located, 10 ml. of a sterile 2% procaine solution (or other local anesthetic) are injected. Anesthesia should occur within 10 minutes. The completeness of anesthesia can be tested by pricking the upper lip on the same side as the injection.

Nerve Block for the Lower Arcade: The right and left mandibular alveolar nerves supply the lower dental arcade. These can be blocked by depositing local anesthetic around the mandibular foramina which are located on the medial sides of the vertical rami of the mandible about 1 inch posterior to the anterior border and closely aligned to an extension of the table surfaces of the lower cheek teeth. To locate the foramen an imaginary line is constructed perpendicular to the lower border of the jaw and passing through the lateral canthus of the eye. A second line extending the table surfaces of the upper cheek teeth is drawn toward the posterior border of the ramus of the mandible. The 2 lines cross at the approximate position of the mandibular foramen.

The point is marked, and a 16-gauge needle of sufficient length (4 to 6 inches depending on the horse) is inserted upward from the angle of the mandible along the medial face,

keeping the needle close to the bone and advancing it along the line dropped from the lateral canthus of the eye. When the point of the needle has reached the spot where the 2 lines cross, inject 20 ml. of sterile 2% procaine solution (or other local anesthetic). The nerve block will be effective in about 10 minutes. Effectiveness can be checked by pricking the lower lip with a sharp needle.

OPERATIVE PROCEDURES

Bishoping: Bishoping is the only dental cosmetic operation that has ever been attempted on a sizable scale. Like much cosmetic surgery in man, it is designed to make the animal appear younger than he really is. It is practiced upon the lower incisor teeth and consists of burning or drilling false dental cups (infundibuli) in the table surfaces and painting their interiors black. Usually large cups are cut in the corners and progressively small cups in the intermediates and centrals (Fig. 36).

The operation was once in vogue among unscrupulous horse dealers and may result in part for the horse traders' not unsullied reputation. The forgery, however, is easily detected by the shape of the table surfaces of the teeth, the angulation of teeth and jaw, the fact that the false infundibulum is not surrounded by enamel, and the presence of residual enamel or of the "dental star." The only reason this is mentioned is that bishoping is still practiced occasionally and should be recognized if encountered. There is neither reason for nor honesty in bishoping and the operation is neither recommended nor condoned.

Floating: Floating usually is done without anesthesia and with minimum restraint. One should keep the anatomy of the mouth in mind. When viewed from the front, the table surfaces of the cheek teeth show a distinct angulation, upward and inward for the lower teeth and downward and outward for the upper. Sharp edges therefore will be found on the buccal borders of the upper arcade and the lingual borders of the lower. Table surfaces must be rough to be efficient. They must be even and compatible with the opposing teeth. With this in mind, the floating or filing procedure is then performed to correct any abnormalities which are found on examination that might hinder proper mastication. A specu-

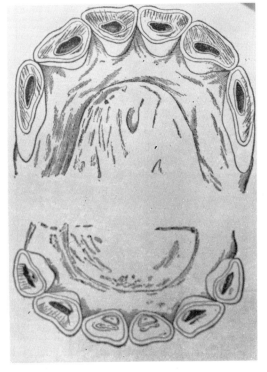

Fig. 36. Bishoping. Note false infundibuli anterior to the enamel remnants. From Huidekoper's *Age of the Domestic Animals.*

lum may be used or the tongue can be grasped and withdrawn to make the horse open his mouth to receive the float. Often this is not necessary as passage of the float itself will cause the horse to open its mouth enough for removal of the sharp edges of the teeth. When more severe floating is necessary, *e.g.* to grind down a protruding tooth, a speculum should be used and the horse should be tranquilized, sedated, restrained, or given general anesthesia as the circumstances warrant.

There is a tendency to overtreat rather than undertreat. The only rasping that is necessary is to remove sharp projections which can abrade or cut the tongue or cheeks and to level any high projections on the table surface which are incompatible with the opposing teeth. With a rasp which is sharp, these projections are usually removed by 4 or 5 strokes over the arcade, depending on how much pressure is placed on the float as well as the consistency of the teeth. To accomplish this removal, the rasp should not be placed flat on the top of the arcade, but should be held at an angle of slightly less than 90° to the lingual surface of the lower arcade and to the buccal surface of the upper. The rasp with the slight angle is used on the lower arcade and the straight rasp is used on the upper arcade (Fig. 37 & 38). When floating the upper arcade be sure that the assistant's arm or the nose band of the halter or speculum is not pressing against the horse's cheek, causing the back side of the rasp to injure the buccal mucosa. If the patient shakes his head or moves it up or down quickly, it is important to give with the movement and not try to restrain the horse with the rasp and cause injury to the inside of the mouth. It is the duty of the assistant to hold the head firm and steady but he should be careful not to take too firm a hold over the soft part of the nose and thus hinder the passage of air through the nostrils.

If the horse is in training or is being ridden or driven, the anterior premolars should be dressed to remove any sharp projections

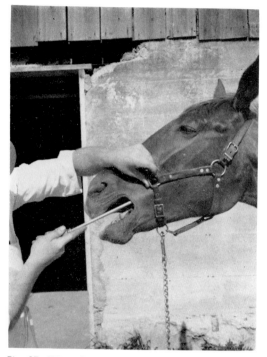

Fig. 37. Filing the upper arcade. Halter is held from cheek.

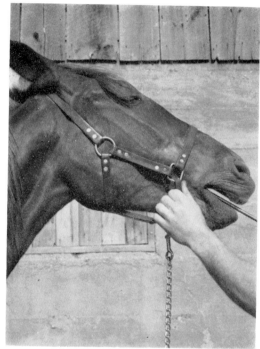

Fig. 38. Filing the lower arcade.

or edges that may cut or abrade the cheeks or the tongue from the action of the bit. This is best accomplished with the 45° float, using a file blade rather than a rasp. By taking a very short hold on this instrument most of the procedure can be accomplished with relative ease. Lingual and buccal edges of the anterior premolars are rounded off to prevent injury to the adjacent soft tissues. In yearlings, it sometimes is necessary to remove enough of the tooth surface to prevent the teeth from contacting one another at all, as some snaffle bits will force a portion of the mucosa of the cheek between these teeth and pieces may be actually bitten out, resulting in a sore mouth and excessive objection to the bit or any attempt at its manipulation. This is of great importance in young saddle horses in training for the rack and slow gaits, when there is excessive manipulation of the bit. In many of these cases, corrective dentistry will have to be done before the training can be resumed.

Cutting of Teeth: Cutting forceps with hardened jaws have been designed to remove projecting portions of molar teeth. Forceps with a compound fulcrum offer the easiest method of applying sufficient force to the cutting edge to sever the tooth cleanly, although for operators with strong arms a simple forceps is satisfactory.

Teeth should be cut under local or general anesthesia as there is a certain amount of strain placed on the tooth that is uncomfortable for the horse. A speculum should be used in this operation. There are no particular refinements of technic that are worth mentioning. The tooth is merely engaged in the jaws of the cutter and severed in much the same way as one cuts steel bolts with a bolt cutter. The technics are virtually identical. Undesirable sequelae include loosening or splitting of the tooth. Teeth of old animals tend to be more fragile than those of young, and should be treated with caution insofar as cutting is concerned.

After the tooth has been cut, it should be dressed with a float and any loose fragments or sharp corners removed. Postsurgical care involves examination to see that infection does not occur. An oral antiseptic may be applied to the gum line of a tooth that has been amputated.

Extraction of Teeth: Extraction always should be performed under local or general anesthesia with a speculum in place. Local anesthesia is preferable, but if normal restraint cannot control the horse, it probably is better to resort to general anesthesia than to cast and forcibly immobilize the animal.

One must determine the firmness of the attachment of the tooth in the alveolus. In cases of alveolar periostitis, the molar may be loose enough to be extracted with forceps. If it is determined that the extraction of a tooth can be accomplished in this way, place the forceps on the affected tooth with the edge of the jaws close to the gum line and gently start a rotating motion with the handles of the forceps, moving them in an arc subtended by the long axis of the forceps, gradually increasing the arc as the tooth loosens. Progress can be determined by a sucking sound around the alveolus and by palpation.

When the tooth has been thoroughly loosened, a fulcrum may then be placed on the table surfaces of the teeth anterior to the affected one and the forceps used as a pry to pull the tooth from the alveolus. As the tooth is raised, it is well to move the forceps down on it and obtain a shorter hold to facilitate removal. If the tooth is too long to be removed without coming into contact with the table surfaces of the opposing teeth, it sometimes can be moved medially to find the necessary room. If this is not possible, the top of the tooth must be cut off with molar cutters to allow enough room for its removal. After the tooth is removed, the alveolar cavity should be carefully searched to be sure all loose pieces of the tooth and its roots have been removed.

The cavity is then flushed with a mild antiseptic solution and packed with gauze or cotton soaked with a suitable antiseptic. Gelfoam or dental wax also may be used to prevent feed from packing in the alveolar space. The horse should be fed mash or ground feed, and hay should be withheld for 2 or 3 days until granulation tissue begins to form.

Repulsion of Teeth: Repulsion of teeth should be resorted to only when extraction is not possible. The operation should be performed under general anesthesia with a speculum in place.

The repulsion of teeth involves trephining to gain access to the base of the tooth and using a dental punch and mallet to drive the tooth from its socket. The principal difficulties are gaining access to the base of the tooth without producing unnecessary damage to the supporting bone, and driving the tooth from its socket without fracturing the jaw, splintering the tooth, or causing unnecessary damage to the alveoli of adjacent teeth.

Repelling is confined to the cheek teeth and can be applied to teeth in either the upper or the lower jaw. Postoperative care may be required from a few days to several weeks, depending upon how soon the infection is overcome, possible involvement of adjacent tissues, and how rapidly healthy granulation tissue fills the vacated alveolus. The owner should be warned that the removal of the tooth will result in elongation of the opposing tooth in the other jaw, and that the horse will need yearly dental care. The basic technics of repulsion are similar, but their application is considerably different and the various approaches for teeth of the upper and lower jaws will be considered separately.

Repulsion of the Upper Cheek Teeth: It is essential to position the trephine opening properly to avoid damage to the nasolacrimal duct and the lacrimal canal which run from the medial canthus of the eye downward and forward to the floor of the nasal cavity near the external nares. A base line constructed from the medial canthus of the eye through the infra-orbital foramen and extending forward to the nares will mark the location of the nasolacrimal duct. Trephined openings should be made below this line. In young animals, due to the length of the teeth, the trephine opening must be kept as close to the line as possible. In older animals it may be made some distance below the line to compensate for shortening of tooth length and sharpening of the facial contours.

Each tooth requires a different location of the trephine opening. For the first and second cheek teeth a line is drawn through the center of the tooth and the opening is made along this line and just below the baseline. For the third through the fifth cheek teeth, the opening is made below the base line along a line passing upward parallel to the posterior border of the tooth. For the sixth cheek tooth the opening should be made over the fronto-maxillary opening and a curved punch used to contact the roots of the tooth. It is fortunate that this tooth seldom needs to be repelled as it is not easily accessible, particularly in young animals where the base of the tooth lies under the floor of the orbit. It should be mentioned that as a horse becomes older the teeth become progressively easier to reach via trephine openings since the gradual eruption of the teeth leaves more space between the baseline and the trephined opening.

Technic: After surgical preparation of the area and application of a speculum to the horse's mouth, an X-shaped incision is made over the spot where the trephine will be placed. The center of the incision should mark the center of the opening. The skin flaps are reflected and are held back from the surgical field with stay sutures or Backhaus forceps. The subcutaneous tissues are dissected until the periosteum is reached. The periosteum is incised with an X-shaped incision and is carefully cleaned from the bone and pushed back under the soft tissues, leaving enough bone exposed to accommodate the trephine. The

center punch of the trephine is set in the center of the field, and with a firm pressure on the handle the instrument is rotated back and forth in an arc of a circle until the blades cut through the exposed bone. The instrument should not be tipped as it is being rotated, as the cutting drum may be broken by this action. The disk of bone usually comes away with the trephine when the instrument is removed, but in some cases the underlying attachments may require that the disk be freed with forceps and a bone chisel.

Once the trephined opening has been made, the base of the tooth to be repelled is carefully located by palpation of the exposed portion of the tooth inside the jaw and projecting the direction of the tooth into the jaw. The punch is then placed upon the base of the tooth and an assistant strikes the end of the punch with a mallet according to directions. The first few blows should be only sufficiently hard to seat the punch against the base of the tooth. If there is insufficient room to do this, the opening should be enlarged with rongeurs or a bone chisel. The accuracy of the punch setting is determined by palpation of impact with a finger on the tooth to be repelled (and on adjacent teeth). If the punch is properly placed, mallet blows subsequent to seating will have a characteristic ring and rebound not found when the punch is penetrating soft tissues. The tooth should then be loosened by blows hard enough to loosen but not hard enough to splinter the base. When the tooth has been loosened, the subsequent blows can be lighter as the tooth is repelled from its alveolus.

After removal, examine the base of the tooth carefully to determine if it is complete. Any dental fragments remaining in the alveolus should be removed with splinter forceps. Occasionally it may be necessary to curette the alveolar cavity. When it has been cleaned it should be packed with antiseptic gauze or dental wax. The periosteum and skin flaps should be approximated over the incision. If a tied packing is used a small central portion of the skin flap should be removed to allow the tie to pass through. An alternative procedure is to remove the skin over the trephine opening.

It may be necessary when repelling the fourth, fifth, and sixth cheek teeth to cut the tooth off with a molar cutter when it is partially repelled as there may not be sufficient space between the table surfaces to allow the tooth to be repelled all the way and movement medially may not be possible without causing undue injury to the alveolus.

Repulsion of the Lower Cheek Teeth: The trephine openings for repulsion of the lower cheek teeth are made on the latero-ventral border of the mandible, using similar surgical technic for placing the trephine as is employed in the upper jaw. The opening for repelling the first cheek tooth is located directly below the table surface of the tooth. For the second through the fifth cheek teeth of horses less than 9 years old, the opening is made below the posterior border of the tooth. In horses more than 9 years old, the opening is aligned more closely with the center of the table surface until the animal is 12 years old. From that age onward, the opening should be under the table surface.

The trephined opening for the fourth and fifth lower cheek teeth may involve the ex-

ternal maxillary artery and vein and the parotid duct. These structures should be carefully exposed, freed, and retracted from the surgical field.

Removal of the sixth cheek tooth presents several special problems:

1. The tooth bed, or root, ends approximately midway between the table surface of the tooth and the greatest curvature of the ramus of the mandible. This necessitates trephining on the lateral side of the mandible rather than on the latero-ventral surface.

2. The trephine point underlies the thick and expansive masseter muscle which creates considerable difficulty in exposing the operative site properly.

3. The curvature of this tooth is greater than any other and requires careful attention during repulsion since the line of force established by the mallet and punch must be at an angle rather than a straight line.

A 3- to 4-inch incision is made just through the skin and parallel to the fibers of the masseter muscle. The center of this incision should lie midway between the table surface of the tooth and the greatest curvature of the mandible. The muscle fibers are then bluntly separated until the bone is reached. A wound retractor, inserted at this time into the muscula-

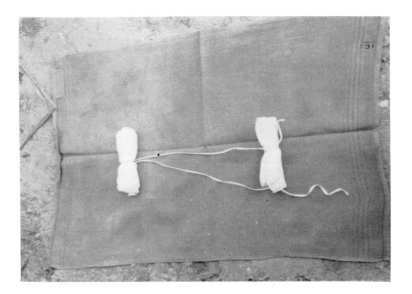

Fig. 39. Gauze packs prepared for insertion after tooth has been repelled.

ture, is a valuable aid in providing exposure of the site. The lowest part of the tooth bed is located by finding the bulging bony prominence of the root, and the trephine opening is made at this point.

The entire tooth can rarely be repelled into the mouth in one piece since the upper sixth tooth is so close. Therefore, the lower tooth must be cut once or twice with a suitable instrument during removal. Care should be taken to avoid injury to major branches of the facial nerve and the masseteric artery which are found between 1 and 2 inches above the ventral border of the mandibular ramus.

As in the upper jaw, the punch should be placed, as nearly as possible, in alignment with the long axis of the tooth. The technic of repulsion is the same. A method of identifying the root of the tooth when excessive enlargement of the mandible is present, is to apply forceps to the tooth and rotate it slightly while palpating through the trephine opening with the finger or the dental punch.

Postoperative Care

Packing: Various methods have been used for packing cavities after tooth extraction. The oldest method, and one still frequently used, is the insertion of a tied gauze roll.

After removal of the tooth and debris, a gauze pack is made by forming several 4 x 4 gauze sponges into a roll and tying it in the center with umbilical type (Fig. 39). The ends of the tape should be left long enough to reach through the trephine opening and to accommodate a second roll which is placed on the outside. The rolls are saturated with a suitable antiseptic or antibiotic solution and the ends of the tape are inserted through the alveolar and trephined openings to the outside. The inner pack is pulled firmly over the mouth of the alveolus and palpated to be sure the opening is completely covered to prevent food from entering the alveolus. The pack should not be drawn into the alveolar cavity. It is secured in place by tying the tapes firmly around the second pack outside the trephine opening.

These dressings may be changed daily or every second day, as the case indicates. When changing the packs, the outside roll is removed and a cord or a length of umbilical tape is attached to the free ends of tape from the alveolar dressing. As the alveolar pack is removed, the new tape is pulled through the alveolus and out of the mouth, and is used to facilitate seating the new pack. If one is trained to work without a speculum as described earlier in this chapter, the changing of dressings is accomplished simply and quickly. Dressings should be used until sufficient granulation has occurred to prevent passage of the tapes.

A. R. Skewes

Dental Wax: In the opinion of the editor, of all the materials and methods used for closing an alveolus from which a tooth has been removed, dental wax is the most satisfactory.

Truwax dentsply baseplate wax is used. It has a melting point of 100 F. which is above the temperature of the mouth and thus it remains solidified when placed in the oral cavity.

After the tooth has been removed and the alveolus cleansed of fragments, 2 sheets of the wax measuring 3" x 6" x ⅛" each are submerged in hot water (95 to 100 C.) Within a few seconds the wax becomes soft and pliable and can be molded roughly in the shape of the tooth just extracted. This should be done hurriedly so that the molded shape may be placed in the alveolus before the wax has "set." As the soft wax plug is inserted into the alveolus it conforms to the shape of the cavity, and the little irregularities therein give the plug a stability which prevents its dislodgment during mastication.

The entire plug should be about half the length of the root of the removed tooth. This allows room for the development of granulation tissue in the root socket. The plug should extend only slightly above the top of the gingiva so that it does not become actively engaged in the process of chewing and thus sacrifice some of its holding qualities. After the wax is in place its surface is molded carefully with a finger to build a slight flange over the gum line. This effectively seals the alveolus.

If it is necessary to remove the plug post-operatively for drainage of a sinus, medication, or inspection, it is done by inserting a hemostat through the trephine opening and dislodging the wax. A new plug may be inserted without anesthesia since its application is attended by little or no discomfort. It will be noticed that at each replacement of the plug less wax is needed because of the rapidly developing granulation tissue.

After the need for treatment has ended a final plug, of appropriate size, is inserted. As granulation tissue fills the alveolus it gradually pushes the wax plug into the oral cavity until it is finally expelled. During convalescence, a gauze dressing is used over the exterior trephine wound.

L. E. Johnson

REFERENCES

1. Frank, E. R.: Veterinary Surgery Notes, revised ed. Burgess Publishing Co., Minneapolis, Minn., 1949.

2. Guard, W. F.: Surgical Principles and Technics, revised ed. W. F. Guard, Columbus, Ohio, 1951.

3. Huidekoper, R. S.: Age of the Domestic Animals, Alexander Eger, Chicago, Ill., 1904.

4. O'Connor, J. J.: Dollar's Veterinary Surgery, 3rd ed. Alexander Eger, Chicago, Ill., 1946.

5. Sisson, S. S. and Grossman, J. D.: The Anatomy of the Domestic Animals, 3rd ed. Saunders, Philadelphia, Pa., 1938.

6. Smith, H. A., and Jones, T. C.: Veterinary Pathology, 2nd ed. Lea and Febiger, Philadelphia, Pa., 1961.

7. Special Report on Diseases of the Horse, revised ed. USDA, United States Government Printing Office, Washington, D. C., 1942.

8. The Merck Veterinary Manual, 2nd ed. Merck and Co., Rahway, N. J., 1961.

CHAPTER 28

SPECIAL PROBLEMS OF PONY PRACTICE

INTRODUCTION

During the past decade the number of ponies in the United States has increased steadily. In 1959, the number registered for the Shetland breed was exceeded only by the American Quarter Horse and the Thoroughbred registrations.[1] A count of registered ponies of recognized breeds can be obtained but there is no way to number the thousands of unregistered ponies of questionable ancestry who serve as pets and sources of amusement for "kids" from 4 to 94. This surge of popularity has reached such proportions that the pony's habitat is no longer restricted to the farms and ranches of America but now includes the backyards of thousands of suburbanites.

A pony, by general definition, is any equine under 14-2 hands in height but different breeds have their own limitations; for example, the registered Shetland may not be more than 46 inches. There are many breeds of ponies: the Shetland, Welsh, and Hackney are most common in America. The Shetlands (and a few other breeds) most closely resemble the ancestral horse of 100,000 years ago. In comparing archaeologic data with the present Shetland, Icelandic, and Exmoor breeds a striking resemblance, if not complete conformity, may be noted. There is little doubt that ponies have been able to survive and to retain this ancestral resemblance only because of their strength, vitality, adaptability, intelligence, and assiduity.[3] These attributes still are demonstrable in the ponies of today.

The acquisition of a pony, in many instances, causes a number of problems for the new owner and his veterinarian. Often, both have had little or no experience in the care, feeding, and management of an equine. Because of his urban or semiurban location and his consideration of the pony as a pet rather than as a large animal, the owner frequently calls upon a small animal or general practitioner rather than an equine specialist concerning his animal. Frequently, there is unnecessary reluctance on the part of veterinarians to accept these calls because of their insufficient experience with ponies. Yet many pony problems may be successfully mastered by the use of common sense and the application of basic medical principles used in other species. A show of genuine interest and a moderate display of initiative often will serve very effectively as a counter-balance to a lack of experience. The application of this approach usually will result in gratifying results on behalf of the client and his pet.

A pony basically is an equine animal and should be so treated. Almost every drug, medical technic, surgical procedure or management practice successful in horses may be applied with equal success in ponies. Of course, size and weight differences must be taken into consideration. Generally, however, the pony has a slightly greater tolerance to drugs (anthelmintics, tranquilizers and anesthetics) on a pound per body weight basis than has the horse.

As may be noted from the preceding paragraph, the author acknowledges a great similarity between the pony and the horse, and believes that, essentially, their ills are the same and can be handled identically. The information to follow, therefore, will be confined to discussions of those conditions and problems most commonly encountered in the pony. An effort will be made to point out where the treatment or the approach to it differs from that applied in the horse.

NUTRITION

Directly or indirectly, no other phase of pony husbandry constitutes so much of a problem to the owner and his veterinarian as does proper nutrition. Many owners inquire about correct feeding practices as soon as they obtain a pony. Too often, however, it is not until the neophyte's animal is in serious trouble that the veterinarian is asked for his professional advice. At this time, permanent and irreversible damage such as chronic laminitis, rickets, etc., may have occurred.

Comparatively little research has been done on the nutritional requirements of the horse and even less information concerning these is available for the pony. It is necessary, therefore, to extrapolate most of the information concerning the correct feeding of these animals. Many times this information, so authoritatively given, is only a "good guess." The feeding of ponies, as the feeding of any other animal, is an "art," mastered usually only after long years of study and experience. The requirements of one animal are not necessarily the same for all. A ration adequate for one individual may starve a second or overfeed a third. However, there are some sound, basic general principles which should be followed.

PASTURE

In the interests of adequate nutrition and of economy, fresh roughage should comprise the major portion of the pony's diet. Except for the addition of hay in winter, pasture roughage often serves as the sole diet for many ponies in the Southeast. Good quality green grass produced under a sound program of fertilization will provide adequate protein and mineral levels and will compensate for many of the deficiencies found in concentrates and dry roughages.[9]

A legume or legume-grass pasture is best. Blue grass and white clover constitute a very satisfactory mixture. Bermuda grass (common or coastal), Kentucky blue grass, alfalfa, clover, fescue, and prairie grass are all suitable for grazing. Alfalfa is highly palatable and nutritious, thus it is especially good for yearlings and broodmares. Because of its palatability, animals often will overeat if permitted. This can be prevented by seeding grass pastures with alfalfa.[9]

Freshly cut grass can be fed safely if not allowed to wilt. In the wilted state, it may cause digestive disturbances. Yard clippings frequently are fed but this practice should be discouraged because too often the grass is allowed to wilt and perhaps heat before it is fed. Also, the clippings may be contaminated with the foliage of ornamental shrubs, trees or bushes, some of which are toxic (*e.g.*, oleander).

DRY ROUGHAGE

It is important that all hay be of reasonably high quality and free of mold and excessive dust. Sprinkling with water or lime water just before feeding will help control dust.

For many years timothy hay has been considered ideal for horses. Unquestionably, it is satisfactory roughage but it is difficult to procure in many areas, and it usually is quite expensive when available. The most desirable dry roughage is a legume-grass mixture.[8] The legume hays (clover and alfalfa) and the legume-grass mixtures (alfalfa and timothy) generally are higher in protein, more readily obtainable, but harder to cure.

Alfalfa hay is especially good for feeding broodmares, foals, and growing stock because of its high protein, carotene, and mineral content. Alfalfa is highly palatable and ponies will overeat unless the quantity is limited. Hay should not be fed free choice regardless of its type because this is a wasteful and needless expenditure. There also is a tendency for animals fed free choice to overeat, thereby predisposing to digestive disturbances. A daily allowance of one pound of alfalfa per 100 pounds of body weight is sufficient. Caution must be exercised in feeding coarse or stemmy alfalfa, for impaction of the bowel is a frequent sequela.

Grass hays such as Bermuda, prairie, oat, orchard, and brome are satisfactory for ponies although they are somewhat lower in protein than are the legumes.

GRAINS

Oats, corn, barley, wheat bran, and sorghum grains (milo) are suitable for feeding ponies. Regardless of the type of grain selected, it should be always of high quality, of good weight, and free of mold. The digestibility of oats, barley, and the grain sorghums is enhanced by rolling or grinding, but for ponies whose teeth are in good condition there is little need to grind or crush corn. Finely ground grain or grain mixtures (chicken feed) should not be fed for they may cause intestinal colic, other digestive disorders, and laminitis.

Wheat bran is highly palatable and slightly laxative. Often it is used as a protein supplement but it is doubtful whether a pony requires any protein supplementation unless undergoing rigorous training, racing or hard daily riding. If additional protein is required soybean oil meal, cottonseed meal and linseed oil meal are better sources. When used, such meals must be fed sparingly if digestive disturbances are to be prevented. It is recommended that only 1 to 1.5 pounds per day be fed to a 1,000-pound horse.[9] These foodstuffs have been credited with improving the bloom of the haircoat but such changes are difficult to evaluate because grooming and care of the animal probably have more influence on the animal's appearance than has the ration.[12]

"Sweet feed" commonly is fed by owners of 1 or 2 ponies because it is convenient. This is a mixture of several grains to which molasses has been added. It can safely be fed to ponies, but it must be remembered that the mixture is no better than the quality of its component grains.

One of the more recent innovations in equine feeding practices is the use of a pelleted feed. Grains, meals, minerals, and hay are ground, mixed and compressed into a pellet. One producing company reports this to be a completely balanced ration and that when fed at 1½ pounds per 100 pounds body weight no other roughage is needed. It may offer the suburban pony owner a convenient way of feeding his animal and alleviate his problem of formulating a ration if the product proves successful. However, there is some question about whether the equine can be maintained free of digestive disturbances on a ration totally devoid of roughage other than that contained in the pellet. Cattle feeding trials in which a pelleted grain-hay ration was given in the absence of other roughage revealed a decreased feed consumption, slower gains and a significantly lower rumen pH.[4]

VITAMIN SUPPLEMENT

There is no evidence that a pony receiving an ordinary ration containing plenty of good quality hay or pasture requires vitamin supplementation.

MINERAL SUPPLEMENT

With the possible exception of broodmares, mature ponies do not need additional minerals except salt, when fed an ordinary ration containing plenty of good quality hay or pasture. Pregnant mares, lactating mares, foals and yearlings should have calcium and phosphorous added to their ration. Steamed bone meal and dicalcium phosphate are good sources of both minerals.

In areas of iodine deficiency, pregnant mares should be fed iodized salt during the latter half of gestation to prevent goiter in their foals.

Although the actual requirements for sodium chloride are not known, it is unlikely that natural feeds supply the daily needs. Salt should be supplied free choice, either as a part of a mineral mix or separately in free form. This practice is superior to feeding in the block form.

Wood chewing by ponies is encountered sometimes. Its etiology is not definitely known and it probably is not identical in each instance. A commonly advanced theory is that this is a manifestation of a mineral deficiency but this conjecture is difficult to support because the addition of a vitamin-mineral supplement does not always eliminate the signs. Other theorists say that wood chewing begins as a nervous mannerism brought about by insufficient exercise, neglect, and boredom and develops into a stable vice; this theory too, cannot be proved or disproved conclusively.

WATER

Clean fresh water should be available constantly. The only time a pony should not have water is immediately after working, when he is hot. Cold or excessive water consumption at this time can produce laminitis.

RATIONS

The idle, mature pony can be maintained on good quality pasture alone. Under poor grazing conditions, 1½ pounds of hay per 100 pounds of body weight should be fed.

Pregnant mares can be maintained on a good legume or legume-mix pasture until the last quarter of gestation; then their ration should be supplemented with approximately ¾ pound of concentrate and ¾ pound of roughage per 100 pounds body weight. Mineral supplements should also be added.

Lactating mares have a high energy requirement. They must meet their own maintenance requirements plus those of milk production. Shetland mares may produce approximately 3 gallons of milk per day.[10] A mare on excellent legume pasture may be able to maintain such production, but usually a concentrate and a protein supplement are necessary. In the absence of pasture, 1 to 1½ pounds each of concentrates and roughage per 100 pounds of body weight should be fed. A vitamin-mineral mixture should be included in the ration.

Foals should be allowed to go to pasture with their dams as soon as they are sufficiently strong to walk. Their diet will consist largely of milk for the first 2 months but often they will nibble grain as early as 3 weeks of age. Allowing the foal to eat from the dam's tub before the mare eats is a satisfactory practice where mares are handled separately, but under band conditions it is desirable to establish a creep feeder to allow the foal to eat when it wants and as much as it needs. A concentrate ration suitable for creep feeding is 5 parts ground oats, 4 parts wheat bran, and 1 part linseed oil meal.

Frequently, pony owners feed carrots, apples, turnips, sugar, bread, etc. as tidbits or rewards. These foodstuffs are not particularly nutritious but are in no way injurious to the animals unless one becomes choked on a large apple or turnip. However, such a practice may spoil animals. Often they become pests, constantly searching the handler's person for such goodies and becoming difficult to bridle, saddle, groom or examine.

PARASITE CONTROL

The control and treatment of parasites in ponies differs little from that in horses. Good stable and corral sanitation must be practiced. Animals should not be fed off the ground and foodstuffs should be protected from fecal contamination. Overgrazing is to be avoided and, where possible, rotation of pastures should be practiced. Periodic chain-harrowing of pastures will scatter fecal deposits and, by the exposure of parasite eggs to the destructive forces of the elements, will help to prevent reinfection.

It is not uncommon to encounter a heavily parasitized pony, usually the result of the owner's ignorance of the parasitic problem or due to his negligence. Such an animal usually is weak, dehydrated, and anemic. Great care must be exercised in treating such animals. The dose of anthelmintic should be decreased or administered in divided doses. Supportive therapy of injectable iron, fluids, whole blood, amino acids, etc., may be indicated.

The anthelmintic to be used is determined upon identification of the infecting parasite, best determined by a fecal examination. Often, however, it must be chosen without the benefit of laboratory findings. Under such circumstances, it is selected on the basis of such considerations as: the patient's age, the clinical signs, and the prevalence of the various parasites of ponies.

Ascarids are the most common parasites of foals and yearlings. In the order of their efficacy, the drugs and their dosages (per 100 pounds body weight) recommended for the treatment of ascarids are: piperazine citrate, 10 Gm.; piperazine-carbon disulfide complex (Parvex: Upjohn Co.), ½ fluid ounce; and carbon disulfide, 2 to 3 ml.

Strongyles, bots, and pinworms usually are a problem only in long yearlings and adults. For the most effective removal of strongyles, a full therapeutic dose of 2.5 Gm. per 100 pounds body weight of phenothiazine and 1 fluid ounce per 100 pounds body weight of piperazine-carbon disulfide complex should be administered at one time.[11] Carbon disulfide, 2 to 3 ml. per 100 pounds body weight, is

most specific for bot removal. A full therapeutic dose of both phenothiazine and piperazine adipate is recommended for removing
pinworms.[11]

Usually, anthelmintics are not as effective
when administered in or on the feed as when
given directly by stomach tube. Fasting the
animal overnight enhances their efficacy. Administration via the intranasal stomach tube
using liquid preparations is preferred. This
technic will prevent stomatitis produced by irritant drugs when capsules are broken in the
mouth, choke from large boluses that lodge in
the esophagus, and the possible waste of expensive liquid medicants not swallowed when
administered by a dose syringe.

Low level phenothiazine feeding has been effective in curtailing reinfestation of strongyles
once these parasites have been removed or
when they have been reduced by treatment. It
is no substitute for full-dose therapy of animals
already heavily parasitized, and the practice
will not eliminate completely the need for
further full-dose treatments. Low level feeding is practiced where ponies are individually
fed a concentrate ration daily but since most
ponies are not so fed, this procedure is not
as popular with pony owners as it is with
horse owners.

PREGNANCY EXAMINATIONS

When the novelty of owning, riding, and
caring for the new pony abates, the owner
may wish to breed the mare and to raise a
foal. The veterinarian may be called upon by
the inexperienced owner to diagnose pregnancy from one week to one year after the
mare has received service. Unlike those for
hot-blooded mares, most requests for pony
mare examinations usually are made relatively
late in the gestation period. The fetus often is
large enough to be palpated readily. Because
the pony mare is smaller and usually less frac-
tious, examination is easier and harm to the
examiner is less likely.

Judiciously performed, rectal examinations
can be routinely used on all pony mares, including Shetlands. This diagnostic procedure
is safe for both the mare and the examiner if
the usual practices of control, protection, and
restraint are observed. When the rectal sphincter is large enough to accommodate the coned
and well-lubricated hand of the examiner
and will allow it to pass with moderate pressure, the technic is not hazardous. Some small
and/or maiden mares cannot be examined
rectally because of anatomic incompatibility.
Of course, the ease or difficulty of diagnosing
pregnancy by rectal examination is dependent
upon the number of examinations performed
by the diagnostician.

COMMON DISEASES

STRANGLES

Strangles is an acute disease of horses and
ponies caused by *Streptococcus equi*. It is
characterized by inflammation of the upper
respiratory tract and abscessation in the adjacent lymph nodes.[2] Its etiology and clinical
signs are identical with those observed in the
horse.

Newly purchased additions to the band or
ponies recently returned from the show circuit are the usual sources of infection. A
strict quarantine program should be followed
on all farms to prevent the introduction of
strangles and other diseases in this way.

Infected ponies should be isolated as soon
as detected, for the nasal discharges are highly
infectious. Most cases respond well to sulfamethazine (1 grain per pound body weight)
and aqueous procaine penicillin G (3000 units
per pound body weight) in combination. If improvement is not noticeable in 24 to 48 hours,
chlortetracycline (2 to 5 milligrams per pound
body weight) should be substituted.

Enlargement of the lymph nodes of the
throat region and acute pharyngitis often produce labored and stertorous breathing. The
noise can be heard at a distance of several
yards. Hot antiphlogistic packs applied to the
throat may alleviate the dyspnea, but occasionally it is necessary to perform a tracheotomy to prevent collapse and death from
anoxia.

After the disease gains entrance into a
band, it usually spreads to all members (with
the possible exception of the older members
who probably are immune). Recent research

has shown that a bacterin prepared from pure cultures of *Streptococcus equi* will control outbreaks in bands of horses.[11] The bacterin is not now available commercially but it should be marketed in the near future.

LAMINITIS

Laminitis, both acute and chronic, occurs very commonly in ponies. Directly or indirectly, it produces more lameness than any other disease.

One of the most frequent causes of acute laminitis is improper feeding through either ignorance or negligence. The overeating of any ration may precipitate an attack but the consumption of finely ground grains (as chicken feed) or spoiled foodstuffs is the common etiology. Spontaneous laminitis sometimes occurs in animals whose only ration is pasture grass. Under such circumstances, the pasture usually is lush, highly palatable, and often of the leguminous type.

The signs of acute laminitis in the pony are the same as those in the horse. The administration of antihistamines, corticosteroids, laxatives, antiferments, cold water to the feet, and sedatives or tranquilizers (when indicated) constitutes the usual treatment.

Chronic laminitis probably is seen more frequently than is the acute form. When owners fail to recognize acute laminitis or when they delay before seeking professional assistance, chronicity results. In the absence of proper treatment or if there is no response to treatment, permanent damage is produced. Many ponies are overly conditioned and their increased body weight contributes further to the breakdown of the foot. Concentric hoof rings, dropped sole, rotation of the coffin bone, seedy toe, overgrown horn wall and malformed feet are common sequelae.

Animals with such foot pathology frequently show constant lameness. The correction of these deformities and the successful treatment of the associated lameness are extremely difficult and, often, are impossible. However, many such affected individuals can be salvaged for broodmares or pets by the application of palliative measures.

Periodic corrective trimming of the feet is necessary. Trimming is made easier and the quality of the horny tissue may be improved by the daily application of neat's foot oil, lanolin or a commercial hoof dressing to the foot wall and sole. Soaking the feet in water or mud for several days prior to trimming may be necessary. It is not uncommon to encounter individuals with such an extensive overgrowth of horn wall, especially at the toe, that their feet have the appearance of skis. Shortening of the horn wall in these animals is limited only by the degree of convexity of the dropped sole. Enough wall must be left so that weight is not brought to bear on the dropped sole or the lameness will be accentuated. Corrective shoeing with a convex boiler plate shoe often will afford some relief.

Neurectomy, if performed on selected patients, may prolong an animal's serviceability. Such surgery is recommended only for individuals who are to serve as broodmares or pets. When sensation no longer exists in the lower leg, stumbling is likely to occur with concomitant degeneration of the foot. These animals are not safe mounts for children or for inexperienced riders and should not be so used.

To be sure that a neurectomy will be effective, a nerve block should first be performed. The neurectomy should be done no higher up the leg than is necessary to remove the lameness, a site best determined by an initial digital nerve block. If, upon exercise, the lameness is not relieved, a volar block should be performed. In the absence of relief from the volar block it may be necessary to block either the median and/or ulnar nerves to render the animal insensitive to pain.

Ponies suffering from milder forms of chronic laminitis frequently find their way into trading circles. Such individuals usually can be "bought right"; a young child and his benevolent father are prime subjects for such a sale. If a veterinary examination is requested, special attention should always be given to the feet. Corticosteroids, phenylbutazone or recent trimming of the feet temporarily may mask a lameness but nothing can remove the concentric "founder rings," the dropped sole or the seedy toe which are positive proof of previous damage and signify the likely occurrence of lameness in the future.

INDIGESTION AND COLIC

Indigestion with colic often is encountered in ponies. Poor care and shoddy feeding practices, the results of negligence or ignorance, probably are the primary causes. Many pony owners "kill 'em with kindness the first month and with neglect thereafter." The new pony often is overfed, given improper feeds (dry mash), or fed spoiled foodstuffs, all of which commonly produce colic. Children, particularly, are irresponsible about overfeeding a new pony. When the novelty of ownership disappears, however, the animal is likely to be fed irregularly, and frequently is offered such indigestible feeds as coarse alfalfa hay (which may produce impactions). Foreign matter (bread wrappers, cardboard, and paper sacks) has been found as the cause of intestinal obstruction.

Generally, the signs exhibited by the "colicky" pony are the same as those seen in the horse. Treatment, too, is similar. It is advisable to administer laxatives, antiferments, etc., via stomach tube. An injectable substance found to be useful in pony indigestion is Coecolysin Bengen*, an organic extract which stimulates gastrointestinal peristalsis while simultaneously increasing gastric secretions. Best results are obtained by the administration of 5 to 10 ml. intramuscularly, followed by 5 ml. at 3- to 4-hour intervals until 3 to 5 doses have been given.

MAMMARY EDEMA

Pregnant mares in late gestation may develop a rather extensive edema of the udder and/or the ventral belly wall 2 to 3 weeks before foaling. The condition is seen most commonly in primiparous mares although it may occur in older broodmares. The udder enlarges and becomes hard and painful; usually there is no milk in the glands. As the condition pro-

*Coecolysin Bengen: Bengen and Company, Hannover, Germany. Distributed through Dr. S. Jackson, Washington, D. C.

gresses, the udder becomes edematous; subcutaneous edema forms along the ventral body wall beginning at the udder and extending forward sometimes as far as the sternum. It pits characteristically with moderate digital pressure.

Moderate exercise, alternate hot and cold water applications and topical liniments, although helpful, will not completely remove the edema. The administration of a diuretic such as acetazolamide sodium (Vetamox: American Cyanamid Co.) may bring about a diminution of signs.

If the edema persists after parturition the mare may not allow the foal to nurse because of the pain caused by the youngster's suckling. However, if the mare is nursed, the edema usually will subside. Some edematous mares fail to experience a letdown of milk. Whether this is due to pain or to some other cause is unknown.

Administration of a tranquilizing drug (100 to 250 mg. of promazine hydrochloride intravenously) usually will render the mare sufficiently docile to allow the foal to nurse. Continous tranquilization for several days may be necessary; this state may be induced by incorporating tranquilizer pellets in the feed. Oxytocin should be given to mares without milk; it may stimulate milk letdown in some individuals but a small percentage of edematous mares never lactate. Most of these mares do lactate satisfactorily following the birth of their second and successive foals.

COMMON SURGICAL PROCEDURES

CASTRATION

Owners constantly inquire as to the best age at which to castrate pony colts. The choice of time is dependent upon several factors. It is best always to wait until the testicles have descended completely before attempting surgery. The opinion has been expressed that the testicles of Shetland ponies are later in their descent than are those of other breeds.[5] Whether this is true because of a breed characteristic or because of the higher incidence of cryptochidism in Shetlands—or if in fact it is true at all—has not been substantiated.[7] As long as the colt is manageable, surgery can be postponed until the descent of the testicles. The probability of a testicle's descent after a colt reaches 18 to 24 months of age is rather unlikely.

The longer the colt is allowed to remain intact the greater and more complete will be the development of the secondary sex characteristics. If a well-muscled, heavily necked, more robust individual is desired, he should not be castrated before he has reached an age of 18 to 24 months. However, unfavorable and undesirable behavior patterns may make earlier castration necessary.

The surgical technic and restraint of the patient are matters of individual preference. Most surgeons find that casting is preferable to the standing method because of the patient's stature. Because the testicles often are small and frequently have but incompletely descended, these annoying obstacles can be handled with greater dexterity in the casted position.

DORSAL PATELLAR FIXATION

A common lameness of ponies, particularly in Shetlands, is produced by a dorsal fixation of the patella. This condition has been confused with lateral luxation of the patella, an entirely different entity much less frequently seen. In dorsal fixation, the patella rides dorsally when the stifle is extended and the medial patellar ligament becomes "hooked" over the medial ridge of the trochlea of the femur. When progression is attempted, the leg is held in a state of posterior overextension for an instant before it is flexed with a quick and often exaggerated movement. In some cases the affected leg is held in posterior extension for several steps and the toe is dragged. The lameness may be present for several steps and then disappear completely until the animal is pivoted or forced to back. Occasionally, an abnormal movement of the patella can be seen and sometimes a distinct popping noise may be heard when the stifle is flexed.

There are several suggested causes of this condition and probably 2 or more are usually involved in each patient. Because the incidence is higher in animals with straight legs and fine

bones, it has been considered a conformation defect. The high occurrence of this disturbance in certain families of the Shetland breed indicates a probable hereditary influence. Poor bone quality and pulled tibial tuberosities have been demonstrated radiographically on affected yearlings, suggesting a possible nutritional deficiency or mineral imbalance.[7]

Stall rest, improvement of the nutrition by feeding a balanced ration fortified with a mineral supplement, and the topical application of liniments or counterirritants often will bring about recovery in young individuals who are but slightly to moderately affected. In older and more severely affected animals, some veterinarians have recommended the use of injectable counterirritants. One-half to 1.0 ml. of Lugol's iodine solution in a 1 to 5 aqueous dilution is injected into both the origin and insertion of each of the 3 patellar ligaments; hyperemia and some tissue destruction thus are induced. When tissues are destroyed, scar tissue formation occurs and consequent shrinking and shortening of the structure take place. If the patellar ligaments, particularly the medial, are shortened, the condition is improved or corrected. Regrettably, such therapy has not been unqualifiedly effective. Some patients so treated improve and others may show complete recovery, but frequently the favorable response is transitory.

Because of these experiences, many equine specialists prefer to perform a medial patellar desmotomy which produces a complete and permanent correction. Since the condition usually is unilateral only the medial ligament on the affected side need be severed. Some surgeons prefer to sever the medial ligament in both legs to prevent the occurrence of the condition in the opposite member.[7] The operation can be performed in the standing position under local anesthetic. A one-half inch skin incision is made over the medial patellar ligament near its insertion on the tibial tuberosity. A blunt pointed bistoury should be used to free and elevate the ligament after which it is parted surgically as close to the tibial tuberosity as possible. The incision should be closed with 1 or 2 interrupted sutures which may be removed in a week. Daily walking exercise should be provided for 5 to 7 days.

EQUIPMENT AND TECHNICS

TWITCH

The pick-handle length chain horse twitch is cumbersome when used on ponies. A smaller twitch, 24 inches in length with a nylon rope anchored in the end, is easier to handle and draws fewer objections from the client.

CASTING HARNESS

Ponies vary so widely in size that it virtually is impossible to fashion any type of a leather casting harness which will fit all animals. Two 25-foot lengths of ½ or ⅜ inch cotton rope and 2 leather or web pastern hobbles can be used as double sidelines to cast and securely tie a pony of any size. The technic has been well-described by Leahy and Barrow.[6]

VAGINAL SPECULUMS

Depending upon the size of the mare and the objectives of the examiner, several types of vaginal speculums can be used. Caslick's equine vaginal speculum usually can be used on older and larger mares. A bovine vaginal speculum of similar design but of smaller size often can be substituted in medium-size mares. A plastic or glass tube speculum is useful for smaller mares for visual examination of the vagina and cervix and/or for the collection of bacterial cultures. For the unusually small mare none of the aforementioned types may be suitable, and the glass barrel from a 50-ml. metal-jacketed syringe may be substituted.

STOMACH TUBES

Difficulty usually is encountered if the standard size equine stomach tubes are used on any but the largest of ponies. However, the colt size (outside diameter ½ inch) tube can be used successfully on nearly all adults. It may be necessary to substitute a horse catheter in small individuals and foals. Industrial air or brake hoses, obtainable in assorted diameters and wall thicknesses, provide a small diameter tube without the usual concomitant loss of stiffness.

CULTURES

Bacterial cultures may be collected inexpensively and quickly from the cervix or uterus by inserting the end of a sterile swab into the end of a plastic artificial insemination pipette. When withdrawn, the swab can be placed into a sterile tube, the end of the applicator stick broken off, and the plastic tube discarded.

ADMINISTRATION OF MEDICATION

The equine balling gun has little use in the administration of medicine to ponies. Even though the mouth, teeth, and pharynx appear large and well-developed, the esophagus is relatively small. Boluses, capsules, and even large tablets are capable of producing choke. Most of these dissolve in time and pass, but the antics of a choked pony in the presence of its owner can lead only to embarrassment and humiliation for the veterinarian. And, if the choke-producing capsule contains an irritant or caustic compound, considerable esophageal necrosis may result. These calamities may be prevented by administering all drugs in liquid form through an intranasal stomach tube.

Difficulty may be encountered in passing a tube because of the small size of the esophagus or the dryness of the mucosa. The subcutaneous injection of pilocarpine or arecoline, small doses of lentin or of other parasympathetic stimulators will facilitate its passage. A similar response often can be obtained in the healthy animal by teasing it with grain. The secretion liberated by the salivary glands acts as a lubricant and simplifies the passage of the tube. These drugs are helpful especially in animals who are anorectic or dehydrated, or those who have high fevers. These medicaments may be of benefit if administered preceding the administration of a bolus or capsule.

On occasion, it may be necessary to dispense powdered drugs in divided doses. The mechanics of administration may raise a problem with many owners. An electuary will resolve the difficulty. To the prescribed amount of the medicament is added corn syrup, honey or molasses until a thick paste is formed. When it is smeared on the gums, lips, and muzzle, ponies — even very sick ones — will lick this sweet material and consume the drug.

P. E. HOFFMAN

REFERENCES

1. Bedell, L. Frank: The Shetland Pony. The Iowa State University Press, Ames, Iowa (1959) 2.

2. Blood, D. C. and Henderson, J. A.: Veterinary Medicine. The Williams and Wilkins Co., Baltimore, Maryland, 1960.

3. Bruns, Ursula: Ponies. D. Van Nostrand Co., Inc., Princeton, New Jersey, 1961.

4. Cullison, A. E.: Effect of physical form of the ration on steer performance & certain rumen phenomena. J. Anim. Sci. 20 (1961) 478-483.

5. Hoffman, P. E.: Pony problems. Georgia Veterinarian, 11 1, 1959.

6. Leahy, J. R. and Barrow, Pat: Restraint of Animals. Cornell Campus Store, Inc., Ithaca, New York, 1953.

7. Lundvall, R. S.: Problems in a Pony Practice. Proceedings of the Fifth Annual American Assn. of Equine Practitioners Convention, December 1959.

8. Morrison, F. B.: Feeds and Feeding. The Morrison Publishing Company, Ithaca, New York, 1956.

9. Nelson, Albert Wendell: Nutrient Requirements of the Light Horse. American Quarter Horse Assn., 1961.

10. Neseni, R., Flade, E., Heidler, G. and Steger, H.: Yield and Composition of Mare's Milk in the Course of Lactation. Arch-Tierzucht, 1 91-129, Nutrition Abstracts and Reviews, 29 (1959) 1374.

11. Anonymous: Bull. of Grayson Foundation, Inc., Lexington, Kentucky, November 1961.

12. Anonymous: Nutritional Horse Sense. Nutritional News Bull., Vol. 17, No. 3, (July 1961), Ralston Purina Company.

CHAPTER 29

HORSESHOEING

INTRODUCTION

Under most conditions shoeing is necessary. Although shoeing does not make walking easier or improve agility, and except in the case of rubber or rope shoes, minimize concussion, it does protect the foot from excessive wear and provides increased traction. In some instances, it also may be used to correct defects in gait, or alleviate pain from an injury.

Poor shoeing may lead to a number of disorders of the leg and foot, or aggravate existing troubles and promote irregularities of gait which can impair a horse's usefulness. The principles of proper shoeing have not changed appreciably in the Twentieth Century, and many "tricks of the trade" available in older horse books still are sound and practical, despite the fact that "ready-to-wear" shoes are available which tend to simplify normal shoeing.

Space does not permit a detailed study of corrective shoeing, nor is such a subject of sufficient interest, except to the specialist, to warrant a detailed and exhaustive treatment. Principles of horseshoeing, however, are of interest to any veterinarian who intends to pursue equine practice, as he should be able to advise clients about shoeing in order to prevent, minimize, or correct foot disorders or injuries.

BASIC CONSIDERATIONS

ANATOMY OF THE FOOT

A sound knowledge of the anatomy of the foot and leg is essential. In addition to information already given in this text, a few details peculiarly applicable to the foot and its horny covering should be mentioned as a guide to proper examination and shoeing technics.

The bony tissues of the foot consist of the distal epiphyses of the cannon bones, the proximal, intermediate and distal phalanges, and 1 distal and 2 proximal sesamoids. The metacarpo-phalangeal and interphalangeal

joints essentially are hinges. Their principal movements are flexion and extension. However, slight rotary and lateral movement is possible. The elastic tissues of the foot are composed principally of the lateral cartilages and the digital cushion. The lateral cartilages (Fig. 1) are 2 rhomboidal plates of fibrocartilage extending backward and upward from the medial and lateral alae of the distal phalanx. Their dorsal borders are located an inch or more above the coronary band. Normal lateral cartilages are flexible to pressure, but may become ossified through disease or repeated concussion. The digital cushion is a wedge-like mass of mixed fibro-elastic

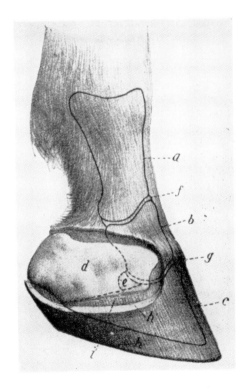

Fig. 1. Digit of horse, showing surface relations of bones and joints. The cartilage is largely exposed. a. proximal phalanx, b, intermediate phalanx, c. distal phalanx, d. lateral cartilage, e. distal sesamoid (navicular), f. pastern joint, g. coffin joint, h. wall of hoof, i. laminar corium. From Sisson after Ellenberger, in Leisering's Atlas.

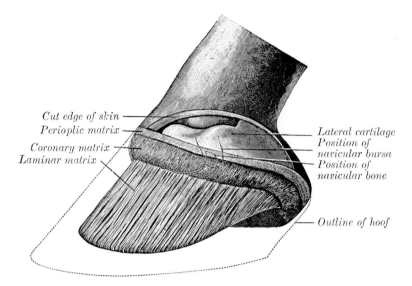

Cut edge of skin
Perioplic matrix
Coronary matrix
Laminar matrix

Lateral cartilage
Position of
navicular bursa
Position of
navicular bone

Outline of hoof

Fig. 2. Lateral view of foot of horse after removal of hoof and part of skin. Dotted lines in front of navicular bone indicate position of coffin joint. From Sisson and Grossman, *The Anatomy of the Domestic Animals* after Schmaltz, *Atlas d. Anat. d. Pferdes.*

and fatty tissue filling the space between the lateral cartilages and forms the heels and the soft tissue portion of the frog. This structure is one of the primary shock absorbers of the foot and extends forward underneath the distal sesamoid (navicular) and deep digital flexor tendon. It helps protect the last 2 structures from shock and pressure from below.

The nutritive structure, or corium (Fig. 2), closely invests the distal phalanx, the lateral cartilages, and the digital cushion, and is divided into 4 parts according to its anatomical location, *i.e.*, the perioplic corium, the coronary corium, the laminar corium, and the corium of the sole. It is covered by the horny portion of the hoof. The corium is an epidermal derivative but differs from normal skin in that it contains no sweat nor sebaceous glands. It is richly supplied with nerves and blood vessels. Its external surface is continuous with the stratum germinativum, or matrix, which proliferates to form the surface layers of horn that cover the bulk of the foot.

The 3 major parts of the hoof, *i.e.* wall, sole, and frog (Fig. 3) are readily distinguished from one another. The wall consists of 3 parts: an external layer, a middle layer, and a laminar layer. The external layer contains the periople and the stratum tectorium. The periople is a narrow band of tissue less than ⅛ inch wide, composed of soft tubu-

lar horn covering the coronary band. The periople is continued by the stratum tectorium, a thin, varnish-like layer of glistening horn which forms the outermost covering of the hoof and whose purpose probably is to retard evaporation of moisture from the remainder of the horny layers. The middle layer forms the bulk of the wall and is composed of a dense mass of horn tubes running parallel to one another. The horn of the middle layer is the hardest portion of the hoof and is produced by the matrix of the coronary corium.

The coronary corium or coronet, is a prominent fleshy ring encircling the foot just below and parallel to the periople. At the heels, the coronet is reflected forward along the sides of the fleshy portion of the frog and becomes lost near the anterior end of that structure. The coronet furnishes nutrition to the middle layer of the wall of the foot, and the portions in the region of the frog supply the bars which are reflected portions of the wall.

The laminar layer (Fig. 4) is composed of approximately 500 to 600 leaves of non-tubular horny tissue lying parallel to one another and to the horn tubes of the middle layer of the wall. They run downward from the lower edge of the coronary band to the margin of the sole. The light-colored horny leaves (the horny laminae) form the deepest layer of the wall and serve to unite the wall to the under-lying soft tissues.

The corium of the sole: This tissue covers the entire inner sole surface of the foot and is continuous with the corium of the frog and bars. It furnishes nutrition to the layer of horn forming the horny sole. Deeply, it is attached to the sole surface of the distal phalanx by a highly modified periosteum.

The corium of the frog: This structure covers the inner surface of the frog and furnishes nutrition to the horny portion of the frog.

The hoof is composed entirely of horn and consists of 4 parts: the wall (and bars), sole, frog, and periople. It is avascular and does not possess nerves.

The wall is all of the hoof which is visible when the foot is on the ground. The lateral sidewall of a normal hoof slants at a greater angle than the medial portion and is somewhat thicker. In front hooves, the wall is thickest at the toe and gradually thins toward the quarters. In hindfeet, there is less difference in the thickness between the toe, sidewalls and quarters. The horny sole is concave and about as thick as the toe portion of the wall. It is round and uneven and usually covered with flakes of exfoliating horn. At the rear, the sole

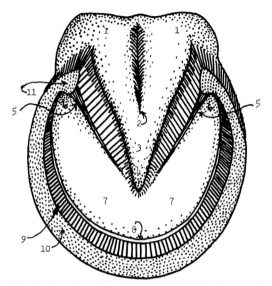

Fig. 3. Ground surface of the hoof. 1. Bulbs, 2. central sulcus of frog, 3. frog, 4. apex of frog, 5. bars, 6. angle of sole, 7. sole, 8. white line (zona lamellata), 9. laminae of wall, 10. wall, 11. angle of wall. Adapted from Bone, *Animal Anatomy and Physiology*.

bears a "V"-shaped notch which receives the bars and the frog. This notch divides the sole into a body and 2 wings. The peripheral rim of the sole is united to the lower border of the wall and bars via the "white line", or zona lamellata (Fig. 3), which is a region of

Fig. 4. Cross-section of foot of horse, cut parallel with the coronary border. The wall appears much thicker at the angles than it actually is, because it is cut very obliquely. Adapted from Sisson and Grossman, *The Anatomy of the Domestic Animals*.

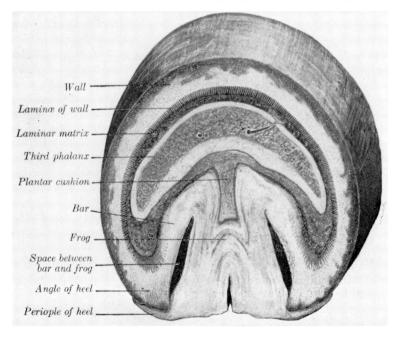

Wall

Laminæ of wall

Laminar matrix

Third phalanx

Plantar cushion

Bar

Frog

Space between bar and frog

Angle of heel

Periople of heel

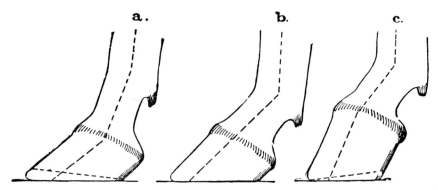

Fig. 5. a. Side view of foot with the foot-axis broken backward as a result of too long a toe. The amount of horn to be removed from the toe in order to straighten the foot axis is denoted by a dotted line; b. side view of a properly balanced foot, with a straight foot-axis of desirable slant; c. side view of stumpy foot with foot-axis broken forward, as a result of overgrowth of the quarters. The amount of horn to be removed in order to straighten the foot-axis is shown by a dotted line. Adapted from U.S. Dept. of Agric., *Diseases of the Horse.*

lighter colored horn composed of the horny lamella of the wall and interleaving plates of horn derived from the sole which fill the interstices. This white line is important since it marks the line along which nails should be driven.

The frog (Fig. 3), is a wedge-shaped mass of soft horn that forms an elastic structure between the bars and the edge of the sole immediately anterior to the bars. The base of the frog unites laterally with the angles of the wall and the apex fills the tip of the "V"-shaped notch in the sole. A broad shallow depression, the central sulcus, divides the frog into 2 halves, which unite anteriorly to form the body and apex. Internally the central sulcus is continued as a ridge, the "frog stay" or spine, which penetrates the soft tissues. Between the frog and the bars lie 2 deep, narrow depressions, the collateral sulci.

With respect to hardness and density, the different parts of the hoof vary considerably. The middle layer of the wall is the hardest. The white line and the frog are the softest, but the horn that composes them is more elastic and does not become hard or brittle under ordinary conditions. The horn of the sole is intermediate in hardness between the wall and the frog. In general, the horn of the wall is fine-grained and tough, although coarse-grained, friable, brittle or granular areas may be found in damaged or abnormal feet. All horn is a poor conductor of heat and the drier

it becomes, the less able it is to transmit extremes of temperature.

In considering the shape of the foot, an imaginary line known as the foot axis is constructed (Fig. 5). This line passes through the central axes of the phalanges and should always be straight whether it be observed from the front or the side. Viewed from the side, the long axis of the proximal phalanx, if prolonged to the ground, should be parallel to the external surface of the toe of the hoof. When viewed from the front, the line of the foot axis should cut the hoof into equal halves. Defects in the shape of the foot or the hoof will cause deviations in the foot axis. A raised heel or a short toe tilts the distal phalanx forward, loosens the flexor tendons, and allows the fetlock joint to sink downward and backward, and the first phalanx to become more nearly parallel to the ground. The foot axis, when viewed from the side, is now broken forward, since the angle of the proximal phalanx is less steep than that of the intermediate or distal. If the toe is long, or the heels short, the intermediate and distal phalanges are tilted backward and lie more nearly parallel to the ground. This tenses the deep digital flexor tendon and forces the fetlock joint forward and upward. The angle of the proximal phalanx to the ground becomes steeper. The foot axis, as seen from the side, is broken backward.

A hoof which supports weight has a different form and arrangement of internal structures than when it is not under load. Since the amount of weight carried by a foot continually changes and the relations of pressures continuously vary, the foot, from a physiologic standpoint, is never at rest. The most pronounced changes of form occur when the hoof bears the greatest weight. Briefly, these changes include:

1. Expansion or widening of the posterior half of the foot from the coronet to the lower edge of the quarters, 2, narrowing of the front half of the foot measured at the coronet, and 3, sinking of the heels and flattening of the wings of the sole.

As weight is placed upon the foot, it is transmitted through the bones and the soft tissues to the wall. The intermediate and distal phalanges and the navicular bone are forced backward and downward. The intermediate phalanx moves downward between the lateral cartilages and presses the deep flexor tendons on the digital cushion. The cushion, compressed from above and unable to expand downward because of the ground pressure against the frog, expands toward the sides pushing the lateral cartilages outward and exerting force against the quarters. The quarters spread and expand the heels. This expansion is assisted by a concomitant flattening and lateral expansion of the horny frog which tend to push the bars apart. If the lateral cartileges are ossified, there is little or no expansion of the heels and frog pressure may lead to painful compression of the digital cushion. As the weight is taken up by the distal phalanx, the sole flattens.

PHYSIOLOGY OF THE FOOT

Physiologic changes in the shape of the foot are greatest in sound, unshod horses, and tend to be more prominent in the forefeet than in the hind. The movements of the various structures within the foot and the associated changes in shape are indispensable to foot health. Not only do they give exercise to the foot, but the expansion and contraction act as a blood pump to aid venous return to the heart, thus permitting a better circulation and increased nutrition and removal of waste products, resulting in a healthier foot. The foot tis-

sues should be kept active by regular exercise. Long rests in the stable or excessive drying of the hoof should be avoided. The periople and the stratum tectorium should never be rasped off during the shoeing process as these structures tend to conserve moisture in the foot and their loss will contribute to dry brittle walls. In any event, a good hoof paint is helpful to retain horn moisture and prevent chipping. Since the movements described here are complete only in unshod animals, shoeing must be regarded as a detriment. But it is a detriment which must be accepted if horses are to be kept at work upon surfaces that produce great amounts of wear.

The entire wall grows outward from the matrix at an equal rate, which is largely dependent upon the state of nutrition of the animal and the amount of blood supplied to the deep tissues of the foot. A number of factors including exercise, grooming, hoof care, feed, and going without shoes tend to increase the blood supply and nutrition to the hoof and favor a more rapid growth of good quality horn. Lack of exercise, extended periods of going shod, dryness of the horn, poor hoof care, and poor nutrition will inhibit the rate of hoof growth. The average rate of growth is approximately 3/8″ per month. The time required for the horn to grow from the coronet to the ground surface varies in proportion to the distance the coronet is from the ground. It takes longer for the hoof to grow from the coronet to the toe than from the coronet to the heels. The difference in time is considerable, being approximately 11 to 13 months for the toe, 6 to 8 months for the sidewalls, and 3 to 5 months for the heels. Hind hooves tend to grow faster than fore, and unshod hooves tend to grow faster than shod.

CARE OF THE FOOT

Irregular growth is fairly common. The principal causes of this are navicular disease, laminitis, improper distribution of the body weight on the hoof, and improper trimming of the foot. Young animals kept stabled for long periods or allowed to run on soft pasture without attention, frequently grow hooves of excessive length. The toes becomes concave from the coronet downward, the quarters curl forward and inward, contraction of the heels may occur and the whole hoof become distorted. Crooked feet can result in crooked legs if the abnormal foot remains uncorrected and is allowed to exert leverage for a few months upon developing bones and ligaments. All colts are not born with straight legs but much of the damage can be corrected by proper care of the feet. Many knuckled-over, knock-kneed, cow-hocked, splayfooted, pigeon-toed, interfering, paddling and winging horses are the results of improper foot care.

In general, unshod animals should have plenty of room for exercise on dry ground. If the animal is stabled, the hooves should be checked every 4 weeks and the lower edge of the wall trimmed to a normal conformation. The soles and clefts of the frog should be cleaned every few days and the entire foot washed. A good hoof paint will prevent excessive drying. In the stable, good straw bedding or shavings should be provided. Any deviations from normal in the foot should be checked and corrected with the intent to straighten the foot axis. Diseases of the foot should be promptly and effectively treated.

EXAMINATION OF THE FOOT

In checking a hoof for health, the following points should be noted:

1. The foot should be equally warm at all parts and should not be tender to palpation or to moderate compression with hoof testers. 2. The coronet should be soft and elastic and should not project beyond the outer surface of the wall. 3. The wall of the foot should be straight from coronet to the ground so that a ruler laid against it at any point parallel to the direction of the horn tubules will touch the wall at every point. 4. The wall should be covered with an outer varnish-like layer of stratum tectorium and show no cracks, clefts, or soft places.

Although every hoof shows a certain amount of irregular growth ("ring formation"), the rings should not be strongly marked and should run parallel to the coronary band. The bulbs of the heels should be full, rounded and of equal height. The sole should be concave, the white line solid, the frog well-developed, and the central sulcus of the frog broad and shallow. The spaces between the bars and the frog should be straight and clean; the bars should be straight from the angle toward the point of the frog, and the angles themselves should be far enough apart so as not to crowd the base of the frog. The horn should have a normal coloration. The color, of course, varies in different animals, but can be considered abnormal when the horn shows a reddish color or where there are cracks along the wall, white line, bars, or frog, or when there are such conditions as thrush, corns, seedy-toe, contraction, or displacement of the heels. The lateral cartilages should be firm and resilient, and yield readily to palpation.

No 2 hooves are exactly alike but all should tend to conform to a general plan. Deviations in natural hoof shape tend to fall into 3 classes when viewed from the front, and into 3 additional classes when viewed from the side. Since the form of the foot determines the pecularities of the shoe which must be applied to it, a knowledge of the natural forms of feet is essential for proper shoeing of normal feet and for corrective shoeing of abnormal. When observed from the front, a horse's feet tend to fall into 3 general categories: regular, base wide, and base narrow. By use of the imaginary line of the foot axis, the type can be determined. In the normal or regular foot, the foot axis is straight and vertical and passes through the center of the foot. In the base wide position, the axis runs downward and outward, and in the base narrow stance, downward and inward. In profile, a normal foot has an angulation of approximately 45 to 50° to the horizontal, a steep foot has an angulation above 50°, and a shallow, or acute angled foot has an angulation below 40°. The shape of the hoof gives some indication of the angulation. Shallow angulation will be characterized by a foot having a relatively long toe and a somewhat shortened heel. The angle made by the front of the wall to the ground usually will be below 35°. A regular angulation will be in the vicinity of 45°. A steep angulation will be characterized by a short, stumpy foot and the angle of the toe to the ground will be in excess of 50°. In regular feet, the lateral side of the wall has a trifle more slope than the medial when seen from the front.

In a base wide hoof, the lateral wall is considerably more slanted than the medial and the lateral quarter is more curved. The weight falls largely upon the medial portion of the hoof, and in flight the hoof tends to move in an inward arc as it is carried forward. From its position on the ground, it breaks over on the inner portion of the toe, is carried forward and inward close to the supporting leg, and then outward to the ground. Such a hoof will tend to cause the horse to interfere.

A hoof of the base narrow type shows an inner wall slightly more slanted than the lateral, and the medial quarter more curved. The lateral quarter is often flat and drawn in at the bottom. The weight falls principally upon the lateral portion of the hoof and, in flight, the hoof tends to move in an outward arc as it is carried forward. The hoof breaks over on the outer portion of the toe and is carried forward, outward and then inward to the ground. This action gives the horse a type of gait known as "paddling" or "winging." A pigeon-toed horse seldom interferes, but a base narrow horse whose toes point straight ahead, frequently will do so.

In a regular hoof, the toe points straight ahead, and when the horse is moving in a straight line the hooves are picked up and carried forward parallel to the long axis of the body and are set down flat. Coming straight toward an observer, the feet seem to rise and fall perpendicularly.

Regarding the hooves themselves, these fall into 2 types, narrow and wide. The narrow hoof has a strongly concave sole with the quarters tending to be parallel and a small frog with nearly perpendicular sidewalls. The horn in such feet tends to be fine-grained and tough. The wide hoof has an almost circular bearing surface with slight concavity of the sole and a large wide frog. The quality of the horn is somewhat coarser. Hind hooves, in general, tend to be narrow and fore hooves tend to be wide.

EXAMINATION FOR SHOEING

After one understands normality it is possible to study proper shoeing. An examination is made prior to shoeing to ascertain the conformation and stance of the horse, the position of the limbs, the shape and quality of the feet, and such faults as may be observed in its manner of movement. The animal must be observed both at rest and in motion. The wear of the old shoe should be carefully noted before it is removed. It is permanent evidence of the manner in which the hoof has been placed on the ground since the shoe was applied, and gives valuable indications for levelling or correcting the hoof and its flight.

Since wear is the effect of friction between the shoe and the ground, and since the properly levelled hoof is set flat to the ground, wear should be uniform at every point except at the toe which will show some rounding of the edge through the act of breaking over. Factors which tend to lengthen the stride also tend to make wear more pronounced in the heels of the shoe, but factors which shorten the stride tend to bring the wear nearer the toe. Laminitis, however, will produce very pronounced wear at the heels. If one branch of the shoe is worn much thinner than the other, the thinner branch has either been set too close to the midline of the foot and has borne the greater load, or the section of wall above the thinner branch is too long or the opposite section too short. One-sided wear and unnatural conformation of the wall of the hoof usually occur together.

After the horse has been observed standing and at walk, trot, or pace and the carriage and the flight of the feet duly noted, necessary recommendations for shoeing can be given. Until this time, no one should feel competent to direct corrective shoeing of a horse.

The shoe, being an artificial support which is by no means ideal, should be applied with great nicety to eliminate some of the detrimental effects of shoeing. It should always be remembered that the shoe, no matter how light it may be, tends to decrease the speed of flight of the foot and thus decrease the speed and agility of the horse.

Every shoe should be shaped to the hoof for which it is intended, providing, of course, that the hoof is of reasonably normal shape. If the hoof has undergone changes in shape, one must attempt to restore the original shape as much as possible. No two shoes are quite alike. Fronts and hinds, rights and lefts, are different and distinguishable. All shoes should be wider at the toe than at the ends of the branches. The average width should be about double the thickness of the wall at the toe. The thickness of the shoe should be sufficient to make it last for about 4 weeks and this thickness should be uniform throughout the shoe except in special cases. The length depends upon the length of the bearing surface of the hoof. The acutely slopping hoof has long, overhanging heels and a considerable portion of the weight falls upon its posterior parts. For such a hoof, the branches of the shoe should extend back to the angles a distance nearly double the shoe thickness. For a hoof of regular shape, the branches should project an amount equal to the thickness of the shoe. In a short stumpy hoof, the shoe should not project more than one-eighth of an inch. In all cases, however, the shoe should cover the entire bearing surface of the wall.

The upper surface of the shoe is known as the hoof surface. That part which is in contact with the horn is called the bearing surface. The bearing surface of both hoof and shoe should be perfectly level from side to side and the shoe should be wide enough to support the full thickness of the wall, the white line, and about one-eighth inch of the sole. The bearing surface of the shoe should be perfectly flat except for the toe which may be slightly turned up. The surface of the shoe between the bearing surface and the inner edge may need to be concaved to prevent pressure extending too far inward upon the sole. This "seating" of the shoe should be deeper or shallower depending upon whether the sole is less or more concave. Strongly concave soles such as found on narrow feet or hindfeet require little or no concaving.

The shoe should be so formed that the nail holes fall directly upon the white line. The holes should be confined to the anterior half of front shoes and the anterior two-thirds of hind shoes. For a medium- or light-weight shoe, 3 nail holes in each branch are sufficient but for heavier shoes, 4 on each side are about right although, in some cases, 4 on the lateral and three on the medial side are sufficient.

To prepare the foot for shoeing, the clinches of the nails of the previous shoe should be straightened with a dull clinch cutter and the nails drawn one at a time. After the nails are drawn, the old shoe is removed and laid aside. Remaining stubs of nails are then drawn or punched out and the hoof is freed of dirt and partially freed of loose horn. The hoof is now dressed to form a base of support in conformity with observations of the flight of the foot and such corrections as may be necessary to turn the foot into a more efficient bearing surface are now made.

A careful preliminary examination should show what parts of the wall require removal and what parts must be left. A greatly overgrown hoof may be shortened with nippers and the sole freed of partially detached flakes of horn. The concave sole of a thick, strong hoof may be pared out around the point of the frog but not so much as to remove all evidence of flaking or exfoliation. The wall should be levelled finally with a rasp until its full thickness is in a single horizontal plane. The bars, if too long, may be shortened but should never be pared on their sides. The wings of the sole and the angle between the bars and the quarters should be trimmed a little low so as not to press upon the hoof surface of the shoe. Corns or bruises of the sole usually are the result of leaving a mass of dry, unyielding horn at this point.

The frog should not be touched other than to remove tags of horn or layers so loose as to form no protection. A soft frog will tend to shorten itself spontaneously but if the frog is dry and hard, it is better to soften it by applying moisture in some form and allow it to wear down naturally than to pare it. It is advantageous to have the frog project slightly

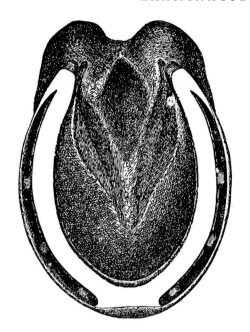

Fig. 6. A left fore hoof of regular form shod with a plain shoe. From U.S. Dept. of Agric., *Diseases of the Horse.*

below the level of the wall, an amount to the thickness of the shoe, although rarely frogs of such size will be seen. The lower border of the wall should be rounded with the rasp to prevent its being bent out and broken. The foot is then set on the ground and again observed from all sides to make sure that the hoof is properly trimmed and shaped.

The shoe is now fitted to the hoof. A shoe fits when its outer border follows the outer edge of the wall in the region of the nail holes, and from the last nail hole to the termination of the branch gradually projects from the surface of the wall until it is about an eighth of an inch beyond the wall at the angle. The shoe should extend beyond the angle for the distance previously described for the various shaped hooves. The shoe should be straight, firm, and fit closely at all points against the wall of the foot. The nail holes should be directly over the white line and the branches of the shoe far enough away from the frog base to permit the passage of a foot pick. The branches of the shoe should be of equal length (Fig. 6, 7).

In fitting a shoe to a hoof of regular form, the shape of the hoof is followed closely but in base wide and base narrow feet, attention must be paid not only to the form of the foot but also to the direction of the pasterns and the distribution of weight. Where most of the weight falls, the hoof surface of the shoe should be widened, and where the least weight falls, the surface should be narrowed. In this way, the weight within the hoof is evenly distributed over the supporting surface. A shoe for a base wide hoof should be fitted full on the inner side of the foot and close on the outer side because the inner side bears most of the weight. The nails in the lateral branch should be placed well back, but on the medial branch should be crowded forward toward the toe. A shoe for a base narrow foot should be the reverse of the given description and the lateral branch of the shoe should be somewhat longer than the medial. A shoe, for an acutely angulated hoof, should have long branches since most of the weight falls on the posterior half of the foot. The support at the toe should be reduced, either by turning the shoe up at the toe or by bevelling it under the toe.

A shoe for a stumpy hoof should have short branches and, in marked stumpiness, should increase the support of the toe where most of the weight falls. To do this, the shoe should be bevelled downward and forward. In cases where the coronet of the lateral quarter extends beyond the lower border of the hoof, the lateral branch of the shoe from the last nail backward must be fitted so full that an imaginary perpendicular dropped from the coronet will just meet the outer border of the shoe. The medial branch, however, should be fitted

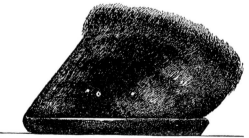

Fig. 7. Side view of a regular hoof showing proper shoeing. Note the slight roll at the toe. From U.S. Dept. of Agric., *Diseases of the Horse.*

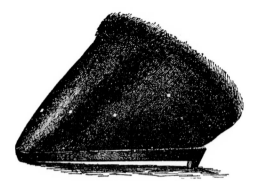

Fig. 8. Side view of a fore hoof shod to quicken "breaking over" action to correct forging. Note the roll of toe and short branches with heel calks to incline the foot forward. From U.S. Dept. Agric., *Diseases of the Horse.*

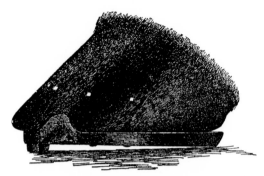

Fig. 9. Side view of a short shod hindfoot to correct for forging. Note the elevation of the toe by a calk and the projection of the horny toe beyond the hoof. When the toe has grown more, the toe calk can be eliminated and the toe set farther forward. From. U.S. Dept. of Agric., *Diseases of the Horse.*

as close as possible. The principle here is to set the new shoe farther toward the side having the greatest wear. In fitting the shoe full at the lateral quarter, care should be taken to see that the bearing surface of the hoof in this region is still supported. It should not be so incompletely covered as to be pinched or squeezed inward against the frog. This can be accomplished by forming the lateral branch of the shoe wider than the medial and punching it so that the nails will fall upon the white line.

In the days when the horse was more common on the streets and farms, only a few blacksmiths had the skill necessary to fit a cold shoe tightly to the foot. Today, with the increase in light horse use and the decrease in good blacksmiths, the statement is more true than ever. Hot fitting, if properly done, is just as accurate, considerably easier, and no more damaging to the horse. To hot fit a shoe, the iron should be at a dark heat and pressed briefly against the dressed hoof. It should be allowed to remain only long enough to produce mild scorching. The marks left upon the foot then indicate what portions of the horn must be trimmed in order to gain a perfect fit.

Nails should always be driven low. They should pierce the wall at approximately 1⅝ inches above the shoe. A nail which penetrates the white line and emerges low upon the wall damages the least possible amount of horn, has a strong clinch, and the strongest possible hold upon the wall because the clinch is pulling more nearly at a right angle to the horn tubes. Nails should be clinched alternately from side to side since this tends to give a closer fit between shoe and horn. The clinched nail should be rasped, but the rasp should not be allowed to remove any portion of the wall above the clinch.

SPECIAL SHOEING

The only limits to corrective and surgical shoeing are the knowledge and ingenuity of the operator, the skill of the blacksmith and the physiology of the horse. Within these limits a large number of corrections can be made, a few of which will be listed. It should always be kept in mind that the lightest shoe which can do the job is the shoe of choice.

Weight always is a problem in shoeing. Not only does it slow the action and decrease the length of the stride, but it may also accentuate faults in gait. Theoretically, the addition of weight will correct a fault such as interfering. Adding weight to the medial branch of a shoe should make the horse carry the foot outward from the median plane of the body. It does, at least in the initial phases of the stride, but during the flight of the hoof, the excess weight tends to pull the foot inward and thus compound the fault one wishes to avoid. Weighting the toe of a shoe should theoretically increase the length of the stride, but this is again compensated by the fact that the weight slows the action and sacrifices speed. One of the classic blunders in horseshoeing was made in the development of a shoe with branches appreciably thickened at the heels and having a marked roll at the toe. The idea was to induce a higher action and a quicker breaking over of the foot. The actual result was not that at all. Though weighting the heels should give a higher action, and rolling the toe should cause quicker breaking over, the marked toe roll lowered the action and the weight slowed it. The 2 factors of weight and roll cancelled each other and all that resulted was a low, slow action and a shorter stride.

The problem of corrective shoeing still is one of weighting and shoe design. Thickening, broadening, thinning, narrowing, lengthening and shortening parts of the shoe to correct or compensate for defects in breaking over action, hoof flight, and hoof landing are all accepted and worthwhile methods of corrective shoeing which have stood the test of time and use. The essential part of the problem is to keep weight at a minimum while obtaining maximum corrective effects. The closer the weight of the shod hoof approaches an unshod one, the more efficiently a horse will move.

In general, the principles involved in corrective shoeing are as follows: A foot shod with a raised heel and rolled toe quickens breaking over and forces the foot to leave the ground slightly earlier than it would if it were unshod or possessed conventional shoes (Fig. 9). A hindfoot shod short, *e.g.*, where a portion of the horny toe extends beyond the shoe, prevents the iron from impacting against the front foot (Fig. 9). A rear shoe with its anterior portion raised either by a toe caulk or by thickening the shoe, raises the toe and tends to shorten the action, slow it, and cause a delayed breaking over of the foot. Proper weighting of the shoes also may be beneficial. Half-shoes, three-quarter shoes and

toe plates have been used, partially for weighting effects and occasionally to permit freedom from wear and allow portions of the horn to lengthen. After sufficient growth of the horn has taken place, the hooves are trimmed and shod properly.

A number of shoes designed to diminish concussion and improve traction on hard, smooth-surfaced roads have been tried. Of these, the rubber-soled shoe, the rope-soled shoe, and the rubber pad shoe have been shown to be effective and practical on wet or dry surfaces. The outstanding fault of all these devices is that they usually are too heavy.

Certain shoes have been used widely to correct defects in stance or gait. Of these, the bar shoe (Fig. 10) is perhaps the most important. It is very helpful in correcting tendonitis involving the flexor tendon, and it is useful to apply frog pressure to hooves with damaged frogs and/or contracted heels. A properly fitted bar shoe can restore a frog to an

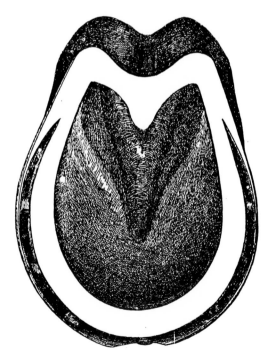

Fig. 10. An example of a bar shoe showing the position of the bar to produce frog pressure. From U.S. Dept. of Agric., *Diseases of the Horse*.

original state of activity even after it has become partially atrophied. A bar shoe also will give the hoof additional support that can be utilized to relieve quarters of excessive pressure induced by inflammation. The bar of the shoe should equal the average width of the branches and should press lightly upon the base of the frog. A leather sole or a metal plate may be placed under the shoe and the space between plate and shoe filled with pine tar and oakum. This packing will permit better distribution of weight along the ground surface of the hoof.

Corrective shoeing is particularly important in gait defects such as forging, crossfiring, and interfering. Forging, a common fault, occurs when the toe of the hindfoot strikes the heel of the front foot. Three things must be accomplished in correction: the forefoot must be made to break over more quickly and be lifted from the ground sooner; the heel of the forefoot and toe of the hind must be shortened to reduce chances of contact; and the hindfoot must be made to break over more slowly and take a shorter stride. The front feet should be shod with a short branched shoe that has a definite roll at the toe and a rise at the heel. The hindfoot should be shod with a short, square-toed shoe that has a rise at the toe.

Crossfiring is essentially the same type of defect as forging, except that it occurs in pacers and is marked by the toe of the hindfoot striking the heel of the opposite forefoot. Correction depends upon weighting and forming shoes that will make the horse advance its feet in a straight line.

In interfering, the medial surface of the foot or lower leg is struck by the opposite foot. This usually occurs in base wide horses which toe out ("splay-footed"), base narrow horses whose feet point straight ahead, in horses with deformed hoofs that give a splay-footed stance, and in animals which have been improperly shod. The fault usually affects the forelegs, but the hindlegs also may be affected, and in rare cases all 4 legs may be involved.

Correction depends upon straightening the flight of the foot. Mild interfering may be stopped by simply squaring off the toe of the striking hoof and applying a shoe with a square toe. In more severe cases, the portion of the foot which does the striking should be identified, rasped off, and fitted with an appropriately shaped shoe. A heavier weighted shoe also may be needed in this case. By careful study of the type of interfering it is possible to gain some advantages from weights, but care should be taken not to overcome the advantage by creating another disadvantage.

Paddling is a gait defect that is more unsightly than detrimental. It occurs occasionally in young horses worked on a longe line, or may be aggravated by this form of training. It may be corrected in young horses with proper foot care and a change of the training regimen. In older horses, shoeing with square-toed shoes that have lateral extensions on both sides of the toe may correct the action.

Chronic laminitis and other hoof deformities can be helped, if not corrected, by special shoeing, trimming, and grooving of the wall of the hoof.

Sand crack and quarter crack can be effectively helped by special shoeing in conjunction with trimming, hoof clamps, and transverse grooving of the cracked portion of the wall.

Dropped sole, corns, and seedy toe can be helped by a surgical-type shoe which consists essentially of a plate covering a surgical packing of pine tar and oakum. There are a number of variations of this technic ranging from a leather pad, which is applied together with the shoe, to small strips of metal inserted between the shoe and the wall and passing across the sole of the foot to hold the packing in place. Specially formed shoes which give localized support and relieve pain also are a part of corrective shoeing. These are, however, as numerous as the types of foot injury which can occur, and their design is predicated upon a specific injury to a specific animal. A listing of the multiplicity of shoes which have been forged for particular purposes has no place in this book. Usually they are made to order upon the recommendations of a specialist. In the course of ordinary practice, a knowledge of all types of corrective shoes would have no practical significance, and blacksmiths with sufficient skill to make them would be hard to find.

A discussion of corrective shoeing would be incomplete without mentioning the Vachette clamp which has been in use for more than 50 years without substantial changes in form, or without substantial improvement in design or function. This device effectively immobilizes sand, toe, or quarter cracks, or other fissures in the wall of the hoof.

The fissure should first be thoroughly cleaned and dried. A cautery is then used to burn 2 notches in the wall, 1 on either side of the crack. The length of the crack determines the number of clamps which must be used. Generally, the clamps are placed one-half to three-quarters of an inch apart. Although principally used in cracks involving the toe, the clamps can be effectively employed in quarter crack providing the wall is of good quality horn and sufficiently thick to stand the strain. The clamps are applied with a special clamping tool and will hold the fissure together and prevent any motion of the crack under normal conditions of strain. The new tissue adhesives offer an interesting and potentially useful method of supplementing the clamps and further immobilizing the fissure, filling the crack, and promoting healing.

J. F. BONE

REFERENCES

1. Armistead, W. W.: Horseshoeing, Veterinarian, Massachusetts, V.M.A. 6 3 (1961) 9-26.
2. Hunting, W.: The Art of Horse-shoeing. Revised ed. American Veterinary Publishing Co., Chicago, Ill., 1920.
3. Ruth, H.: Der. Huf. Gustav Fischer Verlag, Jena, 1959.
4. Sisson, S. S., and Grossman, J. D.: The Anatomy of the Domestic Animals. 3rd ed. W. B. Saunders Co., Philadelphia, Pa. 1938.
5. U.S.D.A., B.A.I.: Diseases of the Horse, Revised ed. Gov't. Printing Office, Washington, D. C., 1942.

ADDITIONAL COMMENTS ON CORRECTIVE SHOEING

The placing of any kind of shoe on a horse is to accomplish one or more of the following purposes:

1. Protection against simple wear.

2. Improvement or correction of the manner of walking.

3. Protection of a diseased or injured foot or some part thereof.

4. Immobilization of the foot or limb.

5. Improvement or restoration of circulation.

6. Restoration of use of foot or limb.

The application of shoes for the last four reasons is the responsibility of every equine practitioner. Many conditions can be remedied or alleviated by proper shoeing only, so we should be able to make or instruct how to make corrective shoes and know how to put them on.

The veterinarian must have a basic understanding of the anatomy, physiology, and the most frequently encountered lesions of the foot and limb in order to understand the reasons for use of a particular shoe.

The circulation of the foot is dependent on many factors both intrinsic and external. Failure of any one factor will deprive the foot of adequate circulation and one or more disease processes will result. The mechanics as well as anatomy of the check ligaments and stay apparatus must be fully understood in order to achieve desired results with some therapeutic shoes. With this information, improvements can be made on the shoes described here, and others can be designed as need for them arises.

PROTECTION OF A DISEASED OR INJURED FOOT

Cracking of the wall of the hoof is commonly seen by veterinarians but, unfortunately, only after an unsuccessful attempt has been made by the owner to remedy it. Complete rigidity of the hoof case is mandatory in these cases. Since a nonflexible wall impairs circulation, provisions must be made to compensate for this. A simple bar shoe with a leather pad under which oakum is placed will be helpful. The nails should be driven at an angle that will tend to keep the sides of the crack in apposition. Addition of pine tar beneath the pad will help keep the sole flexible so that normal pressure on the pad will pump adequate blood through the foot. This will not suffice, however, if the horse is kept on a hard surface and only the shoe comes in contact with the ground. Bedding and soft dirt, when walked on, will create pressure on the pad through the oakum pack to the sole of the foot and thus aid circulation.

Frequently I find that the horse owner has attempted to halt the upward cracking by rasping a notch at the end of the crack. Usually this process results in failure because such a groove does not go through the entire wall. Should it be grooved deeply enough, the wall in that area would be so weakened that it will pull away from its attachments as the groove grows nearer to the ground surface. To stop this process I have had good results from cauterizing a small hole above such cracks. I use a $\frac{1}{2}$- or $\frac{3}{8}$-inch steel rod which has been ground with a lathe to a point $\frac{1}{4}$ inch long and $\frac{1}{8}$ inch in diameter. With the digital nerves blocked, and the iron heated to red heat, I force the point of this rod into a point above the crack until it is halted by the hub of the rod. The resulting wound, being round, prevents further cracking. Even when a horse is sedated and the nerves are blocked the animal often resists the procedure, presumably because of the odor of burnt hoof. To avoid this, I routinely smear the nostrils with some aromatic, such as mentholatum, or squirt a few ml. of camphorated oil into the nostrils to mask the odor.

We often are forced to thin the sole to the sensitive tissues when establishing drainage for a puncture wound, or so-called "gravel," or even for abscesses that may develop following acute laminitis. The owner invariably wants to work this horse before the sole has had sufficient time to repair. In such cases I have welded a light-gauge, steel plate to the inside of a bar shoe level with the bar. A heavy pad of oakum then is placed under the plate, and medication can be administered through a needle forced between the bar of the shoe and the frog of the hoof. The heel nails should be omitted from such a shoe to allow the hoof to spread. This shoe should not be left on the foot too long because the absence of sole pressure will impair the circulation.

When large pieces of the wall are broken or pulled off by a shoe, a sensitive area may be exposed. To prevent foreign material from being forced into such an area, I fill the space with one of the quick-hardening plastics. There are many such preparations available now that will not shrink when dried as the plastic woods do.

IMMOBILIZATION OF FOOT OR LIMB

Many common injuries of the foot or limb will not heal properly unless immobilized. Whenever possible, casting is the procedure of choice, but this is not always practical. Lacerations that involve the tendons below the carpus or around the hock usually suppurate; a cast is impractical in these instances. I use a shoe brace for such cases. Lacerated tendons can be quite easily repaired, and, if a minimum of tension is placed on them, they will heal completely.

The value of such a shoe so far removed from the injury in cases of hock lacerations may be questioned, but consideration of the limb's mechanics will justify the procedure. I have obtained excellent results in horses which were walking on their fetlocks following cuts through tendons and into the navicular bursa. Similar experience has been observed in animals which were walking on the anterior surface of the pastern due to severance of the extensor tendons on the anterior surface of the hock joint.

The shoe brace used is simply an open shoe with a heavy piece of strap steel welded across the volar surface of the shoe, and extending laterally about $\frac{1}{2}$ inch from the shoe. Perpendicular to this extension, 2 additional steel bars are welded to a round padded ring at an angle approximating the angle of the leg. The ring must remain below the carpal or hock joint. The angle of the bars going to the ring will be determined by the position in which the foot is to be maintained. When the extensor tendons are cut, the angle of the brace to the level surface should approximate 90° so that the hoof is extended as much as possible to relieve tension on the sutured tendons. Conversely, the brace to shoe angle will be more oblique to maintain the foot in flexion when the flexor tendons have been severed.

Figures 11 and 12 show the construction of such a shoe, and its application for severed extensor tendons. Doubtlessly, a similar brace

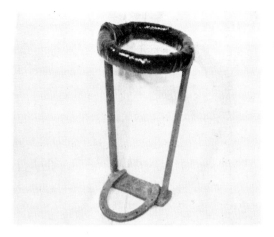

Fig. 11. Shoe brace designed by author.

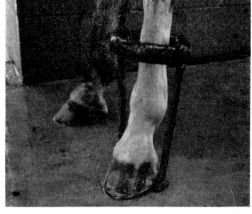

Fig. 12. Application of shoe brace.

could be devised with adjustments to fit different conditions, but making an individual apparatus for each case has merit.

Oddly enough, even unbroken colts do not resist wearing such an apparatus. The length of time the animal must wear this shoe will depend on its age, the amount of trauma to the tissues, and the rate of healing. As a general rule, 6 weeks are sufficient.

When the flexor tendons have been severed, the animal will stand with a very acute pastern angle after the brace is first removed. The owner should be forewarned because in some cases it may appear that no improvement has been achieved. If the tendons have healed, however, they will regain proper tone and, in a matter of 2 or 3 months, the horse will stand as erect on the injured limb as on the opposite one.

RESTORATION OF CIRCULATION

The lesions related to a poorly nourished foot are by far the most common conditions encountered in the riding horse. Laminitis most frequently is responsible, but inadequate hoof trimming or leaving the shoes on for excessive periods causes just as much of this trouble. A poorly nourished foot is dry and scaly. There is little or no elasticity to the hoof case and separation between the sole and wall or dropped sole or seedy toe will result. These conditions are more often the aftereffects of acute laminitis. In my location many cases of laminitis occur in the spring when the horse is fed nothing but native pasture. The cause can be eating too much high carbohydrate grass seed, or the condition may result from obesity. All too often horses are "killed with kindness." The animal's weight is increased to the point that the foot cannot support it.

Infrequent trimming or shoeing also can cause serious lameness, which usually will manifest itself in a different manner. Thrush, in my opinion, is due to poor circulation combined with external factors favorable for growth of bacteria and molds that feed on necrotic hoof tissue before invading healthy tissue. When trimming is neglected, the heels become contracted as a direct result of poor circulation. Sidebones are seen more often with contracted heels than as separate disease entities, because as the horse advances in years the lateral cartilages ossify. If the heels are contracted, this new bone does not have sufficient room within the hoof case and pressure between the newly ossified cartilage and the inner surface of the coronary band will cause lameness.

To restore circulation, the bar shoe with a leather pad, oakum, and pine tar will be helpful if it is remembered to omit the heel nails. Before applying this shoe, the sole should be thinned so that it will give to digital pressure. Thinning of the wall also will help by allowing the hoof to spread slightly with each step the animal takes. Such a procedure should be resorted to only in the most severe cases as the glossy periople found on a healthy foot helps to retain moisture and should not be disturbed unless necessary. Too many farriers deliberately rasp off this covering when shoeing a horse in order to "dress up" the foot. Such a procedure only speeds the drying out and hardening of the hoof.

In arid climates the hooves become very hard, dry, and brittle. This makes it difficult to restore their normal elasticity. Simply soaking the hoof in mud or water does more to soften it than any of the hoof dressings sold commercially. When hooves are badly dried, I force the horse to stand in water for several hours each day. Where the climatic conditions predispose drying, a mud hole around the watering trough will keep the hooves sufficiently moist to prevent the condition from occurring.

Owners often object to use of a pad and bar shoe for treatment of so-called thrush. If the shoe is applied properly with plenty of sole pressure and sandy or soft footing is provided, one can be certain that when the shoe is removed after about 30 days, healthy, odorless tissue will have replaced the moist necrosis. If the patient has undergone a neurectomy, the results will be disappointing.

Restoration of Use of the Limb

A long-lasting, severe unilateral lameness from almost any cause often will lead to the contraction of the flexor tendons. This particularly occurs in young animals. Such an animal may walk apparently normally, but will stub his toe often and limp for several steps afterward. If this animal is on soft sand, he may stand with the anterior surface of the hoof approximating 90°. The diagnosis can be most easily made when the colt is in an extended trot as he often is when playing. He will have his head up, tail high, and as each foot is placed on the ground it seemingly hesitates a fraction of a second before striking the ground. While traveling in this manner the colt will invariably stub his toe and limp for several steps. The diagnosis can be confirmed by extending the hoof with considerable pressure. The stretching of the shortened flexor tendons will cause pain.

Rather than partially severing contracted tendons to lengthen them I apply a shoe that will extend beyond the toe about an inch. This will cause a longer contact of the bottom of the hoof with the ground. Care must be taken that the shoe is not extended too far, and the animal should not be kept on a hard surface. If these precautions are not taken, the extension of the tendons will occur too rapidly and a bowed tendon may result.

The age of the animal and the severity of the contraction will determine how long an extended shoe must be applied. I attempt to keep the hoof angle the same as the opposite hoof and never exaggerate the angle by using toe calks or leaving the toe longer than normal for the individual. Results in these cases will be gratifying, but only if the condition predisposing the contraction has been removed.

In conclusion I will emphasize that therapeutic shoeing has many and varied applications and only a few conditions for it have been mentioned. A thorough understanding of the anatomy and physiology of the limb, the physical principles involved in the gait of the horse, and a basic understanding of horseshoeing will enable veterinarians to design shoes which will restore many horses to usefulness.

C. D. Cooper

CHAPTER 30

VICES

INTRODUCTION

In its broadest aspect, a vice in a horse may be defined as any habit of the animal which serves no useful purpose, but which instead may cause damage to property, or injury to the animal, his stable-mates, or his attendants.

A vice may be a reflection of the animal's basic personality, acquired or inherited. It may indicate nervousness, viciousness, fear, curiosity or excessive energy. It may be copied from other horses or it may be a reaction to poor management. It may be a side reaction to physiologic irritation or a metabolic disturbance or deficiency. Vices may simply be elaborations of ways to dissipate the urges of excess energy. Or they may be due to plain "cussedness."

Whatever its original cause, any vice, once it has become established, is almost impossible to eradicate. The seriousness of a vice depends largely on its effects and on the steps necessary for its suppression. When its importance approaches or exceeds the value of the animal to the owner, it may be advisable to consider disposing of the horse.

Vices range in their effects from social embarrassment to the owner to actual physical damage to life and property. Apparently harmless activity may be the forerunner of harmful behavior. Because of the strength time will give to any habit, the sooner a vice is recognized and combated, the greater is the possibility of its suppression. The most ingenious corrective measures devised by man often are met with equally ingenious and often more persistent countermeasures on the part of the horse. Moreover, horses, as far as most veterinarians are concerned, are no longer simply beasts of burden; they are extremely delicate and financially valuable animals or they are pets, and consequently it no longer is advisable to resort to drastic and/or dangerous remedies in an attempt to eliminate their vices.

In addition to the utilization of various devices and technics for the elimination of vices,

regular daily exercise is of great importance. Most vices thrive on boredom and inactivity. Furthermore, if the circumstances which originally led to the acquisition of a vice are re-established, an animal which has apparently been cured may be expected to resume that vice.

Though a horse may exhibit a vice under almost any conditions, the vices of greatest concern to the veterinarian are seen in the stall or in the paddock. The greatest number of vices will occur in the stall, for it is here that the horse is confined to idleness for hours or even days at a time. The same forces which make a caged lion pace in his cell are then operating on the horse.

CLINICAL ENTITIES

Cribbing

One of the most common of vices is that known variously as "cribbing," "crib biting," "wind swallowing," or "wind sucking." (The last term should perhaps be reserved to designate the act of vaginal insufflation by mares.) Cribbing is the unpleasant habit of force-swallowing gulps of air. To do this, the horse will grasp any suitable or available object with his incisor teeth, pull back and up with an arching movement of the crest of the neck, meanwhile depressing the base of the tongue so that a gulp of air is passed into the esophagus and swallowed. Though the term "cribbing" may have had its origin in the performing of this act on the hay crib or manger, the edge of the door, a water trough, fence post, nail, or any other object will serve equally well. Horses will even use their own lower lips as cribbing objects.

A horse may acquire this vice while seeking relief from the irritation of dentition, or he may copy it from another horse in the same stable. Most often, however, cribbing develops as an elaboration of chewing or biting anything handy, just to pass time.

Anatomically it is far easier for the horse to swallow air than it is to eructate. As the swallowed air must pass from the stomach into the intestines, it is conceivable that the swallowing of large volumes of air can give rise to tympanitic gastritis or enteritis.

Corrective measures are aimed more at prevention of the act than at eradication. Several types of commercially available cribbing straps produce fairly good results. Such a strap may be a wide, stiff, often reinforced leather belt the edges of which press uncomfortably against the trachea whenever the neck is arched. Another type of strap may have several spring-recessed metal prongs which press into the ventral throat region when the neck is arched. A plain leather belt wrapped tightly around the upper throat will sometimes be effective.

Removal of as many projecting objects as possible in the stall or paddock, and electrically wiring those remaining, have been tried in an effort to eliminate this vice. Results usually are discouraging. Horses learn very quickly which objects produce shock, and keep looking for objects which do not. They even learn to recognize the "hot" wire and, if a wire fence voltage machine is the electrical source, will listen for the pulsating noises of the machine to ascertain whether the current is on.

A drastic surgical operation for removal of muscles used in the neck-arching phase of the cribbing act has been resorted to as a cure for this vice. Such treatment may have merit as a last resort, but in most cases it is impractical.

It is emphasized that whatever the method used to combat cribbing, it should be supplemented with ample and regular exercise, for this is a vice arising from boredom and excess energy. Also, there is great probability that this vice will recur if the preventive measures are discontinued and the original environment reestablished.

Weaving

Weaving is a vice seen commonly on the race track, especially among high-strung fillies in racing condition. It may be the simple swaying of the head and neck over the stall door; or it may be the complete lifting and side-to-side swinging of the anterior half of the body, with the wide, pendulum-like arc of the head occupying an entire wall of the stall.

This vice also is a product of nervousness and excess energy. It may be developed independently or it may be copied. In young animals, it often is seen shortly after the horse first races or after the animal has first been subjected to the excitement of working from the starting gate.

The harmful results of this vice are numerous. The front legs often break down under the constant strain. Holes develop in the dirt of the stall floor where the front feet lift and pound, and hence the footing becomes dangerously uneven. The weaver usually will lose weight both from the prolonged exercise and from the suppression of appetite caused by the nervousness. This may lead to such deterioration of physical condition that the horse actually is too exhausted and weak to stand training. For this reason, bad weavers usually are poor racing prospects. Moreover, a pronounced weaver is a threat to neighboring horses who may develop the vice by observation.

This vice has its effects on the grooms as well, for the maintenance of the stall bedding entails extra work, and personnel unfortunate enough to be housed in a room next to a weaver may have sleeping problems.

Correction of this vice is directed toward the relaxing of tensions in the animal. Intravenous administration of calcium gluconate and the B vitamins, particularly B_1, are of some benefit. Tranquilizers and sedatives are effective, but are frowned upon by the racing commissioners in most states if the animal is to be raced.

Since most weavers perform at certain times of the day, they may be effectively restrained by haltering with a short chain during those periods. Hobbles applied to the front feet will shorten the swing of the weaving motion. Short, heavy iron chains attached to the halter and intended to slap the horse's face with each swing may produce some success, but too often the horse merely works the chain into the weaving rhythm. Short, heavy chains attached above each knee will slap the horse's legs, but this, too, can be worked into the rhythm. Suspending water-filled cans from the ceiling and in the doorway so that water spills on the horse's head when he weaves may help for a while, but as with automobile tires or any other objects suspended for the same reason, the animal usually extends the weaving to include these items in the swing. Dividing the stall doorway with ropes or chains will not stop a determined weaver, for he simply will weave against a wall, or he will alter the pattern of the swing to include ducking in and out of the divided sections.

Cohabitation with a docile mascot sometimes will induce sufficient relaxation to stop weaving. Goats are used most often for this purpose. Placing the horse in a small open pen where visibility is unrestricted in all directions likewise will often cause sufficient relaxation to eliminate weaving.

STALL WALKING

Stall walking is a vice closely related to weaving. The afflicted animal makes circular trips around the stall for hours at a time, usually at a walk though occasionally at a trot. As in the case of weaving, the causes of this vice are mainly nervousness and excess energy. Similarly, the occurrence of fatigue, constant irritation to existing leg injuries, loss of flesh and condition and the additional bedding-maintenance problems, are comparable to the consequences of weaving.

The logical initial attempt to correct this vice is to tie the animal with a short chain during the hours he most frequently walks, which may be day or night, or both. Placing the animal in a narrow stall will accomplish the same thing. Some success has come from placing impediments to walking in the stall, such as 3 or 4 bales of straw or 4 or 5 automobile tires suspended from the ceiling. The company of a docile mascot also may be helpful. Some benefit may be achieved from the administration of calcium gluconate and vitamins, and tranquilizers. The results, however, usually are not permanent. Recurrence of this vice may be expected with relaxation or discontinuance of whatever measures have been effective in preventing it.

DIGGING

Digging is another vice arising from excessive nervous energy, though in some instances it may begin as an instinctive attempt to escape confinement. The animal will dig one or several large holes, sometimes 3 feet deep, in the stall. The excavated dirt usually is well-mixed with the bedding and the entire mess must be thrown out, the hole filled with clean dirt, and the bedding replaced. This vice thus creates considerable extra work for the animal's handlers. More important, it endangers the limbs of the digging horse. Sound limbs become injured and leg injuries are aggravated. The same nervousness which causes the animal to dig often causes him to run and jump in his stall, in spite of the hazards he has created. So if he is not hurt while digging, he may well accomplish this by tripping or falling in one of the holes or over one of the mounds of dirt.

Probably the best approach to this vice is to fill the holes with water (before they get too large) and then leave the horse in the stall. Horses usually do not like to walk in water, and dislike digging in water even more. These lakes cut down the area of activity of the animal and it is hoped he will associate causally the digging and the additional confinement. If the vice is not yet well-established, this association may occur and the vice cease.

Other corrective measures are based on other forms of restraint. The most practical is that of bedding the animal on a hard surface, such as a wooden floor. A few futile attempts to dig may suffice. Hobbles placed on the front legs occasionally are used, but this type of restriction is too confining and generally is unsatisfactory. Careful watching and stern punishment at the first signs of digging may produce good results. But unless the horse is caught in the act of digging, there is little chance for association and results will be poor.

MASTURBATION

Masturbation is a vice seen fairly commonly in colts. The ill effects of this act usually are overrated by complaining horsemen at the race track, but it can admittedly be very embarrassing to owners at times. Horses masturbating in the saddling paddock or in the parade to the post in front of the grandstand may cause a few red faces, and this activity certainly does not increase the animal's "will to win," which should be the foremost thought in his mind at this time. The horseman's most common complaint about the act itself is that it causes loss of condition in the animal because of repeated exertion. This vice often is accompanied by an overamorous inclination to breed any fat horse at the race track, especially lead ponies and mares. Occasionally, a horse may misdirect his advances toward a groom. It is such deviations rather than the actual act of masturbation that makes this vice significant.

On the breeding farm, however, the repeated loss of semen can affect the stallion's sperm count and breeding efficiency. Early detection and correction are imperative in this instance.

The simplest and most reliable method of correction is castration. Trainers usually are very much in favor of this, but the owners often balk, regardless of the animal's pedigree or racing achievements, on the ground that their colts may be destined for greatness at the stud.

A number of corrective devices are available, ranging from a simple plastic ring to a complex "Man O' War" harness. The plastic rings come in various diameters and are about ¼ inch wide. A ring of proper size is lubricated and inserted on the penis just behind the glans. Upon erection, the penis enlarges to the confines of the ring, at which point the resulting discomfort brings about a change in mental outlook. A similar device is the cage, a wire basket-like contraption of 2 slightly different sized rings separated about 1 inch by 3 or 4 wire staves. This fits over the glans, and functions much as does the single ring. The "Man O' War" harness is a metal keyhole about 8 inches long, with saw-tooth edges, which is suspended by a leather harness to fit just below and in front of the penis. In normal extension for urination, the penis will fall

through the enlarged area of the keyhole without difficulty. During erection, however, it will be pressed upward and into the saw-tooth projections. Several modifications and simplifications of this harness employ the same principle. The main objections to any harness apparatus are the complications which may arise when an animal lies down, and the extra work involved in putting the harness on and off and in keeping it clean.

Estrogens have been used with some success to control this vice. This remedy must be repeated at regular intervals and has the disadvantage of upsetting the horse's natural hormone balance and possibly causing sexual immaturity and breeding difficulties later.

Regardless of the type of restraint used, it is important that the penis, the sheath, and the device be kept clean to prevent added stimulation through irritation. Mild soap and water make a good cleanser. Much simpler and equally effective is the use of 2 ounces of baby oil or mineral oil irrigated into the sheath with a dose syringe; the scale and dirt will fall off within 1 or 2 days after the oil is applied.

CHARGING

Charging, or savaging, is a dangerous vice when encountered in the stall or paddock. Stallions, or mares with cystic ovaries, most commonly exhibit this vice, although it occurs occasionally in geldings. The animal may charge the groom as he enters the stall with a tub of food or when he turns his back to leave the stall. An unsuspecting passerby who ventures too close to the stall door may be attacked. The attack may vary from a playful nip to a diving charge with ears flat and mouth open. The cause of this vice may be overanxiety at meal time, meanness or fear induced or aggravated by poor handling, or hormone imbalance.

Correction should be directed toward elimination of the cause. Of primary importance is the ability of the groom, for he must be able to anticipate a charge and avoid it. A mean horse will very quickly recognize fright in a groom, and a mean groom will be of no help to a frightened horse. While in the stall, the groom should maintain as much halter control of the horse as is necessary. He should never turn his back on the horse, especially when entering or leaving the stall.

Attacks which come at feed time may be avoided by leaving an empty feed tub inside the stall near the door so that a small can of feed can be tossed into the tub. The groom can then enter the stall unmolested with the rest of the feed ration.

A water pistol may be a very effective means of stopping a charger. The sudden blast in the horse's face usually will so surprise the animal that he immediately will stop and then retreat. Each subsequent charge should be stopped by a blast from the water gun, which should be concealed as much as possible, for otherwise the horse soon will charge only those persons who pass empty-handed.

If the use of a water pistol does not solve the problem, the next step is for the groom to carry a switch for his own protection when entering the stall. A closed wire screen at the door will protect passers-by. If the horse continually attacks attendants working with him, it may be necessary to muzzle him while he is being handled.

If the vice is caused by hormone imbalance, castration or follicular rupture should be considered.

STRIKING OR REARING

Striking and/or rearing, a vice which may develop in fearful or mean horses, is seen when an attendant working on the ground does something to the horse which the horse does not like. The stimulus may be the act of administering a drug or applying a twitch, or some other treatment. It consists in a sudden slap at the attendant with either or both front feet. When this is accompanied with a forward leap, the results can be disastrous. The attendant's best defense is the horse's naturally poor aim, for there is no time for the attendant to escape.

This vice should be handled promptly and thoroughly. It is imperative that the motivation be determined immediately. If it is fear, kind but firm handling is called for. If the

motive is aggressive meanness, punishment should be administered. This can be accomplished best by placing a chain lead shank through the halter rings and under the upper lip to fashion a war bridle. Then, standing near the horse's shoulder, the attendant should make the horse back into a corner, walk to the center of the stall, and then back into the corner again. If the horse strikes again, a flat-footed kick to the underside of the horse's belly by the groom often will so surprise the animal that after another session of backing and leading the horse will not attack again.

Occasionally, there are horses large enough, strong enough, and mean enough to resist stern treatment by becoming even meaner than before. These are cases which, if they cannot be handled, would be better left alone; often, however, the realization that handling is impossible comes only after the battle has begun and retreat is most awkward and difficult.

If the administration of any form of punishment to a horse entails a fight with the animal, the attendant must make every effort to insure that it is not a fair fight and that the horse always is the loser. Pound for pound, man has no chance against the horse; it is only man's brain and his use of it that give him superiority. By maintaining halter control and a position close to the horse's shoulder, the attendant will be out of striking reach of the horse and in a position to keep the animal off balance. If it is at all possible, fights should be anticipated and avoided.

Kicking a horse in the belly may seem to be abusive treatment, but if the kick is properly administered by the flat surface of the upper arch of the foot, there is little chance of hurting the animal. The principal benefits of this form of punishment come from the complete surprise to the horse, and his realization that rearing will expose the belly even more to such punishment. This actually is one of the most effective methods of chastisement without injury. The end of the halter shank can be substituted for the foot if the administrator prefers.

It should be mentioned here that the veterinarian, before he undertakes to administer such corrective measures, should be very certain of his status with the client, and should realize that such treatment is not part of his professional obligations but merely a means of permitting completion of the task he came to perform. If there is any doubt in the veterinarian's mind concerning any of these points, he had better administer a heavy dose of a tranquilizer to the animal and leave the correction of the vice to the animal's attendants.

If striking is the result of fear because of incomplete training, it cannot be considered to be a true vice. Kind but firm treatment, accompanied by the use of tranquilizers, should be used in lieu of any punitive measures.

Cow-Kicking

Cow-kicking is a vice which, as the term implies, is the forward and sideward kicking with either of the animal's hindfeet. Like the vices of charging and striking, it is an act of meanness or fear with injury to the victim as the intent. The cow-kick may be directed at an attendant or at a passerby while the animal is on the tow ring, in the stall, or during the administration of medication or treatment. Occasionally, it is motivated by fear; when this is so, the act may be anticipated.

When the motive is considered to be meanness, the corrective measures must be prompt and thorough. Treatment similar to that for striking is effective. Likewise, the same precautions should be taken.

Fence Chewing

Fence chewing is a costly nuisance seen especially in horses confined within redwood fences. Horses have been known literally to chew themselves out of a paddock overnight. Most of the chewed wood falls to the ground, but some may be swallowed and mouth and lip slivers are not uncommon. Possible causes of this vice are the irritation of dentition, dietary deficiencies (especially of basic minerals), endoparasitic infection, the example of other fence chewers, or simply too much time, energy and inactivity. This undesirable behavior may lead to buccal infections, colic,

premature dental wear, and a lot of fence repairing.

The simplest corrective measures are those of applying metal strips to the top edges of the fence, or transferring the animal to metal-, cement-, or wire-fenced paddocks. If none of these procedures is practical, any of several distasteful liquids may be painted on the fences; these include creosote, pepper and water, or various commercial products. (If the fences are clean and white, the objection to painting is obvious.) The installation of a "hot" wire along the top board, or set off inside it, usually produces good results. Adequate, regular exercise and a constant supply of high-quality feed are important supplements to any treatment.

Dirt Eating

Dirt eating is a vice which may indicate either a systemic deficiency of a basic mineral or a parasitic infection. It causes excessive dental wear and may lead to colic from the ingestion of large quantities of dirt and sand. In the pasture, dirt eating is very difficult to control, although soaking favorite spots with distasteful liquids, such as pine oil, sheep dip, etc., may provide some discouragement. Assuring adequate, regular exercise and the constant availability of good supplemental hay will help.

Fighting

Fighting with other horses is a vice which cannot be anticipated by the guilty animal's behavior toward his handlers. The most gentle animal in the stall may be a terror to his companions in the pasture. Most of the fighting, however, occurs when new members are introduced into a group in the pasture. Usually after a few days the aggressive have convinced the meek, and the one-sided battle will be ended. The judicious administration of tranquilizers to aggressive horses, when such animals are to be pastured with other horses, may alleviate the hostilities.

J. L. Temple

CHAPTER 31

THE VETERINARIAN AND HORSE FARM MANAGEMENT

INTRODUCTION

One of the greatest failings in animal husbandry education today is a tendency for the schools to teach the veterinary aspect of disease control in terms of what a farmer can do to avoid paying veterinary fees. They fail to teach a system of farm management in which the veterinarian and the manager combine their talents to develop a program which prevents disease and produces sound, healthy animals economically. It therefore is the lot of the veterinarian to teach such practices. In this chapter, I intend to discuss veterinary practices and treatment only as they fall into an equine farm management program.

Regardless of how we flatter ourselves about our personal proficiencies and our years of experience, there is little about the treatment of horses that cannot be mastered by any competent practitioner. Just as accurate diagnosis results from systematic examination and elimination of possible conditions which might appear similar, good farm management recognizes possible difficulties and by a system of prevention and elimination will result in economical production of healthy animals. A good farm manager with a system of management which includes a good veterinarian will have markedly better results than will the poor manager using the best of practitioners. It is, therefore, my opinion that to succeed in equine practice you must have a management routine which you and the client understand and follow.

Equine practice tends to have peak demands on one's time, particularly during the foaling, breeding, and sale periods. Some of the routine work can be completed at other times of the year, however, with better results for the horseman and a better balanced work-year for the practitioner. There will be minor changes for various areas of the country and some variation from breed to breed, but the following routine should have application in most practices.

SEASONAL PROGRAMS

Fall Program

Weaning: It has been demonstrated that prolonged nursing of the pregnant mare results in anemia. To give next year's foal the best chance, nursing foals should be removed from the mare between the sixth and seventh months of age. It is quite important to treat foals for parasites a week prior to weaning. This avoids the double stress of weaning and parasites and gives the foal a better start on its own. The essential point in weaning is to insure complete separation of the mare and foal in as near injuryproof surroundings as possible. (The importance of other factors including the signs of the zodiac are subject to personal preference.)

A nice method of weaning in a large band of mares is accomplished by driving into the field with a van, loading one or more mares, and departing for a field some distance away. At weaning age, foals usually are so occupied by their buddies and personal interests that they hardly miss their dams, and in a few days there is only a field of weanlings left.

The majority of people put the mare and foal into a large stall, and then lead the mare out (closing the door behind her) and remove her to a field on a distant part of the farm. Foals may be quieter if placed 2 to a stall. They generally are kept confined for a few days. Tranquilizers may help the nervous mare or foal to survive the stress of weaning. Care of the mare after weaning involves exercise, a reduced ration (usually only grass), removal to a site beyond the sound of the foals, and safe fencing. Since the cessation of milk production depends on the pressure of accumulated milk, they are milked only in case of mastitis. The use of irritants such as camphorated oil, is not recommended.

The number of injuries can be minimized by good fencing and housing. We find that fewer horses are injured when held behind tightly woven wire fences than those constructed of board or stone. Ordinary wire or barbed wire fences and poorly hung or badly designed gates are a menace.

Mares that are in foal require little special attention at this time, other than prophylaxis for tetanus, virus abortion, salmonellosis, and other bacterial infections. Barren mares should be teased, cultured while in heat, treated if infected, and sutured when necessary. Better results follow 4 to 6 months of normalcy before breeding, and this rest will enable a better conception rate than treatment during the breeding season.

Parasites are a year-round problem and must not be neglected. Egg counts give an indication of the severity and spectrum of infection. It may be necessary to treat as often as every 60 days in cases of infection. Low level phenothiazine medication also may be used.

Winter Program

Housing is a controversial subject, and should be considered in terms of space, ventilation, and minimum of hazards. Horses do well in "Madden Sheds" or run-out barns. It is important that the doors are large enough, however, and that there are no corners in which a horse can be cornered by a kicker. There must also be enough trough and hay space so that the more timid animals can get access to feed. Drenching rain or sleet probably is harder on horses than any environmental condition other than small stalls and poor ventilation. More respiratory infection is associated with confinement in small, tight, poorly ventilated stalls than in horses confined by gates in drafty barns.

The treatment of infected mares should be continued until they show a clean culture. Clean barren mares are managed according to individual requirements. Easy keepers may be wintered on little feed, but some old or poorly doing mares must receive special care. Conditions such as thyroid deficiences or other endocrine disorders are best corrected at this time in order to get the reproductive tracts as near normal as possible by the breeding season.

Stallions are carried through the winter in thrifty but not optimum condition in order to start the breeding season while gaining weight. Mares in foal should have plenty of exercise, should not be overcrowded, and should be fed sufficiently to maintain good condition. The use of vitamins, minerals, and other supplements will depend upon soil deficiencies and the quality of feeds.

Yearlings must of necessity be well-fed for they cannot be sold until they have grown and filled out, and this cannot be accomplished without good feed and plenty of it.

Good pasture will maintain horses and fatten most of them. Alfalfa hay and corn approximate a balanced ration, as do timothy and oats. Special rations are based on these combinations. Adequate water must be available at all times. This is equally true in very cold weather as well as in very hot weather. Plenty of roughage is essential. Feeding of grain must be consistent and in keeping with the demand of the individual. The practice always should be to feed the highest quality of roughage, pasture, and grain available (Table 1).

Parasite Control: Bots are controlled by treatment 30 days or more after a hard freeze. Ascarids are primarily a problem in young horses. The parasite thrives in crowded conditions and is encouraged by moving weanlings onto land vacated by yearlings. A study of the life cycle reveals that ascarids lay enormous numbers of eggs and under optimum conditions complete the egg to egg cycle in about 60 days. Treatment must be given at 60-day intervals, beginning at 6 to 9 weeks of age and continued until ascarids are eliminated or the youngsters are sold.

Strongyles are one of the greatest problems. Foals are born free of strongyles, yet may die of verminous aneurysms at 5 weeks of age. Once foals acquire an aneurysm it may take 6 to 9 months for the worms to make their way

Table 1.—Physiologically Equivalent Ages, Body Weights, and Nutrient Allowances.

	KIND OF HORSE	PERCENT OF MATURE WEIGHT						
		10%	20%	30%	40%	50%	60%	100%
Average Age in Months	Lightweight	0.5	2.0	4.0	6.0	10.0	14.0	44
Average Weight in Pounds	Lightweight	100	200	300	400	500	600	1000
Total Daily Feed, Pounds (Maintenance)	Lightweight	—	8.3	9.7	11.0	12.3	13.5	12.6
Daily Feed Intake, Percent of Body Weight (Maintenance)	Lightweight	—	4.2	3.2	2.8	2.5	2.2	1.3
Daily Intake of Digestible Nutrients, Pounds (Maintenance)	Lightweight	—	5.2	6.1	6.9	7.7	8.4	7.9
Digestible Nutrients, Percent of Total Feed	All weights	—	62.5	62.5	62.5	62.5	62.5	62.5
Digestible Protein, Percent of T.D.N.	Lightweight	—	20.0	16.2	13.6	11.0	9.2	7.8
Calcium, Percent of T.D.N.	Lightweight	—	0.52	0.47	0.43	0.38	0.35	0.25
Phosphorus, Percent of T.D.N.	Lightweight	—	0.45	0.42	0.40	0.37	0.35	0.27

back into the digestive tract so that they can be killed by anthelmintics. Therefore, control centers on the older horses on the farm. The parasite program carried out in adults during fall and winter is far more important to the foal than his individual treatment. It must be remembered that the egg hatches and the larva crawls in moist plant material before being ingested by the horse or foal. Damp bedding in stalls can be just as readily a source of contamination as lush pasture.

Year-round treatment with low level phenothiazine contained in the feed of the mares for 21 days of every month is a proven solution for the strongyle problem. Some farmers do not medicate mares all year and must resort to individual therapy. There is some question as to the efficiency of phenothiazine alone in such a program, and better results are obtained by the addition of a piperazine.

A satisfactory routine of parasitic control is as follows: Treat mares and foals one week prior to weaning, using phenothiazine and one of the piperazines. Treat all animals one month after a hard freeze, using carbon disulfide followed by phenothiazine, or carbon disulfide-piperazine combinations and phenothiazine. Worm mares 3 days after foaling and, if possible, move mares and foals to clean fields not contaminated by horses during the previous year. Treat mares and foals at 6 to 8 weeks after foaling. Worm foals at 60-day intervals

until weaning. This may be modified with limited numbers of horses on extensive acreage.

Because of the possible tolerance acquired by parasites to existing vermifuges, one must be constantly considering the use of new drugs. Parasitic control must be a year-round program based on a system of management, therapy, and religious adherence to the program. Never forget that manure is the source of the eggs.

SPRING PROGRAM

Barren Mares: Teasing and teasing records often spell success or failure for a farm management program. They must be carried out every day or on a 3-day per week schedule. Barren mares must be recultured before breeding to be certain that they still are free of genital infections. Maiden mares (those not previously bred) may be bred any time after the middle of February when they have shown consistent and regular heats. In the case of a barren mare with a history of low conception or genital infection, it often is wise to wait until the mare has established a regular pattern of estrus and until her general condition is excellent. This should include complete shedding of the winter hair which usually will follow the appearance of good spring grass and warm weather. Mares showing unsatisfactory heats may be more susceptible to infection at the time of breeding. There may be some effect of sunlight on the anterior pituitary as many mares seem to perform much better after bright sunny weather prevails, and the reverse may be observed during cloudy periods.

Mares recently returned from training often are slow to establish a regular estrual cycle. This is particularly true of those trained by individuals who use hormones frequently in their training routine. It usually is best to allow these mares to make their physiologic adjustments even though this will, on occasion, require as long as a year. Some mares, often referred to as "spec mares," may require speculum examination or rectal palpation to discover or confirm estrus.

With mares in foal, parasitic control is of tremendous importance. Bear in mind that strongyle larvae may thrive and become infective in a damp stall as well as outside. Pregnant mares must have good feed, adequate exercise, and plenty of room.

Yearlings require good feed, parasitic control, attention to their feet, exercise, and safe housing and fencing. Fillies and colts must be separated as spring approaches, and well-developed colts may have to be separated to prevent injury or blemishes acquired during play and fighting.

Foaling facilities must include large, dry, well-lighted stalls, 16 or more feet square. There should be readily available adequate bedding, plenty of water, and a simple water heater. A warm room from which the attendant can watch at foaling time is a tremendous help.

The foaling attendant must be dependable, sober, sensible, able to follow instructions, and smart enough to realize his own limitations. His instructions should be to bandage the mare's tail and wash the hindquarters when labor becomes apparent, and then to leave the mare alone. If there is sufficient help, sutured mares may be opened just prior to foaling. It is a safer policy, however, to open them one week prior to the anticipated foaling unless earlier signs increase the urgency.

Once the placental fluid appears, the foaling attendant should, after thorough personal cleansing, pass a hand inside the fetal membranes and determine that both the front feet and the nose of the foal are presented properly. Beyond this, the mare should be left alone. The mare is much better equipped than the attendant to conduct a normal delivery. Traction on the foal before dilation of the cervix can cause bruising and tearing of the mare, and since mares have inherited several million years' experience in delivering foals, it is best to let them do the necessary work. If anything is wrong or suspicious, however, labor can be suspended temporarily by getting the mare up and walking her. It often is the practice to call the veterinarian at the onset of labor. If the foal is normal it usually will arrive before the veterinarian does. But if there is something amiss, help will arrive before things are out-of-hand. Most adjustments or corrections are made quite easily early in labor.

The mare and new foal should be allowed to lie quietly with the umbilical cord still intact. This will break when either the mare or the foal rises. It should not be broken until after all pulsation has ceased. It has been estimated that as many as 400 to 800 ml. of blood returns to the foal from the placenta shortly after birth and this blood is necessary to give the foal a good start. Iodine is used on the stump as soon as the cord breaks. The foals usually are given tetanus antitoxin, and may be given antibiotics. The latter is a matter of personal choice but in some cases is important. The foal generally begins to nurse within 4 hours and little concern need be shown before that time unless unusual signs are evident. Cleaning often occurs within a few minutes after parturition, but it may take longer, and manual removal of the placenta should not be attempted before 8 to 12 hours have passed. If the placenta does not come away readily, the mare breaks out in a sweat or exhibits nervousness and straining. It is best to wait a few hours before interfering. Some mares evidence great distress over a piece of placenta a few inches in diameter, though others have been observed to pass pieces on the seventh day without manifesting signs of distress.

Hemorrhage is one of the greatest concerns, especially in older mares. Attendants should be advised to watch for colicky pain, profuse sweating, rapid pulse, pale membranes, and high-pitched whinny. This sound is almost diagnostic. Since most hemorrhaging mares die while trying to remain on their feet, care must be taken to protect the foal from being crushed.

Suturing of windsuckers usually is done the morning following foaling.

Observation of the New Foal: Bowel movements usually occur in the first few hours. If the foal is observed to raise its tail and strain excessively, it may be necessary to administer an enema of soapy water or glycerine. Some may even require oil by stomach tube. Care should be taken in administering enemas or purges since the foal's intestines are fragile and subject to rupture.

Infection may appear as a septicemia with signs of drowsiness, inappetence, weakness, temperature either elevated or subnormal, exaggerated movements, or prostration. It is well to obtain both blood cultures and blood counts, but, in addition, to start immediately with administration of broad-spectrum antibiotics. Other aids, such as fluid and blood transfusions, should be used as required.

Foals with circulatory defects often exhibit similar signs but these cases usually can be differentiated by clinical examination and laboratory tests, or at postmortem examination.

Knuckling and contractions can often be corrected early by casts or splints. These should not be applied too tightly nor left on so long as to cause necrosis. Weak pasterns and hocks often correct themselves, particularly with good sunshine; however, dramatic results follow vitamin D therapy.

Foals should be examined twice daily through the first 7 days of life for evidence of anemia or jaundice. This condition can be remedied if detected early. The navel should be observed daily for any indication of infection or discharge. Many small hernias disappear as the animal grows. Larger ones must be repaired if it is apparent that it is best not to wait until weaning. A good indication of the foal's general condition can be obtained by observing the mare's mammae. Full glands indicate that something is wrong.

Mares are examined at 7 days with a speculum to determine the condition of the vagina and cervix as well as to examine the discharges which emanate from the uterus. When doubt exists, a cervical sample is taken for culture. As the conception rate for 9-day breedings is low except at the end of the season, it is wise to wait until the 27th to 30th day before breeding.

GENERAL COMMENTS ON BREEDING

Stallions should be housed in cheerful surroundings with company. Roomy, well-ventilated, substantial stalls with large, well-fenced paddocks are desirable. Rations should be the best available, so fed as to have the stallion go into the breeding season while improving in condition. Supplementation will depend on deficiencies which exist in the soil, or on the available roughage and grain. The stallion must be protected from the mare. The following considerations are important to the owner of the stallion:

1. A health certificate should be required which indicates that the mare is not in foal, is free from genital infection, and is in condition for breeding.

2. Be sure that the mare is in heat. Mares should be teased before breeding. Those that seem unruly can be jumped with a teaser. Make certain that the teaser has no opportunity to serve the mare.

3. The stallion must be given physical protection. Mares usually are twitched, and a forefoot is strapped up until the stallion has mounted. If preferred, hobbles will limit the mare's ability to kick.

4. As the stallion dismounts, the mare's head should be brought around to the left. This will protect the stallion, the stud groom, and the veterinarian, if semen is being collected.

Breeding Sanitation: It has been felt since the studies of Dr. Dimock that a large percentage of genital infections in mares are acquired at breeding time, therefore a routine of sanitation must be followed. The following regimen has proved to be effective:

1. Tease the mare and induce urination to eliminate as much vulvar discharge as possible.

2. Bandage the mare's tail with a fresh clean bandage (3-inch gauze).

3. Thoroughly wash the mare's entire hindquarters with mild soap and water.

4. Rinse with clean water.

5. Bring in the stallion, induce an erection, and wash the external genitalia thoroughly. If the stallion is dirty, do not hesitate to use a mild soap, but be sure to rinse thoroughly and remove all the soap.

6. Handlers and attendants should scrub their hands and arms since all cleaning of mare and stallion is useless if a groom, with manure on his hands, assists the stallion in making entry.

7. After service, the stallion is again washed and rinsed with a mild antiseptic.

If the service is reinforced with insemination, there is no excuse for any breach of sanitation on the part of the veterinarian. It is advisable to have stainless steel equipment, plenty of cotton, mild soap, plenty of clean, warm water, and clean towels. No breeding program can be effectively managed without strict attention to cleanliness. Sanitation must follow a routine and be practiced continually. One mistake can nullify all effort.

Teasing and Confirmation of Pregnancy: Teasing is continued after breeding on the chance that conception did not occur. Further information can be obtained by examination of the mare with a speculum on the 18th, 27th and 35th days postcoition. If any suggestion of heat is observed, further observations are made every other day. Rectal examination is made on the 45th day. In the event that no fetus is found, it is wise to recheck the mare in a few days and if she again appears to be barren, attempt to induce estrus. Mares may be bred on any satisfactory show of estrus. Since a small percentage of mares abort or reabsorb the fetus, it is wise to recheck for pregnancy at 60 to 75 days postcoition. If the examination is negative, and it is still the breeding season, the mare should be rebred if estrus can be induced.

SUMMER PROGRAM

Summer management is a continuous operation. The amount of feed and housing particularly is subject to change. Remember that a broodmare, like a cow, cannot give adequate milk without enough feed. Also, feed is necessary for the growth of the foal *in utero*.

Parasites do greater damage in foals, but a program which ignores parasitism in the adult ignores the source of the foal's infection. Worming of foals is begun at 42 to 60 days of age, and may have to be repeated every 60 days until their sale. Older horses are wormed as egg counts in the feces rise.

From the time they are weaned, yearlings are handled with an eye to their future, *e.g.* sale, racing, show, or work. It is desirable that they grow rapidly and soundly. The essential requirements are good feed, parasitic control, protection from injury, care of the feet, and whatever handling and training are required. Parasite treatment and foot-trimming are done on schedules. In hot weather, as sale time approaches, yearlings usually are kept in during the day to protect them from flies and sunburn, and are turned out at night. Since they are active and impetuous, good fencing and safe pastures are important.

GENERAL CONSIDERATIONS FOR YEAR-ROUND MANAGEMENT

1. Provide for quarantine of new arrivals. Determine the parasite load of all new arrivals. Their treatment may prevent parasite build-up.

2. Examine all mares for pregnancy on arrival. This will prevent later embarrassments as failure to foal, foaling in the barren mare field, or foaling a few days after being bred.

3. Identify all animals on arrival (a hoof brand is helpful). If possible, animals should carry halter plates giving their name, the owner's name, and, if available, the breeding.

4. Stall doors should have the mare's name, expected foaling date, stallion's name, and stallion for the coming season. Other pertinent notes, such as whether she is sutured, should also be included. Mares leaving the farm for breeding should be accompanied by a data sheet containing the name of mare,

the stallion to which she is to be bred, and the owner's name and address. All necessary health certificates and breeding contracts should accompany the mare.

5. Accurate records of each animal are important. Records should give owner's name, address and telephone, insurance data, and previous breeding records, which should include as much information as possible about foals. Records of any sensitivities, dormant conditions, or disorders which may recur are helpful. Teasing records must be complete. It is of great help to have available the records of previous years. These are often helpful in interpreting patterns of behavior which the mare may show.

H. H. SUTTON

TO CHAPTER 8 CONCERNING THIABENDAZOLE

Subsequent to preparation of the discussion in Chapter 8 about the treatment of endoparasites, reports have appeared concerning the efficacy of a newly synthesized anthelmintic called thiabendazole. A commercial preparation, Equizole (Merck & Co.), containing this chemical has been tested extensively. Its antiparasitic action against both large and small strongyles and pinworms of horses is impressive. Effective dosages range from 25 to 100 mg. per kg. of body weight. Toxicity studies indicate that this compound has an unusually wide margin of safety for the horse.

On the basis of preliminary studies it appears that thiabendazole also may provide effective control of ascarid infection when used at a dose level of 100 mg. per kg. of body weight.

INDEX

INDEX

D

X